Radiographic Atlas of Colon Disease

Radiographic Atlas of COLON DISEASE

Edward I. Greenbaum, M.D.
Section of Gastrointestinal Radiology
Long Beach (Calif.) Veterans Administration Hospital
Associate Adjunct Professor
Department of Radiologic Sciences
University of California, Irvine

YEAR BOOK MEDICAL PUBLISHERS, INC.
CHICAGO · LONDON

Library of Congress Cataloging in Publication Data
Main entry under title:

Radiographic atlas of colon disease.

Includes index.
1. Colon (Anatomy)—Radiography—Atlases. 2. Colon (Anatomy)—Diseases—Diagnosis—Atlases. I. Greenbaum, Edward I. [DNLM: 1. Colon—Radiography—Atlases. WI17 R129]
RC804.R6R33 617'.5547'0757 79-19979
ISBN 0-8151-3923-3

To my wife, Carol, the "editor-in-chief" whose remarkable patience and excellent common sense helped make this book possible.

Preface

The price of wisdom is above rubies.—Old Testament, Job 28:18

*To know that we know what we know,
and that we do not know what we do not know,
that is true knowledge.*—Thoreau, *Walden* (quoting Confucius)

THE PURPOSE of this book is to fill a gap in the current literature on the radiology of colon disease. For many years, the subject matter in this volume has been spread throughout the world literature; nowhere was it available within the covers of a single textbook. An atlas approach has been utilized that covers every major disease process involving the colon; many minor and less common diseases have also been included. Over 2,000 illustrations demonstrate in pictorial form the nuances and subtleties of each disease process. We have attempted to show not only the basic findings within the disease process but also the minor variations that can often cause confusion in diagnosis. In certain instances, line drawings, graphs, and endoscopic and correlative gross pathologic material have been added to fully amplify the radiologic findings. Chapters on angiography, ultrasound and computed axial tomography explain how these modalities can best be used in specific instances.

The chapters in this book have been arranged in alphabetical order by subject so that the reader can rapidly find the information he seeks.

I invite criticism and comment from my colleagues. In 1871, Emerson stated in one of his lectures, "If a man can write a better book, preach a better sermon, or make a better mousetrap than his neighbor, though he builds his house in the woods, the world will make a beaten path to his door." The only way I can make this a better book is with your help. I hope that you will beat a path to my door and tell me what you like and what you don't like. I hope you will send me interesting case reports that you think should be included. Every effort will be made to include such material, and all criticisms will be seriously considered for future editions.

Both the contributors and I hope that this atlas will be a thorough, practical and useful reference for the physician in his everyday practice.

EDWARD I. GREENBAUM, M.D.

Contributors

DENIS C. ADLER, M.D.,
Clinical Professor of Radiology, Los Angeles County/University of Southern California Medical Center, Los Angeles

KOSHI ANDO, M.D.,
Department of Surgery, Shizuoka Red Cross Hospital, Japan

J. FRANK ARGUELLO, M.D.,
Department of Gastroenterology and Infectious Diseases, San Clemente (Calif.) General Hospital

SHOZO BABA, M.D.,
Associate Professor, Department of Surgery, Hamamatsu University School of Medicine, Hamamatsu, Japan

JEANNE W. BAER, M.D.,
Department of Radiology, St. Luke's Hospital Center; Assistant Professor of Clinical Radiology, College of Physicians and Surgeons, Columbia University, New York

ERNEST M. BASS, M.D.,
The Medical Centre, Randwick, Australia

LAWRENCE W. BASSETT, M.D.,
Department of Radiological Sciences, University of California, Los Angeles, Center for Health Sciences

SAMUEL L. BERANBAUM, M.D.,
Attending Radiologist, University Hospital, New York, and Bellevue Hospital, New York; Clinical Professor of Radiology, New York University Medical School

ROBERT N. BERK, M.D.,
Professor and Chairman, Department of Radiology, University of California, San Diego, School of Medicine

DAVID G. BRAGG, M.D.,
Professor and Chairman, Department of Radiology, University of Utah Medical Center, Salt Lake City

PHILIP A. BRODEY, M.D.,
Department of Radiology, Mt. Zion Hospital and Medical Center, San Franciso; Clinical Instructor, Department of Radiology, University of California, San Francisco

KEITH BURNETT, M.D.,
Department of Radiological Sciences, University of California, Irvine

S. CHAWLA, M.D.,
Lady Hardinge Medical College, New Delhi, India

MICHAEL H. CHILDRESS, M.D.,
Department of Radiology, University of Michigan Medical Center, Ann Arbor

JAMES L. CLEMENTS, JR., M.D.,
Director, Gastrointestinal Radiology, Grady Memorial Hospital, Atlanta; Professor of Radiology, Emory University School of Medicine

ALLEN J. COHEN, Ph.D., M.D.,
Assistant Professor, Department of Radiology, University of California, Irvine, Orange, California

DAVID K. CROMWELL, M.D.

DONALD N. DYSART, M.D., F.A.C.R.,
Department of Radiology, Scott and White Clinic, Temple, Texas

S. BOYD EATON, JR., M.D.,
Chief, Department of Radiology, West Paces Ferry Hospital, Atlanta

IWAO ENDO, M.D.,
Associate Professor, Department of Surgery, Ryuku University School of Medicine, Japan

CHARLES J. FAGAN, M.D.,
Professor of Radiology, University of Texas Medical Branch, Galveston

LEO S. FIGIEL, M.D., F.A.C.R.,
Vice-Chairman, Radiology, Harper-Grace Hospitals; Clinical Assistant Professor of Radiology, Wayne State University School of Medicine, Detroit

STEVEN J. FIGIEL, M.D.,
Director, Nuclear Medicine, Harper-Grace Hospitals; Clinical Assistant Professor of Radiology, Wayne State University School of Medicine, Detroit

GERALD J. GELFORD, M.D.,
Kettering (Ohio) Medical Center

GARY G. GHAHREMANI, M.D.,
Chairman, Department of Diagnostic Radiology, Evanston (Ill.) Hospital; Professor of Radiology, Northwestern University Medical School, Chicago

LOUIS A. GILULA, M.D.,
Co-Chief, Musculoskeletal Section, Barnes Hospital, St. Louis; Associate Professor of Radiology, Edward Mallinckrodt Institute of Radiology, Washington University School of Medicine, St. Louis

PETER E. GIUSTRA, M.D.,
Penobscot Bay Medical Center, Rockland, Maine

SETH N. GLICK, M.D.,
Assistant Professor of Radiology, Department of Diagnostic Radiology, Hahnemann Medical College and Hospital, Philadelphia

LAWRENCE E. GOLDBERGER, M.D.,
Assistant Professor of Radiology, University of California Medical Center, San Diego

HOSSEIN GOLJI, M.D.,
Chief, Spinal Cord Injury Service, Long Beach (Calif.) Veterans Administration Medical Center; Associate Clinical Professor, Department of Surgery, Division of Urology, University of California, Irvine

EDWARD I. GREENBAUM, M.D.,
Section of Gastrointestinal Radiology, Long Beach (Calif.) Veterans Administration Hospital; Associate Adjunct Professor, Department of Radiologic Sciences, University of California, Irvine

JAMES M. HALLS, M.B., F.R.C.P. (C),
Chairman, Department of Radiology, Los Angeles County/University of Southern California Medical Center, Los Angeles

STEPHEN J. HANDLER, M.D.,
Chief, Diagnostic Ultrasound, Department of Radiology, Long Beach (Calif.) Veterans Administration Hospital

JEFFERSON O. JANES, M.D.,
Chief, Radiology Service, Veterans Administration Medical Center, Salt Lake City; Assistant Professor of Radiology, University of Utah College of Medicine, Salt Lake City

BARBARA M. KADELL, M.D.,
Department of Radiological Sciences, University of California, Los Angeles, Center for Health Sciences

WILLIAM KIRKPATRICK, M.D., (retired),
Assistant Professor of Radiology, Baylor College of Medicine, Houston

P. RUBEN KOEHLER, M.D.,
Professor of Radiology, Chief, Diagnostic Division, University of Utah College of Medicine, Salt Lake City

ROBERT E. KOEHLER, M.D.,
Associate Professor of Radiology, Edward Mallinckrodt Institute of Radiology, Washington University School of Medicine, St. Louis

IGOR LAUFER, M.D.,
Department of Radiology, University of Pennsylvania School of Medicine, Philadelphia

THOMAS L. LAWSON, M.D.,
Milwaukee County Medical Complex; Associate Professor of Radiology, Medical College of Wisconsin

FRED A. LEE, M.D.,
Department of Radiology, Childrens Hospital of Los Angeles; University of Southern California School of Medicine, Los Angeles

JOSEPH F. LINSMAN, M.D., F.A.C.R., F.A.C.P.
Associate Visiting Radiologist, U.C.L.A. School of Medicine; Emeritus Associate Clinical Professor of Radiology, Loma Linda University; Emeritus Attending Physician, Department of Diagnostic Radiology, Cedars-Sinai Medical Center, Los Angeles

WILLIAM MARTEL, M.D.,
Department of Radiology, University of Michigan Medical Center, Ann Arbor

MORITO MARUTA, M.D.,
Assistant Professor, Department of Surgery, Fufita Gakuen University Hospital, Japan

LESLIE S. MENUCK, M.D.,
Radiologist, Palomar Memorial Hospital, Escondido, California; Assistant Clinical Professor of Radiology, University of California, San Diego, School of Medicine

HARVEY L. MEYERS, M.D., (deceased),
Professor of Radiology, University of Southern California School of Medicine, Los Angeles; Acting Head, Department of Radiology, LAC-USC Medical Center, Los Angeles

MORTON A. MEYERS, M.D.,
Professor and Chairman, Department of Radiology, State University of New York at Stony Brook

ROSCOE E. MILLER, M.D.,
Distinguished Professor of Radiology, Indiana University School of Medicine, Indianapolis

L. B. MORETTIN, M.D.,
Department of Radiology, University of Texas Medical Branch, Galveston

H. MULDER, M.D.,
Director of Diagnostic Radiology, Red Cross Hospital, The Hague

STANLEY NOVY, M.D., M.A.C.R.,
Department of Radiology, St. Joseph Hospital, Houston

P. E. S. PALMER, F.R.C.P., F.R.C.R.,
Department of Diagnostic Radiology, University of California, Davis

REED P. RICE, M.D.,
Department of Radiology, Duke University Medical Center, Durham, North Carolina

LEE F. ROGERS, M.D.,
Chairman, Department of Radiology, Northwestern Memorial Hospital, Chicago

BERNARD ROSWIT, M.D.,
Chief, Radiation Therapy Service, Veterans Administration Hospital, Bronx, New York; Professor, Radiation Therapy, Mt. Sinai Medical School, New York

WELLAND F. SHORT, M.D.,
Radiologist, Memorial Hospital, Albany, New York; Visiting Associate Professor of Clinical Radiology, University of Pittsburgh School of Medicine

H. SHULMAN, M.D., F.R.C.P. (C),
Department of Radiology, Sunnybrook Medical Centre, University of Toronto

BRUCE D. SMITH, M.D.,
Assistant Professor, Department of Radiology, University of Texas Health Science Center at San Antonio

STEVEN K. TEPLICK, M.D.,
Associate Professor of Radiology, Department of Diagnostic Radiology, Hahnemann Medical College and Hospital, Philadelphia

TATSUO TERAMOTO, M.D.,
Assistant, Department of Surgery, Keio University School of Medicine, Tokyo

WILLIAM M. THOMPSON, M.D.,
Department of Radiology, Duke University Medical Center, Durham, North Carolina

MARVIN WEINER, M.D.,
Department of Radiological Sciences, University of California, Los Angeles, Center for Health Sciences

Contents

Chapter 1

Abnormalities of Colonic Haustration

MICHAEL H. CHILDRESS, M.D.
WILLIAM MARTEL, M.D.

THERE IS considerable variation in the degree of haustration encountered in the colon in asymptomatic individuals. The haustral pattern is most pronounced and regular in the transverse segment and is less obvious in the ascending colon. It is frequently minimal or completely absent in the descending and sigmoid segments. Alteration of colonic haustration has been reported in chronic ulcerative colitis, granulomatous colitis, cathartic colon, scleroderma, dermatomyositis, myotonic dystrophy, amyloidosis, Fabry's disease (angiokeratoma corporis diffusum) and various infectious diseases such as strongylosis, schistosomiasis and amebiasis.[1-12]

Haustra rèpresent colonic outpouchings and are a manifestation of two types of folds: muscular or functional and crescentic or anatomical. When the teniae coli are severed, the muscular folds disappear but the anatomical folds persist. Both types of folds can be symmetric or asymmetric.[13] Most authors have attributed the presence of haustration to contraction of the teniae coli, but Dick et al.[1] have emphasized that contraction of the circular muscle also plays a role.

Loss of haustration has been variously attributed to functional change in the muscularis mucosa and muscularis propria, functional neurosis,[14] and submucosal damage—often associated with fibrosis.[1] Circumstantial evidence suggests that loss of haustra is functional in many cases. Reappearance of the haustra in ulcerative colitis, frequently reported as "reversibility" of ulcerative colitis (Fig 1–1), is an example. In addition, one often observes haustra in one phase of a single examination but not in another. It is possible that haustration is influenced by intracolonic pressure; this would explain why it occasionally appears diminished on a barium enema examination but not on a small bowel examination (with barium in the colon). This is particularly frequent in elderly patients.

Ulcerative Colitis

The classic condition associated with complete loss of colonic haustration is chronic ulcerative colitis (see Fig 1–1, A–C). Such loss of haustration has been attributed to submucosal damage, usually with fibrosis,[1] but submucosal changes are not invariably present.[14] The possibility that the haustral alteration in this disease is functional is suggested by cases in which the colon reverts to a normal haustral pattern after a period of disease inactivity (see Fig 1 – 1, D). It is of interest that in such cases, narrowing of the rectosigmoid, often slight, persists even though the haustra "reappear." Occasionally the effects of colonic distention may be observed in this disease (Fig 1 – 2). In ulcerative colitis not only is there loss of haustration, but the lumen is reduced and there is foreshortening. Often the entire colon is affected, but in a significant number of patients the changes are most obvious in the transverse and the left side of the bowel. Thus the disease may appear to be segmental, but the segment involved is invariably quite long and usually associated with involvement of the rectum and rectosigmoid. Skip lesions, frequent in granulomatous colitis, are virtually never seen in this condition and the segment involved shows changes throughout its circumference.

Granulomatous Colitis

Eccentric mural involvement, skip areas and discrete ulcers have been emphasized as features of granulomatous colitis. The rectosigmoid often appears normal. Granulomatous colitis is characterized by transmural involvement and consequently reversibility is probably less frequent than in ulcerative colitis. Occasionally, it is not possible to distinguish between ulcerative and granulomatous colitis. In most patients with the latter condition, the small bowel, in addition to the colon, is affected. The appearance of haustration in the "less distended colon" (as during small bowel examination) is not likely to be encountered in this condition (Fig 1 – 3), in contradistinction to chronic ulcerative colitis.

Cathartic Colon

Cathartic colon has been infrequently analyzed pathologically, but mucosal atrophy, disruption of the muscularis mucosa and minimal submucosal change have been described.[2] Reappearance of haustration has been noted following cessation of laxative abuse.[3] The right side is affected more commonly and to a greater degree than the left, and narrowing of the rectosigmoid is typically absent (Fig 1 – 4).

Scleroderma

Scleroderma may be confused with ulcerative colitis when it is associated with an ahaustral appearance (Fig 1 – 5). The presence of "diverticula" or sacculations (Fig 1 – 6) and the lack of foreshortening and narrowing are helpful distinguishing features. The cause of loss of haustration in this disease is not clear. Histologic findings that have been cited are atrophy and fibrosis of the muscularis propria.[4, 5] Whether there truly is a relationship between these changes is uncertain. It is possible that in this condition too the loss of haustration is functional. For example, the loss of haustration may not be as obvious in patients in whom the colon is not fully distended (see Fig 1 – 6).

Amyloidosis

The roentgen features of amyloidosis of the colon include loss of haustration (Fig 1 – 7, A), mucosal ulceration, polyps and luminal stenosis.[6] Involvement of the small bowel may cause diffuse thickening of the valvulae conniventes or generalized dilatation associated with the roentgen findings of malabsorption (see Fig 1 – 7, B). Histologically, one may observe amyloid deposition in small blood vessels and atrophy of the tunica muscularis.[6]

Other Conditions

Loss of colonic haustration has been reported in dermatomyositis,[5] myotonic dystrophy,[7] and Fabry's disease.[8] Reports of such involvement in these diseases are rare. In Fabry's disease one often also finds narrowing, shortening and a granular-appearing mucosa. Thickening of the colonic wall may occur, probably secondary to ceramide trihexoside deposition in smooth muscle.[8]

Rarely, infectious diseases such as strongylosis, schistosomiasis and amebiasis may be associated with loss of haustration, but in these conditions there often are strictures and mucosal ulcerations. Furthermore, generalized loss of haustration, as occurs in chronic ulcerative colitis, is uncommon in these conditions, although it has been reported.[9-12] It should be recognized that although reports of such lesions relate the changes to a specific parasite, more than one parasite is frequently present in the feces in these cases.[10] Occasionally additional features suggest the nature of the lesions, e.g., calcification in the colonic wall in schistosomiasis.[11]

REFERENCES

1. Dick, A. P., Berridge, F. R., and Grayson, M. J.: The pathologic basis of the radiological changes in ulcerative colitis. A study of cases treated by colectomy, Br. J. Radiol. 32:432, 1959.
2. Urso, F. P., Urso, M. J., and Lee, C. H.: The cathartic colon: Pathological findings and radiological/pathological correlation, Radiology 116:557, 1975.
3. Heilbrun, N.: Roentgen evidence suggesting enterocolitis associated with prolonged cathartic abuse, Radiology 41:486, 1943.
4. Martel, W., Chang, S. F., and Abell, M. R.: Loss of colonic haustration in progressive systemic sclerosis, Am. J. Roentgenol. 126:704, 1976.
5. Robinson, J. C., and Teitelbaum, S. L.: Stercoral ulceration and perforation of the sclerodermatous colon: Report of two cases and review of the literature, Dis. Colon Rectum 17:622, 1974.
6. Ritvo, M., and Litner, C.: Roentgen manifestations of primary amyloidosis of the colon. Case report, Am. J. Roentgenol. 89:760, 1963.
7. Krain, S., and Rabinowitz, J. G.: The radiologic features of myotonic dystrophy with presentation of a new finding, Clin. Radiol. 22:462, 1971.
8. Flynn, D. M., Lake, B. D., Boothby, C. B., et al.: Gut lesions in Fabry's disease without a rash, Arch. Dis. Child. 47:26, 1972.
9. Drasin, G. F., Moss, J. P., and Cheng, S. H.: Strongyloides stercoralis colitis: Findings in four cases, Radiology 126:619, 1978.
10. Chait, A.: Schistosomiasis mansoni: Roentgenologic observations in a nonendemic area, Am. J. Roentgenol. 90:688, 1963.
11. Lehman, J. S., Jr., Farid, Z., Bassily, S., et al.: Colonic calcification and polyposis in schistosomiasis. Report of a case, Radiology 98:379, 1971.
12. Kolawole, T. M., and Lewis, E. A.: Radiologic observations on intestinal amebiasis, Am. J. Roentgenol. 122:257, 1974.
13. Torsoli, A., Ramorino, M. L., and Crucioli, V.: The relationships between anatomy and motor activity of the colon, Am. J. Dig. Dis. 13:462, 1968.
14. Bockus, H. L.: *Gastroenterology,* Vol. II (2d ed.; Philadelphia: W. B. Saunders Co., 1964).

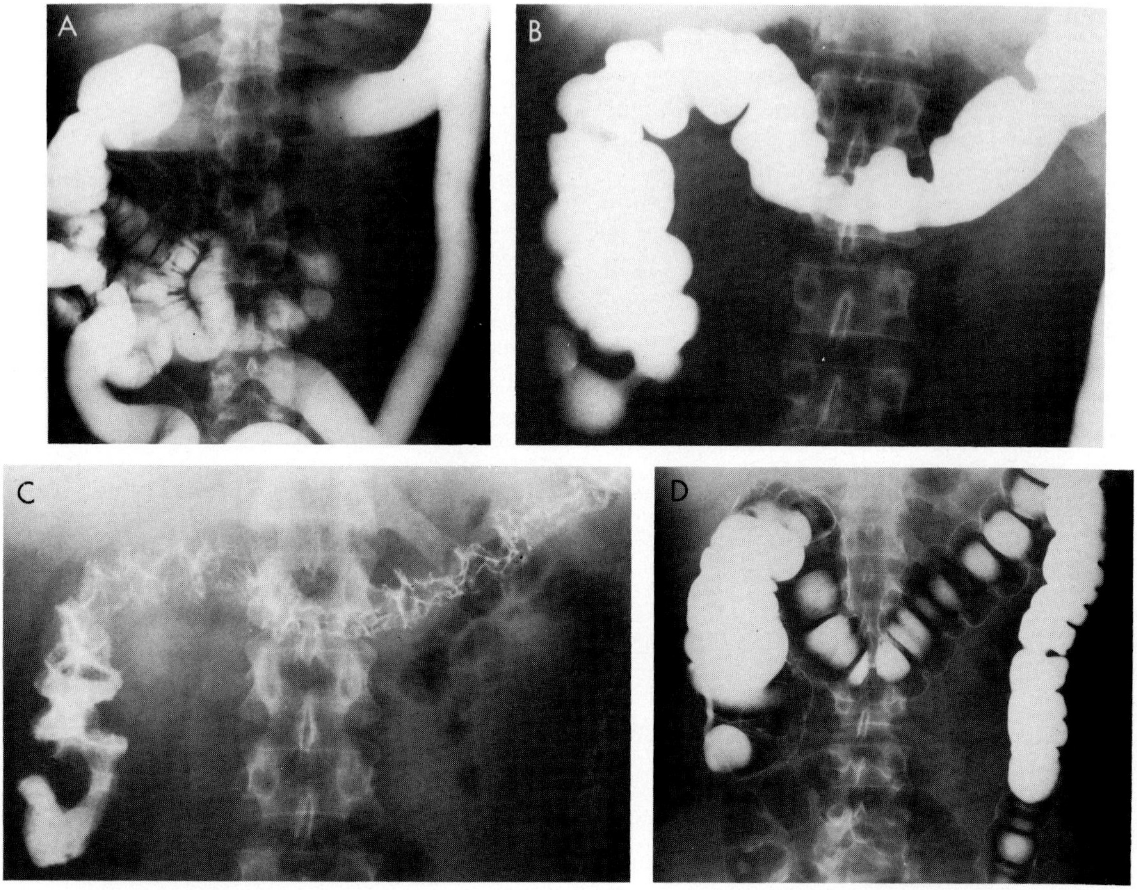

Fig 1–1.—Chronic ulcerative colitis. **A,** barium enema shows "distorted" haustral pattern of right colon, loss of haustration in transverse and descending colon and sigmoid narrowing. **B** and **C,** pre- and postevacuation films, respectively, 3 years later show abnormal irregular haustral pattern in ascending and transverse segments and distorted mucosal pattern. **D,** barium air contrast (6 months after study shown in **B** and **C**) shows normal haustral pattern. Patient was asymptomatic for several years.

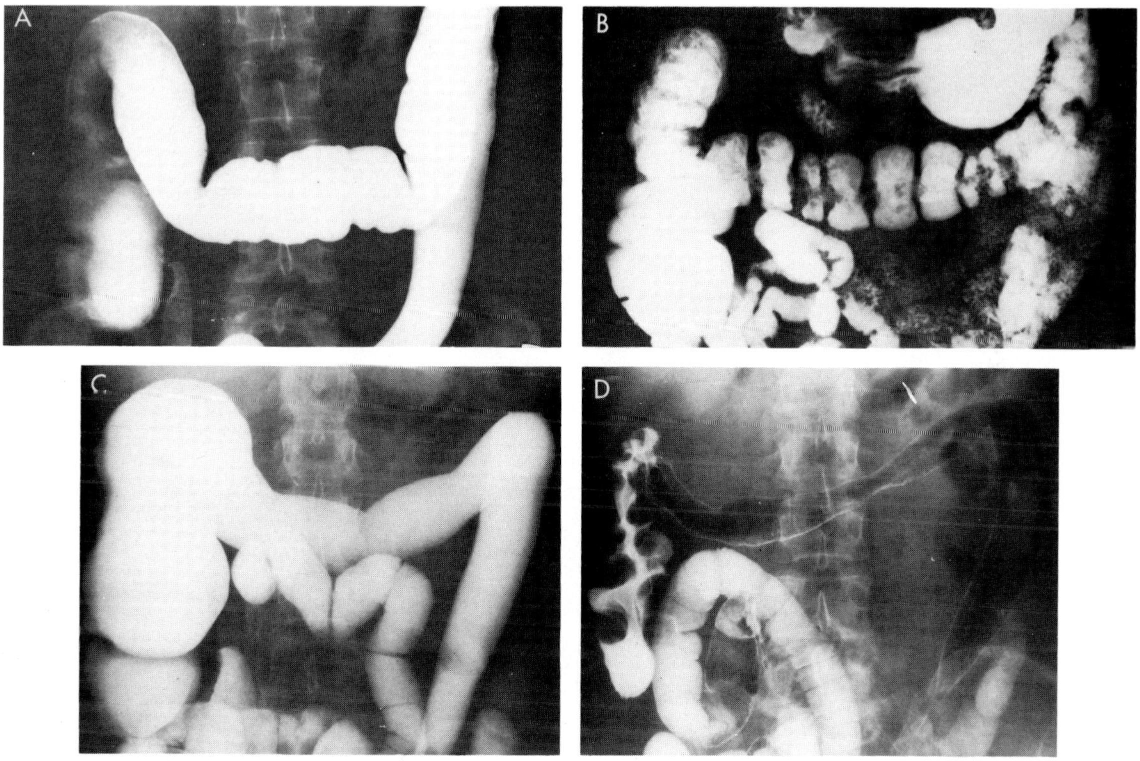

Fig 1–2. – Chronic ulcerative colitis. **A,** barium enema with full colonic distention shows almost complete loss of haustration. **B,** small bowel examination, 2 days later with less colonic distention, shows normal haustral pattern. **C** and **D,** 5 years later, pre- and postevacuation films show diffuse loss of haustration and abnormal mucosal pattern.

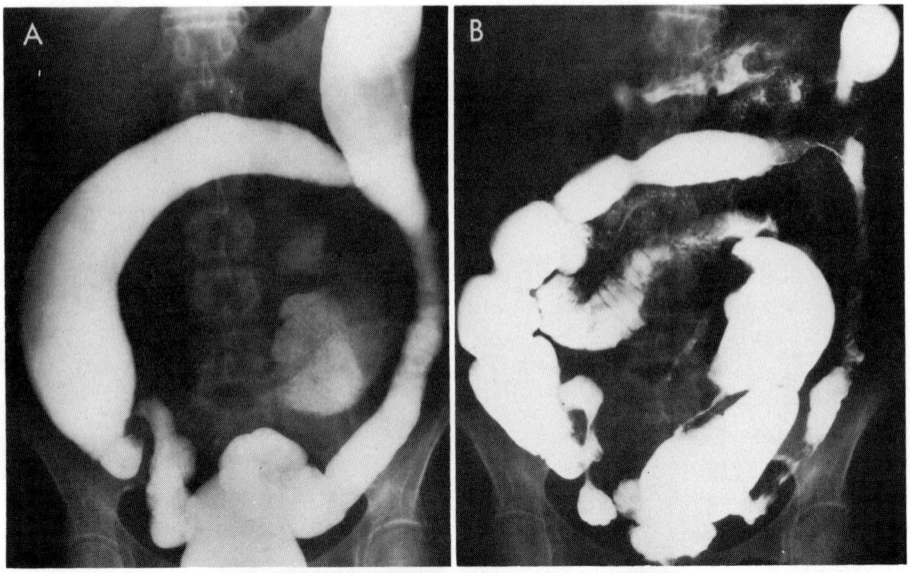

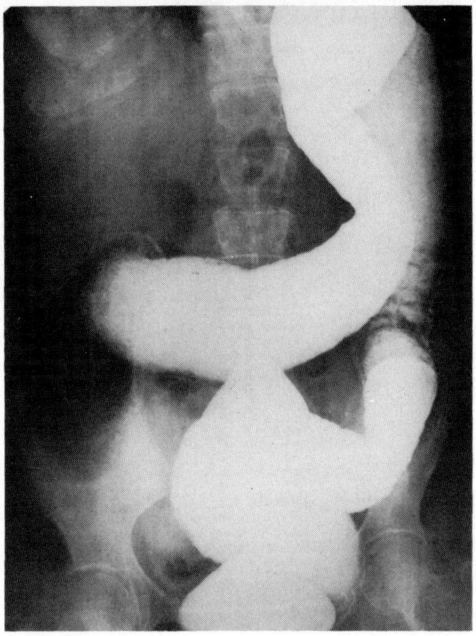

Fig 1–3 (top).—Granulomatous colitis. **A,** barium enema reveals narrowed, foreshortened and ahaustral colon with distensible rectosigmoid. Note involvement of small bowel and cecum. **B,** loss of haustration is evident in colon during small bowel examination. Note small bowel involvement, with partial obstruction.

Fig 1–4 (bottom).—Cathartic colon. Loss of haustration is most marked in ascending and transverse colon. Cecum and ascending colon are outlined by gas and barium. Rectosigmoid is normal.

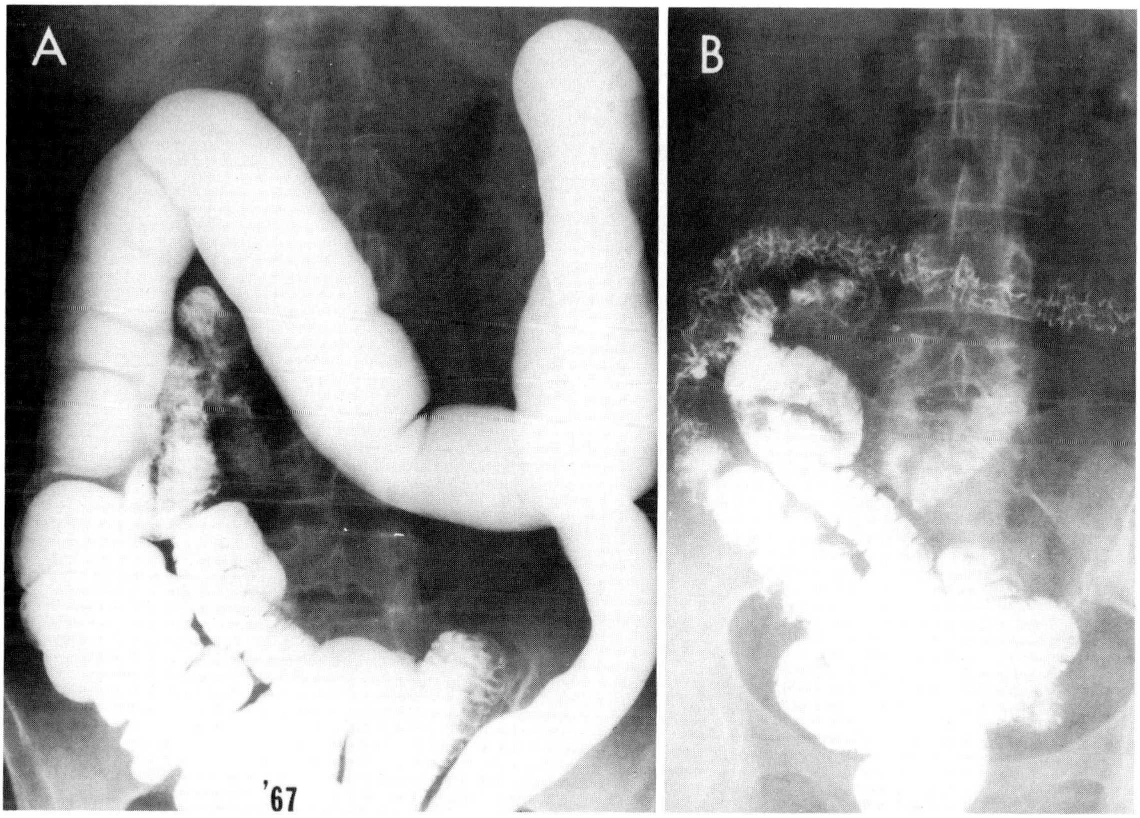

Fig 1–5.—Scleroderma. **A** and **B,** pre- and postevacuation films. There is loss of haustration in transverse colon but no foreshortening, and mucosal pattern is normal. (From Martel et al., Am. J. Roentgenol. 126:704, 1976, with permission.)

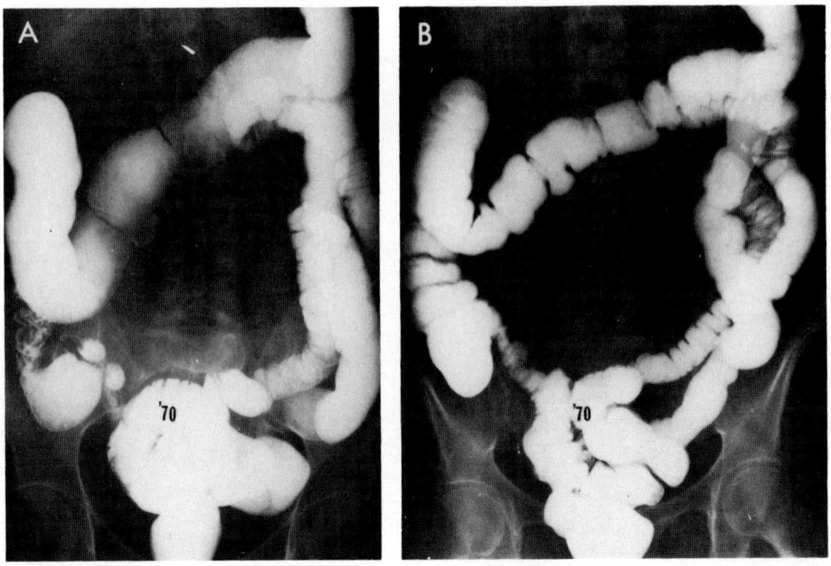

Fig 1–6.—Scleroderma. **A,** anteroposterior projection. **B,** posteroanterior projection with less colonic distention. Loss of haustration appears somewhat more marked when transverse colon is fully distended.

Fig 1–7.—Intestinal amyloidosis in patient with multiple myeloma. **A,** loss of colonic haustration. **B,** small bowel examination. Dilatation, retained fluid and delayed transit are present. Both large and small bowel were affected by amyloidosis. (From Gompels, B. M., Votaw, M. L. and Martel, Wm. Radiology 104:509, 1972, with permission.)

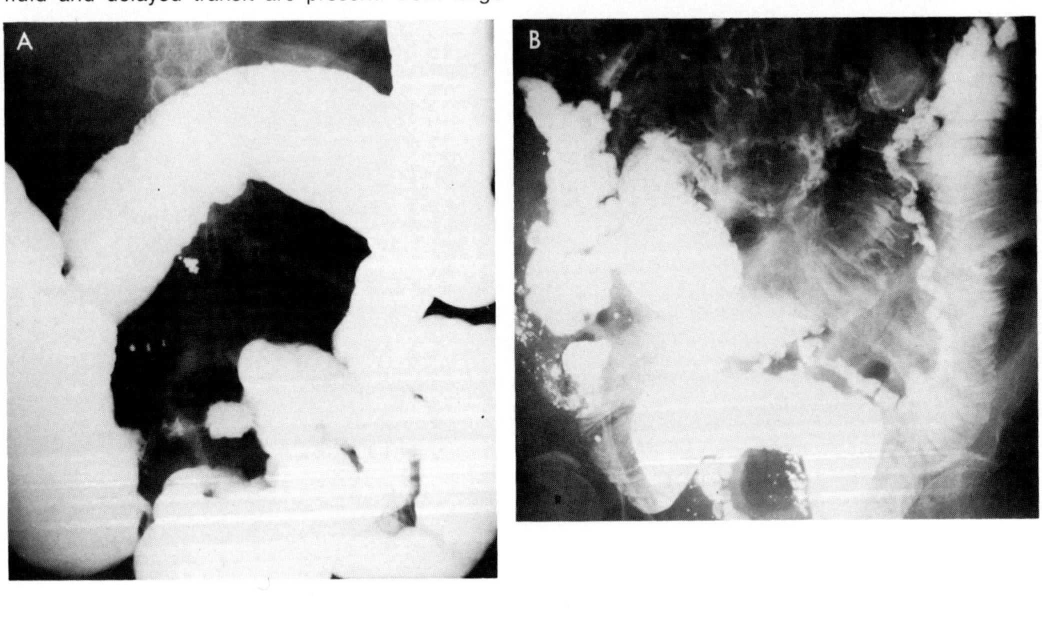

Chapter 2

Amebiasis and Tropical Diseases of the Colon

P. E. S. PALMER, F.R.C.P., F.R.C.R.

IT IS TEMPTING to describe the "tropical" colon as being the same as the colon anywhere else, with the added problems of diseases such as schistosomiasis, trichuriasis and a superabundance of amebiasis. But this is not so, and a clear distinction must be made between the colons of visitors to the tropics, be they temporary residents or travelers, and the colons of those who are indigenous to tropical countries. The latter are much less likely to be afflicted with ulcerative colitis, regional enteritis or diverticulosis; malignant disease also will be unlikely to occur and the patterns of tropical infections will be modified by repeated contact and partial immunity. Thus, the differential diagnosis of a colonic stricture, for example, depends on an accurate clinical history: if found in an elderly traveler from North America or Europe after a brief stay in the tropics, the stricture probably will be due to a carcinoma. The brief visit will not significantly have altered the differential probabilities. But in an emigrant from the tropics, such a stricture probably will be amebic or tuberculous and most unlikely to be malignant.

There are similar differences in the pattern of intestinal obstruction, and—to make it more complicated—the causes of intestinal obstruction vary in their relative frequency even within the tropics. For instance, wherever there is a high roughage diet, volvulus is common; intussusception has a similar, but different geographic, variation in incidence. Both have different frequencies in males and females, adults and children. And both vascular disease and diverticulosis are unlikely considerations in differential diagnosis.

Amebiasis (Figs 2–1 to 2–9)

Infection by the protozoan *Entamoeba histolytica* is worldwide, although particularly common in the tropics and subtropics. It is transmitted either by water or food that has been contaminated by carriers of cysts. When swallowed, the amebic cyst passes unharmed through the stomach and releases trophozoites in the small bowel. Although many of these are destroyed, others produce strong proteolytic enzymes and hyaluronidases, which are capable of lysing the intestinal epithelium. The trophozoites burrow into the mucosa and are always associated with bacteria: this results in the classic flask-shaped ulcer. However many cysts there are within the intestine, no symptoms occur until there has been tissue invasion. Only then is there clinical amebiasis (Figs 2–1 to 2–9), and only after invasion will the amebae stimulate sufficient antibody reaction to make the serologic test positive. These reactions remain positive after treatment and thus indicate past infection as well as current invasion: when the serologic results are negative, amebiasis can be virtually excluded.

The earliest recognizable lesion is a small abscess in the submucosa, usually of the cecum; such ulcers are usually multiple and diffuse. Deeper penetration occurs and necrosis follows, with the amebae migrating to the adjacent mucosa and submucosa, causing marked edema and, later, perforation. When the vessels and lymphatics are involved, embolization occurs and there is further spread of the disease. The colon is the most frequently affected organ, but the liver and any part of the body, including lung, pericardium and brain may become infected. Thoracic amebiasis is almost always (but not invariably) secondary to hepatic involvement, following spread of rupture or a liver abscess through the diaphragm.

The clinical spectrum of amebiasis is very wide, from desperately ill health to virtually no symptoms. There may be acute dysentery with abdominal pain, tenderness and fever or, alternatively, constipation or even no bowel symptoms. A liver abscess may be the cause of pain, and pyrexia an almost incidental finding, or it may be identified when it ruptures into the chest or abdomen. An amebic lung abscess may develop without other evidence of amebic disease.

Radiologically the pathologic changes of edema and ulceration are identified by a thickened, rigid bowel wall with swollen and irregular mucosa and multiple tiny ulcers. These may be seen anywhere throughout the length of the large bowel, although the cecum is the primary site of involvement. Amebiasis is almost always multifocal, and a careful search throughout the length of the colon for other areas of infection is an important aspect of differential diagnosis. Depending on the reaction of the patient, the radiologic findings may be those of acute colitis, even producing sufficient bowel distention to mimic the megacolon of ulcerative colitis. There may be strictures, but these are almost always associated with an area of colitis elsewhere. There may be tumorlike amebomas, which can be mistaken for malignancy. In the end stages of the disease, the colon becomes fibrotic.

Schistosomiasis (Fig 2–10)

Schistosomiasis is an infection caused by a parasitic blood fluke: all the major varieties (Fig 2–10) (*Schistosoma mansoni, Schistosoma haematobium* and *Schistosoma japonicum*) can affect the large bowel, but *S. mansoni* does so most frequently. Schistosomiasis mansoni is most common in Egypt, Arabia, the northern part of South America, Puerto Rico and the Caribbean. Thousands of Puerto Ricans in New York harbor *S. mansoni,* although, fortunately, climatic differences are unlikely to let the parasite spread and become a North American problem! *S. mansoni* requires a specific snail to complete its cycle, and these survive only where the water temperature does not fall below 60 F (15 C).

Schistosomiasis is an infection of the vascular system. The blood flukes live and copulate in the portal vein and are strictly intravenous parasites. They migrate along the vessel wall, usually within the liver. The eggs are deposited (in the case of *S. mansoni*) in the large bowel or rectum but may be found anywhere else. They stimulate multiple granulomas, with hyperplastic mucosal edema. Rarely, solitary and relatively large granulomas occur, particularly in individuals who suffer repeated infections and who have developed some immunity. Allergy also may occur. The whole pathologic process is extremely complex.

Clinically, the traveler returning from the tropics will often remember redness and an itchy skin after contact with fresh water (swimmer's itch) and will have blamed this on "sunburn." Three or four weeks later headache, backache, chills, fever, abdominal discomfort and anorexia develop, with fever varying from 99 to 105 F (38.5–40.5 C). There usually is a marked eosinophilia. Serologic tests will then become positive in most patients, although a negative test does not exclude infection. In those not previously exposed to schistosomiasis, the illness can be severe and life threatening, but none of these prodromal symptoms are likely to be recognized in patients who have had a lifetime contact with the infection. *S. mansoni* goes on to produce bloody diarrhea with much mucus, cirrhosis, portal hypertension and splenomegaly. Pulmonary hypertension is an added complication. In the colon there will be widespread granulomatous disease with mucosal polyps and strictures.

The radiologic findings in *S. mansoni* infection in the colon vary from edematous mucosa with tiny ulcers, usually with a segmental distribution, to multiple polyps 1–2 cm in size found particularly in the left colon and rectum. They may become sufficiently large to cause obstruction, intussusception or rectal prolapse. Eventually there will be a stenosing granulomatous colitis. Rarely, pericolic schistosomal abscesses may develop.

Trichuriasis or Whipworm Infection

The whipworm, *Trichuris trichiura,* infects the human cecum and colon and rarely the distal ileum. It is found throughout the world but particularly in warm, moist tropical climates, e.g., the southern United States and countries such as Brazil (an incidence of up to 40%) and Costa Rica (25–50%). In endemic areas it may be an almost normal inhabitant of the colon. Infection occurs by ingesting contaminated food or water and, in the case of small children, by playing with contaminated soil. The worm after ingestion gathers some nourishment in the small bowel but eventually settles in the cecum and large intestine where, in heavy infections, it may be spread throughout the whole colon. It may be totally unsuspected until found by chance in the stool or after treating the patient for ascariasis (with which it is often associated). It may cause severe chronic diarrhea, particularly in those who are undernourished. It is a frequent cause of rectal prolapse. Repeated infections may give rise to allergic reactions such as urticaria.

The radiologic diagnosis (Fig 2–11) is usually incidental to investigation of some other colonic problem. The excess mucus may flocculate around the hundreds of small whipworms, but an air contrast examination demonstrates the wavy radiolucent outlines of the Trichuris worms within the colon and rectum. The female worm is uncurled and whiplike, whereas the male is tightly coiled.

Bacillary Dysentery and Typhoid

Bacillary dysentery is unlikely to be a radiologic diagnosis, but it causes an acute diffuse inflammation of the colon and when it becomes chronic, neither the patient, the bowel nor the feces return to normal for many months. It is one of the causes of heavy content of gas in both small and large bowel on plain x-ray examination, and a film in the erect position may demonstrate fluid levels simulating obstruction. In the acute stage there may be edema and spasm throughout the length of the colon, and focal ulceration may occur. In the more chronic infections, transient spasm with loss of haustration, and eventually rigidity and fixation, will be found. Most cases will be mistaken radiologically for ulcerative colitis or regional enteritis.

Typhoid may affect the proximal colon, causing hyperplasia of the lymphoid tissue (particularly paratyphoid B) and an inflammatory swelling of the ileocecal valve. However, it is mainly a small bowel infection. It is one of the causes of bowel perforation and pseudo obstruction.

Chagas' Disease (South American Trypanosomiasis)

This infection (Fig 2-12) is entirely confined to South America, where it is extremely common. It has many different manifestations and is unlikely to be seen as an acute problem in the returned traveler. It results from infection with *Trypanosoma cruzi*, which is transmitted by several species of bugs. The insects are found in the mud walls and surroundings of rural homes, particularly those that are dimly lit. It is carried by several species of animals. The disease has also been transmitted by blood transfusion, very rarely by contaminated food. The acute disease affects the heart and central nervous system particularly. Chronic infections affect the esophagus, heart and colon. The underlying physiologic abnormality is disturbance or absence of peristalsis, resulting in motor incoordination. In the colon the clinical symptom is chronic constipation with bowel movements at intervals from one week to several months. The colon becomes dilated (megacolon), and because of the impacted fecal contents, inflammation and stasis ulceration develop. Sigmoid volvulus may occur. Radiologically the colon is enormously dilated and elongated and may be identified on plain radiographs. Unlike other causes of megacolon, the distribution may be segmental with a few relatively normal and unaffected segments intervening.

Helminthoma

The resident of the tropics and very rarely the returned traveler may develop a granulomatous reaction around a worm that has perforated the bowel. This forms a helminthoma. Any parasite may induce this, but the most common cause is the Oesophagostomum species of West and East Africa, Southeast Asia and parts of South America. It is one of the additional causes of a tumor in the bowel, particularly around the cecum and sigmoid (Fig 2-13).

Tuberculosis

Tuberculous colonic infection (Fig 2-14) is not common in any part of the world, but it must be recognized as one of the causes of a contracted and shrunken cecum, of colonic strictures and of colitis. Tuberculous peritonitis is relatively frequent in many parts of the tropics and may result in adhesions, causing intestinal obstruction.

Lymphogranuloma Venereum

Lymphogranuloma venereum (Fig 2-15) should be considered a possible infection in those who have lived in the tropics or in the visitor who has indulged in the more lurid pastimes of a tropical port. It is frequently seen in prostitutes of both sexes. The primary genital lesion is often unnoticed but the inguinal buboes and the proctocolitis are unlikely to be ignored. There will be associated diarrhea or constipation, rectal bleeding and excess mucus. In the chronic stage there is extensive fibrosis, particularly in the female, with development of rectovaginal fistula. The radiologic findings are essentially those of the strictures, which usually are long and tubular, located in the anorectal area or involving the whole rectum and sigmoid colon. They can be mistaken for regional enteritis or tuberculosis. Fistulas and perirectal abscesses are extremely common.

Malignant Disease

Carcinoma of the colon is uncommon in many parts of the tropical world: lymphoma does not have any particular geographic distribution. In children, Burkitt's lymphoma frequently affects any part of the alimentary tract. The Kaposi sarcoma may occasionally present as a largely solitary tumor within the bowel, particularly in the cecum. Intestinal polyps are more likely to be caused by infection (particularly *S. mansoni*) than by malignancy, although familial polyposis may be seen in any region.

Since many details of a very extensive subject have been omitted in this brief summary, perhaps the most important aid to diagnosis is to remember that these diseases exist, that they behave differently in the traveler and in the immigrant and that either individual may be suffering only from an ordinary, common or garden variety Western affliction.

REFERENCES

AMEBIASIS

Cain, G. D., *et al.*: Extensive stenosis of the colon and fistula formation following amoebic dysentery, Gastroenterology 61:898, 1971.

Cardoza, J. M., *et al.*: Radiology of invasive amebiasis of the colon, A. J. R. 128:935, 1977.

Faegenburg, D., *et al.*: Toxic megacolon in amebic colitis, A. J. R. 99:74, 1967.

Juniper, K., Jr.: Acute amebic colitis, Am. J. Med. 33: 377, 1962.

Lewis, E. A., and Antia, A. U.: Amoebic colitis: review of 295 cases, Trans. R. Soc. Trop. Med. Hyg. 63:633, 1969.

Radke, R. A.: Ameboma of the intestine: an analysis of 78 collected and 41 previously unreported cases, Ann. Intern. Med. 43:1048, 1955.

Recio, P. M.: Ameboma of the colon, Dis. Colon Rectum 8:205, 1965.

Reeder, M. M., and Palmer, P. E. S.: *The Radiology of Tropical Diseases* (Baltimore: Williams & Wilkins Co., in press), chap. 1.

Shaff, B. L., and Wolfowitz, J.: Enterocolic amoebic fistulae, Br. J. Surg. 49:535, 1962.

SCHISTOSOMIASIS

Chait, A.: Schistosomiasis mansoni: roentgenologic observations in a nonendemic area, A. J. R. 90:688, 1963.

Cheever, A. W., *et al.*: Pathological lesions associated with Schistosoma mansoni infection in man, Trans. R. Soc. Trop. Med. Hyg. 61(5):626, 1967.

El-Sallab, R. A., *et al.*: Angiographic appearances of bilharzial mass of the colon, Br. J. Radiol. 40:151, 1967.

Garcia-Palmieri, M. R., and Marcial-Rojas, R. A.: The protean manifestations of schistosomiasis mansoni: A clinicopathological correlation, Ann. Intern. Med. 57:763, 1962.

Medina, J., *et al.*: The roentgen appearance of schistosomiasis mansoni involving the colon, Radiology 85:682, 1965.

Reeder, M. M., and Palmer, P. E. S.: *The Radiology of Tropical Diseases* (Baltimore: Williams & Wilkins Co., in press), chap. 2.

TRICHURIASIS

Fisher, R. M., and Cremin, B. J.: Rectal bleeding due to Trichuris trichiura, Br. J. Radiol. 43:214, 1970.

Reeder, M. M., Astacio, J. E., and Theros, E. G.: Case of the month from the AFIP: massive Trichuris infestation of the colon, Radiology 90:382, 1968.

Reeder, M. M., and Palmer, P. E. S.: *The Radiology of Tropical Diseases* (Baltimore: Williams & Wilkins Co., in press), chap. 14.

TYPHOID & DYSENTERY

Bohrer, S. P.: Typhoid perforation of the ileum, Br. J. Radiol. 39:37, 1966.

Farman, J., *et al.*: Roentgenology of infectious colitis, A. J. R. 119:375, 1973.

Reeder, M. M., and Palmer, P. E. S.: *The Radiology of Tropical Diseases* (Baltimore: Williams & Wilkins Co., in press), chap. 13.

CHAGAS' DISEASE

Reeder, M. M., and Palmer, P. E. S.: *The Radiology of Tropical Diseases* (Baltimore: Williams & Wilkins Co., in press), chap. 4.

HELMINTHOMA

Reeder, M. M., and Palmer, P. E. S.: *The Radiology of Tropical Diseases* (Baltimore: Williams & Wilkins Co., in press), chap. 17.

Welchman, J. M.: Helminthic abscess of the bowel, Br. J. Radiol. 39:372, 1966.

TUBERCULOSIS

Abrams, J. S., and Holden, W. D.: Tuberculosis of the gastrointestinal tract, Arch. Surg. 89:282, 1964.

Barson, A. J., and Kirk, R. S.: Colonic tuberculosis with carcinoma, J. Path. 101:289, 1970.

Brenner, S. M., Annes, G., and Parker, J. G.: Tuberculous colitis simulating nonspecific granulomatous disease of the colon, Am. J. Dig. Dis. 15:85, 1970.

Hancock, D. M.: Hyperplastic tuberculosis of the distal colon, Br. J. Surg. 46:63, 1958.

McDonald, J. B., and Middleton, P. J.: Tuberculosis of the colon simulating carcinoma, Radiology 118(2): 293, 1976.

Reeder, M. M., and Palmer, P. E. S.: *The Radiology of Tropical Disease* (Baltimore: Williams & Wilkins Co., in press), chap. 5.

Werbeloff, L., *et al.*: The radiology of tuberculosis of the gastrointestinal tract, Br. J. Radiol. 46:329, 1973.

LYMPHOGRANULOMA VENEREUM

Annamunthodo, H., and Marryatt, J.: Barium studies in intestinal lymphogranuloma venereum, Br. J. Radiol. 34:53, 1961.

Klein, I.: Roentgen study of lymphogranuloma venereum: report of 24 cases, A. J. R. 51:70, 1944.

Reeder, M. M., and Palmer, P. E. S.: *The Radiology of Tropical Diseases* (Baltimore: Williams & Wilkins Co., in press), chap. 16.

MALIGNANT DISEASE

Reeder, M. M., and Palmer, P. E. S.: *The Radiology of Tropical Diseases* (Baltimore: Williams & Wilkins Co., in press), chap. 35.

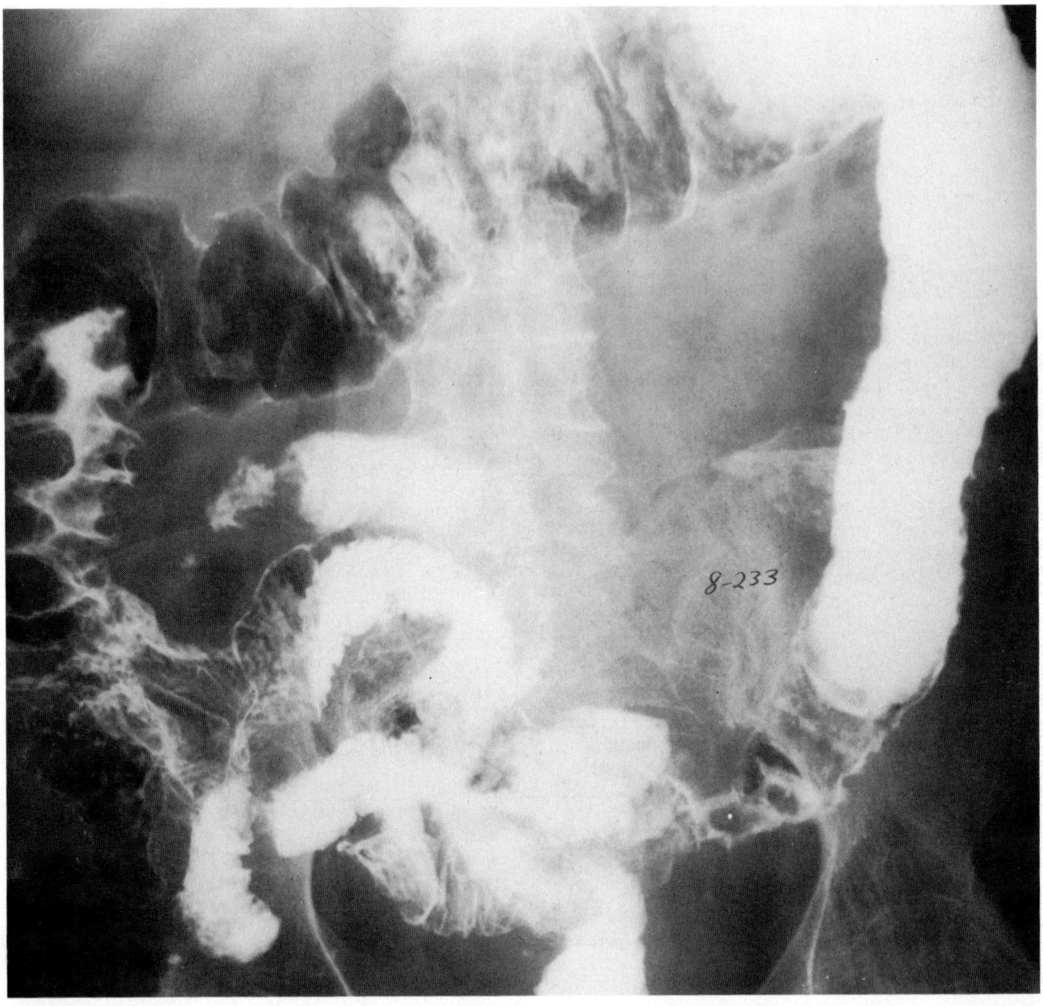

Fig 2–1.—Spectrum of amebiasis. Lower part of cecum shows mucosal edema; in ascending colon, edema is so severe that there is "thumbprinting." Proximal transverse colon has granular pattern due to multiple small ulcers and is beginning to dilate. Descending colon shows ulceration in silhouette on both sides, with loss of normal haustration; lower down there is edema of sigmoid colon. Pelvic portion of sigmoid colon is quite narrow, probably due to an early ameboma. Remainder of sigmoid loop and rectum show marked ulceration and edema.

It is unusual to see all these changes at the same time. Mucosal ulceration (as seen in descending colon in this radiograph) is one of the earliest pathologic findings. Dilatation (shown in transverse colon) usually indicates severe, acute inflammatory process. Thumbprinting (shown in ascending colon) reflects marked mucosal edema. The ameboma (in the sigmoid) is a hyperplastic granuloma resulting from secondary bacterial infection of an amebic abscess in bowel wall. This section of colon will be thickened and rigid. It probably will be palpable. (Courtesy of Dr. Philip Palmer and Armed Forces Institute of Pathology, Neg. No. 68-3558–1 (229498-233). Reproduced with permission.)

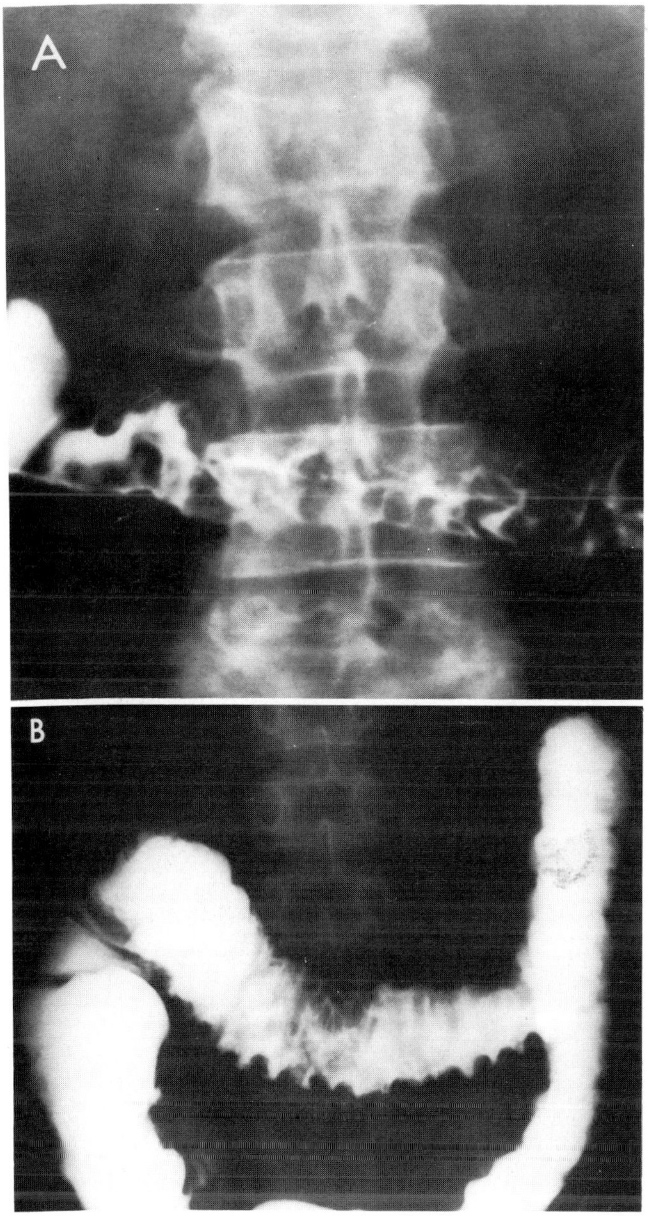

Fig 2–2.—Mucosal pattern in amebic infection of the colon may vary considerably. **A,** transverse colon is nodular with fine ulceration. This section of bowel will be thickened because of edema: peristalsis will be reduced and there will be local tenderness on palpation. **B,** edema of transverse colon, resulting in thick transverse folds surrounding affected area. This easily could be mistaken for early diverticulitis, and associated edema of descending colon could occur in any type of colitis. In many such patients, the diagnosis must be made by clinical and laboratory means. *(Continued.)*

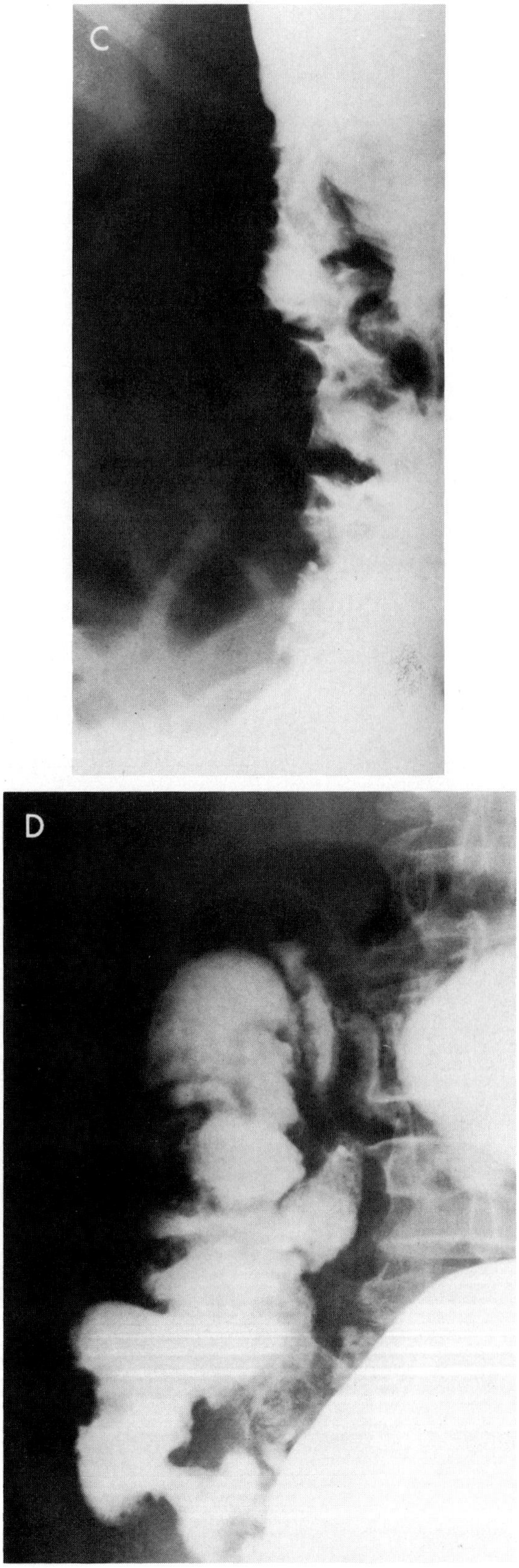

Fig 2–2 *(cont.)*. – **C,** ulceration causing serration of edge of colon. Amebic ulcers may be so small that radiologic appearance is merely that of a hazy and indistinct bowel wall. In other cases, ulceration is more obvious, and associated edema causes rigidity and loss of normal haustral pattern, as seen in this patient. A double contrast examination is preferred for demonstrating ulceration, particularly in early stages. **D,** severe mucosal edema of cecum and ascending colon completely destroying normal radiologic pattern, obliterating haustration and associated with decreased motility. Macroscopically the bowel in this patient would be thick and edematous with multiple ulcers of all sizes, excess mucus and blood and, because of bacterial invasion, obvious pus as well. Patient's bowel was acutely inflamed and necrotic. However, rest of bowel in amebiasis may be surprisingly normal or may exhibit much earlier invasion in some other segment: the stage of disease is not consistent throughout length of bowel. (Courtesy of Dr. Philip Palmer. **D** from Armed Forces Institute of Pathology, Neg. No. 1069804. Reproduced with permission.)

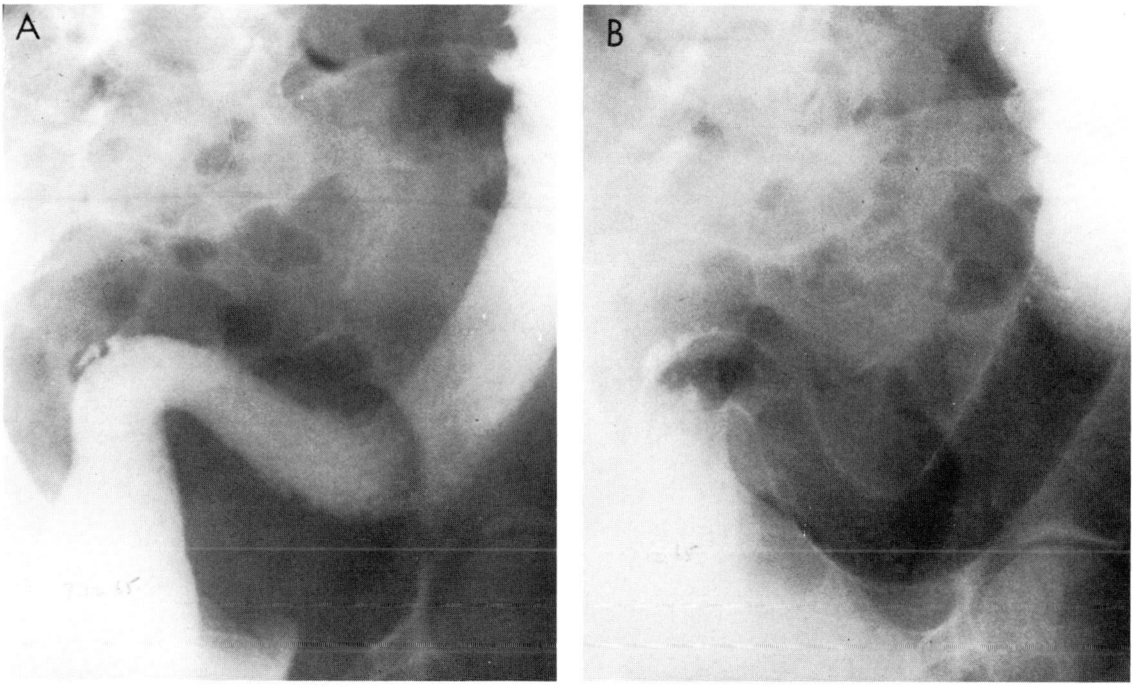

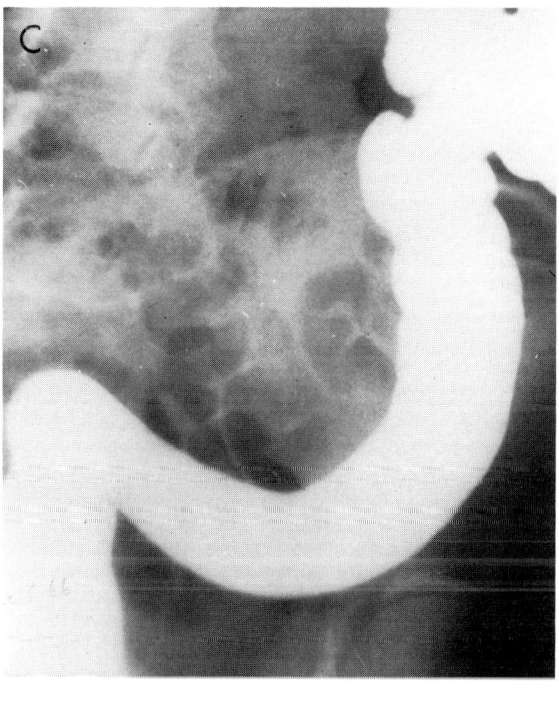

Fig 2–3.—Amebiasis mimicking ulcerative colitis. **A,** sigmoid colon of patient complaining of diarrhea, with blood and mucus in stools and lower abdominal pain and tenderness. Film shows severe local colitis, with ulceration and edema. Normal segmented pattern of sigmoid has been completely obliterated by swelling of mucosa and submucosa. **B,** air contrast study on same day shows numerous mucosal ulcers, causing granular pattern typical of ulcerative colitis. However, following treatment for amebiasis, there was considerable improvement. Ulceration healed but fibrosis followed, and 6 months later **(C)** bowel was rigid, smooth and fibrotic, as may also follow ulcerative colitis. It can be extremely difficult radiologically to differentiate the various patterns of colitis, and errors may arise if clinical examination of stool and mucosa is insufficient. Steroid or surgical therapy aimed at ulcerative colitis may be disastrous if the true diagnosis is amebic infection. (From Reeder and Palmer, *The Radiology of Tropical Diseases* [Baltimore: Williams & Wilkins Co., 1979], with permission. Original radiographs courtesy of Dr. J. Farman.)

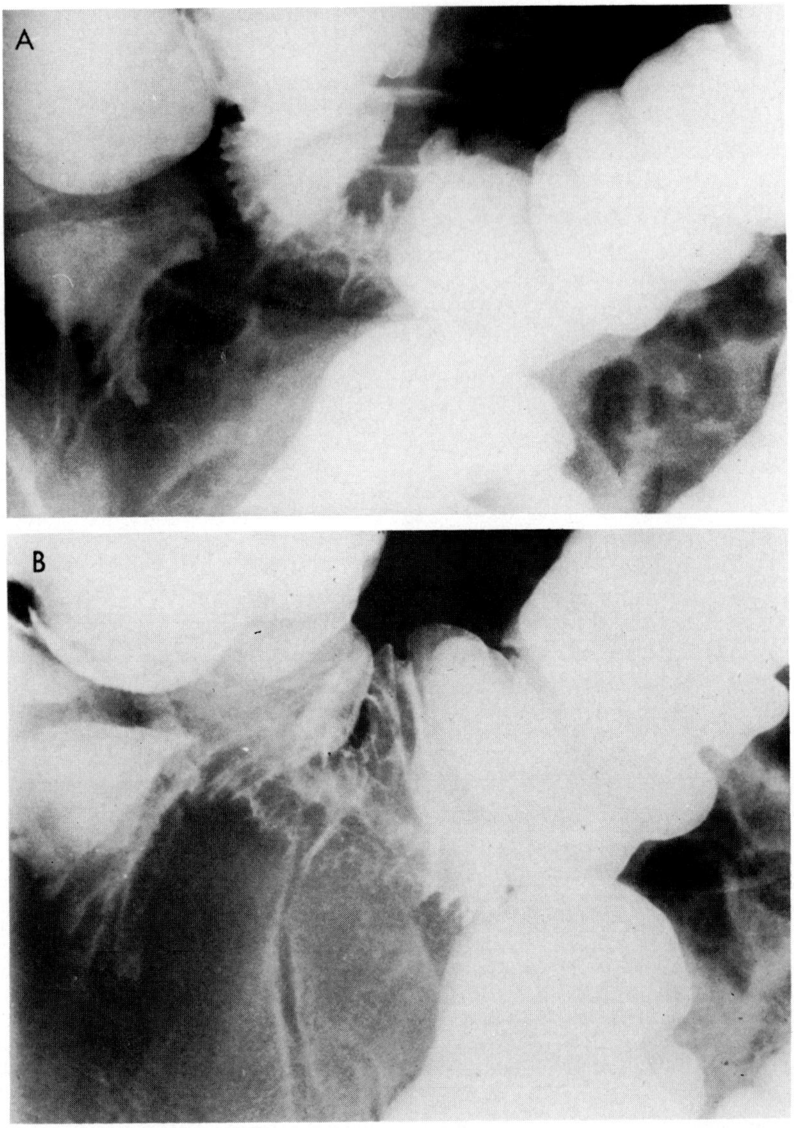

Fig 2–4.—Amebiasis particularly affects the cecum. However, a very careful search should be made for area of infection elsewhere in colon because in this way it is sometimes possible to distinguish between tumor in cecum and ameboma. **A** and **B,** two views showing obliteration of normal tip of cecum by large "tumor," which pathologically was granulomatous mass caused by amebiasis. Nearby transverse colon shows typical segment of ulcerated and edematous bowel with inflammatory saw-toothed edge. Cecum and colon were not adherent; these were two separate lesions, making the diagnosis of amebiasis very probable. (From Reeder and Palmer, *The Radiology of Tropical Diseases* [Baltimore: Williams & Wilkins Co., 1979], with permission.)

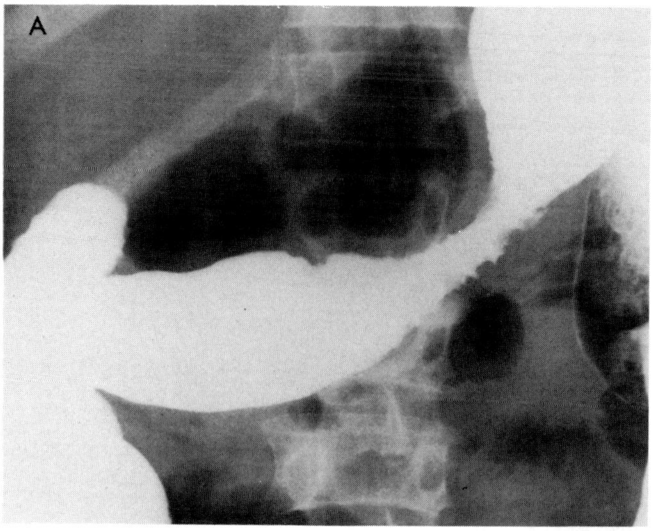

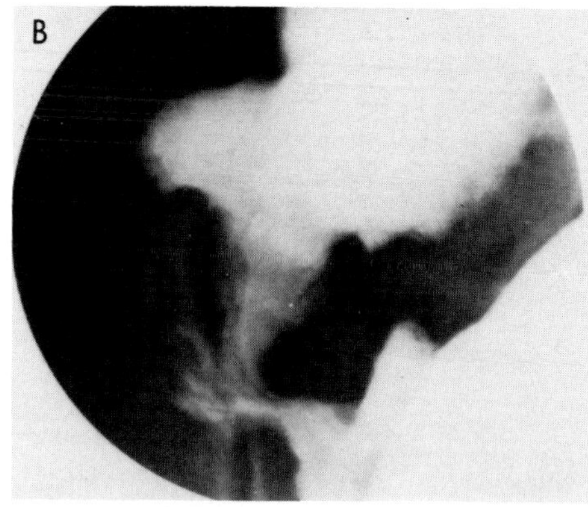

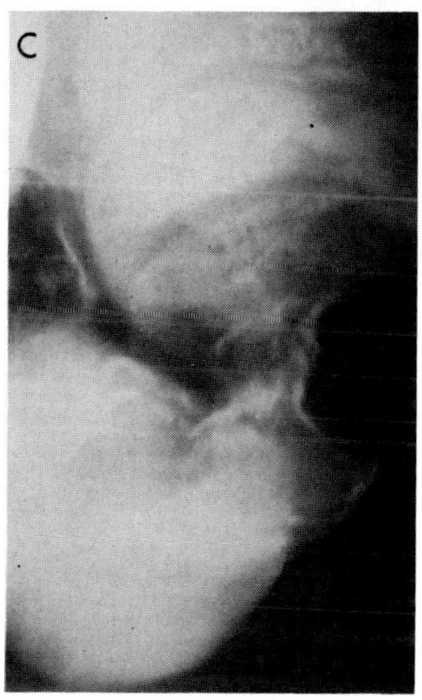

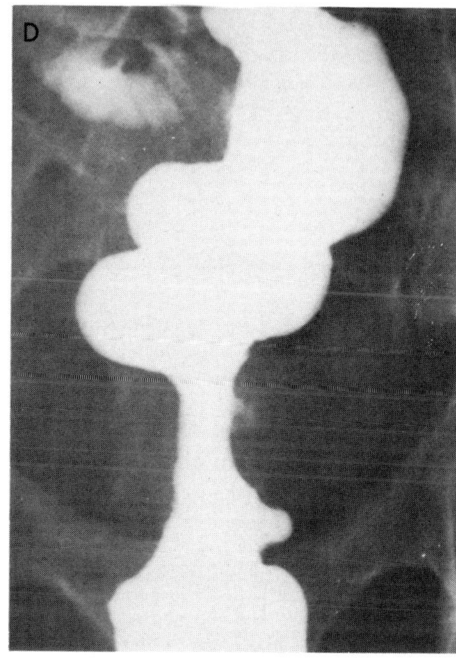

Fig 2–5.—An ameboma may exhibit a variety of patterns and may occur anywhere throughout the bowel. Although more common in the cecum and ascending colon, they are also found in the transverse colon or sigmoid. Although very characteristic of amebiasis, the radiologic diagnosis is not dependent on demonstration of an amebic tumor because there is a geographic variation in the frequency of ameboma (for reasons so far unexplained), and thus amebic granuloma may be common in some parts of the world and relatively rare in others. **A,** long, narrow segment of transverse colon proximal to splenic flexure, showing edema and mucosal ulceration. Transition from normal to abnormal bowel is gradual, with extensive adjacent peripheral ulceration: this is characteristic of amebomas. There is marked thickening of bowel wall, clearly seen against contrast of gas-filled viscera. The "tumor" was easily palpable and disappeared with amebic therapy. This elongated ameboma could occasionally be mistaken for a lymphoma or, where appropriate, other parasitic bowel involvement. **B, C** and **D,** three examples of "apple core" type of ameboma: **(B)** in ascending colon, **(C)** in sigmoid and **(D)** in rectum. In each there is a narrow constriction with edematous edges: the constriction may be sufficiently tight to present clinically as intestinal obstruction, and the radiologic appearances may be indistinguishable from a carcinoma. When, as often happens, there are other areas of colitis in the bowel, an ameboma may be suspected. Characteristically, there is more associated inflammation and ulceration adjacent to an ameboma than in malignant disease, and true obstruction is less common in amebiasis than in malignancy. Radiologically it is often possible to demonstrate distention of the stenosed area when it is due to amebiasis, whereas malignant infiltration seldom can be distended. It is noteworthy that a barium enema rarely causes pain in amebiasis, whereas in obstructive malignancy the enema is often painful. In case of doubt, specific treatment for amebiasis may cause rapid regression over a period of 3 or 4 weeks; in malignancy there will be no change. When amebiasis is as close to the rectum as in **D,** cutaneous ulceration may occur either through fistula formation or through direct contamination of the skin around the anus. Intact skin is not invaded by the amebae. Similar rectal strictures and fistulas may occur in lymphogranuloma venereum and tuberculosis. (**A** and **D,** from Reeder and Palmer, *The Radiology of Tropical Diseases* [Baltimore: Williams & Wilkins Co., 1979], with permission. **B,** Armed Forces of Pathology, neg. no. 10698071; **C,** neg. no. 9-432. Reproduced with permission.)

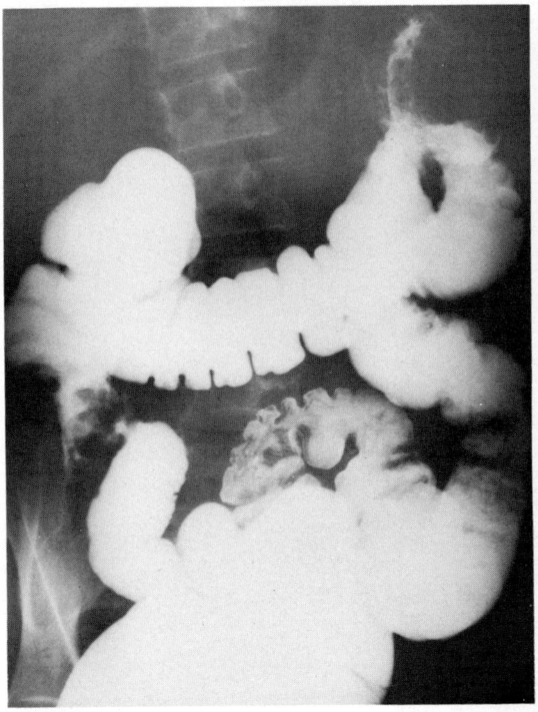

Fig 2–6 (above).—Amebic infection in a West African. Cecum has lost its normal saclike appearance and has narrowed to a coneshape, shrinking so that ileocecal valve appears to be close to tip of cecum. Valve in this case is thickened, rigid and fixed in open position so that reflux occurs in almost all barium enema examinations. (This is a helpful feature, distinguishing amebic infection from tuberculosis, in which reflux seldom occurs.) It would be impossible to distinguish this cecum from malignant disease if the obvious colitis in the splenic flexure were not recognized. There is marked mucosal edema also in upper part of descending colon, with loss of normal haustral pattern and with obvious ulceration. When two areas of bowel are involved in this way, amebiasis becomes very likely. (Courtesy of Professor S. B. Lagundoye and Radiology Library, University of Ibadan, Nigeria.)

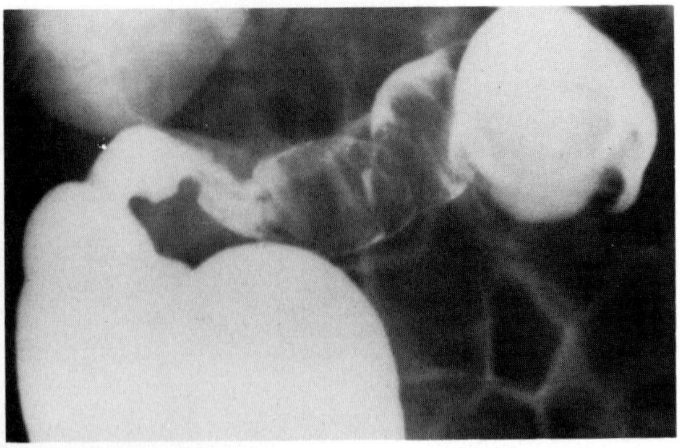

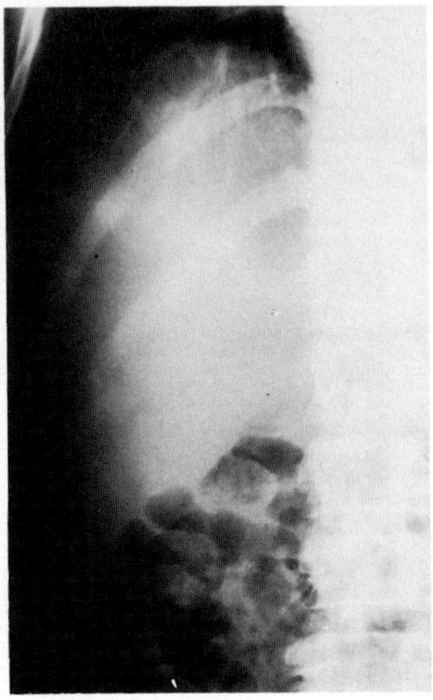

Fig 2–7 (above, right).—Intussusception due to amebiasis. This is particularly common in children but may occur at any age. Intussusception may occur because of stricture due to an ameboma, or because of thickening of part of bowel wall, which becomes rigid and is forced downward with normal bowel peristalsis. This possibility must be remembered in children wherever there is a likelihood of amebic infection. Risks of reduction by barium enema are probably no more than from surgery, but if antiamebic treatment can be instituted first, the whole process is less traumatic for both radiologist and patient. (From Reeder and Palmer, *The Radiology of the Tropical Diseases* [Baltimore: Williams & Wilkins Co., 1979], with permission.)

Fig 2–8 (below, right).—Enlargement of liver in acute amebiasis reflects underlying pathologic change of "amebic hepatitis." It also may indicate one or more amebic abscesses. It may be found in a patient whose main complaint is constipation and who has no history of "dysentery." Assessment of size of liver clinically may be very misleading because liver may extend upward into chest rather than downward into abdomen. (From Reeder and Palmer, *The Radiology of Tropical Diseases* [Baltimore: Williams & Wilkins Co., 1979], with permission.)

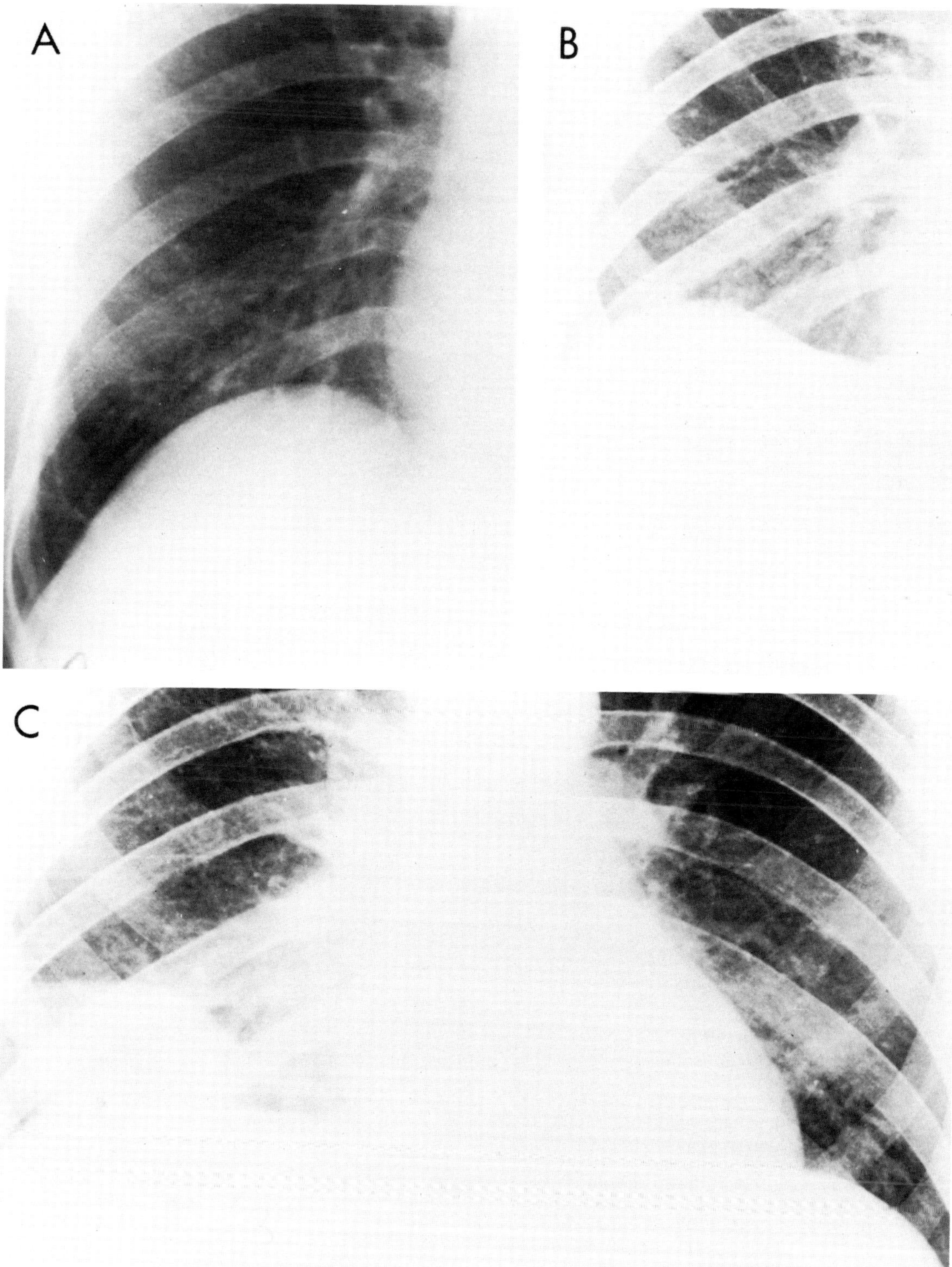

Fig 2–9.—Spectrum of amebic liver disease affecting chest. **A,** elevation of right side of diaphragm. This may be the only abnormal finding. Lung may be entirely normal, and costophrenic angle may remain clear. This may be unchanged for many weeks. **B,** bulge in diaphragm may be central or lateral and cannot be accurately associated with position of underlying abscess, nor does a localized deformity clearly indicate that such an abscess exists. When process is acute, the earliest change in lung above diaphragm is slight increase in haziness and small pleural effusion. **C,** later, lung may become edematous and resemble pneumonia. In some cases there has been lymphatic spread through diaphragm and there is truly an amebic lung infection. In many other cases, diaphragm has become immobile and the "cloud" is result of local stasis and edema. *(Continued.)*

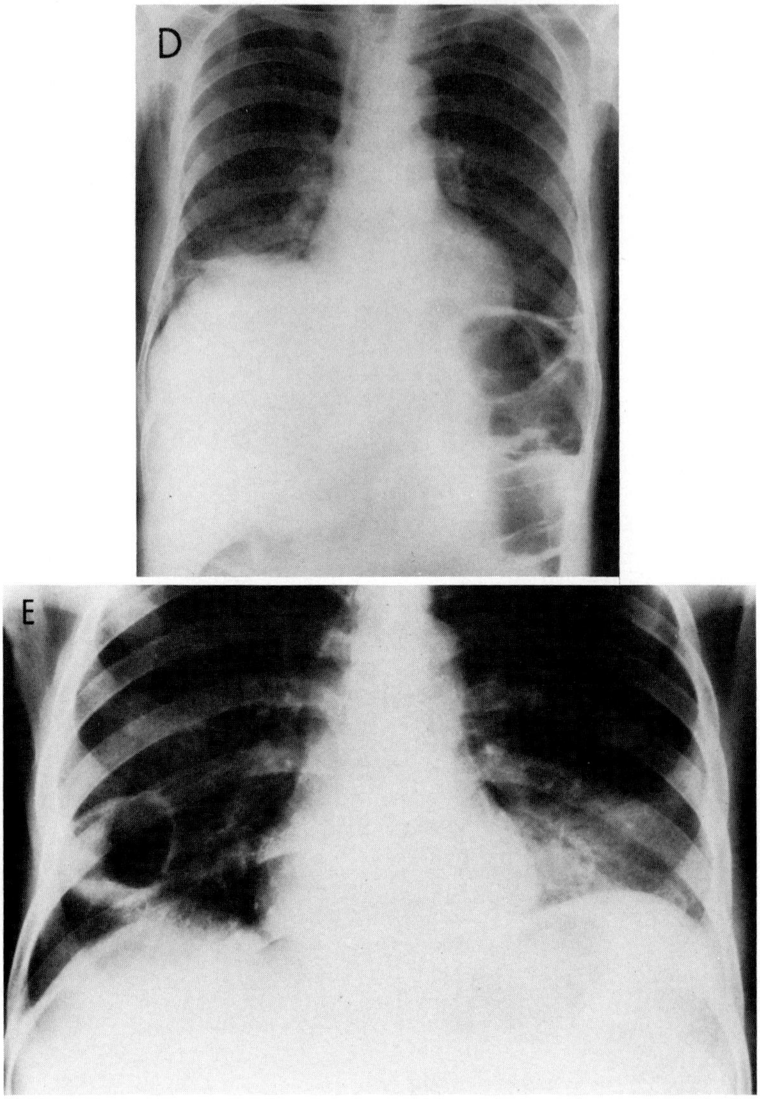

Fig 2–9 ***(cont.).*** – **D,** in other patients, lung above diaphragm becomes atelectatic, again because of lack of movement of elevated diaphragm. It may be mistaken for pulmonary infarction or infection. In many patients a pleural effusion will be predominant finding, but in others, as in this case, costophrenic angle may remain clear and no effusion develops. **E,** lymphatic spread of infection through diaphragm may cause localized lung abscess, with a fluid level. Costophrenic angle may remain clear, and cavity may resemble simple pyogenic abscess. A similar abscess may occur anywhere in lung field, even when amebic infection has not been clinically suspected and liver is normal. In other patients, lung abscess develops rapidly into amebic empyema, with more severe prognosis. Note in this case **(E)** a cloud above left diaphragm and small left pleural effusion. Infection in left side of liver may reproduce identical changes in left side of chest, and amebic abscess may rupture into pericardium, causing acute pericarditis and very severe illness. Although in this patient, sputum contained amebae, this finding is not consistent and diagnosis must be suspected when liver is enlarged or there is lack of response to standard therapy for pyogenic lung abscess. (From Reeder and Palmer *The Radiology of Tropical Diseases* [Baltimore: Williams & Wilkins Co., 1979], with permission.)

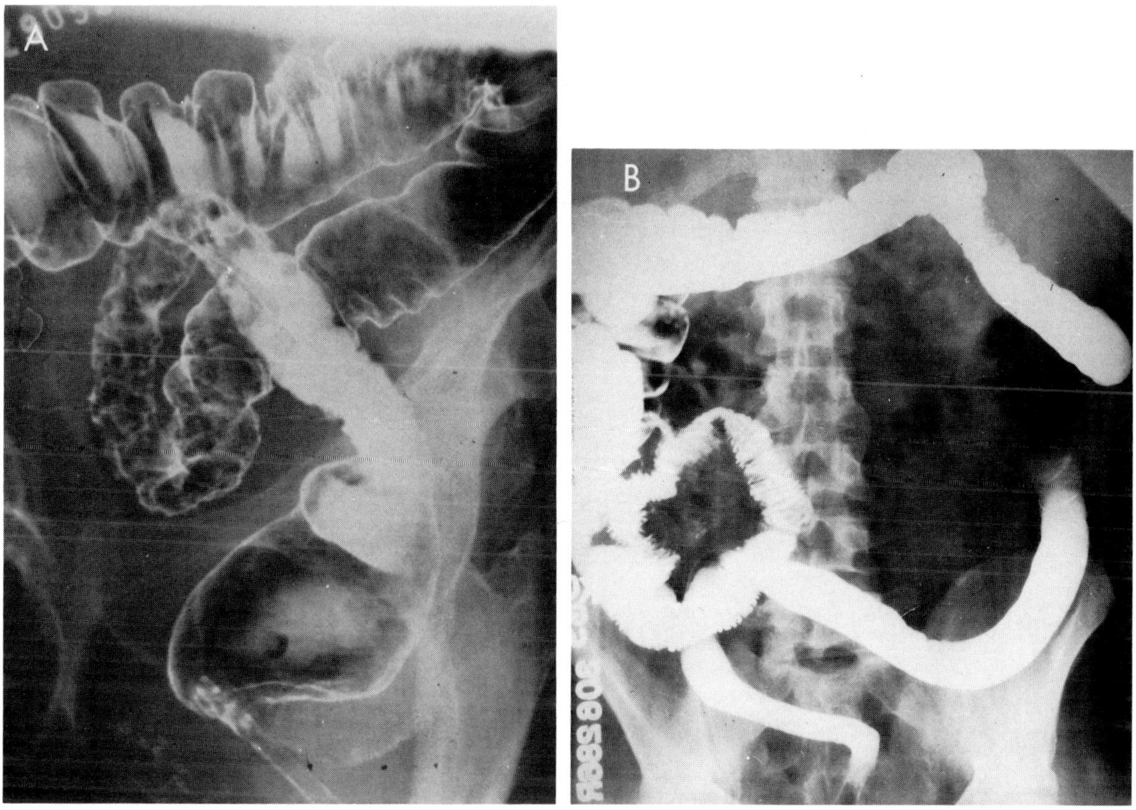

Fig 2–10. – Schistosomiasis. All varieties of schistosomiasis may affect colon, but only *S. mansoni* consistently does so. **A,** earliest change is edema of bowel mucosa, often with tiny ulcers or spiculation. Affected area of bowel will be in spasm, and distention with barium enema will be difficult. This is well shown in sigmoid loop in this double contrast examination. In lower descending colon tiny ulcers and loss of normal mucosal pattern may be seen. As infection progresses **(B),** there is complete loss of haustration, typically, as shown here, in descending and sigmoid colon. No part of bowel is exempt. *(Continued.)*

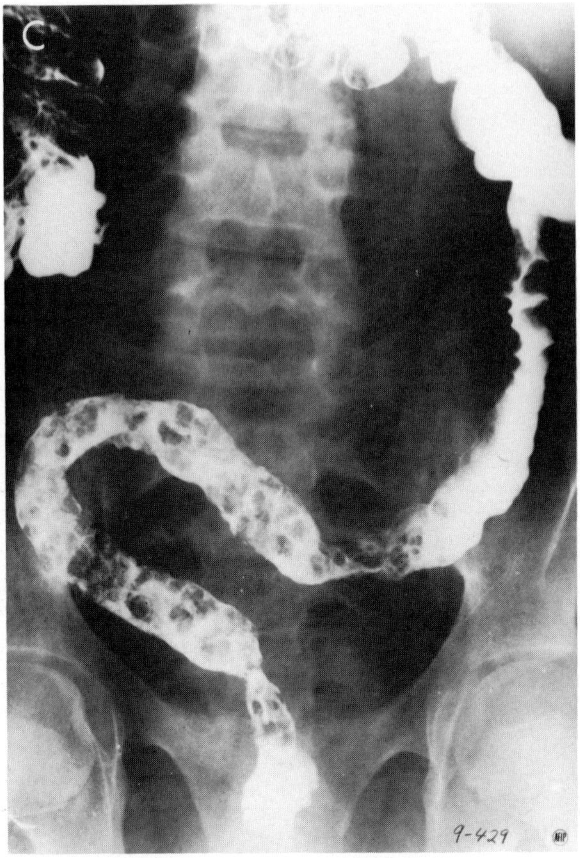

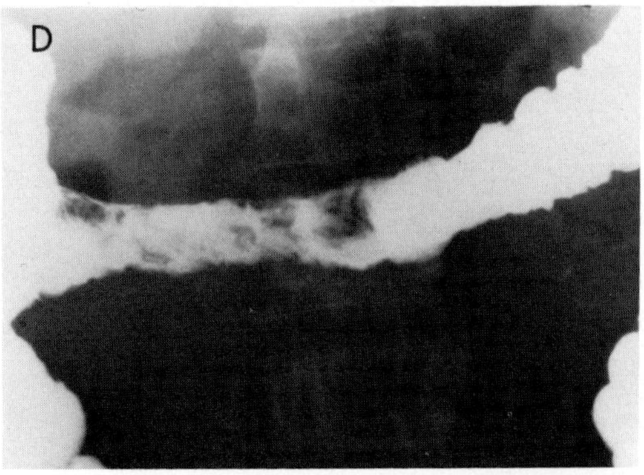

Fig 2–10 *(cont.).* – **(C),** when infection is heavy and chronic, multiple polyps develop. Although these are usually 1–2 cm in diameter, they may become so large that obstruction or intussusception occurs. Polyps result from submucosal granulomas, which eventually acquire a short stalk. They are very vascular and friable and bleed easily. Polyp formation is most common where there are combined *S. mansoni* and *S. hematobium* infections; there is thus a geographic variation in their frequency. Polyp formation is not common in Europe and North America. Schistosomal granulomatous colitis may heal with stenosis and pericolic infiltration and is then indistinguishable from any other form of granulomatous colitis: it may even progress to form strictures. Large solitary "bilharziomas" have been reported lying in bowel wall or mesentery. These are uncommon.

Differential diagnosis of *S. mansoni* colitis is difficult at all stages, unless this possibility is remembered. Early in disease, infection will be mistaken for regional enteritis and, later, if there is a solitary granulomatous tumor, radiologic diagnosis may be malignancy. It is not always sufficient to merely examine the stool to exclude *S. mansoni:* mucosal biopsy is essential. Radiologists should remember that all schistosomal infections are likely to involve liver and many other parts of body. *S. mansoni,* for example, produces significant change in lung and may result in pulmonary hypertension. **D,** colonic infection with *S. haematobium* (without *S. mansoni*) is unusual but results in an edematous granular mucosa, as demonstrated here in transverse colon. (**A** and **D** from Reeder and Palmer, *The Radiology of Tropical Diseases* [Baltimore: Williams & Wilkins Co., 1979]. **B,** Armed Forces Institute of Pathology, neg. no. 9779 (68–9019–11); Fig 2–10, **C,** neg. no. 68-7498 (229499–429, used with permission.)

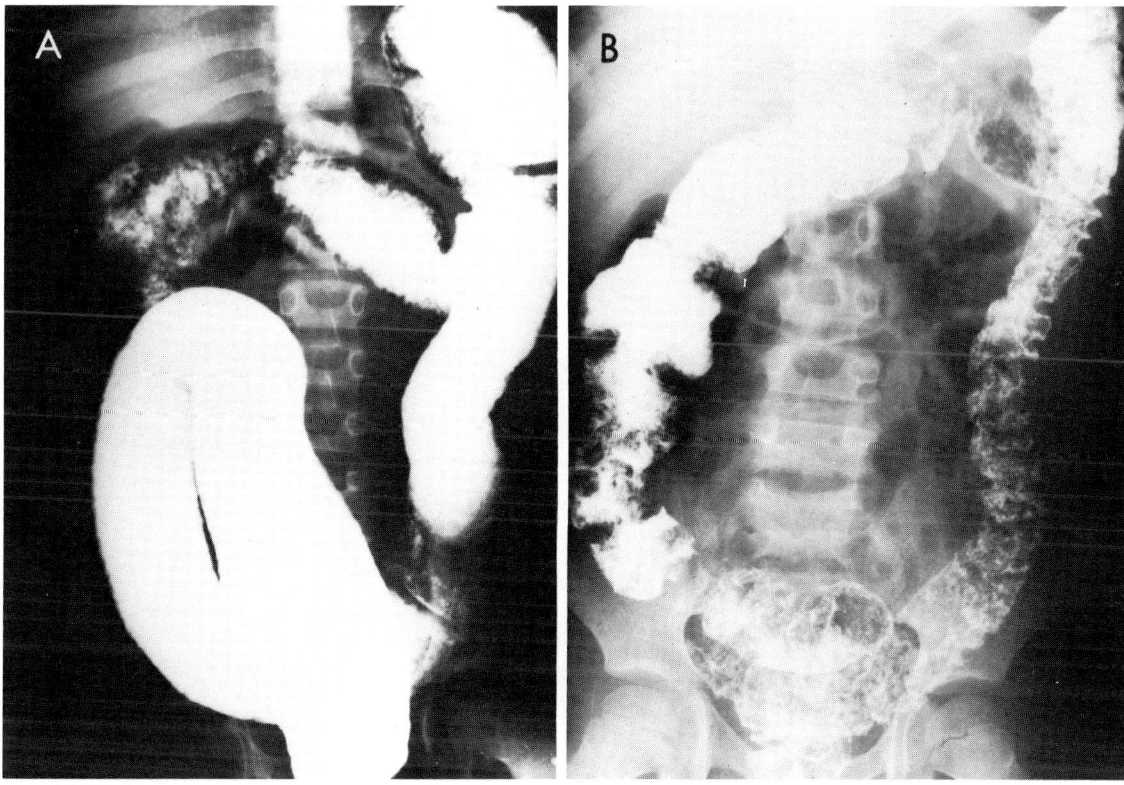

Fig 2–11.—Whipworm. Infection with whipworm, *Trichuris trichiura,* is likely to be an incidental finding radiologically during the investigation of rectal bleeding or other colonic symptoms. The barium enema may be completely normal, or may show **(A)** a granular mucosal pattern. **B,** excess mucus, together with edematous mucosa, may produce quite severe and extensive changes mimicking severe colitis. *(Continued.)*

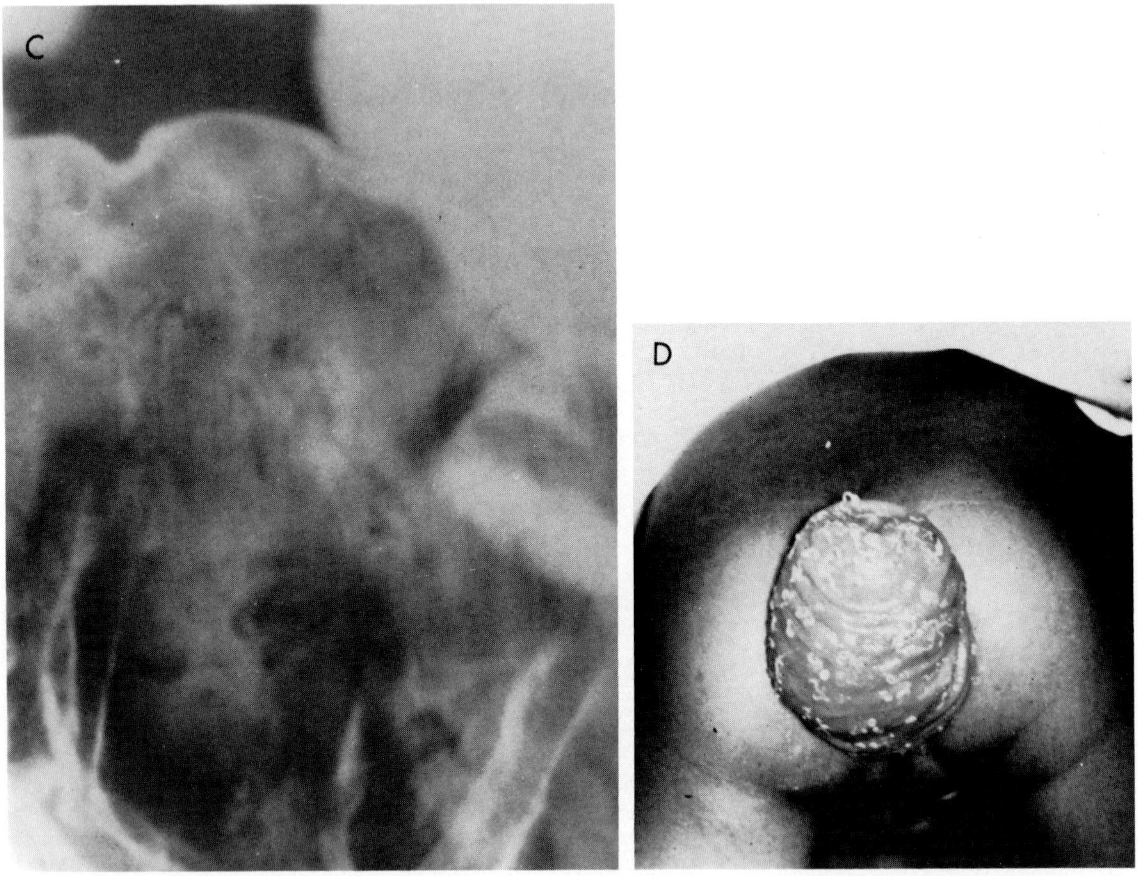

Fig 2–11 *(cont.)*. – **C,** double contrast examination will show wavy pattern of small Trichuris worms. The uncurled whiplike worms are female; the more tightly coiled, resembling a target, are male. **D,** trichuriasis is a common cause of rectal prolapse in children. The bowel may be infected by hundreds of worms when prolapse occurs because of swollen edematous mucosa and resulting dysfunction. (**A,** Armed Forces Institute of Pathology, neg. no. 67–9998–8; **B,** neg. no. 67–9998–4. **C,** from Reeder and Palmer, *The Radiology of Tropical Diseases* [Baltimore: Williams & Wilkin Co., 1979], with permission.)

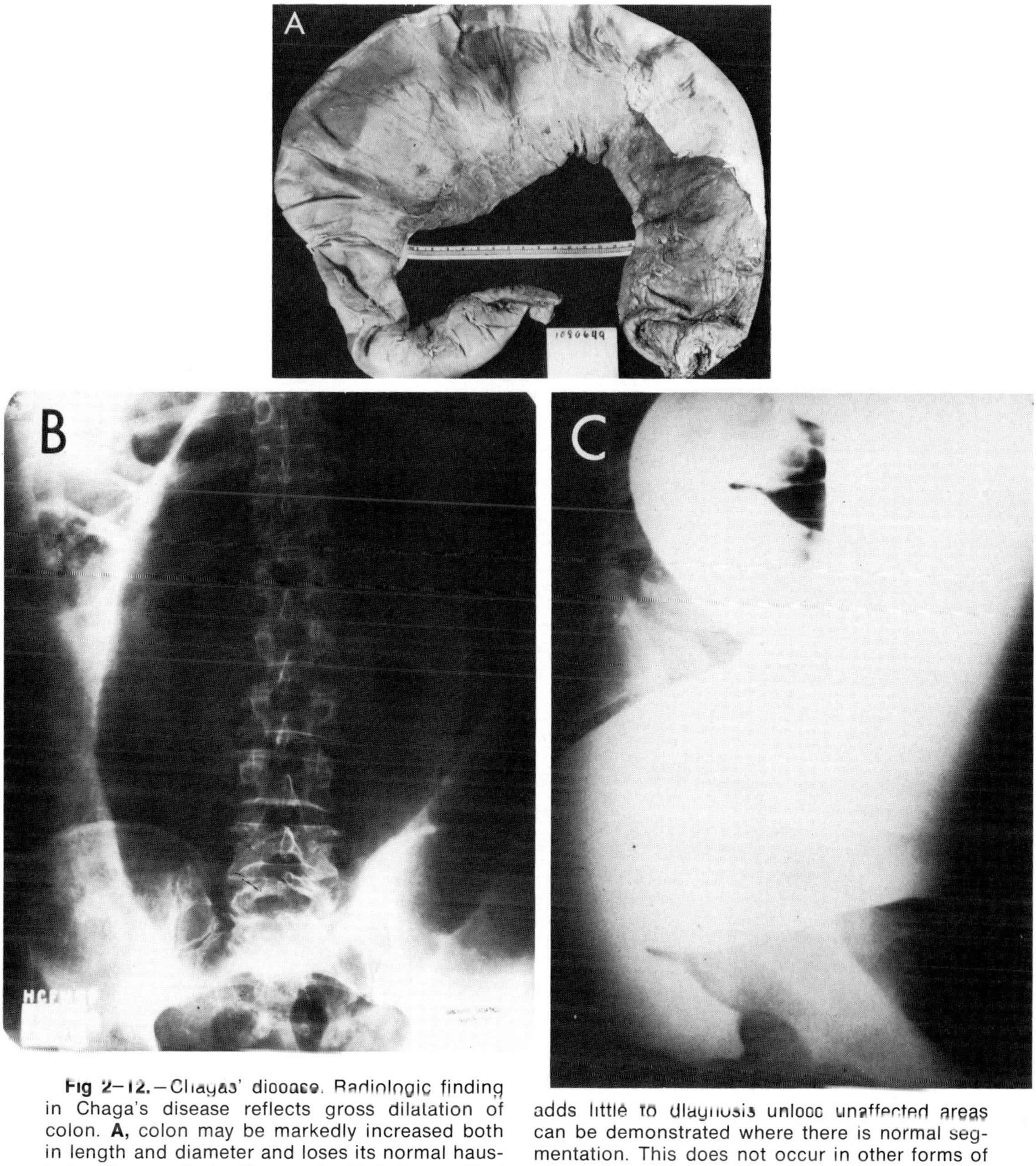

Fig 2–12.—Chagas' disease. Radiologic finding in Chaga's disease reflects gross dilatation of colon. **A,** colon may be markedly increased both in length and diameter and loses its normal haustral pattern entirely. **B,** grossly dilated, gas-filled loops of colon in Chagas' disease—a true "megacolon." **C,** filling enormous colon with barium adds little to diagnosis unless unaffected areas can be demonstrated where there is normal segmentation. This does not occur in other forms of megacolon. (**A,** Armed Forces Institute of Pathology, neg. no. 67–5314 (1080649), used with permission.)

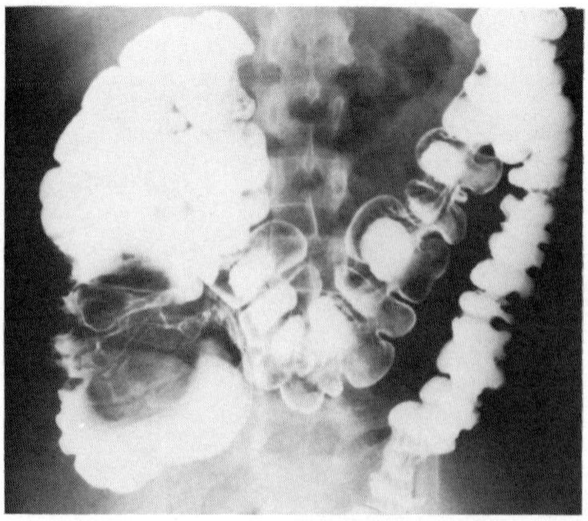

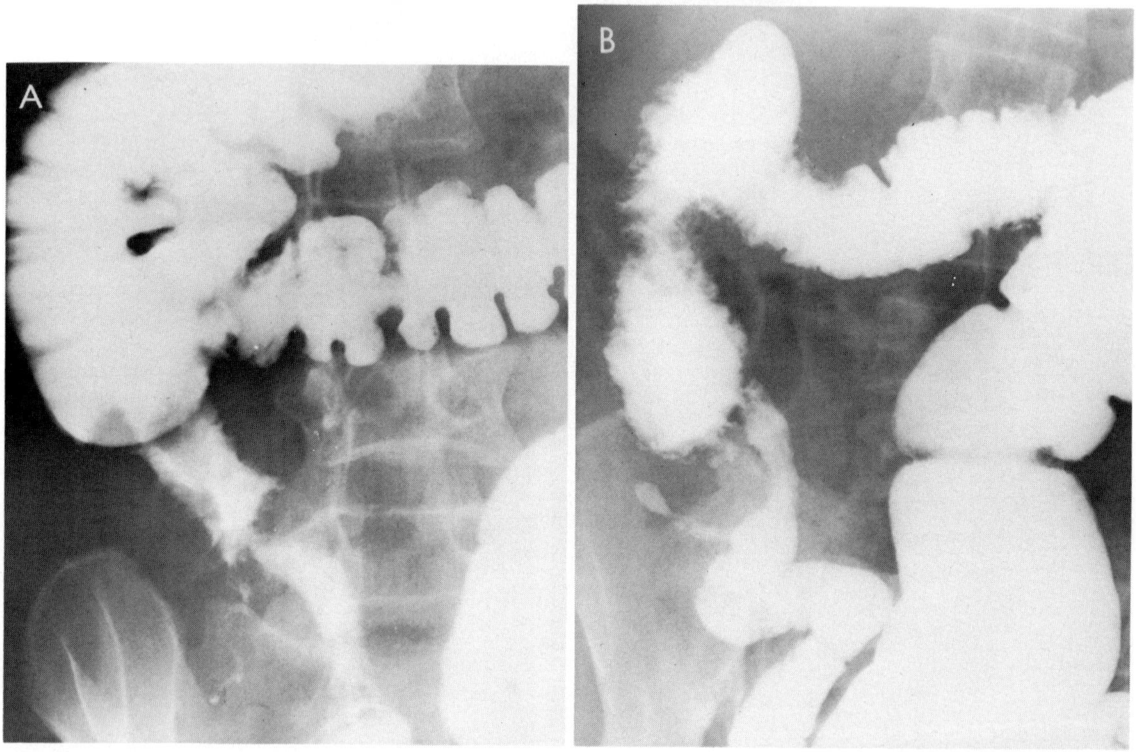

Fig 2–13 (top).—Helminthoma. Large "tumor" in cecum caused by hypertrophic granulomatous reaction around a worm that has perforated wall of gut. Although most common in this region of bowel, the tumors may occur anywhere throughout colon and may be eccentric. Differential diagnosis will include an amebic infection, lymphoma, carcinoma and only very rarely helminthoma. (From Reeder and Palmer, *The Radiology of Tropical Diseases* [Baltimore: Williams & Wilkins Co., 1979], with permission.)

Fig 2–14 (bottom).—Tuberculosis. Tuberculous infection of cecum and colon may cause constriction and shrinkage or resemble colitis. **A,** contracted and constricted cecum, with ulceration and mucosal edema, which is one of the more common varieties of alimentary tuberculosis. In this case there is pericecal abscess, and also infection of terminal ileum. **B,** more extensive tuberculous infection in which there is ulceration extending from terminal ileum and involving cecum and most of ascending colon and proximal transverse colon. Bowel wall is edematous, rigid and ulcerated and there is a pericecal abscess. Similar areas of infection, ulceration, edema and constriction may occur anywhere within colon. Differential diagnosis must include amebiasis, malignancy, fungus infections (also actinomycosis) and, around the cecum, an appendicular abscess. Reflux from cecum into ileum is uncommon in tuberculosis, although terminal ileum also may be primarily involved. (**A** and **B** courtesy of Professor S. B. Lagundoye and Radiology Library, University of Ibadan, Nigeria. **B,** reproduced from Reeder and Palmer, *The Radiology of Tropical Diseases* [Baltimore: Williams & Wilkins Co., 1979], with permission.)

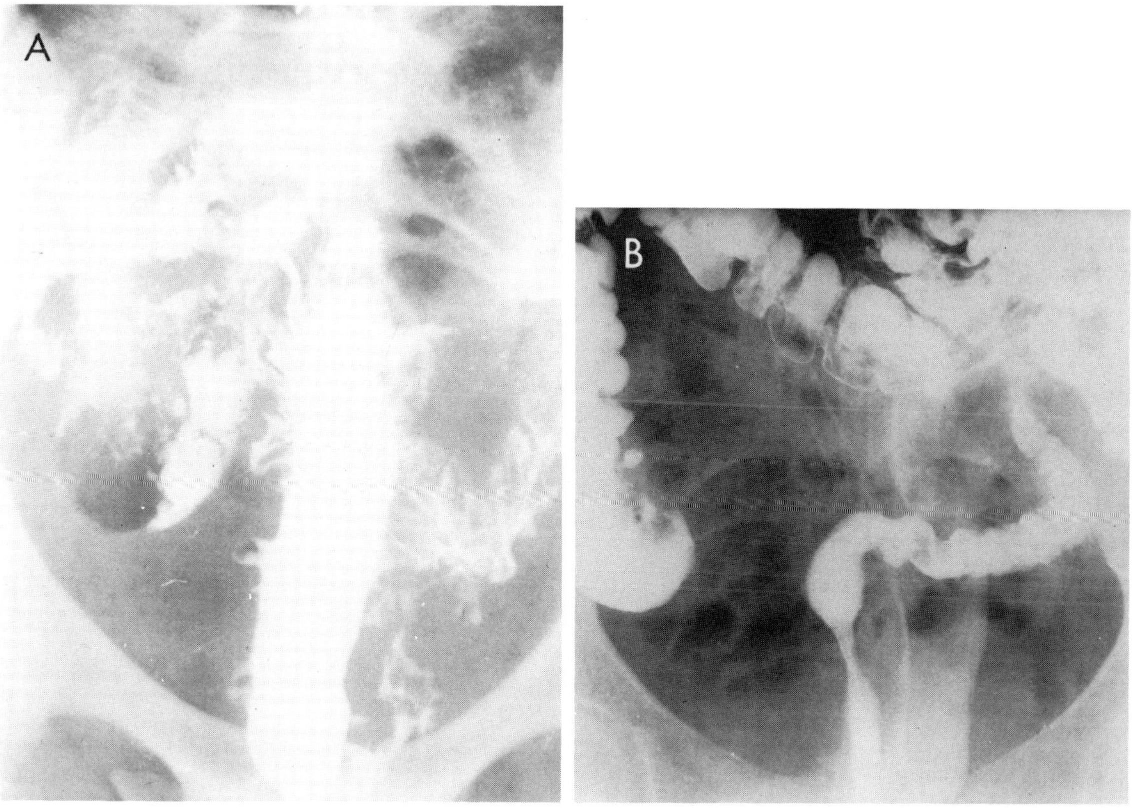

Fig 2–15.—Lymphogranuloma venereum (LGV), is essentially an infection of the lower colon, sigmoid and rectum. It causes strictures, fibrosis and fistulas. **A,** narrow, rigid, ulcerated, fistulous rectum and rectosigmoid in chronic case of LGV. **B,** less severe infection, but with same pattern of narrowing and elongation of rectal sigmoid. A stricture is developing at rectosigmoid junction, and there are ulceration and colitis above it. Eventually this may narrow and cause obstruction. (**A,** Armed Forces Institute of Pathology, neg. no. 625903, used with permission. **A** and **B** from Reeder and Palmer, *The Radiology of Tropical Diseases* [Baltimore: Williams & Wilkins Co., 1979], with permission. **B,** courtesy of the Radiology Teaching Library of the University of Cape Town, Cape Town, South Africa.)

Chapter 3

Angled Sigmoid View

DONALD N. DYSART, M.D.

THE SIGMOID and rectosigmoid regions of the colon are at times the most difficult areas in the gastrointestinal tract for the radiologist to visualize adequately. Anatomical variations such as a low lying ptotic mid-transverse colon, a pelvic cecum or a markedly redundant sigmoid often preclude a clear, unobstructed view of these areas. When barium refluxes into the distal small bowel, this may also interfere with a clear look. Because of these variations, the recording and documentation of pathology, or the lack of pathology, in these areas on overhead films can prove frustrating. In practices where the services of a physician skilled in the use of a sigmoidoscope are not available, the burden of an adequate study falls entirely on the radiologist, and it behooves him to use any and all techniques available to help verify his findings. Spot films, 70-mm roll films, cineradiography or videotape recording during fluoroscopy are often helpful in documenting what the radiologist sees while he is performing the examination. Occasionally the spot films may be the only films that document adequately the pathology identified by the fluoroscopist.

The number of overhead films and the projections in which they are taken vary widely according to the practice and experience of the examiner,[1] and he should determine during the fluoroscopic examination which overhead views he needs, pre- and postevacuation, to demonstrate the findings. Many times special views such as oblique, decubitus, lateral, upright and/or angled views will be necessary to show a lesion.

The angled views are helpful to show lesions in the sigmoid and rectosigmoid regions. The technique used in obtaining these angled views may vary depending upon the experience of the examiner. The Chassard-Lapiné view[2] is helpful but is somewhat uncomfortable for the patient and should not be used during reproductive age because of high exposure to the pelvic organs.[3] The angled view may be obtained either in a supine or prone position. In the supine position, the tube is angled 30 degrees cephalad.[4] In the prone position, the tube is angled 30–35 degrees caudad, depending on the patient's thickness.[5] Most of our experience has been with the PA, or prone angled view, of the sigmoid. On some occasions, slightly oblique (about 10 degrees angle LAO or RAO) angled views have been helpful to separate redundant sigmoid loops or to rotate the cecum or ileum out of the way.

REFERENCES

1. Margulis, A. R.: Examination of the Colon, in Margulis, A. R., and Burhenne, H. J. (eds.): *Alimentary Tract Roentgenology,* Vol. II (2d ed.; St. Louis: C. V. Mosby Co., 1973).
2. Chassard, and Lapiné, M. M.: Étude radiographique de l'arcade pubienne chez la famme enceinte; une nouvelle méthode d'appréciation du diamètre bi-ischiatique, J. Radiol. Electrol. 7:113, 1923.

3. Margulis, A. R.: Roentgenographic Examination of the Colon, in Bockus, H. L. (ed.): *Gastroenterology*, Vol. II (3d ed.; Philadelphia: W. B. Saunders Co., 1976).
4. Ettinger, A., and Elkin, M.: Study of the sigmoid by special roentgenographic views, Am. J. Roentgenol. 72:199, 1954.
5. Dysart, D. N., and Stewart, H. R.: Special angled roentgenography for lesions of the rectosigmoid. Five year survey, 1959–1963, Am. J. Roentgenol. 69:285, 1966.

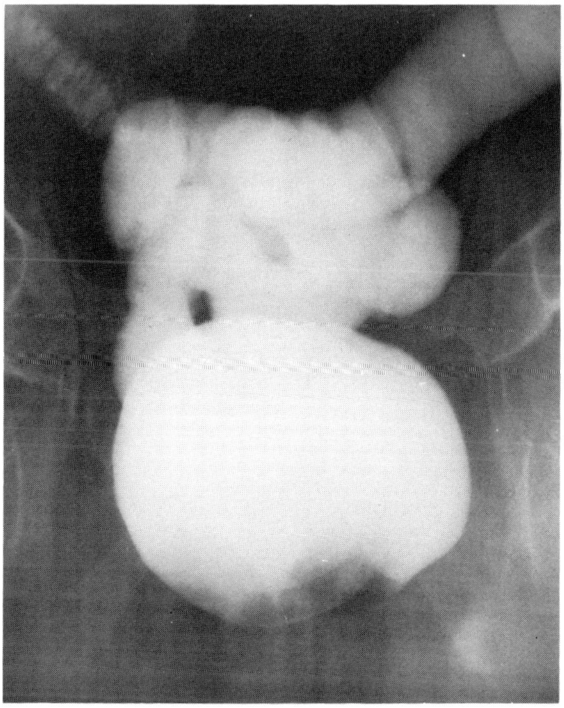

Fig 3–1.—Redundant sigmoid, difficult to visualize on filled PA angled view.

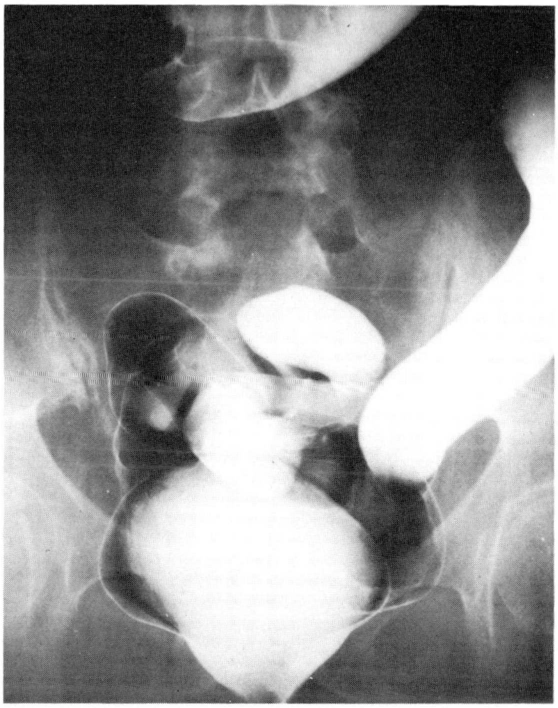

Fig 3–2.—Same patient as Fig 3–1 with double contrast technique, which permits a "see-through" look at the redundant loops.

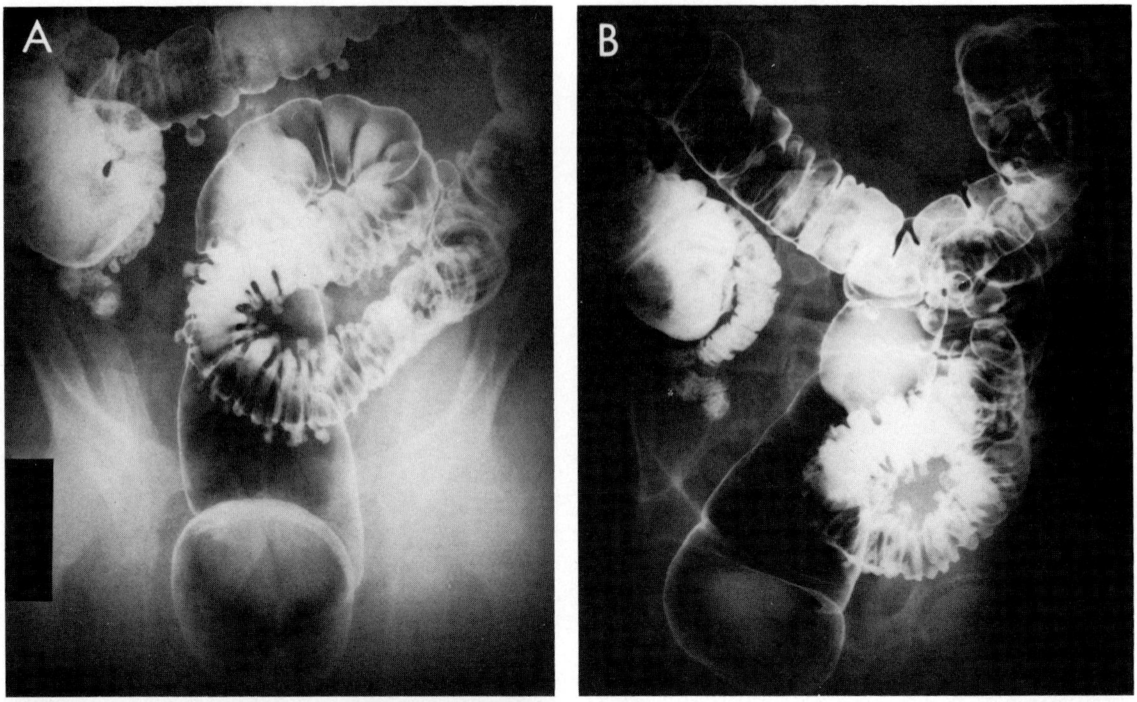

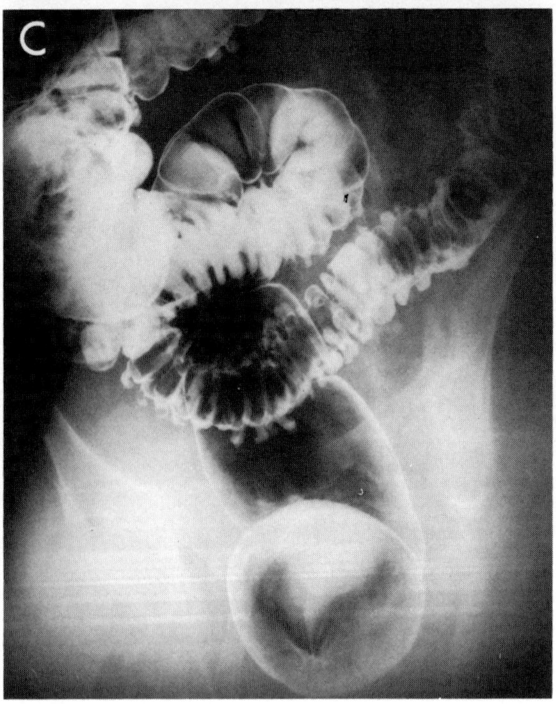

Fig 3–3.—Redundant sigmoid with diverticula. **A,** PA angled view shows a dilated, elongated, slightly redundant sigmoid with multiple diverticula in mid- and upper sigmoid regions; **B,** RAO angled view; **C,** LAO angled view. Oblique angled views give different looks at various areas of sigmoid and rectum.

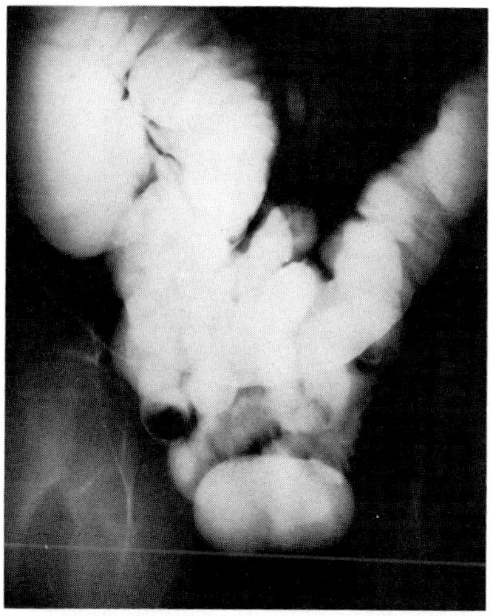

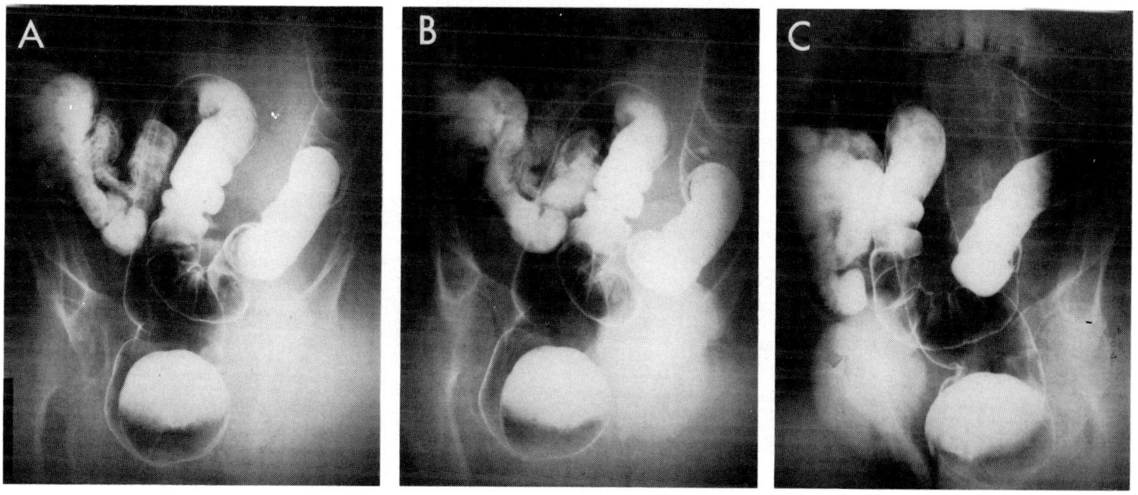

Fig 3–4 (top).—Redundant sigmoid and ptotic midtransverse colon. Barium refluxed into terminal ileum, and low lying ptotic midtransverse colon completely obscured sigmoid on PA angled view.

Fig 3–5 (bottom).—Redundant sigmoid. **A**, PA angled view showed portion of redundant sigmoid obscured by barium refluxed into terminal ileum. **B**, RAO angled view showed portion of sigmoid still obscured. **C**, LAO angled view clears obscured portion of sigmoid.

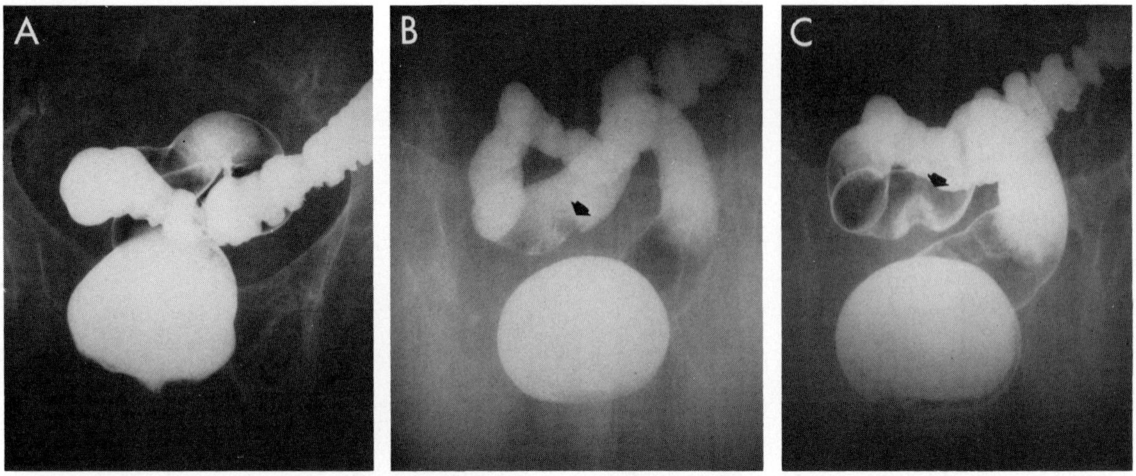

Fig 3–6.—Polypoid adenocarcinoma of sigmoid. Patient several years after operation for bladder malignancy presented with rectal bleeding. Proctosigmoidoscopy reported negative. **A,** PA view showed no lesion in sigmoid. **B,** PA angled view was only view to show polypoid lesion in midsigmoid *(arrow).* Resigmoidoscopy again did not identify a lesion. Patient returned about 1 year later, again with rectal bleeding; sigmoidoscopy showed no lesion. **C,** PA angled view demonstrated polypoid lesion in midsigmoid *(arrow),* slightly larger than on prior examination. Pathology revealed grade II adenocarcinoma with infiltration into base of polypoid lesion.

Fig 3–7.—Polypoid adenocarcinoma of sigmoid. **A,** PA view showed no lesion in sigmoid but did show two other benign adenomatous polyps *(single arrows)* in colon and a carcinoma *(double arrows)* in ascending colon. **B,** PA angled view was only view to show large polypoid carcinoma in midsigmoid *(arrow).*

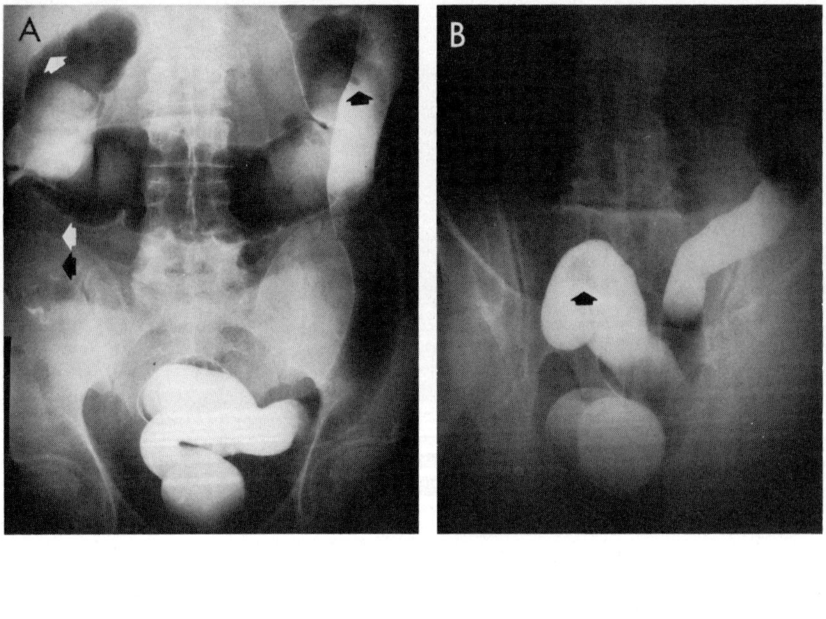

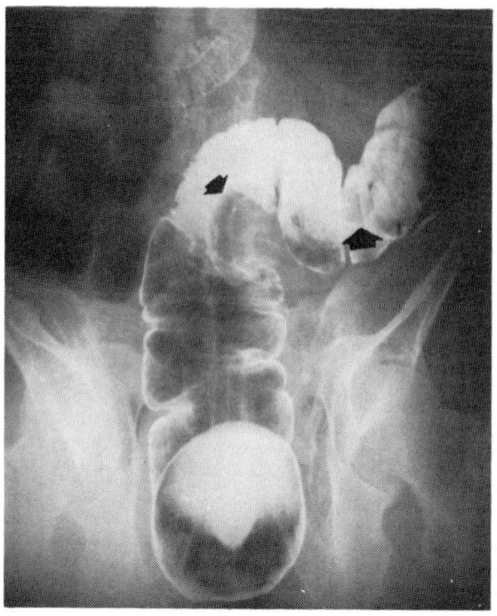

Fig 3–8 (left).—Polypoid adenocarcinoma and benign pedunculated adenomatous polyp of sigmoid. The PA angled view was only view to show well the large polypoid adenocarcinoma *(small arrow)* in distal sigmoid and large pedunculated benign adenomatous polyp in midsigmoid *(wide arrow).*

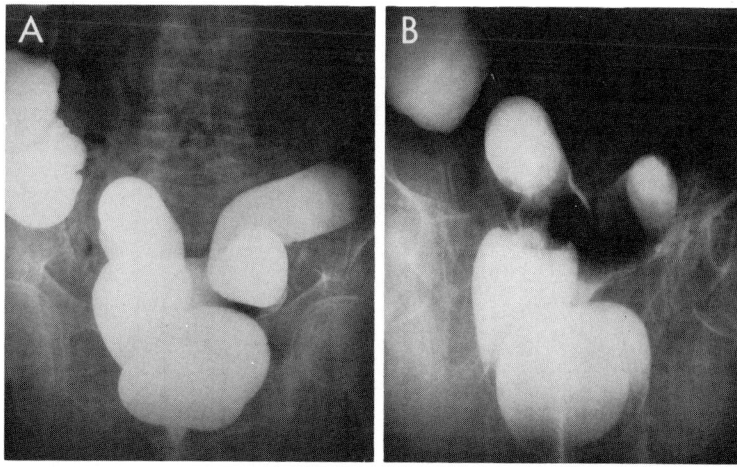

Fig 3–9 (right).—Annular adenocarcinoma of sigmoid. **A,** PA view showed no lesion in colon. **B,** PA angled view showed well an annular carcinoma in distal sigmoid. Pathologic examination showed grade III adenocarcinoma.

Fig 3–10.—Annular adenocarcinoma of sigmoid. **A,** routine pre-evacuation film showed a few diverticula in sigmoid and a poorly prepared colon. **B,** routine pre-evacuation PA angled views showed annular lesion in midsigmoid. This lesion was not appreciated during fluoroscopy by an experienced radiologist. **C,** on repeat examination, filled pre-evacuation angled view again showed annular lesion in midsigmoid. Radiologist stated that, even knowing where to look, he was unable to identify lesion during fluoroscopy.

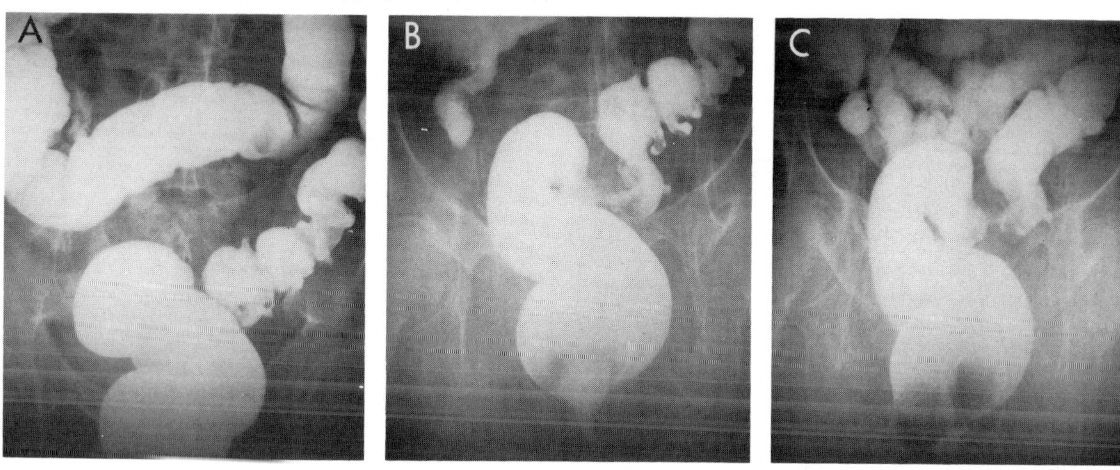

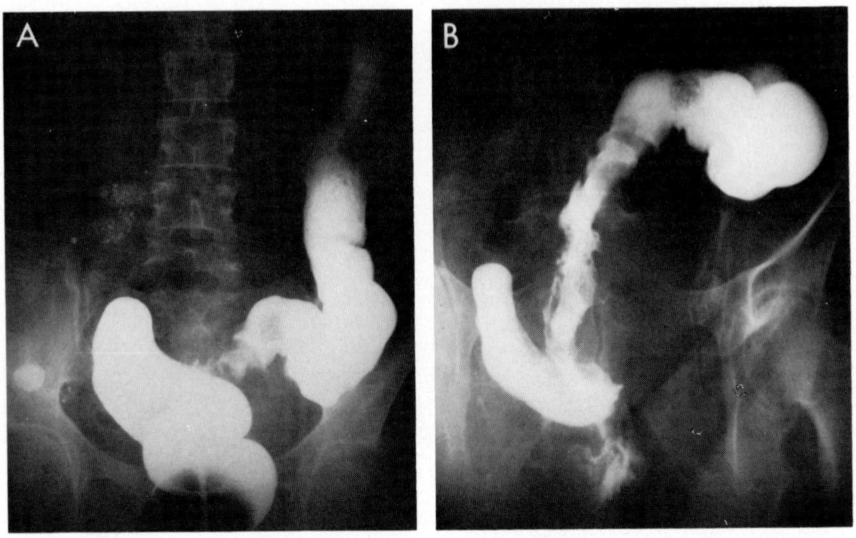

Fig 3–11.—Annular adenocarcinoma with chronic perforation of sigmoid. **A,** PA view shows partially a lesion in midsigmoid. **B,** PA angled view showed well the entire lesion involving midsigmoid. Pathologic examination showed a grade III adenocarcinoma with chronic perforation.

Fig 3–12.—Inflammatory stricture of sigmoid. **A,** PA view shows only some diverticula in sigmoid. **B,** PA angled view showed well an inflammatory stricture in upper sigmoid *(arrow).*

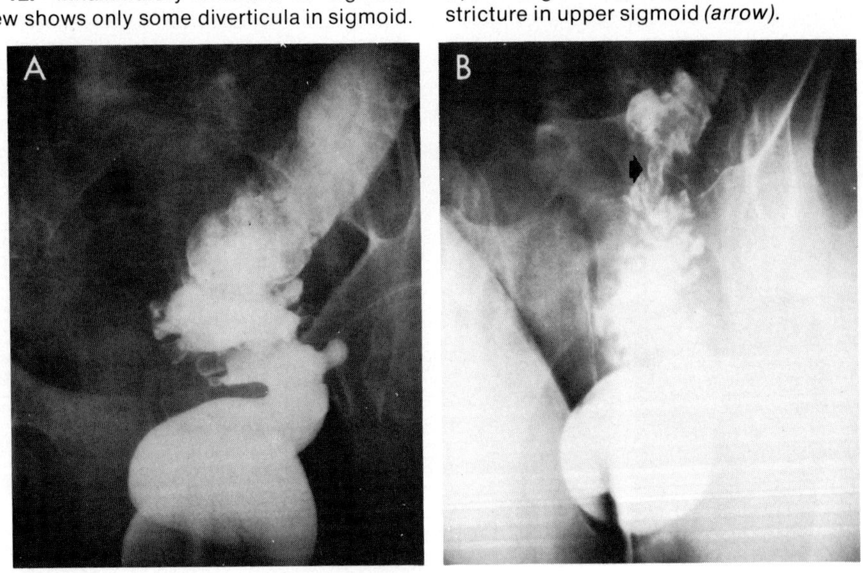

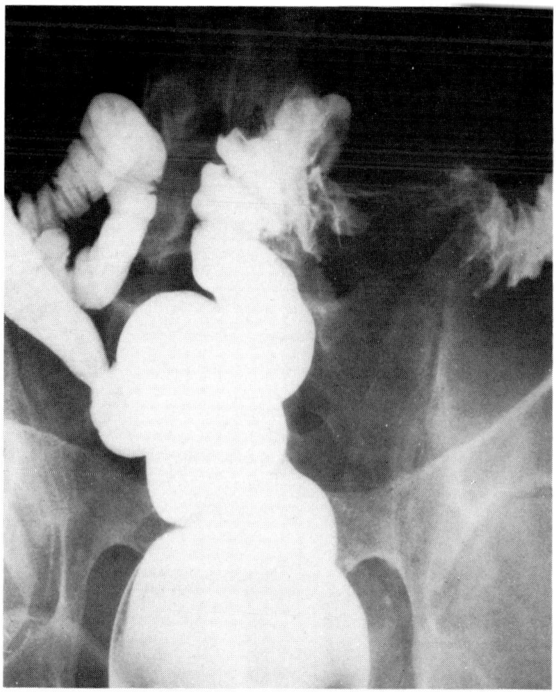

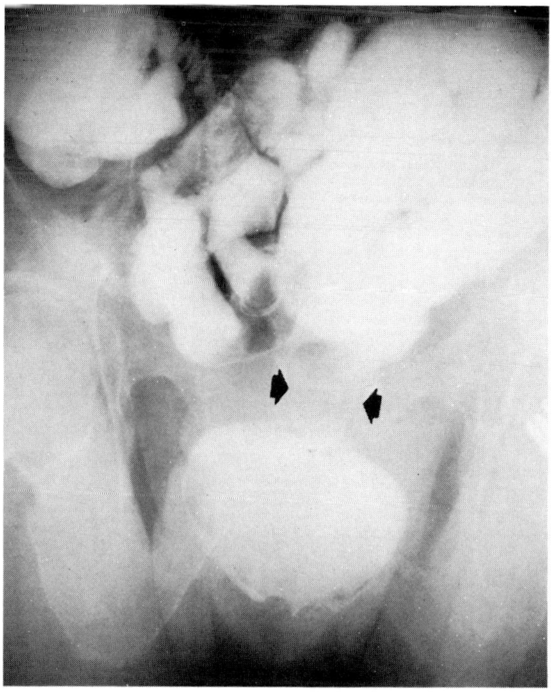

Fig 3–13 (left).—Pericolic abscess in sigmoid area. Pre-evacuation PA angled view showed many diverticula in upper sigmoid with narrowed segment due to extrinsic pressure from chronic perforation of a diverticulum, with pericolic abscess formation.

Fig 3–14 (right).—Ischemic bowel disease. Pre-evacuation PA angled view showed a narrowed segment in upper rectum *(arrows)*. Many biopsies revealed only inflammatory tissue. This was called carcinoma but at surgery and pathologically only inflammatory tissue could be demonstrated. Clinically this was thought to be ischemic bowel disease.

Fig 3–15 (left).—Endometriosis of sigmoid. Pre-evacuation PA angled view showed irregular narrowed area in midsigmoid with no evidence of mucosal destruction *(arrows)*. Pathologic results showed this to be endometriosis involving bowel wall.

Fig 3–16 (right).—Granulomatous ileocolitis of sigmoid and ileum. Pre-evacuation PA angled view showed extent of involvement of sigmoid by granulomatous ileocolitis.

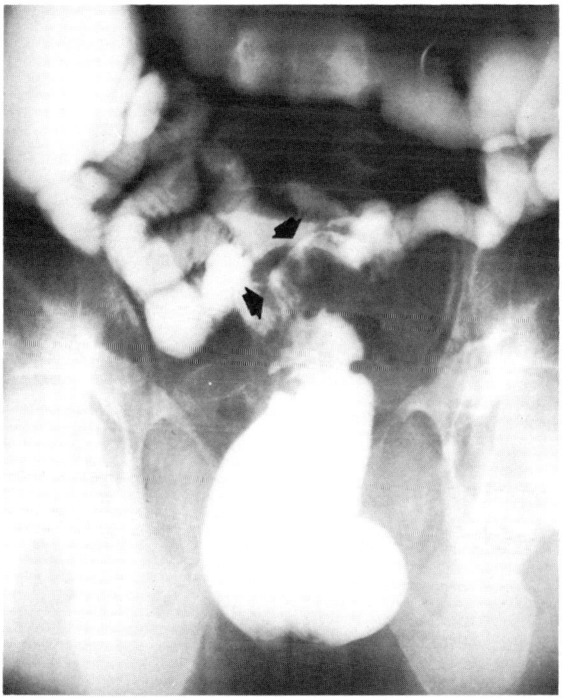

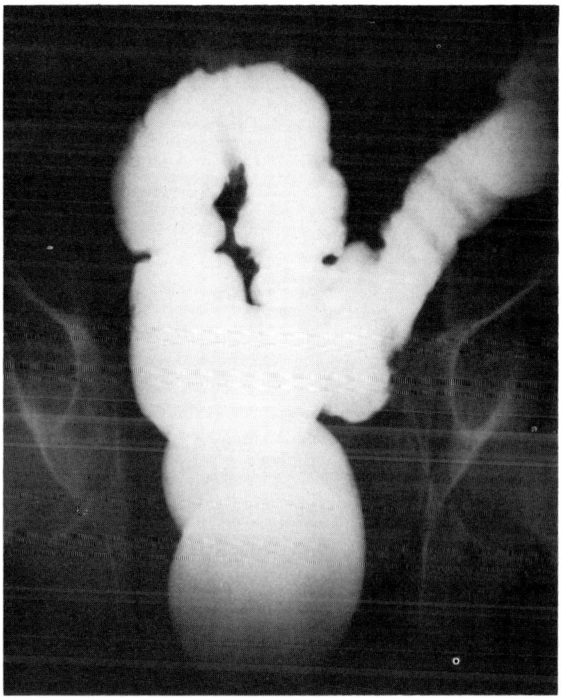

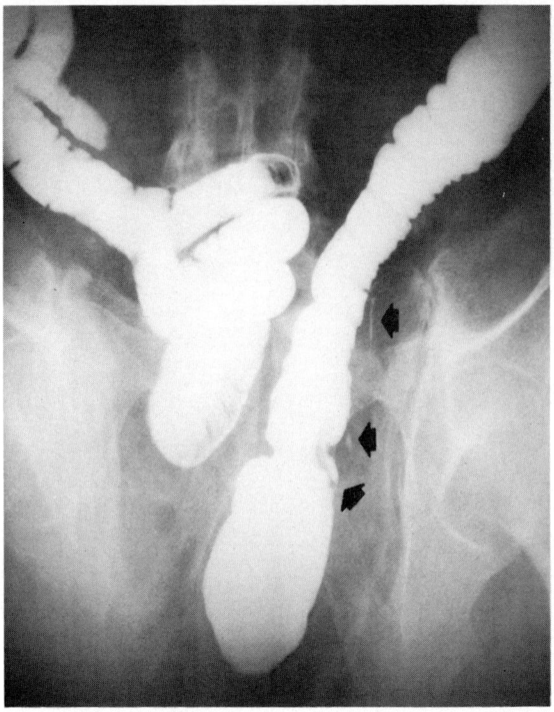

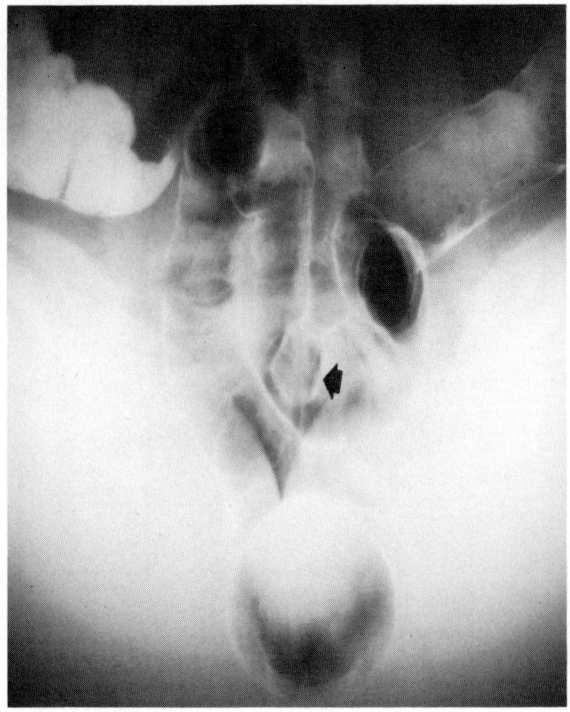

Fig 3–17 (left). – Anastomotic fistula of sigmoid. Routine follow-up colon examination on patient 1 year post resection of carcinoma of sigmoid. Pre-evacuation PA angled view showed fistulous tract with origin of tract at site of anastomosis *(arrows).*

Fig 3–18 (right). – Polypoid adenocarcinoma of sigmoid. PA angled view on double contrast study showed polypoid lesion *(arrow)* in midsigmoid. The other four views obtained in air study only suggested the presence of a lesion in this area.

Fig 3–19. – Pelvic lipomatosis. **A,** Pre-evacuation angled view showed elongation, elevation and narrowing of distal sigmoid and upper rectum due to pelvic lipomatosis. **B,** intravenous pyelogram obtained shortly after colon examination showed normal-appearing mucosa in sigmoid and upper rectum. Approximated pelvic ureters, small bladder and relative radiolucency of pelvis are well seen.

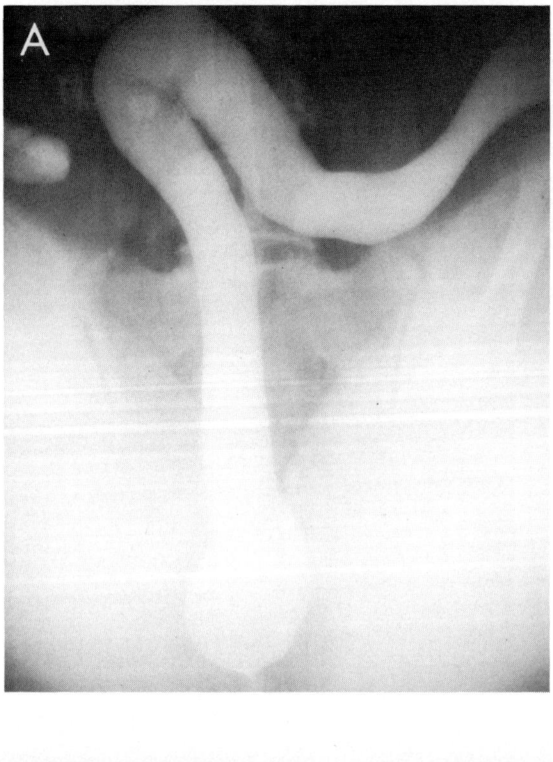

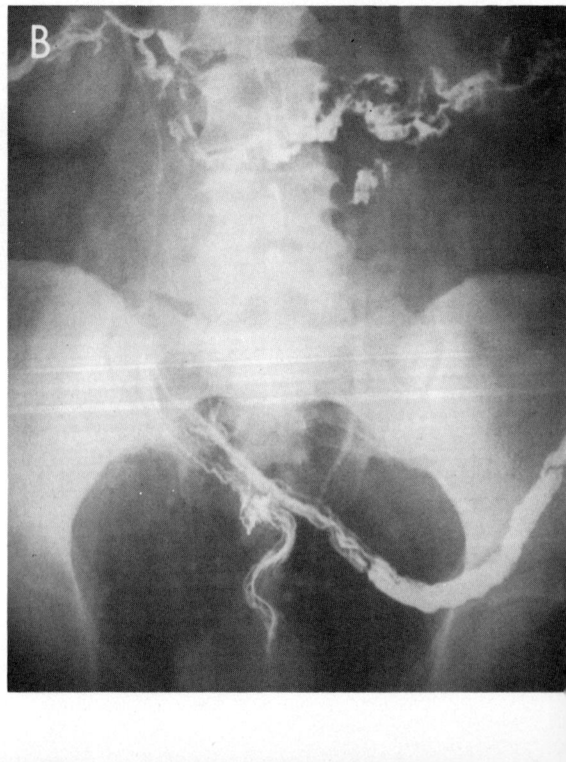

Chapter 4

Autonomic Dysreflexia During Barium Enema

KEITH BURNETT, M.D.
HOSSEIN GOLJI, M.D.

Etiology

DURING RADIOLOGIC EXAMINATION of the colon in spinal cord injury patients, the radiologist may encounter a phenomenon known as autonomic dysreflexia. This entity, a serious medical emergency, was described by Head and Duddoch[1] in 1917 as a "mass reflex" below the level of the cord lesion in patients with spinal cord injury.

The uncontrolled autonomic hyperactivity can originate from stimulation of the skin, genitourinary tract manipulation, ejaculation, uterine contraction, instrumentation of the urethra, distention of the bladder and urinary stones and infection. Also, it can originate from stimulation and/or distention of the lower gastrointestinal tract, including anus, rectum and distal colon. This fact is of direct concern to examiners attempting barium enemas. Recently, abdominal angiography has been blamed as another possible cause of hyperreflexia.[6]

Signs and Symptoms

The symptoms of autonomic hyperreflexia include pounding headache, flushing and/or sweating of the face and neck, apprehension, blockage of nasal passages, nausea and/or vomiting, vague abdominal pain, goose flesh, blurred vision and convulsion. Paroxysmal hypertension is the rule, sometimes greater than 300/150.[7] The average quadriplegic blood pressure is 90/60; therefore, "normal" pressures (i.e., 145/90) may signify a hypertensive crisis. Bradycardia usually is present and is of diagnostic importance.

Complications

The attacks of paroxysmal hypertension may cause cardiac failure and retinal and/or cerebral hemorrhage. Also, acute ischemic renal, myocardial and cerebral insult should be considered a potential complication of overzealous treatment of hypertension.

Neuropathology

The pathophysiology of autonomic dysreflexia has been well described by Kurnick.[2] Stimulation of skin or of the genitourinary or gastrointestinal tracts (i.e., distention of the rectum during barium enema) activates the afferent sensory nerve endings of the sympathetic pathways that ascend in the spinothalamic tracts and posterior columns to the posterior roots of gray matter of the spinal cord below the level of injury[8] (Fig 4–1). At this time a reflex sympathetic arc is activated and the motor efferent outflow produces spasm of the pelvic viscera, pilo-erection and arteriolar spasm, causing systemic hypertension. The baroreceptors in the carotid sinus and aortic arch are stimulated by systemic hypertension, and the generated impulses activate a reflex arc, causing bradycardia through vagus nerve hypertonia. Intact afferent fibers from the aortic arch and carotid sinus to the vasomotor center in the medulla result in vasodilatation above the level of the cord lesion, with generation of heat, perspiration and flushing of the head and neck. However, in 85% of patients with spinal cord lesions at or above the level of T6, the normal inhibitory efferent sympathetic outflow from the higher centers cannot reach below the level of injury. Therefore, hyperreflexia ensues and the vascular system innervated by the isolated cord below the lesion remains in spasm, the skin being pallid and cold.

Treatment

The constellation of symptoms that constitute autonomic hyperreflexia should be recognized immediately and treated as an emergency. First, the stimulus should be eliminated, e.g., termination of the enema, removal of the rectal tube and/or unclamping of the bladder Foley catheter. Then the patient is placed in sitting position or at least with the head elevated. Also, the vital signs should be checked and the blood pressure taken at 5-minute intervals. The radiologist should immediately consult with personnel trained in hypertensive crises to keep the patient under close observation and continue medical treatment.

HYPOTENSIVE DRUGS

Recent radiologic literature suggests intravenous administration of a 300 mg bolus of diazoxide (Hyperstat) to control the hypertension.[6] However, this therapy may lead to acute hypotension with attendant possibilities of renal failure, cerebral ischemia and/or myocardial ischemia with infarct.

At the spinal cord injury center of the Long Beach Veterans Administration Hospital, largest in the U. S. A., considerable experience has resulted in a separate protocol[7]: while the above nonmedication measures are under way, the patient is asked to breath amyl nitrite released from breakage of an ampule under his nose. This inhalation of amyl nitrite may be repeated or reinforced with sublingual nitroglycerin (1/150 grain). If this treatment is unsuccessful in reducing the blood pressure to safe limits, hydralazine (Apresoline) should be administered as a slow intravenous injection. The starting dose is 4 mg (0.25 cc), which may be repeated every 15 minutes to a total dose of 20 mg. In persistent cases, the same course of treatment may be repeated, with close observation of blood pressure. Mild cases of autonomic dysreflexia may be treated with multiple 0.25 cc (4 mg hydralazine) intramuscular injections. Contraindications to hydralazine therapy include coronary artery disease and known hypersensitivity to the drug. Spinal anesthesia is advocated only in the most severe and persistent forms of autonomic dysreflexia.

An important point in the treatment of dysreflexia is diagnostic differentiation from the usual radiologic contrast reaction. Although confusion of the two is unlikely during barium examination, treatment measures for anaphylaxis would be counterproductive and possibly dangerous in dysreflexia.

Prophylaxis

The occurrence of autonomic dysreflexia during barium enema studies is uncommon, but predictability is not possible. The literature reports the efficacy of premedication with phenoxybenzamine (Dibenzyline) and mecamylamine (Inversine) in patients with histories of previous episodes of autonomic dysreflexia. However, conclusive evidence of the effectiveness of prophylactic treatment regimens is lacking.[4, 6] In our experience, the most effective preventive measures are gentle manipulation of the patient; use of lubricants containing local anesthetic agents; slow, gentle infusion; and prevention of unnecessary dilatation of the rectum.

Summary

Barium enema examination may precipitate autonomic dysreflexia, an emergency in patients with high spinal cord injuries. The hyperreflexia is characterized by exaggerated autonomic symptoms and potentially dangerous hypertension. Advocated treatment consists of supportive measures and use of hypotensive drugs. The differential diagnosis is fairly easy and preventive measures are mostly mechanical.

REFERENCES

1. Head, H., and Duddoch, J.: Autonomic bladder, excessive sweating and some other reflex conditions in gross injuries, Brain 40:188, 1917.
2. Kurnick, N. B.: Autonomic hyperreflexia and its control in patients with spinal cord lesions, Ann. Intern. Med. 44:678, 1956.
3. Pollock, J. J., et al.: Defects in regulatory mechanisms of autonomic function in injuries in spinal cord, J. Neurophysiol. 12:85, 1951.
4. Sizemore, G. W., and Winternitz, W. W.: Autonomic hyperreflexia—suppression with alpha-adrenergic blocking agents, N. Eng. J. Med. 282:795, 1970.
5. Barbaric, Z. L.: Autonomic dysreflexia in patients with spinal cord lesions: Complication of voiding cystourethrography and ileal loopography, Am. J. Roentgenol. 127:293, 1976.
6. Fleischman, S., and Shah, P.: Autonomic dysreflexia: An unusual radiologic complication, Radiology 124:695, 1977.
7. Protocol of Spinal Cord Injury Center, Long Beach Veterans Administration Medical Center, Long Beach, California.
8. Nathan, P. W., and Smith, M. D.: Centripetal pathway from the bladder and urethra within the spinal cord, J. Neurol. Neurosurg. Psychiatry 14:262, 1951.

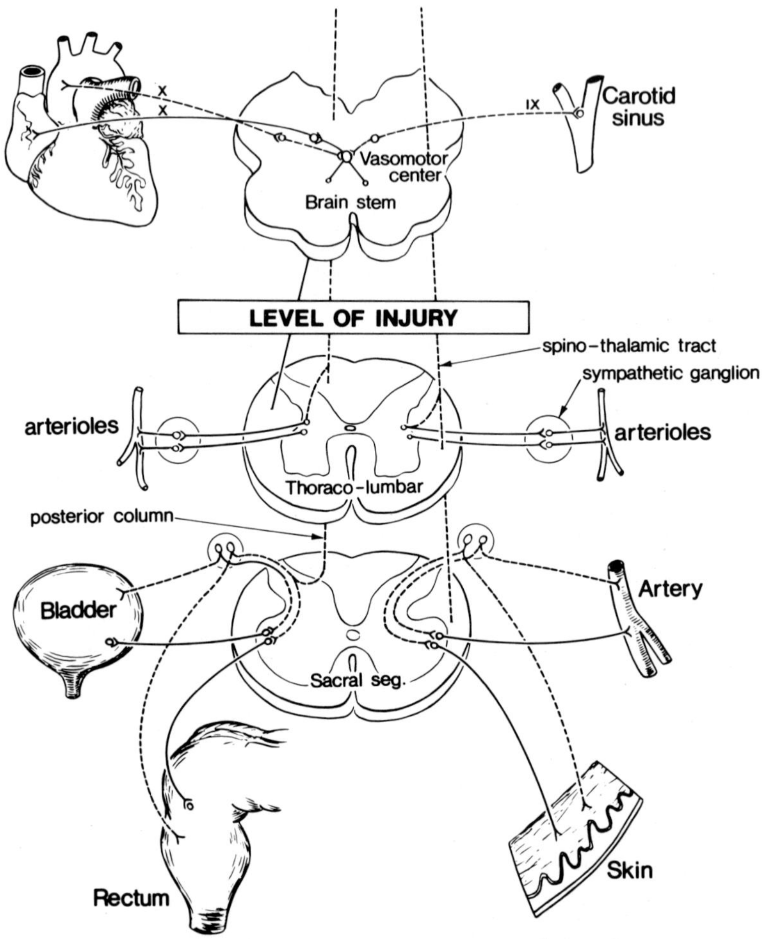

Fig 4–1.—Pathophysiology of autonomic dysreflexia. (From Fleischman and Shah, Radiology, 124:695, 1977, with permission.)

Chapter 5

Behçet's Disease

SHOZO BABA, M.D.,
MORITA MARUTA, M.D.,
KOSHI ANDO, M.D.,
TATSUO TERAMOTO, M.D.,
IWAO ENDO, M.D.

BEHÇET'S DISEASE is characterized by a mucocutaneo-ocular triple-symptom complex first described by Behçet in 1937. Behçet's disease accompanied by vascular, intestinal or neural involvement is called vasculo-Behçet, intestinal Behçet and neuro-Behçet disease, respectively.

In Japan the incidence of Behçet's disease has been increasing significantly and it has now become a social problem. In a nationwide investigation, 2,520 cases were registered.

Intestinal Behçet's Disease: Five Cases

In five patients studied with the intestinal form, the ulcers tended to perforate at multiple sites, especially in the ileocecal region. Perforation or penetrating ulcers were found in all patients. Two were operated on due to repeated perforations.

In two of the five patients, the preoperative diagnosis was established by observing the ulcer colonofiberoscopically. A deep, round ulcer was observed. It had a sharp, slightly reddened, elevated margin.

Skin eruptions, aphthous stomatitis and ocular lesions also occur in ulcerative colitis. Distribution of the ulcers in the two diseases differs: in ulcerative colitis the ulcers usually start at the rectum; in intestinal Behçet's disease, the ileocecal region is most frequently involved. Another difference lies in the depth of the ulcers: ulcers in intestinal Behçet's disease are much deeper. In performing colonofiberoscopy, the utmost care is necessary because the intestinal wall is edematous and the ulcer is deep enough to perforate. A healed ulcer in the sigmoid colon is recognized by its discolored, patchy appearance.

Compared with Crohn's disease, there is less inflammatory process surrounding the ulcer (e.g., less thickening of the intestinal wall and no stenotic area). Granulomas were not found in the five patients. Fistula formation has been occasionally reported. Ulcers are multiple and scattered and tend to perforate more easily than those in Crohn's disease, in which perforation rarely occurs.

Characteristic radiographic findings of the colon in Behçet's disease are demonstrated in Figure 5 – 1. En face, the ulcers appeared ring shaped and, in profile, falciform shaped. Haustra usually are present, whereas they do not occur in ulcerative colitis.

REFERENCE

1. Baba, S., et al.: Intestinal Behçet's disease: Report of 5 cases, Dis. Colon Rectum 19:428, 1976.

This article originally appeared in Diseases of the Colon and Rectum 19:428, 1976, and is reprinted with permission of the authors and the J. B. Lippincott Company.

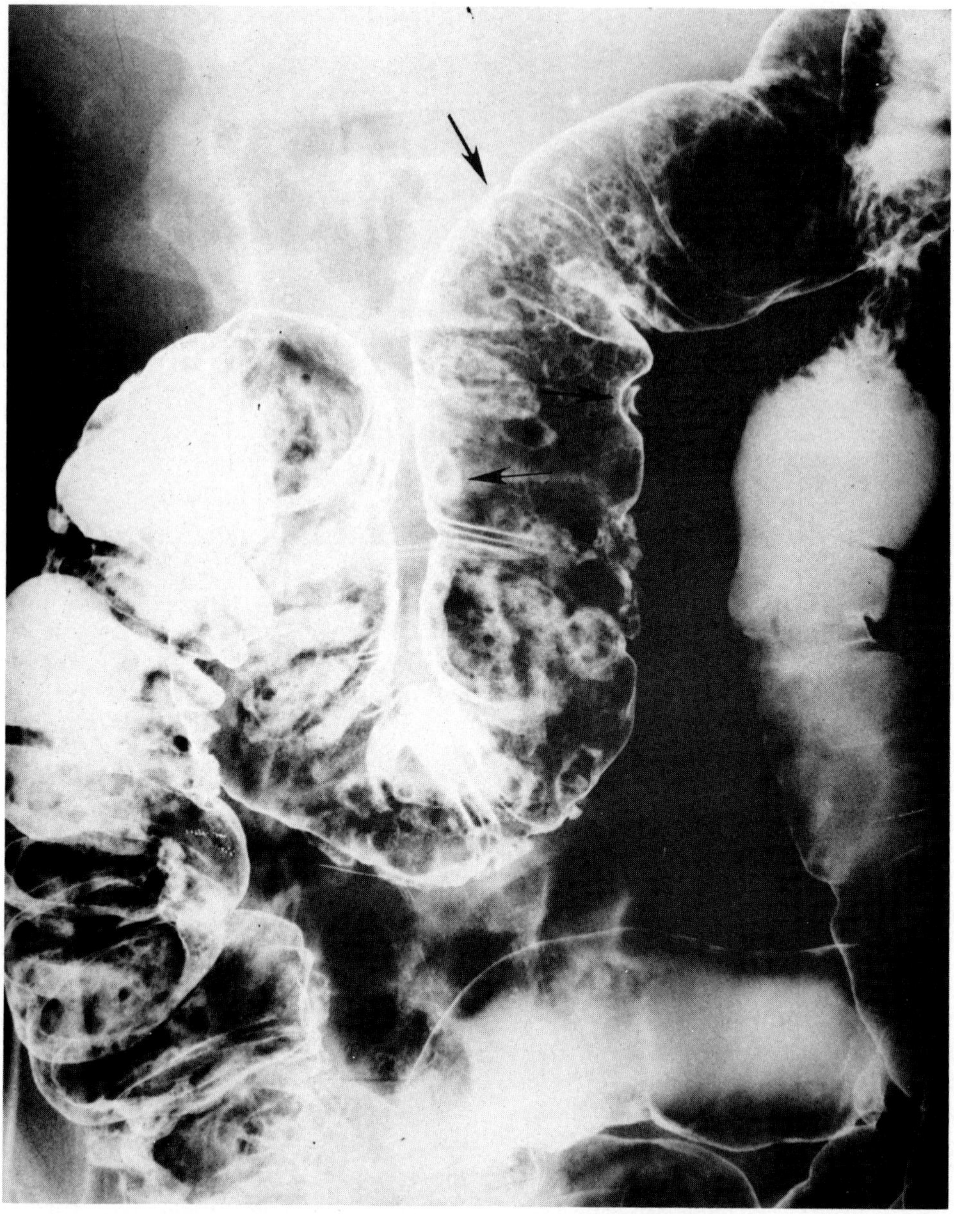

Fig 5–1.—Behçet's disease. Multiple ring-shaped ulcers seen en face *(arrows)* on air contrast barium examination. Ulcers can also be seen projecting beyond coutour of colon *(arrows)*.

Chapter 6

Carcinoids of the Colon and Rectum

H. SHULMAN, M.D. F.R.C.P. (C)
P. GIUSTRA, M.D.

CARCINOID TUMORS have been reported in lung, ovary, pancreas, gallbladder and teratomas.[7] However, over 90% originate in the gastrointestinal tract, the majority in the terminal ileum or appendix (Table 6-1).[10] Only 15-20% of gastrointestinal carcinoids are found in the rectum.[7] Seven percent or less occur in the colon where they constitute about 1-2% of all colonic tumors (Fig 6-1).[26] These carcinoids were long believed to be benign, but Pearson and Fitzgerald[23] (1949) and MacDonald[16] (1956) clearly demonstrated the malignant nature of extra-appendiceal carcinoids. The malignant nature of the colonic carcinoid is reflected by the 60% incidence of metastases at the time of discovery of the primary lesion—the highest in the gastrointestinal tract.[2, 29, 30]

Although there is some debate regarding whether the first carcinoid tumor was reported by Merling[17] in 1838 or Langhans[14] in 1867, it is generally agreed that the classic microscopic description can be credited to Lubarsch[15] (1888). The term "karzinoide" was first used in 1907 by Oberndorfer[20], who believed it to be a benign lesion. In 1912, Saltykow[28] reported the first carcinoid of the colon (sigmoid), whereas Corten[8] probably described the first clearly malignant colonic carcinoid in 1932. The carcinoid syndrome was first described as part of one disease entity in 1952[3] and was reported in association with a carcinoid tumor of the colon in 1960.[5]

TABLE 6-1.—GASTROINTESTINAL CARCINOIDS, 3000 CASES (AFTER ORLOFF)

SITE	INCIDENCE	METASTASES %
Appendix	47	3
Ileum	27.5	35
Rectum	17	12
Colon*	2	60

*In Godwin's review of 2,837 carcinoids, 6.5% were colonic with 70% metastases.

Pathology

Enterochromaffin cells, from which carcinoid tumors arise, are found in tissue derived from the primitive gut, specifically the bronchial tree and gastrointestinal tract. In the gastrointestinal tract, these cells—formerly called Kulchitsky or argentaffin cells—are found in the crypts of Lieberkuhn. It is now recognized that there is more than one type of enterochromaffin cell and that the staining and biochemical characteristics of the cell, as well as the tumor arising from that cell, will vary with the site of origin.[4, 12, 21, 22]

Grossly the rectal carcinoid most often

presents as a small, submucosal, sessile or polypoid nodule less than 2 cm in size.[7, 24] In the remainder of the colon (excluding the appendix), the carcinoid tumor is rarely less than 2 cm and may present as a bulky polypoid mass, as an annular encircling lesion or less commonly as a large ulcerating tumor. The appearance on inspection is indistinguishable from adenocarcinoma, except perhaps for the frequently accompanying extensive mesenteric component—a result of both direct invasion and the tumor's propensity for desmoplastic reaction.[29, 30] The resulting extraluminal mass may be several times larger than the primary lesion.

Microscopically the small, uniform, round or polygonal epithelial cells are found in columns or masses within fibrous stroma with no evidence of true gland formation. Anaplasia and frequency of mitoses, the usual histologic indications of malignancy, are not valid for carcinoid tumors. The most widely accepted criteria for malignancy are (1) evidence of invasion by the neoplastic cells into or beyond the muscularis and/or (2) metastases to regional nodes or beyond.

Examples of these carcinoids are shown in Figures 6–2 to 6–14.

Appendix

The appendix is the commonest site of gastrointestinal carcinoids and the carcinoid is the commonest tumor of the appendix.[7] Muscularis and lymphatic invasion are common findings but metastases are rare, which is reflected in the 99% 5-year survival.[18] When carcinoid is found in acute appendicitis, it is the cause of it in about one third of cases and an incidental finding in the remainder.[7] The appendiceal tumor is rarely, if ever, demonstrated radiographically.

Rectum

Based on the more than 1,200 rectal carcinoids reported to date,[10, 11] 80–90% are under 2 cm in size, benign, asymptomatic and usually an incidental finding. Rectal carcinoids over 2 cm have an 80–90% incidence of malignancy and behave like adenocarcinomas[1, 11, 21, 24] (Table 6–2). The clinical manifestations are the same as with any rectal lesion, with bleeding the commonest presentation.

TABLE 6–2.—RECTAL CARCINOIDS—RELATIONSHIP OF SIZE TO MALIGNANCY*

NO. OF CASES	SIZE	% MALIGNANT
234	<1 cm	1.7
77	1–2 cm	10
45	>2 cm	82

*After Bates.

The treatment advised is local resection if the lesion is under 2 cm and there is no evidence of muscularis invasion.[21, 24] Because of the increasing incidence of malignancy and metastases with increasing size,[11, 19, 21] carcinoids over 2 cm (or with evidence of muscularis invasion) require radical resection.

Colon

The signs and symptoms of colonic carcinoids include abdominal pain, a palpable mass, diarrhea, rectal bleeding, weight loss and constipation[21, 25, 27]; i.e., the clinical presentation (in the absence of the carcinoid syndrome) is indistinguishable from that of adenocarcinoma. Although some authors continue to present colonic carcinoids as slow-growing malignancies,[2] the 5-year survival reported by Kuehn et al.[13] was 15%. It is apparent that, given sufficient time, colonic carcinoids enlarge, invade and ultimately metastasize.[27, 31] The sites of predilection for metastatic disease are liver, bone, lung and brain.[29]

Radiology

The radiographic appearance of colonic carcinoids reflects the gross pathology and in general is indistinguishable from carcinoma.[2, 7] These tumors are large, averaging 5 cm when first detected.[2, 30] They may appear as a polypoid filling defect, an annular "apple-core" lesion, an obstructing or partially obstructing mass and, occasionally, with ulceration.[2, 5, 30] Smooth, round calcifications associated with the tumor or its accompanying fibrous mass have been described in the small bowel[6] but have not been reported in the colon.

The angiographic findings outlined below are based on reports of ileal carcinoids,[6] as there has been no report of angiography performed on a colonic carcinoid. The most consistent angiographic abnormality is arterial wall infiltration, ranging from minor irregularity to complete occlusion. Other reported findings include stellate arterial appearances, narrowing of peripheral mesenteric branches and the presence of tortuous collaterals. Accumulation of contrast medium may occur but is not a common finding. Arteriovenous shunting has not been described.

Associated Malignancy

The incidence of an associated (usually gastrointestinal) malignancy varies from series to series (Table 6-3). The true incidence is probably considerably lower than reported, as many carcinoids (particularly rectal) without an associated neoplasm must go undetected.[10]

TABLE 6-3.—INCIDENCE OF MALIGNANCY ASSOCIATED WITH CARCINOID OF RECTUM AND COLON

	NO. OF CASES	INCIDENCE OF ASSOCIATED MALIGNANCY (%)
Rectum		
Greenwood	661	6.1
Morgan	37	32
Orloff	38	3
Colon		
Godwin	113	10
Rosato	22	22
Morgan	10	0

Carcinoid Syndrome

The carcinoid syndrome is found in less than 10% of patients with a gastrointestinal carcinoid[9] and is characterized by flushing, cyanosis, wheezing, crampy abdominal pain, intermittent diarrhea and right-sided valvular disease.[7, 25] Once thought to be caused by a single hormone (serotonin) produced by the enterochromaffin cell, it is now known that the biochemistry of the "malignant carcinoid spectrum" is far more complex. There are many excellent reviews on the subject.[7, 9, 25, 29] The carcinoid syndrome is most often seen in patients with ileal primary tumors and hepatic metastases.[18] Colonic carcinoids in association with the syndrome are unusual but have been reported.[2, 5, 7]

REFERENCES

1. Bates, H. R., Jr.: Carcinoid tumors of the rectum—a statistical review, Dis. Colon Rectum 9:90, 1966.
2. Berardi, R. S.: Carcinoid tumors of the colon (exclusive of the rectum): Review of the literature, Dis. Colon Rectum 15:383, 1972.
3. Biörck, G., Axen, O., and Thorson, A.: Unusual cyanosis in a boy with congenital pulmonary stenosis and tricuspid insufficiency. Fatal outcome after angiocardiography, Am. Heart J. 44:143, 1952.
4. Black, W. C., III: Enterochromaffin cell types and corresponding carcinoid tumors, Lab. Invest. 19: 473, 1968.
5. Bluth, I.: Gastrointestinal carcinoid tumors: Roentgen features, Radiology 74:573, 1960.
6. Boijsen, E., Kaude, J., and Tylén, U.: Radiologic diagnosis of ileal carcinoid tumors, Acta Radiol. Diag. 15:65, 1974.
7. Cheek, R. C., Wilson, H., Sherman, R. T., and Storer, E. H.: Carcinoid tumors, Curr. Probl. Surg., Nov., 1970.
8. Corten: Demonstrationen 4.2 Felle von Malignem Karzinoid, Beitr. Pathol. 56:364, 1932–33.
9. Crowder, B. L., II., Judd, E. S., and Dockerty, M. B.: Gastrointestinal carcinoids and the carcinoid syndrome: Clinical characteristics and therapy, Surg. Clin. North Am. 47:915, 1967.
10. Godwin, J. D., II.: Carcinoid tumors: An analysis of 2837 cases, Cancer 36:560, 1975.
11. Greenwood, S. M., Huvos, A. G., Erlandson, R. A., and Malt, S. H.: Rectal carcinoid and rectal adenocarcinoma: A case report and review of the literature, Dis. Colon Rectum 17:644, 1974.
12. Hosoda, S.: Carcinoid tumors: Review of literature with special references to sites of origin and humoral substances produced, Acta Pathol. Jpn. 22:533, 1972.
13. Kuehn, P. G., Coley, G. M., and Christine, B.: Carcinoid tumors—A study of 535 cases. Presented at

the 26th Annual Meeting of the James Ewing Society, Louisville, Ky., April 26–28, 1973.
14. Langhans, T.: Ueber einen Drüsenpolyp im Ileum, Arch. Pathol. Anat. 38:559, 1867.
15. Lubarsch, O.: Ueber den primären Krebs des Ileum nebst Bemerkungen über das gleichzeitige Vorkommen von Krebs und Tuberculose, Arch. Pathol. Anat. 3:281, 1888.
16. MacDonald, R. A.: A study of 356 carcinoids of the gastrointestinal tract, Am. J. Med. 21:867, 1956.
17. Merling: Cited by Elting, A. W.: Primary carcinoma of the vermiform appendix, with a report of three cases, Ann. Surg. 37:549, 1903.
18. Moertel, C. G., Dockerty, M. B., and Judd, E. S.: Carcinoid tumors of the vermiform appendix, Cancer 21:270, 1968.
19. Morgan, J. G., Marks, C., and Hearn, D.: Carcinoid tumors of the gastrointestinal tract, Ann. Surg. 180: 720, 1974.
20. Oberndorfer, S.: Ueber die kleinen Dünndarmcarcinome, Verh. Dtsch. Pathol. Ges. 11:113, 1907.
21. Orloff, M. J.: Carcinoid tumors of the rectum, Cancer 28:175, 1971.
22. Pearse, A. G. E.: The APUD cell concept and its implications in pathology, Pathol. Annu. 27, 1975.
23. Pearson, C. M., and Fitzgerald, P. J.: Carcinoid tumors—a re-emphasis of their malignant nature: Review of 140 cases, Cancer 2:1005, 1949.
24. Peskin, G. W., and Orloff, M. J.: A clinical study of 25 patients with carcinoid tumors of the rectum, Surg. Gynecol. Obstet. 109:673, 1959.
25. Postlethwait, R. W.: Gastrointestinal carcinoid tumors. A review, Postgrad. Med. 40:445, 1966.
26. Powell, J., and Barlow, J. F.: Clinicopathological conference. Seventy-seven year old Caucasian female with cecal mass demonstrated on x-ray, SD J. Med. 29(5):7, 1976.
27. Rosato, F. E., and Rosato, E. F.: Carcinoid tumors of the large bowel, CA 29:353, 1970.
28. Saltykow, S.: Über die Genese der "karzinoiden Tumoren," sowie der "Adenomyone" des Darmes, Beitr. Pathol. 54:559, 1912.
29. Sanders, R. J., and Axtell, H. K.: Carcinoids of the gastrointestinal tract, Surg. Gynecol. Obstet. 119: 369, 1964.
30. Shulman, H. S., and Giustra, P. G.: Invasive carcinoids of the colon, Radiology 98:139, 1971.
31. Swensen, S. R., Snow, E., and Gaisford, W. D.: Carcinoid tumors of the gastrointestinal tract, Am. J. Surg. 126:818, 1973.

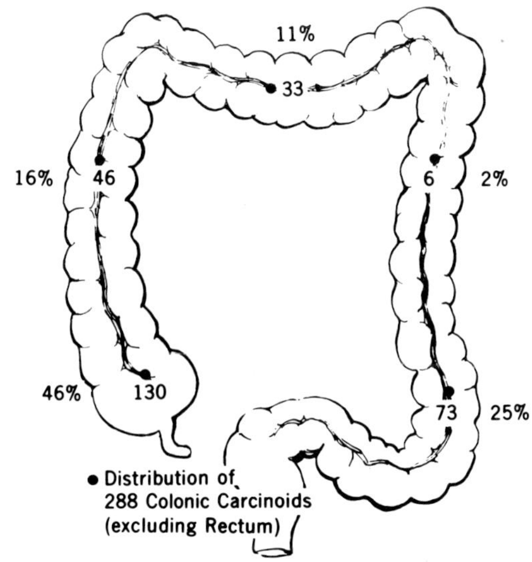

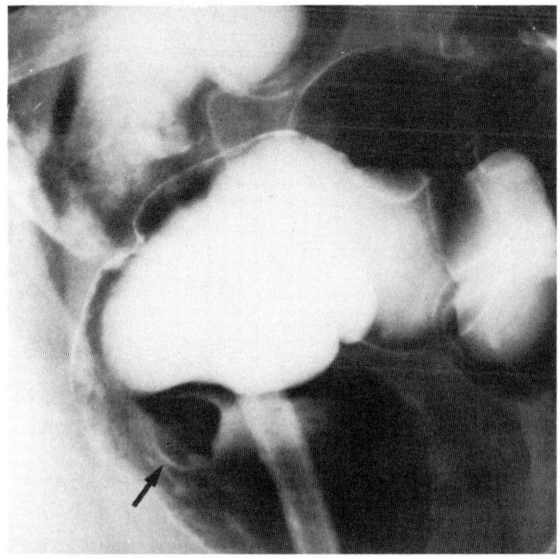

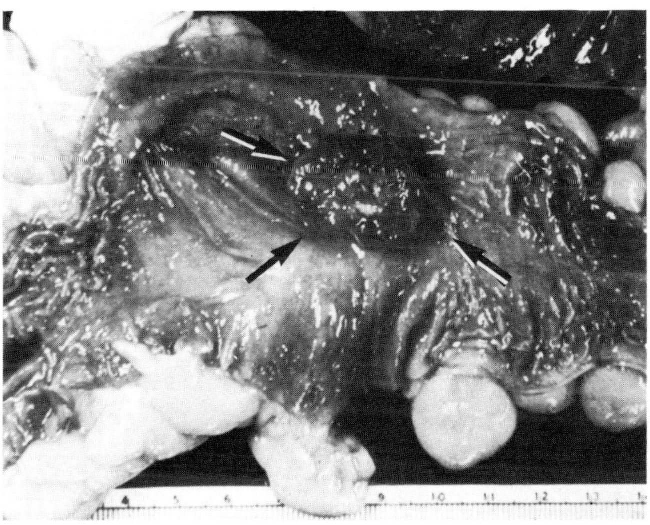

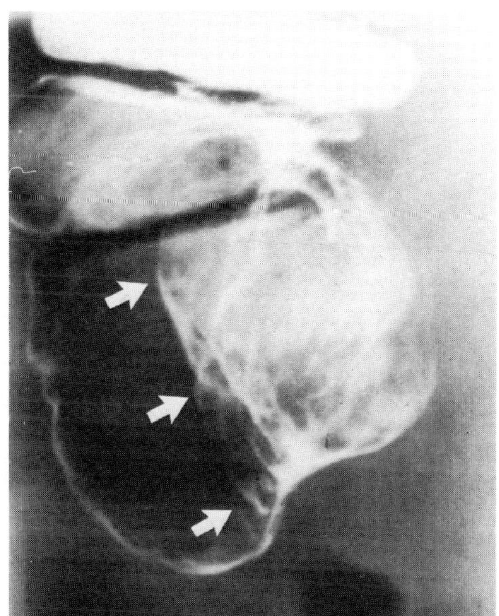

Fig 6–1 (top left).—Distribution of colonic carcinoids from review of literature.[2, 10, 19, 30]

Fig 6–2 (top right).—Smooth, round, sessile 2-cm lesion of rectum *(arrow)* was histologically a noninvasive carcinoid tumor. Over 80% of rectal carcinoids are under 2 cm in size and seldom demonstrated radiographically. As with most rectal carcinoids of this size, this lesion was an incidental finding. (From Shulman and Giustra, Radiology, 98:139, 1971, with permission.)

Fig 6–3 (bottom left).—This 2.5-cm superficially ulcerated lesion *(arrows)* of the rectosigmoid was found incidentally at autopsy. Although smaller than usual malignant colonic carcinoid tumor, its appearance is typical of polypoid form of lesion. Although patient died of unrelated disease, mesenteric abdominal nodes and liver were both involved with metastatic carcinoid tumor. (From Shulman and Giustra, Radiology 98:139, 1971, with permission.)

Fig 6–4 (bottom right).—This 4-cm smooth, polypoid lesion *(arrows)* of cecum was attached to medial wall by small stalk, an unusual finding in colonic carcinoids. Although there is no deformity of medial wall, mesenteric invasion was present. (From Shulman and Giustra, Radiology 98:139, 1971, with permission.)

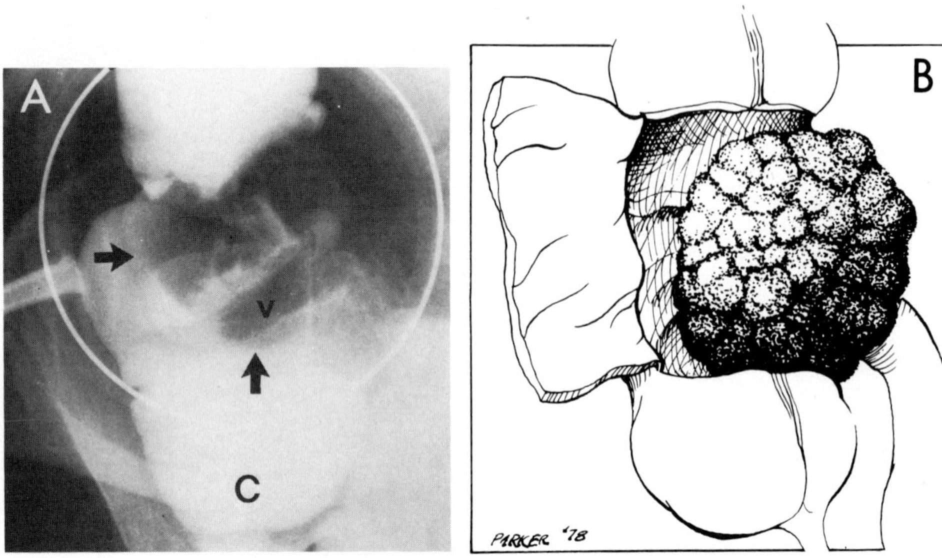

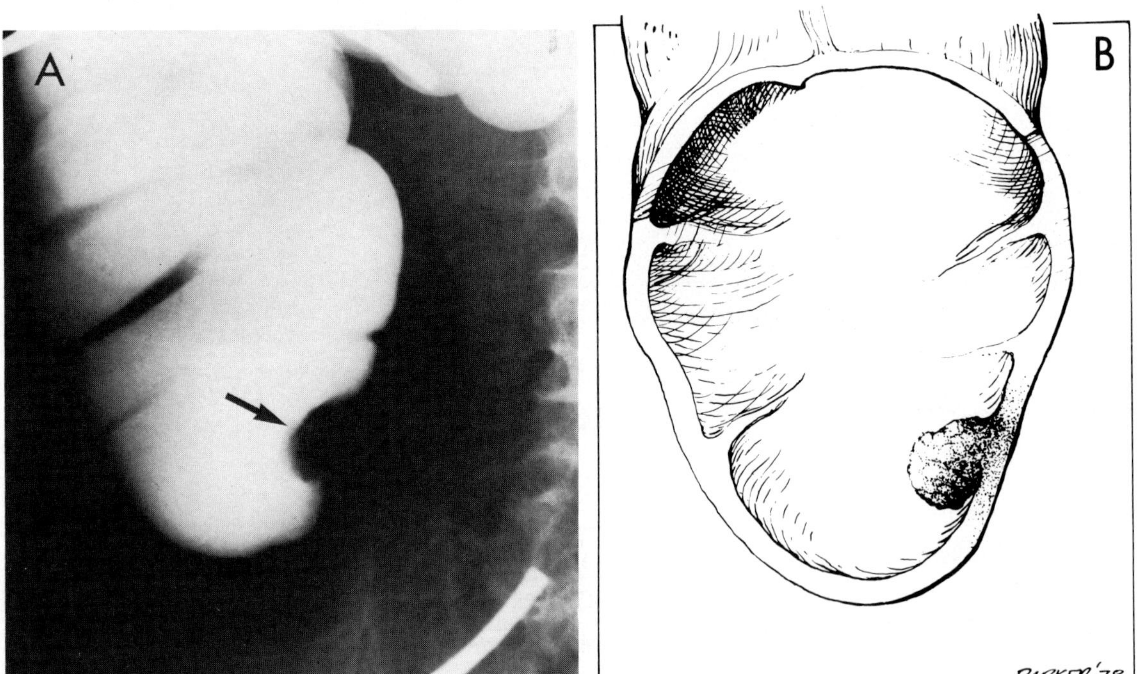

Fig 6–5 (top).—**A,** 5-cm mass outlined above arose mainly from medial surface of ascending colon. As is common with most right-sided tumors, it is polypoid, with large sessile base **(B),** tumor was invading wall and extending into mesentery *(arrows)*. *C* = cecum; *V* = ileocecal valve. (**A** from Shulman and Giustra, Radiology 98:139, 1971, with permission.)

Fig 6–6 (bottom).—**A** and **B,** proved carcinoid tumor *(arrow)* of cecum is considerably smaller than the 5-cm average colonic carcinoid.[2] Right-sided lesions of this size are usually asymptomatic. (Courtesy Dr. E. I. Greenbaum, Los Angeles, California.)

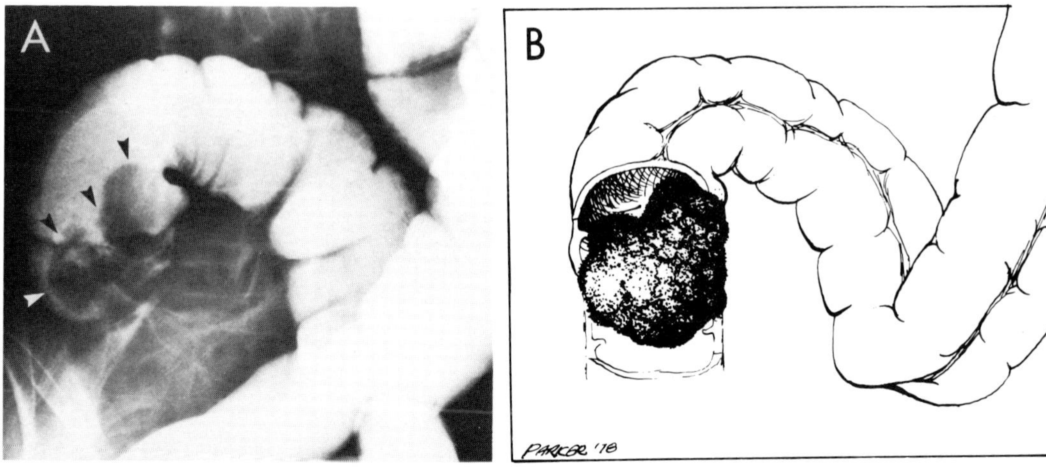

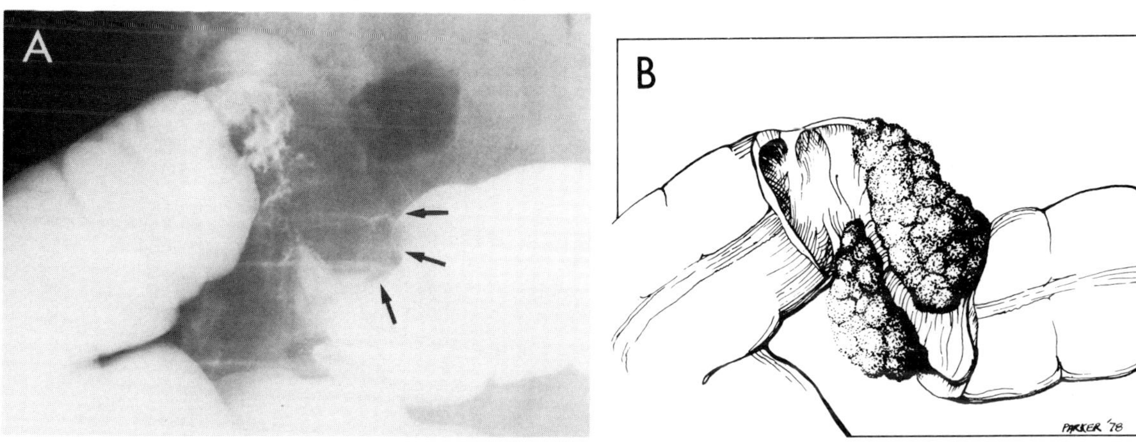

Fig 6–7 (top). – **A** and **B**, lobulated tumor mass *(arrowheads)* in *the* distal ascending colon is basically polypoid, but was also found to be partially encircling bowel. Clinical presentation was that of incomplete obstruction.

Fig 6–8 (bottom). – **A** and **B**, apple core type of defect produced by this annular carcinoid is commonest presentation in transverse colon. As accompanying diagram illustrates, this 5-cm-long tumor had extended beyond bowel into mesentery. "Shoulder" defect *(arrows)* is typical of commoner adenocarcinoma, from which this is indistinguishable. (**A** from Shulman and Giustra, Radiology 90:100, 1071, with permission.)

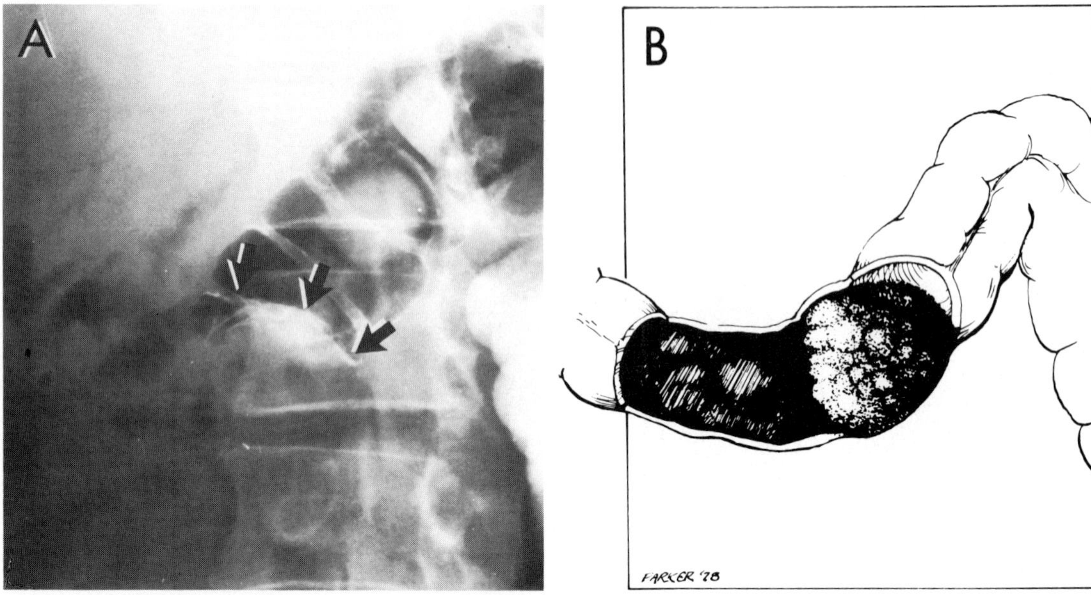

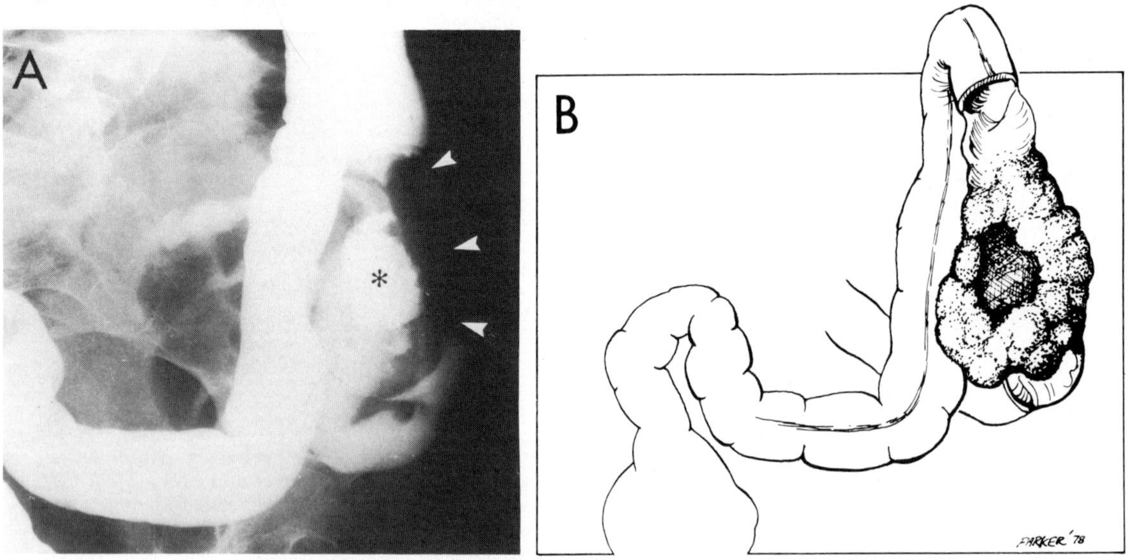

Fig 6–9 (top).—**A** and **B,** radiograph and accompanying diagram illustrate polypoid form of carcinoid *(arrows),* which has resulted in obstruction of transverse colon. Proximal bowel has been decompressed. Intussusception of colon may occur with this type of lesion.[5]

Fig 6–10 (bottom).—**A** and **B,** 7-cm carcinoid tumor of distal (redundant) transverse colon has large, central ulcer (*) in addition to extraluminal mass *(arrowheads).* In spite of size of tumor and degree of narrowing of lumen, there was no clinical evidence of obstruction. Provisional diagnosis was lymphosarcoma. Tumor had invaded mesentery, and regional nodes were involved with metastatic disease. (**A** from Shulman and Giustra, Radiology 98:139, 1971, with permission.)

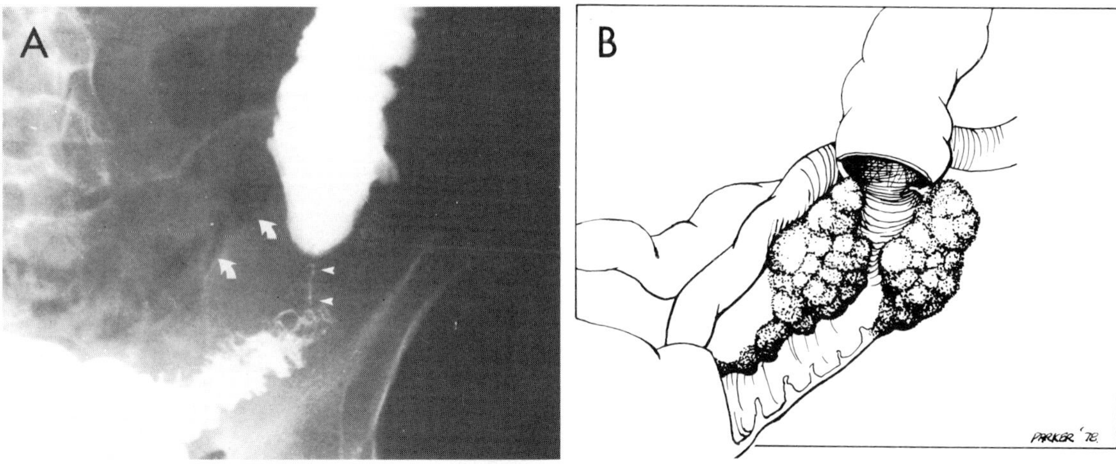

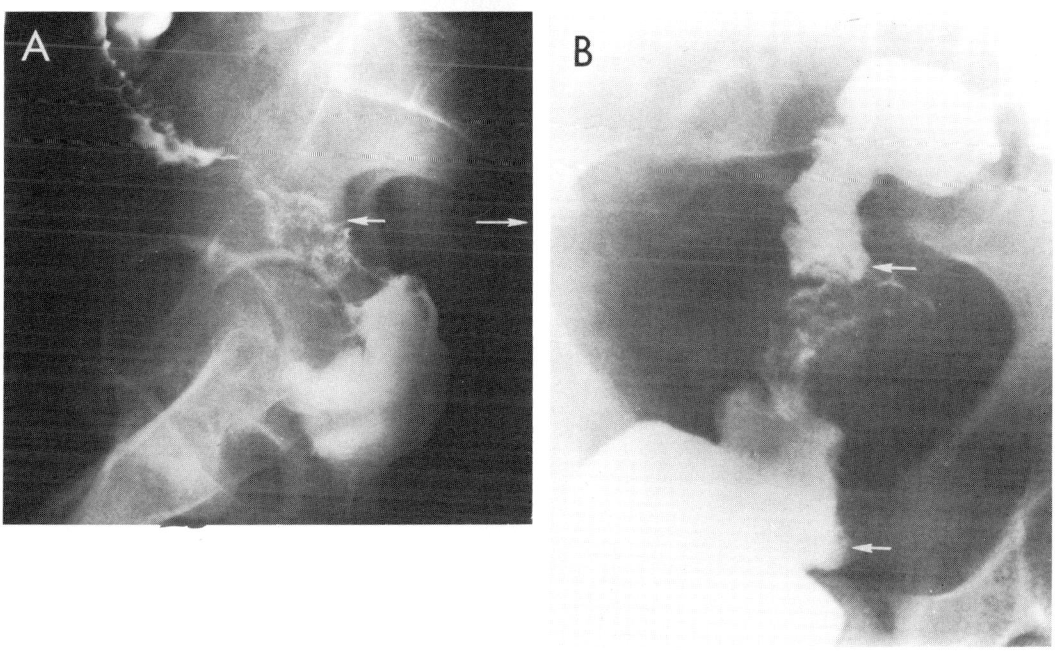

Fig 6–11 (top) – **A** and **B**, 5-cm mass was partially encircling distal descending colon *(arrowheads)*. Extent of extraluminal component can be inferred by displaced adjacent small bowel *(arrows)*. (**A** from Shulman and Giustra, Radiology 98:139, 1971, with permission.)

Fig 6–12 (bottom). – **A** and **B**, rectosigmoid is second commonest site for carcinoid tumors of colon (after cecum). Extensive infiltrating lesion of rectosigmoid *(arrows)* illustrated above extended to within 3 cm of anal verge. At surgery, tumor had invaded mesentery, and metastases were noted in regional nodes and liver. Widening of presacral space is result of considerable extracolonic mass associated with tumor. (From Shulman and Giustra, Radiology 98:139, 1971, by permission.)

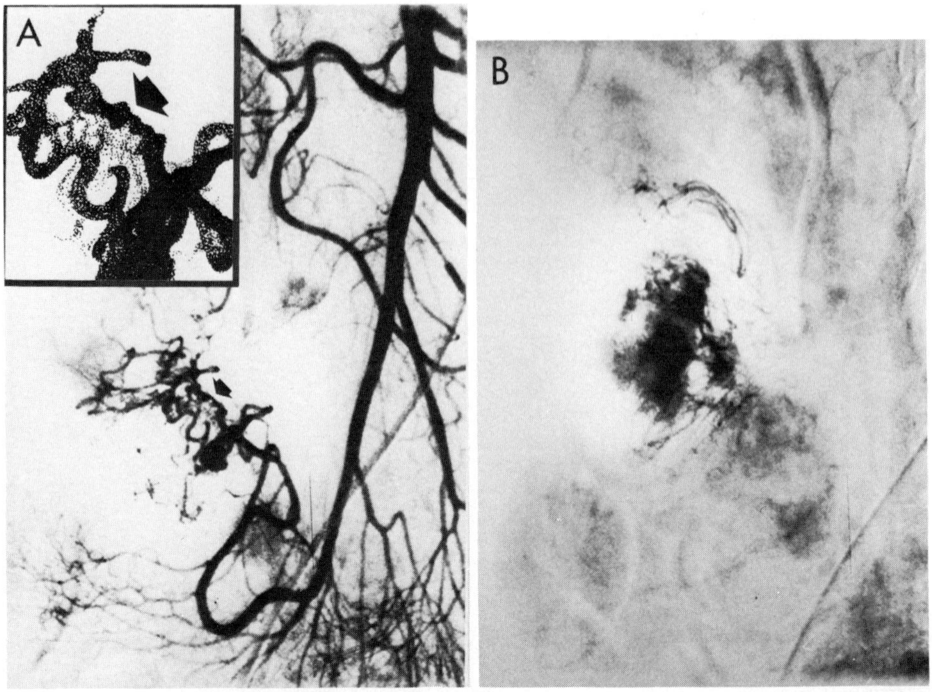

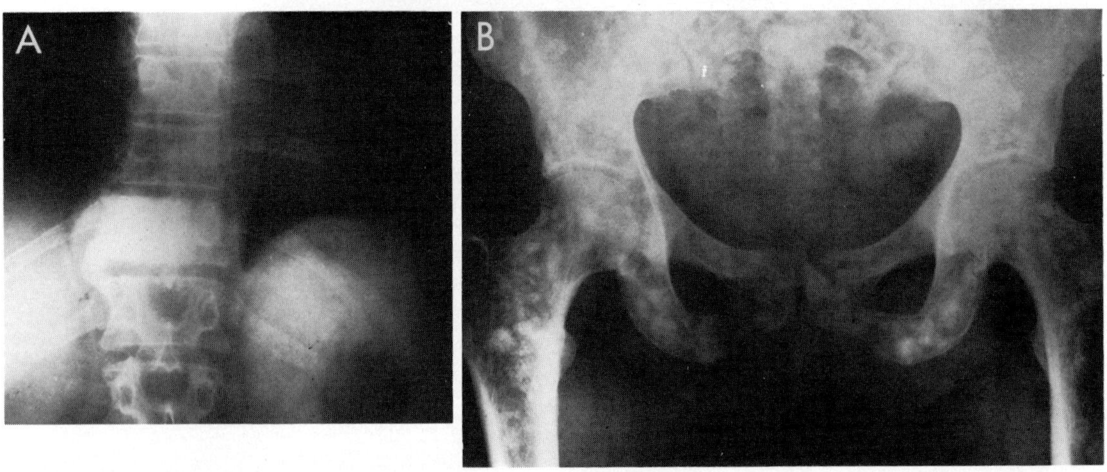

Fig 6–13 (top).—**A** and **B,** selective superior mesenteric arteriogram in patient who presented with large right lower quadrant mass and obstruction. An infiltrating, malignant carcinoid involving cecum and terminal ileum was found at surgery. Precise origin of tumor was not clear due to extent of disease. Irregular narrowing of peripheral mesenteric branches (*arrow,* inset) is typical. Stellate arterial appearance described with ileal carcinoids is not demonstrated. **B,** dense accumulation of contrast medium in late phase is uncommon finding in small bowel carcinoids. Its presence in this case may be due to size of tumor mass. (Courtesy of Dr. E. Lansdown, Department of Radiology, Toronto General Hospital, Toronto, Ontario, Canada.)

Fig 6–14 (bottom).—**A** and **B,** radiographs from two different patients with malignant colonic carcinoid. Both blastic and lytic metastases have been described, but as with carcinoid tumors of the lung, blastic lesions are more common. Bony metastatic disease may be isolated, as in "ivory vertebra" **(A),** or take the more familiar appearance of widespread blastic nodules **(B).** (**B** courtesy of Dr. E. Lansdown, Department of Radiology, Toronto General Hospital, Toronto, Ontario, Canada.)

Chapter 7

Carcinoma of the Colon and Rectum

SETH N. GLICK, M.D.
IGOR LAUFER, M.D.

CARCINOMA OF THE COLON is the most common form of malignancy, accounting for 15% of all carcinomas and 75% of all malignant gastrointestinal tumors. Current methods of treatment have not improved the 5-year survival statistics in patients with advanced tumors. Therefore, the major hope for decreasing the mortality of this disease lies in early detection. Currently available radiographic techniques allow detection of colonic carcinoma in its earliest stages.

The purpose of this chapter is to illustrate the spectrum of radiographic abnormalities found in patients with carcinoma of the colon and rectum, starting with the appearance of early carcinoma and progressing to advanced cancer and its complications.

Early Carcinoma

Although there is continuing controversy regarding the relationship between benign polyps of the colon and carcinoma, there is no doubt that most early colonic carcinomas present as polypoid lesions[1, 2] (Fig 7–1). In most cases the early carcinoma is found as a malignant focus in an otherwise benign adenomatous polyp or villous adenoma (Fig 7–2). Therefore, detection of early colon cancer is to a large extent an exercise in polyp detection,[3, 4] in the realization that a great many benign polyps will be detected for every early cancer.

There are no absolute criteria for the detection of malignancy in a colonic polyp. However, the radiographic appearance of the polyp may be analyzed with respect to several features to give an estimate of the likelihood of malignancy.[5, 6] The most important factor is the size of the polyp. Malignancy is virtually unheard of in polyps under 5 mm in diameter. The vast majority of these polyps are hyperplastic rather than neoplastic. Even in polyps 5–10 mm in size, the incidence of carcinoma is very low, probably of the order of 1% or less. At 1–2 cm, there is a 10% incidence of malignancy, whereas polyps greater than 2 cm have a 40–50% likelihood of malignancy.[1, 7]

The next significant feature is the growth pattern of the polyp. Carcinoma tends to be sessile rather than pedunculated, its width being greater than its height (Fig 7–3). The presence and nature of a stalk provide important diagnostic information. Polyps with a long, thin stalk rarely contain carcinoma, although occasionally a focus of carcinoma is found in the head of the polyp. Even more rarely does the carcinoma invade the stalk (Fig 7–4).[8] However, the presence of a short, thick stalk frequently is associated with carcinoma (Fig 7–5).

Indentation or puckering of the wall of the colon at the base of the polyp is also suggestive of malignancy (Fig 7–6). Although this was described as being due to invasion of the colonic wall by the tumor, this finding may be simulated by benign pedunculated tumors with traction on the colonic wall. Surface irregularity is described as a feature suggestive of malignancy. However, we have not found this to be a reliable sign. Irregularity of the surface may be seen in villous tumors or may be caused by ulceration or irregular growth of the tumor at the mucosal surface.

Advanced Carcinoma

The predominant radiologic feature of the advanced carcinoma depends on the pattern of growth of the tumor. Intraluminal growth results in a polypoid appearance; intramucosal spread results in a plaque-like carcinoma; circumferential spread around the lumen of the bowel produces the typical annular carcinoma; submucosal spread results in linitis plastica or scirrhous carcinoma; and extracolonic growth may result in an extraluminal mass, perforating carcinoma and many of the complications discussed later in this chapter.

POLYPOID

When the predominant pattern of growth is intraluminal, a polypoid tumor results. This form of tumor is found most frequently in the right side of the colon, and patients usually present with occult rectal bleeding or anemia. The radiographic appearances of an advanced polypoid carcinoma may vary from a relatively small, smooth-surfaced polyp to a bulky, fungating, lobulated mass with an irregular ulcerated surface (Fig 7–7). Frequently, polypoid carcinomas are mucinous on histologic examination. These carcinomas may contain an area of calcification or ossification that may be visible on the plain radiograph[9, 10] (Fig 7–8). They may appear as discrete densities of variable size and shape. In some cases there is fine, punctate calcification or a hazy, poorly defined area of increased density. Mucinous carcinomas represent about 50% of all colon carcinomas in patients under age 17. The prognosis is poor.

PLAQUE-LIKE CARCINOMA

This form is the precursor of the annular carcinoma (Fig 7–9). The vast majority present with bleeding.[11] This is observed in the barium-filled colon as a contour defect, often with central ulceration (Fig 7–10, A). On double contrast examination this may be seen as a surface irregularity or as a linear density if only part of the lesion is caught in tangent (see Fig 7–10, B and C).[12, 13]

ANNULAR CARCINOMA

This is the most common appearance of carcinoma of the colon (Fig 7–11, A–C). The growth is predominantly circumferential with a variable intraluminal component. On contrast examination there is a segment of luminal narrowing, which is usually less than 4 cm in length. At least one and usually both margins of the lesion demonstrate an abrupt transition between the intraluminal component and the adjacent normal mucosal surface. This is termed the tumor shoulder or overhanging edge. The normal fold pattern is obliterated within the narrowed segment, and ulceration is frequent. Occasionally, retrograde obstruction of the flow of barium may occur because of a ball-valve mechanism in a patient without clinical bowel obstruction (Fig 7–11, D). The narrowing may be so severe that the mucosal features cannot be evaluated. Differential diagnosis is rarely a problem if the entire lesion can be outlined. Occasionally the lesion may be appreciated on the plain radiograph of the abdomen as an area of soft tissue density interrupting the continuity of the colonic gas pattern (Fig 7 – 12).

LINITIS PLASTICA OR SCIRRHOUS CARCINOMA

This is a specific histologic entity with a high predilection for longitudinal invasion within the colonic wall. Histologic examination characteristically reveals a combination of sheets of anaplastic cells, mucin-secreting signet ring cells and an abundant fibrous stroma infiltrating the submucosa. The mucosa and lumen are relatively spared. Long segments of colon, at least 3 cm and usually greater than 10 cm in length, are involved (Fig 7 – 13). There is a significant degree of extracolonic invasion. Mesentery and lymph nodes are usually involved, and peritoneal seeding is the rule. This lesion is usually (two-thirds) in the rectosigmoid, and over two thirds of the patients are men. Linitis plastica is a rare lesion occurring in about 0.1% of colonic carcinomas.[14, 15, 16] Twenty to thirty-three percent of the reported cases have been associated with ulcerative colitis. The lumen usually is mildly narrowed, and muscular invasion results in a rigid, fixed caliber. The surface of the segment may be straight or convex toward the lumen. The segment of loop is straightened or sharply angulated because of the mesenteric involvement. The mucosa in the center is usually effaced by submucosal infiltration. Occasionally, small ulcerations are present in the mucosa. The folds may be thickened toward the periphery of the lesion. The margins are tapered and the typical overhanging edges are not seen. Rarely there are no detectable features to differentiate this from an inflammatory stricture or from serosal metastases (Fig 7 – 14).

EXTRACOLONIC GROWTH

It is extremely unusual for the predominant growth pattern to be exophytic. When this occurs, the initial radiographic observation may be a soft tissue mass on a plain radiograph of the abdomen. Contrast examinations of the urinary system or upper gastrointestinal tract may show displacement of adjacent viscera. Once a barium enema is performed, the true nature of the problem is revealed (Fig 7 – 15). The extracolonic growth may extrinsically narrow the lumen of an adjacent colonic segment or the lumen of the segment in direct contiguity with the carcinoma. The latter observation may obscure the diagnosis owing to the atypical length of luminal narrowing. Most of the complications of colonic carcinoma, as well as the prognostic determinants, relate to the extraluminal growth of the malignancy.

Associated and Predisposing Lesions

In the barium enema in patients with carcinoma of the colon, other abnormalities are sometimes observed. These lesions occasionally may obscure the diagnosis of carcinoma either by distracting the radiologist from its detection or by producing confusion in interpretation of the malignant segment. The types of pathology vary from diseases that predispose to malignancy to alterations that have a high statistical association because of common etiologic factors or a predilection for the same age group. Some other unusual lesions have been reported with carcinoma but these are probably chance occurrences. This last category includes leiomyosarcoma,[17] carcinoid tumor,[18] carcinoma of the appendix[19] and serosal metastases from extracolonic primary malignancies.

The two most obvious premalignant disorders are inflammatory bowel disease and the polyposis syndromes.[20-22] Familial polyposis usually presents with gastrointestinal symptoms in the third decade, the average age of diagnosis being 25 years. Two thirds of patients presenting with symptoms have carcinoma at the time of diagnosis (Fig 7 – 16). Fifty percent have carcinoma by the age of 30, and 65% by the fifth decade.[23] The average age of death from carcinoma of the colon is 40. The incidence of carcinoma in familial polyposis is virtually 100% unless colectomy is performed. Gardner's syndrome has similar statistical data;[20] however, the soft tissue changes usually precede the gastrointestinal findings. When the Peutz-Jeghers syndrome involves the colon, there is a slightly increased risk of colonic carcinoma, although unlike the prior syndromes, the lesions themselves are not premalignant.[20]

The increased risk of colonic carcinoma in patients with chronic ulcerative colitis has been well documented.[24] The risk of carcinoma increases with duration of the disease and becomes significant after 10 years, although a few carcinomas are found in patients with disease of shorter duration. The average age at the time of detection of carcinoma is 35 years. In at least 50% of patients, the colitis is quiescent, most of the remaining cases showing only mild or moderate activity.[25, 26] The risk of carcinoma is related to the duration of the disease and its extent. With total colonic involvement for 30 years, carcinoma will develop in 56% of patients. Carcinoma is uncommon when colitis is confined to the left colon or rectum. Although there are varying reports concerning the segmental distribution of the carcinoma, most observers believe that the distribution is uniform around the colon. Whereas, in general, 50–60% of carcinomas of the colon are within the range of the 25 cm sigmoidoscope, most carcinomas in ulcerative colitis are proximal to the sigmoid colon. Multiple carcinomas are more common in ulcerative colitis, with a reported incidence of 25–33%.

The multiple lesions usually have the same morphology. The gross appearance in ulcerative colitis also differs from the typical colonic carcinoma.[26, 27] Over 50% are long segments (greater than 6 cm) of concentric or eccentric luminal narrowing with areas of nodular elevation or plaque formation on the surface (Fig 7–17, A). The transition zone may be tapered, although occasionally a small edge may be seen. About one-fourth have the typical annular, plaque-like or polypoid appearance (see Fig 7–17, B), and 20% have the linitis plastica configuration, which may be difficult to distinguish from a benign stricture (see Fig 7–14). Fifty percent of carcinomas are the mucinous variant, and calcification may occasionally be seen.[28] Obstruction is rare. The poor prognosis probably relates to the delay in detection, with an initial false negative rate on barium enemas of 30–50%.[29]

There is also an increased incidence of colon cancer in patients with granulomatous colitis, but the increase is much less dramatic than in patients with ulcerative colitis.[30] The few cases we have seen have presented as fairly typical annular carcinomas (Fig 7–18), but too few such cases have been reported to draw conclusions regarding the morphology, distribution and risk factors for carcinoma in granulomatous colitis.

Other types of inflammatory bowel disease have also been associated with carcinoma. These include infections such as schistosomiasis,[31] lymphogranuloma venereum[32] and amebiasis.[33] Carcinoma has also been reported in patients with radiation-induced colitis following treatment for carcinoma of the cervix.[34] Rectal carcinoma has been reported in patients with chronic anal fistula.[35]

Patients with ureterosigmoidostomy have a definite risk of carcinoma at the site of anastomosis. The latency interval is 10–30 years if the procedure was performed for a benign disorder and 5–10 years if the initial problem was malignancy. The average interval is 17 years.[36]

Patients with a single carcinoma of the colon show a higher risk of having a second colonic carcinoma.[37, 38] This lesion may be either synchronous, i.e., a lesion found at the same time as the first lesion, or metachronous, i.e., a lesion developing some time after the first lesion was discovered. Multiple primary carcinomas are found in 3–4% of patients with colonic carcinoma. The tumors may be found adjacent to each other (Fig 7-19, A) or in different segments of the colon (see Fig 7-19, B). The risk of a second carcinoma is related to the presence of adenomatous polyps. Sentinel polyps are found in 25-30% of patients with colonic carcinoma (Fig 7-20). These patients are at higher risk for development of a second carcinoma and the risk increases with the number of coexisting polyps. When synchronous carcinomas are present, benign adenomatous polyps are found in 75% of patients[9] (see Fig 7-19, A). The prognosis in patients with multiple carcinomas is basically that associated with the most aggressive lesion.

Diverticula are frequently present in association with carcinoma (Fig 7-21, A). This is not surprising considering that the age group involved is similar, and there may be common dietary etiologic factors. However, there is no direct relationship. The problem that arises is that massive diverticulosis may obscure a carcinoma or that diverticular disease and its complications may simulate carcinoma.

The relationship between colonic carcinoma and inguinal hernia has been debated. In a study of patients with colonic carcinoma, 22.5% had an inguinal hernia either at the time of diagnosis or within the preceding 2 years.[39] Like diverticula, the relationship is most likely to be related to their relative frequencies. In another series, all patients having both inguinal hernia and colonic carcinoma had symptoms or signs pertaining to the malignancy; there was no higher incidence of occult carcinoma in patients with inguinal hernia.[40]

Complications of Carcinoma

The radiographic appearance of the carcinoma is frequently altered by the presence of local complications. The five major complications are (1) bleeding, (2) obstruction, (3) perforation, (4) intraperitoneal spread and (5) local recurrence.

BLEEDING

Some form of bleeding occurs in most patients with colon carcinoma. Most commonly this is manifest as either anemia or occult blood in the stool. Rarely is there massive bleeding[41] such that mesenteric angiography is performed as the initial diagnostic procedure.

OBSTRUCTION

Carcinoma can cause obstruction of the colon by several different mechanisms. Most commonly this is due to growth of the tumor. The site of the obstruction is usually easily identified on plain films of the abdomen by the presence of dilated colon containing fluid levels (Fig 7-22). If the ileocecal valve is incompetent, there may be considerable distention of the small bowel, and the plain film may actually suggest a small bowel obstruction[42-43] (Fig 7-23).

Colonic obstruction may also be produced by colocolic intussusception owing to a polypoid carcinoma.[44, 45] These are usually due to tumors originating in the cecum, and the intussusception may extend as far as the splenic flexure (Fig 7-24). The barium enema study shows the classic features of an intussusception. If the intussusception can be reduced, the polypoid tumor can be demonstrated.

Chronic obstruction of the left colon by carcinoma may result in several additional complications. These include cecal volvulus[46] and diastatic rupture of the cecum.[47] The latter diagnosis is suggested by the triad of massive intraperitoneal air, generalized bowel distention and massive cecal distention. This complication should be anticipated when the diameter of the cecum approaches 10 cm.

The segment of colon proximal to an obstructing lesion may suffer ischemic changes.[48] This complication is thought to be related to intermittent elevations of intralu minal pressure, resulting in a decrease in intramural blood flow. The affected segment of colon demonstrates the typical features of colonic ischemia with mucosal thickening and thumbprinting. Occasionally, diffuse small serration may be seen (Fig 7–25). With extensive disease, intramural or portal vein gas may be evident. With progression of this complication, colonic gangrene and perforation may result.

PERFORATION

Extracolonic growth of the tumor with necrosis rarely results in free perforation with communication between the colonic lumen and the peritoneal cavity (Fig 7–26). More commonly a pericolic abscess develops so that the radiographic features are more suggestive of an inflammatory process such as diverticulitis[49] (Fig 7–27). With resolution of the inflammation, the underlying carcinoma may become more evident. The extracolonic tumor may affect adjacent organs, resulting in a wide variety of manifestations including small bowel obstruction, ureteral obstruction, splenic vein occlusion or invasion of the inferior vena cava.[50] With progression of this process, a fistula may develop. The most commonly affected organs are the bladder,[51] greater curvature of the stomach,[52] (Fig 7–28) and postbulbar segment of the duodenum (Fig 7–29).[53]

INTRAPERITONEAL SPREAD

Peritoneal carcinomatosis may produce ascites by causing lymphatic obstruction. Seeded metastases tend to settle in the region of the ileocecal valve and along the superior aspect of the sigmoid colon. However, they are probably most common in the pouch of Douglas where they produce a typical extrinsic defect on the anterior wall of the rectosigmoid junction[54] (Fig 7–29).

LOCAL RECURRENCE

Carcinoma has a particular tendency to recur at the suture line. For some reason, this is found with colocolic anastomoses but is rarely found in patients with an ileocolic anastomosis. It may frequently be difficult to distinguish between a normal anastomosis and a local recurrence. For this purpose, it is essential to get a baseline study at 2–3 months following surgery for future comparisons. The normal anastomosis demonstrates smooth, symmetric narrowing, usually less than 1 cm in length, with smooth overlying mucosa. On the other hand, recurrent carcinoma produces an asymmetric, nodular anastomosis, and the overlying mucosa may be irregular or ulcerated[55] (Fig 7–30).

REFERENCES

1. Morson, B. C.: The polyp-cancer sequence in the large bowel, Proc. R. Soc. Med. 67:451, 1974.
2. Lane, N., and Fenoglio, C. M.: Observations of the adenoma as precursor to ordinary large bowel carcinoma, Gastrointest. Radiol. 1:111, 1976.
3. Ott, D. J., and Gelfand, D. W.: Colorectal tumors: Pathology and detection, Am. J. Roentgenol. 131: 691, 1978.
4. Laufer, I.: *Double Contrast Gastrointestinal Radiology, with Endoscopic Correlation* (Philadelphia: W. B. Saunders Co., 1979).
5. Youker, J. E., Dodds, W. J., and Welin, S.: Colonic Polyps, in Margulis, A. R., and Burhenne, H. J. (eds.): *Alimentary Tract Roentgenology,* Vol. II (St. Louis: C. V. Mosby Co., 1973), pp. 1037–1067.
6. Ekelund, G., Lindstrom, C., and Rosengren, J. E.: Appearance and growth of early carcinomas of the colon-rectum, Acta Radiol. (Diag) 15:670, 1974.
7. Laufer, I.: The double contrast enema: Myths and misconceptions, Gastrointest. Radiol. 1:19, 1976.
8. Smith, T. R.: Pedunculated malignant colonic polyps with superficial invasion of the stalks, Radiology 115:593, 1975.
9. Seaman, W. B.: Unusual Roentgen Manifestations of Large Bowel Cancer, in Felson, B. (ed.): Semin. Roentgenol. (New York: Grune & Stratton, Inc., 1976), pp 89–100.
10. Ghahremani, G. G., Meyers, M. A., and Port, R. B.: Calcified primary tumors of the gastrointestinal tract, Gastrointest. Radiol. 2:331, 1978.
11. Dreyfuss, J. R., and Benacerraf, B.: Saddle cancers of the colon and their progression to annular carcinomas, Radiology 129:289, 1978.
12. Kressel, H. Y., and Laufer, I.: Principles of Double Contrast Diagnosis, in Laufer, I. (ed.): *Double*

Contrast Gastrointestinal Radiology, with Endoscopic Correlation (Philadelphia: W. B. Saunders Co., 1979).
13. Ho, C. S., and Rubin, E.: Linear shadows in the air contrast enema, Radiology 127:621, 1978.
14. Raskin, M. M.: Some specific radiologic findings and considerations of linitis plastica of the gastrointestinal tract, CRC Crit. Rev. Clin. Radiol. Nucl. Med. 7:87, 1976.
15. Raskin, M. M., Viamonte, M., and Viamonte, M., Jr.: Primary linitis plastica carcinoma of the colon, Radiology 113:17, 1974.
16. Greenbaum, E. I., and Freedman, S: Neoplasia of the colon over a long segment, Clin. Radiol. 24:416, 1973.
17. Alfonso, A. E., and Hertz, R. E.: Synchronous leiomyosarcoma and adenocarcinoma of the rectum: Report of a case and review of the literature, Dis. Colon Rectum 18:228, 1975.
18. Greenwood, S. M., Huvos, A. G., Erlandson, R. A., et al.: Rectal carcinoid and rectal adenocarcinoma—A case report and review of the literature, Dis. Colon Rectum 17:644, 1974.
19. Birla, R. K., Nolan, R. B., and Birla, S. R.: Synchronous adenocarcinoma of the vermiform appendix and the rectosigmoid: Case report and review of the literature, Dis. Colon Rectum 18:687, 1975.
20. Dodds, W. J.: Clinical and roentgen features of the intestinal polyposis syndromes, Gastrointest. Radiol. 1:143, 1976.
21. Bussey, H. J. R.: Familial polyposis coli: Family Studies, Histopathology, Differential Diagnosis and Results of Treatment (Baltimore: Johns Hopkins Press, 1975).
22. Bartram, C. I., and Laufer, I.: Polyposis Syndromes, in Laufer, I. (ed.): *Double Contrast Gastrointestinal Radiology—With Endoscopic Correlation* (Philadelphia: W. B. Saunders Co., 1979).
23. Winawer, S. J., Sherlock, P., Schottenfeld, D., et al.: Screening for colon cancer, Gastroenterology 70:783, 1976.
24. Lennard-Jones, J. E., Morson, B. C., Ritchie, J. K., et al.: Cancer in colitis; assessment of the individual risk by clinical and histological criteria, Gastroenterology 73:1280, 1977.
25. Bartram, C.: Radiology in the current assessment of ulcerative colitis, Gastrointest. Radiol. 1:383, 1977.
26. Hodgson, J. R., Sauer, W. G.: The roentgenologic features of carcinoma in chronic ulcerative colitis, Am. J. Roentgenol. 86:91, 1961.
27. Fennessey, J. J., Sparberg, M. B., and Kirsner, J. B.: Radiological findings in carcinoma of the colon complicating chronic ulcerative colitis, Gut 9:388, 1968.
28. Shockman, A. T.: Calcified carcinoma of the colon superimposed on chronic ulcerative colitis, Am. J. Dig. Dis. 14:683, 1969.
29. James, E. M., and Carlson, H. C.: Chronic ulcerative colitis and colon cancer: Can radiographic appearance predict survival patterns?, Am. J. Roentgenol. 130:825, 1978.
30. Lightdale, C. J., Sternberg, S. S., Posner, G., et al.: Carcinoma complicating Crohn's disease: Report of seven cases and review of the literature, Am. J. Med. 59:262, 1975.
31. Shindo, K.: Significance of schistosomiasis japonica in the development of cancer of the large intestine: Report of a case and review of the literature, Dis. Colon Rectum 19:460, 1976.
32. Levin, I., Romaro, S., Steinberg, M., et al.: Lymphogranuloma venereum: Rectal stricture and carcinoma, Dis. Colon Rectum 7:129, 1964.
33. Camacho, E.: Amebic granuloma and its relationship to cancer of the cecum, Dis. Colon Rectum 14:12, 1971.
34. Black, W. C., III, and Ackerman, L. V.: Carcinoma of the large intestine as a late complication of pelvic radiotherapy, Clin. Radiol. 16:278, 1965.
35. Heidenreich, A., Collarini, H., Paladino, A. M., et al.: Cancer in anal fistulas: Report of two cases, Dis. Colon Rectum 9:371, 1966.
36. Preissig, R., Barry, W. F., et al.: The increased incidence of carcinoma of the colon following ureterosigmoidostomy, Am. J. Roentgenol. 121:806, 1974.
37. Fishel, R. E., Dermer, R.: Multifocal carcinoma of the large intestine, Clin. Radiol. 26:495, 1975.
38. Schottenfeld, D., Berg, J. W., and Vitsky, B.: Incidence of multiple primary cancer. II Index cancers arising in the stomach and lower digestive systems, J. Natl. Cancer Inst. 43:77, 1969.
39. Davis, W. C., Jackson, F. C.: Inguinal hernia and colon carcinoma, CA 18:143, 1968.
40. Juler, G. L., Stemmer, E. A., and Fuelleman, R. W.: Inguinal hernia and colorectal carcinoma, Arch. Surg. 104:778, 1972.
41. Wallace, H. W., Stremp, E. E., and Davis, W. C.: Massive gastrointestinal hemorrhage—An unusual resultant of cecal malignancy, Am. J. Surg. 106:989, 1963.
42. McIver, J. R., and Don, C.: The fluid filled colon in acute large bowel obstruction, Am. J. Roentgenol. 94:410, 1965.
43. Kent, K. H., and Raskowski, H. J.: Colon lesions masquerading as small bowel obstruction on the plain roentgenogram of the abdomen, Am. J. Roentgenol. 88:671, 1962.
44. Dick, A., and Green, G. J.: Large bowel intussusception in adults, Br. J. Radiol. 34:769, 1961.
45. Weilbaecher, D., Bolin, J. A., Hearn, D., et al.: Intussusception in adults: Review of 160 cases, Am. J. Surg. 121:531, 1971.
46. Ritvo, M., Farrell, G. E., Jr., and Shauffer, I. A.: The association of volvulus of the cecum and ascending colon with other obstructive colonic lesions, Am. J. Roentgenol. 78:587, 1957.
47. Novy, S., Rogers, L. F., and Kirkpatrick, W.: Diastatic rupture of the cecum in obstructing carcinoma of the left colon: Radiographic diagnosis and surgical implications, Am. J. Roentgenol. 121:281, 1975.

48. Schwartz, S. S., and Boley, S. J.: Ischemic origin of ulcerative colitis associated with potentially obstructing lesions of the colon, Radiology 102:249, 1972.
49. Laufer, I., and Joffe, N.: Roentgenologic aspects of chronic perforating carcinoma of the colon, Dis. Colon Rectum 16:127, 1973.
50. Atwood, H.D., and Giles, P. F. H.: Direct intracardiac extension of a carcinoma of the cecum, J. Pathol. 91:266, 1966.
51. Aldrete, J. S., and ReMine, W. H.: Vesicocolic fistula. A complication of colonic cancer—long-term results of its surgical treatment, Arch. Surg. 94: 627,1966.
52. MacMahon, C. E., and Lund, P.: Gastrocolic fistulae of malignant origin: A consideration of its nature and report of five cases, Am. J. Surg. 106:333, 1963.
53. Vieta, J. O., Blanco, R., and Valentini, G. R.: Malignant duodenocolic fistula: Report of two cases, each with one or more other synchronous gastrointestinal cancers, Dis. Colon Rectum 19:542, 1976.
54. Meyers, M. A.: *Dynamic Radiology of the Abdomen—Norman and Pathologic Anatomy* (New York: Springer-Verlag, Inc., 1976). pp 37–82 and 333–345.
55. Bartram, C., and Hale, J. A.: Radiological diagnosis of recurrent colonic carcinoma at the anastomosis, Gut 2:778, 1970.

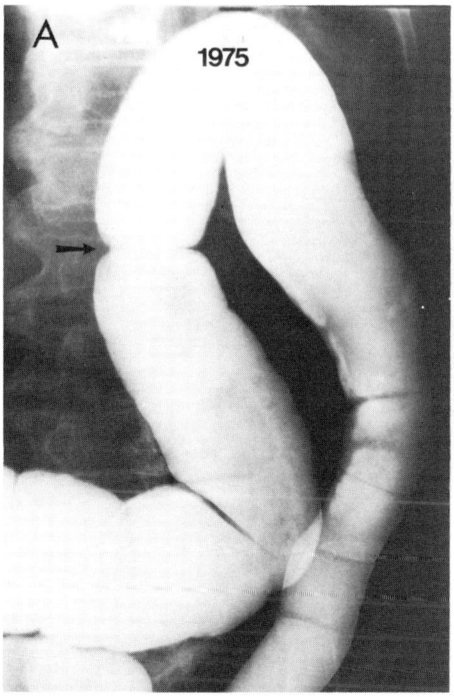

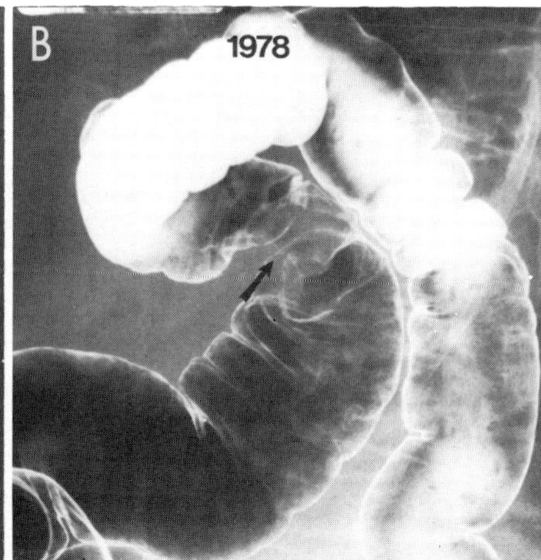

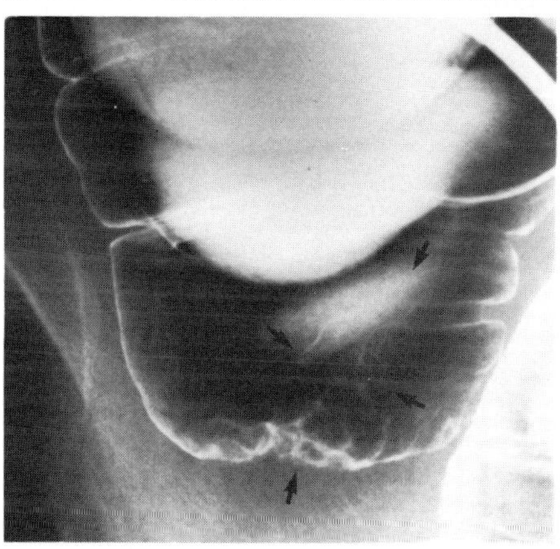

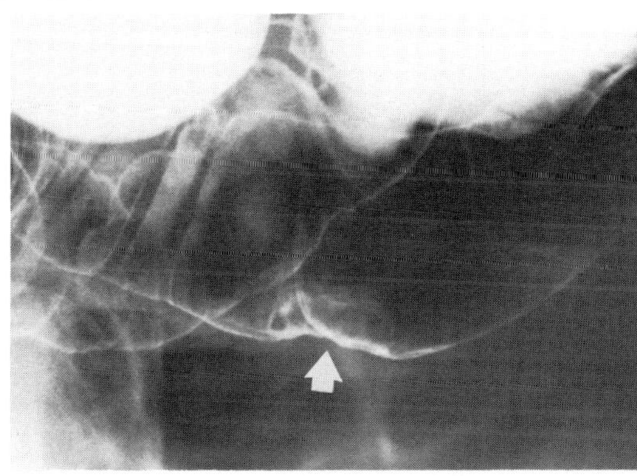

Fig 7–1 (top).—Development of colonic carcinoma. **A,** barium enema shows very small polypoid lesion *(arrow)* on superior aspect of distal transverse colon. This was not appreciated at the time. **B,** 3 years later, this small lesion *(arrow)* has progressed to become a typical annular carcinoma. (From Laufer, I.: *Double Contrast Gastrointestinal Radiology, with Endoscopic Correlation* [Philadelphia: W. B. Saunders Co., 1979]. Reprinted with permission.)

Fig 7–2 (bottom left).—Mucosal carcinoma arising in villous adenoma. There is a flat, lobulated tumor at tip of cecum *(arrows).* At surgery this was a villous adenoma with intramucosal carcinoma. (From Laufer, I.: *Double Contrast Gastrointestinal Radiology, with Endoscopic Correlation* [Philadelphia: W. B. Saunders Co., 1979]. Reprinted with permission.)

Fig 7–3 (bottom right).—Polypoid carcinoma. Sessile polyp *(arrow)* in which width is greater than height. This growth pattern suggests carcinoma.

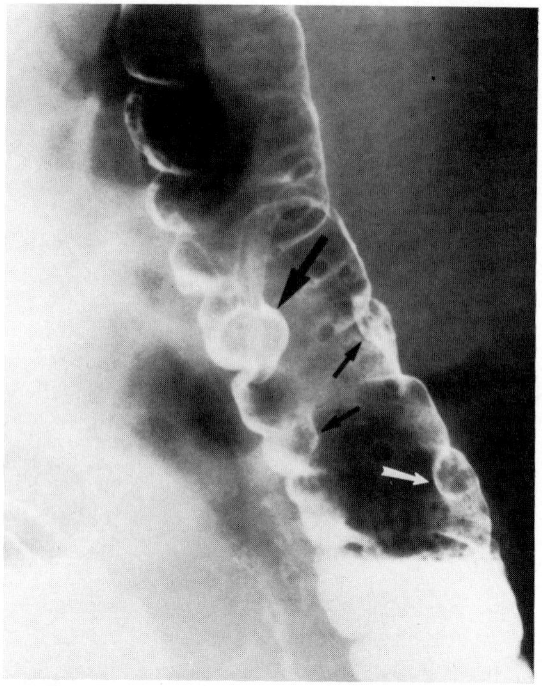

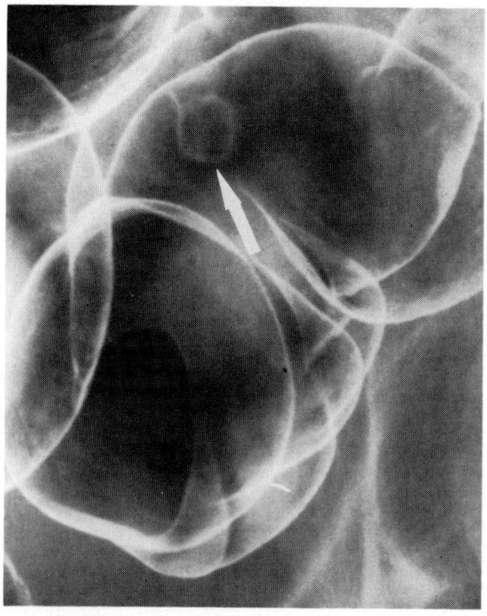

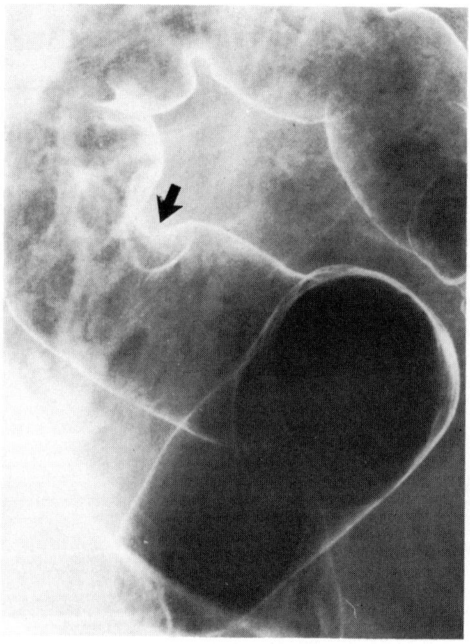

Fig 7–4 (top).—Unusual pedunculated carcinoma. Note 1.5 cm polypoid lesion with long, thin stalk *(large arrow)*. This proved to be adenocarcinoma with invasion of stalk. Smaller polypoid lesions *(small arrows)* were metaplastic polyps. (From Laufer, Gastrointest. Radiol. 1:19, 1976, with permission.)

Fig 7–5 (bottom left).—Pedunculated carcinoma. Polypoid lesion with short, thick stalk present in sigmoid colon, suggestive of a malignant polyp. (From Laufer, I.: *Double Contrast Gastrointestinal Radiology, with Endoscopic Correlation* [Philadelphia: W. B. Saunders Co., 1979]. Reprinted with permission.)

Fig 7–6 (bottom right).—Indrawing *(arrow)* of base of polyp due to carcinoma. (From Laufer, I.: *Double Contrast Gastrointestinal Radiology, with Endoscopic Correlation* [Philadelphia: W. B. Saunders Co., 1979]. Reprinted with permission.)

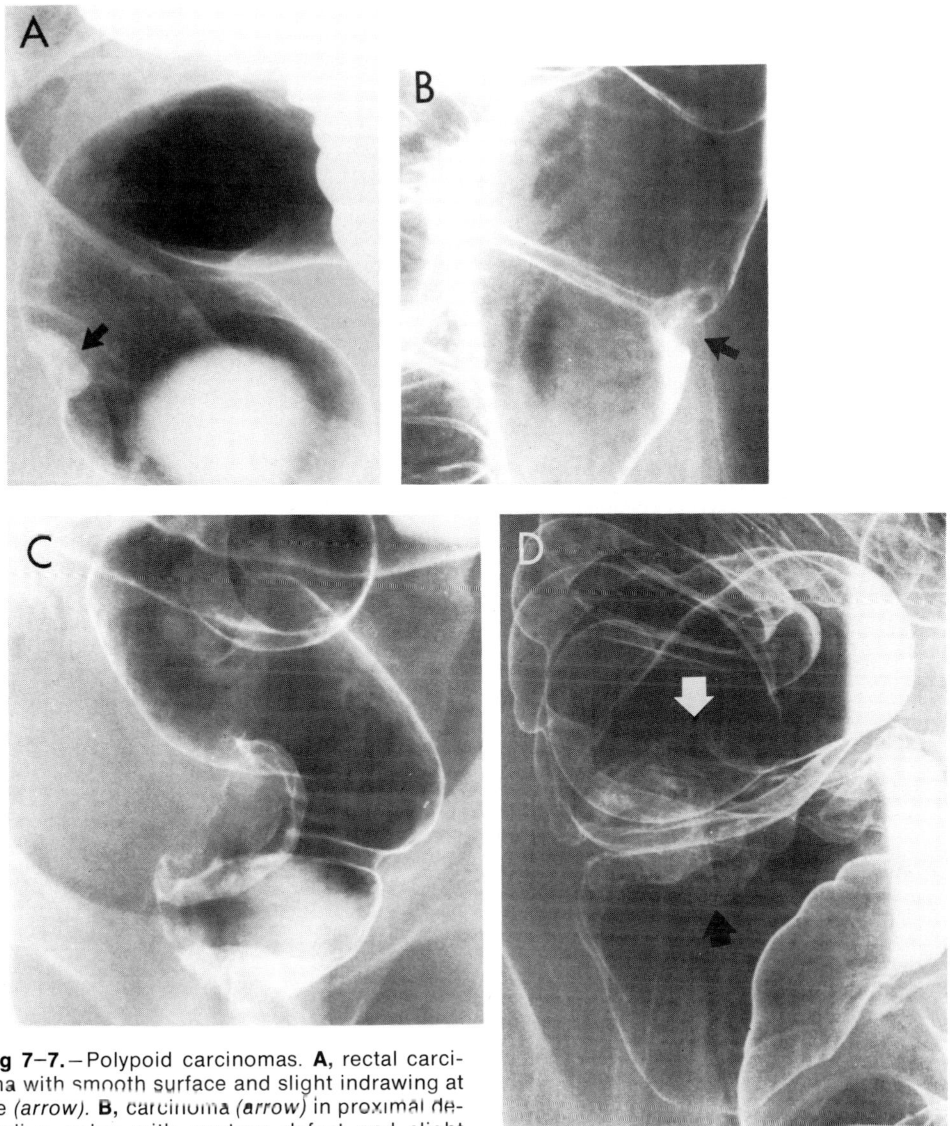

Fig 7–7.—Polypoid carcinomas. **A,** rectal carcinoma with smooth surface and slight indrawing at base *(arrow).* **B,** carcinoma *(arrow)* in proximal descending colon with contour defect and slight irregularity of surface. **C,** polypoid carcinoma arising from right lateral wall of rectum. **D,** large, lobulated polypoid carcinoma *(arrows)* arising in cecum, adjacent to ileocecal valve. (**A** from Laufer, Gastrointest Radiol. 1:19, 1976. **B** and **C** from Laufer, I.: *Double Contrast Gastrointestinal Radiology, with Endoscopic Correlation* [Philadelphia: W. B. Saunders Co., 1979]. Reprinted with permission.)

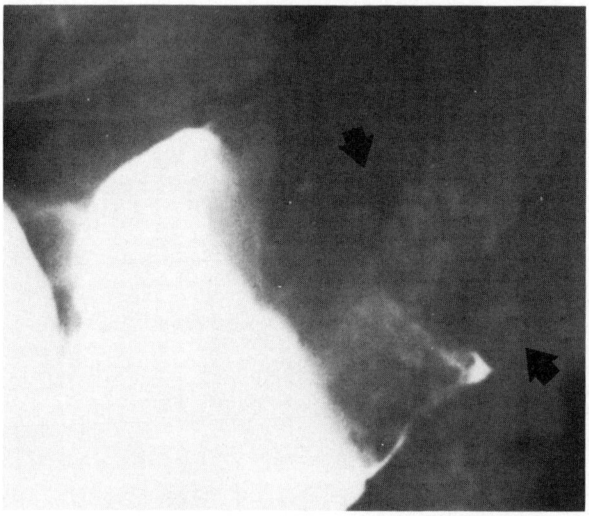

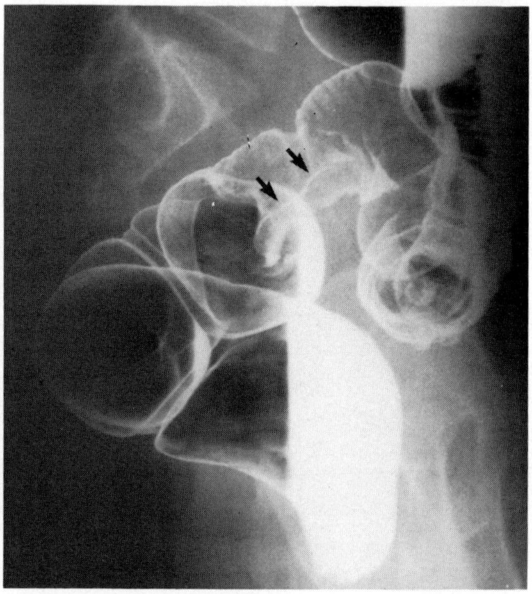

Fig 7–8 (left).—Mucinous adenocarcinoma with mottled calcification *(arrows).*

Fig 7–9 (right).—Plaque-like carcinoma. Cross table lateral film of rectosigmoid shows plaque-like tumor on anterior wall at rectosigmoid junction *(arrows).* (From Laufer, I.: *Double Contrast Gastrointestinal Radiology, with Endoscopic Correlation* [Philadelphia: W. B. Saunders Co., 1979]. Reprinted with permission.)

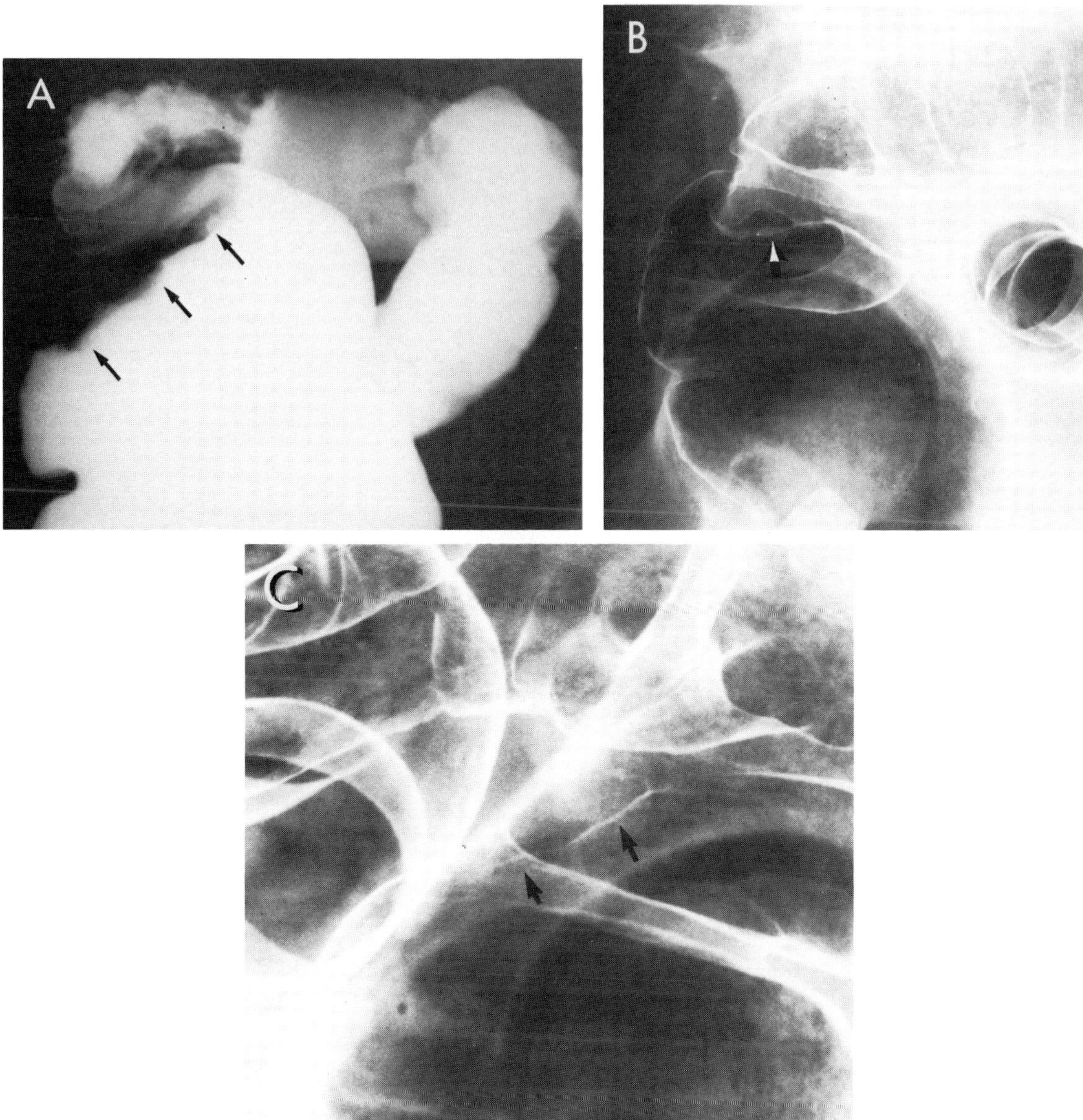

Fig 7–10.—Plaque-like carcinoma. **A,** barium-filled film shows irregularity of contour at recto-sigmoid junction *(arrows).* **B,** double contrast film in lateral projection shows plaque-like lesion en face *(arrow).* **C,** in oblique projection, tumor *(arrows)* is seen only as faint white line, as part of lesion is caught in tangent.[9] (From Laufer, I.: *Double Contrast Gastrointestinal Radiology—with Endoscopic Correlation* [Philadelphia: W. B. Saunders Co., 1979]. Reprinted with permission.)

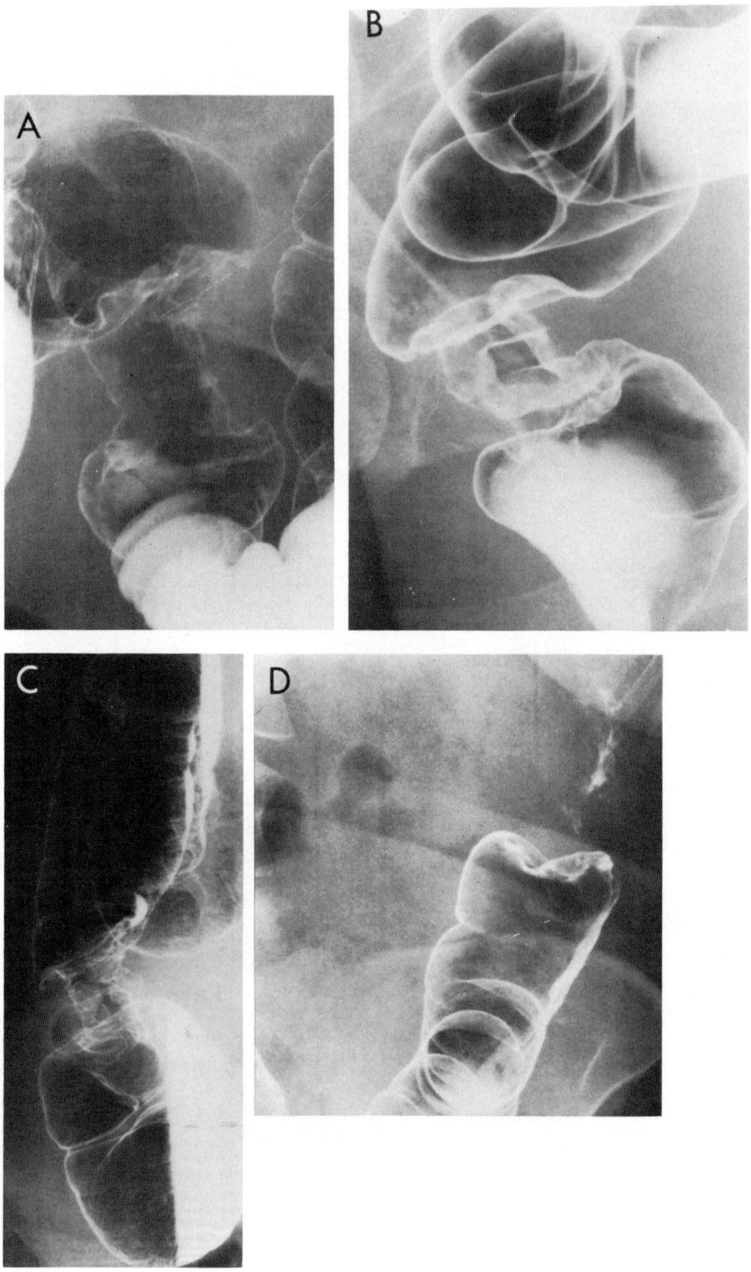

Fig 7–11.—Annular carcinoma. Typical annular or apple core lesions in **A,** sigmoid; **B,** rectum; **C,** ascending colon; and **D,** annular carcinoma of descending colon with retrograde obstruction. (From Laufer, I.: *Double Contrast Gastrointestinal Radiology, with Endoscopic Correlation* [Philadelphia: W. B. Saunders Co., 1979]. Reprinted with permission.)

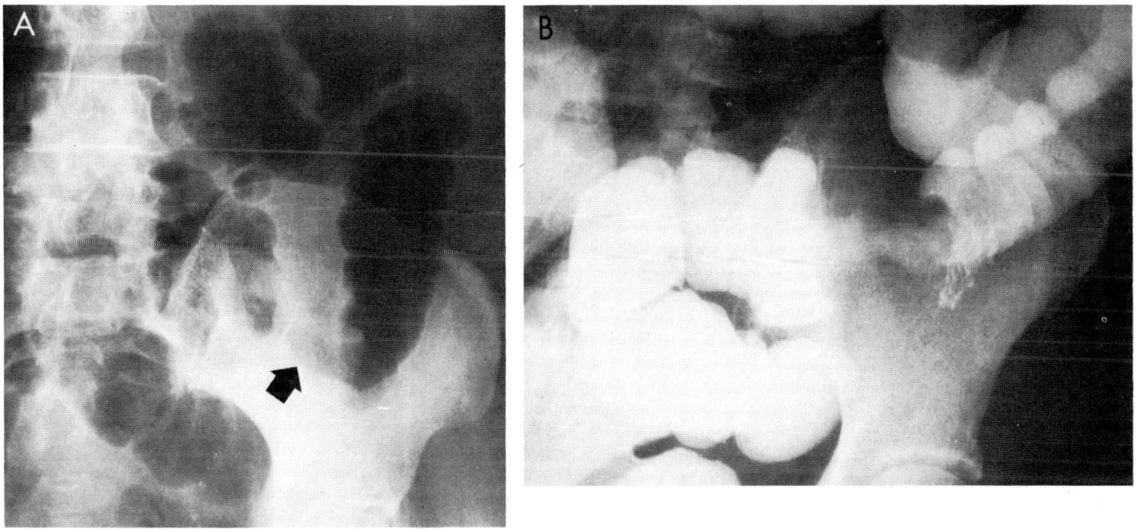

Fig 7–12.—Plain film diagnosis. **A,** plain film of abdomen shows narrowing of gas-filled distal descending colon *(arrow)*. **B,** barium enema confirms that finding was due to annular carcinoma.

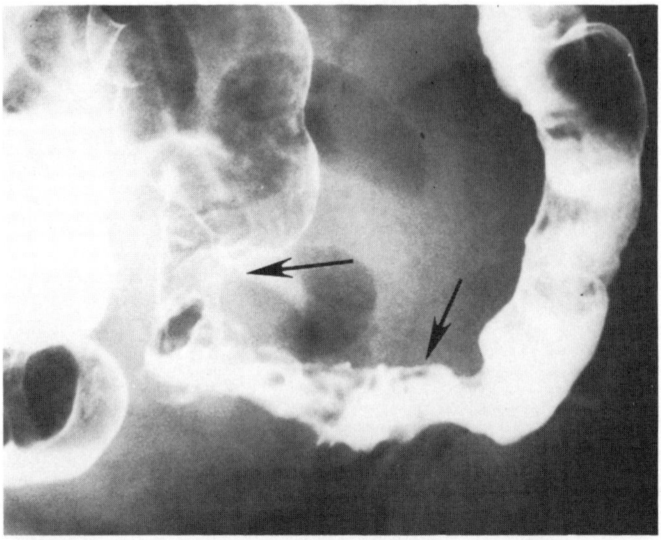

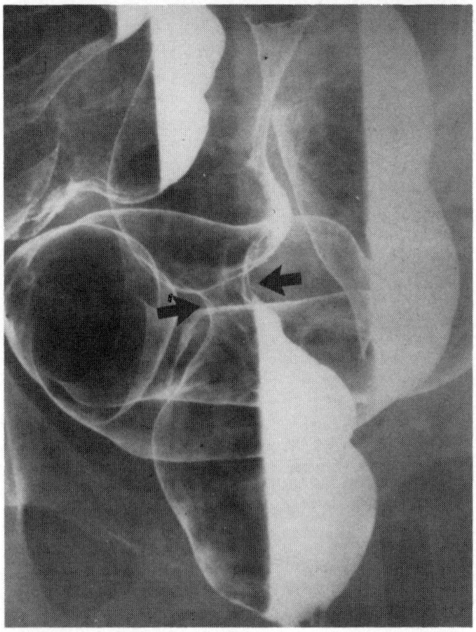

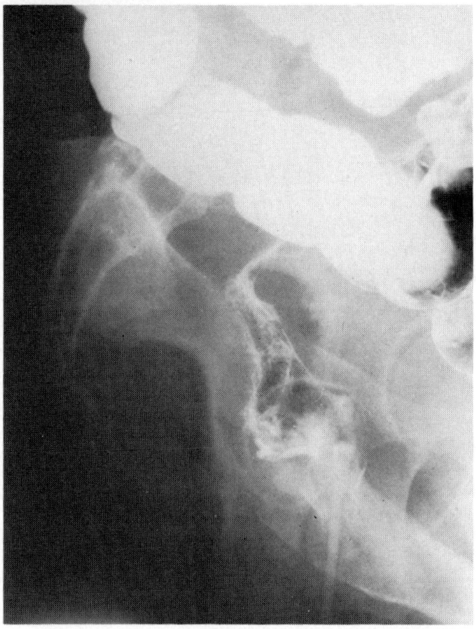

Fig 7–13 (top).—Scirrhous carcinoma causing long narrowed segment in sigmoid colon with an irregular contour. (Courtesy of Dr. A. Megibow, New York.)

Fig 7–14 (left).—Tapered stricture at rectosigmoid junction due to carcinoma *(arrows)*. Patient had previous history of ulcerative colitis. Appearance is indistinguishable from a benign stricture. (Courtesy of Dr. Clive Bartram, London, England.) (From Laufer, I.: *Double Contrast Gastrointestinal Radiology, with Endoscopic Correlation* [Philadelphia: W. B. Saunders Co., 1979]. Reprinted with permission.)

Fig 7–15 (right).—Exophytic carcinoma. Moderate narrowing of rectum with marked increase in retrorectal space due to exophytic growth of carcinoma. Mucosal irregularity of rectum is due to ulcerative proctitis. (Courtesy of Dr. Edward Greenbaum, Los Angeles.)

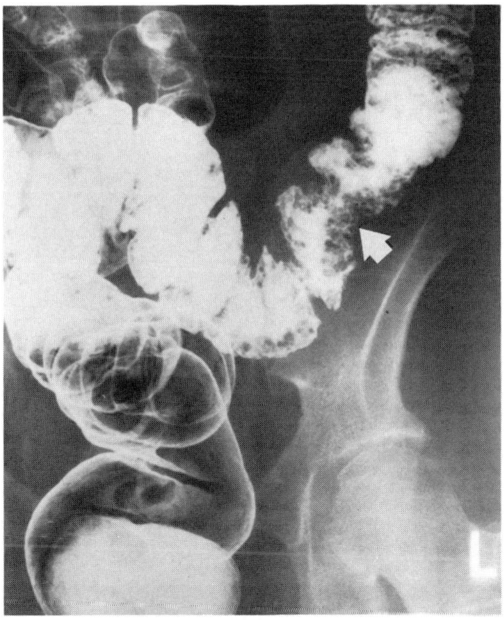

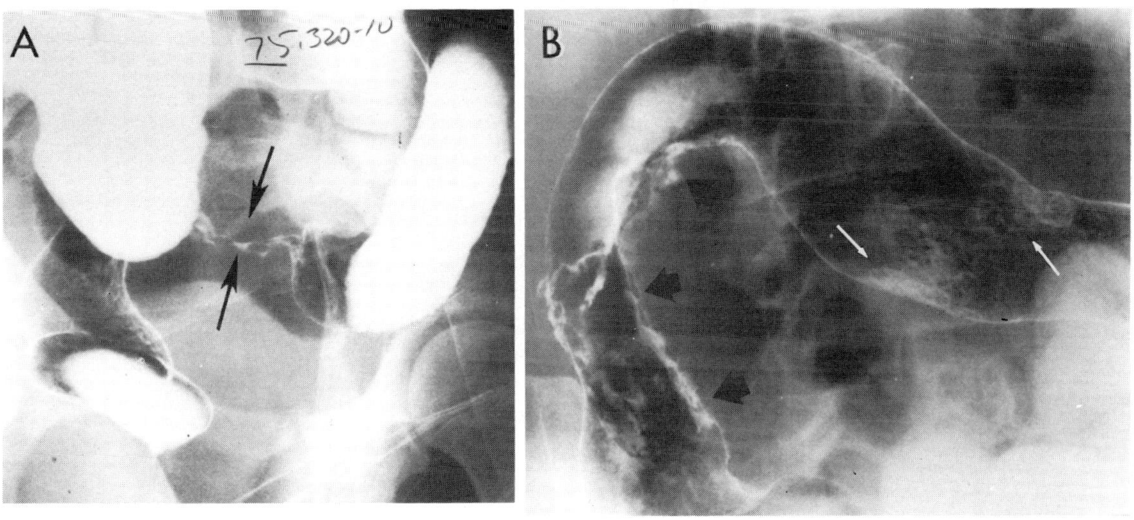

Fig 7–16 (top). – Carcinoma in familial polyposis. Mucosal surface is studded with tiny polyps, best seen in descending colon. Irregular narrowing *(arrow)* was due to carcinoma.

Fig 7–17 (bottom). – Carcinoma in ulcerative colitis. **A,** long stricture of rectosigmoid due to carcinoma. Note granular appearance of mucosa due to ulcerative colitis. (Courtesy of Dr. Clive Bartram, London, England.) **B,** there is a large irregular carcinoma *(large arrows)* involving right colon in patient with 12-year history of ulcerative colitis. *Small arrows* indicate additional areas of adenomatous change. (From Laufer, I.: *Double Contrast Gastrointestinal Radiology, with Endoscopic Correlation* [Philadelphia: W. B. Saunders Co., 1979]. Reprinted with permission.)

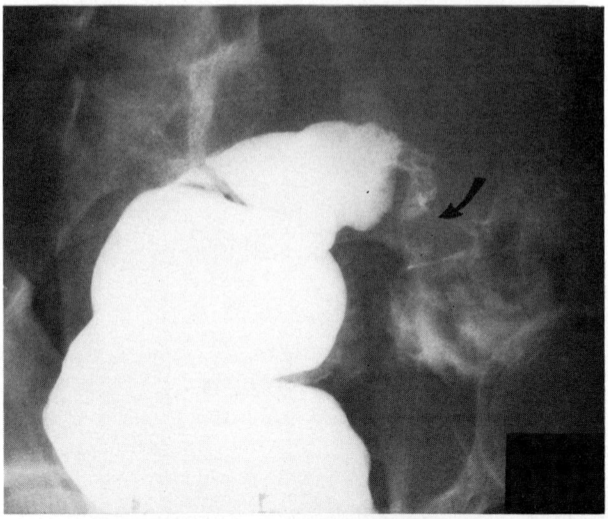

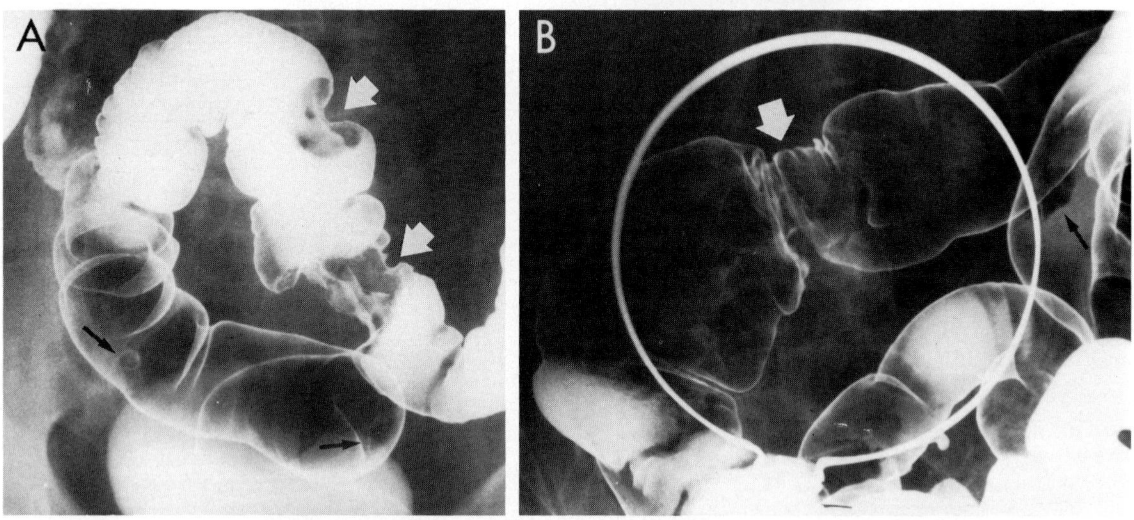

Fig 7–18 (top).—Carcinoma in granulomatous colitis. High-grade obstruction at sigmoid colon due to carcinoma in patient with long history of granulomatous colitis.

Fig 7–19 (bottom).—Multiple carcinomas and adenomatous polyps. **A,** two carcinomas in sigmoid colon *(large arrows).* Distal lesion is annular carcinoma, whereas more proximal lesion is polypoid carcinoma. In addition, there are two adenomatous polyps *(small arrows).* **B,** annular carcinoma at hepatic flexure *(large arrow)* and smaller polypoid carcinoma in descending colon *(small arrow).* (**B** from Laufer, I.: *Double Contrast Gastrointestinal Radiology, with Endoscopic Correlation* [Philadelphia: W. B. Saunders Co., 1979]. Reprinted with permission.)

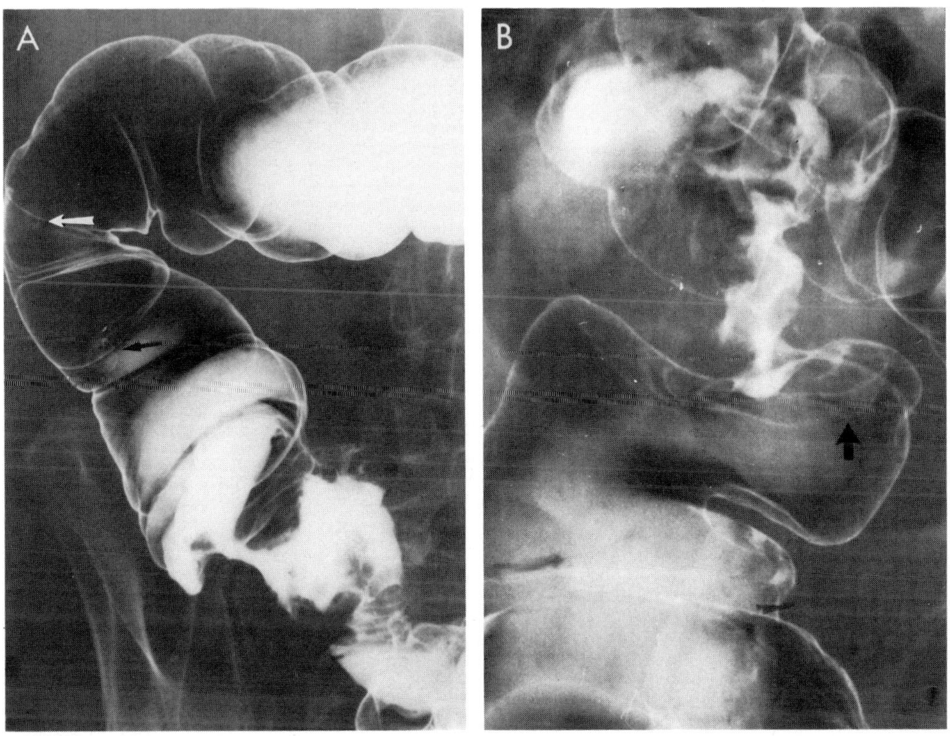

Fig 7–20.—Carcinoma with sentinel polyps. **A,** carcinoma of cecum with two adenomatous polyps *(arrows)* in the right colon. **B,** carcinoma of rectosigmoid with sentinel polyp *(arrow)*. (**B** from Laufer, I.: *Double Contrast Gastrointestinal Radiology, with Endoscopic Correlation* [Philadelphia: W. B. Saunders Co., 1979]. Reprinted with permission.)

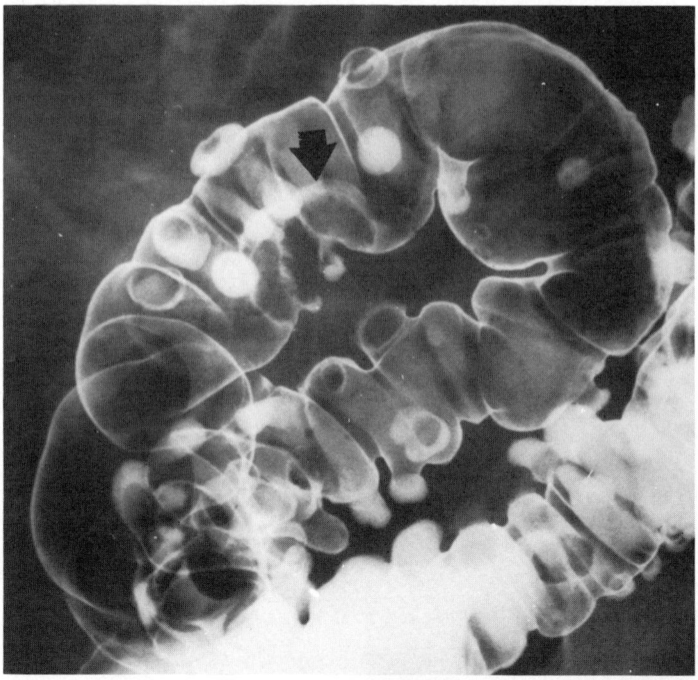

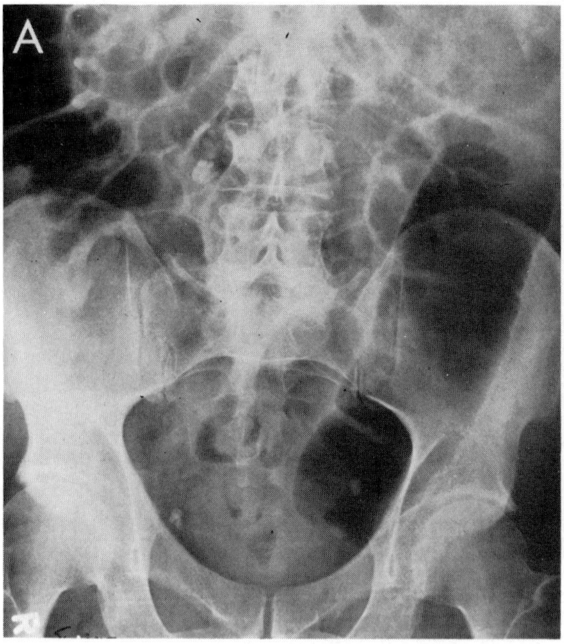

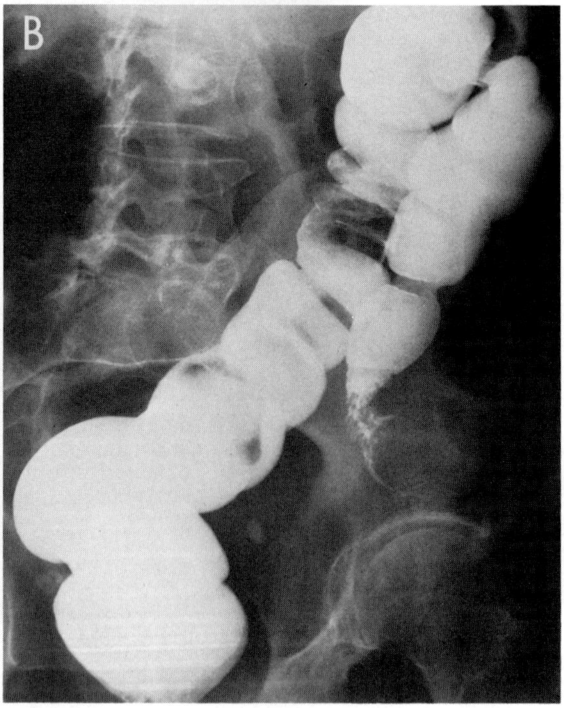

Fig 7–21 (top).—Diverticular disease and carcinoma. A polypoid carcinoma of sigmoid colon *(arrow)* is extensively involved by diverticulosis. (From Laufer, I.: *Double Contrast Gastrointestinal Radiology, with Endoscopic Correlation* (Philadelphia: W. B. Saunders Co., 1979, with permission.)

Fig 7–22 (bottom).—Colonic obstruction due to carcinoma. **A,** plain film shows gaseous distension extending to distal descending colon. **B,** barium enema confirms presence of obstructing carcinoma at this level. (Courtesy of Dr. Herbert Y. Kressel, Philadelphia.)

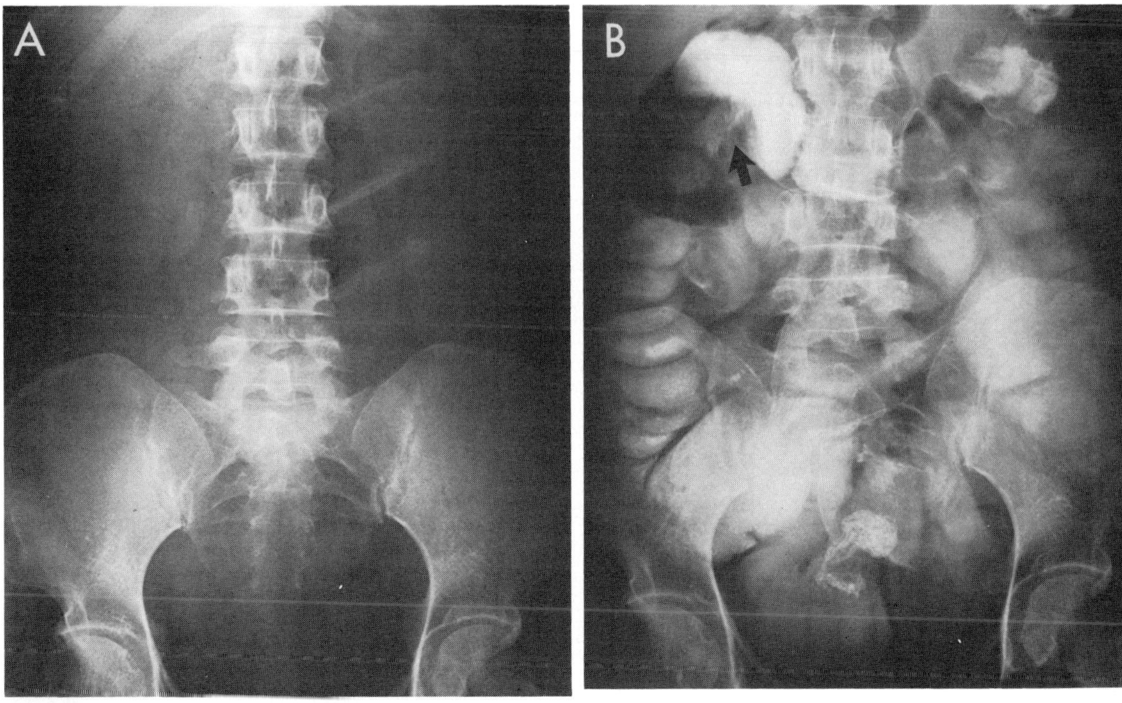

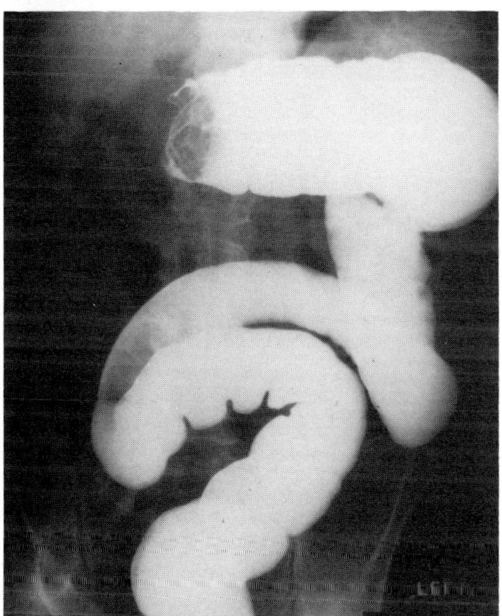

Fig 7–23 (top).—Colonic carcinoma simulating small bowel obstruction. **A,** plain film of abdomen shows dilated loops of small bowel, suggestive of small bowel obstruction. **B,** late film from small bowel follow through examination shows obstructing carcinoma *(arrow)* at hepatic flexure.

Fig 7–24 (bottom).—Colocolic intussusception. Barium enema shows polypoid filling defect in midtransverse colon due to cecal carcinoma that has intussuscepted to transverse colon. (Courtesy of Dr. Edward Greenbaum, Los Angeles.)

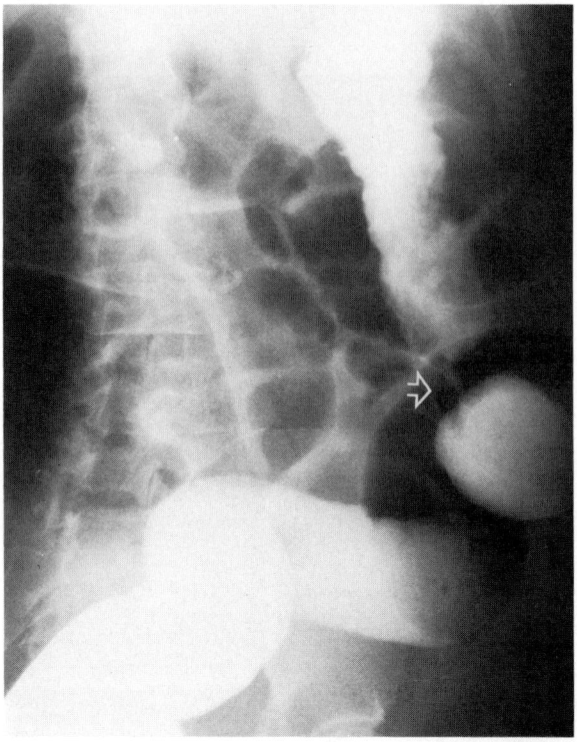

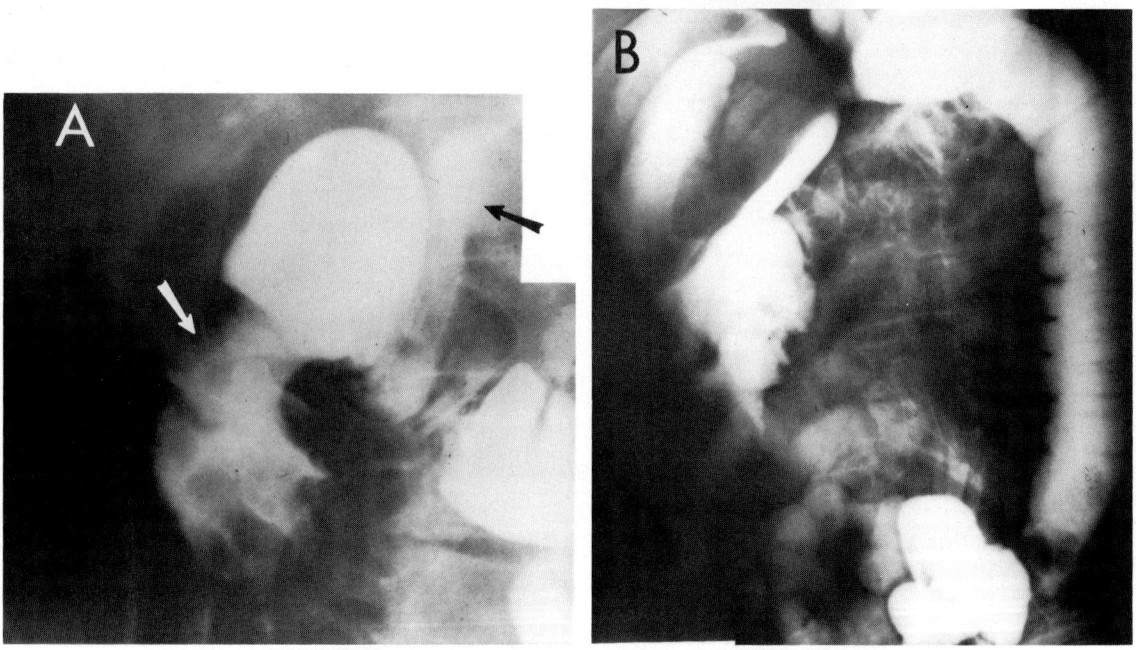

Fig 7–25 (top).—Colonic ulceration proximal to carcinoma. There is an annular carcinoma of distal descending colon *(arrow)* with marked irregularity of mucosa proximal to lesion, secondary to ulceration. These ulcerations are believed to be due to ischemia.

Fig 7–26 (bottom).—Free perforation, secondary to carcinoma. **A,** spot film of hepatic flexure shows carcinoma (white arrow) and extravasation (black arrow) of contrast from hepatic flexure. **B,** later film shows contrast extravasating into subphrenic and subhepatic spaces from carcinoma at hepatic flexure. Patient presented with gross amount free air on upright PA chest. (Courtesy of Dr. Edward Greenbaum, Los Angeles.)

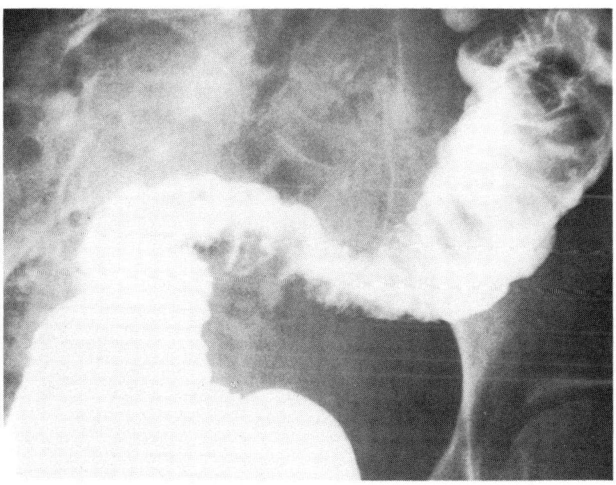

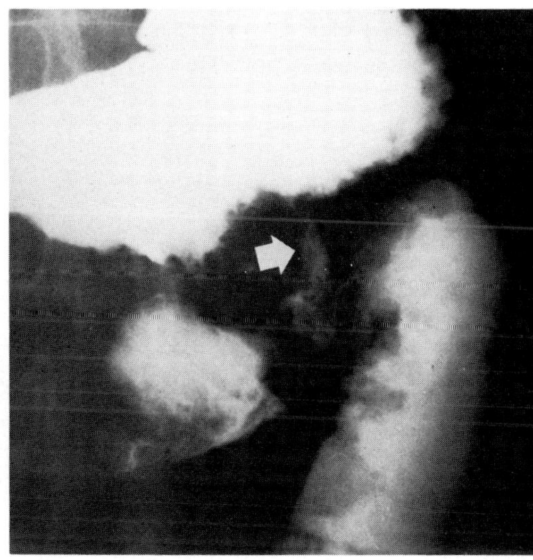

Fig 7–27 (left). – Pericolic abscess secondary to carcinoma. Note long area of narrowing in sigmoid. Appearance is most suggestive of inflammatory process. At operation there was a carcinoma with a pericolic abscess.

Fig 7–28 (right). – Carcinoma of hepatic flexure with cologastric fistula *(arrow)*.

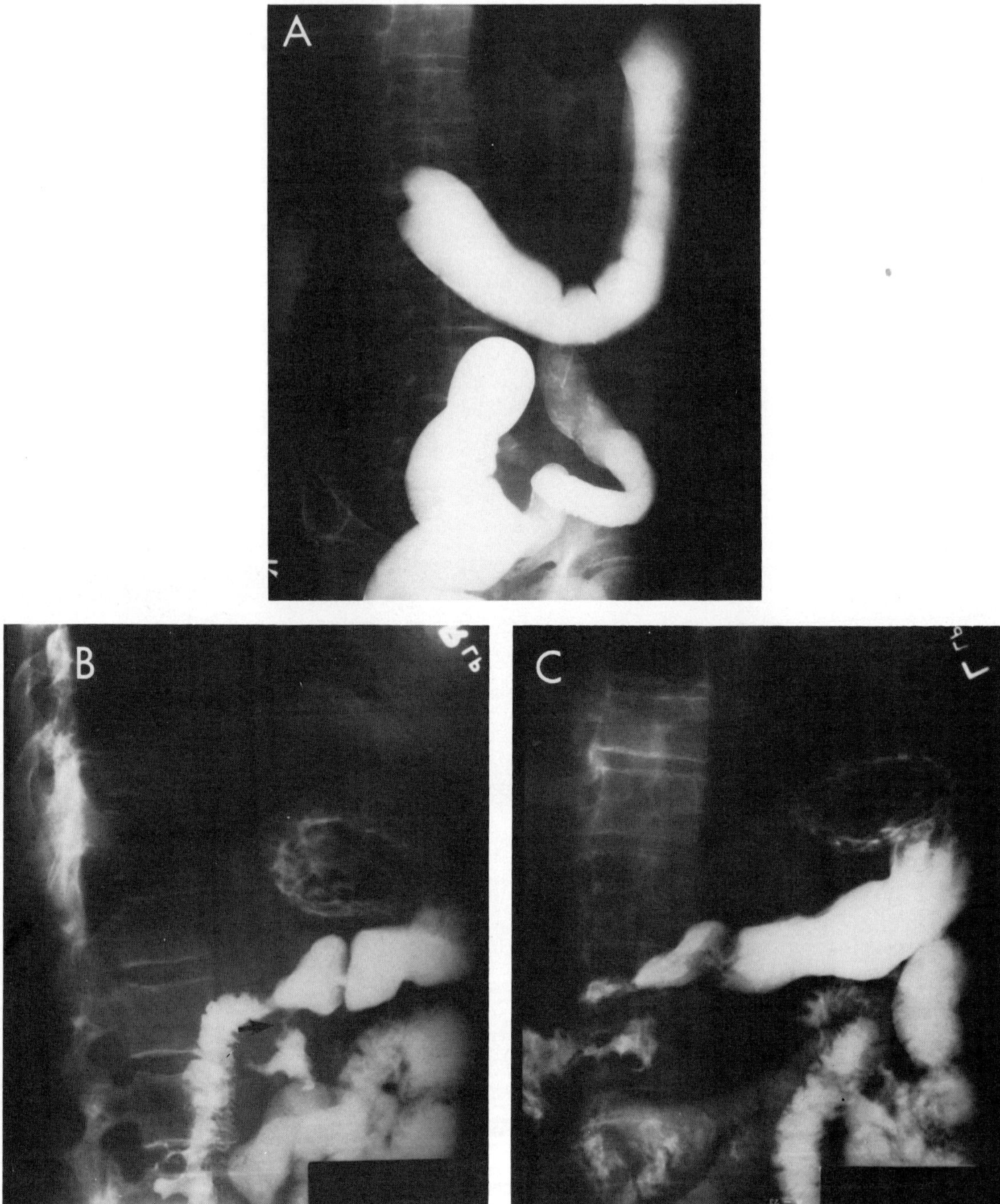

Fig 7–29.—Coloduodenal fistula. **A,** Barium enema shows obstructing carcinoma at proximal transverse colon. **B** and **C,** films from upper gastrointestinal series show fistula from proximal duodenum *(arrow)* into colon at hepatic flexure. (Courtesy of Dr. Edward Greenbaum, Los Angeles.)

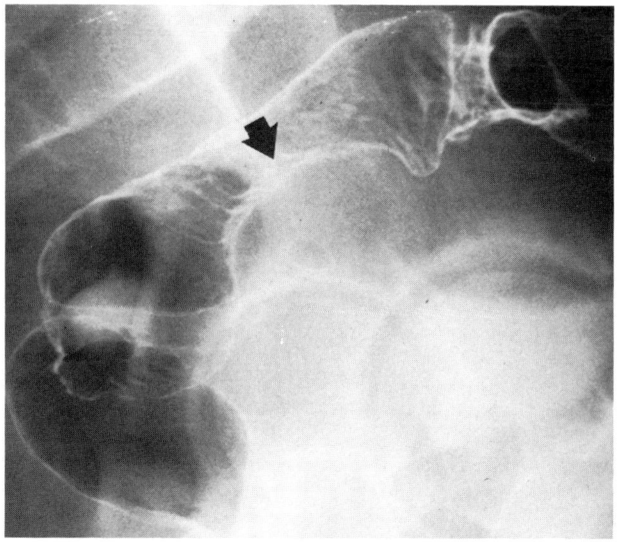

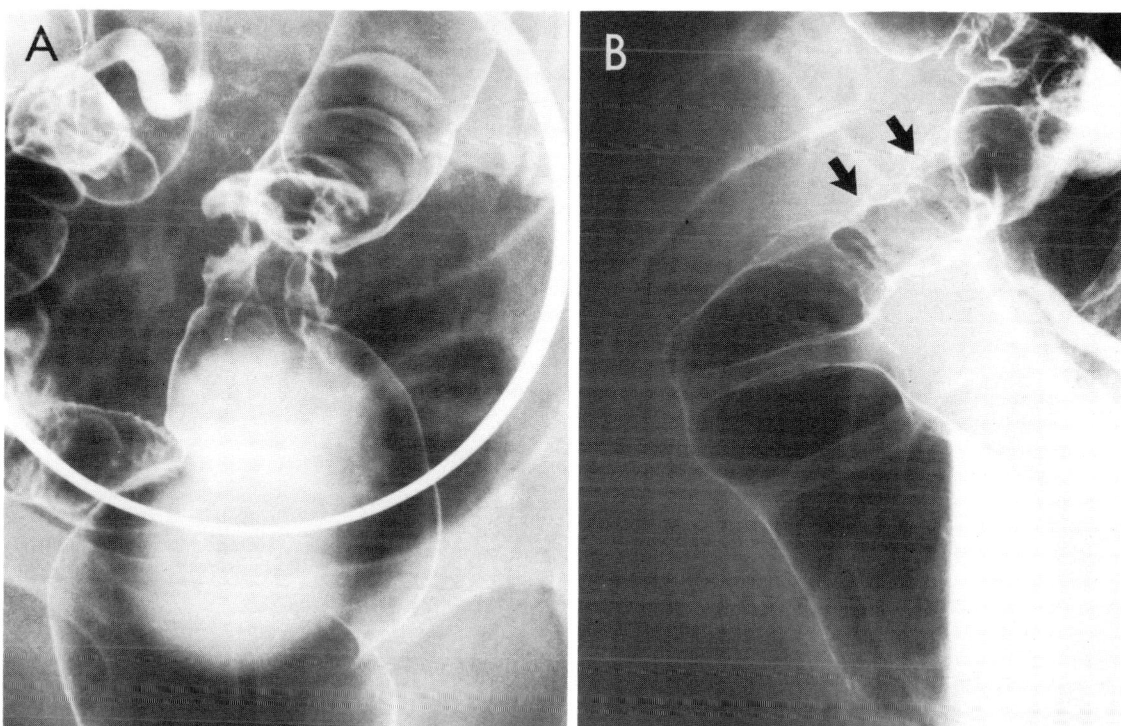

Fig 7–30 (top).—Carcinoma of colon with metastases to pouch of Douglas. There is a smooth impression on anterior aspect of rectosigmoid junction *(arrow)* due to peritoneal seeding of metastases to pouch of Douglas.

Fig 7–31 (bottom).—**A** and **B,** two examples of marked irregularity *(arrows)* at anastomotic line due to local recurrence of colonic carcinoma.

Chapter 8

Colitis Cystica Profunda

H. MULDER, M.D.

COLITIS CYSTICA PROFUNDA is a rare condition of unknown cause characterized by the presence of mucous cysts deep in the muscularis mucosae.[3] The patients usually are young adults,[4, 7] who often present with nonspecific complaints of rectal bleeding, diarrhea or rectal prolapse.[2] In the pediatric age group, the condition is extremely rare.[5] The bowel wall appears thickened, and nodular polypoid tumors are seen; sometimes small ulcerations are present. The condition is almost always localized to the rectosigmoid region.

In addition to large mucous cysts, biopsy specimens show features of chronic inflammation, accompanied by marked fibrosis and disorganization of the mucosa and submucosa.

Radiographic Features

The barium examination may show a solitary intraluminal defect (Figs 8–1 to 8–3), but usually there are multiple intraluminal, nodular, space-occupying lesions (Figs 8–6, 8–9 and 8–10). Almost always these lesions are present only in the rectosigmoid region, but sometimes they are found in the rest of the colon.[8] One or more shallow ulcer niches may be present (Fig 8–5). On postevacuation films, the intraluminal filling defect gives rise to local inability of the rectal wall to collapse completely (Fig 8–4). The mucosal folds usually are moderately to extremely enlarged (Fig 8–7). In some cases the retrorectal space is thickened.[5] Sometimes one is able to follow up a lesion with an initial ulcerative appearance to the state of intraluminal filling defects, as shown in Figures 8–5 to 8–7. The described features are not exclusive to this condition. Radiographically a solitary intraluminal filling defect should be differentiated from polyps and other benign tumors that are occasionally observed at this age. With multiple nodular, space-occupying lesions and extremely enlarged mucosal folds, the possibility of carcinoma and lymphosarcoma as well as granulomatous colitis, endometriosis and submucosal hemorrhage must be considered. The scanty literature on this subject repeatedly indicates that adenocarcinoma of the rectum is too hastily diagnosed. This is especially the case with superficial biopsies.[6, 7] Only sufficiently deep biopsy specimens reveal the characteristic mucous cysts (Fig 8–11).

Pathogenesis

The pathogenesis of colitis cystica profunda is obscure. It is frequently thought that a local congenital anomaly of the muscular tunics gives rise to herniation of colonic mucosa through the muscularis mucosae.[2] Most likely, however, the mucous cysts are the result of an extension of regenerating surface epithelium into the submucosa tracking down through mucosal ulcerations, as to some extent confirmed by follow up in some patients.

The microscopic features of colitis cystica profunda match those described in 1966 by Allen[1] as hamartomatous inverted polyps and also those of a solitary ulcer in the rectum described in 1969 by Madigan and Morson.[6]

REFERENCES

1. Allen, M. S., Jr.: Hamartomatous inverted polyps of the rectum, Cancer 19:257, 1966.
2. Epstein, S. E., Ascari, W. Q., Ablow, R. C., Seaman, W. B., and Lattes, R.: Colitis cystica profunda, Am. J. Clin. Pathol. 45:186, 1966.
3. Goodall, H. B., and Sinclair, I. S. R.: Colitis cystica profunda, J. Pathol. 73:33, 1957.
4. Grant, K. B., and Roller, G. J.: Colitis cystica profunda, Radiology 89:110, 1967.
5. Ledesma-Medina, J., Reid, B. S., and Girdany, B. R.: Colitis cystica profunda, Am. J. Roentgenol. 131: 529, 1978.
6. Madigan, M. R., and Morson, B. C.: Solitary ulcer of the rectum, Gut 10:871, 1969.
7. Mulder, H., and Te Velde, J.: Colitis cystica profunda, Radiol. Clin. Biol. 43:529, 1974.
8. Wayte, D. M., and Helwig, E. B.: Colitis cystica profunda, Am. J. Clin. Pathol. 48:159, 1967.

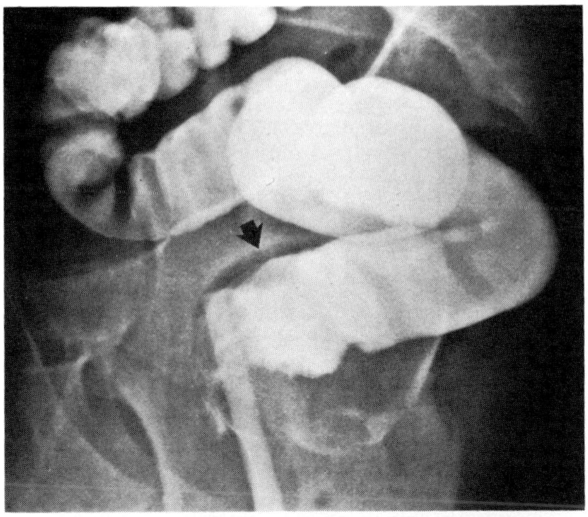

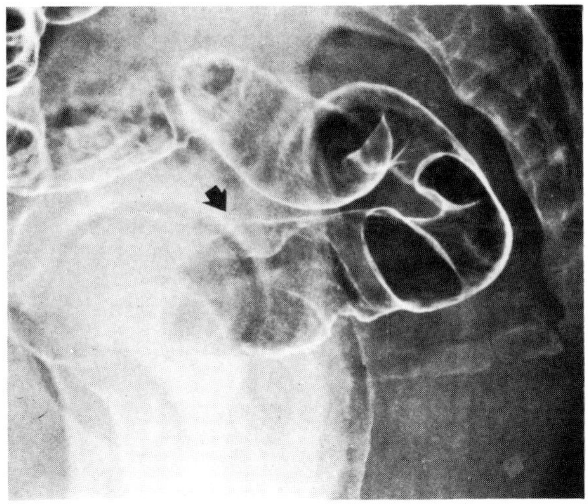

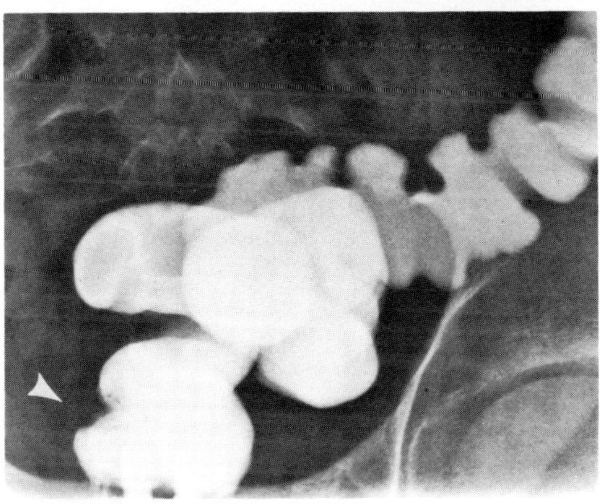

Fig 8–1 (top left).—Man, age 19, with complaints of frequent rectal blood loss. Lateral view at barium enema examination. Semicircular filling defect on anterior wall of rectum *(arrow)*. No other abnormalities present in colon.

Fig 8–2 (top right).—Same patient as in Figure 8–1. After air insufflation, a semicircular defect is seen, with coating of contrast medium on surface of this structure. Biopsy specimen at first suggested malignancy. Later a deep biopsy revealed characteristic mucous cysts.

Fig 8–3 (bottom).—Follow-up examination 2 years later of same patient as in Figures 8–1 and 8–2. Recurrence of frequent rectal bleeding. AP spot film of rectosigmoid. Small nodular polypoid lesion on right-hand wall of rectum *(arrow)*.

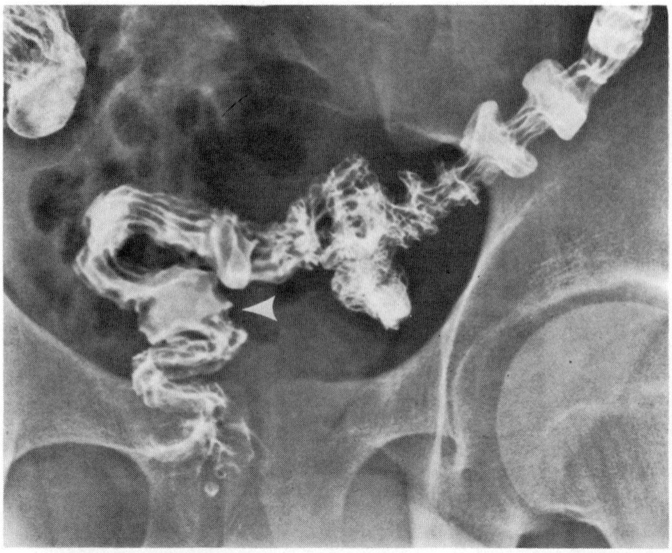

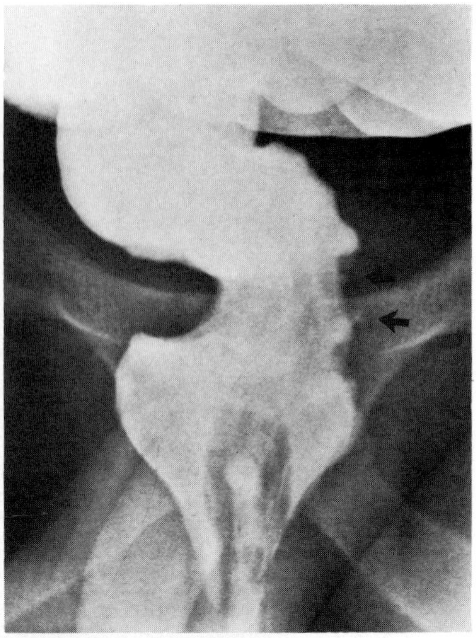

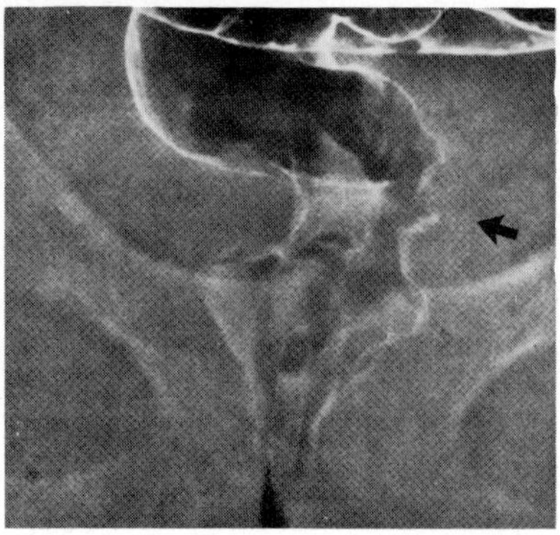

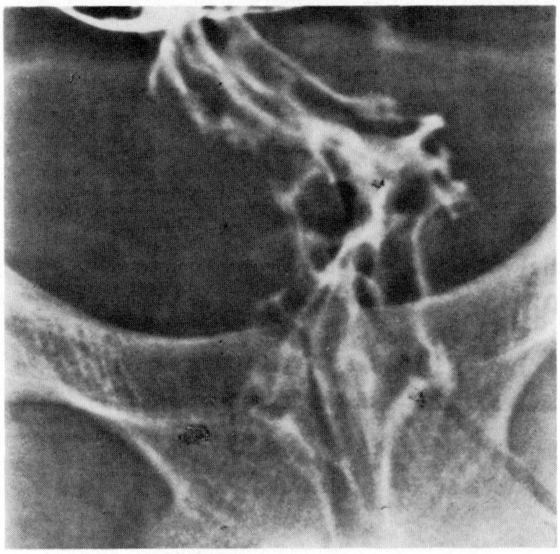

Fig 8–4 (top left).—Same patient as in Figures 8–1 to 8–3 after evacuation. There is local inability of wall of distal sigmoid to collapse completely *(arrow)*. At same spot, plicae show local effacement.

Fig 8–5 (top right).—Man, age 24, with 1-year history of diarrhea, often with blood and mucus in stools. AP spot film of rectum. Irregular surface of left-hand wall of rectum with at least two ulcers *(arrow)*. Opposite this area a constriction is seen, possibly as result of a spasm.

Fig 8–6 (bottom left).—Radiologic follow-up 2 years later in same patient as in Figure 8–5. AP double contrast view of rectum reveals two distinct filling defects at same spot that ulcers were found in patient in Figure 8–5 *(arrow)*.

Fig 8–7 (bottom right).—Same patient. Post-evacuation AP spot film. Mucosal folds in rectum are markedly thickened and irregular. Without previous films, a malignant process might be considered.

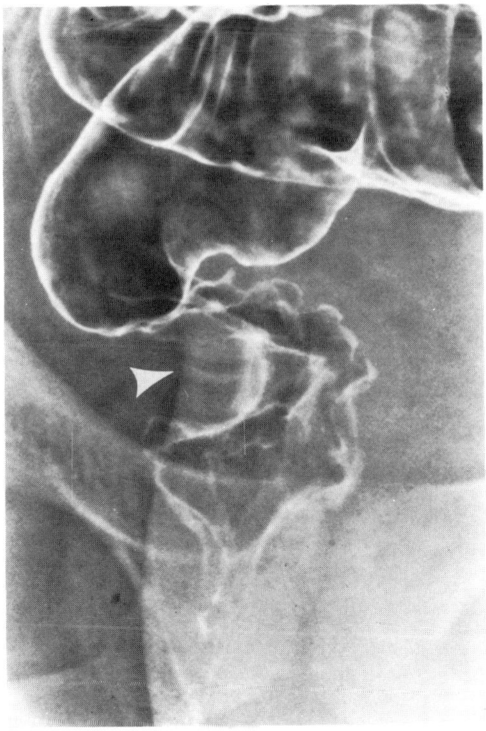

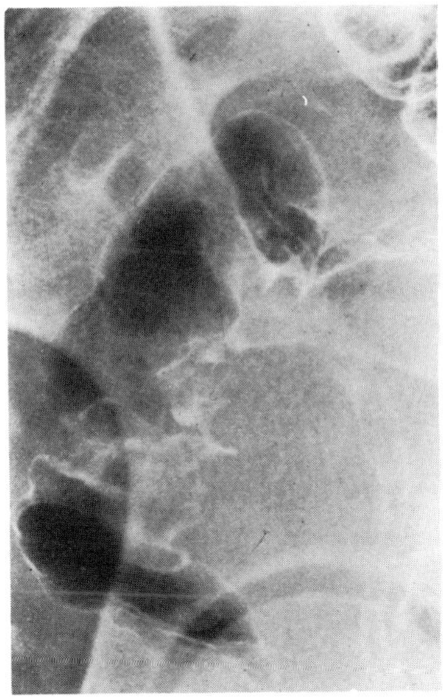

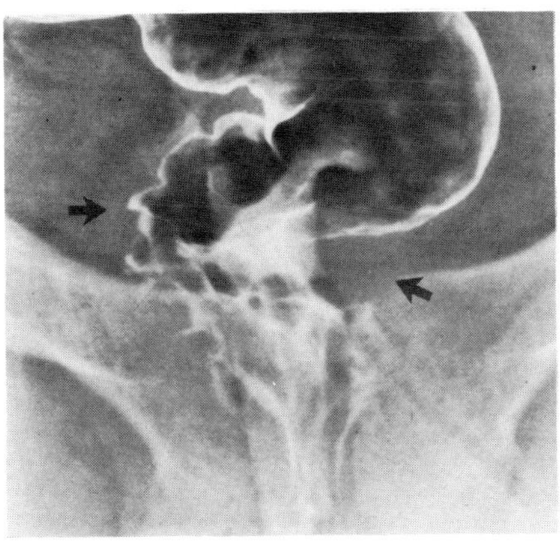

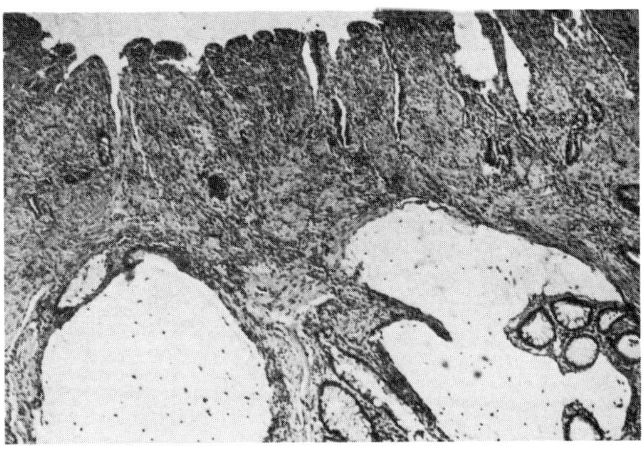

Fig 8–8 (top left).—Follow-up study of same patient as in Figures 8–5 to 8–7. PA spot film of rectum shows same area as in Figures 8–5 and 8–6. Area of constriction is more indurated *(arrow)*. Mucosal folds are enlarged.

Fig 8–9 (top right).—Woman, age 27, who during more than 3 years had complaints of diarrhea and blood in stools. Lateral double contrast spot film of rectum reveals multiple nodular polypoid lesions and ulcerations on anterior wall of rectum.

Fig 8–10 (bottom left).—Man, age 20, with frequent rectal blood loss and local pain at evacuation. Both rectoscopy and barium enema suggested malignancy. Deep biopsy specimens revealed true nature of multiple filling defects *(arrows)*.

Fig 8–11 (bottom right).—Biopsy specimen showing submucosal mucus-filling cysts with marked fibrosis and atrophy of mucosa.

Chapter 9

Colon Complications Following Renal Transplantation

REED P. RICE, M.D.
WILLIAM M. THOMPSON, M.D.

PATIENTS WHO HAVE UNDERGONE renal transplantation are prone to develop a variety of colon complications. These include ileus, obstruction, diverticulitis, ischemic colitis, necrotizing enterocolitis and ulceration with massive hemorrhage. Uremia and immunosuppression play a role in the cause of some of these entities; certainly the steroids, which are part of the posttransplant regimen, may mask the symptoms associated with some of the more serious complications (e.g., bowel perforation, abscess and peritonitis).[5-7, 19] As a result, there frequently is a delay in recognition of the major complications, with resultant increased morbidity and mortality.[19]

Colon Obstruction

The differential diagnosis between ileus and obstruction generally offers the same problems as in other postoperative situations. One cause of obstruction rarely encountered in other circumstances, but well documented in renal transplant patients, is massive impaction associated with the use of nonabsorbable aluminum hydroxide gel antacids. Undoubtedly, uremia and dehydration contribute to the development of obstructing impactions, predominantly in the right colon. Localization to the right colon has not been adequately explained.[1, 3] Impaction may be so severe that perforation results[2, 19] (Fig 9–1). Impactions resulting from the use of nonabsorbable aluminum antacids can be minimized by substituting some magnesium-containing antacids.[9]

Colon Perforation

There is a significant incidence of spontaneous colon perforation in renal transplant patients.[1, 2, 5, 7, 10, 11, 13, 17, 19] Many of these perforations are associated with diverticular disease[16]; and there is a high incidence of free peritoneal perforation compared to the nontransplant patient, in whom most diverticular perforations remain localized.[2, 5, 6, 10, 13, 19] Colon perforations associated with diverticulitis generally occur months or years after successful transplantation and in our experience usually are not associated with transplant rejection (Fig 9–2). The steroids and other immunosuppressive agents apparently interfere with the body's natural defense mechanism.[4] These agents contribute to the increased incidence of diverticulitis in the renal transplant patient as well as to poor localization of the inflammatory process.

Colon necrosis and perforation also have resulted from ischemic colitis and pseudomembranous colitis.[2, 10, 13-15] Sepsis is a common problem in transplant patients, and colon perforations and/or fistulization have been attributed to involvement by intra-abdominal abscesses. This complication is more likely to occur in the immediate postsurgical period. (Fig 9–3)[19]

In addition to these causes of spontaneous perforation, traumatic perforations of the colon have resulted from the overzealous use of exchange resin enemas.[5, 19] Peritoneal dialysis trocars also have penetrated the colon.[19]

Whatever the cause, colon perforation is more common than gastroduodenal perforation in patients who have undergone renal transplantation. In our series of patients, perforations of the colon outnumbered gastroduodenal perforations by about two to one.[11, 20] Colon perforation is associated with a very high mortality. This is undoubtedly related to delay in diagnosis and treatment as well as to diminished ability of the immunosuppressed patient to withstand infection.

In renal transplant patients who present with abdominal pain or any sign of peritonitis, an aggressive diagnostic evaluation is indicated. Depending on plain film and clinical findings, it is important to proceed immediately with appropriate ultrasound, computerized tomography or water-soluble contrast examinations of the upper or lower gastrointestinal tract. In the Duke University series of 24 patients with gastrointestinal perforation, the diagnosis was established by plain films or contrast examination of the gastrointestinal tract in most patients prior to surgery.[10, 19, 20] In many of these patients, the possibility of perforation was initially suggested on the basis of the plain abdominal film finding of extraluminal gas, either localized in an abscess or free in the peritoneum (Fig 9–4). Most of these patients were evaluated prior to the availability of modern Gray scale ultrasonography and body computerized tomography. Both of these techniques have a well-established role in the diagnosis and localization of abscess, though the precise localization of the point of perforation would still depend on appropriate contrast examination of either the colon or upper gastrointestinal tract.

Colon Hemorrhage

Hemorrhage from the gastrointestinal tract is the most common life-threatening gastrointestinal complication of renal transplantation.[8] In most instances the bleeding site will be located in the upper gastrointestinal tract, but significant colon hemorrhage may also occur. Cecal ulcers are a recognized source of bleeding and have been cited by several authors.[2, 10-18] Significant colon hemorrhage may also be associated with pseudomembranous colitis and ischemic episodes. In some patients no specific cause for a significant hemorrhage can be determined.

As in other patients with massive, red rectal bleeding and negative nasogastric aspirations, emergency arteriography is the procedure of first choice for diagnosis of the bleeding site. Not only is angiography the most accurate means of diagnosing the site of hemorrhage, but in most instances catheter techniques are successful in controlling the hemorrhage. Emergency barium enema and colonoscopy have very little role in the assessment of massive colon bleeding.[12]

REFERENCES

1. Aguilo, J. J., Zincke, H., Woods, J. E., and Buckingham, J. M.: Intestinal perforation due to fecal impaction after renal transplantation, J. Urol. 116: 153, 1977.
2. Bernstein, W. C., Nivatvongs, S., and Tallent, M. B.: Colonic and rectal complications of kidney transplantation in man, Dis. Colon Rectum 16:255, 1973.
3. Brettschneider, L., Monafo, W., and Osborne, D. P.: Intestinal obstruction due to antacid gels, Gastroenterology 49:291, 1965.
4. Canter, J. W., and Shorb, P. E., Jr.: Acute perfora-

tion of colonic diverticula associated with prolonged adenocorticosteroid therapy, Am. J. Surg. 121:46, 1971.
5. Hadjiyannakis, E. J., Evans, D. B., Smellie, W. A. B., and Calne, R. Y.: Gastrointestinal complications after renal transplantation, Lancet 2:781, 1971.
6. Hognestad, J., and Flatmark, A.: Colon perforation in renal transplant patients, Scand. J. Gastroenterol. 11:289, 1976.
7. Julien, P. J., Goldberg, H. I., Margulis, A. R., and Belzer, F. O.: Gastrointestinal complications following renal transplantation, Radiology 117:37, 1975.
8. Lewicki, A. M., Saito, S., and Merrill, J. P.: Gastrointestinal bleeding in the renal transplant patient, Radiology 102:533, 1972.
9. Lipschutz, D. E., and Easterling, R. E.: Spontaneous perforation of the colon in chronic renal failure, Arch. Intern. Med. 132:758, 1973.
10. Meyers, W. C., Harris, N., Stein, S., Brooks, M., Jones, R. S., Thompson, W. M., Stickel, D. L. and Seigler, H. F.: Alimentary tract complications after renal transplantation. Submitted to Ann. Surg.
11. Misra, M. K., Pinkus, G. S., Birtch, A. G., and Wilson, R. E.: Major colonic diseases complicating renal transplantation, Surgery 73:942, 1973.
12. Oddson, T. A., Johnsrude, I. S., Jackson, D. C., and Rice, R. P.: The diagnostic evaluation of patients with acute gastrointestinal hemorrhage—with special attention to the changing role of barium examinations, Radiol. Clin. North Am. 16:123, 1978.
13. Penn, I., Brettschneider, L., Simpson, K., Martin, A., and Starzl, T. E.: Major colonic problems in human homotransplant recipients, Arch. Surg. 100: 61, 1970.
14. Perloff, L. J., Chon, H., Petrella, E. J., Grossman, R. A., and Barker, C. F.: Acute colitis in the renal allograft recipient, Ann. Surg. 183:77, 1976.
15. Powis, S. J. A., Barnes, A. D., Dawson-Edwards, P., and Thompson, H.: Ileocolonic problems after cadaveric renal transplantation, Br. Med. J. 8:99, 1972.
16. Renshaw, T. S., and Phelps, D. B.: Perforation of colonic diverticula, J. Bone Joint Surg. (Am) 54: 1070, 1972.
17. Sawyerr, O. I., Garvin, P. J., Codd, J. E., Graff, R. J., Newton, W. T., and Willman, V. L.: Colorectal complications of renal allograft transplantation, Arch. Surg. 113:84, 1978.
18. Sutherland, D., Frech, R. S., Weil, R., Najarian, J. S., and Simmons, R. L.: The bleeding cecal ulcer: Pathogenesis, angiographic diagnosis, and nonoperative control, Surgery 71:290, 1972.
19. Thompson, W. M., Seigler, H. F., and Rice, R. P.: Ileocolonic perforation: A complication following renal transplantation, Am. J. Roentgenol. 125:723, 1975.
20. Thompson, W. M., Seigler, H. F., and Rice, R. P.: The gastrointestinal complications of renal transplantation, Semin. Radiol. 13:319, 1978.

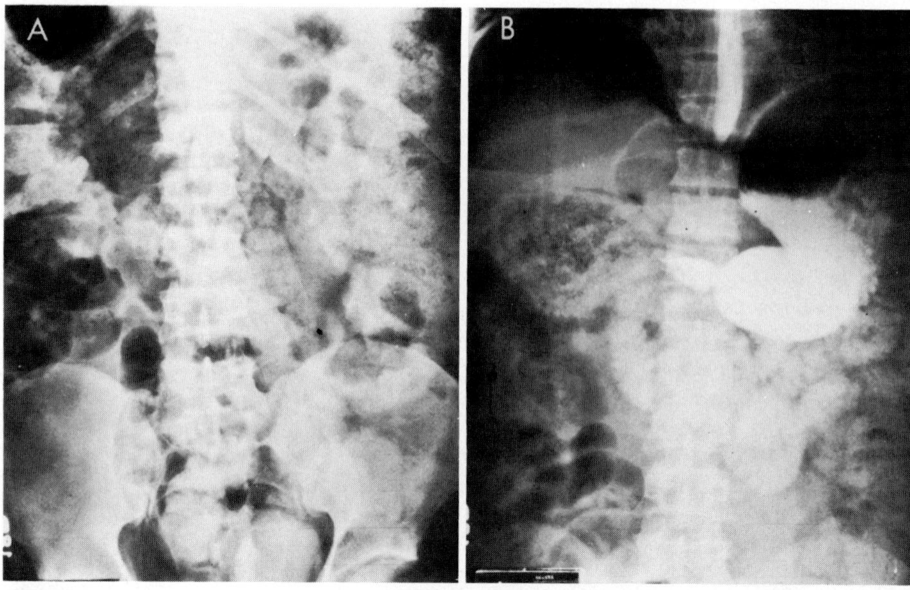

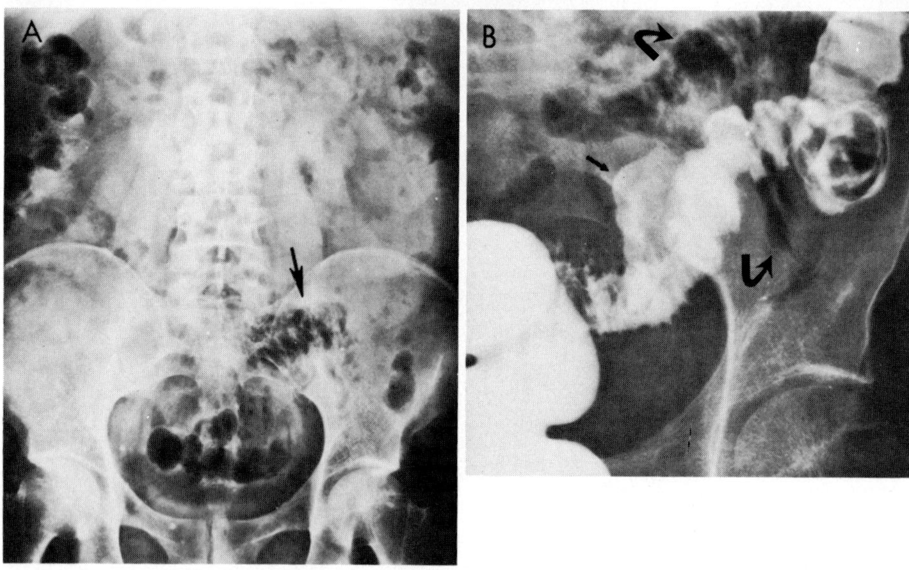

Fig 9–1 (top). – **A,** supine film of abdomen shows impaction filling virtually entire colon in man age 43 with abdominal pain 7 days post renal transplantation. **B,** upright film from upper gastrointestinal series done with water-soluble contrast medium several hours later during episode of acute abdominal pain. Massive pneumoperitoneum is present in addition to previously described colon impaction. Patient was taking aluminum hydroxide gel, and at laparotomy the impaction was largely composed of this material. Perforation in ascending colon was secondary to pressure necrosis. Patient died 14 days following partial colon resection and colostomy. (From Thompson et al., Am. J. Roentgenol. 125:723, 1975, with permission.)

Fig 9–2 (bottom). – **A,** supine film of abdomen shows mottled gas lucency in left lower abdomen *(arrow)* in man age 31 with 5-day history of left lower quadrant pain and fever. This acute abdominal episode occurred 3 years after successful renal transplantation. **B,** emergency contrast enema using water-soluble contrast media shows localized extravasation of contrast medium *(small arrow)* as well as extraluminal mottled gas collection *(curved arrows).* Patient's diverticular perforation and abscess remain well localized and the patient survived a colostomy and abscess drainage. (From Thompson et al., Am. J. Roentgenol. 125:723, 1975, with permission.)

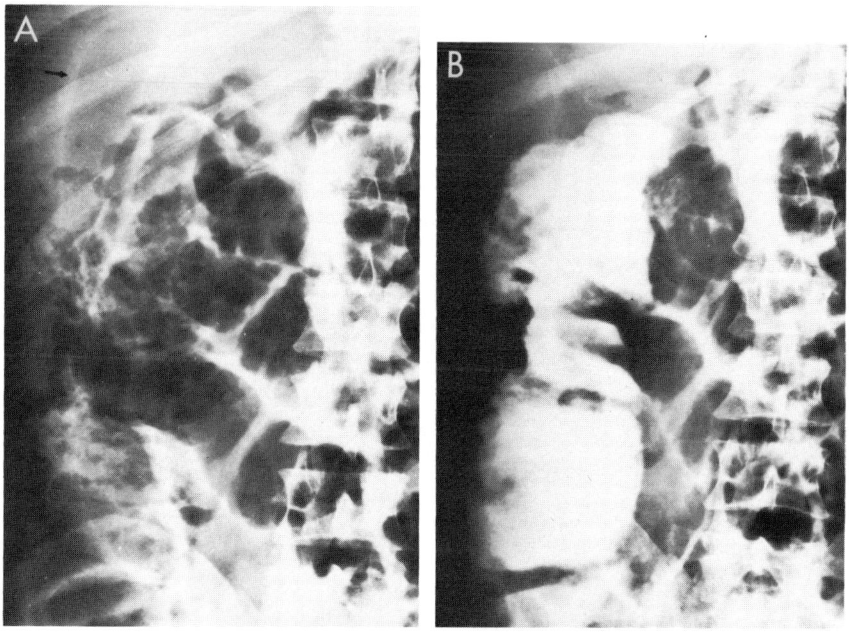

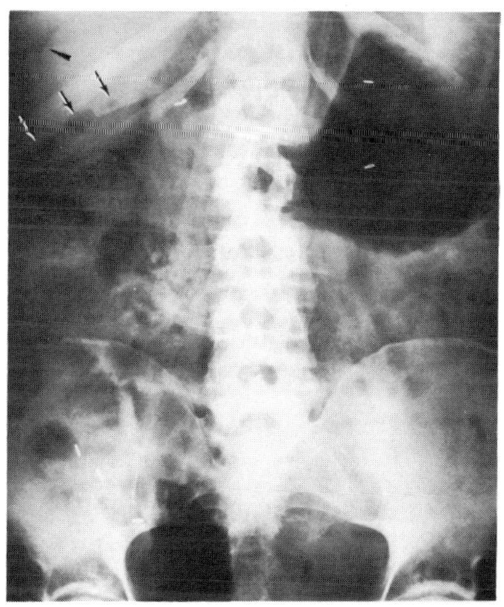

Fig 9–3 (top). – **A,** detailed view from supine film of abdomen in a man age 38 (who was experiencing increasing abdominal distention and symptoms of peritonitis) 9 days post renal transplantation. *Small arrow* indicates localized homogeneous gas collection in subhepatic space. There is also evidence of mottled collection of gas occupying right pericolic area and evidence of gas within right colon wall. **B,** emergency contrast enema confirmed extraluminal gas collection in subhepatic space and presence of pneumatosis coli. Film is a detailed view from postevacuation film. There was no emptying of right colon, which was completely necrotic at time of surgery, immediately following this examination. Pathologic examination revealed ischemic necrosis of colon and ileum with multiple perforations. Patient died 48 hours after partial colectomy. (From Thompson et al., Am. J. Roentgenol. 125:723, 1975, with permission.)

Fig 9–4 (bottom). – Supine film of abdomen in man, age 45, shows extraluminal gas in right upper quadrant 9 months following renal transplantation. For 12 days patient had experienced mild abdominal distention and pain, which had become suddenly worse a few hours prior to film. Extraluminal gas indicates pneumoperitoneum with localization anterior to liver as well as to subhepatic space *(small arrows).* Urgent surgery followed this examination and demonstrated a diverticular perforation with generalized peritonitis. (From Thompson et al., Semin. Roentgenol. 13:319, 1978, with permission.)

Chapter 10

Colonic Ileus

MORTON A. MEYERS, M.D.

SIGNIFICANT ADYNAMIC ileus of the colon, also described as pseudo-obstruction or as Ogilvie's syndrome,[1] is characterized by selective or disproportionate gaseous distention of the large intestine in the absence of an organic obstruction. Its clinical importance lies in its distinction from true mechanical obstruction and in the fact that it can progress to perforation.

Pathogenesis

The basic etiologic features of colonic ileus are not known but it is apparently related to imbalance between the sympathetic and parasympathetic innervation.[2-4] It usually accompanies or follows some major systemic abnormality. These include acute appendicitis, cholecystitis, gastroenteritis, and pancreatitis, extra-abdominal trauma, cardiac disease and respiratory and extraperitoneal infection. It also occurs occasionally in patients with sepsis, shock, lead intoxication, morphine overdosage, ganglionic blocking agents, renal failure or electrolyte imbalance. It also has been encountered following pelvic operation, including hysterectomy, cesarean section and prostatic surgery.[5-8]

Clinical Presentation

The clinical picture is that usually associated with mechanical obstruction of the colon. Progressive abdominal distention occurs, first clinically apparent within 2–7 days in patients who have undergone surgery, although there may be passage of liquid feces and gas. Bowel sounds, although perhaps diminished, tend to remain evident.

Radiologic Features

Abdominal radiographs demonstrate often striking dilatation of the colon with gas (Figs 10–1, A, and 10–2). The dilatation is typically localized to the large intestine but is clearly out of proportion to any distended small bowel loops that may accompany the process. There usually is much less gas in the rectum, sigmoid and portions of the descending colon than in the right and transverse colon. Massive distention of the cecum, which may be horizontally oriented (see Fig 10–1), characteristically dominates the radiographic presentation. A cecal diameter as great as 18–20 cm has been observed.[5, 19] Serial films over several days may show no further cecal distention or mild progression.[5]

Bryk and Soong[10] noted that the plain film appearance of colonic ileus is frequently that of acute dilatation of a previously normal colon. These authors emphasize that preserved haustrations; thin, well-defined septae; and smooth inner colonic contours are the cardinal features of the acuteness of the process. In colonic obstruction, in contrast, the mucosal edema and adherent fecal matter and secretions lead to an accentuation of haustrations, with numerous closely packed septae or loss or shallowness of haustrations; large amounts of fecal retention; thickened, ill-defined, irregular septae; and a ragged inner colonic contour. Although predominant fluid distention of the colon may be somewhat more indicative of colonic obstruction, erect films in many instances of colonic ileus have demonstrated considerable intraluminal fluid.[5]

The differential diagnosis of plain film abdominal findings includes—in addition to mechanical obstruction of the descending colon—volvulus of the sigmoid, mesenteric vascular disease and toxic dilatation of the colon. Ileus of the right and transverse colon in association with acute pancreatitis is explained by the effects of the liberated pancreatic enzymes within the phrenicocolic ligament on the anatomical splenic flexure.[11] When the dilatation is restricted particularly to the cecum, cecal volvulus and cecal bascule[12] also must be considered.

Despite the plain film features indicating adynamic ileus of the colon, barium enema study usually is necessary to completely exclude the possibility of an obstructive lesion.[5] This often documents that the left colon distal to the splenic flexure is not as distended as are the ascending and transverse colon (see Fig. 10–1, B). Even in the face of massive dilatation, an incompetent ileocecal valve with ready reflux into the terminal ileum may be present. Colonic evacuation typically is sluggish.

In evaluating mechanical obstruction of the colon, Lowman and Davis[14, 15] stressed the possibility of cecal necrosis and perforation when the cecal diameter reaches 9 cm. In the instance of cecal rupture due to colonic ileus, the cecal diameter has always been 9 cm or larger, ranging from 9 to 20 cm.[5, 13] However, the fact that the cecum may remain distended to diameters of 14–18 cm for a few days in colonic ileus without inevitable perforation is supported by several series.[5] The law of Laplace states that the pressure required to distend the walls of a hollow viscus is inversely proportional to its radius; the greater the radius the less the pressure required. Since the portion of the colon with the largest diameter is the cecum, its tensile strength is exceeded first. The increasing distention may impede blood flow, further leading to necrosis and perforation of the cecum. The intraluminal pressure needed to produce rupture is between 20 and 55 mm Hg.[16] The perforations almost invariably occur on the anterior surface of the cecum and are diastatic in nature. There is, first, splitting of the serosa followed by a separation of the muscular layers through which the mucosa herniates and ultimately ruptures.[17] An incompetent ileocecal valve does not guarantee against cecal rupture.[18, 19]

Free intraperitoneal air is apparent in only about 50% of cases, and barium enema examination may not be helpful in making the diagnosis of perforation.[9] Surprisingly, even after perforation, there may be no appreciable decompression of the cecum.

Complication of Cecal Perforation

More than 20 patients with cecal perforation in severe or protracted colonic ileus, with a mortality of 43%, have been described (Fig 10–3).[6, 8, 9, 13] These perforations were probably attributable to delay in recognition of the cecal necrosis as well as of the primary disease state.

Treatment

Management of colonic ileus is generally conservative, directed to correction of any electrolyte and fluid imbalance and to aspiration with a nasogastric tube and a rectal tube. When a short term of conservative therapy is unrewarding, cecal distention reaches a 9 cm diameter or right lower quadrant symptoms or findings develop, operative decompression by cecostomy has been advocated to prevent peritonitis.[6, 13, 20]

REFERENCES

1. Ogilvie, H.: Large-intestine colic due to sympathetic deprivation, Br. Med. J. 2:671, 1948.
2. Stephens, F. O.: Syndrome of intestinal pseudo-obstruction, Br. Med. J. 1:1248, 1962.
3. Melamed, M., and Kubian, E.: Relationship of the autonomic nervous system to "functional" obstruction of the intestinal tract, Radiology 80:22, 1963.
4. Wanebo, H., Mathewson, C., and Conolly, B.: Pseudo-obstruction of the colon, Surg. Gynecol. Obstet. 133:44, 1971.
5. Meyers, M. A.: Colonic ileus, Gastrointest. Radiol. 2:37, 1977.
6. Morton, J. H., Schwartz, S. I., and Gramiak, R.: Ileus of the colon, Arch. Surg. 81:425, 1960.
7. Millar, D. R., and Ovlisen, B.: Two cases of spontaneous perforation of the caecum following caesarean section, Acta Obstet. Gynecol. Scand. 45:254, 1966.
8. Jensen, H. K.: Spontaneous perforation of the caecum following caesarean section, Acta Obstet. Gynecol. Scand. 51:381, 1972.
9. Wojtalik, R. S., Lindenauer, S. M., and Kahn, S. S.: Perforation of the colon associated with adynamic ileus, Am. J. Surg. 125:601, 1973.
10. Bryk, D., and Soong, K. Y.: Colonic ileus and its differential roentgen diagnosis, Am. J. Roentgenol. 101:329, 1967.
11. Meyers, M. A., and Evans, J. A.: Effects of pancreatitis on the small bowel and colon: Spread along mesenteric planes, Am. J. Roentgenol. 119:151, 1973.
12. Bobroff, L. M., Messinger, N. H., Subbarao, K., and Beneventano, T. C.: The cecal bascule, Am. J. Roentgenol. 115:249, 1972.
13. Gierson, E. D., Storm, F. K., Shaw, W., and Coyne, S. K.: Caecal rupture due to colonic ileus, Br. J. Surg. 62:383, 1975.
14. Lowman, R. M., and Davis, L.: An evaluation of cecal size in impending perforation of cecum, Surg. Gynecol. Obstet. 105:711, 1956.
15. Davis, L., and Lowman, R.: Roentgen criteria of impending perforation of the cecum, Radiology 68: 542, 1957.
16. Carrasquilla, C., Arbulu, A., Fromm, S., and Lucas, C.: Cecum perforation due to adynamic ileus, Dis. Colon Rectum 13:252, 1970.
17. Ravid, J. M.: Diastasis and diastatic perforation of gastrointestinal tract. A clinical, pathologic, and experimental study, Am. J. Pathol. 27:33, 1951.
18. Eckman, W. G., Wenzke, F., and Abramson, W.: Perforation of the cecum complicating adynamic ileus, Am. J. Surg. 96:718, 1958.
19. Robertson, J. A., Eddy, W. A., and Vosseler, A. J.: Spontaneous perforation of the cecum without mechanical obstruction, Am. J. Surg. 96:448, 1958.
20. Adams, J. T.: Adynamic ileus of the colon: An indication for cecostomy, Surgery 109:503, 1974.

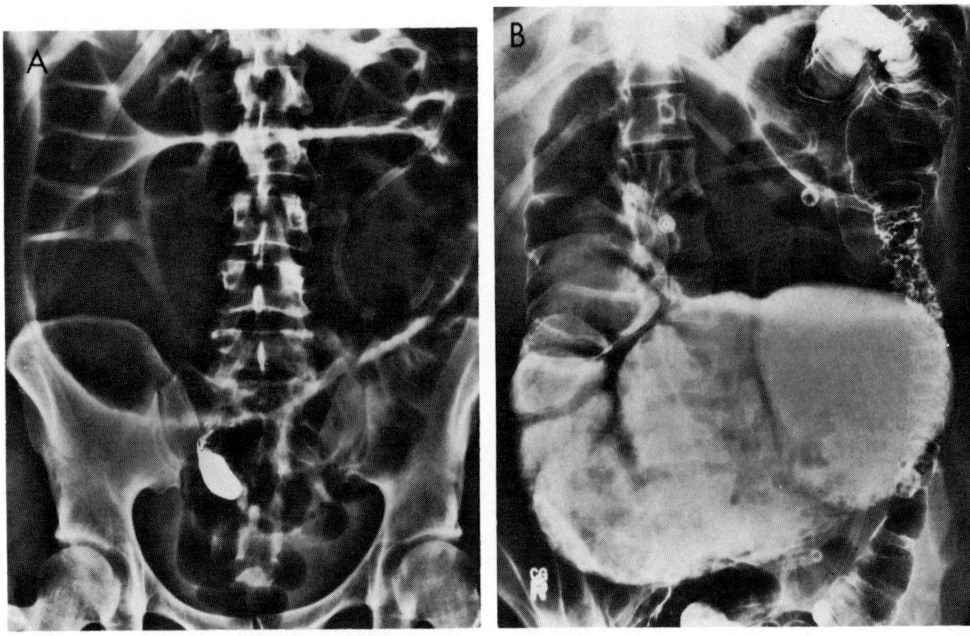

Fig 10–1.—**A,** plain film of abdomen 6 days after pelvic surgery demonstrates gas throughout colon with dilatation up to region of anatomical splenic flexure. Cecum, horizontally oriented, is disproportionately distended. **B,** barium enema study excludes possibility of mechanical obstruction. Cecal diameter measures 16 cm. (From Meyers, Gastrointest. Radiol. 2:37, 1977, with permission.)

Fig 10–2 (left).—Marked distention of ascending colon with cecal diameter of 17 cm 1 week following right hip nailing. There is minimal small intestinal dilatation. (From Meyers, Gastrointest. Radiol. 2:37, 1977, with permission.)

Fig 10–3 (right).—**A,** marked distention of colon to distal descending level, with cecal dilatation to 10 cm, in patient with generalized lymphosarcoma. **B,** barium enema study 4 days later demonstrates cecal perforation, with extravasation up paracolic gutter to subhepatic and subphrenic spaces *(arrows).* (From Meyers, Gastrointest. Radiol. 2:37, 1977, with permission.)

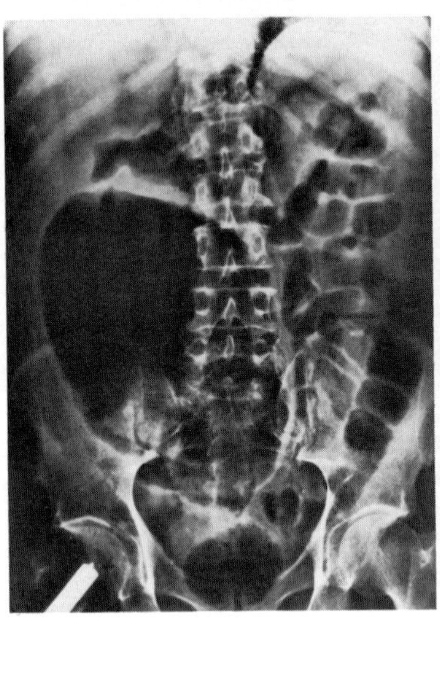

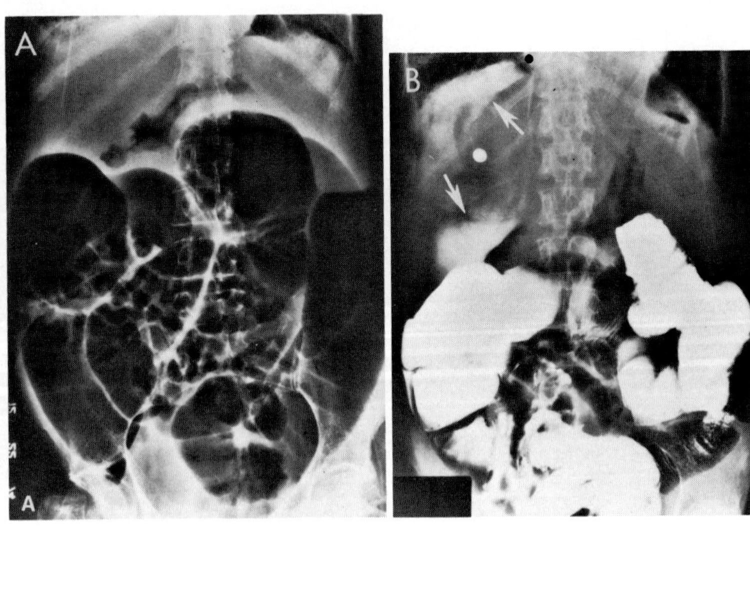

Chapter 11

Complications of Colonoscopy

MORTON A. MEYERS, M.D.
GARY G. GHAHREMANI, M.D.

FIBEROPTIC COLONOSCOPY is being used increasingly for endoscopic visualization of the large intestine, particularly in the removal of colonic polyps using an electrosurgical snare advanced through the biopsy channel of the colonoscope. Despite the relative flexibility of the instrument and the removal of polyps by cauterization under direct visualization, several complications have been encountered (Table 11–1). Radiologic examination plays a decisive role in the initial identification and documentation of many complications. The one that occurs most frequently and requires prompt diagnostic evaluation is perforation of the colon. Rupture of a diverticulum is occasionally produced by instrumentation or colonic insufflation. Cauterization of a polyp at its base or pedicle may result in coagulation necrosis of the colonic wall, producing perforation.

Technical Considerations

Fiberoptic colonoscopes of varying lengths permit endoscopic evaluation of the colon from the rectum to the cecum. Passage through the rectum is performed under direct vision, but negotiation through the sigmoid usually is accomplished without complete visualization of the lumen.[1] Visualization of the entire wall of the colon is carried out primarily during withdrawal. Not infrequently some difficulty in passage of the instrument is encountered at the points of curvature of the rectosigmoid and the junction of the sigmoid and descending colon, and too much "persuasive pressure"[2] in advancing the scope may result in mural perforation. Marked redundancy of the colon and narrowing or angulation due to diverticulosis, previous inflammatory processes or extrinsic compression of the lumen by pelvic masses may make negotiation difficult. The colonoscope may be advanced into a prominent diverticulum, causing its orifice to be mistaken for the proximal continuation of the colonic lumen. Insufflation of the colon by gas has also been incriminated in diverticular perforation. Although advancement of the colonoscope may be monitored fluoroscopically, most endoscopists use fluoroscopy or abdominal radiography only when difficulty is met.[1,3,4]

TABLE 11–1.—MAJOR COMPLICATIONS OF COLONOSCOPY

Mural perforation and serosal laceration
Rupture of a diverticulum
Bleeding
Abscess secondary to perforation in passing through a stricture
Mesosigmoid hematoma
Splenic avulsion and rupture in withdrawing the instrument
Incarceration of the instrument in hernia

Colonoscopic Perforations

The 1974 American Society for Gastrointestinal Endoscopy survey showed that the most common complication of diagnostic colonoscopy was perforation (0.22%). Furthermore, colonoscopic polypectomies resulted in perforation in 0.29% of cases, although its most common complication was hemorrhage (1.9%).[5] Other workers have reported a perforation rate as high as 1.9% with initial experience in colonoscopy.[6]

The most common sites of mural perforation during diagnostic colonoscopy include the rectosigmoid and the junction of the sigmoid and descending colon.[5, 7] Many perforations occur during mechanical manipulations, including the techniques of slide-by, alpha maneuver and straightening of the sigmoid loop. Friability of the wall from inflammatory colitis is a recognized hazard.[5, 7]

The colonoscope may also be advanced into a prominent diverticulum, causing its orifice to be mistaken for the proximal continuation of the colonic lumen. Insufflation of the colon by gas has also been incriminated in diverticular perforation.

Colonoscope fulguration of polyps has wide application but may also result in serious complications. A loop of wire is advanced through the biopsy channel of the colonoscope, and an electric current is applied while the snare is closed around the pedicle or base of the polyp. Large, sessile lesions may have to be removed in piecemeal fashion.[8] Overzealous application of heat, inadvertent inclusion of a portion of the colonic wall in the cautery snare or unclear visualization of the snare in the center of the bowel lumen while touching a point on the opposite wall may produce coagulation necrosis and resultant perforation.[7]

Free (intraperitoneal) perforation is about four times more frequent than closed (extraperitoneal) perforation, both in diagnostic colonoscopy and following polypectomy.[5]

Clinically, perforation may be recognized immediately or there may be considerable delay. Intraperitoneal rupture is usually immediately apparent but may be initially overlooked, particularly in the aged or infirm patient.[7] Prompt surgical closure is generally indicated. A few reports suggest that some cases may be treated conservatively without the need of emergency laparotomy.[9, 10] Extraperitoneal perforation may be masked for several hours or days[7] and is often not evident by the usual clinical methods of auscultation, palpation and percussion. Indeed, it may not be until the extraperitoneal gas extends to the abdominal wall, mediastinum or cervical tissues that it first becomes clinically apparent. One report cites the death of a patient who had an uneventful polypectomy and was well upon discharge 3 days later.[11] He was in a moribund state when he returned on the eighth postoperative day. Autopsy revealed a perforated diverticulum. However, extraperitoneal rupture generally follows a more benign course and may be treated conservatively. We have recommended routine abdominal radiography following diagnostic and therapeutic colonoscopy.[7] Because the colon is distended for easier endoscopic passage and visualization, considerable extraluminal gas is usually apparent if rupture has occurred.

Free intraperitoneal air is indicated on a supine film by increased radiolucency, visualization of the falciform ligament and perhaps the umbilical folds, and demonstration of both sides of the bowel wall (Figs 11–1, 11–2 and 11–3). The latter may be the main finding but can be somewhat subtle, with the wall outlined as a white strip ("bas relief" sign).[12] Erect or decubitus films readily demonstrate free intraperitoneal air (Fig 11–4). With procedures limited commonly to the left half of the colon, intraperitoneal gas indicates perforation of the sigmoid colon (usually at its junction with the rectum or descending colon) or at the site of an anterior polypectomy.

Extraperitoneal perforation most commonly involves the rectum or the posterior wall of the descending colon. It is also important to recognize that fully 75% of colonic diverticula face the extraperitoneal tissues,[13] so that acute diverticular perforation usually gives rise to extraperitoneal gas (Fig 11-5) and only occasionally to intraperitoneal air. Perforation of the sigmoid or transverse colon into the mesentery also extends posteriorly as indicated by extraperitoneal gas.[14] Recent correlative anatomical-radiologic studies have established the characteristic distribution and localization of extraperitoneal gas depending on its source.[14] The extraperitoneal structures are divided by fascial planes into three distinct compartments: (1) anterior pararenal, (2) perirenal and (3) posterior pararenal. Extraperitoneal gas within each compartment has been shown to have a distinctive spread and localization.

Rectal perforation is indicated by gas ascending the posterior pararenal spaces bilaterally, with lucent areas paralleling the lateral borders of the psoas muscles; superiorly, it sometimes extends as high as the upper renal pole and adrenal gland, the medial border of the spleen and liver, the medial crus of the diaphragm and the immediate subphrenic tissues (Figs 11-6 and 11-7). Extension into the flank fat stripes, anterior abdominal wall, scrotum and mediastinum may occur.

Extraperitoneal (posterior) perforation of the sigmoid, descending or ascending colon results in a unilateral collection of gas within the anterior pararenal space, shown by a collection of mottled lucent areas with a generally vertical axis. These characteristically extend medially over the psoas muscle to approach the spine but usually do not infiltrate the flank stripe (Fig 11-8). Perforation of the sigmoid colon at a site between the leaves of the mesocolon may give rise to extraperitoneal gas within the anterior pararenal spaces bilaterally. Both intra- and extraperitoneal gas may be seen, depending upon the site and size of the colonic perforation. These plain film observations become particularly crucial when one realizes that emergency enemas with water-soluble contrast material may not directly demonstrate the site of colonic perforation (see Fig 11-7, B). Radiologic localization of the precise site is important, when the site of perforation is clinically uncertain, in order to initiate proper treatment and anticipate possible complications.

Other Complications

A spectrum of other complications has also been experienced. Insufflation of gas to facilitate passage of the colonoscope occasionally may cause massive, prolonged dilatation of the small intestine in patients with a patulous ileocecal valve[16] (Fig 11-9). Mural perforation by the colonoscope at the site of a stricture may result in a localized abscess. A hematoma may develop in the sigmoid mesentery as the result of difficulty in passing the instrument or attempts to alter or bypass the redundant curvature of the sigmoid loop (Fig 11-10). Serosal lacerations or seromuscular tears, often clinically occult, have also been encountered due to mechanical pressures of the instrument.[17-19] Problems may also be encountered during withdrawal of the instrument. Reported complications include incarceration of the colonoscope in an unsuspected inguinal hernia and avulsion and rupture of the spleen, presumably secondary to instrumental intussusception of the colon.[7]

REFERENCES

1. Waye, J. D.: Colonoscopy, Surg. Clin. North Am. 52:1013, 1972.
2. Overholt, B. F.: Flexible fiberoptic sigmoidoscopy. Technique and preliminary results, Cancer 28:123, 1971.

3. Gaisford, W. D.: Gastrointestinal polypectomy via the fiberendoscope, Arch. Surg. 106:458, 1973.
4. Wolff, W. I., and Shinya, H.: Polypectomy via the fiberoptic colonoscope. Removal of neoplasms beyond reach of the sigmoidoscope, N. Engl. J. Med. 288:329, 1973.
5. Rogers, B. H. G., Silvis, S. E., Nebel, O. T., Sugawa, C., and Mandelstam, P.: Complications of flexible fiberoptic colonoscopy and polypectomy, Gastrointest. Endosc. 22:73, 1975.
6. Spencer, R. J., Coates, H. L., and Anderson, M. J., Jr.: Colonoscopic polypectomies, Mayo Clin. Proc. 49:40, 1974.
7. Meyers, M. A., and Ghahremani, G. G.: Complications of fiberoptic endoscopy. II. Colonoscopy, Radiology 115:301, 1975.
8. Wolff, W. I., and Shinya, H.: Polypectomy via the fiberoptic colonoscope. Removal of neoplasms beyond reach of the sigmoidoscope, N. Engl. J. Med. 288:329, 1973.
9. Ecker, M. D., Goldstein, M., Hoexter, B., Hyman, R. A., Naidich, J. B., and Stein, H. L.: Benign pneumoperitoneum after fiberoptic colonoscopy, Gastroenterology 73:226, 1977.
10. Taylor, R., Weakley, F. L., and Sullivan, B. H., Jr.: Non-operative management of colonoscopic perforation with pneumoperitoneum, Gastrointest. Endosc. 24:124, 1978.
11. Geneen, J. E., Schmitt, M. G., Jr., and Hogan, W. J.: Complications of colonoscopy (Abst.), Gastroenterology 66:812, 1974.
12. Meyers, M. A., and Oliphant, M.: Pitfalls and pickups in plain-film diagnosis of the abdomen, Curr. Probl. Radiol. 4:1, 1974.
13. Meyers, M. A., Volberg, F., Katzen, B., et al.: Haustral anatomy and pathology: A new look. II. Roentgen interpretation of pathological alterations, Radiology 108:505, 1973.
14. Meyers, M. A.: Radiological features of the spread and localization of extraperitoneal gas and their relationship to its source. An anatomical approach, Radiology 111:17, 1974.
15. Lezak, M. B., Goldhamer, M.: Retroperitoneal emphysema after colonoscopy, Gastroenterology 66:118, 1974.
16. Meyers, M. A., and Ghahremani, G.: Complications of gastrointestinal fiberoptic endoscopy, Gastrointest. Radiol. 2:273, 1977.
17. Livstone, E. M., Cohen, G. M., Troncale, F. J., and Touloukian, R. J.: Diastatic serosal lacerations: An unrecognized complication of colonoscopy, Gastroenterology 67:1245, 1974.
18. Wu, T. K.: Occult injuries during colonoscopy, Gastrointest. Endosc. 24:236, 1978.
19. Sjögren, R. W., Johnson, L. F., Butler, M. L., Heit, H. A., Gremillion, D. E., and Cammerer, R. C.: Serosal laceration: A complication of intra-operative colonoscopy explained by transmural pressure gradients, Gastrointest. Endosc. 24:239, 1978.

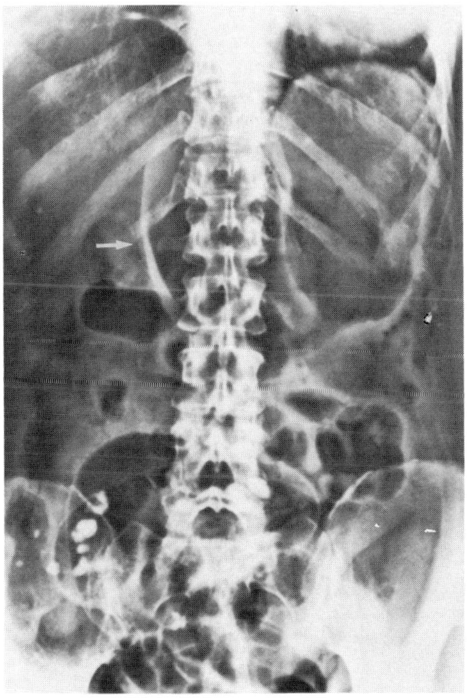

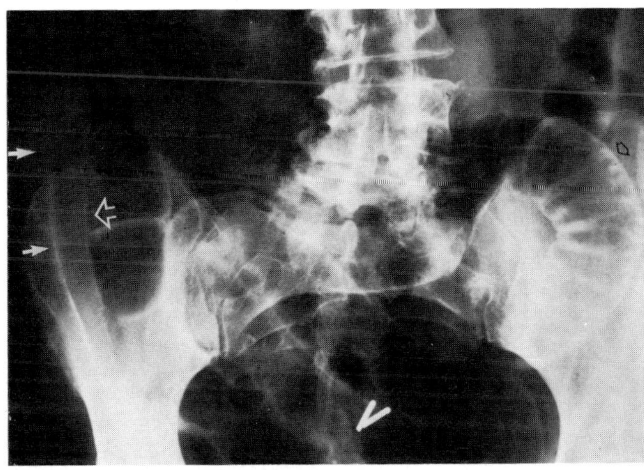

Fig 11–1 (left).—Sigmoid perforation secondary to coagulation necrosis of colonic wall at colonoscopic polypectomy. Gross free intraperitoneal air causes lucent distention of abdomen and allows visualization of falciform ligament *(arrow)*. (From Meyers and Ghahremani, Radiology 115:301, 1975, with permission.)

Fig 11–2 (right).—Sigmoid perforation due to coagulation necrosis, despite creation of pseudopedicle by colonoscopic traction on a sessile polyp. Free intraperitoneal air *(closed arrows)* is revealed by visualization of bowel wall *(open arrows)*. (From Meyers and Ghahremani, Radiology 115:301, 1975, with permission.)

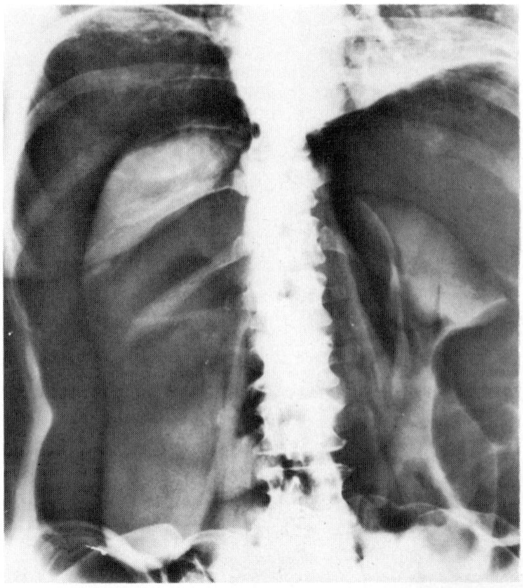

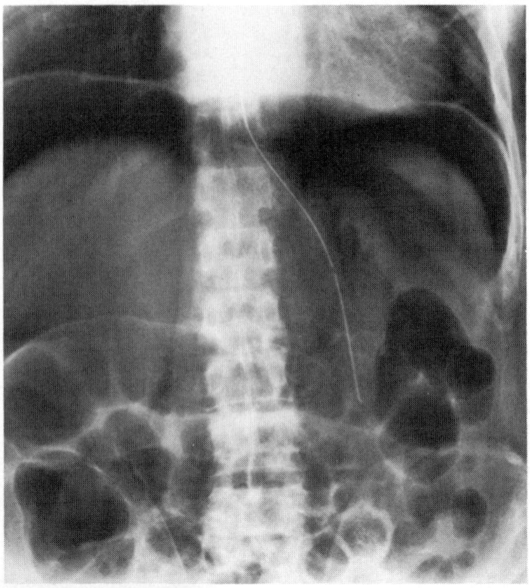

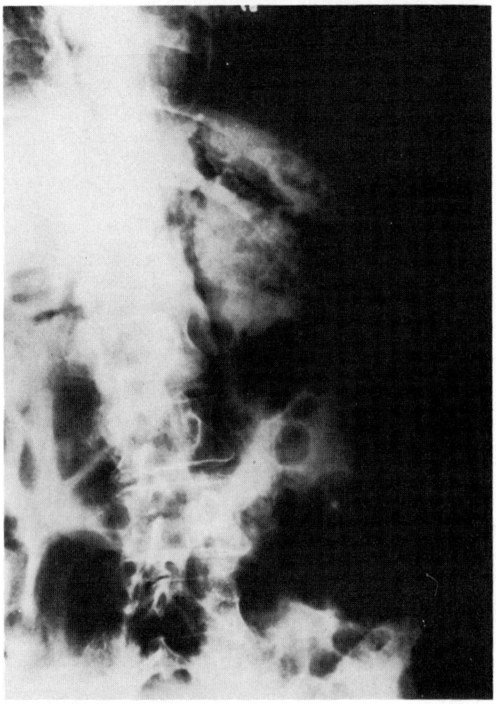

Fig 11–3 (left).—Sigmoid perforation in patient with chronic ulcerative colitis, thought to be secondary to insufflation of large intestine by air. Massive free intraperitoneal air. (From Meyers and Ghahremani, Radiology 115:301, 1975, with permission.)

Fig 11–4 (right).—Sigmoid perforation occurring during alpha maneuver. Erect abdominal film demonstrates free subdiaphragmatic gas bilaterally, with visualization of bowel wall. (From Meyers and Ghahremani, Radiology 115:301, 1975, with permission.)

Fig 11–5 (bottom).—Perforation of diverticulum of descending colon during colonoscopy. Extraperitoneal gas outlines left kidney and medial border of spleen. No free air or extraperitoneal gas on right side was seen. (From Meyers and Ghahremani, Gastrointest. Radiol. 2:273, 1977, with permission.)

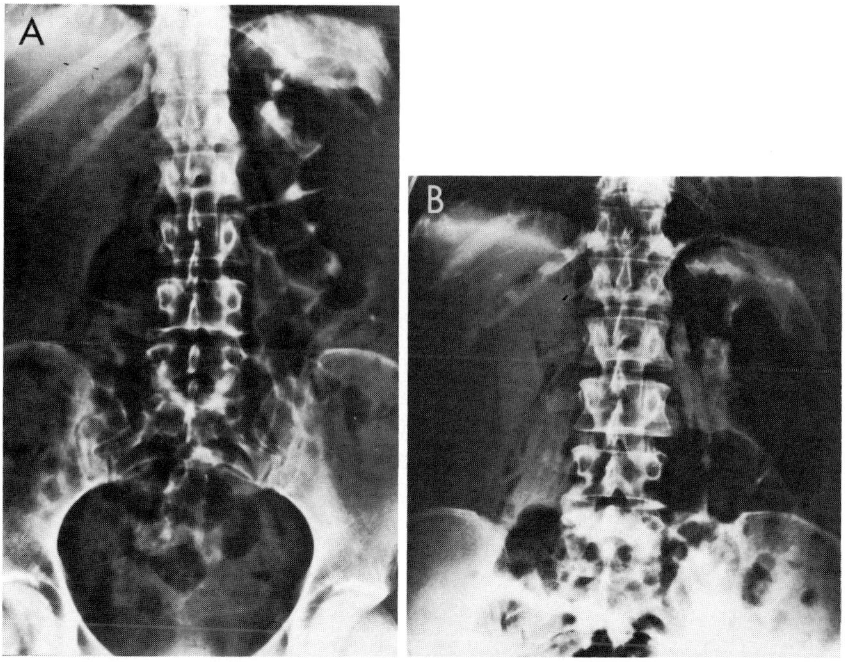

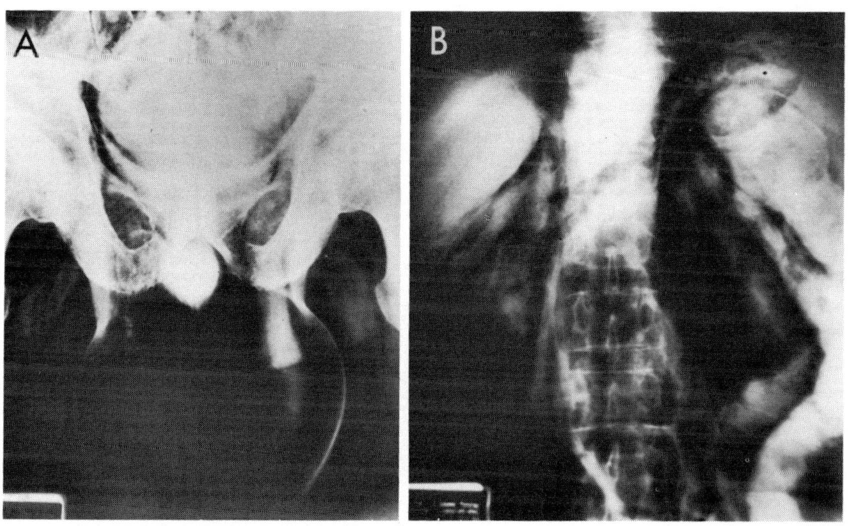

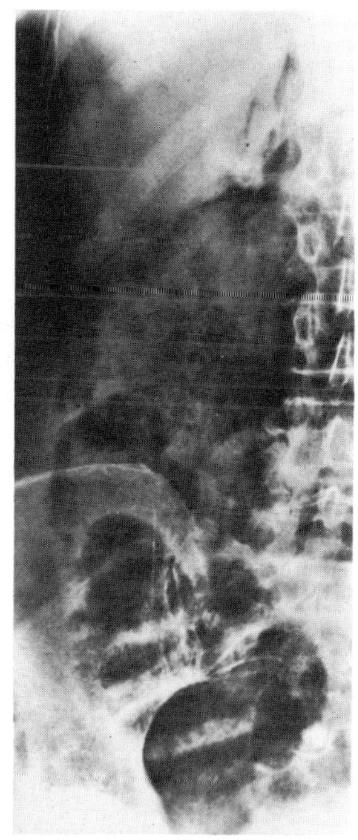

Fig 11–6 (top). – Rectal perforation secondary to colonoscopy. Supine **(A)** and erect **(B)** films demonstrate extraperitoneal gas paralleling lateral borders of psoas muscles. Cephalad extension on left outlines upper pole of kidney, adrenal gland, medial border of spleen, medial crus of diaphragm and immediate subphrenic tissues. These findings localize gas to posterior pararenal compartments. (From Meyers and Ghahremani, Radiology 115:301, 1975, with permission.)

Fig 11–7 (bottom left). – Rectal perforation secondary to colonoscopy. **A,** massive scrotal and extraperitoneal gas. **B,** gas within both posterior pararenal spaces outlines lateral borders of psoas muscles, upper renal poles and adrenal glands, medial borders of liver and spleen, medial crura of diaphragm and immediate subphrenic tissues. Gastrografin enema study of left colon demonstrated no extravasation. (**A** from Lezak and Goldhammer, Gastroenterology 66:118, 1974, with permission. **B** from Meyers and Ghahremani, Radiology 115:301, 1975, with permission.)

Fig 11–8 (bottom right). – Perforation of hepatic flexure following colonoscopic polypectomy. Mottled lucent areas on right represent collections of gas extending medially over psoas muscle and approaching spine. Flank stripe is intact. These changes localize extraperitoneal gas to anterior pararenal space. (From Meyers and Ghahremani, Radiology, 115:301, 1975, with permission.)

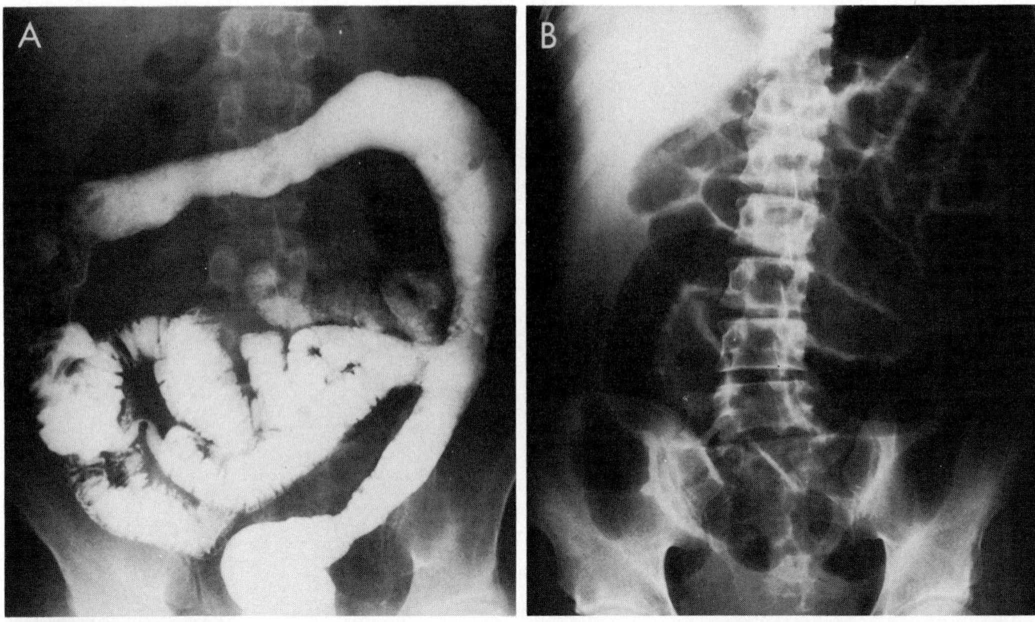

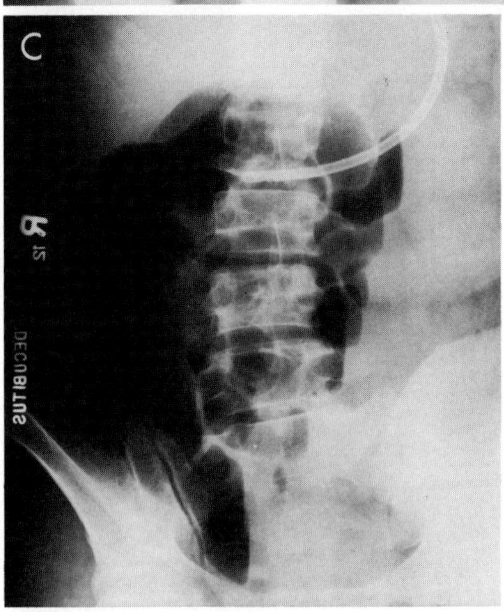

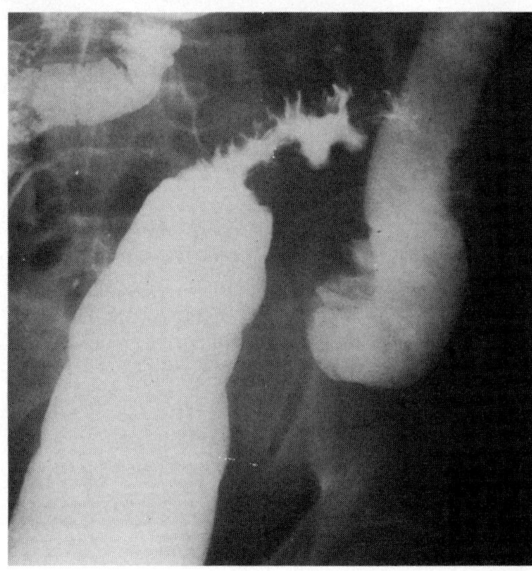

Fig 11–9 (top and **bottom left).**—Prolonged gaseous distention of small intestine following fiberoptic colonoscopy. **A,** barium enema examination shows diffuse chronic ulcerative colitis and patulous ileocecal valve. **B,** supine radiograph of abdomen immediately after colonoscopy demonstrates marked distention of small intestine. **C,** left lateral decubitus film obtained 2 days later shows persistent dilatation and fluid levels within small intestine. Bowel gas pattern became normal on fourth day after colonoscopy. (From Meyers and Ghahremani, Gastrointest. Radiol. 2:273, 1977, with permission.)

Fig 11–10 (bottom right).—Barium enema examination 3 days after colonoscopic removal of a polyp shows evidence of intramural hematoma localized to segment of sigmoid colon. (From Meyers and Ghahremani, Gastrointest. Radiol. 2:273, 1977, with permission.)

Chapter 12

Diastatic Rupture of the Cecum in Obstructing Carcinoma of the Left Colon

STANLEY NOVY, M.D.
LEE F. ROGERS, M.D.
WILLIAM KIRKPATRICK, M.D.

THE CECUM may rupture as a result of mechanical obstruction of the distal large bowel. This has been termed a diastatic rupture in reference to the mechanism of injury. It is thought that the distention of the cecal wall leads to a separation of the muscular layers through which the mucosa protrudes and at this site ultimately ruptures. The most common cause of the distal obstruction with cecal perforation is carcinoma of the colon.[2, 6, 7] This results in a characteristic radiologic triad of a massive pneumoperitoneum, a gastrointestinal air pattern indicative of a distal obstruction of the large bowel and marked dilatation of the cecum (Figs 12–1 to 12–3). It is curious and seemingly contradictory that the cecum is dilated in the presence of a perforation.

Discussion

PATHOMECHANICS

An obstruction of the intestinal tract produces distention of the bowel proximal to the point of obstruction. Given equal pressure throughout the colon, the greatest distention will occur in that portion of the colon with the largest diameter, the cecum. This is explained by the law of Laplace,[10] which states that the pressure required to distend the walls of a hollow viscus is inversely proportional to its radius; the greater the radius, the less pressure required. This is mathematically stated in the formula $T = PD$ (where T equals wall tension, P equals intraluminal pressure and D equals diameter of the viscus). The tensile strength of the colon wall will be exceeded sooner in that portion of the colon that has the greatest diameter.[10] The intraluminal pressure needed to produce perforation is between 20 and 55 mm Hg.[3, 7, 9]

The resultant perforation is most commonly found on the anterior surface of the cecum. It may vary in length from 5 to 40 mm, its longest diameter parallel to the longitudi-

---

Diastatic Rupture of the Cecum in Obstructing Carcinoma of the Left Colon: Radiographic and Surgical Implications, by S. Novy, originally appeared in Am. J. Roentgenol. 123:281, 175. Reprinted by permission of the author and of American Roentgen Ray Society.)

nal axis of the intestine.[8] The margins of the rupture are sharp and show no evidence of previous inflammation. The tear in the outer longitudinal muscle layer is wider than the tear in the inner circular muscle layer. There may be multiple tears in the same segment of a tear, or tears through the entire wall may be seen in association with other areas, where the mucosa is seen to protrude through the diastasis of the muscle layers of the cecum, as described above. Microscopically, atrophy of all layers, with only a minimal degree of edema or round cell infiltration indicative of inflammation, is seen. In almost all reported cases, no gross or microscopic evidence of preexisting mucosal inflammation or ulceration could be seen in the distended or ruptured bowel.

Three theories have been proposed to explain the cecal perforation.[8] (1) A vascular theory states that, as the lumen of the intestine distends, the blood vessels within its walls become obliterated and the area supplied by these vessels becomes necrotic. A hemorrhagic infarction is thus produced, which, in turn, is followed by perforation. Although the tear is usually situated on the anterior mesenteric border or the anterior wall of the cecum, which has a poor blood supply, there appears to be little, if any, microscopic evidence to support this theory. (2) A toxic infectious theory states that there is an increase in the virulence of bacterial flora in the closed loop obstruction of the intestine and an increase in the permeability of the intestinal wall. This leads to bacterial invasion of the mucosa with subsequent necrosis, ulceration and extension of the process to the outer layers of the wall, with a resultant transmural perforation. As in the first theory, there is little microscopic support for such a course of events. (3) The mechanical theory appears to best explain the perforation: progressive distention of the cecum leads to a diastasis of the muscular wall through which the mucosa protrudes and ultimately ruptures.

ROENTGENOGRAPHIC FINDINGS

Roentgenograms of the abdomen in the presence of a ruptured cecum secondary to a distal colonic obstruction were first described by Rack.[7] He stated that the combination of large quantities of free intraperitoneal air in association with greatly distended loops of colon, especially the cecum, with or without distention of the small intestine, would suggest the diagnosis.

It is curious and seemingly contradictory that, following perforation and an accumulation of a large amount of free air in the peritoneum, the cecum would remain greatly distended. A precise explanation as to why the cecum does not collapse or decompress under these circumstances is not available. It has been suggested that a perforation is sealed by the omentum or adjacent bowel,[7] but this is not supported by surgical or autopsy findings when an open perforation is identified. For the cecum to collapse, it might be presumed that the intraperitoneal pressure would have to exceed the intraluminal pressure of the colon. It may be that an equilibrium is achieved between the distended colon and peritoneal cavity and therefore the cecum remains distended.

Surgical Implications

Ruptures of the cecum in association with large bowel obstruction carry a very high degree of morbidity and mortality. The mortality ranges from 36 to 72%.[1, 5] In the face of a distal colonic obstruction, the cecum should be examined at the time of surgery for impending or actual perforation. Some authorities have stated that a cecostomy is preferable to a transverse colostomy in the presence of a distal bowel obstruction or large bowel obstruction.[4] Although we are in no position to argue this point, it would seem wise to examine the cecum thoroughly before perforation. This would obviate or prevent the oversight of such a perforation with its attendant morbidity and mortality.

Some investigators have attempted to relate the transverse diameter of the cecum to the possibility of impending cecal perforation. Davis and Lowman[5] stated that when the transverse diameter is over 9 cm, impending perforation should be suspected. The transverse diameter of the cecum in the present cases measured 11, 10.5, 10.5 and 11 cm, respectively. In our experience, 9 cm seems to be a low figure, since we have encountered numerous cases of cecal distention of this magnitude that did not result in perforation.

REFERENCES

1. Albers, J. H., Smith, L., and Carter, R.: Perforation of the Cecum, Ann. Surg. 143:251, 1956.
2. Byrne, J. J.: Large Bowel Obstruction, Am. J. Surg. 99:168, 1960.
3. Carrasquilla, C., Arbulu, A., Fromm, S., and Lucas, C.: Cecal perforation due to adynamic ileus, Dis. Colon Rectum 13:252, 1970.
4. Clark, D. D., and Hubay, C. A.: Tube cecostomy: Evaluation of 161 cases, Ann. Surg. 175:55, 1972.
5. Davis, L., and Lowman, R. M.: Roentgen criteria of impending perforation of the cecum, Radiology 68: 543, 1957.
6. Desai, M. G., and Rodko, E. A.: Perforation of colon in malignant tumors, J. Can. Assoc. Radiol. 24: 344, 1973.
7. Rack, F. J.: Obstructive perforation of cecum, Am. J. Surg. 84:527, 1952.
8. Ravid, J. M.: Diastasis and diastatic perforation of gastrointestinal tract, Am. J. Pathol. 27:33, 1951.
9. Von Burt, C. A.: Pneumatic rupture of intestinal canal, Arch. Surg. 22:875, 1931.
10. Wojtalik, R. S., Lindenauer, S. M., and Kahn, S. S.: Perforation of colon associated with adynamic ileus, Am. J. Surg. 125:601, 1973.

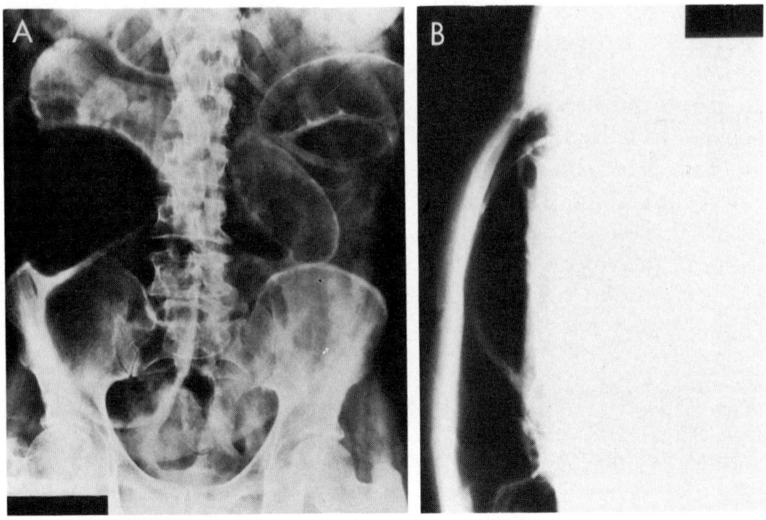

Fig 12–1.—**A,** kidney, ureter and bladder (KUB) film shows distention of cecum measuring 11 cm and dilated loops of bowel. Note "double wall" sign with air on both sides of bowel wall. **B,** massive pneumoperitoneum. (From Novy, Am. J. Roentgenol. 123:281, 1975, with permission by the publisher, American Roentgen Ray Society.)

Fig 12–2.—**A,** dilated loops of bowel with distention of cecum measuring 10.5 cm. **B,** massive pneumoperitoneum. (From Novy, Am. J. Roentgenol. 123:281, 1975, with permission by the publisher, American Roentgen Ray Society.)

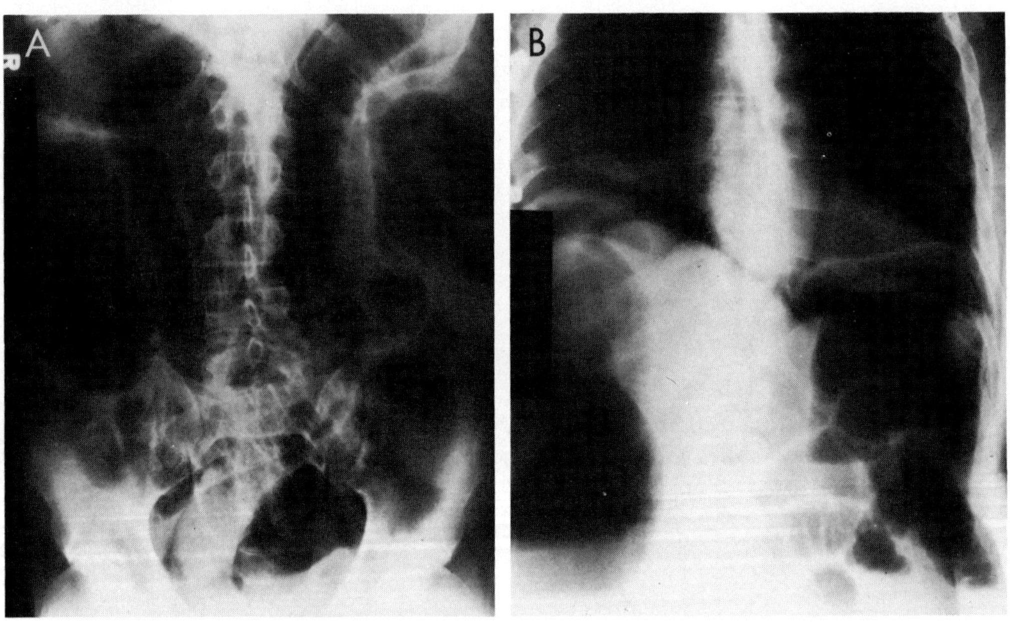

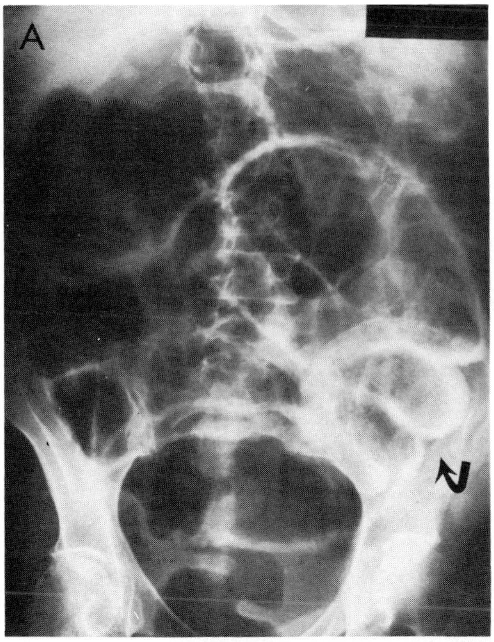

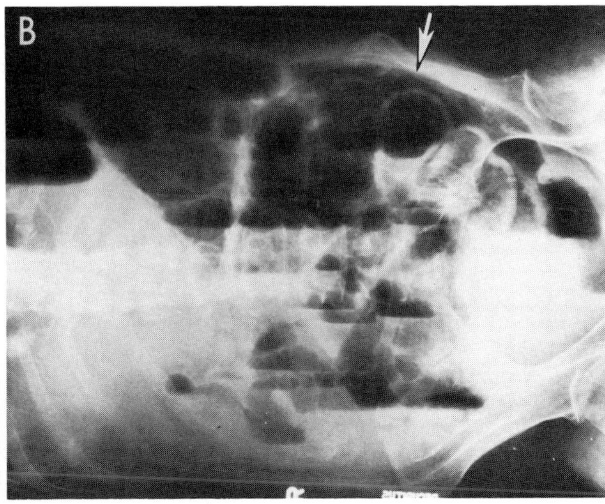

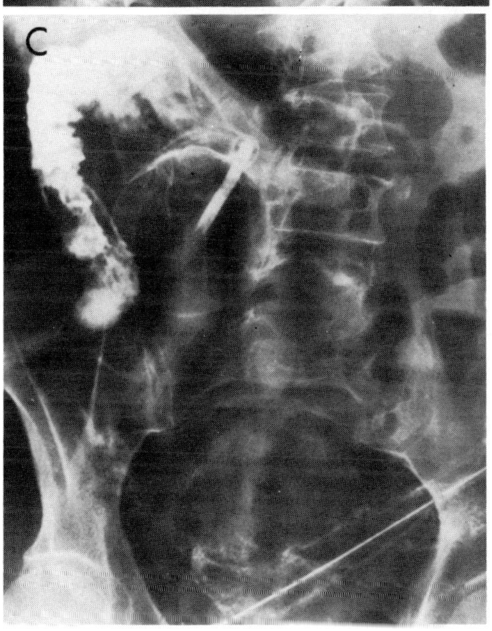

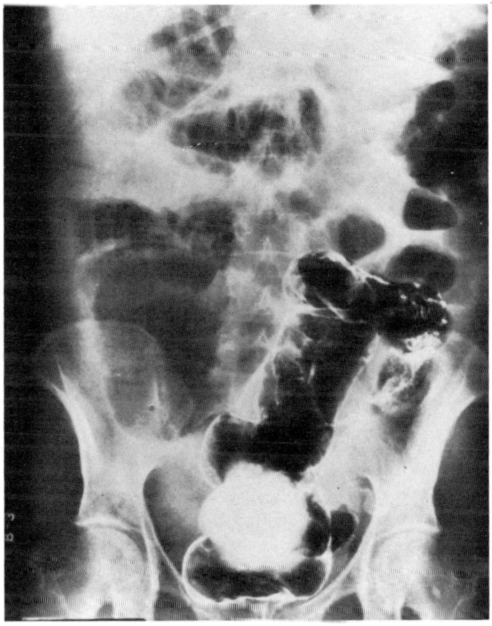

Fig 12–3 (top and **bottom left).** – **A,** dilated loops of bowel with distention of cecum. Air seen on both sides of bowel wall *(arrows).* **B,** decubitus film shows dilated loops of bowel with air-fluid levels and air on both sides of bowel wall *(arrow).* **C,** barium enema examination through colostomy demonstrating perforation of cecum with extravasation of barium. (From Novy, Am. J. Roentgenol. 123:281, 1975, with permission by the publisher, American Roentgen Ray Society.)

Fig 12–4 (bottom right). – Dilated loops of bowel with distention of cecum measuring 11 cm. Barium enema demonstrating obstruction in sigmoid. (Courtesy A. F. Barrell, M. D., Houston.)

Chapter 13

Diverticular Disease of the Colon

ANGIOGRAPHY IN DIVERTICULAR HEMORRHAGE

LAWRENCE E. GOLDBERGER, M.D.

ALTHOUGH COLONIC diverticula have been recognized for almost two centuries, the prevalence and importance of this disease entity have been elucidated much more recently. Currently it is estimated that about 25% of the population between the ages of 60 and 70, and 50% of those over the age of 70, have colonic diverticula.[1-5] The true prevalence is undoubtedly higher because many people with colonic diverticula are asymptomatic.

Only in the past 10–15 years have we begun to truly understand the pathogenesis of colonic diverticula and the causes of their complications, specifically hemorrhage. The work of Painter and associates[6-8] and Arfwidsson[9] has given us a clear understanding of the development of colonic diverticula. They have shown how segmentation of the colon produced by muscular contraction leads to localized increased pressure. This localized increased pressure results in herniation of mucosa and submucosa through natural weaknesses in the colonic wall provided by penetration of the segmental blood vessels. The anatomical and angiographic studies by Meyers et al.[10] and by others[11, 12] have confirmed the relationship of colonic diverticula to penetration of the large vasa recta.

Bleeding in Diverticulosis

Diverticular bleeding is the most common cause of severe rectal hemorrhage of colonic origin, when "severe" is defined as requiring transfusion.[15, 16]

It is now readily accepted that by far the most bleeding in diverticular disease is seen without any evidence of diverticulitis.[1, 13-15] It has been estimated that lower gastrointestinal bleeding of varying magnitude occurs in 20–30% of patients with diverticula and that the hemorrhage is severe enough to require hospitalization and treatment in 5%.[1, 13, 14] The onset of bleeding is usually sudden and accompanied by the urge to defecate. The blood and stool admixture may be bright red, maroon or tarry. The bleeding is usually painless, and symptoms are related to the sudden hypovolemia. The incidence and severity tend to increase with age.[14]

Until quite recently, the mechanism responsible for diverticular bleeding was poorly understood. Meticulous investigation of resected specimens is required to identify the site of bleeding and to understand its cause. The first reported case of massive rectal hemorrhage from an eroded artery in the wall of a diverticulum was by Kocour[17] in 1937. A few additional cases were reported up to

1967 when Salvati et al.[18] presented two additional cases and proposed a mechanism for this complication of diverticular disease. They noted a disproportionate number of patients whose bleeding was from right-sided diverticula despite the predominance of diverticula in the left colon. The absence of significant inflammation in the wall of the eroded artery supported the concept that trauma to the vessel, rather than primary vascular disease, was the cause of bleeding. Salvati et al.[18] proposed that inspissated feces or a true fecalith gradually enlarged the diverticulum until it impinged on the adjacent artery. The constant pulsation of the artery against the feces-filled diverticulum leads to pressure necrosis in the wall of the artery, resulting in hemorrhage into the diverticulum. In support of this theory, two cases of Salvati et al. showed histologic evidence of split and frayed internal elastic membranes only in the portion of the arterial wall that abutted on the diverticulum.

Meyers et al.[10] had clearly shown the relationship of the arterial vessel closely applied to the dome of colonic diverticula. Subsequent publications of Meyers and colleagues[19, 20] in 1976 give us a clear understanding of the mechanism involved in massive diverticular hemorrhage. Serial histologic sectioning of bleeding diverticula showed the cause to be rupture of the underlying vas rectum either at the dome of the diverticulum or along its antimesenteric margin near its orifice. The rupture of the vessel was always eccentric along the side toward the lumen of the diverticulum. The arterial lesion was consistently characterized by eccentric intimal thickening and focal narrowing of the media toward the lumen of the diverticulum. These changes are most consistent with trauma related to mechanical, thermal or chemical causes. The fact that right-sided diverticula have wider necks and domes would allow the vasa recta to be exposed to traumatic factors over a greater length. This may explain the predominance of hemorrhage from right-sided diverticula.

Numerous authors in recent years have shown the predominance of the right half of the colon as the site for massive diverticular bleeding.[13, 18, 20-28] About 70% of the demonstrated bleeding diverticula have been proximal to the splenic flexure, despite the fact that the sigmoid colon harbors the overwhelming majority of colonic diverticula.[29] This predominance of right-sided colonic bleeding in diverticular disease may well explain many of the failures of blind left colon resections for diverticular hemorrhage prior to the advent of angiographic localization.

Role of Angiography

With the prevalence of diverticular disease, and the 5% incidence of bleeding as a complication requiring hospitalization and treatment, it is fortunate that at least 80% of these hospitalized patients respond to conservative therapy of bed rest, sedation and volume replacement.[16, 23] Since many patients with bleeding diverticulosis are in an elderly age group with many concurrent medical problems, it is not surprising that the mortality for emergency surgery is high.[16, 30-34] This fact, coupled with the high rate of recurrent bleeding in patients who have undergone blind segmental colon resection,[30, 31, 35, 36] has led several surgeons to advocate total colonic resection with ileoproctostomy for bleeding diverticulosis.[30, 32, 37] Attempts to localize the site of bleeding at surgery for limited resection have been disappointing and frustrating.[15, 31, 32, 38, 39] Therefore, it is not surprising that angiography has been welcomed eagerly by most surgeons to localize the site of bleeding and, in many cases, to attempt to stop the hemorrhage through transcatheter interventional means (Cases 1–4).

The value and efficacy of angiography in the diagnosis and treatment of gastrointestinal hemorrhage are now well established. First introduced into the American literature in 1963, Nusbaum and Baum[40] reported their experience in selective catheterization, demonstrating the site of bleeding in dogs with rates of blood loss as low as 0.5 cc per minute. Subsequent reports[41-46] of gastrointestinal hemorrhage demonstrated in human patients were soon published, and the technique has been embraced by physicians the world over. The demonstration, and transcatheter therapy of diverticular bleeding, has become relatively common in places where emergency angiography by well-trained personnel is available. Fortunately, the appearance of diverticular bleeding is usually quite characteristic owing to frequent pooling of the contrast medium in the bleeding diverticulum (see Case 1).

Vasopressor and Transcatheter Embolic Therapy

The value of transcatheter vasoconstriction was originally shown for control of variceal bleeding by infusing pituitrin into the superior mesenteric artery to decrease portal venous flow.[47] Subsequently, pituitrin and other vasoconstrictors were used to control arterial bleeding in the upper gastrointestinal tract.[48, 49]

In 1973, and again in 1975, Baum et al.[28, 35, 50] reported successful short-term and long-term control of diverticular hemorrhage by infusion of pitressin. Similar success was reported by others.[23]

It would appear that preoperative diagnosis by angiography and even short-term control of bleeding by vasoconstrictors allow fluid replacement, stabilization and a rational surgical approach. The combination of these factors results in a dramatic decrease in mortality compared to emergency blind segmental resection or subtotal colectomy.[16, 30, 36, 51]

With the advent of angiographic localization of diverticular bleeding sites, we have emerged from the era of empiric left hemicolectomies for hemorrhage, which has often been from the right side of the colon. With the use of vasoconstrictive therapy, most patients can have bleeding successfully stopped. A decision can then be made regarding either elective resection of the offending diverticulum in a stable patient or nonsurgical followup. Repeat episodes of bleeding may be from widely separated diverticula. This knowledge might argue for either nonsurgical treatment or total colectomy (see Case 2). Large series of patients with both nonsurgical and operative resection will need to be observed for longer periods to determine which mode of therapy is better.

There are cases in which vasopressin fails to control diverticular bleeding. In the event that the patient is a poor surgical risk, embolization of the bleeding artery may be carried out[52] (see Cases 2 and 3). Embolization of various organs has been extensively reported,[53, 54-61] but the colon for the most part has not been included in this form of transcatheter therapy. The reluctance to embolize the colon stems from the relative lack of collateral blood supply to the colon compared to that of the stomach and duodenum. Although the potential for collateral supply is not as great in the colon as in the other hollow viscera, the colon does have a rich submucosal plexus.[62-64] The two cases of successful embolization for diverticular bleeding, as well as a case of colon embolization for a bleeding carcinoma[53, 54] and two cases of embolic control of superior mesenteric artery hemorrhage secondary to abdominal abscess, indicate that this technique is feasible. Further experience will be necessary to evaluate the true risk of ischemic injury.

Technique of Angiography

In angiography for gastrointestinal hemorrhage, an aortogram is rarely performed.

Direct selective catheterization of the celiac, superior mesenteric or inferior mesenteric artery is accomplished via the groin using modified Seldinger technique. The choice of catheters and catheter shape varies widely depending on the angiographer's training. Preshaped catheters are now widely available in a variety of sizes, shapes and materials. High quality angiography requires a 1000-ma, three-phase generator, rapid film changer and power injector. Microfocal spot x-ray tubes (0.3 mm and less) are especially necessary for magnification when attempting to identify small vascular lesions. They are not necessary for routine workup in acute gastrointestinal hemorrhage.

In suspected lower gastrointestinal bleeding, the superior mesenteric artery (SMA) should be injected first. This is because of the higher incidence of colonic bleeding from the right side. Injection volumes in the SMA should approximate 40–50 ml of 76% meglumine diatrizoate at a rate of 5–6 ml per second. Filming sequences can vary but should extend well into the venous phase, i.e., 20–24 seconds. An acceptable sequence would be two films per second for 3 seconds, one per second for 3 seconds and then one every 3d second for 18 seconds.

If the source of bleeding is not found on the SMA injection (it may require more than one injection to include all of the bowel supplied by the SMA), then the inferior mesenteric artery (IMA) is studied next. Injection volume here is usually 20–25 ml at a rate of 2–4 cc per second. If an IMA study is performed, it will be necessary to have a Foley catheter to drain the bladder so as not to obscure portions of the colon with opacified urine.

If no bleeding site is found after SMA and IMA studies, a celiac injection should be made, since upper gastrointestinal bleeding occasionally masquerades as lower gastrointestinal bleeding. In Casarella and colleagues' series,[21] three of 27 patients with clinical lower gastrointestinal bleeding had bleeding from peptic ulcer disease identified on a celiac study.

It should also be noted that arteriocapillary bleeding may be sporadic. If no bleeding site is found in a patient who clinically is actively bleeding at the time of angiography, a second injection is probably indicated[21, 65] (see Case 2). It is thought that the first injection of contrast may act as a vasodilator and stimulate the bleeding seen on the subsequent injection. No clear-cut data on the rate of bleeding necessary to visualize at angiography exist for human patients. It is probably in excess of the 0.5 cc per minute seen in the laboratory animal.[40]

The management of vasopressin (Pitressin) infusion will be discussed below. If vasopressin fails and embolization is desired, subselection of the feeding artery from the SMA must be accomplished. This is not a difficult task. The original catheter is exchanged over a guidewire for a thin-walled catheter, preshaped with a gentle curve corresponding to the forward bend of the SMA from the aorta and a second distal curve to engage the desired branch. The distal curve should be short (about 1 cm) and sharp (45 degrees) in the direction of the origin from the SMA of the desired branch. By advancing this catheter all the way out the SMA over the guidewire, selective vessels will be individually engaged as the catheter is slowly retracted. We have used Gelfoam cut into small pieces and soaked in contrast medium. These should be injected by suspending the Gelfoam in a small amount of saline in a 1-cc syringe. Gelfoam should be injected one piece at a time, with intervening hand injections of contrast medium to ascertain the desired embolic result. Other agents (e.g., autologous tissue, autologous clot and Oxycel) have been used applying the same principles.

Pituitrin—Use and Side Effects

Although much more commonly used for control of diverticular bleeding, Pituitrin has several disadvantages compared to embolization. First of all, there are systemic effects of the drug. These include decreased coronary blood flow, decreased cardiac output and a strong antidiuretic response.[66, 67] Cardiac problems such as bradycardia, hypertension, arrhythmia and arrest are potential problems[68-70] but generally are not seen with the low dose intra-arterial infusions used to control gastrointestinal bleeding.

The second set of problems relates to prolonged catheter position. Emboli are always a potential problem, although rarely seen. Bleeding around the puncture site can usually be controlled with a sandbag. Hematoma around the puncture site is the most common complication but rarely requires operative therapy. There is also the need for prolonged bed rest, with immobilization of the catheterized groin. This condition has its own well-known complications.

Therefore, the use of vasopressin infusions should not be embarked upon lightly. The angiography team must take responsibility for the care and management of the catheter as well as the infusion of pressors. This requires close cooperation with the clinical team that is managing the patient.

The initial dose of surgical Pituitrin to be infused is usually 0.1 – 0.2 units per minute. This should be evaluated with a repeat arteriogram after 15 – 20 minutes to see what effect it has had on hemorrhage and flow to the organ involved. Depending on the presence or absence of continued bleeding, and the amount of vasoconstriction, the dose may be adjusted up or down. If the dose rate is changed, another arteriogram in 15 – 20 minutes should be performed for the same reasons. Most bleeding will be controlled at an infusion rate of 0.2 units per minute. Bleeding that does not respond to 0.4 units per minute probably will not respond to higher levels and surgery should be undertaken.

The therapeutic effect of vasopressin is manifested by a local decrease in blood flow from vasoconstriction. It is this decreased flow rate that probably allows time for a stable clot to form. There does not appear to be an escape from the vasoconstrictive effect of vasopressin, as this effect is independent of the autonomic nervous system.[51]

An arterial pump is necessary to continuously and accurately administer the Pituitrin infusion. The simplest method of preparing the drug for infusion is to mix 100 units of surgical Pituitrin (20 units per vial) with 500 cc of normal saline or 5% dextrose. This gives a solution with a concentration of 0.2 units per ml, allowing an infusion rate generally between 0.5 and 2 ml per minute. Because of the antidiuretic effect of vasopressin, this volume must be carefully included in the patient's intake and output. If it becomes necessary to decrease the volume of administered fluids, the concentration of Pituitrin may be increased. The catheter itself should be firmly secured in the groin either with tape or a skin suture. Dislodgment of the catheter is one of the obvious reasons for vasopressin failure.

The schedule of Pituitrin infusion must be varied to fit the individual needs of the patient. In general, however, the following schedule of gradual weaning will be helpful in the patient who has a good response.

1. 0.2 units per minute for 6 hours.
2. 0.1 unit per minute for 24 hours.
3. D5W or saline, 1 cc per minute for 24 hours.
4. Pull catheter if no further signs of bleeding.

If at any time the bleeding recurs, the infusion goes back to 0.2 – 0.4 units per minute until control is reestablished, and the weaning procedure starts over again.

The systemic effects of vasopressin mentioned at the beginning of this section generally are mild with regard to decreased cardiac function. The antidiuretic effects vary greatly from individual to individual and must be carefully watched.

It is necessary to mention that, although use of vasopressin is generally a safe form of therapy, several publications have dealt with severe complications of mesenteric[71-73] and peripheral[67-74] ischemia from vasopressin infusion into the SMA. In most instances these complications resulted from a departure from the management program described.

It is advisable to check catheter position daily with a portable film, or at any time when it is suspected that the catheter may have become dislodged; when bleeding recurs despite continued infusion; or when peripheral ischemic changes become apparent.

The recent interest in *intravenous* pressor infusion requires a brief comment. Although this form of therapy may have some efficacy in control of variceal bleeding, it does not appear useful for arteriocapillary hemorrhage.[75-78]

Summary

The prevalence of diverticular disease and its complications, specifically hemorrhage, makes it quite likely that most radiologists will at one time or another encounter a request for angiography in a patient with suspected diverticular bleeding. The ease of demonstration of the source of bleeding, as well as the potential therapeutic gain from localization of the bleeding site or transcatheter hemostasis, makes this a highly desirable study. Knowledge of the common sites for diverticular bleeding as well as various transcatheter therapeutic methods should allow the radiologist to play a significant role in the diagnosis and therapy of diverticular hemorrhage.

CASE REPORTS

Case 1 (Figs 13–1 to 13–5)

A woman, age 80, with known diverticulosis presented with massive bright red rectal bleeding.

Case 2 (Figs 13–6 to 13–10)

A man, age 69, with known diverticulosis had an initial diverticular hemorrhage in 1974, eventually treated with embolization of right colic artery. No surgery was performed at that time and the patient returned 10 months later with recurrent lower intestinal hemorrhage, demonstrated arteriographically to be from a second diverticulum in distal transverse colon.

Case 3 (Figs 13–11 to 13–14)

A male renal transplant patient, age 52, had had a previous right transverse colostomy for perforated left colon diverticulum. He had acute onset of massive hemorrhage into colostomy bag. The patient was considered a very poor surgical risk.

Case 4 (Figs 13–15 to 13–17)

A woman, age 87, was referred for angiography for second major gastrointestinal hemorrhage in 6 weeks. The patient was markedly hypotensive.

REFERENCES

1. Editorial: Massive bleeding from diverticular disease of the colon, Lancet 1:706, 1963.
2. Morson, B. C.: Pathology of diverticular disease of the colon, Clin. Gastroenterol. 4:37, 1975.
3. Parks, T. G.: Natural history of diverticular disease of the colon, Clin. Gastroenterol. 4:53, 1975.
4. Ellis, H.: Colonic diverticula—pathology and natural history, Br. Med. J. 8:565, 1970.
5. Fleischner, F.: Diverticular disease of the colon. New observations and revised concepts, Gastroenterology 60:316, 1971.
6. Painter, N., Truelove, S., Ardran, G., and Tuckey, M.: Segmentation and the localization of intraluminal pressures in the human colon, with special reference to the pathogenesis of colonic diverticula, Gastroenterology 49:169, 1965.
7. Painter, N., and Burkitt, D.: Diverticular disease of the colon, a 20th-century problem, Clin. Gastroenterol. 4:3, 1975.
8. Painter, N., and Burkitt, D.: Diverticular disease of the colon: a deficiency disease of western civilization, Br. Med. J. 2:450, 1971.
9. Arfwidsson, S.: Pathogenesis of multiple diverticula of the sigmoid colon in diverticular disease, Acta. Chir. Scand. (Suppl.) 342:3, 1964.
10. Meyers, M., Volberg, F., Katzen, B., et al.: The angioarchitecture of colonic diverticula, Radiology 108:249, 1973.
11. Slack, W.: Diverticula of the colon and their relation to the muscle layers and blood vessels, Gastroenterology 39:708, 1960.
12. Slack, W.: The anatomy, pathology and some clinical features of diverticulitis of the colon, Br. J. Surg. 50:185, 1962.

13. Gennaro, A., and Rosemond, G.: Colonic diverticula and hemorrhage, Dis. Colon Rectum 16:409, 1973.
14. Welch, C., and Hedberg, S.: Gastrointestinal hemorrhage, Part I. General considerations of diagnosis and therapy, Adv. Surg. 7:95, 1973.
15. Noer, R., Hamilton, J., Williams, D., et al.: Rectal hemorrhage: Moderate and severe, Ann. Surg. 155: 794, 1962.
16. Behringer, G., and Albright, N.: Diverticular disease of the colon – A frequent cause of massive rectal bleeding, Am. J. Surg. 125:419, 1973.
17. Kocour, E.: Diverticulosis of the colon: Its incidence in 7000 consecutive autopsies with reference to its complications, Am. J. Surg. 37:433, 1937.
18. Salvati, E., Hyun, B., and Varga, C.: Massive hemorrhage from colonic diverticula caused by arterial erosion: A practical theory of its mechanism and causation, Dis. Colon Rectum 10:129, 1967.
19. Meyers, M., Alonso, D., Gray, G., et al.: Pathogenesis of bleeding colonic diverticulosis, Gastroenterology 71:577, 1976.
20. Meyers, M., Alonso, D., and Baer, J.: Pathogenesis of massively bleeding colonic diverticulosis: New observations, Am. J. Roentgenol. 127:901, 1976.
21. Casarella, W., Kanter, I., and Seaman, W.: Right-sided diverticula as a cause of acute renal hemorrhage, N. Engl. J. Med. 286:450, 1972.
22. Casarella, W., Galloway, S., Taxin, R., et al.: "Lower" gastrointestinal tract hemorrhage: New concepts based on arteriography, Am. J. Roentgenol. 121:357, 1974.
23. Eisenberg, H., Laufer, I., and Skillman, J.: Arteriographic diagnosis and management of suspected colonic diverticular hemorrhage, Gastroenterology 64:1091, 1973.
24. Patel, H., Chawla, K., Chawla, S., et al.: Massive rectal hemorrhage from right-sided colonic diverticula, Am. J. Gastroenterol. 66:76, 1976.
25. Ho, K.: Hemorrhagic diverticulosis: Demonstration of source of bleeding – Letter to the editor, Arch. Pathol. Lab. Med. 101:106, 1977.
26. Vega, J., and Lucas, C.: Selective angiography – inadequate guide for surgery in bleeding colonic diverticula, Arch. Surg. 111:913, 1976.
27. Grieske, J., Kahn, P., and Moran, J.: Arterial ligation for control of colonic diverticular hemorrhage, J.A.M.A. 217:1100, 1971.
28. Athanasoulis, C., Baum, S., Rosch, J., et al.: Mesenteric arterial infusions of vasopressin for hemorrhage from colonic diverticulosis, Am. J. Surg. 129: 212, 1975.
29. Havia, T.: Diverticulosis of the colon – A clinical and histological study, Acta Chir. Scand. (Suppl.) 415:7, 1971.
30. Klein, R., and Gallagher, D.: Massive bleeding from diverticular disease, Am. J. Surg. 118:553, 1969.
31. McGuire, H., Jr., and Haynes, B., Jr.: Massive hemorrhage from diverticulosis of the colon: Guidelines for therapy based on bleeding patterns in fifty cases, Ann. Surg. 175:847, 1972.
32. Olsen, W.: Hemorrhage from diverticular disease of the colon: The role of emergency subtotal colectomy, Am. J. Surg. 115:247, 1968.
33. Taylor, F., and Epstein, L.: Treatment of massive diverticular hemorrhage, Arch. Surg. 98:505, 1969.
34. Rigg, B., and Ewing, M.: Current attitudes on diverticulitis with particular reference to colonic bleeding, Arch. Surg. 92:321, 1966.
35. Baum, S., Athanasoulis, C., and Waltman, A.: Angiographic diagnosis and control of large bowel bleeding, Dis. Colon Rectum 17:447, 1974.
36. Ramanath, H., and Hinshaw, J.: Management and mismanagement of bleeding colonic diverticula, Arch. Surg. 103:311, 1971.
37. Drapanas, T., Pennington, D., Kappelman, M., et al.: Emergency subtotal colectomy: Preferred approach to management of massively bleeding diverticular disease, Ann. Surg. 177:519, 1973.
38. Jensen, G.: Massive hemorrhage from diverticulosis of the colon, Am. J. Surg. 95:813, 1958.
39. Sorger, K., and Wacks, M.: Exsanguinating arterial bleeding associated with diverticular disease of the colon, Arch. Surg. 102:9, 1971.
40. Nusbaum, M., and Baum, S.: Radiographic demonstration of unknown sites of gastrointestinal bleeding, Surg. Forum 14:374, 1963.
41. Nusbaum, M., Baum S., Blakemore, W., et al.: Demonstration of intra-abdominal bleeding by selective arteriography: Visualization of celiac and mesenteric arteries, J.A.M.A. 191:389, 1965.
42. Baum, S., Nusbaum, M., Blakemore, W., et al.: The preoperative radiographic demonstration of intra-abdominal bleeding from undetermined sites by percutaneous selective celiac and superior mesenteric arteriography, Surgery 58:797, 1965.
43. Kanter, I., Schwartz, A., and Fleming, R.: Localization of bleeding point in chronic and acute hemorrhage by means of selective visceral arteriography, Am. J. Roentgenol. 103:386, 1968.
44. Koehler, P., and Salmon, R.: Angiographic localization of unknown acute gastrointestinal bleeding sites, Radiology 89:244, 1967.
45. Baum, S., Nusbaum, M., Clearfield, H., et al.: Angiography in the diagnosis of gastrointestinal bleeding, Arch. Intern. Med. 119:16, 1967.
46. Reuter, S., and Bookstein, J.: Angiographic localization of gastrointestinal bleeding, Gastroenterology 54:876, 1968.
47. Nusbaum, M., Baum, S., Kuroda, K., et al.: Control of portal hypertension by selective mesenteric drug infusion, Arch. Surg. 97:1005, 1968.
48. Rosch, J., Gray, R., Grollman, J., et al.: Selective arterial drug infusions in the treatment of acute gastrointestinal bleeding, Gastroenterology 59:341, 1970.
49. Nusbaum, M., Baum, S., and Blakemore, W.: Clinical experience with the diagnosis and management of gastrointestinal hemorrhage by selective mesenteric catheterization, Ann. Surg. 170:506, 1969.
50. Baum, S., Rosch, J., Dotter, C., et al.: Selective

mesenteric arterial infusions in the management of massive diverticular hemorrhage, N. Engl. J. Med. 288:1269, 1973.
51. Baum, S., Athanasoulis, C., Waltman, A., et al.: Angiographic diagnosis and control. Part I of Gastrointestinal hemorrhage, Adv. Surg. 7:149, 1973.
52. Goldberger, L., and Bookstein, J.: Transcatheter embolization for treatment of diverticular hemorrhage, Radiology 122:613, 1977.
53. Goldstein, H., Medellin, H., Ben-Menachem, Y., et al.: Transcatheter arterial embolization in the management of bleeding in the cancer patient, Radiology 115:603, 1975.
54. Cho, K., and Reuter, S.: Embolic control of superior mesenteric artery hemorrhage caused by abdominal abscess, Am. J. Roentgenol. 128:1041, 1977.
55. Bookstein, J., and Goldstein, H.: Successful management of post-biopsy fistula with selective arterial embolization, Radiology 109:535, 1973.
56. Gold, R., and Grace, D.: Gelfoam embolization of the left gastric artery for bleeding ulcer: Experimental considerations, Radiology 116:575, 1975.
57. Newton, T., and Adams, J.: Angiographic demonstration and non-surgical embolization of spinal cord angioma, Radiology 91:873, 1968.
58. Ring, E., Athanasoulis, C., Waltman, A., et al.: Arteriographic management of hemorrhage following pelvic fracture, Radiology 109:65, 1973.
59. Rosch, J., Dotter, C., and Brown, M.: Selective arterial embolization: A new method for control of acute gastrointestinal bleeding, Radiology 102:303, 1972.
60. Sokoloff, J., Wickbom, I., and McDonald, D., et al.: Therapeutic percutaneous embolization in intractable epistaxis, Radiology 111:285, 1974.
61. Stanley, R., and Cubillo, E.: Nonsurgical treatment of arteriovenous malformations of the trunk and limb by transcatheter embolization, Radiology 115:609, 1975.
62. Bockis, J., and Moffat, D.: The intrinsic blood vessels of the pelvic colon, J. Anat. 92:52, 1958.
63. Griffiths, J.: Extramural and intramural blood supply of the colon, Br. Med. J. 1:323, 1961.
64. Ross, J.: Vascular patterns of small and large intestine compared, Br. J. Surg. 39:330, 1952.
65. Stanley, R., and Wise, L.: Arteriography in diagnosis of acute gastrointestinal tract bleeding, Arch. Surg. 107:138, 1973.
66. Ericsson, B.: Hemodynamic effects of vasopressin. An experimental study in normovolemic and hypovolemic anesthetized dogs, Acta Chir. Scand. (Suppl.)414:4, 1971.
67. Twiford, T., Granmayeh, M., and Tucker, M.: Gangrene of the feet associated with mesenteric intraarterial vasopressin, Am. J. Roentgenol. 130: 558, 1978.
68. Conn, H., Ramsby, G., and Storer, E.: Selective intra-arterial vasopressin in the treatment of upper gastrointestinal hemorrhage, Gastroenterology 63: 634, 1972.
69. Conn, H., Ramsby, G., Storer, E., et al.: Intra-arterial vasopressin in the treatment of upper gastrointestinal hemorrhage: A prospective, controlled clinical trial, Gastroenterology 68:211, 1975.
70. Beller, B., Trevino, A., and Urban, E.: Pitressin-induced myocardial injury and depression in a young woman, Am. J. Med. 51:675, 1971.
71. Renert, W., Button, K., Fuld, S., et al.: Mesenteric venous thrombosis and small-bowel infarction following infusion of vasopressin into the superior mesenteric artery, Radiology 102:299, 1972.
72. Roberts, C., and Maddison, F.: Partial mesenteric arterial occlusion with subsequent ischemic bowel damage due to pitression infusion, Am. J. Roentgenol. 126:829, 1976.
73. Berardi, R.: Vascular complications of superior mesenteric artery infusion with pitressin in treatment of bleeding esophageal varices, Am. J. Surg. 127:757, 1974.
74. Motsay, G., Sutherland, D., and Simmons, R.: Reversible pedal ischemia following intra-arterial infusion of vasopressin at a high dosage level required for control of massive bleeding from the small bowel: A case report, Ann. Surg. 178:648, 1973.
75. Barr, J., Lakin, R., and Rosch, J.: Similarity of arterial and intravenous vasopressin on portal and systemic hemodynamics, Gastroenterology 69:13, 1975.
76. Davis, G., Bookstein, J., and Hagan, P.: The relative effects of selective intra-arterial and intravenous vasopressin infusion, Radiology 120:537, 1976.
77. Davis, G., Bookstein, J., and Coel, M.: Advantage of intraarterial over intravenous vasopressin in gastrointestinal hemorrhage, Am. J. Roentgenol. 128: 733, 1977.
78. Naderi, M., and Bookstein, J.: Rectal bleeding secondary to fecal impaction: Angiographic diagnosis and treatment, Radiology 126:387, 1978.

Editor's Note.—A recent report implicates Gelfoam embolization, used in a patient with massive diverticular hemorrhage, as a cause of segmental left colon ischemia. In this patient, the catheter in the inferior mesenteric artery was advanced easily to the branch supplying the area of hemorrhage, and five 2×2-mm pieces of Gelfoam were embolized into the bleeding vessel. The leak was not seen on the postembolization angiogram. A barium enema 4 days following the angiogram showed a short, dilated hypotonic segment about 4 cm long in the descending colon corresponding to the site of the bleeding diverticulum. The patient was treated conservatively; however, 6 weeks after discharge a repeat barium enema showed a strictured area in the descending colon at the site of embolization. The authors conclude that "the risk of ischemia and infarction does not negate the fact that this procedure may be lifesaving in some patients with massive bleeding" (Mitty, H. A., Efremidis, S., and Keller, R. J.: Colonic stricture after transcatheter embolization for diverticular bleeding, Am. J. Roentgenol. 133:519, 1979).

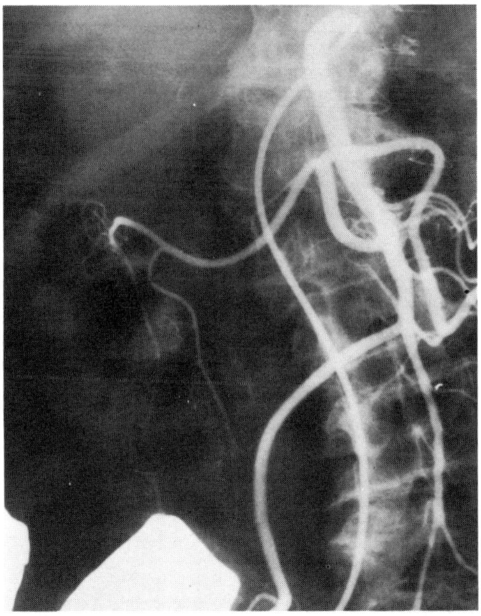

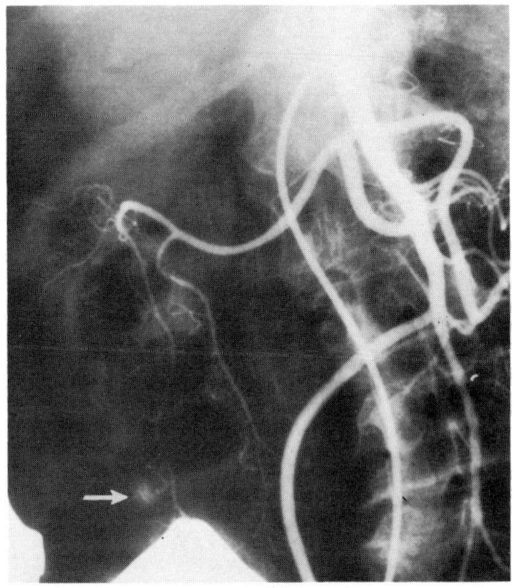

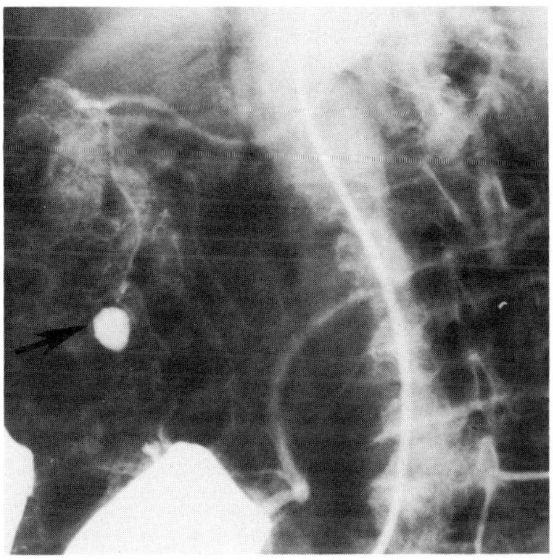

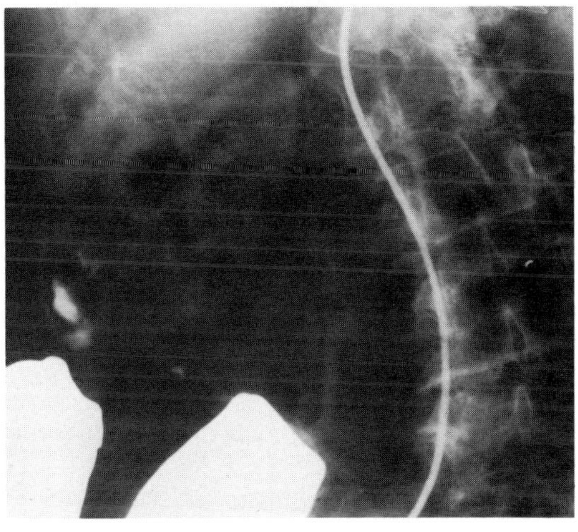

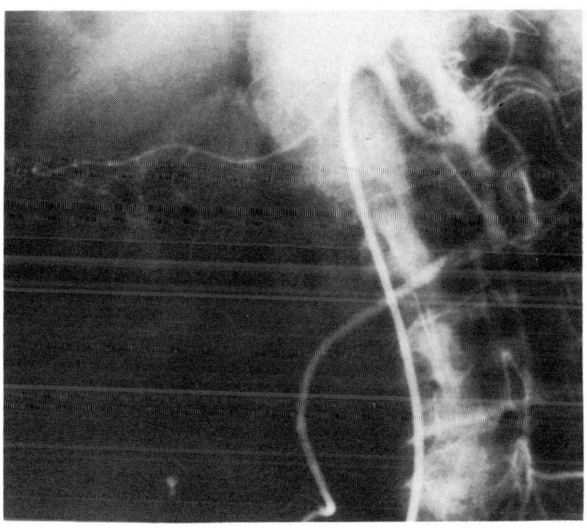

Fig 13–1 (top left). – Case 1: early arterial phase SMA injection. No evidence of extravasation.

Fig 13–2 (top right). – Case 1: film 1 second later shows early extravasation from branch of right colic artery *(arrow)*. Note stretching of branch over large diverticulum in ascending colon.

Fig 13–3 (center left). – Case 1: dense contrast extravasation now seen to be confined to diverticulum, giving characteristic appearance *(arrow)*.

Fig 13–4 (center right). – Case 1: during venous phase, extravasated contrast has spilled out of diverticulum and has begun to spread out in right colon.

Fig 13–5 (bottom left). – Case 1: repeat SMA injection after 20 minutes of vasopressin infusion into the SMA at 0.2 units per minute. Note marked constrictive effect of vasopressin in SMA and all its branches. Extravasation of contrast has ceased. Small dense collection in proximal ascending colon represents residue of barium from previous barium enema.

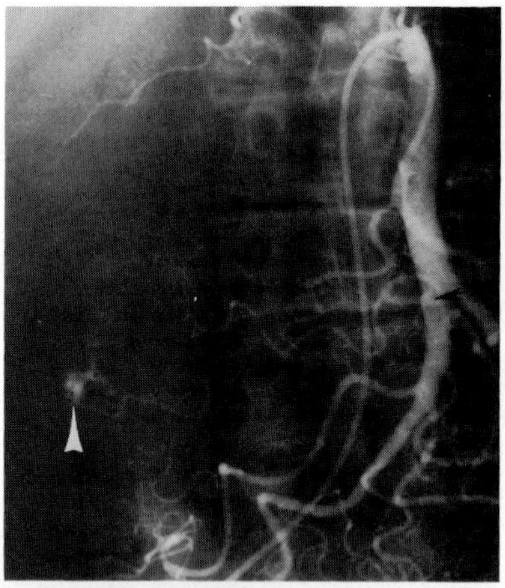

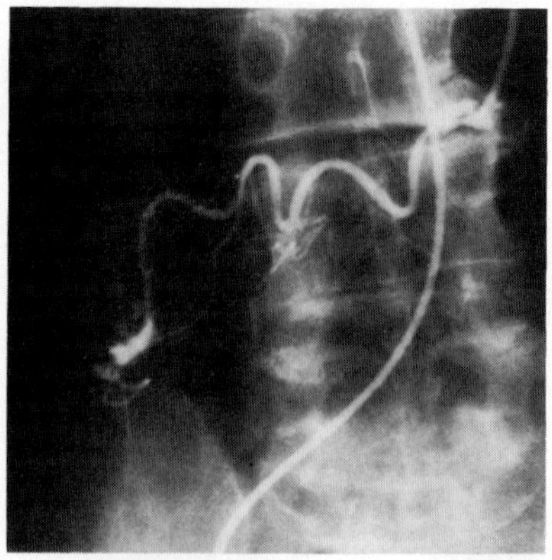

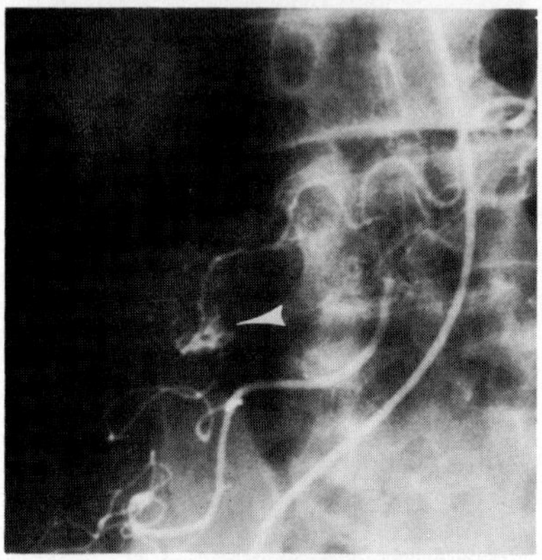

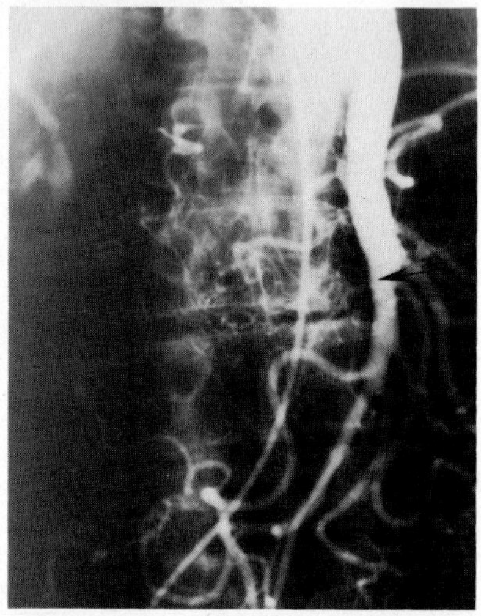

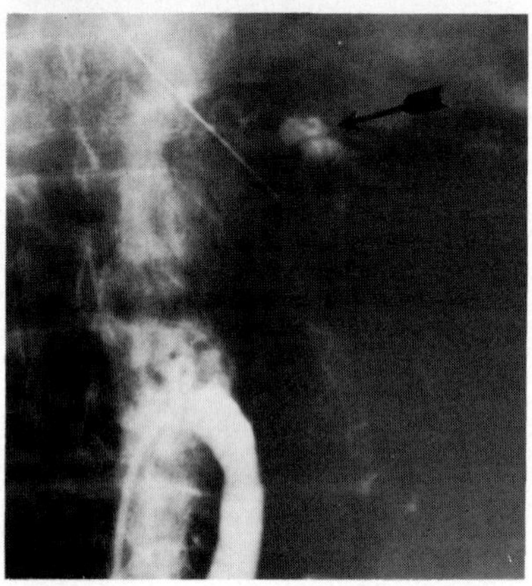

Fig 13–6 (top left).—Case 2: SMA injection during initial bleeding episode demonstrates typical diverticular hemorrhage from branch of right colic artery (*white arrowhead* indicates early extravasation; *black arrow* indicates origin of right colic artery). (From Goldberger, L., and Bookstein, J.: Radiology 122:615, 1977. Reproduced by permission of Radiological Society of North America, publisher.)

Fig 13–7 (top right).—Case 2: after SMA infusion of vasopressin failed to control hemorrhage, catheter was advanced into right colic artery; injection reveals persistent extravasation at distal end of right colic artery. (From Goldberger, L., and Bookstein, J.: Radiology 122:615, 1977. Reproduced with permission of Radiological Society of North America, publisher.)

Fig 13–8 (center left).—Case 2: repeat right colic injection after about 20 minutes of super-selective infusion of vasopressin at 0.4 units per minute. Bleeding has not stopped, although extravasation slowed *(arrowhead);* there is a marked vasoconstrictive effect of vasopressin infusion seen in right colic artery and its branches. Following this, embolization of right colic artery with 0.1 cc of Gelfoam was performed with immediate cessation of bleeding (not shown).

Fig 13–9 (center right).—Case 2: repeat SMA injection 10 months later at time of second lower gastrointestinal hemorrhage shows persistent occlusion of previously embolized right colic artery *(arrow).* No extravasation noted at this time and patient had clinically ceased bleeding. (From Goldberger, L., and Bookstein, J.: Radiology 122:615, 1977. Reproduced with permission of Radiological Society of North America, publisher.)

Fig 13–10 (bottom left).—Case 2: repeat SMA injection, later the same day when profuse rectal bleeding recurred, shows collection of extravasation in transverse colon diverticulum *(arrow).* Vasopressin failed to control bleeding and a right hemicolectomy, including the bleeding site, was performed. Note: surgical specimen contained portion of colon supplied by previously embolized right colic artery. No ischemic changes were noted. (From Goldberger, L., and Bookstein, J.: Radiology 122:615, 1977. Reproduced by permission of Radiological Society of North America, publisher.)

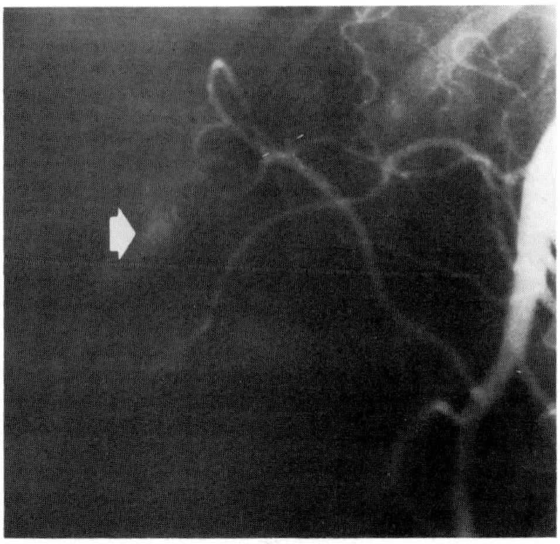

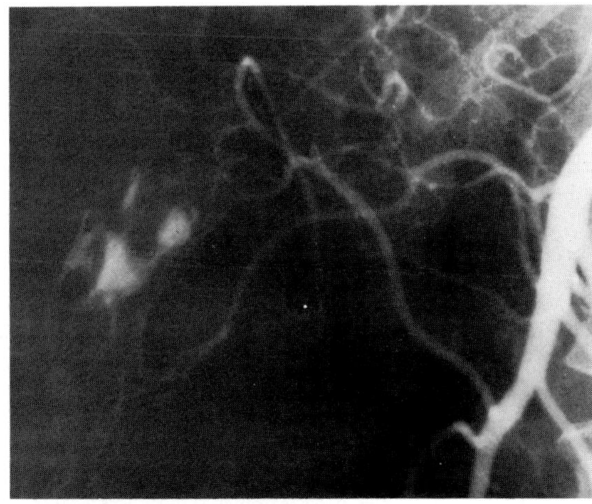

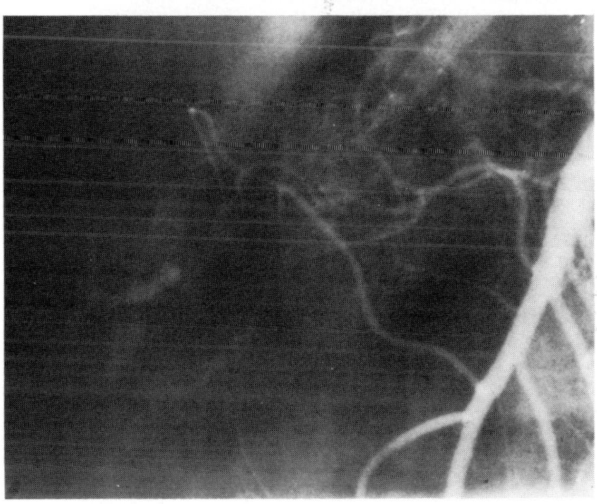

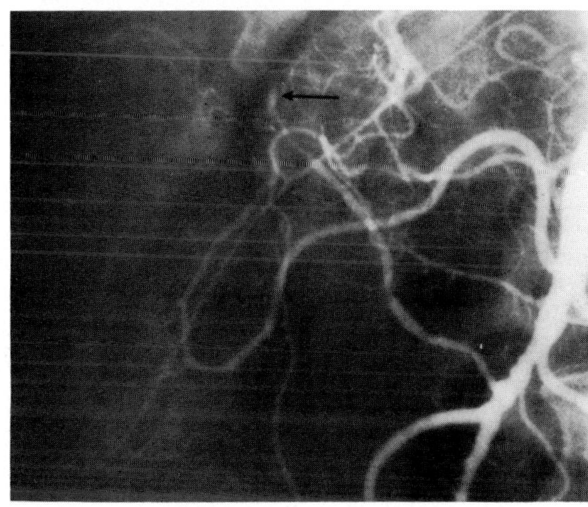

Fig 13–11 (top left).—Case 3: early film from SMA injection shows extravasation of contrast confined in large diverticulum in distal ascending colon *(arrow)*.

Fig 13–12 (top right).—Case 3: later arterial film from same injection shows pooling of contrast in diverticulum as well as spill of contrast beyond diverticulum into surrounding colon. (From Goldberger, L., and Bookstein, J.: Radiology 122:614, 1977. Reproduced with permission of Radiological Society of North America, publisher.)

Fig 13–13 (bottom left).—Case 3: repeat SMA injection following 20 minutes of vasopressin infusion at 0.4 units per minute. This shows mild vasoconstriction of branch vessels and continued, although somewhat diminished, extravasation. (From Goldberger, L., and Bookstein, J.: Radiology 122:614, 1977. Reproduced with permission of Radiological Society of North America, publisher.)

Fig 13–14 (bottom right).—Case 3: SMA injection after embolization of right colic artery with 0.2 cc of Gelfoam. *Arrow* points to opacified Gelfoam embolus. No further extravasation is seen. Beaded appearance of distal SMA is secondary to spasm from guidewire and catheter used to subselectively engage right colic artery for embolization procedure. (From Goldberger, L., and Bookstein, J.: Radiology 122:614, 1977. Reprinted with permission of Radiological Society of North America, publisher.)

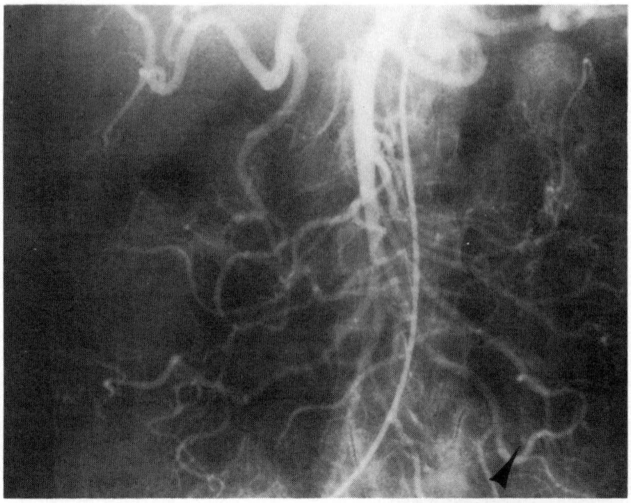

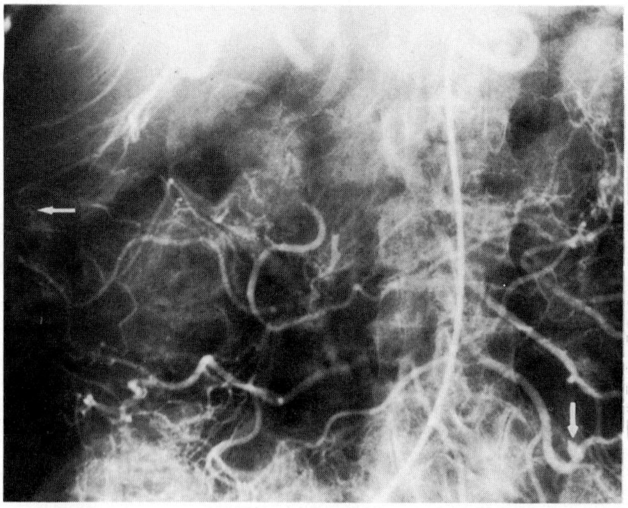

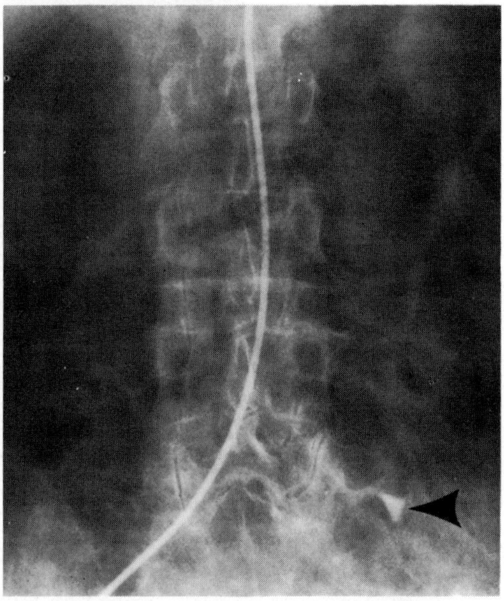

Fig 13–15 (top).—Case 4: early film from SMA injection. Extravasation is noted *(arrowhead)* as very faint triangular collection of contrast in region of distal transverse colon.

Fig 13–16 (bottom left).—Case 4: increasingly dense extravasation contained in irregularly shaped diverticulum *(vertical white arrow)*. Note also small arteriovenous malformation in region of hepatic flexure, as evidenced by irregular tangle of vessels and parallel simultaneous filming of artery and vein *(horizontal white arrow)*.

Fig 13–17 (bottom right).—Case 4: contrast remains in triangular diverticulum *(arrowhead)*, well beyond venous phase of injection. Patient had temporary control of bleeding with vasopressin infusion into the SMA at 0.2 units per minute. When bleeding recurred, patient was electively taken to surgery for partial colectomy. This procedure satisfactorily controlled bleeding, but patient died from postoperative cardiopulmonary complications.

DIVERTICULAR DISEASE OF THE RIGHT COLON

SAMUEL L. BERANBAUM, M.D.

DIVERTICULITIS OF THE CECUM was first described by Potier in 1912. Although much less common than in the sigmoid, diverticulitis of the right colon is not rare. The latter condition frequently is misdiagnosed and often mistreated. Many contributions on this subject have appeared in the surgical and gastroenterologic literature. Review articles date from Anderson's work in 1947[1] and include the reports of Greany and Snyder,[6] Vaughn and Narsete,[15] Lauridsen and Ross,[7] Nissenbaum et al.[11] and Asch and Markowitz.[2] The radiologic material is scanty despite the undisputed fact that the most reliable diagnostic aid is the barium enema examination.[3, 8, 12] Wolf[16] and associates[13] set forth some of the essential roentgenographic features of right-sided diverticulitis.

Right colon diverticulosis consists of two entities. (1) The first type starts in the left colon and progresses to the transverse and ascending portions of the colon. This type is initiated by a muscular dysfunction as a result of spasm, the degenerative process of aging and an increase in intraluminal pressure, eventuating in herniation of the mucosa at the site of vascular perforations where there is a locus of lesser resistance. (2) The second type consists of solitary or multiple diverticula of the cecum (or ascending colon). It is probably congenital, and at least 75% of cases are true diverticula, i.e., contain all the layers of the intestine. This type usually occurs in a younger age group and is close to the ileocecal valve – within 2 cm above or 1 cm below this level. It tends to be larger than other colonic diverticula and its complications require different surgical therapy.[5]

PLAIN FILM ROENTGENOGRAM

The plain film roentgenogram of the abdomen may be the only procedure available to the radiologist if immediate surgery is deemed necessary on clinical grounds.

The findings suggestive of diverticulitis are (1) a paracolic mass, (2) a calcified fecalith (Fig 13 – 18) and (3) a distended loop of the small bowel near the mass (Table 13 – 1). Although Nissenbaum et al.[11] state that one third of the cases are associated with fecalith, only one patient in our original series[4] had a calcified fecalith, and no other similar case has been encountered since publication in 1972. If this triad is noted in the right lower quadrant in a patient who has had an appendectomy, it is strongly indicative of diverticulitis. Since malrotation of the cecum is not an unusual occurrence, these findings may be seen in almost any area of the abdomen (Fig 13 – 19). Perforation may result in partial obliteration of the properitoneal fat

TABLE 13 – 1. – ROENTGEN FINDINGS IN DIVERTICULAR DISEASE OF RIGHT COLON

Plain film roentgenography
Paracolic mass or abscess (extraluminal gas)
Fecalith
Distended loop of small bowel ("sentinel loop")
Retroperitoneal abscess
Free air in abdomen
Barium enema examination
Transverse ridging
Spiculations "pointing toward" abscess
Limited distensibility and extensibility of colonic lumen
Asymmetric narrowing of lumen
No mucosal destruction in adjacent bowel
Paracolic mass, producing a contour defect
Extrinsic fixation usually limited to one wall of bowel
Other diverticula, proximal or distal to abscess
Fistula (uncommon)
Displacement of adjacent organs
Extraluminal gas
Air contrast study – limited distensibility and extensibility of colonic lumen
Angiography
Bleeding site
Hyperemia
Absence of tumor vessels
Extent of granulation tissue

line with localized intraperitoneal fluid similar to that seen in appendicitis. Small collections of extraluminal gas are practically diagnostic of inflammatory disease (diverticular or appendicular). Free perforation of a right-sided diverticulum with pneumoperitoneum is rare.

BARIUM ENEMA EXAMINATION

The barium enema examination is the most reliable procedure in diagnosis of diverticulitis. We prefer barium to water-soluble contrast agents provided the study is done with carefully controlled fluoroscopy.

A barium enema study without preparation in acute cases is not contraindicated in the absence of peritonitis and should be encouraged when appendicitis or right-sided diverticulitis is being considered in the clinical diagnosis. In spite of the difficulties relative to fecal defects, the appearance of the cecum, appendix and terminal ileum may be diagnostic. A barium-filled appendix usually excludes appendiceal pathology, whereas a nonvisualized appendix in the appropriate clinical setting is more suggestive of appendiceal than diverticular pathology. Figure 13–20 illustrates a rare exception to this concept, namely, an appendiceal abscess with a barium-filled appendix.

In order to make a roentgen diagnosis of right-sided diverticulitis, demonstration of a complication of colonic diverticula is essential. Eccentric mural defects, paracolic masses, fistulas or other signs of inflammation must be demonstrated. When the cecum is maximally distended with barium, the lesion may be seen as a localized discrete, eccentric, extracolonic, extramucosal indentation. The contour defect is produced by extrinsic pressure of the paracolic mass adjacent to or attached to the serosal surface or its mesentery. The mucosa is intact. The folds are transverse and crowded and may be edematous. The defect has a wide base and no overhanging edge or tumorous nodulation.

The diseased diverticulum usually is not identified, since it has been obliterated. It is localized in the center of the mass. The closed diverticulum may appear as a spicule. Adjacent diverticula may be seen with variable distortion, and there is obliteration or edema of the properitoneal fat line. The involved wall and adjacent area show limited distensibility (Figs 13–21 to 13–25). Fluoroscopic and roentgenographic technique is most important. The mass may be detectable in only one position. Gravity may help to demonstrate the defects and so decubitus and upright films are routinely employed regardless of whether one uses single contrast or pneumocolon technique (Fig 13–26).

In our original series, the paracolic mass was slightly more frequent on the medial than on the lateral aspect of the right colon.

The intact mucosal folds are puckered and may assume different degrees of pleating or spiculation depending on the position of the patient and extent of filling of the colon. A certain degree of variability is noted fluoroscopically and radiographically, the spikes pointing toward or converging toward the abscess (Fig 13–27). By contrast, extramucosal mural malignant disease owing to metastases produces a more fixed, rigid type of pleating, with shortening of the longitudinal extent of the wall, and the spikes diverge or radiate away from the center of the mass.

Eccentricity is a major diagnostic criterion favoring diverticular versus appendiceal abscess (Fig 13–28, A). If the inflammatory involvement is circumferential, it indicates an abscess surrounding the viscus and is more likely to be secondary to appendiceal disease (see Fig 13–28, B). Such an appearance is less likely in right-sided diverticulitis.

Caput coli changes offer important clues in diagnosis. Eccentric contour defects with or without spiculation may be noted and are frequently associated with functional disturbances. Emptying of the caput is often bizarre with irregular thickened folds. The terminal ileum may be involved by any inflammatory process in the vicinity and thus may superficially mimic granulomatous ileitis.

Extraluminal gas (see Fig 13–27, B) practically assures the diagnosis of inflammatory disease, although rarely a perforated carcinoma may show similar findings. Appendiceal abscess, diverticular abscess, foreign body perforation or an abscess from some other location tracking down (e.g., duodenal ulcer or gallbladder) must all be considered in the differential diagnosis. The extraluminal gas is often minimal and difficult to detect and must be searched for diligently. A black radiolucent smudge within the center of the mass rather than discrete bubbles may be the only clue.

Functional change in or adjacent to an area of diverticulitis of the right colon may involve both the large and small intestines. Irritability, spasm, thickened haustra and eccentric transverse ridging are often seen. At the site of inflammation, the colon cannot elongate completely so that it becomes foreshortened on that wall owing to fixation and spasm (Fig 13–29).

Small extracolonic abscesses may easily be overlooked. A local area of transverse ridging with spiking (Fig 13–30, A) may be the only manifestation. A somewhat larger area of involvement is seen in Figure 13–30, with evidence of an obliterated diverticulum in the center associated with stretching and pressure on the adjacent diverticula. After resolution of such a process, diverticula may be seen. This suggests that adjacent diverticula were temporarily occluded by the mass but not affected by the inflammation. The responsible diverticulum is seen only on rare occasions after complete resolution.

Diverticular disease may mask a tumor. All filling defects must be explained, both mucosal and extramucosal. The most important criterion in differentiation of carcinoma from diverticulitis is the normal intact mucosa in the latter. A pericolic mass may at times simulate the abrupt shelving of carcinoma. A hypotonic study with Glucagon may be of value. Intussusception due to tumor, either benign or malignant, may accompany right-sided diverticulosis (Fig 13–31). This has not been seen in left-sided diverticulosis. If diverticulitis is present, fixation prevents intussusception.

Difficulties in differentiation of tumor from diverticulitis may be just as great in the right colon as in the left. One patient demonstrated this problem most graphically. He was treated conservatively while on vacation in England, based on a clinical diagnosis of subsiding appendicitis. A barium enema performed several weeks after the initial attack revealed diverticular disease with marked spasticity and irritability. Spot filming only in the correct obliquity revealed the presence of a tumor, which was confirmed with contrast technique. At surgery a 2 cm carcinoma was found with liver metastases (Fig 13–32).

AIR CONTRAST STUDY

The air contrast examination is not contraindicated in diverticulitis except in fulminating cases. This is true when performed as a second examination after postevacuation from a barium enema or as a single primary procedure in a pneumocolon study. It presents a better opportunity for evaluation of the affected segment of the bowel with regard to distensibility and contour of the affected wall. It affords confirmation of the findings elicited from the barium study. In addition, it may demonstrate an unsuspected tumor.

Differentiation from primary carcinoma is difficult in those cases of concurrent disease, since the spasticity may obscure an adjacent neoplasm. In diverticulitis the mucosa is intact. Mucosal destruction, tumor nodule, rigidity and absence of distensibility or extensibility are all hallmarks of malignant disease but at times are difficult to elicit. Circumferential narrowing with partial shelving, as in sigmoidal diverticulitis, rarely presents a major problem requiring hypotonic study for differentiation. This usually is not necessary probably because of the wider lumen of the right colon.

Summary

The problems of right-sided diverticular disease are similar to those of left-sided diverticular disease, the variations in features resulting from location. Recognition of the complications and differentiation from appendiceal disease and neoplasia are the most important considerations.

REFERENCES

1. Anderson, L.: Acute diverticulitis of cecum, Surgery 22:479, 1947.
2. Asch, M. J., and Markowitz, A. M.: Cecal diverticulitis: Report of 16 cases and review of literature, Surgery 65:906, 1969.
3. Bahabozorgni, S., Demuth, W. E., and Blakemore, W. S.: Diverticulitis of ascending colon, Am. J. Surg. 115:295, 1968.
4. Beranbaum, S. L., Zausner, J., and Lane, B.: Diverticular disease of the right colon, Am. J. Roentgenol. 115:334, 1972.
5. Fleischner, F. G.: *Diverticular Disease and Irritable Colon,* Margulis, A. R., and Burhenne, H. J. (eds): (St. Louis: C. V. Mosby Co., 1967, pp. 784–810.
6. Greany, E. M., and Snyder, W. H.: Acute diverticulitis of cecum encountered at emergency surgery, Am. J. Surg. 94:270, 1957.
7. Lauridsen, J., and Ross, F. P.: Acute diverticulitis of cecum, Arch. Surg. 64:320, 1952.
8. Localio, A. S., and Stahl, W. M.: Diverticular disease of alimentary tract; 1. Colon, Curr. Probl. Surg., Dec. 1967.
9. Miangolarra, C. J.: Diverticulitis of right colon, Am. J. Surg. 153:861, 1961.
10. Milburn, L. F.: Massive hemorrhage and solitary cecal diverticulum, Georgetown Med. Bull. 17:107, 1963.
11. Nissenbaum, J., Sparks, A. J., and Ellison, G. R.: Cecal diverticulum; report of case diagnosed by roentgen ray and surgically proven; review of original literature, Am. J. Roentgenol. 73:596, 1955.
12. Parks, T. G., and Connell, A. M.: Comparative study of radiological and clinical findings in diverticular disease of colon, Gut 10:414, 1969.
13. Schapira, A., Leichtling, J. J., Wolf, B. S., Marshak, R. H., and Janowitz, H. D.: Diverticulitis of cecum and right colon: Clinical and radiographic features, Am. J. Dig. Dis. 3:351, 1958.
14. Seaman, W. B.: Colon: Old problems, new concepts, Radiology 100:251, 1971.
15. Vaughn, A. M., and Narsete, E. M.: Diverticulitis of cecum, Arch. Surg. 65:763, 1952.
16. Wolf, B. S.: Roentgen findings in diverticulitis of right side of colon, Mt. Sinai J. Med. NY 23:697, 1956.

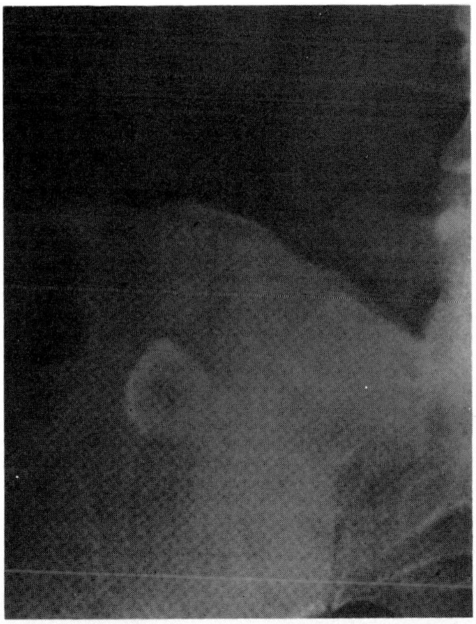

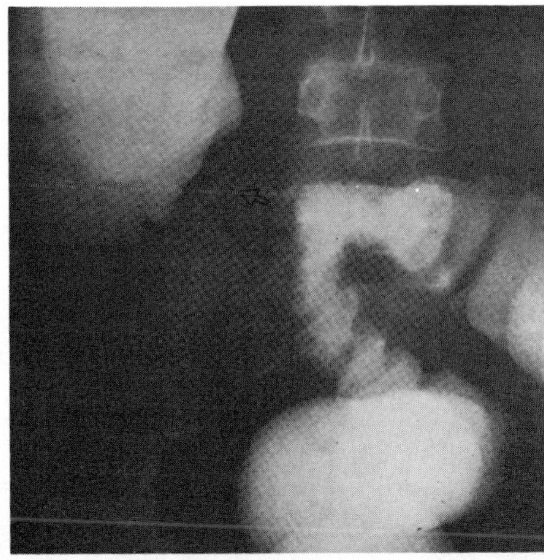

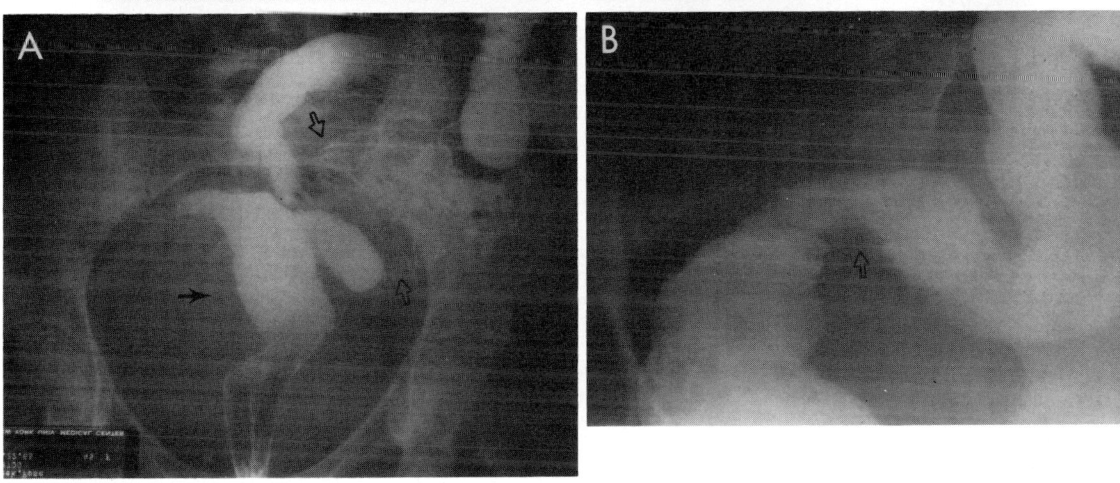

Fig 13–18 (top left).—Right lower quadrant calcification in patient with recurrent abdominal pain, weight loss and history of previous appendectomy. At surgery, a 3 cm inflammatory mass was found originating from narrowed cecal diverticulum containing calcified fecalith. (From Beranbaum et al., Am. J. Roentgenol. 115:334, 1972, with permission.)

Fig 13–19 (bottom).—**A,** postevacuation roentgenogram shows malrotation with entire colon in left side of abdomen. Cecum is above sigmoid (between *open arrows*). Right pelvic mass indents rectosigmoid (*closed arrow*). No diverticula are seen. **B,** oblique exposure. Pelvic mass compresses anterior aspect of rectum *(arrow)*. Note spiking of mucosal folds. At surgery, ruptured cecal diverticulum was found with right pelvic abscess. Terminal ileum was above and to right of cecum.

Fig 13–20 (top right).—Barium enema examination showed an opacified appendix, barely visible on this film, but better defined on other films. Note inflammatory changes in sigmoid with haustral abnormalities and indentation defect consistent with a pelvic abscess, which at surgery was found to be due to perforation of tip of appendix *(arrow)*.

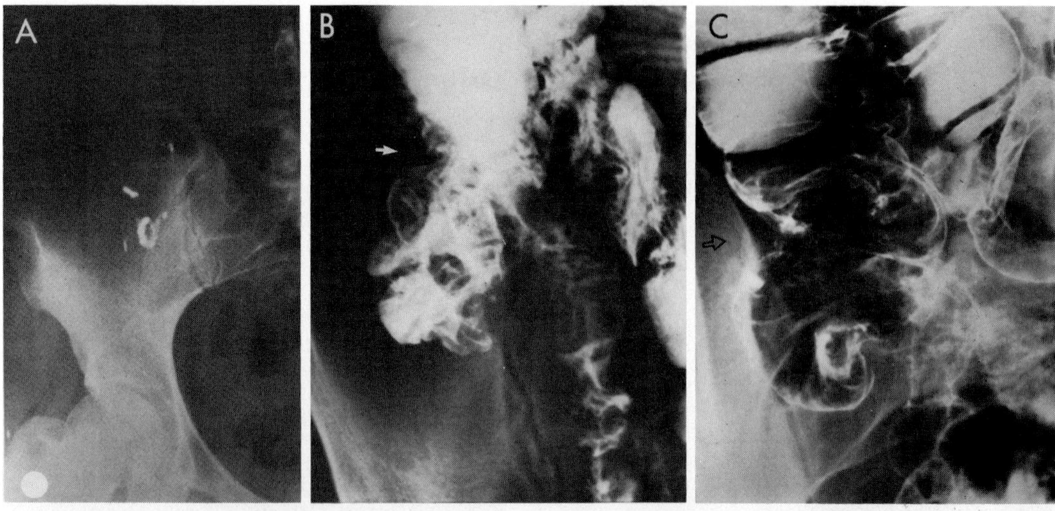

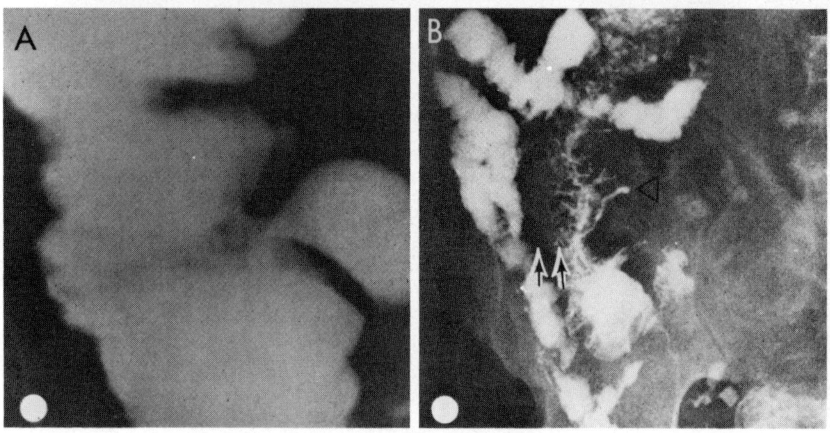

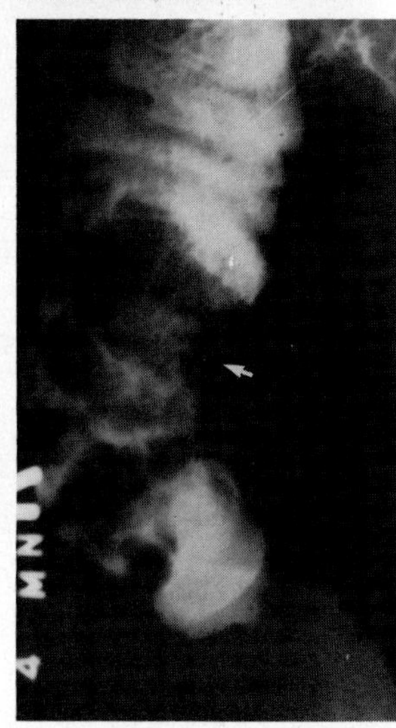

Fig 13–21 (top).—**A,** preliminary roentgenogram shows stasis of barium in irregularly filled appendix from barium enema performed 1 week earlier. Diagnosis of granulomatous disease of terminal ileum and cecum made at that time. **B,** barium-filled study shows laterally located paracolic mass *(arrow)* and cecum which is irritable and incompletely filled. Appendix is partially invaginated and adherent to cecum with tip directed to the mass. No diverticula are demonstrated. Terminal ileum is normal. **C,** double contrast study demonstrates distensibility of walls of cecum, lateral paracolic mass *(arrow)* and partially invaginated appendix. Roentgen diagnosis of appendiceal abscess was made. At surgery an abscess was found, as described, and pathologically proved to be due to ruptured diverticulum.

Fig 13–22 (bottom left).—**A,** cecal spot roentgenogram with filling of normal terminal ileum and appendix. An isolated diverticulum on medial aspect of ascending colon above ileocecal valve is smooth in outline with no sign of inflammatory disease. Lumen of ascending colon is constricted, with irregular lateral border (decreased distensibility). **B,** postevacuation roentgenogram. Laterally located ileum is displaced by abscess *(double arrows)* away from margin of ascending colon. Colonic mucosal folds are coarsened and irregular but not destroyed. Medially located isolated diverticulum is undisturbed *(open arrow).* At surgery, diverticular abscess found indenting lateral surface.

Fig 13–23 (bottom right).—Postevacuation roentgenogram. Fairly large diverticular abscess was found at surgery. Barium enema study was read preoperatively as entirely normal. Retrospectively, the only abnormality is indentation *(arrow)* on medial aspect of cecum and ascending colon (in postevacuation roentgenogram). No detailed spot filming, decubitus, upright roentgenograms or air studies were obtained.

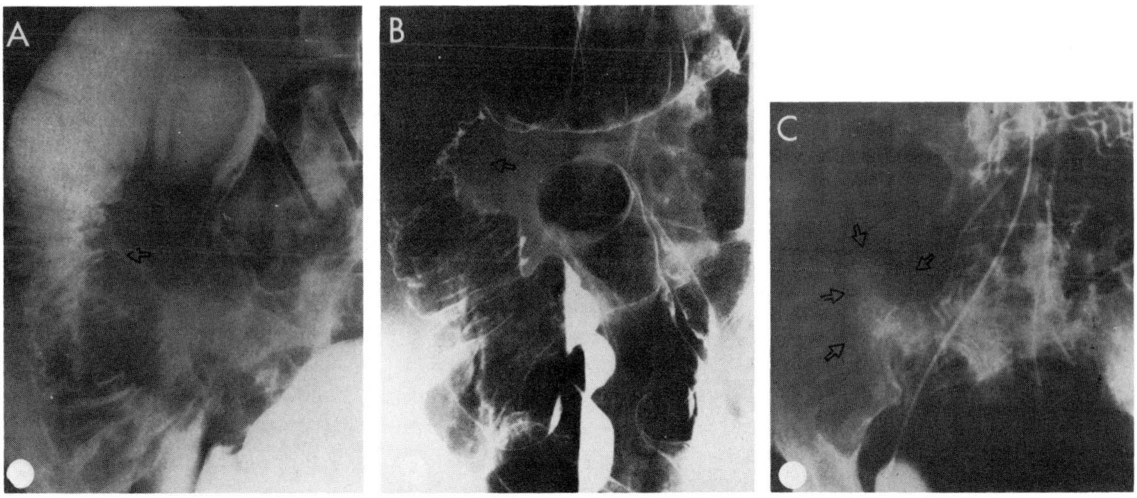

Fig 13–24.—**A,** supine barium air contrast study shows concavity *(arrow)* on medial aspect of mid-ascending colon, with spiculation. On original roentgenogram, smudge of extraluminal gas was noted. **B,** decubitus barium air contrast study demonstrates mass to better advantage *(arrow)* and indicates intact mucosa associated with spiculation. **C,** superior mesenteric angiogram shows mass with vascular blush *(arrows)*. At surgery a perforated right-sided diverticulitis was noted.

Fig 13–25.—Two different patients with medially located cecal diverticular abscess, proved surgically. **A,** double contrast study of cecum shows medial indentation by abscess. Gas-filled terminal ileum is displaced medially. Note very fine spiculations adjacent to abscess *(arrow)*. **B,** cecum is irregularly filled, and an indentation is noted on its medial aspect *(double arrows)*. The appendix is located on lateral aspect *(single arrow)*.

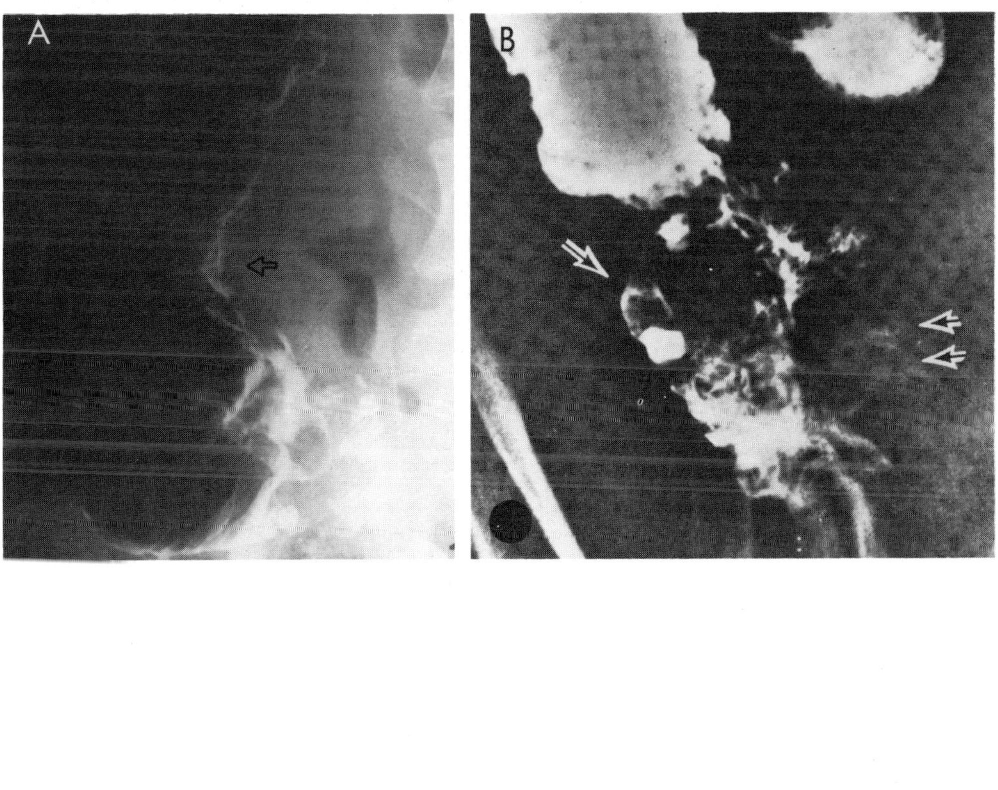

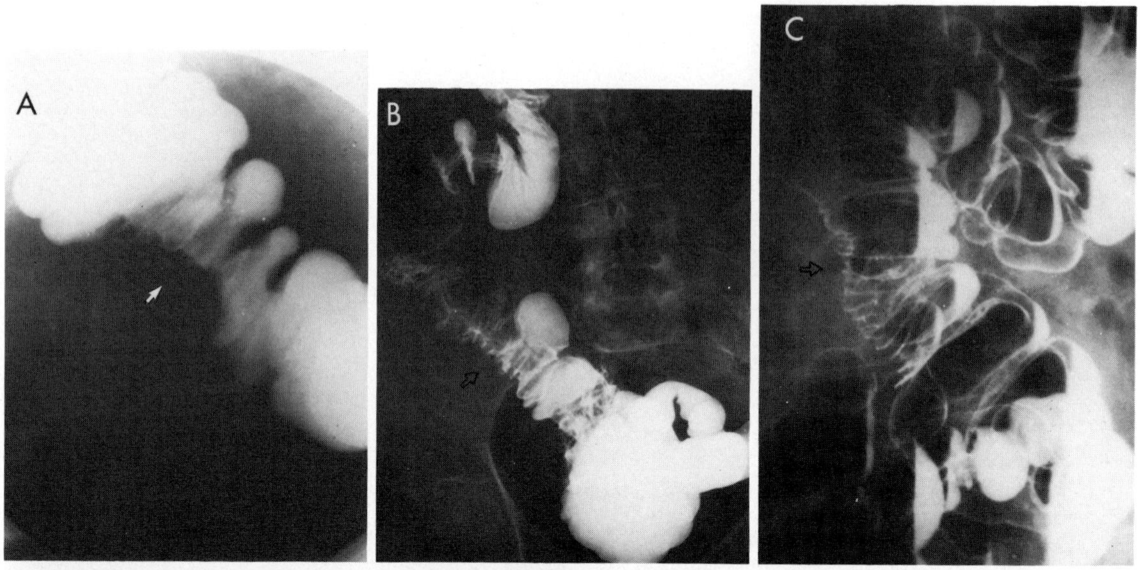

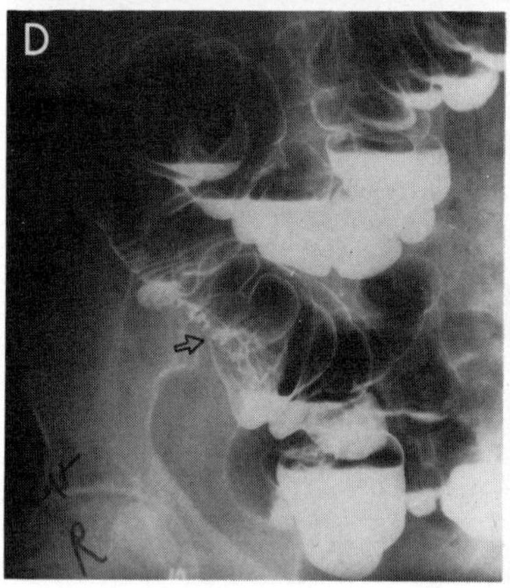

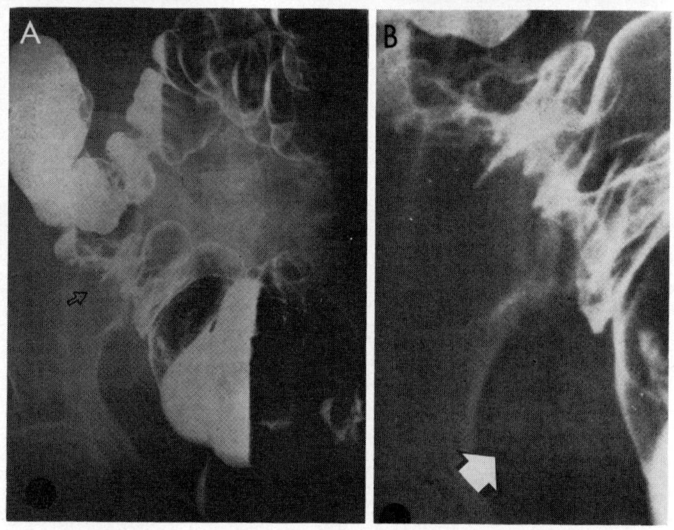

Fig 13–26 (top and **bottom left).** – Diverticular abscess of lateral aspect of ascending colon. **A,** barium-filled colon *(arrow).* **B,** postevacuation *(arrow).* **C,** decubitus *(arrow).* **D,** upright view *(arrow).* Note that spiculations and extent of disease stand out better on postevacuation study than on barium-filled study. Decubitus and upright films use gravity to aid in demonstration of mass effect.

Fig 13–27 (bottom right). – **A,** proved diverticular abscess on lateral aspect of ascending colon *(arrow),* with coarse spiculations best demonstrated on decubitus exposure. **B,** contact print of same case shows small bubbles of extraluminal gas *(arrow)* (better seen on original film).

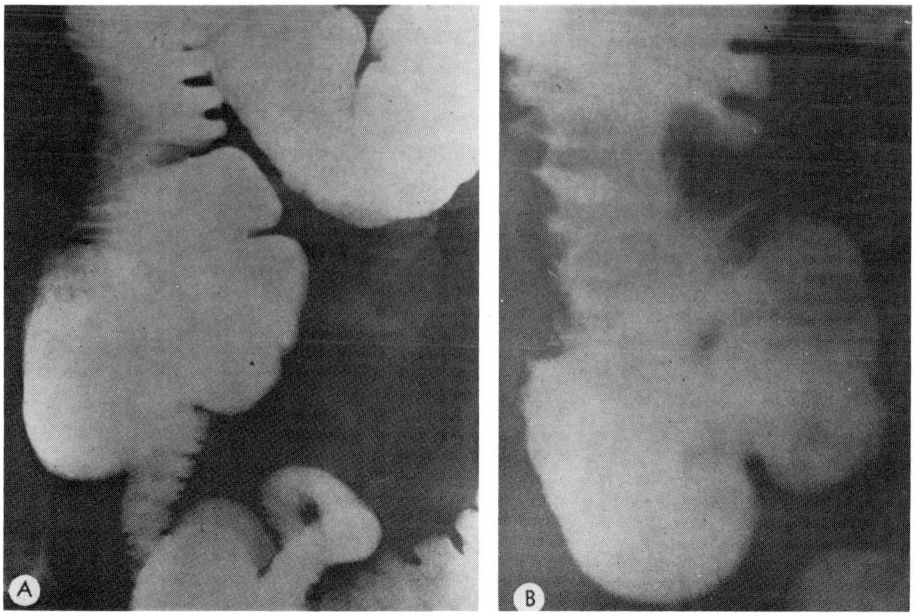

Fig 13–28.—**A,** diverticular abscess found at surgery, with paracolic mass noted at lateral aspect of ascending colon. Note spiculations and transverse ridgings. Indentation of caput coli with terminal ileum posterior and inferior indicates retrocecal appendix (found at surgery). Appendix was not involved. **B,** circumferential mass at ascending colon with mucosal edema and spiking. Similar indentation of caput coli due to retrocecal appendix, which had ruptured and produced abscess.

Fig 13–29.—**A** and **B,** right-sided diverticulitis may present as functional disturbance with eccentric thickened haustral pattern of varying degrees, as seen in two different patients with localized tenderness. No diverticula are seen.

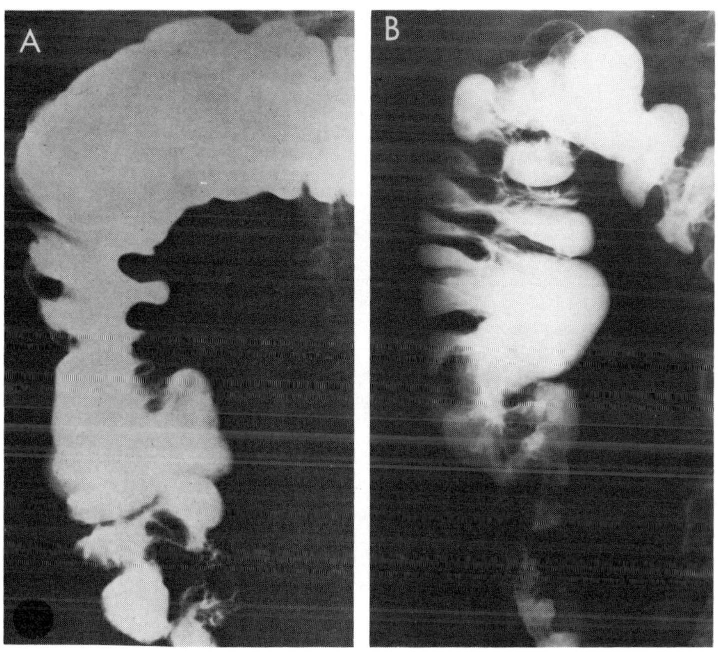

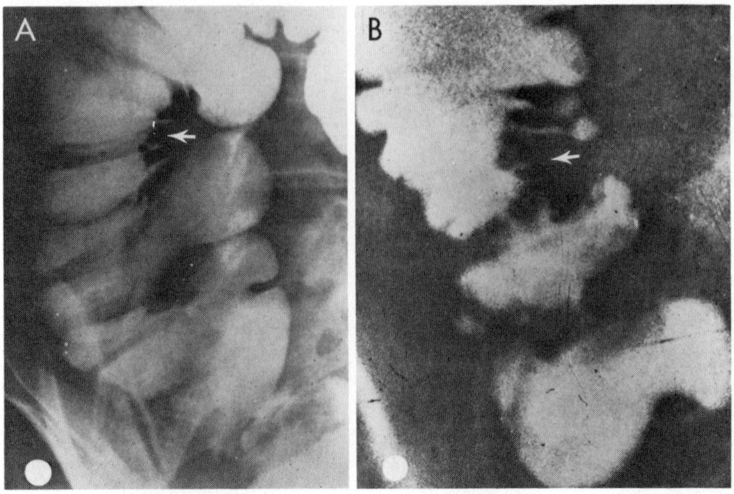

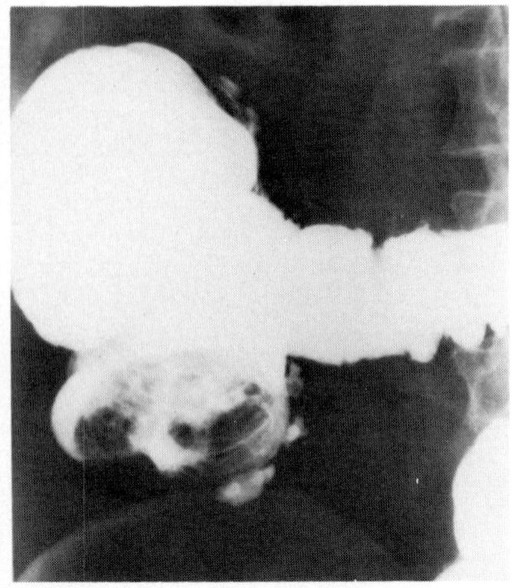

Fig 13–30 (left). – **A,** functional disturbance with spiculations, transverse ridging and lack of elongation of ascending colon *(arrow)*. No diverticula are noted. This patient improved on a medical regimen. Findings are probably ascribable to mild diverticulitis or inflammation of appendices epiploicae. **B,** similar findings in another patient treated medically but with a more definite paracolic mass *(arrow)* associated with diverticula.

Fig 13–31 (right). – Carcinoma of cecum with intussusception and diverticula nearby.

Fig 13–32. – **A,** neoplasm may mimic right-sided diverticulitis. Functional abnormality noted in sequential 70 mm spot filming with diverticula, spasm, incomplete filling and decreased distensibility of medial and lateral walls of ascending colon. **B,** diverticula with spasticity and thickened haustra on medial aspect. Filling defect at lateral aspect ascending colon was a 2 cm tumor *(arrow)*. **C,** Tumor *(arrows)* was confirmed on air study.

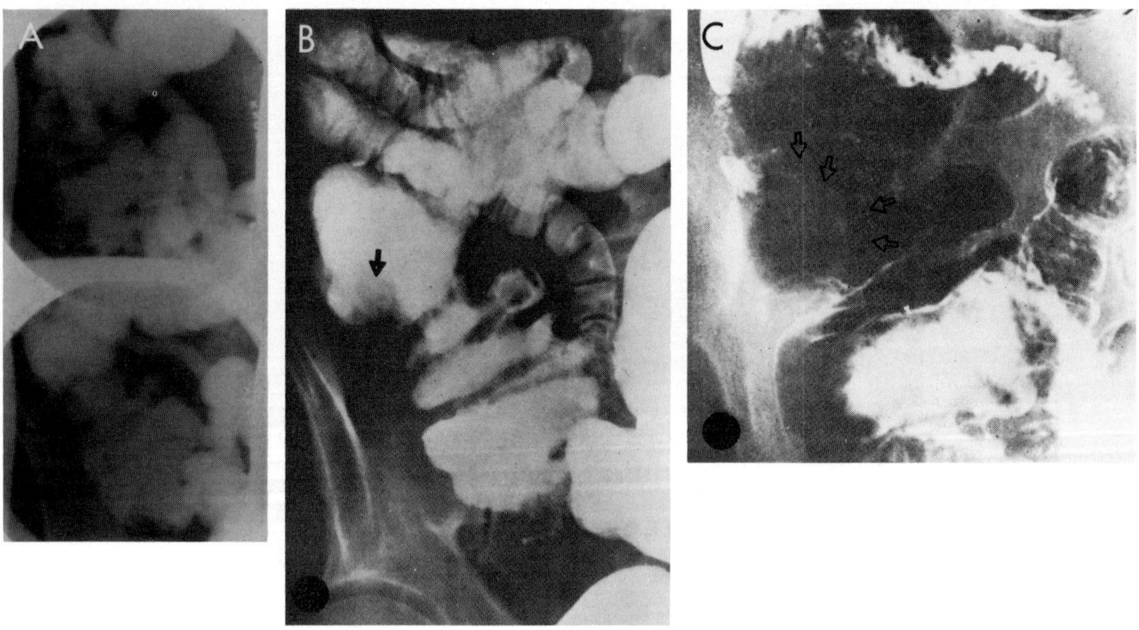

DIVERTICULAR DISEASE OF THE LEFT COLON

EDWARD I. GREENBAUM, M.D.

DIVERTICULA are most commonly found in the sigmoid, but they may occur anywhere in the colon. They represent herniations of the mucosa and submucosa through small defects in the muscularis at the point where vessels enter or leave. They are aligned along the margins of the tenia coli and appear as small flask-shaped sacs, usually 0.5 – 1 cm in diameter, with a slitlike or rounded mouth.[1]

When diverticula are single or few in number, there is no alteration in the haustral configuration. When they are numerous or massive, so much mucous membrane is absorbed in the formation of diverticula that very little is left over for the lining of the main channel. This causes the muscularis to be accordioned in appearance. The tightly crowded haustral folds and narrowed colonic channels, with the resultant sawtoothed appearance on barium enema, is solely a feature of diverticulosis (Fig 13 – 33). In a study of the resected specimens with the described radiographic configuration, Fleischner and Ming[2] concluded that the sawtoothed appearance on the roentgenogram was not correlated with the presence of diverticulitis in the pathologic specimen.

True diverticulitis is a micro- or macroperforation of a diverticulum into or beyond the wall of the colon, with spreading or extradiverticular inflammation. Occasionally, despite the clinical presentation of diverticulitis, the barium enema may be essentially normal (Fig 13 – 34). As the area of extracolonic inflammation increases and/or abscesses develop, the colon examination may reflect an extramucosal, extracolonic mass defect secondary to the abscess formation (Fig 13 – 35). Extracolonic extravasation of barium may be seen in diverticulitis, with complete scaling off at the site of perforation at a later date (Fig 13 – 36). Typically, the resultant inflammatory mass causes a long segmental area of narrowing, with preserved mucosal pattern and tapered margins and at least one or two diverticula in the immediate vicinity (Fig 13 – 37). A sinus tract may be seen extending outward from the area of diverticulitis, which may or may not communicate with the pericolic abscess (Figs 13 – 38 to 13 – 41). Sometimes a short intramural fistula is seen, and in this event careful differentiation from granulomatous colitis must be made (Fig 13 – 42).[3] The linear extent of the tract in diverticulitis is usually short, while the tracts in granulomatous colitis tend to be long, often exceeding 10 cm. Coloenteric (Fig 13 – 43), colovesicular (Fig 13 – 44), gastrocolic[4] (Fig 13 – 45) or colovaginal fistula (Fig 13 – 46) may develop.

Complete occlusion of the lumen may occur owing to the inflammation and spasm (Fig 13 – 47). In this event, 0.5 – 0.75 mg of glucagon by intravenous injection is recommended for relief of the spasm in order to demonstrate the channel and thus differentiate this process from a malignancy.[5] In some cases diverticulitis will mimic carcinoma radiographically (Fig 13 – 48). In other instances, diverticulitis will cause a chronic localized inflammatory change in the wall of the colon, producing an intramural mass that can easily be confused with intramural, extramucosal tumor (e.g., leiomyoma) (Fig 13 – 49). Diverticulitis might present on abdominal series as a large bowel obstruction[6] (Fig 13 – 50), but in other instances it may present as a mechanical small bowel obstruction. Certainly this possibility should be considered in every elderly patient presenting with a combination of small bowel obstruction and left lower quadrant pain[7] (Fig 13 – 51). Free perforation may occur with gross subdiaphragmatic air or in other instances, if the perforation is extraperitoneal, air may be seen under the diaphragm but will not move with changes in position.

There may be free peritonitis, which can easily be diagnosed with meglumine diatrizoate (Gastrografin) enema (Fig 13–52, A–C). With peritonitis, pus may extend along the pericolonic gutters to cause a subphrenic abscess (Fig 13–53).

Rectal diverticulitis with perforation (Fig 13–54) is rare but is extremely important, since several of the reported cases have been misdiagnosed as carcinoma resulting in unnecessary abdominal perineal resections.[8] Retrorectal perforation may be demonstrated by the filling of an abscess cavity with barium (Fig 13–55). Extension of the inflammatory process to the retroperitoneal space occasionally occurs. In one case, the presenting feature was fluctuant flank mass with an air-fluid level noted on the upright position. There was filling of this abscess cavity on barium examination of the colon (Fig 13–56).

Fistulas due to diverticulitis, right-sided diverticulitis and lower gastrointestinal hemorrhage secondary to diverticulosis are covered elsewhere in this chapter.

REFERENCES

1. Robbins, S. L.: *Textbook of Pathology* (1st ed.; Philadelphia: W. B. Saunders Co., 1957).
2. Fleischner, F. G., and Ming, S-C: Revised concepts on diverticular diseases of the colon, Radiology 84: 599, 1964.
3. Marshak, R. H., Lindner, A. E., Pochaczevsky, R., and Maklansky, D.: Longitudinal sinus tracts in granulomatous colitis and diverticulitis, Semin. Roentgenol. 11:101, 1976.
4. Ghahremani, G. G., Olsen, J.: Gastrocolic fistula secondary to diverticulitis of the splenic flexure, Dis. Colon Rectum, 17:98, 1974.
5. Gohel, V. K., Dalinka M. K., and Coren, G. S.: Hypotonic examination of the colon with glucagon, Radiology 115:1, 1975.
6. Love, L.: Large bowel obstruction, Semin. Roentgenol., 8:299, 1973.
7. Figiel, L. S., and Figiel, S. J.: Lesions of the large intestine producing acute symptoms, Radiol. Clin. North Am. 2:33, 1964.
8. Giustra, P. E., Root, J. A., and Killoran, P. J.: Rectal diverticulitis with perforation, Radiology 105:23, 1972.

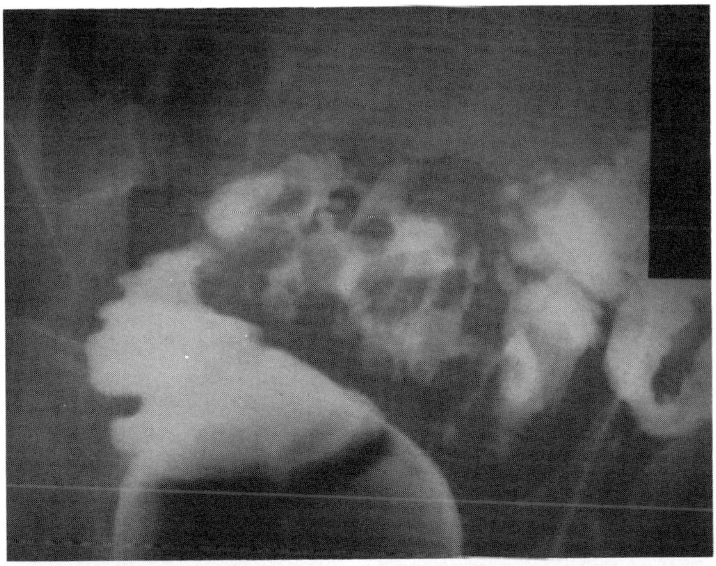

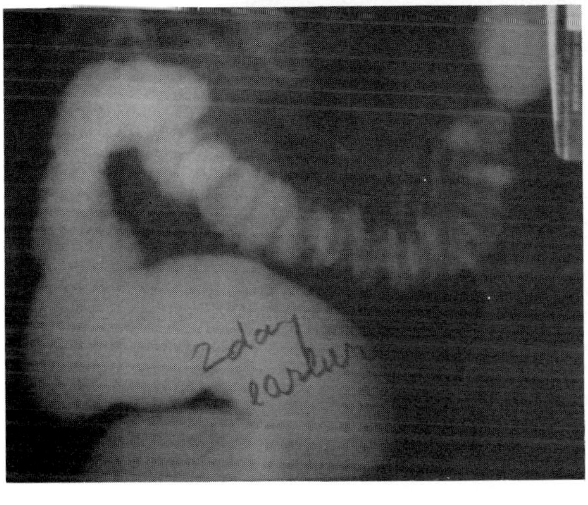

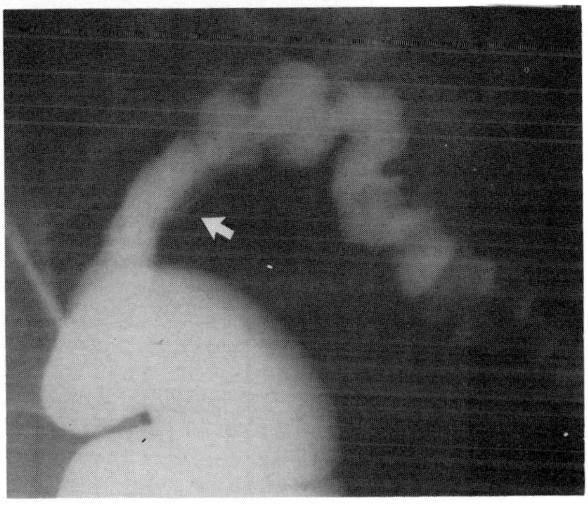

Fig 13–33 (top).—Diverticulosis presenting with tightly crowded haustral folds and narrowed colonic channel, creating sawtoothed appearance on barium enema. This is not a feature of diverticulitis.

Fig 13–34 (left).—Patient had clinical findings of diverticulitis, but colon examination was essentially normal with only scattered diverticula seen in sigmoid colon.

Fig 13–35 (right).—Repeat barium enema performed 2 days later on same patient as in Figure 13–34. Now there is evidence of extrinsic, extracolonic mass indenting rectosigmoid junction at its inferior surface *(arrow)*. The mass contained 150 cc of frank pus. This case demonstrates that a negative barium enema does not preclude presence of diverticulitis.

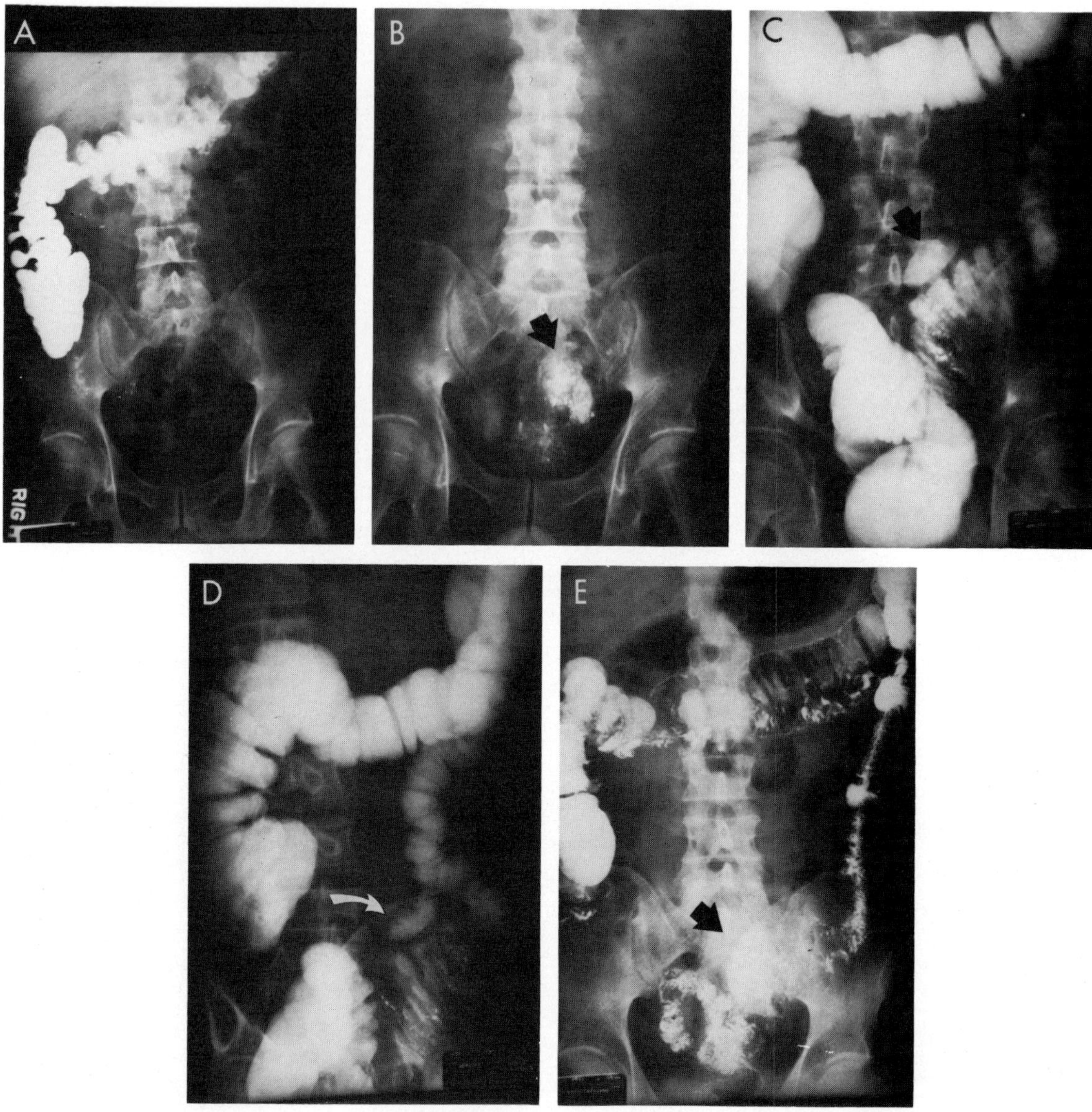

Fig 13–36. – **A,** diverticulitis presenting with generalized abdominal pain. Because of diffuse nature of patient's symptoms, an upper gastrointestinal examination was performed and a normal study was reported. Follow-up KUB revealed barium in right hemicolon with no residual barium in small bowel and no evidence of diverticulitis on plain film. **B,** KUB done 2 days later reveals abnormal collection of barium in left pelvis, amorphous and apparently extracolonic *(arrow).* This prompted the radiologist to be suspicious of diverticulitis and a barium was performed **(C–E).** This confirmed that amorphous collection of barium as seen on KUB (Fig B) was indeed extracolonic *(arrows)* and represented a prior perforated diverticulitis. Absence of extravasation of barium at time of BE examination indicated that perforation had sealed off. Had this colon examination been performed at this particular time there would have been no evidence of extravasation. And the diagnosis of diverticulitis would have been difficult to prove on radiologic grounds alone.

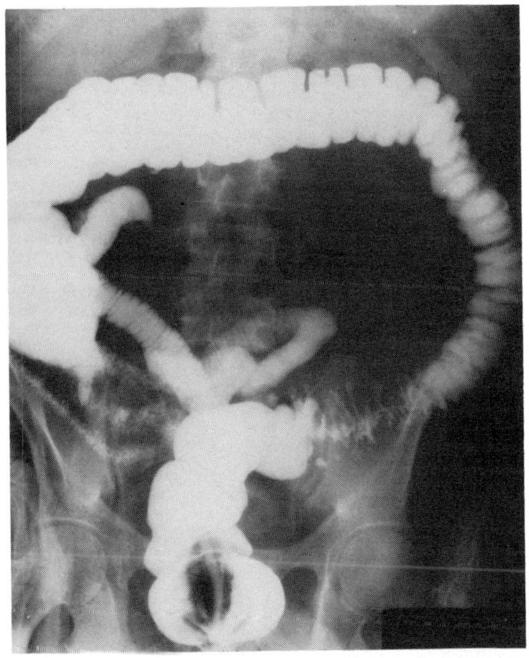

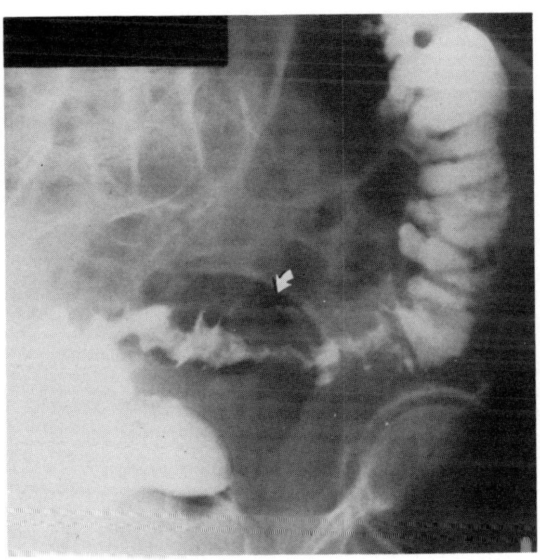

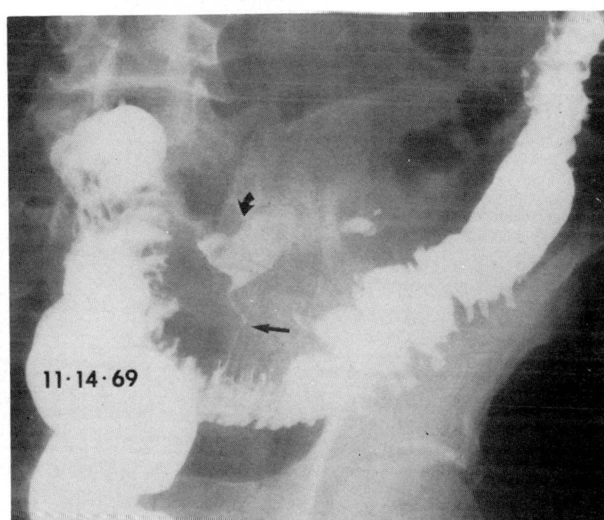

Fig 13–37 (top).—Typical appearance of diverticulitis with narrowing of long segment of colon usually in sigmoid with preserved mucosal pattern, tapered margins and scattered diverticuli in immediate vicinity.

Fig 13–38 (left).—Sigmoid diverticulitis *(arrow)* with sinus tract extending superiorly from its midportion.

Fig 13–39 (right).—Diverticulitis with fistulous communication to an abscess *(arrows)*, which fills with barium at time of examination.

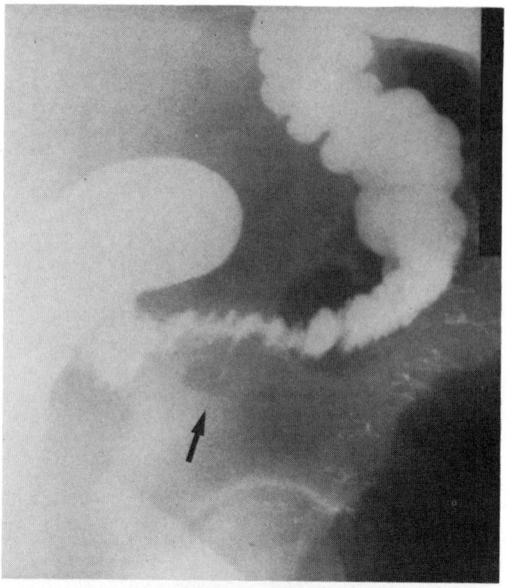

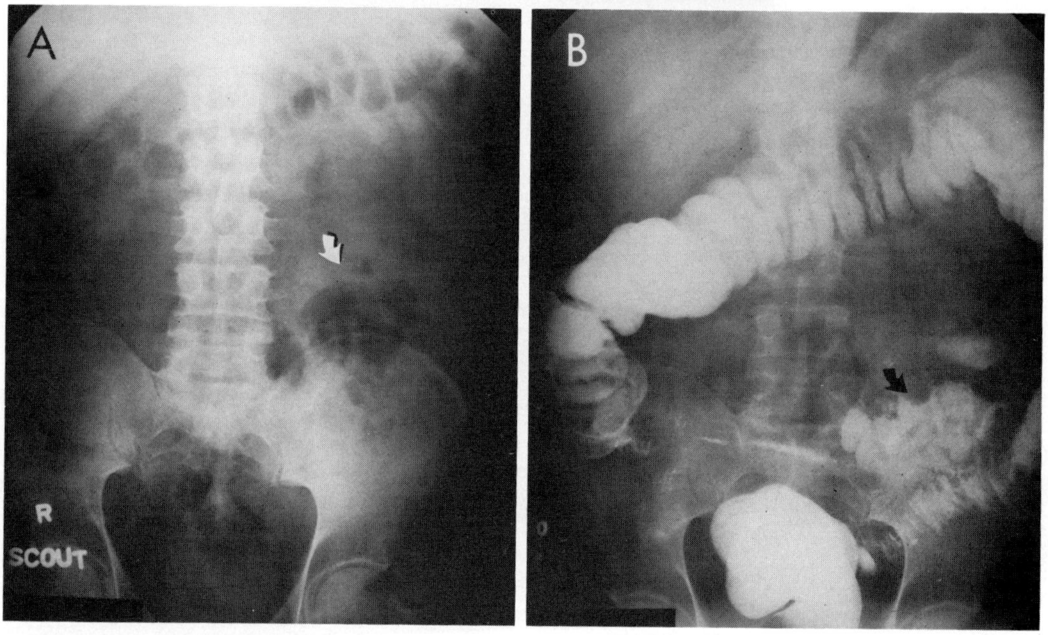

Fig 13–40 (top).—Diverticulitis with small sinus tract extending inferiorly to small round abscess outlined by air and not filled with barium *(arrow).*

Fig 13–41 (bottom).—**A,** diverticulitis presenting on plain film with large extracolonic collection of gas outlining an abscess cavity *(arrow).* **B,** barium enema examination reveals long zone of diverticulitis in sigmoid colon with filling of abscess cavity with barium *(arrow).* (Courtesy of Dr. Gus Bird, Long Beach, Calif.)

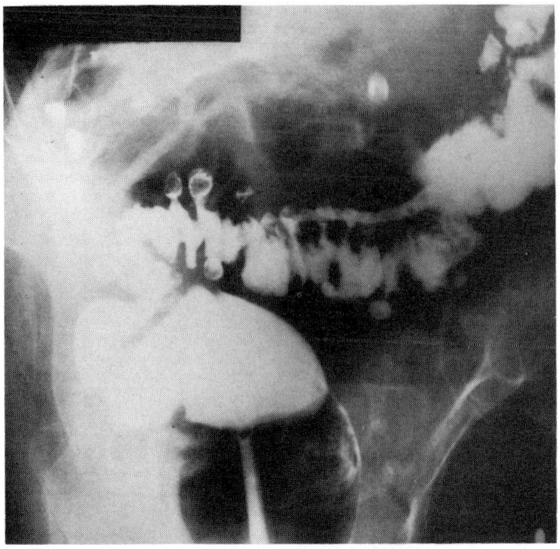

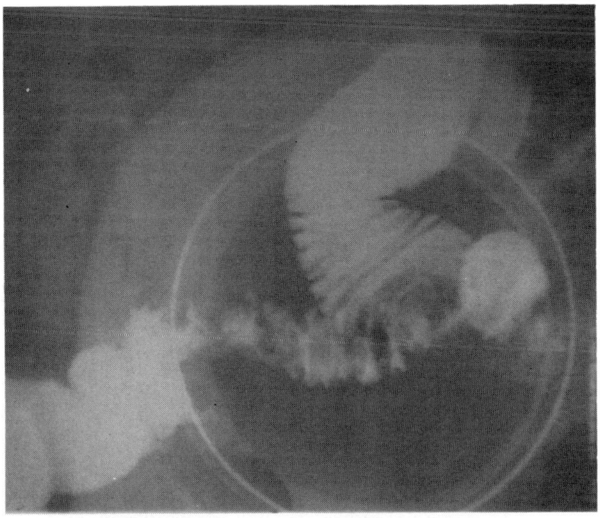

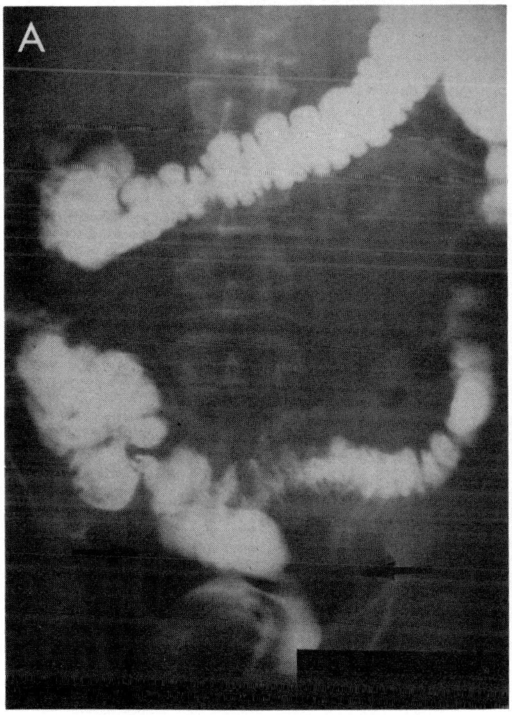

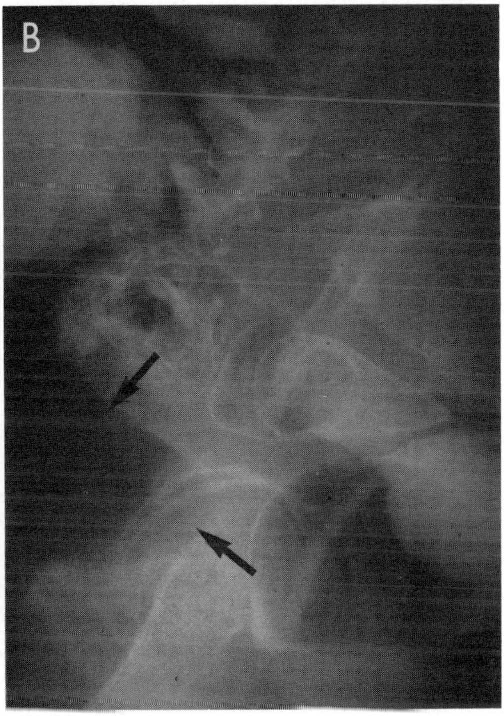

Fig 13–42 (top left).—Focal diverticulitis of midsigmoid with short intramural longitudinal fistulous tract at its superior margin.

Fig 13–43 (top right).—Diverticulitis with coloenteric fistula. During fluoroscopy, barium flowed through sigmoid colon and immediately filled small bowel through fistulous communication. Careful observation during fluoroscopy and early spot filming must be performed in order to exclude the possibility that barium entering small bowel is not filling retrograde through ileocecal valve.

Fig 13–44 (bottom).—**A** and **B,** diverticulitis with colovesicular fistula. AP and lateral views show long segmental zone of diverticulitis of sigmoid colon with air in bladder. Patient was experiencing pneumaturia. At time of examination, fistula had closed and could not be outlined with barium.

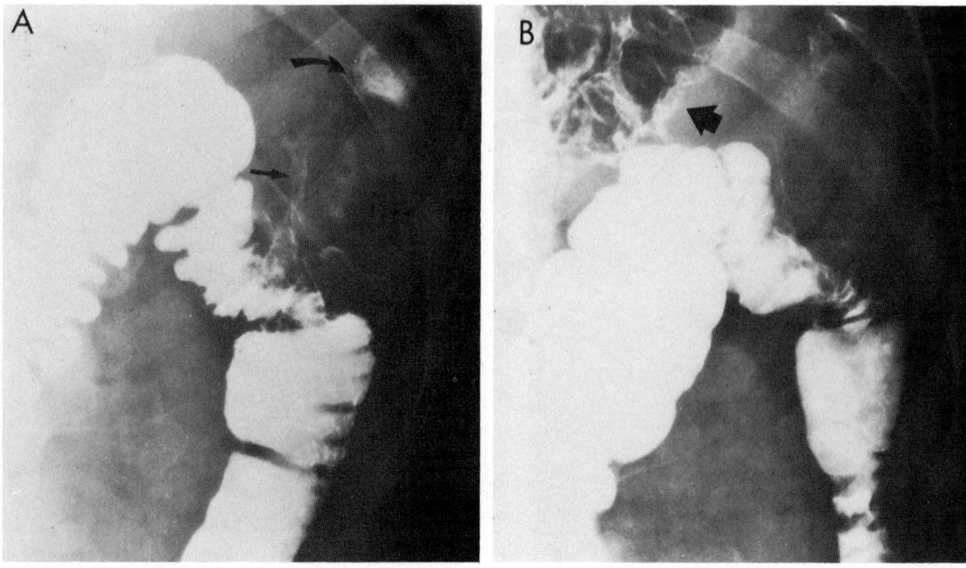

Fig 13–45.—Gastrocolic fistula secondary to diverticulitis of splenic flexure. **A,** splenic flexure in left anterior oblique projection, with demonstration of segmental constriction of colon with ulcerated mucosa and fistulous communication *(small arrow)* with an abscess cavity *(large arrow)*. **B,** subsequent roentgenogram shows opacification of stomach *(arrow)* through gastrocolic fistula. (Courtesy of G. G. Ghahremani, M. D., and reprinted from Dis. Colon and Rectum, 17:98, 1974, with permission of J. B. Lippincott Co.

Fig 13–46.—**A,** diverticulitis presenting with colovaginal fistula. Film taken in left posterior oblique position shows focal area of diverticulitis in midsigmoid colon with extravasation of barium in region of vagina *(arrow)*. **B,** lateral rectal view shows barium in vagina *(arrows)*.

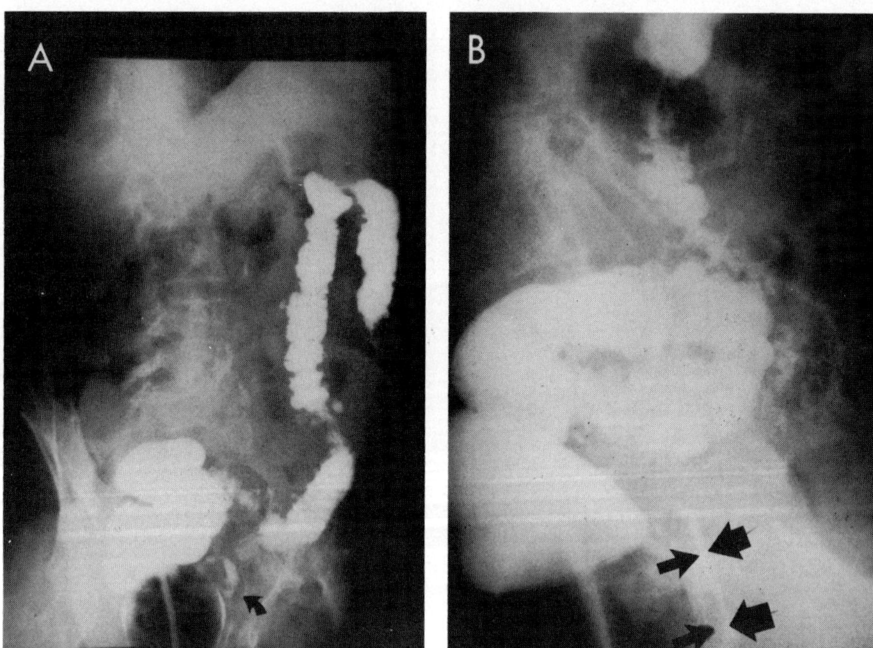

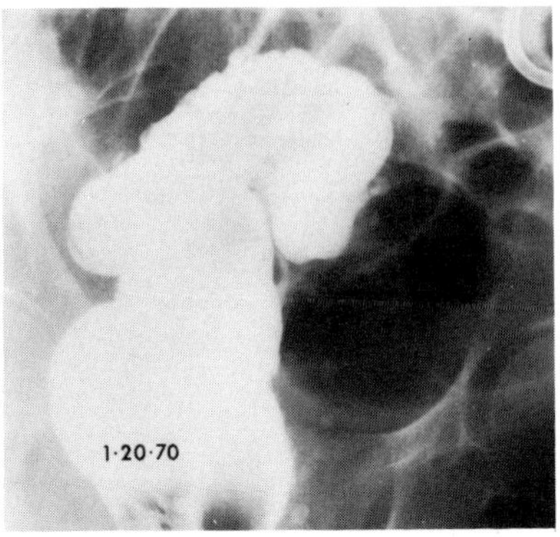

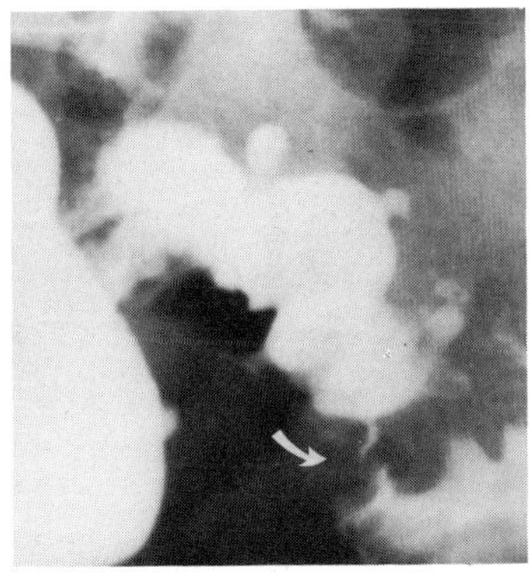

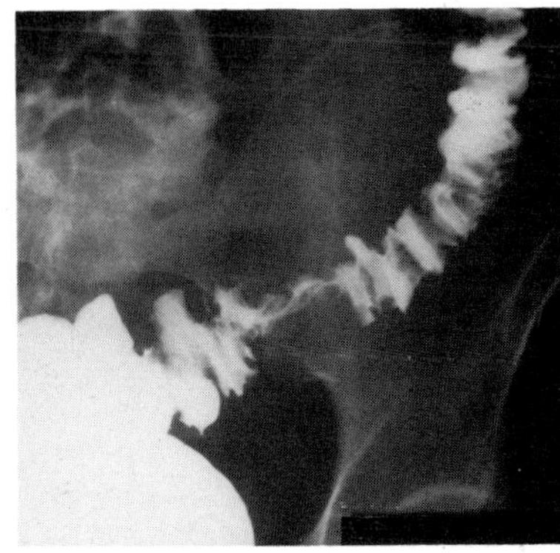

Fig 13–47 (left).—Diverticulitis presenting with occlusion of lumen, which may be due to combination of inflammation and spasm. Glucagon may be used in this instance to relieve spasm in order to demonstrate the channel and help differentiate this process from a malignancy.

Fig 13–48 (center).—Diverticulitis may mimic an annular carcinoma. In this case there is a short stenotic zone with overhanging margins *(arrow)*, but at resection the pathologist found diverticulitis without evidence of malignancy.

Fig 13–49 (right).—Elongated intramural mass indenting inferior aspect of sigmoid colon secondary to chronic diverticulitis. This must be differentiated from other causes of intramural extramucosal masses, e.g., leiomyoma, lipoma.

Fig 13–50.—Diverticulitis presenting with large bowel obstruction. **A,** colon distended to level of sigmoid colon with small amount of gas, as seen in collapsed rectosigmoid distal to obstructing diverticulitis. **B,** right lateral decubitus film shows obstructed colon with air-fluid levels throughout. Small amount of reflux distention of small bowel is noted because of incompetent ileocecal valve. **C,** barium enema was attempted but, in spite of use of glucagon, only a small portion of channel could be outlined with barium. There is evidence of diverticulitis, although entire channel is not completely filled.

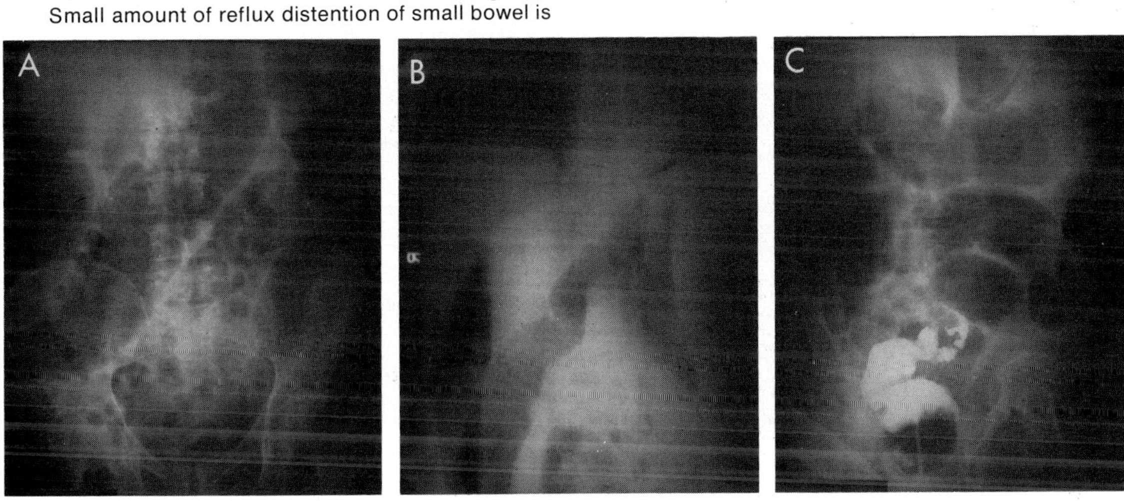

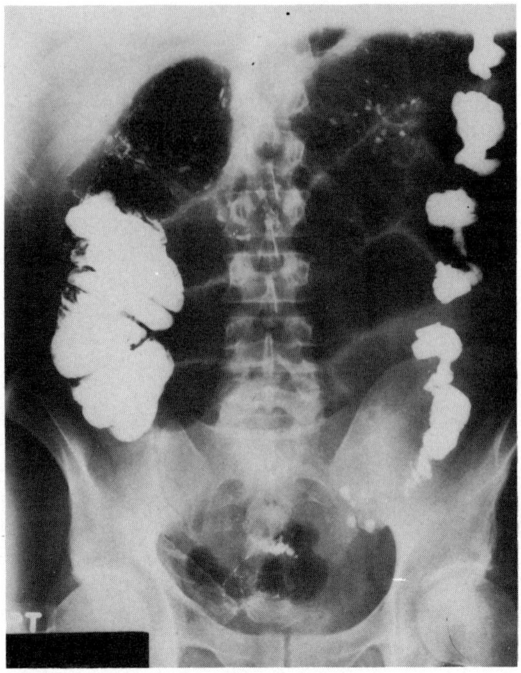

Fig 13–51.—Mechanical small bowel obstruction with multiple dilated loops of small bowel and collapsed distal colon. This, in an elderly patient with left lower quadrant pain, must strongly suggest presence of diverticulitis as underlying cause.

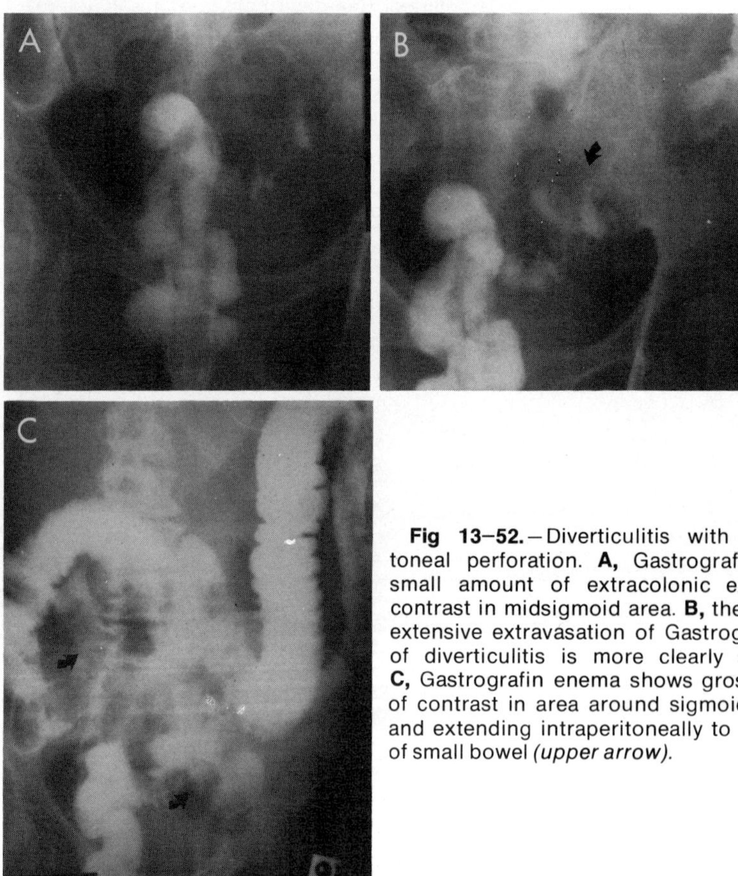

Fig 13–52.—Diverticulitis with free intraperitoneal perforation. **A,** Gastrografin enema with small amount of extracolonic extravasation of contrast in midsigmoid area. **B,** there is now more extensive extravasation of Gastrografin, and area of diverticulitis is more clearly shown *(arrow)*. **C,** Gastrografin enema shows gross extravasation of contrast in area around sigmoid *(lower arrow)* and extending intraperitoneally to surround loops of small bowel *(upper arrow)*.

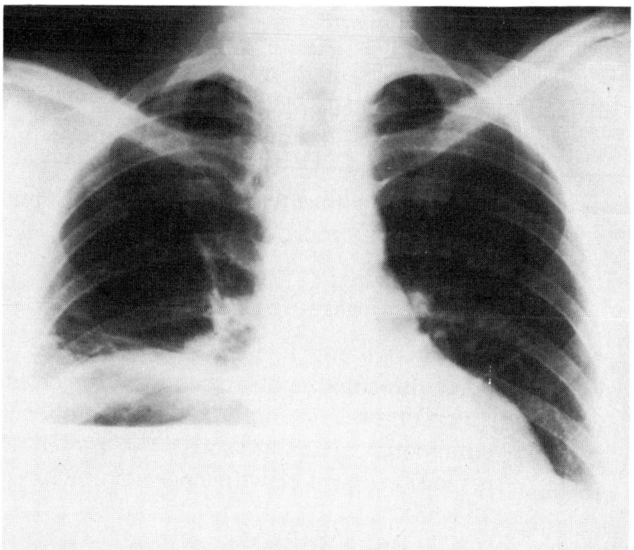

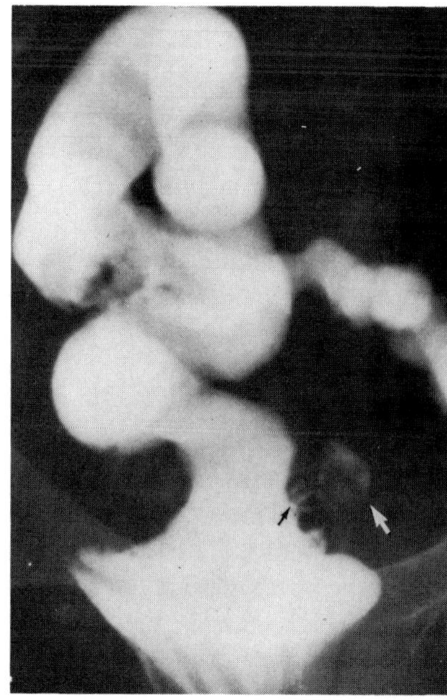

Fig 13–53 (left).—Diverticulitis with secondary right subphrenic abscess. Film shows long air-fluid level in right subphrenic space with elevation of right hemidiaphragm and associated right pleural effusion.

Fig 13–54 (right).—Rectal diverticulitis with perforation. An almost symmetric, bilateral, concave narrowing of midportion rectal ampulla is present with 1 cm collection of barium outside left lateral wall. Fine linear streaks of barium *(black arrow)* mark site of perforation and probably represent fistulous tracts extending to afore-described pericolic abscess *(white arrow).* (Courtesy of P. E. Giustra, M. D., and reprinted from Radiology 105:23, 1972, with permission of the Radiological Society of North America.)

Fig 13–55 (left).—Diverticulitis with perforation at rectosigmoid junction and retrorectal extension. Barium fills large abscess cavity posterior to rectum. There is marked widening of presacral space secondary to associated inflammation.

Fig 13–56 (right).—Diverticulitis with extension to retroperitoneal space. **A,** abscess cavity presenting with air-fluid level in left flank. This was lateral and posterior to left kidney, and could be palpated in the left flank on P.E. **B,** barium enema showing filling of retroperitoneal abscess with barium *(arrows).*

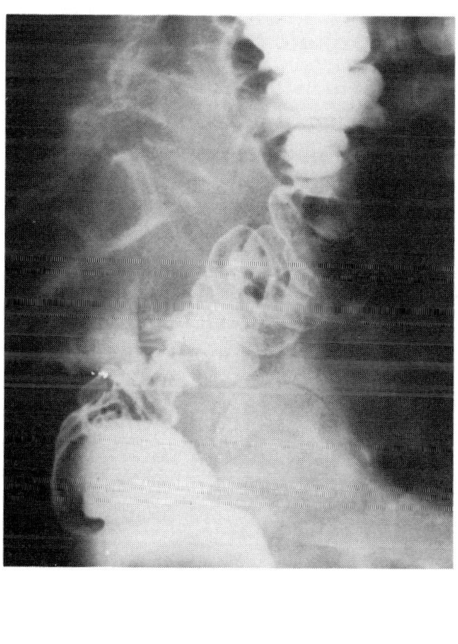

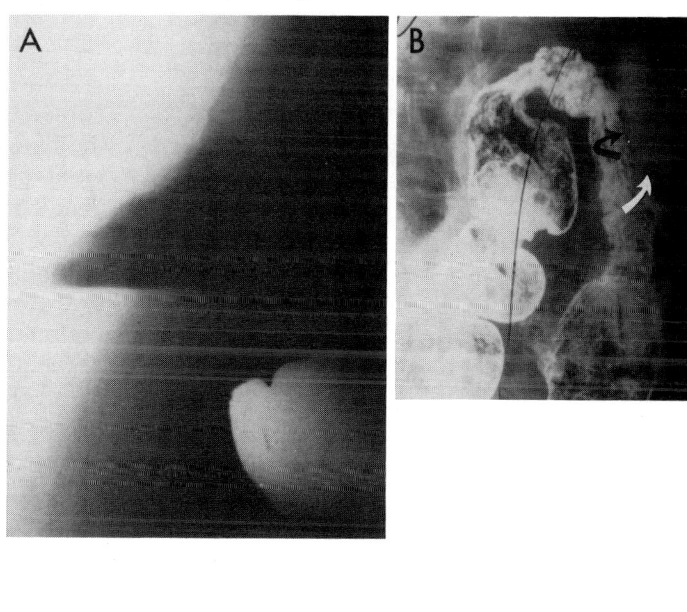

UNUSUAL FISTULAS DUE TO COLONIC DIVERTICULITIS

JEFFERSON O. JANES, M.D.

ALTHOUGH GREATER THAN 90% of fistulas secondary to colonic diverticulitis are communications with the urinary bladder or small intestine,[1] some of the least common have serious sequelae and may be overlooked clinically as the cause of life-threatening disease (Table 13–2).

Colocoxal Fistula

This term encompasses communication between the colon and hip, buttock or thigh. Although this fistula is rare,[2-8] most case reports have stressed delayed treatment, with a resultant high mortality.[3, 5, 9-12] Gas present within the surrounding soft tissues—including the thigh from gangrene and/or soft tissue emphysema, secondary to the forcing of intraluminal colonic gas into soft tissues via the fistula—often is the only early radiographic sign. Barium enema examination may demonstrate extravasation into the pericoxal area (Fig 13–57, A). Although most such fistulas originate from the sigmoid colon,[4] involvement of the right or transverse colon has been described.[11, 13] Clinical and radiographic findings of coxal septic arthritis (see Fig 13–57, B), or osteomyelitis of the femur in the absence of soft tissue gas, make the diagnosis more difficult.[6]

TABLE 13–2.—VARIETIES OF UNUSUAL FISTULAS DUE TO DIVERTICULITIS: SURVEY OF THE LITERATURE

TYPE	NO. OF CASES REPORTED
Colocoxal[3, 9] (to hip, thigh)	14
Colocolic[1, 13, 22]	11
Colovenous[8, 10, 17] (to inferior mesenteric vein)	10
Colocutaneous[11, 14] (spontaneous)	5
Coloureteral[1, 14]	2
Colojejunal[20]	2
Colosalpingeal[1]	1
Colouterine[1]	1
Coloenterovaginal[1]	1
Colovesicovaginal[11]	1
Cologastric[5]	1
Coloperineal/perianal[1]	1

From Smith et al.[8]

Colocutaneous Fistula

Although the incidence of postoperative colocutaneous fistulas secondary to colonic diverticulitis is about 6%, spontaneous colocutaneous fistulas are rare.[8, 14-15] Either type is readily identified with a barium enema (Fig 13–58).

Colovenous Fistula

Diverticular perforation into the inferior mesenteric vein fortunately has been infrequently demonstrated.[8, 16, 17] (Figs 13–59 and 13–60). Communication with the intrahepatic portal system, which can be seen during radiographic examination,[8, 14-15, 17] suggests that a water-soluble enema may be more appropriate in a suspected acute diverticulitis, especially if intrahepatic gas is present on plain films of the abdomen.[8]

Coloappendiceal Fistula

A rare entity, this fistula usually is demonstrated by early filling of the appendix during the barium enema and is secondary to sigmoid diverticulitis[8, 18, 19] (Fig 13–61). Appendicitis almost always causes obstruction without filling of the appendix during the barium enema.[20, 21] Appendiceal diverticula tend to cause bleeding in younger individuals, with periappendiceal inflammation only occasionally seen.[20, 21] A direct communication with the cecum near the appendix has been demonstrated.[22]

Coloepidural Fistula

Perhaps the most bizarre fistula caused by acute diverticulitis is that between the colon and epidural space (Fig 13–62). The mechanism of this complication probably results from involvement of Batson's venous plexus, perineural sheaths and/or direct extension from an adjacent abscess.[8]

Multisystem Fistulas

Although 10% of colonic diverticular fistulas are coloenteric, most of these are sigmoidoileal.[23, 24] Rare enteric fistulous communication resulting from diverticulitis between the splenic flexure and the stomach has been reported.[25] Sigmoidojejunal diverticular fistulas also have been reported.[23] Most coloenteric fistulas are complicated by multiple communications with other organ systems, resulting in intractability, sepsis or severe fluid and electrolyte imbalance caused by loss of succus entericus (Fig 13–63). Since most coloenteric fistulas are secondary to granulomatous bowel disease, radiographic evidence of such bowel disease should be vigorously sought.[18, 23, 24] Complicated diverticular fistulas to the genitourinary tract have been described involving the ureter,[1, 14] fallopian tubes,[1] uterus,[1] and vagina[1, 11], as well as the more common colovesical fistulas.[1]

Summary

Although unusual in occurrence, the fistulas described above secondary to diverticulitis of the colon may represent severe, life-threatening disease with no clue as to the etiology of the disease process. Such events underscore the potential severity of diverticulitis and pose particularly challenging problems in diagnosis and management. It should be emphasized that, whereas most fistulas are best studied with barium enema examination, in certain cases sinography, cystography, intravenous urography and small intestinal examination may provide equal or better demonstration of the presence and location of the cause of fistular disease.[2, 3]

REFERENCES

1. Colcock, B. P., Stahman, F. D.: Fistulas complicating diverticular disease of the sigmoid colon, Ann. Surg. 175:838, 1972.
2. Small, W. P., and Smith, A. N.: Fistula and conditions associated with diverticular disease of the colon, Clin. Gastroenterol. 4:171, 1975.
3. Goldfarb, W. B., Monafo, W., and McAlister, W. H.: Clinical value of fistulography, Am. J. Surg. 108: 902, 1964.
4. Linscheid, R. L., Kelly, P. J., and Symmonds, R. E.: Emphysematous cellulitis of the hip and thigh resulting from enteric fistula, J. Bone Joint Surg. (Am) 45:1691, 1963.
5. Dawson, R. L. G., and Hardy, R. H.: Diverticulitis presenting as emphysematous cellulitis of the leg, Br. Med. J. 1:498, 1948.
6. Farmer, R. G., Weakley, F. L., Klein, H. J. et al.: Colonic diverticulitis with perforation to region of left hip; a rare complication, Cleve. Clin. Q. 37: 161, 1970.
7. Korsten, J., Mattey, W. E., Bastidas, J., et al.: Subcutaneous emphysema of the thigh secondary to ruptured diverticulum of the ascending colon, Radiology 106:555, 1973.
8. Smith, H. J., Berk, R. N., Janes, J. O., Clayton, R. S., and Williams, J. L.: Unusual fistulae due to colonic diverticulitis, Gastrointest. Radiol. 2:387, 1978.
9. Smith, W. S., and Ward, R. M.: Septic arthritis of the hip complicating perforation of abdominal organs, J.A.M.A. 195:170, 1966.
10. Graham, G. A., Bernstein, R. B., and Gronner, A. T.: Gas in the portal and inf. mes. veins caused by diverticulitis of the sigmoid colon, Radiology 114: 601, 1975.
11. Carpenter, W. S., Allaben, R. D., and Kambouris, A. A.: Fistulas complicating diverticulitis of the colon, Surg. Gynecol. Obstet. 134:625, 1972.
12. Pickels, R. F., Karmody, A. M., Tsapogas, M. J., et al.: Subcutaneous emphysema of the lower extremity of gastrointestinal origin, Dis. Colon Rectum 17:82, 1974.
13. Mayo, C. W., and Blunt, C. P.: Surgical management of complications of diverticulitis of the large intestine: Analysis of 202 cases, Surg. Clin. North Am. 30:1005, 1950.
14. Rodkey, G. V., and Welch, C. E.: Diverticulitis of the colon. Evolution in concept and therapy, Surg. Clin. North Am. 45:1231, 1965.
15. Roman, P. W., Wagner, J. H., and Steinbach, S. H.: Massive fatal embolism during barium enema study, Radiology 59:190, 1952.
16. Rosenberg, L. S., and Fine, A.: Fatal venous intravasation of barium during a barium enema, Am. J. Roentgenol. 73:771, 1959.
17. Juler, G. L., Dietrick, W. R., and Eisenman, J. L.:

Intramesenteric perforation of sigmoid diverticulitis with non-fatal venous intravasation, Am. J. Surg. 132:653, 1976.
18. Conlon, P. C., and Lewis, J. R.: Roentgen diagnosis of appendicocolic fistulation, Am. J. Roentgenol. 88:707, 1962.
19. Marshak, R. H., Lindner, A. E., Pochaczevsky, R., and Maklansky, D.: Longitudinal sinus tracts in granulomatous colitis and diverticulitis, Semin. Roentgenol. 11:101, 1976.
20. Diner, W. C., and Barnhard, H. J.: Acute diverticulitis, Semin. Roentgenol. 7:415, 1973.
21. Berk, R. N., and Lasser, E. C.: In *Radiology of the Ileocecal Area* (Philadelphia: W. B. Saunders Co., 1975), pp. 74; 123.
22. Sanowski, R. A., and Costello, J. L.: Sigmoidocecal fistula, Am. J. Gastrointest. 48:56, 1967.
23. Marshak, R. H., and Eliasoph, J.: Inflammatory lesions of the small bowel secondary to colonic diverticulitis, Am. J. Dig. Dis. 6:423, 1961.
24. Kroening, P. M.: Sigmoido-ileal fistulas as a complication of diverticulitis, Am. J. Roentgenol. 96:323, 1966.
25. Ghahremani, G. G., and Olsen, J.: Gastrocolic fistula secondary to diverticulitis of the splenic flexure, Dis. Colon Rectum 17:98, 1974.

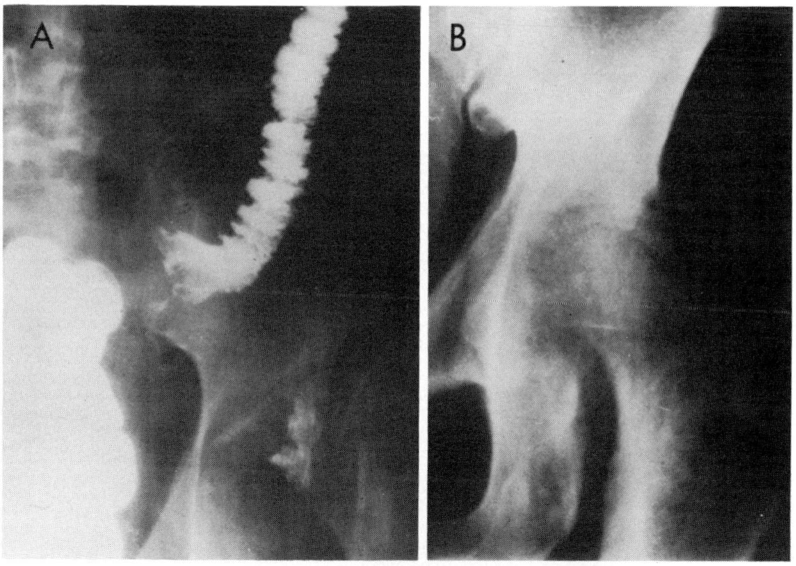

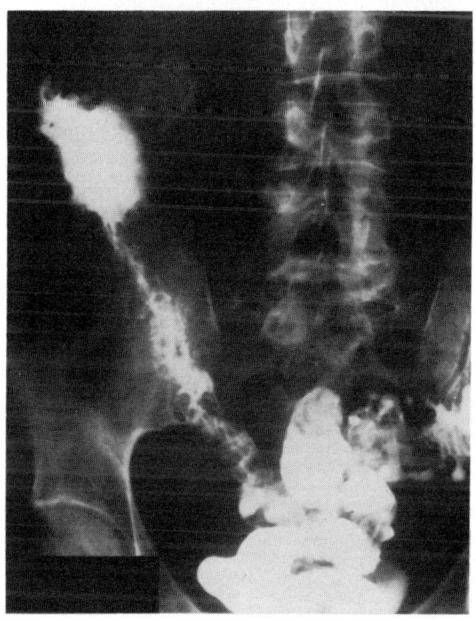

Fig 13–57 (top).—**A,** colocoxal fistula. Radiograph from barium enema examination showing segmental narrowing of sigmoid colon due to acute diverticulitis. Barium has entered hip joint through colocoxal fistula. Fistula due to acute diverticulitis was confirmed at surgery. **B,** colocoxal fistula. Radiograph of left hip showing destruction of hip joint due to septic arthritis. (From Smith et al., Gastrointest. Radiol. 2:387, 1978, with permission.)

Fig 13–58 (bottom).—Colocutaneous fistula. Radiograph from barium enema examination showing irregular narrowing of sigmoid colon due to acute diverticulitis. Diverticulosis also evident. Long subcutaneous tract extending from sigmoid colon to skin of abdominal wall is filled with barium. Colocutaneous fistula confirmed at surgery. (From Smith et al., Gastrointest. Radiol. 2:387, 1978, with permission.)

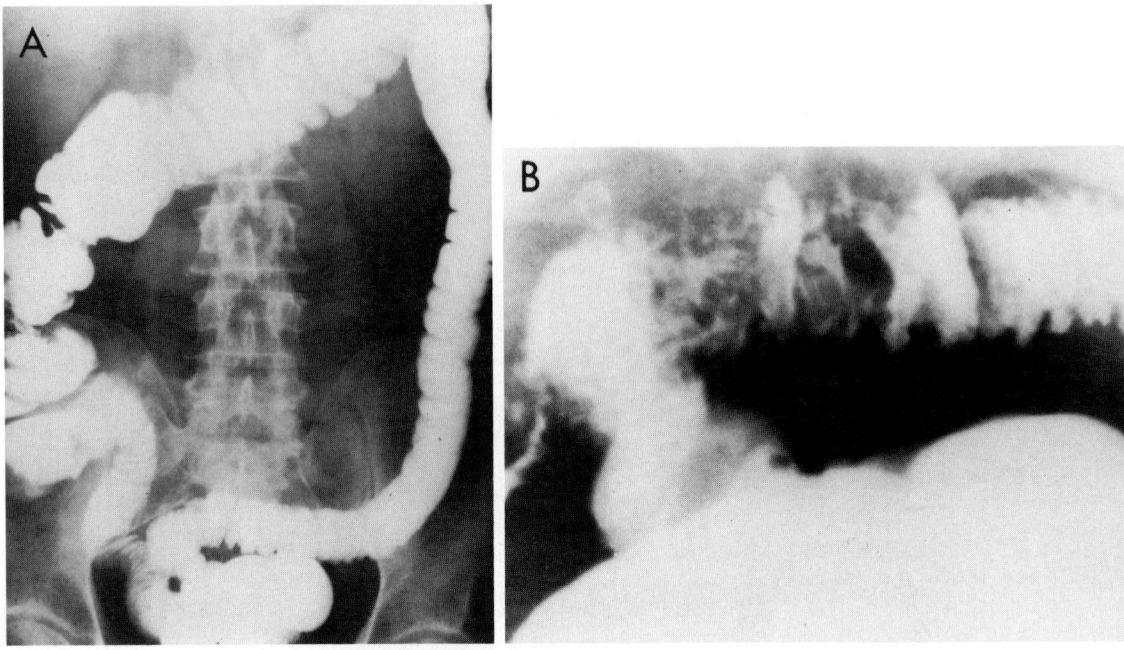

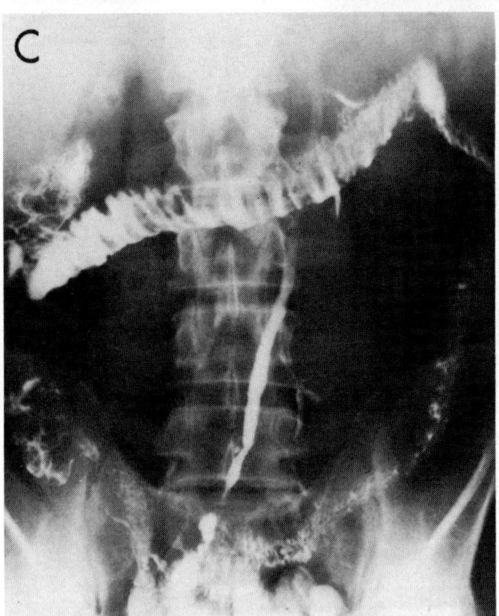

Fig 13–59.—**A,** colovenous fistula. Radiograph from barium enema examination showing only minimal changes of spastic colon disease. **B,** colovenous fistula. Spot film made during barium enema examination showing narrowing of sigmoid colon and fistulous tract. A few diverticula are present. **C,** postevacuation radiograph showing barium in inferior mesenteric vein. Barium and gas are visible in a liver abscess. Barium remained in vein for 3 days after examination and was gradually replaced by gas. At surgery, a small abscess was found due to perforation of sigmoid colon. Patient did well for 8 days following operation but suddenly developed irreversible shock and died. Autopsy confirmed presence of barium in inferior mesenteric vein and showed thrombosis of portal and splenic veins and multiple liver abscesses. (From Smith et al., Gastrointest. Radiol. 2:387, 1978, with permission.)

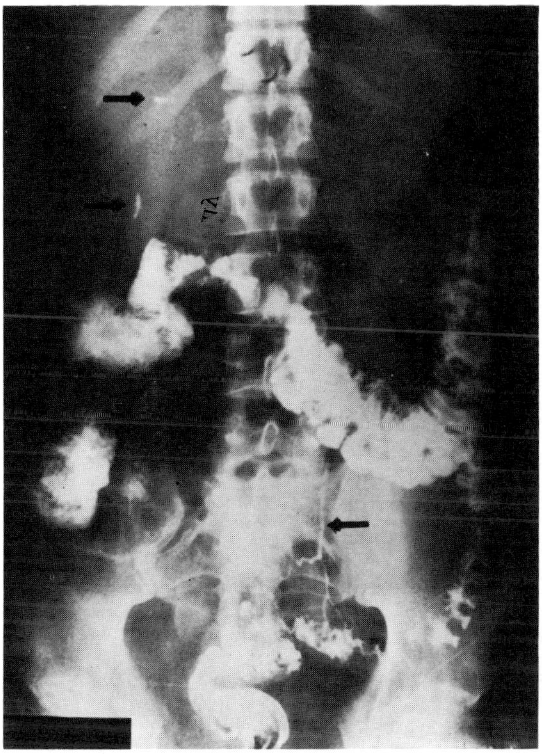

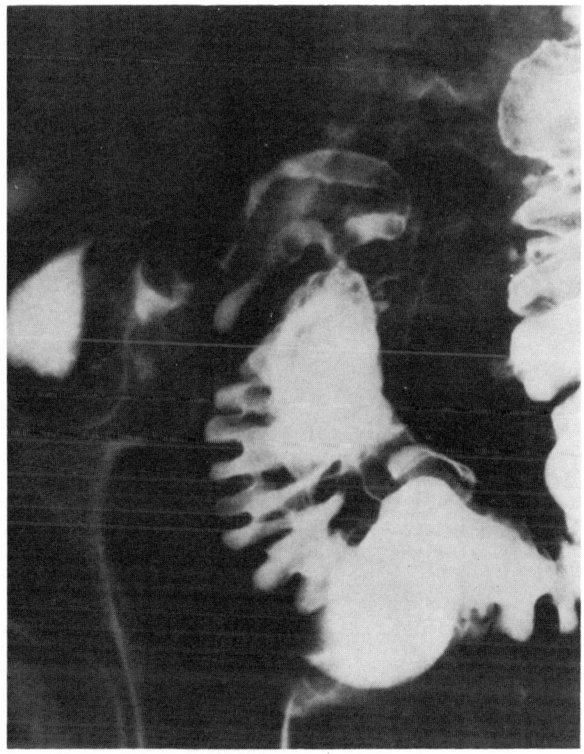

Fig 13–60 (left).—Colovenous fistula. Radiograph from barium enema examination showing barium within inferior mesenteric vein near sigmoid colon *(lower arrow)*. Barium also present in intrahepatic veins *(upper arrows)*. (From Juler et al., Am. J. Surg. 132:653, 1976, with permission.)

Fig 13–61 (right).—Coloappendiceal fistula. Radiograph from barium enema examination showing filling of appendix *via* sigmoid colon. Marked spastic colon disease of sigmoid is apparent, and there is no obstruction of appendix. Coloappendiceal fistula due to diverticulitis was confirmed at surgery. (From Smith et al., Gastrointest. Radiol. 2:387, 1978, with permission.)

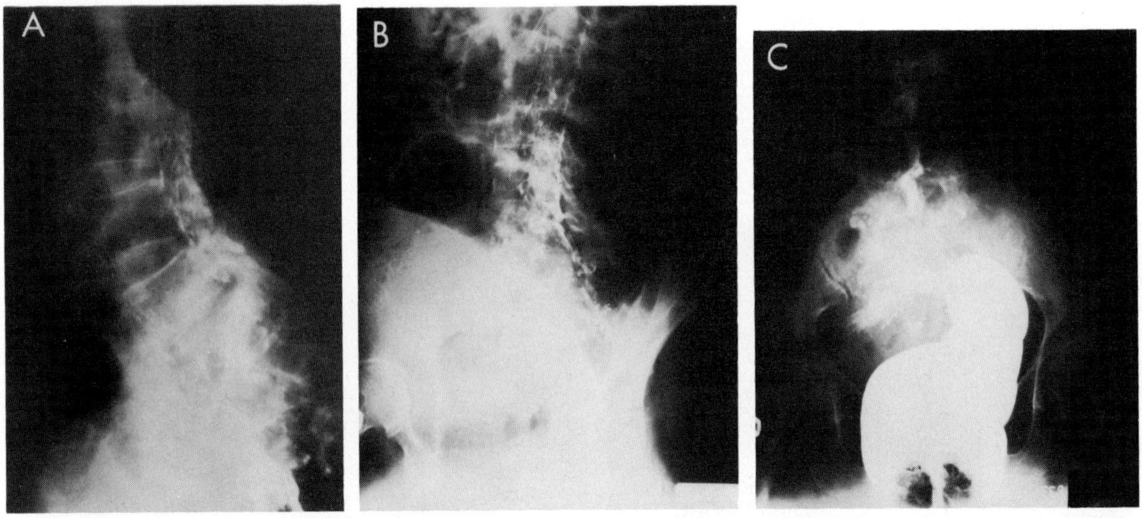

Fig 13–62.—**A,** coloepidural fistula. Lateral radiograph of spine made following barium enema examination showing barium in presacral soft tissues and epidural space. Barium is present in rectum. Presence of acute diverticulitis with perforation was confirmed at autopsy. Large amount of barium present in epidural space. **B,** coloepidural fistula. Oblique view showing epidural barium. **C,** coloepidural fistula. AP view showing filling of abscess and tracking of barium into epidural space. (From Smith et al., Gastrointest. Radiol. 2:387, 1978, with permission.)

Fig 13–63.—**Left,** multisystem fistula. Radiograph from barium enema examination showing barium entering bladder and small intestine via sigmoid colon. **Right,** multisystem fistula. Radiograph from BE showing filling of small intestine and bladder (at *B*). Colovesico-enteric fistula due to acute diverticulitis was confirmed at surgery. (From Smith et al., Gastrointest. Radiol. 2:387, 1978, with permission.)

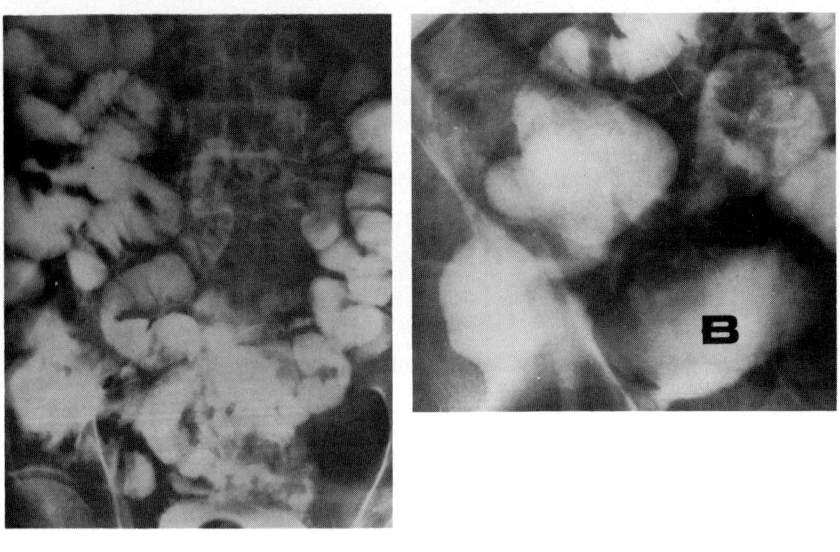

Chapter 14

Duplication of the Colon

E. M. BASS, M.B.Ch.B., D.M.R.D., F.R.C.R.,
M.Med.(Rad.D.), F.R.A.C.R.

DUPLICATION OF THE COLON is an uncommon congenital anomaly usually diagnosed during infancy or early childhood. Although it is less common than small bowel duplication, Kottra and Dodds[4] reviewed 50 reported cases and found a female preponderance but no apparent racial or familial predilection.

Classification

A classification system for colon duplication is shown in Table 14-1 and Figure 14-1. Type I duplication is limited to the colon or rectum and usually is partial. Type II lesions often involve the entire colon and are associated with duplication of the lower urinary or genital tracts or both. Associated congenital anomalies, involving other parts of the gastrointestinal tract and the genitourinary and musculoskeletal systems, are found with both types but are more common with type II lesions. Type IIa lesions, with two separate perineal ani, usually are associated with double genitalia and a double urethra and bladder. These patients usually are continent and have no symptoms; complaints are limited to the cosmetic disfiguration. Most type IIb lesions also have double genitalia and urinary tract duplication, and symptoms are related to the fistula or obstruction from inadequate drainage. Surgery usually is successful in these cases. Patients with type IIc cases usually have single genitals, but all have duplications of the lower urinary tract. These patients have symptoms of obstruction, and operative results are poor.

TABLE 14-1.—CLASSIFICATION OF COLON DUPLICATIONS

Type I.—Duplication limited to alimentary tract (frequently asymptomatic)
- (a) Spherical
- (b) Tubular
- (c) Double barreled: one or more communications with colon
  - Limited to colon
  - Associated ileal duplication
- (d) Multiple duplications: combinations of a, b and c

Type II*.—Colon duplication (usually double barreled) associated with duplications of urinary or genital tract (frequently symptomatic)
- (a) Two separate perineal ani
- (b) Fistulas, i.e., distal portion of one or both duplicates having a fistulous connection with another hollow viscus
- (c) Anorectal agenesis (imperforate anus): one or both rectums imperforate; in the pelvis; no fistula

*Modified from Smith.[7]

Pathologic Features

True intestinal replications must be distinguished from enteric cysts and vitelline remnants[7] and have the following characteristics: (1) intimate attachment to some part of the alimentary tract, (2) smooth muscle coat and (3) mucosal lining similar to stomach, small bowel or colon.

Colon duplications may have a spherical, tubular or double-barreled configuration and usually are located along the mesenteric border of the colon. A patient with colonic triplication has been reported by Gray.[1] As a rule, the duplicates share a mesentery, when present, and a blood supply. The duplication may bulge into the colon lumen if it is restricted by encircling muscle. If a communication exists, the duplication contains feces, whereas noncommunicating duplications contain clear, often mucoid fluid. Enzymatic secretions may cause ulceration and bleeding, with resultant discoloration of the liquid contents.

On histologic examination the outer wall of the duplication has all the tissue layers of a normal colon. The common wall may vary from two mucosal layers with intervening connective tissue to two complete, attached colon walls. The mucosal layer is always alimentary in type, but may not correspond to that of the adjacent bowel, e.g., gastric mucosa may be present in rectal duplication.

Clinical Features

Minor forms of colonic duplication are often asymptomatic and may remain unrecognized unless associated with other congenital anomalies. Symptoms usually are related to obstruction, with resultant constipation, distention and pain. The cause of the obstruction varies. Noncommunicating lesions (types Ia and IIb) often enlarge due to retained secretions and compress the adjacent bowel. Type I lesions projecting into the lumen may cause intussusception.[2] Type II lesions become distended when the distal anomaly prevents adequate emptying. Gastrointestinal bleeding may result from ulceration owing to enzymatic secretions. In addition, stretching of mesenteric vessels around the duplication may cause ischemia,[2] with resultant blood loss.

Pain may result from overdistention and obstruction; rarely, proteolytic enzymes in the secretions cause inflammation.

A palpable abdominal mass may be the presenting feature, especially in children. Ravitch[5] described a case in which the duplication compressed the left ureter with resultant hydronephrosis. A carcinoma may arise in a duplicated colon,[3] and alter the symptomatology.

Radiologic Features

The roentgen features (Figs 14–2 to 14–5) depend on the size, shape, extent and location of the duplication. Small duplications often show no abnormal roentgen findings.

Plain abdominal films may show a nonspecific soft tissue mass. Calcification within a duplication is rare.[8] Large or small bowel obstruction is present when the duplication significantly compresses the adjacent bowel lumen. Communicating duplications may be seen as a gas-filled structure in close apposition to the bowel, often with an air-fluid level on the erect film. Associated congenital anomalies of the lumbar spine or sacrum may be evident.

The diagnosis usually is made by *barium examinations*. The colon or rectum is frequently displaced or compressed by an adjacent mass. Communicating lesions usually show an irregular duplicate lumen, and discrete ulcers may be seen if gastric mucosa is present. Unsuspected double-barreled lesions may be recognized by air-containing haustral markings adjacent to the barium-filled colon; these later fill with barium through the communication. Complete duplications with separate perineal or ectopic anal openings are easily recognized by introducing barium through both openings. A small bowel series may show associated anomalies, especially ileal duplication, malrotation or Meckel's diverticulum. Intravenous pyelography or cystography may demonstrate a double bladder or urethra.

Differentiation from mesenteric cysts or lymph cysts may be difficult on roentgenographic studies, although these cysts have a thinner wall and less tendency to significantly compress the adjacent bowel. Colon duplications in adults may simulate carcinoma, whereas in infants the resultant obstruction, constipation and abdominal distention must be distinguished from Hirschsprung's disease.

Discussion

Knowledge of the varied clinical and roentgenographic features of colon duplication helps the radiologist to make the diagnosis and to suggest appropriate additional studies when indicated. A confident roentgenographic diagnosis may spare an asymptomatic patient an unnecessary exploratory laparotomy. Complete radiologic evaluation of such patients must include examinations of the colon, small bowel, lumbar spine, pelvis and genitourinary tract. Unless the duplications are obstructed or show other significant symptoms, management is conservative. Duplications of the lower genitourinary tract usually are consistent with fertility and good health, and surgery is reserved for patients who are symptomatically or cosmetically disturbed.

REFERENCES

1. Gray, A. W.: Triplication of large intestine, Arch. Pathol. 30:1,215, 1940.
2. Gross, R. E., Holcomb, G. W., and Farber, S.: Duplications of alimentary tract, Paediatrics 9:449, 1952.
3. Heiberg, M. L., Marshall, K. G., and Himal, H. S.: Carcinoma arising in a duplicated colon. Case report and review of literature, Br. J. Surg. 60:981, 1973.
4. Kottra, J. J., and Dodds, W. J.: Duplication of the large bowel, Radiology 113:310, 1971.
5. Ravitch, M. M.: Hind-gut duplication-doubling of colon and genito-urinary tracts, Ann. Surg. 137:588, 1953.
6. Smith, E. D.: Duplication of anus and genitourinary tract, Surgery 66:909, 1969.
7. Smith, J. R.: Accessory enteric formations: Classification and nomenclature, Arch. Dis. Child. 30:87, 1960.
8. Weber, H. M., and Dixon, C. F.: Duplication of entire large intestine (colon duplex): Report of case, Am. J. Roentgenol. 55:319, 1946.

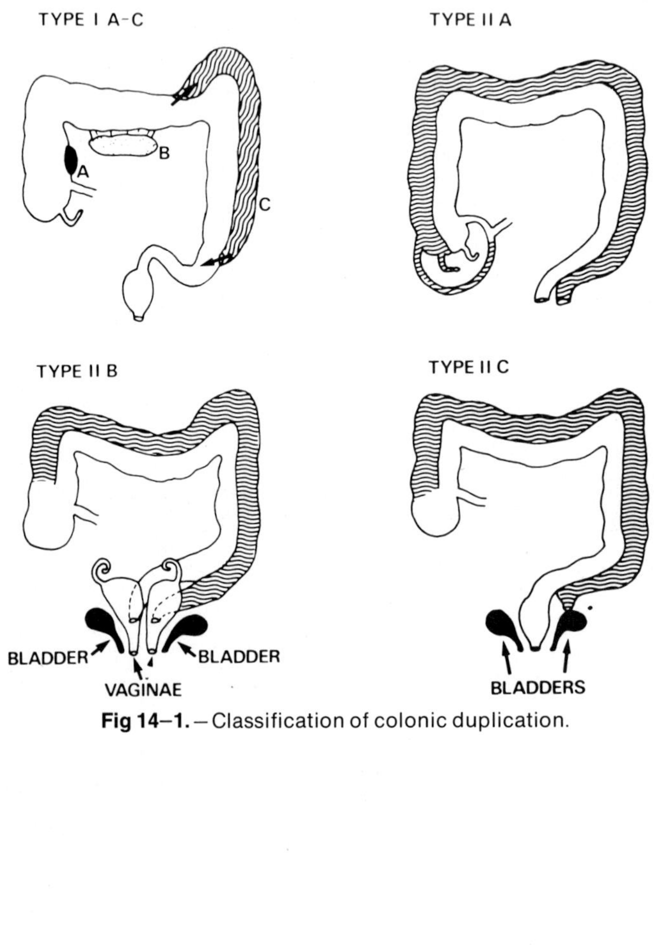

Fig 14–1.—Classification of colonic duplication.

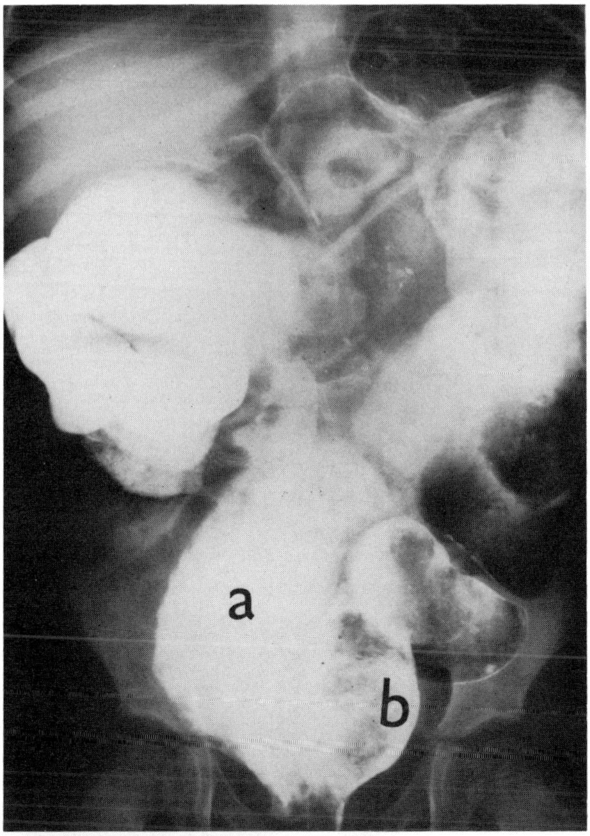

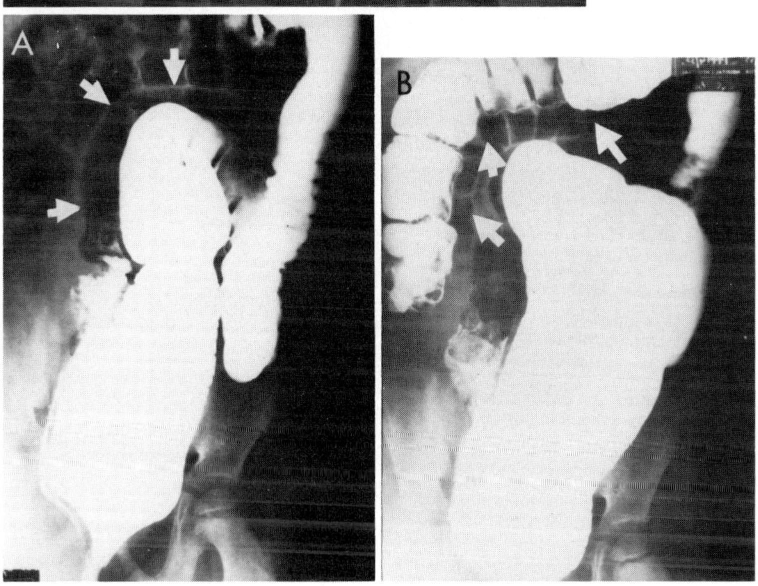

Fig 14–2 (top).—Barium enema through single anal opening on child aged 2 years. Duplicated lumina (*a* and *b*) join distally at rectum and proximally at transverse colon. Note impacted fecal masses in lumen (*b*).

Fig 14–3 (bottom).—**A,** barium enema in child age 6 years with two anal orifices and separate catheterization of each opening. Note air-filled duplicated lumen adjacent to larger barium-filled lumen (*arrows*). **B,** barium has now flowed to cecum in larger lumen. Note air-filled haustra adjacent to transverse and ascending colons (*arrows*).

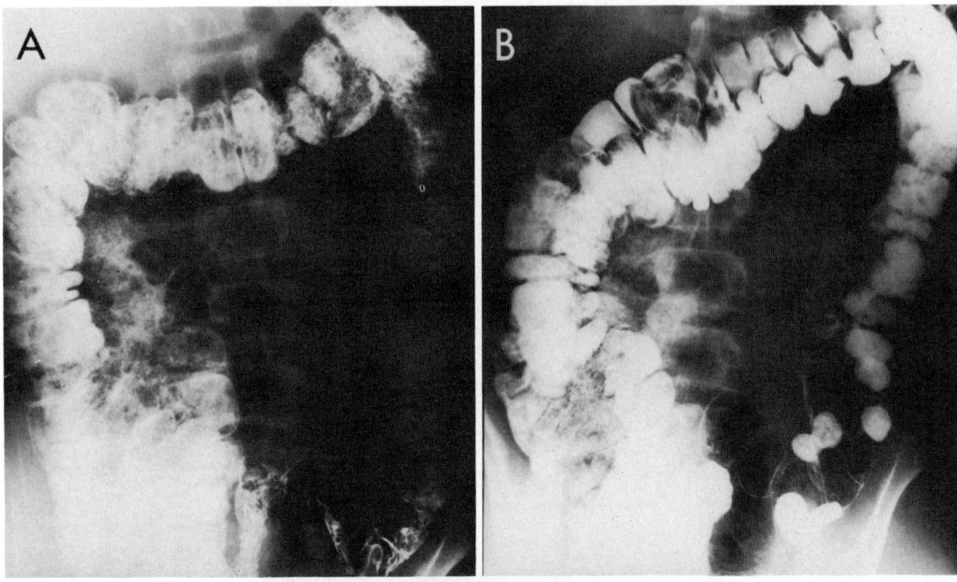

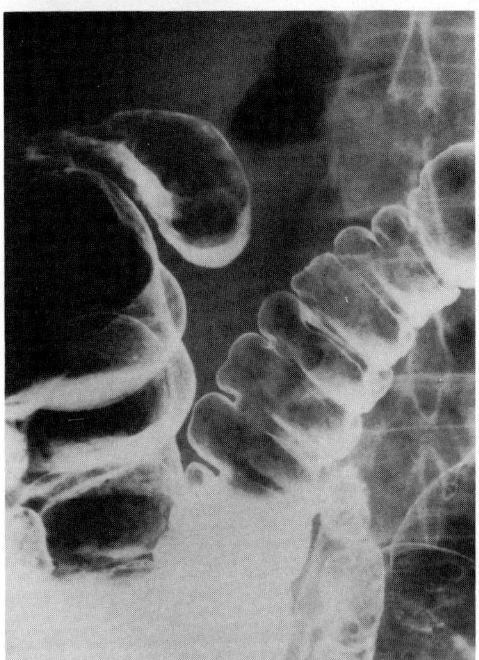

Fig 14–4 (top).—**A,** same patient as in Figure 14–3 nine years later. Barium-filled colon with air-containing haustra seen superior to transverse colon. **B,** both lumina now filled with barium.

Fig 14–5 (bottom).—Woman age 62. Diverticular structure arising from hepatic flexure. Mucosal lining in this small tubular communicating reduplication is continuous with adjacent colon.

Chapter 15

Endometriosis of the Colon

CHARLES J. FAGAN, M.D.

ENDOMETRIOSIS may be defined as the growth of ectopic tissue composed of the epithelial and stromal elements of normal endometrium.

Incidence

The true incidence of endometriosis is difficult to determine. Its frequency at laparotomy has been estimated to be 17%.[1] Other estimates suggest that 5% of women seen by gynecologists and 50% of all women, sometimes during their active menstrual life, have endometriosis.[2, 3]

Intestinal involvement is believed to occur in 12% of patients with pelvic endometriosis. Eighty-five percent of these lesions occur in the rectosigmoid colon, involvement of the small bowel, cecum and appendix accounting for the remainder of the intestinal lesions.[4]

Pathologic Changes

Endometriosis is a nonneoplastic process incapable of autonomous growth. However, its phases of proliferation, necrosis and desquamation are all mediated through an estrogen–progesterone axis. Ectopic glandular tissue trapped within smooth muscle stimulates hypertrophy of that tissue. Also, the marked fibroproliferative reaction incident to the cyclic bleeding that occurs results in cicatrization with ensuing constriction. It is these properties that cause extensive damage not unlike a true neoplasm—enlarging, displacing, distorting, kinking and even obstructing organs, including the intestine.

No completely adequate description of the pathogenesis of endometrial implants is available. Theories proposing transtubal reflux, hematogenous and lymphatic mobilization and coelomic metaplasia have been described.[5]

Clinical Considerations

In general, endometriosis is an illness of women between the ages of 25 and 45. However, involvement of the colon is most common in the fifth decade, and intestinal endometriosis may produce symptoms long after menopause. Conversely, there are case reports in which intestinal endometrial implants involve women under the age of 20 and as young as age 14 years.[6]

The disease is more common in the white nulliparous woman or in women who have become pregnant late in their reproductive years. Absolute or relative sterility is the rule.

Many patients with intestinal endometriosis are asymptomatic, the disease being discovered incidentally during abdominal and pelvic surgery for various conditions. Symptomatic patients may complain of menstrual difficulties, e.g., dysmenorrhea, men orrhagia and intermenstrual bleeding. Pelvic and abdominal pain and dyspareunia are often present. The pain may be unrelated to menstruation and of a chronic, cramping nature when the endometrial process is associated with a partial small bowel or colon obstruction. More typically, the symptoms are exaggerated by menstruation. They are of long duration, are unassociated with weight loss or ill health and abate after menopause. The occurrence of cyclic rectal bleeding does not occur as often as the medical literature would lead one to believe, since the intramural lesions usually spare the mucosa.

Positive physical findings are frequently absent. As a result, many women with pelvic and intestinal endometriosis undergo extensive diagnostic investigations and are eventually labeled as having psychosomatic disease. Infrequently the clinician is able to palpate a tender nodule in the soft tissues of the pelvis or in the wall of the intestine. In contrast, an endometrioma is often detected as a nonspecific pelvic mass during a pelvic examination.

Radiographic Findings

Endometrial lesions of the colon have many faces. Varying proportions of muscle hypertrophy, stimulated by ectopic endometrial tissue, fibrosis and adhesions, account for radiographically apparent intestinal lesions. For the most part the lesions simulate other much more common abnormalities of the colon. Extrinsic pressure on the rectum or displacement of the colon by a large endometrioma represents a nonspecific finding on a barium enema examination (Fig 15–1). Intramural involvement may simulate a variety of lesions, i.e., a large polypoid lesion (Fig 15–2), an inflammatory lesion (Fig 15–3), or a carcinoma (Figs 15–4 and 15–5). The most typical configuration of the colon is the long, scalloped, intramural lesion that involves the antimesenteric side of the colon (Fig 15–6). Even this "characteristic lesion" may be confused with diverticulitis. Endometriosis of the cecum, an uncommon lesion, is usually manifested by an oval, discrete, intramural lesion that spares the mucosa (Fig 15–8). Appendiceal involvement, also an infrequent lesion, is manifested by nonfilling of that structure during a barium enema examination; intussusception of the appendix into the lumen of the cecum has been described as the "inside-out" appendix.[7]

Pelvic ultrasonography is helpful in demonstrating an endometrioma (see Figs 15–1, 15–7 and 15–9) but supplies no diagnostic information about the intramural lesion and about the muscular and fibroproliferative changes, including adhesions, associated with the process.

An intramural lesion of the rectosigmoid colon associated with kinking, segmental narrowing and degrees of obstruction of the ureters on the excretory urogram (see Fig 15–9) should alert one to the presence of pelvic endometriosis. Endometrial seeding of the cul-de-sac with extension to the rectovaginal septum and anterior rectal wall results in barium enema images (Fig 15–10) that should prompt the diagnosis of endometriosis with a high level of confidence.

REFERENCES

1. Tyson, J. A.: Surgical considerations in gynecologic endocrine disorders, Surg. Clin. North Am. 54:425, 1974.
2. Wilson, J. R., Beechman, C. T., and Tarrington, E. R.: *Obstetrics in Gynecology* (3d ed.; St. Louis: C. V. Mosby Co., 1966).
3. Jenkinson, E., and Brown, W.: Endometriosis, J.A.M.A. 122:349, 1943.
4. Elliott, G., Christensen, B., and Elliott, K.: Invasive intestinal endometriosis, Can. J. Surg. 13:387, 1970.
5. Fagan, C. J.: Endometriosis: Clinical and roentgenographic manifestations, Radiol. Clin. North Am. 12: 109, 1974.
6. Sutton, L. A.: The clinical features of endometriosis, NY State J. Med. 41:1343, 1941.
7. Hill, B., Schmitt, K., and Economou, S.: The inside-out appendix, Radiology 95:613, 1970.

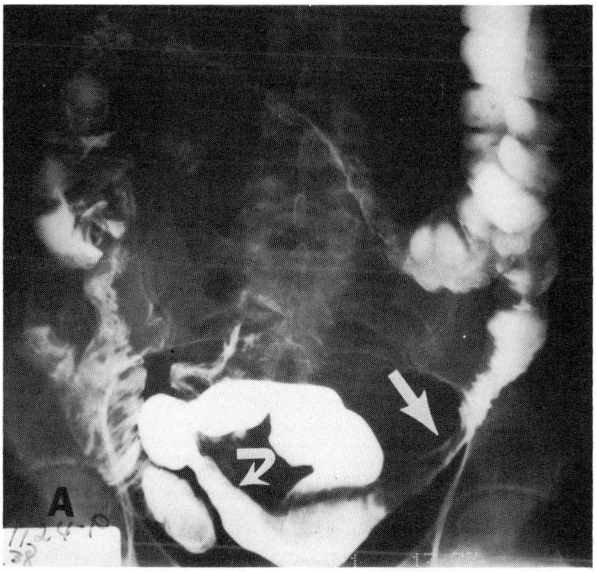

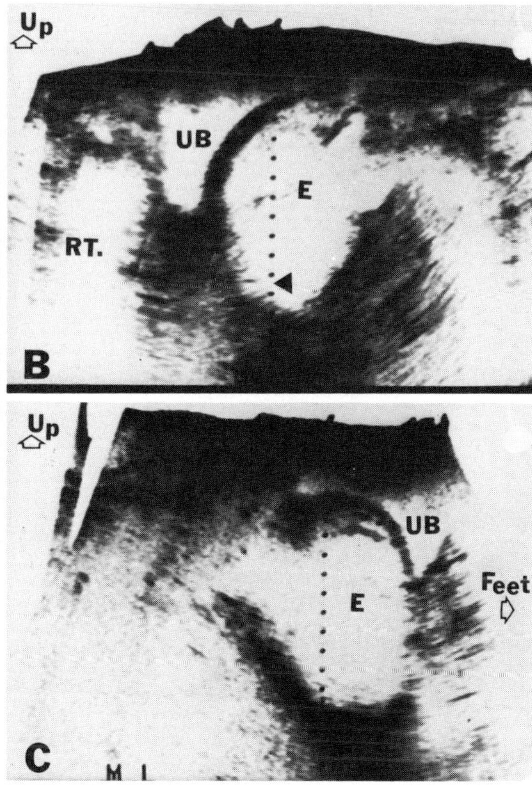

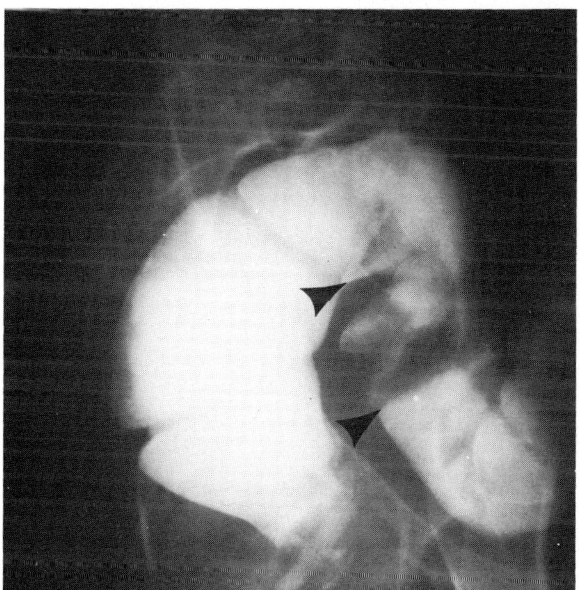

Fig 15–1 (top). – Huge endometrioma displacing rectum and sigmoid colon. **A,** anteroposterior post-evacuation film from barium enema examination. Sigmoid colon is displaced downward and to right and left *(arrows)* by large, readily palpable pelvic mass located in left side of pelvis. No intrinsic involvement of colon is evident. **B,** pelvic ultrasound study, transverse echotomogram made 3 cm above pubic symphysis. Urinary bladder *(UB)* contains small amount of urine and is displaced to right by huge fluid-filled, cystic endometrioma *(E)*. The circular lesion has a diameter of 10 cm (*arrowhead* indicates 1 cm scale). **C,** pelvic ultrasound study, longitudinal echotomogram made in midline of body. Large endometrioma *(E)* seen in **B** fills pouch of Douglas and depresses dome of bladder *(UB)*.

Fig 15–2 (bottom). – Polypoid endometrial lesion. Lateral view of rectum. This 4 cm long broad-based, polypoid lesion *(arrowheads)* extended into lumen and required excisional biopsy to exclude possibility of polypoid carcinoma. Preoperatively, patient complained of constipation, cramping lower abdominal pain and tenesmus. Symptoms were exaggerated during menstruation. The smooth muscle hypertrophy and fibroproliferative reaction associated with endometrial envasion into muscularis can result in a large intramural lesion that mimics an intraluminal polyp. (From Fagan, Radiol. Clin. North Am. 12:109, 1974, with permission.)

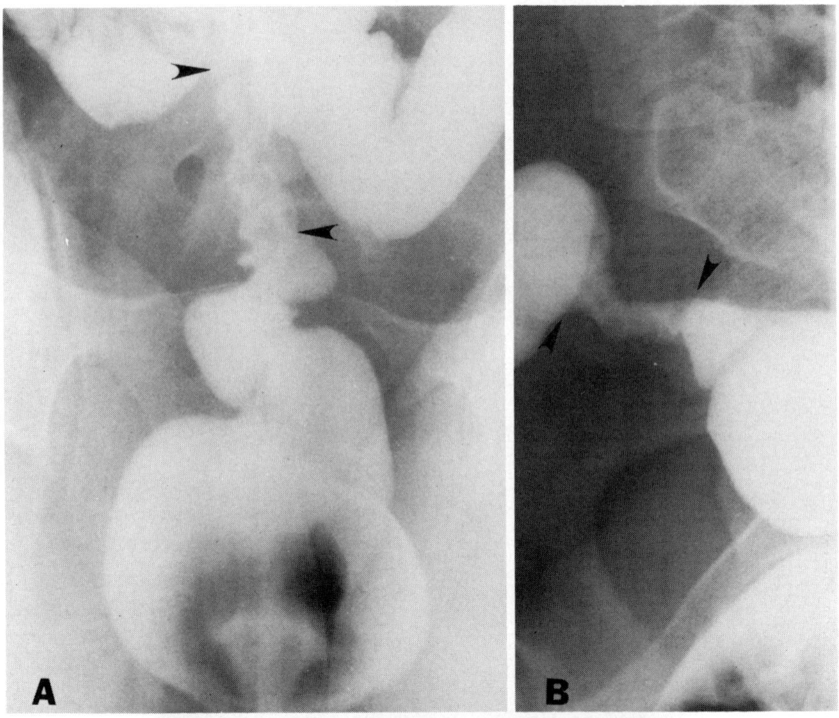

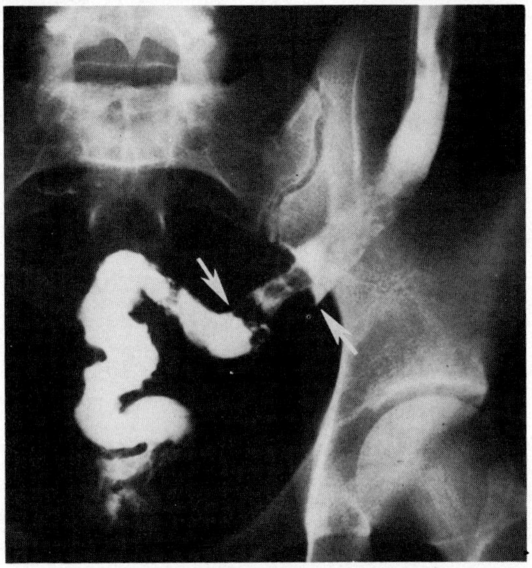

Fig 15–3 (top).—Inflammatory-like endometrial lesion of rectosigmoid colon. Barium enema: **A,** anteroposterior, and **B,** lateral views. A poorly marginated, long, lumen-narrowing, inflammatory-like endometrial involvement *(arrowheads)* of colon just above reflection of peritoneum at level of second sacral segment. Seeding of cul-de-sac, common to pelvic endometriosis, makes this a frequent site of involvement. Encircling configuration of this particular lesion is unusual, and deformity of contour is largely a function of hypertrophy of muscularis. (From Fagan, Radiol. Clin. North. Am. 12:109, 1974, with permission.)

Fig 15–4 (bottom).—Endometriosis simulating carcinoma of sigmoid. AP roentgenogram of lower gastrointestinal tract reveals sharply marginated, short, intramural, lumen-narrowing endometrial lesion *(arrows),* which has several radiographic features of malignancy. Intestinal endometriosis may produce symptoms many years after menopause, making this particular type of lesion a very ominous finding in elderly women. However, most lesions occur in relatively young age group and usually are associated with history of menstrual difficulties and infertility. There is no anemia, rectal bleeding or weight loss. Intact mucosa is only radiographic clue that lesion is benign. (From Fagan, Radiol. Clin. North Am. 12:109, 1974, with permission.)

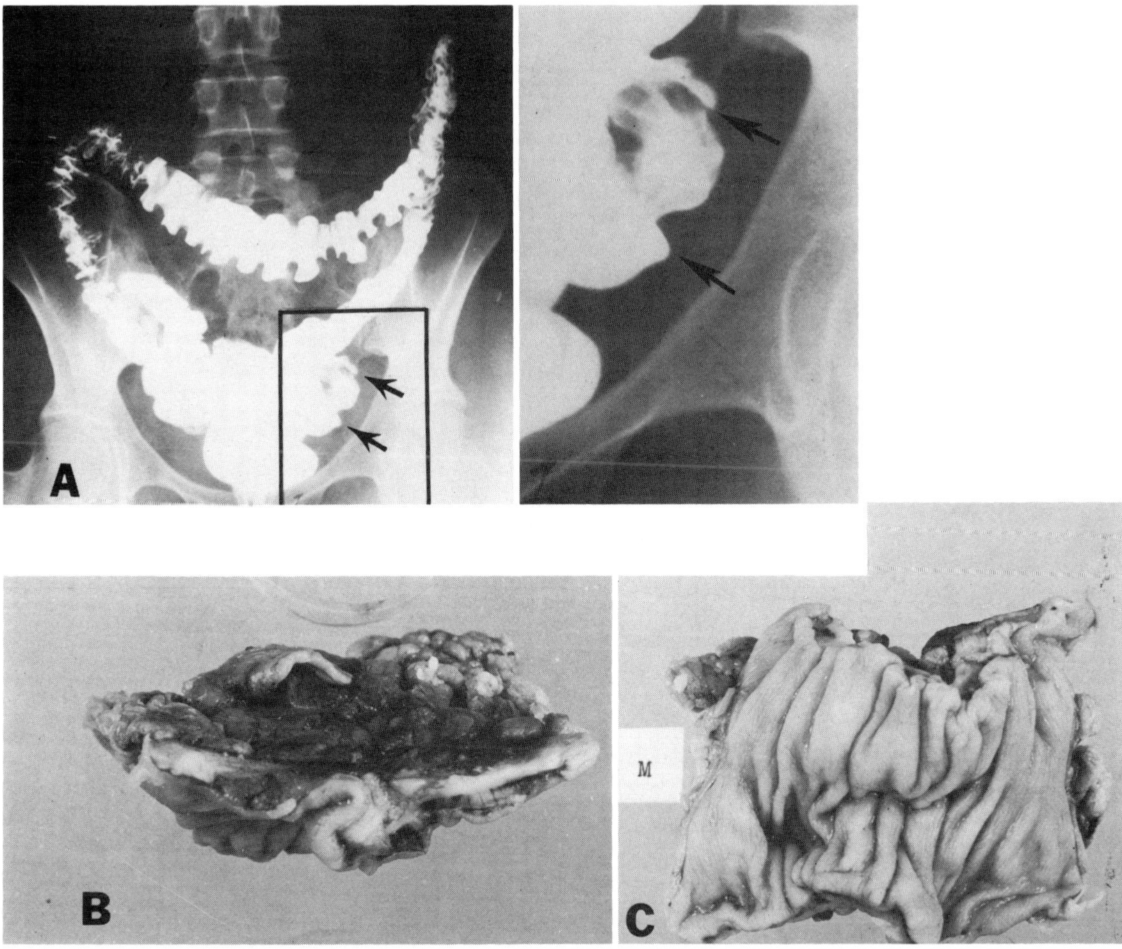

Fig 15–5. – Bulky intramural lesion with an intact mucosa. Ectopic endometrial tissue implanted in mural portion of intestine has decided potential to stimulate hyperplasia of smooth muscle while sparing any reaction or involvement of subjacent mucosa. **A**, barium enema, AP view. A short, bulky, constricting lesion with abrupt margins is shown *(arrows)*. **B**, surgical specimen, serosal side. Bulky lesion presents angry, irregular nodular appearance. **C**, surgical specimen, mucosal side. Mucosa is intact.

Since endometrial implants rarely involve intestinal mucosa, cyclic rectal bleeding as a manifestation of colonic endometriosis has been overstated, although it does occur occasionally (Courtesy of Dr. R. N. Cooley, Galveston; from Fagan, Radiol. Clin. North Am. 12:109, 1974, with permission.)

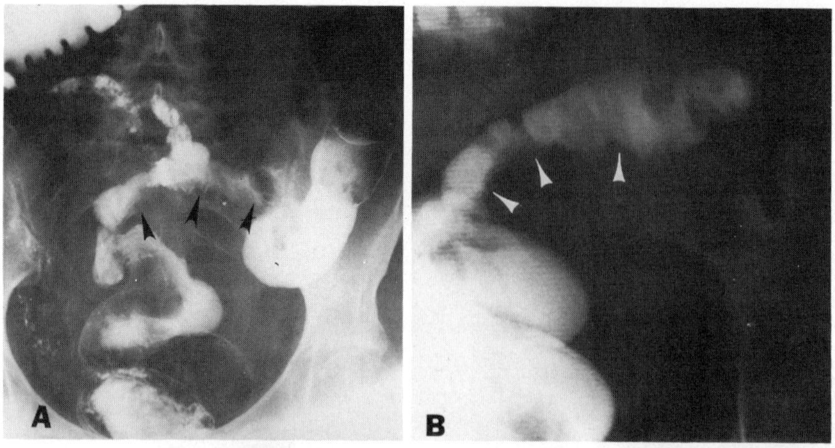

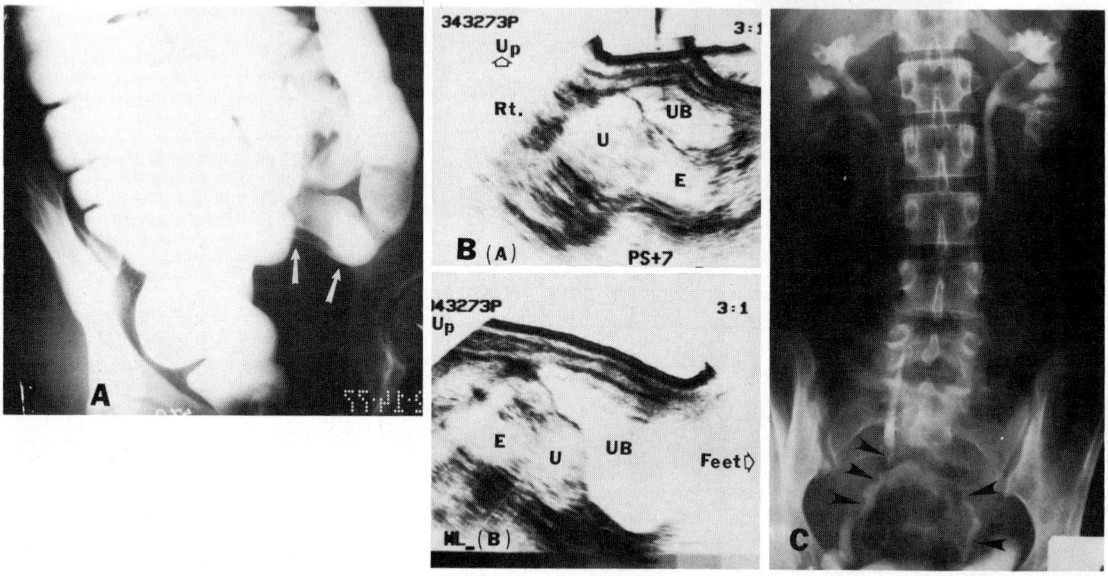

Fig 15–6 (top).—"Typical" intramural colonic lesions of endometriosis. Barium enema examination: **A,** anteroposterior view; **B,** left posterior oblique view. Antimesenteric margin of sigmoid colon is involved by 11 cm long scalloped lesion. Implant, composed of endometrial glands and stroma, and the intense fibrotic reaction it excites, invade bowel wall and extend into muscularis. This creates typical, intramural lesion with smooth surfaces and sharp margins, as depicted above. Tiny spiculations *(arrowheads)* represent lateral margins of intramural implants, not ulcerations. Appearance of lesion may be confused with diverticulitis. (From Fagan, Radiol. Clin. North Am. 12:109, 1974, with permission.)

Fig 15–7 (bottom).—Pelvic endometriosis displacing colon and involving distal ureters. Endometrial involvement of ovaries may result in development of large cystic spaces filled with brown blood debris to form "chocolate cysts" or endometriomas. These lesions often present as nonspecific pelvic masses displacing urinary bladder, uterus and colon. **A,** barium enema examination, left posterior oblique view. Smooth, extrinsic pressure along undersurface of sigmoid colon *(arrows)* resulted from large endometrioma of left ovary. **B,** ultrasound of pelvis, transverse echotomograms *(A)* made 7 cm above pubic symphysis *(PS+7)* and longitudinal echotomogram *(B)* made in the midline of body. Endometrioma *(E),* manifested by sonolucent mass with shaggy margins, is located posterior to urinary bladder *(UB)* and uterus *(U).* The abnormality displaces uterus to the right and is responsible for extrinsic pressure defect on undersurface of sigmoid colon depicted in **A. C,** excretory urogram. In this particular case, pelvic endometriosis, other than endometrioma depicted in **A** and **B,** extrinsically involved pelvic portions of both ureters *(arrowheads),* resulting in mild hydronephrosis of both kidneys.

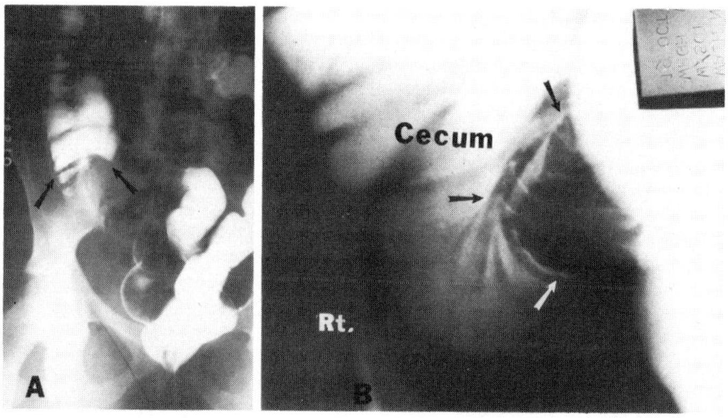

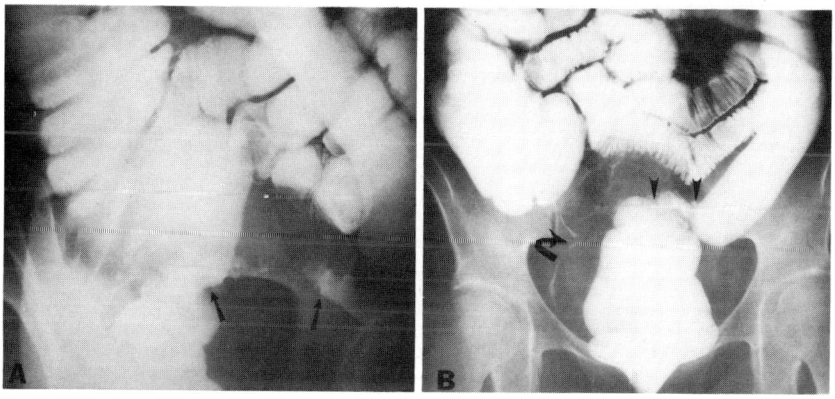

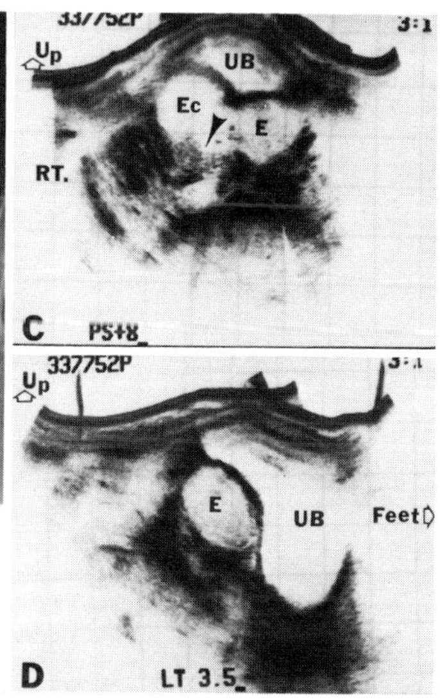

Fig 15–8 (top). – Endometriosis of cecum. Endometrial involvement of cecum rarely occurs. When it does, kinking constricting type of lesion typical of endometriosis in rest of the colon usually is not present. Instead, tip of cecum is imprinted by well-marginated, nodular lesion not unlike that associated with umbilication of an appendiceal stump, or intramural neoplasm of cecum (e.g., carcinoid) or various abnormalities of appendix (e.g., abscess or mucocele). Upper gastrointestinal examination: **A,** anteroposterior view, and, **B,** fluoroscopic spot view. Discrete, circular, intramural lesion of cecal pole is demonstrated *(arrows).* Mucosa is uninvolved. This configuration is typical of cecal endometriosis. (From Felson and West, Radiol. Clin. North Am. 7:83, 1969, with permission.)

Fig 15–9 (bottom). – Endometriosis of sigmoid colon, distal right ureter and pelvic endometrioma. **A,** barium enema examination: left posterior oblique view. Long segment of intramural endometriosis of sigmoid colon *(arrowheads)* associated with narrowing of lumen is projected over left innominate bone. **B,** barium enema examination: AP view. Sigmoid lesion seen in **A** is present *(arrows)* but foreshortened. Narrowing and kinking of distal right ureter, opacified by excretory urogram performed prior to barium enema study, also evident *(curved arrow).* **C,** pelvic ultrasound study: transverse echotomogram made 8 cm above pubic symphysis demonstrates urinary bladder *(UB),* solid endometrioma *(E)* on left and a second, larger, lobulated endometrioma *(Ec)* on right. Latter lesion is primarily cystic but contains debris *(arrowhead)* and is classified as a complex lesion. **D,** pelvic ultrasound study: longitudinal echotomogram made 3.5 cm to left of midline. Solid endometrioma *(E)* on left in **C** is identified behind urinary bladder *(UB).* It is oval, measuring 6 cm across widest diameter.

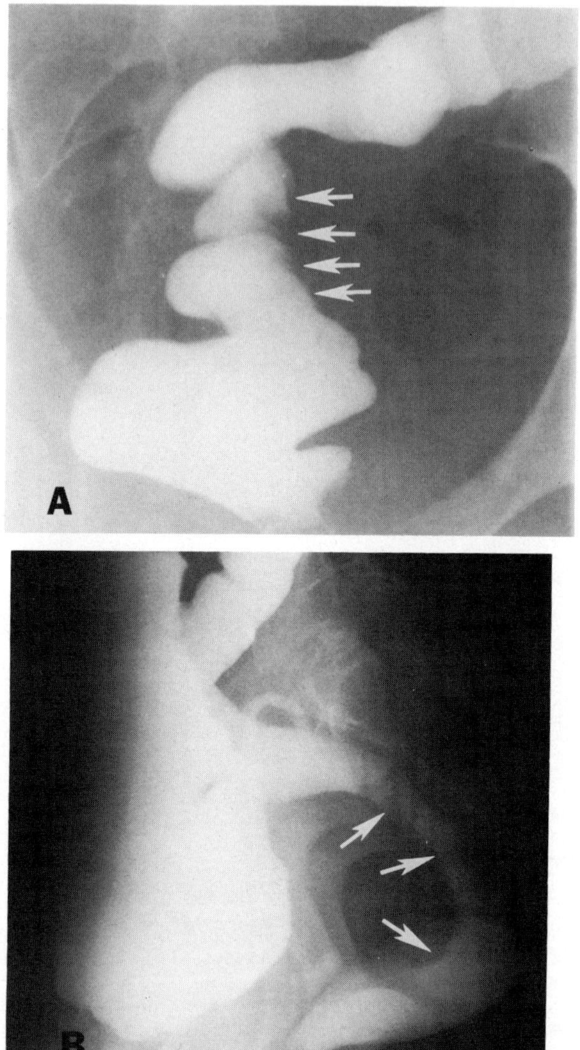

Fig 15–10.—Rectal endometriosis. Cul-de-sac endometrial seeding, with involvement of rectovaginal septum, often results in invasion of rectal wall. Barium enema: **A,** anteroposterior and **B,** lateral views of rectum. Multiple intramural implants resulting in smooth, scalloped defects in lateral and anterior surface of rectum are demonstrated *(arrows).* Lumen is narrowed slightly, mucosa intact. This type of involvement may be overlooked unless barium enema examination includes lateral projection of rectum. (From Fagan, Radiol. Clin. North Am. 12:109, 1974, with permission.)

Chapter 16

Extrinsic Lesions Affecting the Colon

COLONIC MANIFESTATIONS OF GALLBLADDER DISEASES

GARY G. GHAHREMANI, M.D.
MORTON A. MEYERS, M.D.

THE LARGE BOWEL not only occupies a significant portion of the abdominal cavity but its peritoneally mobile segments (transverse colon and sigmoid) and the retroperitoneally fixed parts (ascending and descending colon) are intimately related to most abdominal viscera.[1, 2] Therefore, both inflammatory and neoplastic lesions of adjacent organs easily can involve the large bowel through the established anatomical pathways.[3-7] At times, it is the striking manifestations of such colonic involvement that first bring the patient to medical attention.

Furthermore, barium enema examination often is used as the initial radiologic study in evaluation of a variety of nonspecific abdominal complaints, so that correct identification of the secondary nature of colonic alterations can be crucial in diagnosing the primary source of the problem. In this context, abnormalities of the colon due to gallbladder pathology deserve particular attention because of the prevalence of biliary diseases and because of the often nonspecific or misleading clinical presentation of these abnormalities. For example, symptoms suggestive of large bowel disease, e.g., rectal bleeding and diarrhea, are not uncommonly associated with lesions originating in the gallbladder.[3, 8-17]

This section is therefore intended to illustrate the radiographic spectrum of colonic involvement by gallbladder diseases and to provide differential diagnostic guidelines for the findings noted on barium enema examination.

Cholecystocolic Relationships: Normal Radiographic Anatomy

The right colic or hepatic flexure may be considered as two separate segments with distinguishable topographic features.[1-4] (1) The proximal or ascending part, which represents continuation of the retroperitoneally fixed ascending colon, is in close proximity to the lateral margins of the right kidney. (2) The transverse portion of the flexure is located anteriorly and thereby intimately related to the gallbladder and the right lobe of the liver (Fig 16–1, A). The gallbladder itself is attached superiorly to the undersurface of the liver, but the rest of it is covered by a peritoneal reflection that forms the serosal surface. It has been shown that in 64–78% of individuals, the body and fundus of the gallbladder are virtually in direct contact with the adjacent transverse portion of the hepatic flexure (see Fig 16–1, B).[3, 12] The remaining individuals do not exhibit a close anatomical relationship between the hepatic flexure and the gallbladder because of congenital variations in size, position and degree of mobility of the gallbladder, liver and colon.

Cholecystocholic Relationships: Radiologic Pathologic Aspects

ACUTE CHOLECYSTITIS

The inflammation usually results in diffuse thickening and edema of the wall of the gallbladder, and fibrinous exudates may form on its congested serosal surface. The gallbladder often becomes distended owing to associated obstruction of the cystic duct by an impacted stone or inflammatory edema of the spiral mucosal folds known as valves of Heister.[13] These changes produce several recognizable findings on barium enema examination: extrinsic compression of the hepatic flexure by the distended gallbladder, evidence of localized mucosal edema of the colon and segmental contractions narrowing the lumen (Fig 16–2). Since acute cholecystitis usually results in nonvisualization by oral cholecystogram, the above-noted barium enema abnormalities can provide indirect but useful criteria for the correct diagnosis.[3] Since the changes are transient, the cholecystocolic interface will return to normal following an episode of acute but uncomplicated cholecystitis.

CHRONIC CHOLECYSTITIS

In patients with chronic recurrent cholecystitis, the wall of the gallbladder becomes diffusely thickened, and fibrinous adhesions usually form between its serosal surface and the adjacent organs. Therefore, the often shrunken gallbladder becomes tightly adherent to the neighboring segments of the hepatic flexure, duodenum and greater omentum.[3, 10, 13-16] These adhesions must be removed to make the gallbladder visible and accessible when cholecystectomy is attempted. Such pericholecystic adhesions may present as a localized extrinsic compression on the superior aspects of the hepatic flexure (Fig 16–3, A). On the other hand, chronic cholecystitis and associated adhesions may produce polypoid filling defects or pseudotumors composed of granulation tissue in the involved colon (see Fig 16–3, B), requiring segmental resection at the time of surgery.[8, 17, 18]

PERICHOLECYSTIC ABSCESS

Phlegmonous inflammation of the gallbladder may lead to perforation and generalized peritonitis. In most instances, however, the process remains localized because the greater omentum and the serosa of the neighboring structures become adherent to and effectively seal the gallbladder.[3] Such pericholecystic abscess may encircle the hepatic flexure of the colon and produce an annular lesion closely resembling a primary carcinoma of the colon (Fig 16–4). In several reported cases, the resultant involvement of the colon has been so severe that differentiation from carcinoma on the basis of radiographic or intraoperative findings has not been possible.[8, 9, 16, 17, 19, 20] Nevertheless, careful evaluation of the abnormalities noted on barium enema—particularly the specific location in the anterior segment of the hepatic flexure, the length of the lesion and apparent preservation of the otherwise retracted and crowded colonic mucosal folds—should correctly indicate the secondary nature of the findings.

HYDROPS, EMPYEMA AND OTHER CAUSES OF DISTENDED GALLBLADDER

Obstruction of the cystic duct by impacted stone, inflammatory edema of the spiral folds and scarring may produce a markedly distended gallbladder owing to retention of secretions (hydrops). The gallbladder content may subsequently become infected, causing an empyema. In both instances, a distended gallbladder can be recognized on plain radiographs of the abdomen or barium enema examination by virtue of a localized indentation on the superior aspect of the hepatic flexure (Fig 16–5).[1-4, 21] This segment also would show evidence of mucosal edema and spasm in patients with empyema, whereas the lack of such inflammatory changes and the absence of leukocytosis, jaundice and localized tenderness are highly diagnostic of hydrops.[3]

Porcelain gallbladder denotes diffuse calcifications in the form of large plaques or flakes within the muscular wall of the organ. The condition is often associated with a calcified gallstone occluding the outlet of the gallbladder, as well as marked thickening of the wall owing to long-standing inflammation. Such a chronically diseased gallbladder may become adherent to the hepatic flexure (Fig 16–6) and perhaps induce pressure necrosis and hemorrhage in its wall.[3]

Courvoisier gallbladder refers to the distention of the gallbladder subsequent to obstruction of the common bile duct by carcinoma arising in the head of the pancreas. Barium enema examination of such patients may show extrinsic compression of the hepatic flexure by the distended gallbladder (Fig 16–7). Occasionally the evidence for direct extension of the pancreatic tumor to the transverse colon also may be seen.[4, 22]

Carcinoma of the Gallbladder

This tumor tends to infiltrate the wall of the gallbladder and rapidly invades the adjacent structures. In a series of 78 cases reported by Litwin[23], extension of the malignancy to the colon was present in 22%. About 15% of patients with carcinoma of the gallbladder will demonstrate radiographic evidence of colonic involvement on barium enema examination.[3, 24, 25] Therefore, the cholecystocolic relationships become important factors in the spread of cancer, production of clinical symptoms and feasibility of surgical treatment. Although involvement of the colon usually is a delayed manifestation of the disease, the resultant rectal bleeding and other intestinal complaints also may be the initial presenting symptoms.[3, 4]

The spectrum of barium enema findings associated with carcinoma of the gallbladder primarily depends on the location of the tumor as well as on preexisting cholecystocolic relationships.[3, 24, 25, 26] Therefore, a malignancy originating in or involving the inferior surface of the body and fundus of the gallbladder is most likely to directly involve the adjacent hepatic flexure (Fig 16–8). In contrast, a tumor developing in the neck of the gallbladder tends to obstruct the cystic duct and thereby cause only extrinsic compression of the colon by the distended gallbladder.[3, 24, 25]

Cholecystocolic Fistula

Spontaneous enterobiliary fistulas are a complication of chronic cholecystitis with lithiasis in about 75% of patients. Perforating duodenal ulcer; carcinomas originating in the gallbladder, colon or pancreas; and a few rare entities are responsible for the remainder of the patients.[10, 13, 17, 24] Cholecystocolic fistulas, which account for about one third of all enterobiliary fistulas, usually represent the end result of failure to properly diagnose and treat chronic cholecystitis.[3, 8, 10, 15, 20] In such patients the formation of pericholecystic adhesions permits the gallbladder to subsequently erode and discharge its content into the colon. This may result in impaction of a gallstone in the colon (Fig 16–9). The basic plain film findings are air within the biliary duct and an irregular collection of gas within the shrunken gallbladder. The cholecystocolic fistula itself is best demonstrated on barium enema examination, which can clearly outline the site of communication by reflux of contrast material (see Fig 16–9, A).

Cholecystocolic fistulas also may form as a result of extension of a gallbladder carcinoma into the adjacent hepatic flexure, duodenum or both.[13, 25, 28] Such patients may initially present with diarrhea, melena and loss of weight—symptoms that are more suggestive of intestinal than biliary tract disease.[3] Accordingly, the barium enema examination not only will delineate the fistula but may provide information about the underlying problem (Fig 16–10).[29] Radiologic differentiation of the basic etiologic factors, i.e., cholecystitis from carcinoma, is at times difficult, since the tumor often is superimposed on chronic cholecystitis with or without gallstones. However, demonstration of extensive mucosal destruction and tumefaction of the involved colon, with or without associated cholecystocolic fistula, would suggest the presence of gallbladder carcinoma (Fig 16–10).

REFERENCES

1. Whalen, J. P.: Anatomy of the colon. Guide to intra-abdominal pathology, Am. J. Roentgenol. 125:3, 1975.
2. Whalen, J. P., and Riemenschneider, P. A.: Analysis of normal anatomic relationships of colon as applied to roentgenographic observations, Am. J. Roentgenol. 99:55, 1967.
3. Ghahremani, G. G., and Meyers, M. A.: The cholecysto-colic relationships. A roentgen-anatomic study of the colonic manifestations of gallbladder disorders, Am. J. Roentgenol. 125:21, 1975.
4. Meyers, M. A.: *Dynamic Radiology of the Abdomen. Normal and Pathologic Anatomy* (New York: Springer-Verlag, Inc., 1976).
5. Meyers, M. A., and Evans, J. A.: Effects of pancreatitis on small bowel and colon: Spread along mesenteric planes, Am. J. Roentgenol. 119:15, 1973.
6. Meyers, M. A., and McSweeney, J.: Secondary neoplasms of bowel, Radiology 105:1, 1972.
7. Meyers, M. A., and Whalen, J. P.: Roentgen significance of duodenocolic relationships: Anatomic approach, Am. J. Roentgenol. 117:263, 1973.
8. Kaplan, B. J.: Massive lower gastrointestinal hemorrhage from cholecystocolic fistula, Dis. Colon Rectum 10:191, 1967.
9. Kent, K. H.: Extrinsic lesions affecting transverse colon, Am. J. Roentgenol. 89:779, 1963.
10. Safaie-Shirazi, S., Zike, W. L., and Printen, K. J.: Spontaneous enterobiliary fistulas, Surg. Gynecol. Obstet. 137:769, 1973.
11. Stahl, W. M., Jr.: Gastrointestinal tract hemorrhage due to gallbladder disease, N. Engl. J. Med. 260: 471, 1959.
12. Jacobson, H. G., Shapiro, J. H., Stern, W., and Poppel, M. H.: Positional relation of gallbladder to hepatic flexure, Am. J. Dig. Dis. 1:294, 1956.
13. Glenn, F., and Mannix, H., Jr.: Biliary enteric fistula, Surg. Gynecol. Obstet. 105:693, 1957.
14. Hoffman, G. L., Jr., von Kassel, K. F., and Hoerr, S. O.: Obstruction of small intestine caused by acute cholecystitis, Arch. Surg. 76:412, 1958.
15. Marshak, R. H., and Henkin, W.: Cholecystocolic fistula, Radiology 53:555, 1949.
16. Rockoff, S. D., and Tuddenham, W. J.: Adherent gallbladder simulating intrinsic lesion of right side of colon: Report of a case, Am. J. Roentgenol. 87: 749, 1962.
17. Neville, W. E.: Duodenocolic fistula due to acute cholecystitis, Am. J. Surg. 87:300, 1954.
18. Kyaw, M. M., and Koehler, P. R.: Pseudotumors of colon due to adhesions, Radiology 103:597, 1972.
19. DiRienzo, S., and Mosca, L. G.: Epiplopericolitis: Significance of its roentgenological diagnosis, Am. J. Roentgenol. 66:215, 1951.
20. Waggoner, C. M., and LeMone, D. V.: Clinical and roentgen aspects of internal biliary fistulas: Report of twelve cases, Radiology 53:31, 1949.
21. Scanlan, R. L., and Young, B. R.: Roentgen diagnosis of gallbladder and biliary tract disease without cholecystography, Am. J. Roentgenol. 72:639, 1954.
22. Meyers, M. A., Volberg, F., Katzen, B., and Abbott, G.: Haustral anatomy and pathology: New look. II. Roentgen interpretation of pathological alterations, Radiology 108:505, 1973.
23. Litwin, M. S.: Primary carcinoma of gallbladder: Review of 78 patients, Arch. Surg. 95:236, 1967.
24. Keill, R. H., and DeWesse, M. S.: Primary carcinoma of gallbladder, Am. J. Surg. 125:726, 1973.
25. McConnel, F.: Malignant neoplasm of gallbladder: Roentgenological diagnosis, Radiology 69:720, 1957.
26. Khilnani, M. T., Wolf, B. S., and Finkel, M.: Roentgen features of carcinoma of gallbladder on barium meal examination, Radiology 79:264, 1962.
27. Hall Drake, E. P., and Goodwin, J. F.: Duodenocolic fistula complicating carcinoma coli, Br. J. Surg. 36:204, 1948.
28. Fahim, R. B., McDonald, J. R., Richards, J. C., and Ferris, D. O.: Carcinoma of gallbladder: Study of its modes of spread, Ann. Surg. 156:114, 1962.
29. Overton, R. C., Bolton, B. F., and Usher, F. C.: Extrinsic deformities of colon mimicking carcinoma: Report of three cases, Surgery 36:906, 1954.

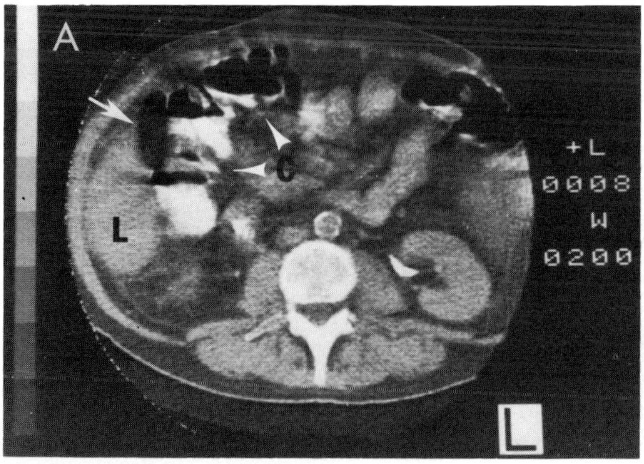

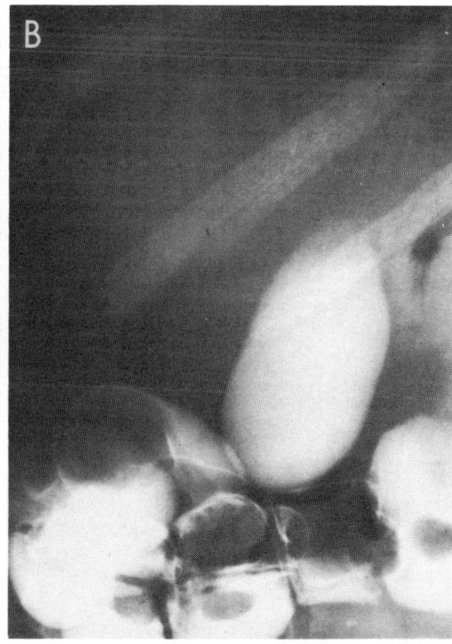

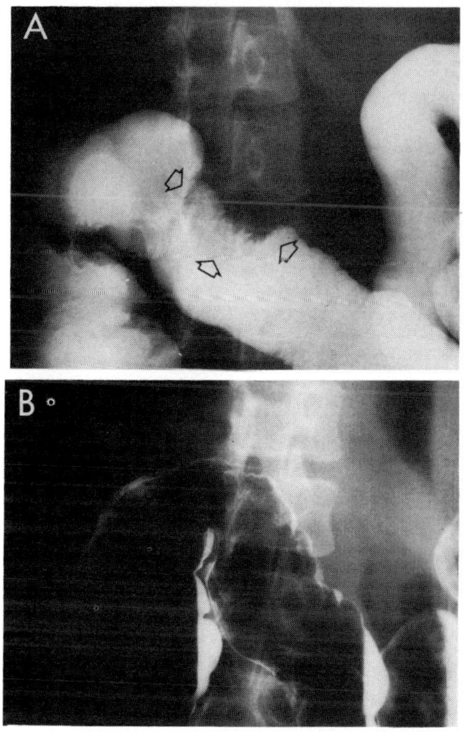

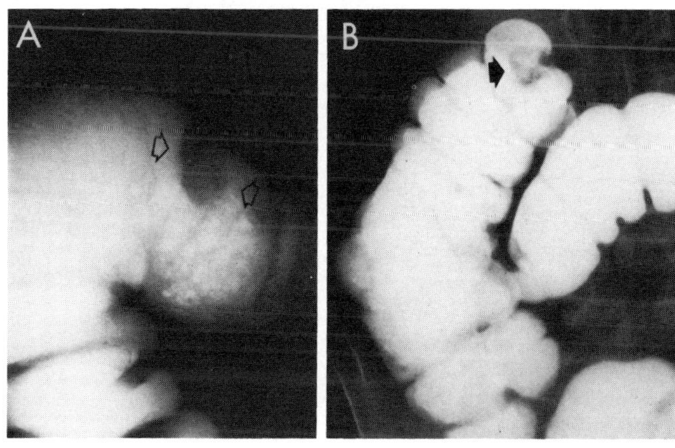

Fig 16–1 (top).—Radiographic anatomy of cholecystocolic relationships. **A,** computerized tomographic cross section of upper abdomen demonstrates position of gallbladder *(arrow)* anteriorly between right lobe of liver *(L)* and hepatic flexure of colon *(C) (arrowheads).* **B,** normal indentation of superior aspect of hepatic flexure by fundus of gallbladder is revealed by combination of oral cholecystogram and barium enema examination.

Fig 16–2 (bottom left).—Acute cholecystitis. **A,** barium enema study during acute episode shows localized mucosal edema and extrinsic compression of colon by enlarged gallbladder *(arrows).* **B,** Air contrast colon examination 2 weeks after remission of symptoms shows return to normal appearance of hepatic flexure. (From Ghahremani and Meyers, Am. J. Roentgenol. 125:21, 1975, with permission.)

Fig 16–3 (bottom right).—Chronic cholecystitis with adhesions causing pseudotumor of hepatic flexure in two patients. **A,** in woman age 60, localized mass in anterior hepatic flexure *(arrows)* was surgically proved to be result of fibrinous adhesions between gallbladder, colon and greater omentum. **B,** barium enema examination of another patient with chronic cholecystitis shows 1.5 cm filling defect *(arrow)* with irregular collection of barium in most superior aspect of hepatic flexure. (From Ghahremani and Meyers, Am. J. Roentgenol. 125:21, 1975, with permission.)

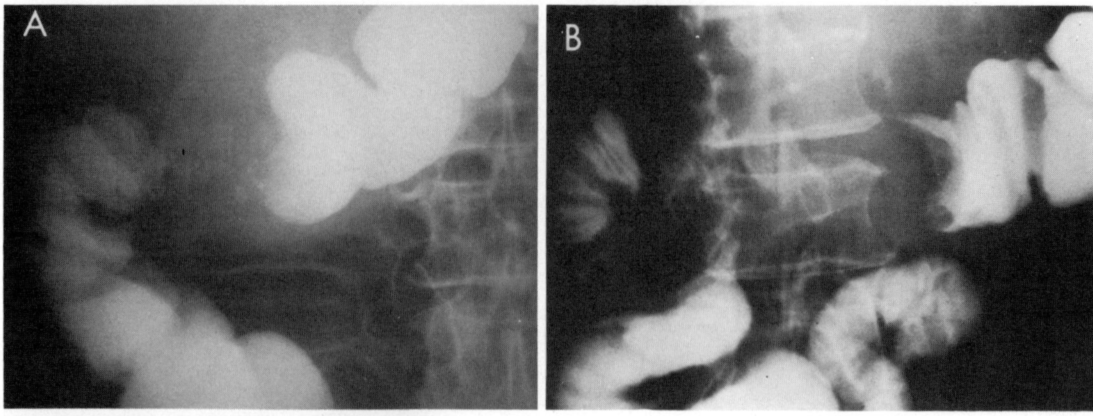

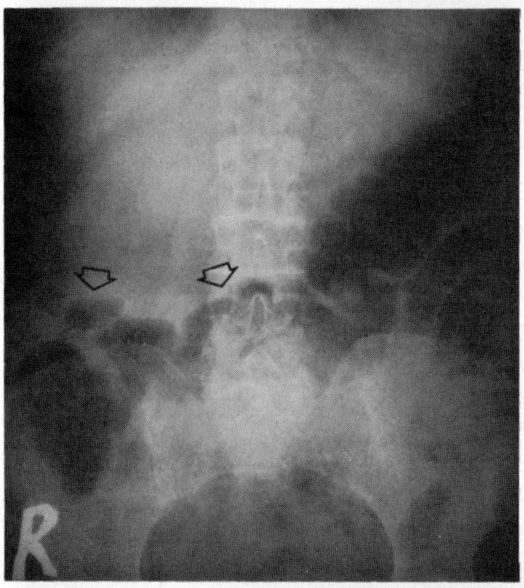

Fig 16–4 (above). – **A** and **B,** pericholecystic abscess in man age 67 with several days' history of fever, right upper quadrant tenderness and rectal bleeding. Barium enema examination shows 6 cm long constricting lesion of anterior hepatic flexure with shelflike distal border resembling carcinoma of colon. Operative findings were those of perforated gallbladder empyema with pericolic abscess. (From Ghahremani and Meyers, Am. J. Roentgenol. 125:21, 1975, with permission.)

Fig 16–5 (left). – Hydrops of gallbladder. Supine film of abdomen demonstrates inferior displacement of hepatic flexure *(arrows)* by markedly distended gallbladder.

Fig 16–6 (below). – Calcified gallbladder in man age 81 who presented with palpable abdominal mass and rectal bleeding. **A,** plain film shows large "porcelain" gallbladder with impacted stone in its neck *(arrow).* **B,** barium enema examination demonstrates medial and upward displacement of gallbladder *(black arrows)* due to its adherence to wall of proximal transverse colon. *White arrow* shows impacted stone.

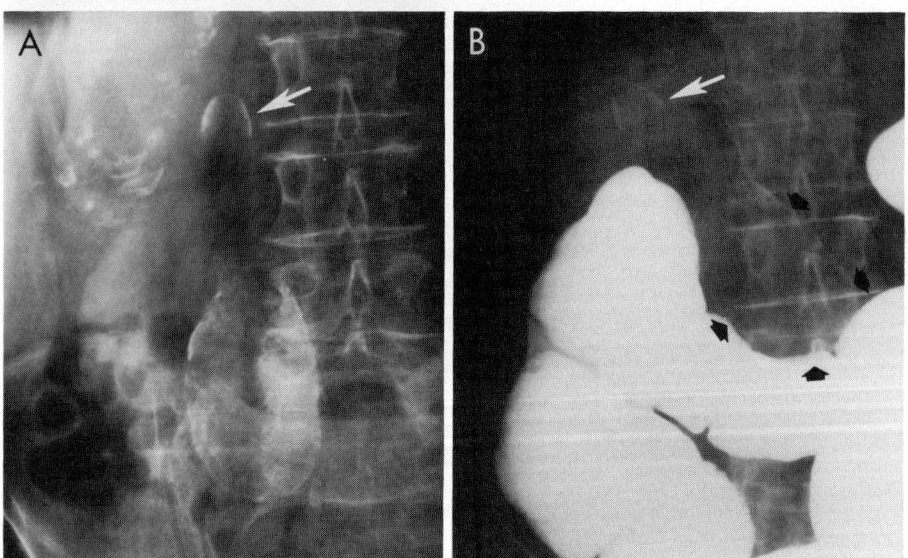

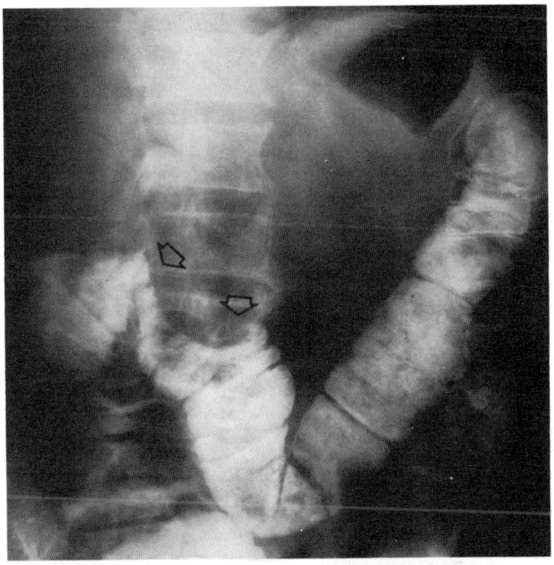

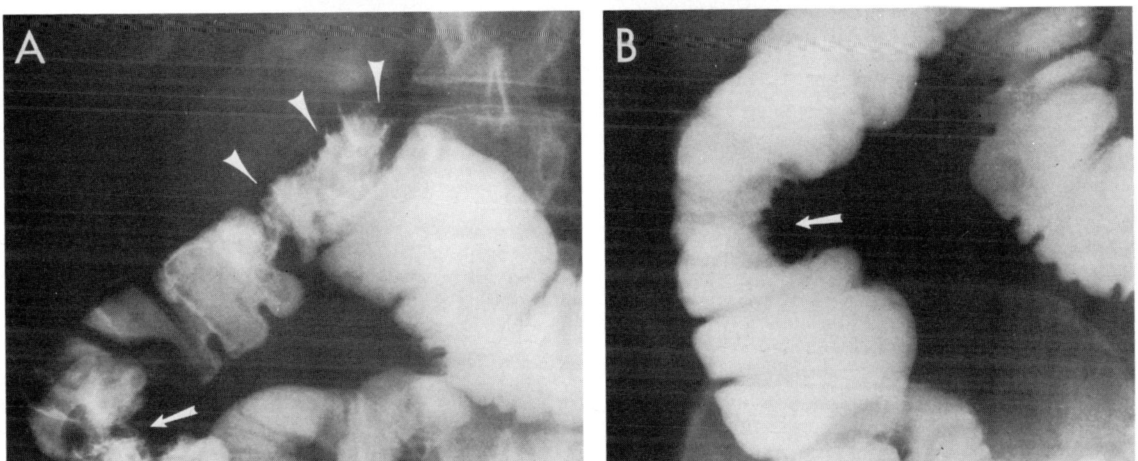

Fig 16–7 (top).—Smooth extrinsic compression of hepatic flexure by distended gallbladder *(arrows)* secondary to obstruction of common bile duct by carcinoma of pancreas. (From Ghahremani and Meyers, Am. J. Roentgenol. 125:21, 1975, with permission.)

Fig 16–8 (bottom).—**A** and **B,** carcinoma of gallbladder involving colon. Two spot films show extensive tumor infiltration of superior border of hepatic flexure *(arrowheads),* as well as metastatic deposit *(arrow)* in wall of ascending colon. (From Ghahremani and Meyers, Am. J. Roentgenol. 125:21, 1975, with permission.)

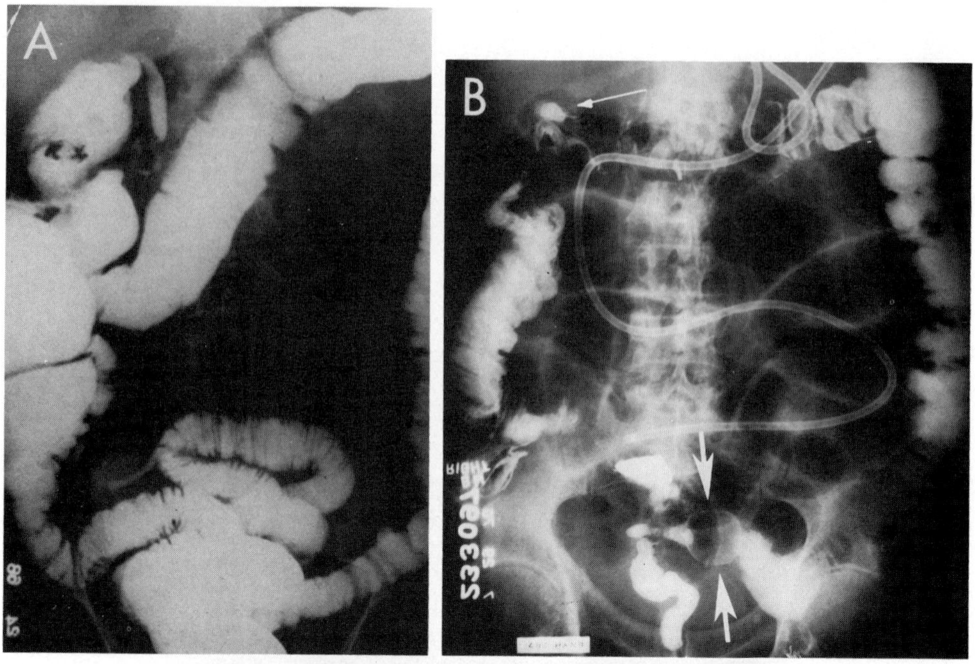

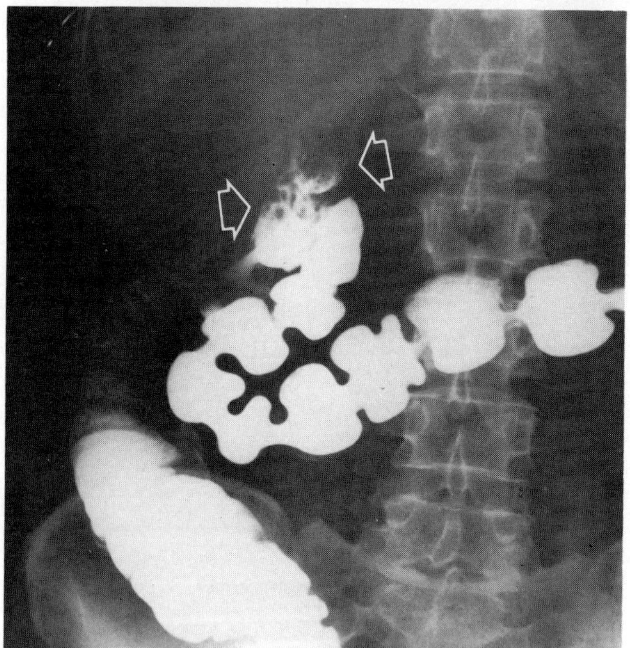

Fig 16–9 (top).—Cholecystocolic fistula complicating chronic cholecystitis in two patients. **A,** barium enema examination demonstrates wide communication between gallbladder containing small stones and adjacent hepatic flexure. **B,** gallstone ileus due to impaction of large radiolucent gallstone *(large arrows)* in sigmoid colon. There is marked dilatation of intestinal loops, and shrunken gallbladder *(small arrow)* is partially filled with barium. (From Ghahremani and Meyers, Am. J. Roentgenol. 125:21, 1975, with permission.)

Fig 16–10 (bottom).—Cholecystocolic fistula caused by carcinoma of gallbladder. Tumor is seen projecting within gallbladder lumen *(arrows)* and infiltrating the adjacent segment of hepatic flexure.

DIRECT EFFECTS OF RENAL DISEASES ON THE COLON

MORTON A. MEYERS, M.D.

MANY PATIENTS with renal disease present with symptoms that seem to arise from the digestive tract. Almost every case of urinary tract disease is known to be accompanied by some gastrointestinal complaint of a transitory or permanent character.[1] Clinical investigation of such patients is often started with barium enema studies. It is thus important to recognize that characteristic effects on specific portions of the colon may uncover the primary renal disease and redirect the course of evaluation.[2, 3]

Basic to a radiologic appreciation of the characteristic colonic changes is an understanding of the anatomical relationships.

Anatomical Considerations

RIGHT KIDNEY

The right kidney is in intimate relationship to a particular segment of the colon as it courses obliquely over the lower pole (Fig 16–11). This occurs precisely at its level between (1) the distal ascending colon and the posterior hepatic flexure, which is related superiorly to the deep inferior visceral surface of the liver, and (2) the anterior hepatic flexure as it crosses the descending duodenum—this segment marks the beginning of the transverse mesocolon and is related superiorly to the gallbladder.

Figure 16–11 further illustrates that, whereas the upper two thirds of the right kidney are related to the right colon between its two flexures, the lower pole is inframesocolic and is related laterally and anteriorly to the distal ascending colon.

LEFT KIDNEY

The relationships of the left kidney to the bowel are most intimate to the distal transverse and proximal descending colon. Figure 16–12 illustrates these relationships and the complex peritoneal reflections in the left flank. The reflections of the transverse mesocolon cross the left kidney anteriorly, along a narrow "bare area" at the junction of its middle and lower thirds, to continue with the peritoneal reflections over the descending colon. At the junction of the transverse and descending colon, the peritoneum reflects from the anatomical splenic flexure to form the phrenicocolic ligament,[4] which inserts on the left diaphragm at the level of the 10th and 11th ribs. The distal transverse colon is related to the anterior surface of the lower half of the left kidney, although at variable distances, depending on the length of the transverse mesocolon. The lower pole is fully inframesocolic. The extraperitoneal descending colon passes downward along the lateral border of the left kidney, turning somewhat medially toward the lower border of the psoas muscle at the lower pole. Other peritoneal reflections account for the splenorenal ligament, within which the tail of the pancreas inserts.

Radiologic Observations

The intimate anatomical relationships of the kidneys to specific portions of the colon precisely account for characteristic changes of deformity or distortion.[2, 3]

CHARACTERISTIC MASS DISPLACEMENTS

Right Kidney (Figs 16–13 to 16–19)

In masses originating within the upper two thirds of the right kidney, the right colon segment most typically involved is that extending between the posterior and anterior hepatic flexures. This demonstrates displacement, respectively, inferiorly and anteriorly

Extrinsic pressure may be further shown by flattening and compression of the superior and posterior haustral rows at this site. Extension of a renal mass laterally into the flank displaces the posterior hepatic flexure inferiorly. Further progression may result in striking displacement of the ascending colon medially and anteriorly. Maintenance of the lateral haustral contours with extrinsic flattening of the posterior haustral sacculations characterizes the mass effects as extraperitoneal, rather than sited within the intraperitoneal lateral paracolic gutter.[5, 6]

A mass originating in the lower pole of the right kidney characteristically elevates the colon between the two hepatic flexures. Extrinsic compression occurs on the inferior haustral rows at this site, and the process may affect adjacent segments of the transverse and ascending colon. Oblique projections document that the affected colon also is usually displaced anteriorly and medially. At times, very discrete pressure changes, selectively on the posterior haustra of this segment, may be recognizable even on frontal projections—an observation further substantiating the extraperitoneal nature of the mass.[6]

Left Kidney

Left renal masses usually come into relationship with the colon before they attain a size that displaces the stomach, duodenojejunal junction or small bowel. Masses arising in the upper half may displace the distal transverse colon inferiorly and anteriorly. Those originating in the lower half are often first revealed by typical effects on specific portions of the left colon. The descending limb of the distal transverse colon appears compressed and displaced laterally and anteriorly (Fig 16–20). Significantly, the landmark of the anatomical splenic flexure is preserved. Masses projecting from the lower pole displace the descending colon laterally and anteriorly (Fig 16–21). Again, the anatomical splenic flexure is unaffected.

INVASIVE HYPERNEPHROMA

Renal neoplasms may directly invade adjacent segments of colon. On the left, characteristically affected are the distal transverse and proximal descending segments.[3, 7] They may be seen as recurrences many years after the primary tumor has been resected. They tend to produce bulky intraluminal masses without significant obstruction, since they generally elicit no desmoplastic response (Fig 16–22).

PERINEPHRITIS AND RENOINTESTINAL FISTULAS

Advanced perirenal infection may break through fascial boundaries to involve overlying colon.[8] The descending colon passes downward along the lateral border of the left kidney, turning somewhat medially toward the lateral border of the psoas muscle at the lower pole (Fig 16–23). At this level the descending colon lies within areolar tissue in the anterior pararenal space behind the posterior parietal peritoneum. Normally it is separated posteriorly from the kidney and perirenal fat by the anterior renal fascia.

The pathogenesis involves a site of renal infection that breaks through the capsule of the kidney to contaminate the perirenal space. Fulminating infections erupt through the fascial boundaries and spread to the overlying structures. On the left, the distal transverse colon, and particularly the proximal or mid-descending colon, and on the right, the ascending colon are involved. Changes reflecting at least inflammatory adherence may affect principally the medial or posterior contour of the colon or they may be circumferential. They are manifested primarily by spastic narrowing, scalloped induration and inflammatory mucosal thickening[3, 8] (Figs 16–24 to 16–26). In the descending colon, localization to the area distal to the splenic flexure overlaps the site involved in the extension of pancreatitis to the colon,[3, 9] but lack of associated changes involving the flexure itself is a helpful differential point.

A gross extraperitoneal sinus communication represents advanced transmural erosion. Most renocolic fistulas are secondary to an underlying chronic kidney infection.[3, 8]

RENAL AGENESIS AND ECTOPIA

Agenesis or ectopia of the kidney is frequently accompanied by characteristic malposition of specific portions of the colon.[3, 10]

These anomalies are not rare. Unilateral renal agenesis and renal ectopia have been found more frequently on roentgen examination (1 in 500) than in autopsy series (1 in 700 – 1,500).[3] There is a male to female ratio of 3:2, and the anomalies are more common on the left side.[11] In unilateral agenesis, the opposite kidney has been found to be diseased in one third of cases, usually secondary to chronic pyelonephritis.[11] Compensatory hypertrophy of the solitary kidney renders it more susceptible to injury. In an ectopic kidney or crossed renal ectopia with fusion, the incidence of complications such as lithiasis, infection and hydronephrosis approaches 50%. Pelvic ectopy is important in obstetrics because it may complicate delivery. Anomalies of structures arising from the urogenital ridge are associated with these renal conditions in almost 20% of cases.[11]

Right Side

On the right side, barium enema study may first reveal the condition by demonstrating that the posterior portion of the hepatic flexure of the colon occupies the area of the renal fossa.[12]

Left Side

With agenesis or ectopia of the left kidney, the mesenteric distal transverse colon may be deflected posteriorly and medially into the "empty" renal fossa area. Similarly, the anatomical splenic flexure of the colon may be deflected toward the same site (Figs 16 – 27 and 16 – 28). The anatomical splenic flexure normally is not only the most posterior but also the most fixed portion of the large intestine, being restrained by the phrenicocolic ligament.[4] The colonic malposition may be evident as a finding on plain films (Fig 16 – 29).

In left renal agenesis or ectopia, the colonic changes should not be confused with displacement by an enlarged spleen. Splenomegaly may depress the anatomical splenic flexure of the colon but does not displace it medially.

These changes in intestinal position have not been seen after acquired atrophy of the kidney. Presumably, adipose replacement between the intact perirenal fascial layers contributes to this. However, colonic malposition may be noted after anterior nephrectomy[3] (Fig 16 – 30).

DIRECT COLONIC EFFECTS UNIQUE TO RENAL ECTOPIA

In cases of ectopic kidney in the true pelvis, there is usually no definite pressure effect on the sigmoid colon, presumably because the kidney within the sacral hollow does not come into relationship with the anteriorly directed sigmoid loops.[10]

However, renal ectopia in the iliac fossa or lower abdomen may result in a characteristic mass effect on or displacement of the ascending or descending colon[10] (Fig 16 – 31). Failure to recognize the characteristic mass effects and displacements as secondary to renal ectopia may lead to unnecessary surgery.

REFERENCES

1. Katz, A. B.: Gastrointestinal manifestations of urinary tract disease, J. Urol. 69:726, 1953.
2. Meyers, M. A.: The reno-alimentary relationships: Anatomic-roentgen study of their clinical significance, Am. J. Roentgenol. 123:386, 1975.
3. Meyers, M. A.: *Dynamic Radiology of the Abdo-*

men: Normal and Pathologic Anatomy (New York/Heidelberg/Berlin: Springer-Verlag, 1976).
4. Meyers, M. A.: Roentgen significance of the phrenicocolic ligament, Radiology 95:547, 1970.
5. Meyers, M. A., Volberg, F., Katzen, B., et al.: Haustral anatomy and pathology: A new look. II Roentgen identification of normal pattern and relationships, Radiology 108:497, 1973.
6. Meyers, M. A., Volberg, F., Katzen, B., et al.: Haustral anatomy and pathology: A new look. II. Roentgen interpretation of pathologic alterations, Radiology 108:505, 1973.
7. Meyers, M. A., and McSweeney, J.: Secondary neoplasms of bowel, Radiology 105:1, 1972.
8. Meyers, M. A.: Colonic changes secondary to left perinephritis: New observations, Radiology 111: 525, 1974.
9. Meyers, M. A., and Evans, J. A.: Effects of pancreatitis on the small bowel and colon: Spread along mesenteric planes, Am. J. Roentgenol. 119:151, 1973.
10. Meyers, M. A., Whalen, J. P., Evans, J. A., et al.: Malposition and displacement of bowel in renal agenesis and ectopia: New observations, Am. J. Roentgenol. 117:323, 1973.
11. Doroshow, L., and Abeshouse, B. S.: Congenital unilateral solitary kidney: Report of 37 cases and review of the literature, Urol. Surv. 11:219, 1961.
12. Curtis, J. A., Sadhu, V., and Steiner, R. M.: Malposition of the colon in right renal agenesis, ectopia, and anterior nephrectomy, Am. J. Roentgenol. 129: 845, 1977.

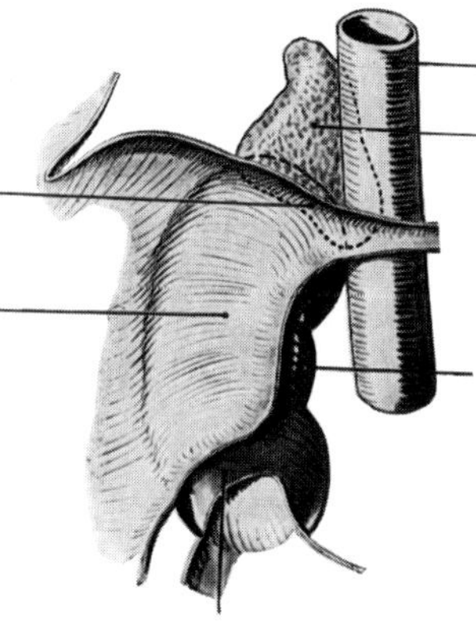

Fig 16–11.—Frontal drawing emphasizing relationships of right kidney to hepatic flexure of colon by virtue of its peritoneal reflections. I.V.C. = Inferior vena cava. (From Meyers, A. M.: *Dynamic Radiology of the Abdomen: Normal and Pathologic Anatomy* [New York: Springer-Verlag, Inc., 1976], used by permission.)

Fig 16–12.—Frontal drawing emphasizing relationship of left kidney to colon by virtue of their peritoneal reflections. (From Meyers, M. A.: *Dynamic Radiology of the Abdomen: Normal and Pathologic Anatomy* [New York: Springer-Verlag, Inc., 1976], used by permission.)

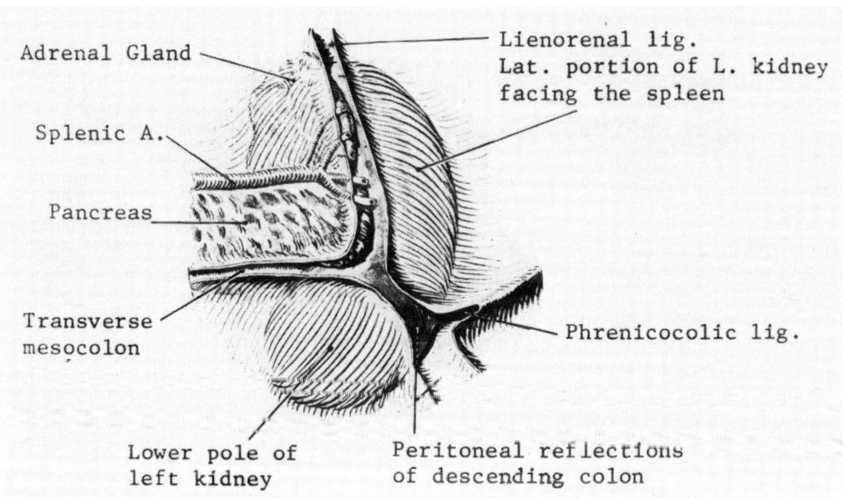

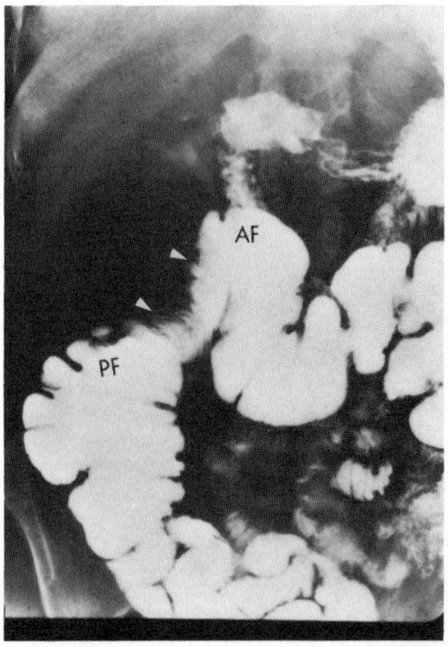

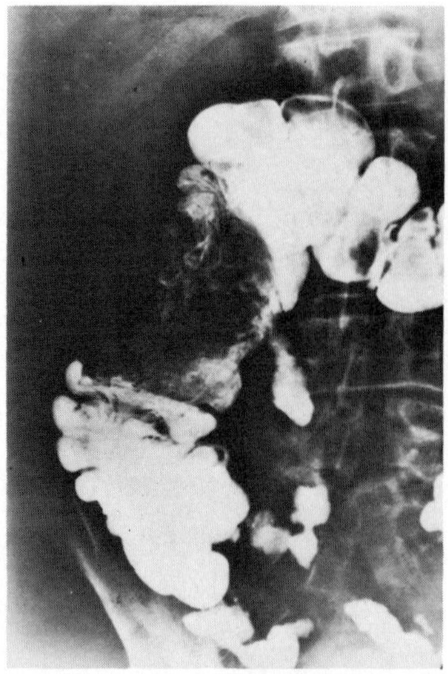

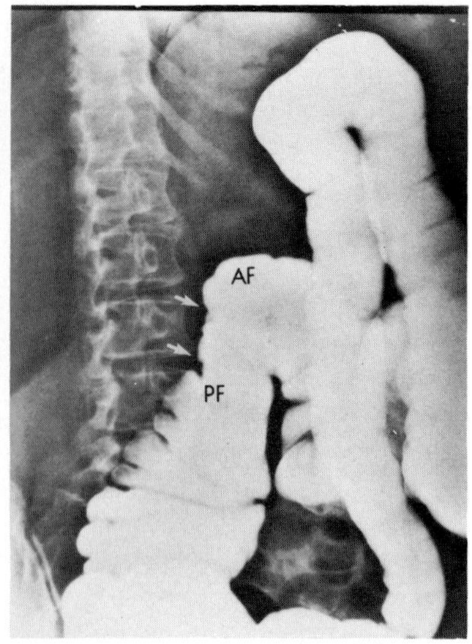

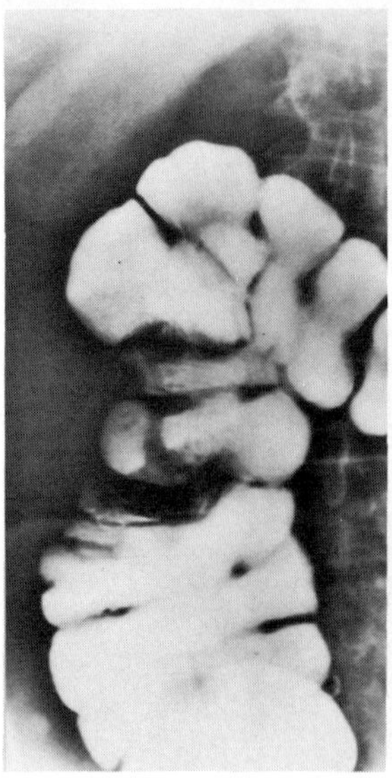

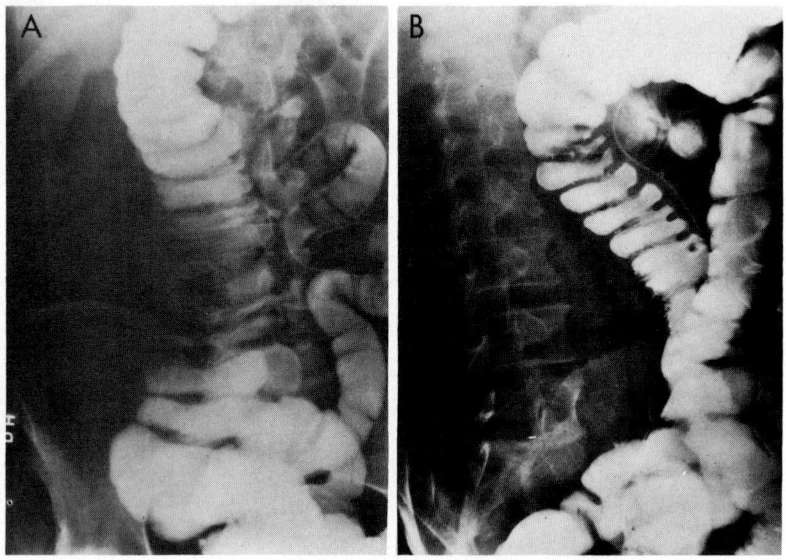

Fig 16–13 (top left).—Displacement of right colon by right renal cyst. Large intestine between posterior *(PF)* and anterior *(AF)* hepatic flexures is displaced inferiorly and medially, with extrinsic compression of its superior haustral row *(arrowheads).* Posterior flexure is mildly displaced downward, as the mass, originating in the middle third of kidney, extends laterally into flank. Note that there is no displacement of descending duodenum. (From Meyers, et al., Am. J. Roentgenol. 123:386, 1975, with permission.)

Fig 16–14 (top center).—Displacement of right colon by hydronephrotic right kidney. Segment between the two hepatic flexures is displaced inferiorly and medially. There is extrinsic flattening of its superior haustral border and marked compression of the lumen by the hugely dilated renal pelvis. (From Meyers, et al., Am. J. Roentgenol. 123:386, 1975, with permission.)

Fig 16–15 (top right).—Displacement of right colon by right renal cyst. Oblique view shows large intestine between posterior *(PF)* and anterior *(AF)* hepatic flexures displaced anteriorly and medially, with extrinsic flattening of its posterior haustral row *(arrows).* (From Meyers et al., Am. J. Roentgenol. 123:386, 1975, with permission.)

Fig 16–16 (bottom left).—Displacement of right colon by right multicystic kidney. Medial displacement and mass effect upon distal ascending colon. (From Meyers, M. A.: *Dynamic Radiology of the Abdomen: Normal and Pathologic Anatomy* [New York: Springer-Verlag, Inc., 1976], used by permission.)

Fig 16–17 (bottom right).—**A** and **B,** displacement of right colon by right renal hypernephroma. The mass extends deeply in flank and markedly displaces ascending colon medially and anteriorly. (From Meyers, et al., Am. J. Roentgenol. 123:386, 1975, with permission.)

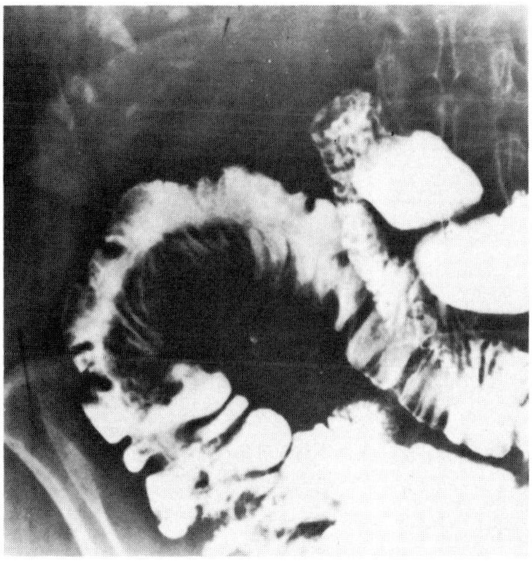

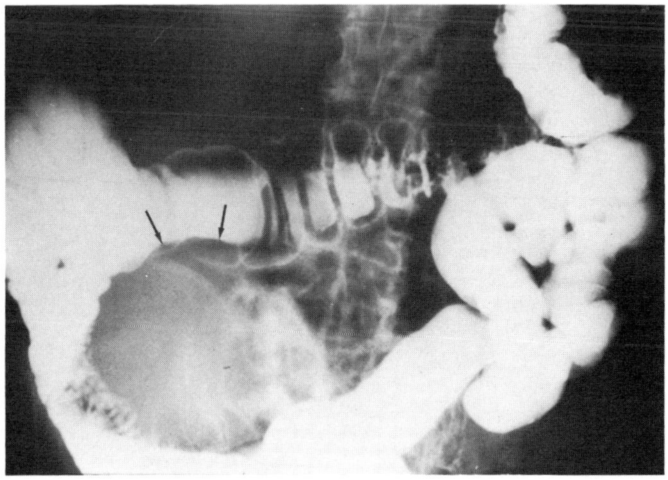

Fig 16–18 (left). — Displacement of right colon by inframesocolic renal cyst. Superior displacement of segment between two hepatic flexures, with extrinsic compression of its inferior haustral row. The mass also affects ascending colon. (From Meyers, et al., Am. J. Roentgenol. 123:386, 1975, with permission.)

Fig 16–19 (right). — Displacement of right colon by right renal sarcoma. There is mild extrinsic pressure on inferior border of segment between the two hepatic flexures by inframesocolic mass projecting from lower renal pole. Note that pressure effects can be localized particularly to posterior haustral rows *(arrows)*. (From Meyers, et al., Am. J. Roentgenol. 123:386, 1975, with permission.)

Fig 16–20. — **A** and **B,** displacement of left colon by left renal cyst. Anatomical splenic flexure *(SF)* is maintained, but there is lateral and anterior displacement of descending colon *(arrows)*. Mass enlargement of lower pole of kidney is identifiable *(large arrows)*. (From Meyers, AJR 123:386, 1975, with permission.)

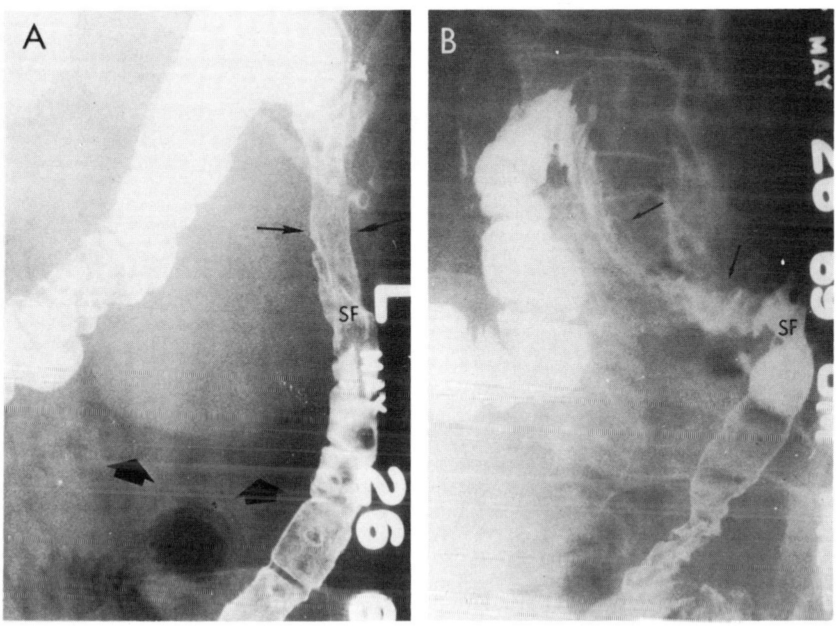

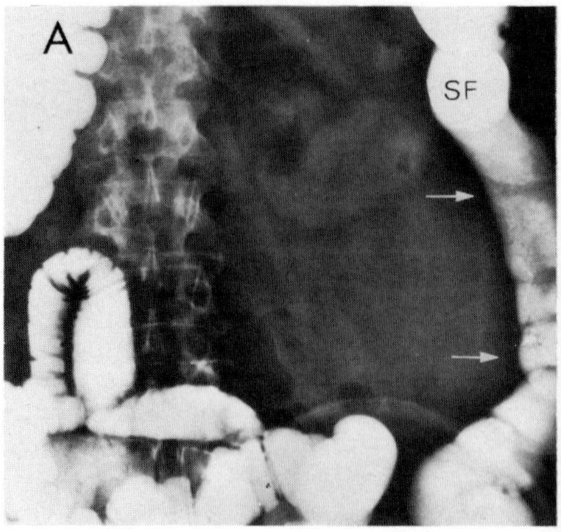

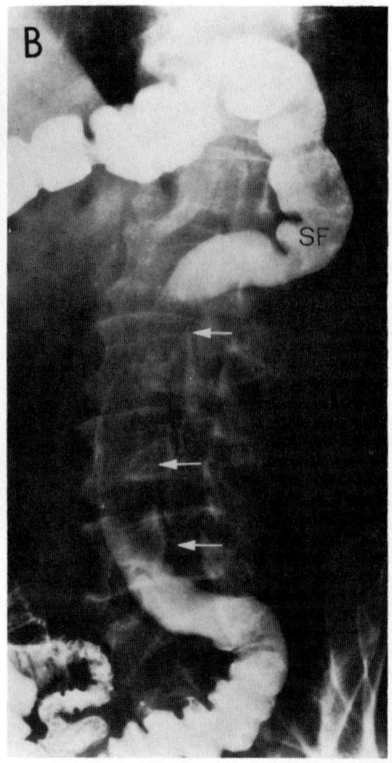

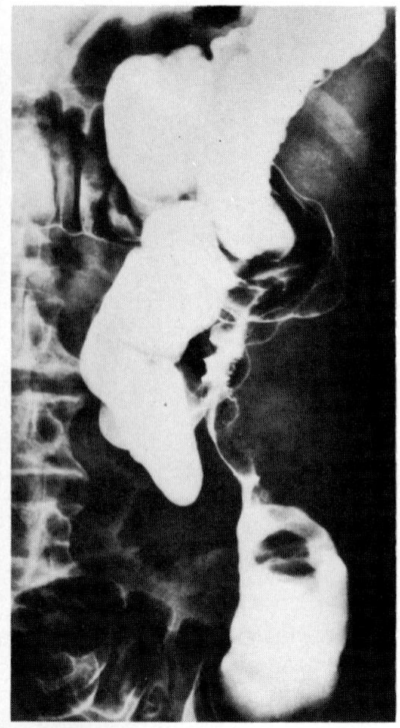

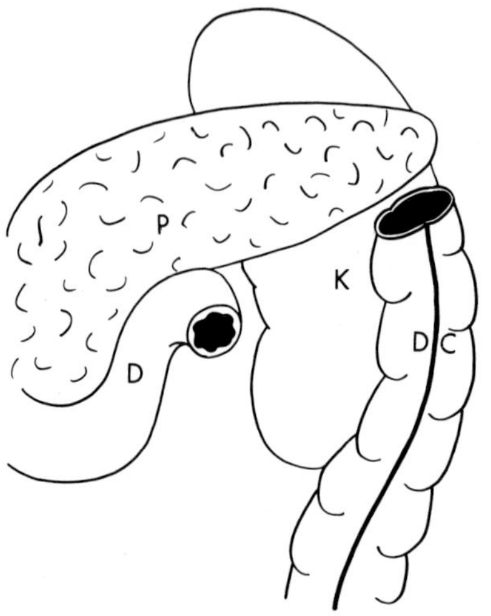

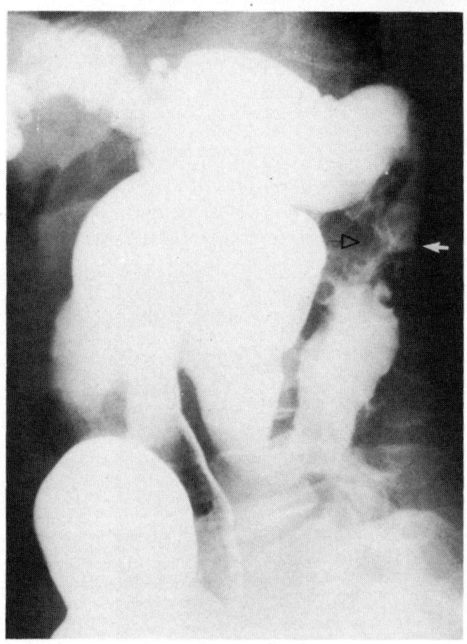

Fig 16–21 (top left).—**A** and **B,** displacement of left colon by left renal cyst. Descending colon is displaced laterally and anteriorly *(arrows)* by large cyst originating from lower renal pole. Anatomical splenic flexure *(SF)* is unaffected. (From Meyers, M. A.: *Dynamic Radiology of the Abdomen: Normal and Pathologic Anatomy* [New York: Springer-Verlag, Inc., 1976], used by permission.)

Fig 16–22 (top right).—Direct invasion of colon by left renal carcinoma. Extrinsic and intramural masses of descending colon with bulky polypoid intraluminal extensions.

Fig 16–23 (bottom left).—Frontal drawing illustrating relationship of descending colon *(DC)* to left kidney *(K)* distal to splenic flexure. *P* = pancreas; *D* = duodenum.

Fig 16–24 (bottom right).—Colonic changes secondary to left perinephritis. Lateral radiograph demonstrates persistent irregular narrowing 5 cm in length *(arrows)* just distal to splenic flexure. Mucosal folds are intact and there is no significant obstruction. Attention was then directed to the kidney, and a radiologic workup revealed multiple perirenal abscesses. At nephrectomy, lateral surfaces of masses were adherent to descending colon. (From Meyers, Radiology 111:525, 1974, with permission.)

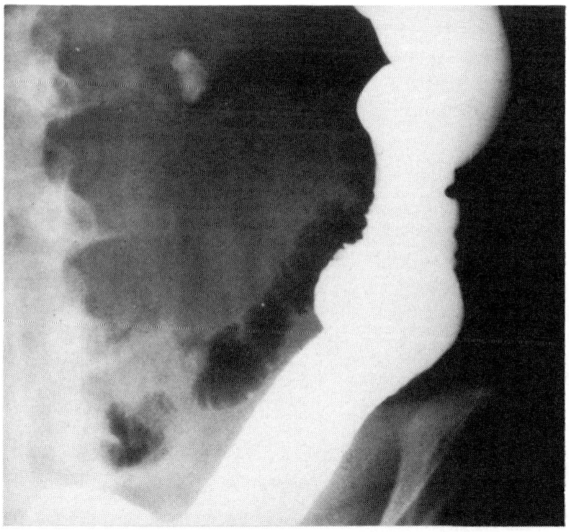

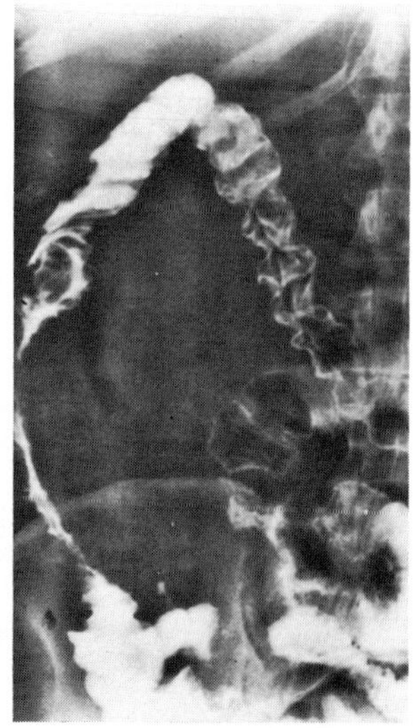

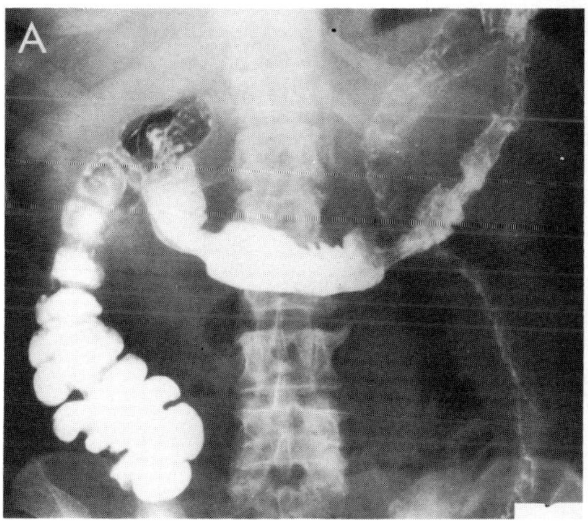

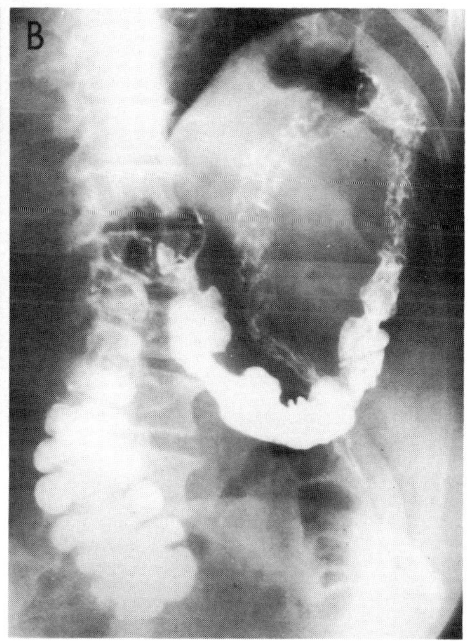

Fig 16–25 (top left).—Colonic changes secondary to left perinephritis. Barium enema study reveals localized rigidity and scalloping along medial wall of middescending colon. Left renal calculus is evident. Left xanthogranulomatous pyelonephritis and diffuse perirenal abscess were confirmed at nephrectomy, which also revealed inflammatory process adhering to medial wall of descending colon. (From Meyers, Radiology, 111:525, 1974, with permission.)

Fig 16–26 (top right).—Colonic changes secondary to right perinephritis. Barium enema study shows mass displacement and inflammatory mucosal thickening of ascending colon. Intravenous urography demonstrated no function in enlarged right kidney containing opaque calculus. Nephrectomy confirmed presence of xanthogranulomatous pyelonephritis with perirenal abscess adherent to ascending colon. (From Meyers, M. A.: *Dynamic Radiology of the Abdomen: Normal and Pathologic Anatomy* [New York: Springer-Verlag, Inc., 1976], used by permission.)

Fig 16–27 (bottom).—Colonic malposition in left renal agenesis. **A** and **B,** barium enema demonstrates marked posterior malposition of distal transverse colon and anatomical splenic flexure in area of left renal bed. (From Meyers, M. A.: *Dynamic Radiology of the Abdomen: Normal and Pathologic Anatomy* [New York: Springer-Verlag, Inc., 1976], used by permission.)

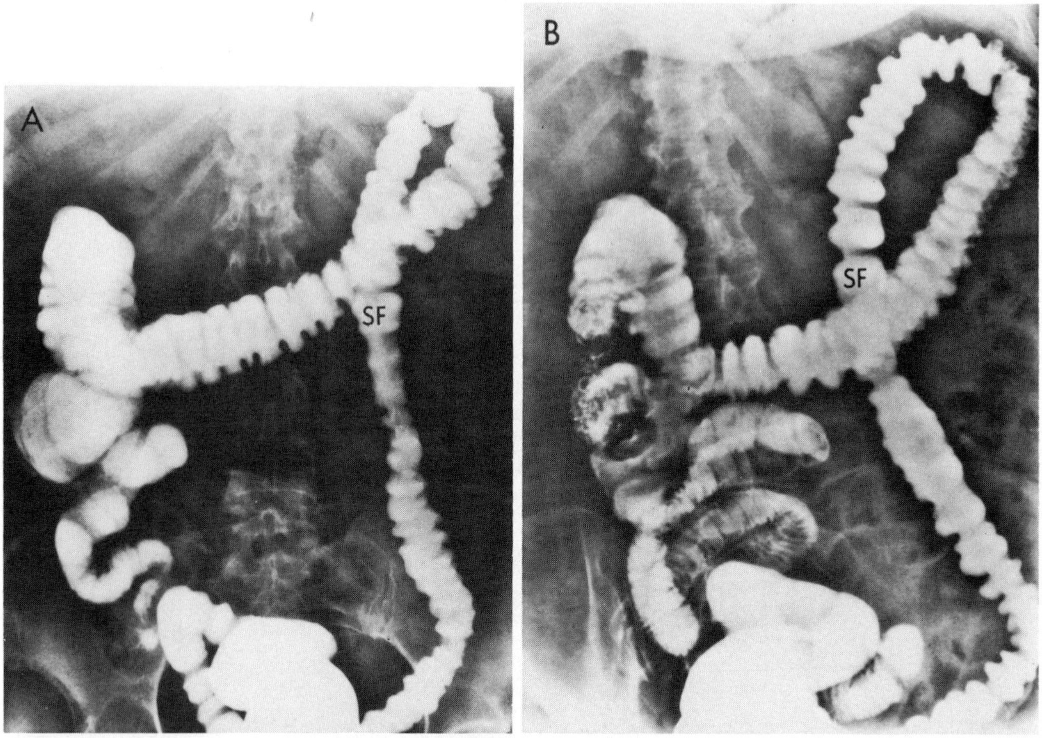

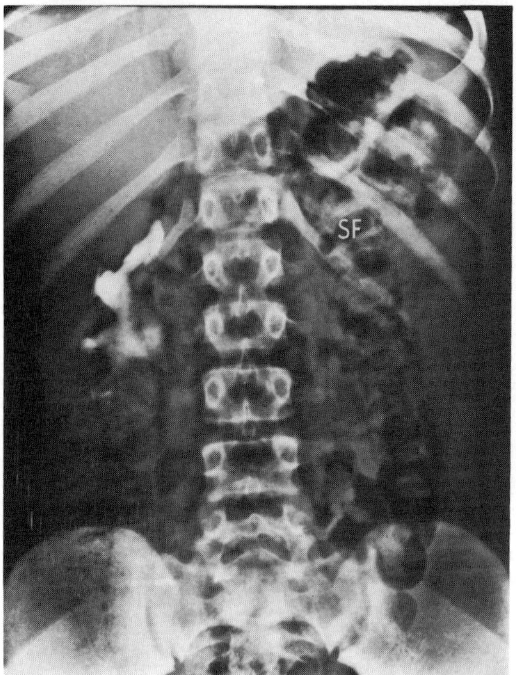

Fig 16–28 (above).—Colonic malposition in left renal agenesis. **A** and **B,** anatomical splenic flexure *(SF)* is deflected medially and posteriorly, occupying position of "empty" renal fossa. (From Meyers, M. A.: *Dynamic Radiology of the Abdomen: Normal and Pathologic Anatomy* [New York: Springer-Verlag, Inc., 1975], used by permission.)

Fig 16–29 (left).—Colonic malposition in left renal agenesis. Excretory urogram. In this child the anatomical splenic flexure *(SF)* occupies "empty" renal fossa. There is compensatory hypertrophy of right kidney. (From Meyers, M. A.: *Dynamic Radiology of the Abdomen: Normal and Pathologic Anatomy* [New York: Springer-Verlag, Inc., 1976], used by permission.)

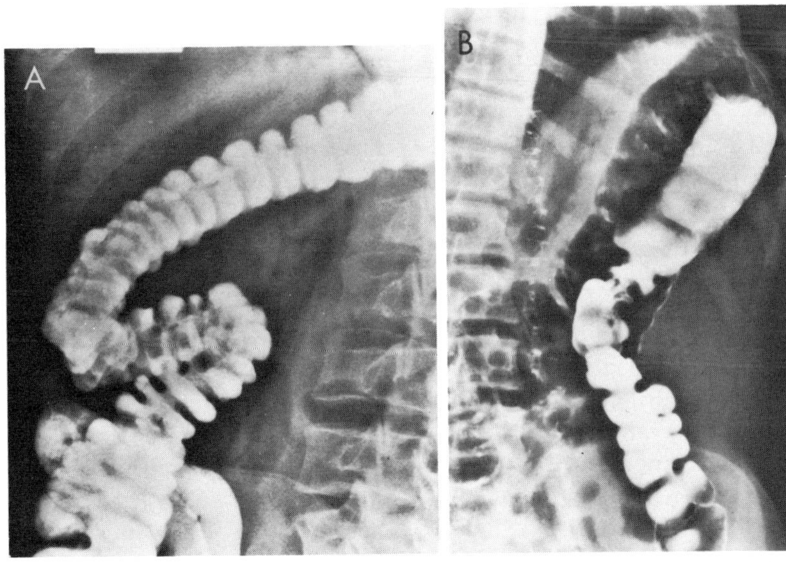

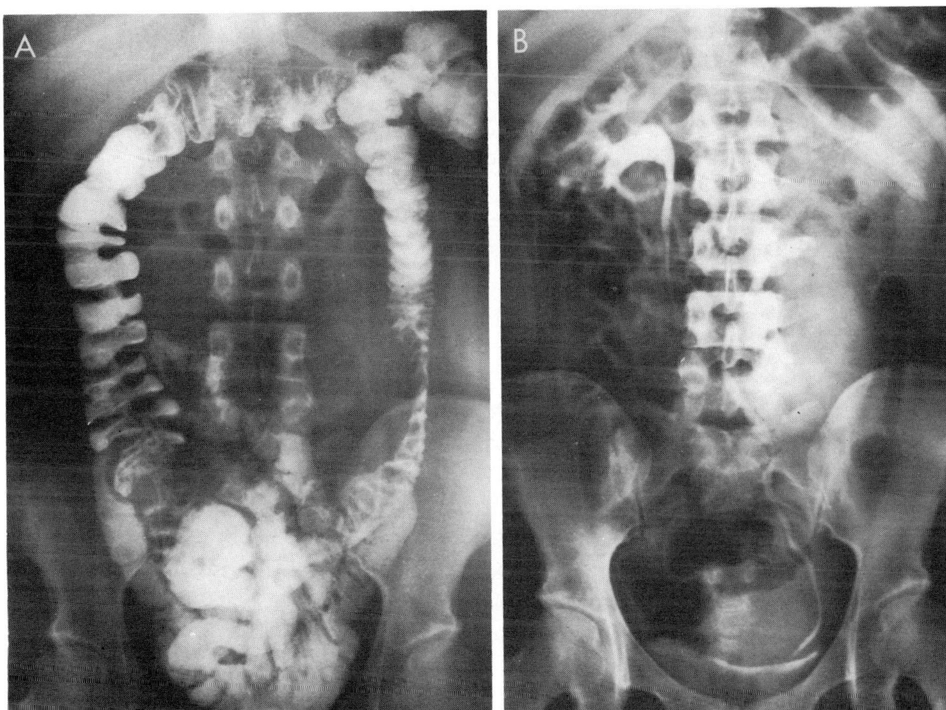

Fig 16–30 (top). – **A** and **B,** malposition of colon following right and left nephrectomy. In two patients, hepatic and splenic flexures are deviated into "empty" renal fossa. (From Meyers, M. A.: *Dynamic Radiology of the Abdomen: Normal and Pathologic Anatomy* [New York: Springer-Verlag, Inc., 1976], used by permission.)

Fig 16–31 (bottom). – Ectopic kidney in woman age 24 with left lower quadrant mass. **A,** barium enema examination demonstrates extrinsic mass impression on medial aspect of lower descending colon. Note that anatomical splenic flexure is medially directed into "empty" left renal fossa. **B,** intravenous urogram documents left ectopic kidney with marked anterior malrotation in relationship laterally to descending colon. (From Meyers, et al., Am. J. Roentgenol. 117:323, 1973, with permission.)

DISEASES OF PANCREAS AS THEY AFFECT THE COLON

JAMES L. CLEMENTS, JR., M.D.
S. BOYD EATON, JR., M.D.

PANCREATIC INFLAMMATORY disease producing radiologically demonstrable colonic abnormalities is encountered less commonly than disease affecting the more intimately associated stomach and duodenum. When changes in the colon secondary to pancreatic inflammation are encountered, they may be a source of diagnostic confusion since they can mimic primary or secondary neoplasm, segmental inflammatory bowel disease or ischemic changes.

Radiographic evidence of colonic involvement secondary to pancreatic inflammation is seen in the transverse colon and splenic flexure most commonly because of the anatomical relationship of the pancreas to the transverse mesocolon and phrenicocolic ligament.[1, 2] These mesenteric planes provide a route of spread for extravasated pancreatic enzymes to the transverse colon from the hepatic to splenic flexures. The small bowel mesentery continues with the transverse mesocolon so that enzymes also may spread to involve the jejunum and ileocolic region.

In addition, pancreatic exudates may extend retroperitoneally into the paracolic gutters and pelvis where reactive changes in the ascending, descending or sigmoid colon can be produced.

Structural abnormalities that may be detected on barium enema examinations in patients with pancreatic inflammatory disease include diffuse and localized displacement, mucosal edema and spiculation, and segmental stricture formation.[3] Signs of colonic necrosis and perforation may be encountered.[4]

In our experience, carcinoma of the pancreas has involved the colon more rarely than inflammatory disease. Advanced neoplastic disease may extend directly to the transverse colon or splenic flexure. Intraperitoneal seeding of pancreatic carcinoma to the pouch of Douglas, sigmoid mesocolon, lower small bowel mesentery and right paracolic gutter—with involvement of the rectum, sigmoid and right colon by metastatic masses—may occur.[5, 6]

It should be emphasized that the colonic findings secondary to pancreatic disease are often nonspecific. The clinical setting should influence the radiologist's index of suspicion, particularly with lesions detected in the transverse colon and splenic flexure. The readily available barium contrast examination of the upper gastrointestinal tract and more specialized methods of ultrasound and computerized tomography of the abdomen should be used to confirm or rule out pancreatic disease.

REFERENCES

1. Meyers, M. A., and Evans, J. A.: Effects of pancreatitis on the small bowel and colon: Spread along mesenteric planes, Radiology 119:151, 1973.
2. Meyers, M. A.: Roentgen significance of the phrenicocolic ligament, Radiology 95:539, 1970.
3. Eaton, S. B., Jr., and Ferrucci, J. T., Jr.: *Radiology of the Pancreas and Duodenum* (Philadelphia: W. B. Saunders Co., 1973).
4. Thompson, W. M., Kelvin, F. M., and Rice, R. P.: Inflammation and necrosis of the transverse colon secondary to pancreatitis, Am. J. Roentgenol. 128: 943, 1977.
5. Salik, J. O.: Extrarectal tumors caused by silent carcinomas of the stomach and pancreas, J.A.M.A. 175:457, 1961.
6. Meyers, M. A.: Distribution of intra-abdominal malignant seeding: Dependency on dynamics of flow of ascitic fluid, Radiology 119:198, 1973.
7. Weens, H. S., and Walker, L. A.: The radiologic diagnosis of acute pancreatitis and cholecystitis, Radiol. Clin. North Am. 2:89, 1964.
8. Atkinson, G. O., Clements, J. L., Jr., Milledge, R. D., and Weens, H. S.: Pancreatic disease simulating urinary tract disease, Clin. Radiol. 24:185, 1973.

9. Clements, J. L., Jr., Bradley, E. L. III, and Eaton, S. B., Jr.: Spontaneous internal drainage of pancreatic pseudocysts, Am. J. Roentgenol. 126:985, 1976.
10. Shapiro, J. H., Beneventano, T. C., Feldman, F., Lalli, A. F., Reilly, B. J., and Viamonte, M., Jr.: Film interpretation session, R.S.N.A., November 27, 1977.
11. Shapiro, J. H., Beneventano, T. C., Feldman, F., Lalli, A. F., Reilly, B. J., and Viamonte, M., Jr.: Film interpretation session. Summary of discussion and diagnoses, Radiology 125:829, 1977.

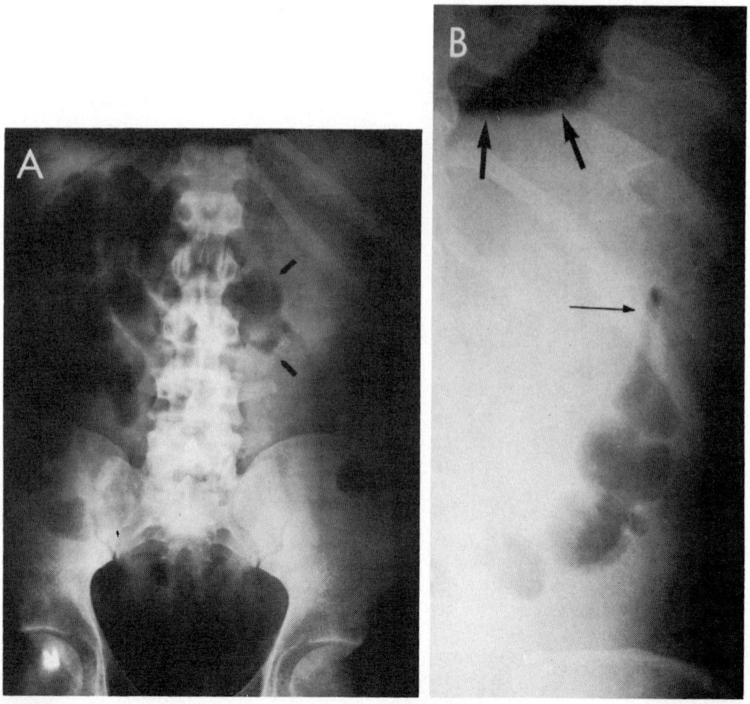

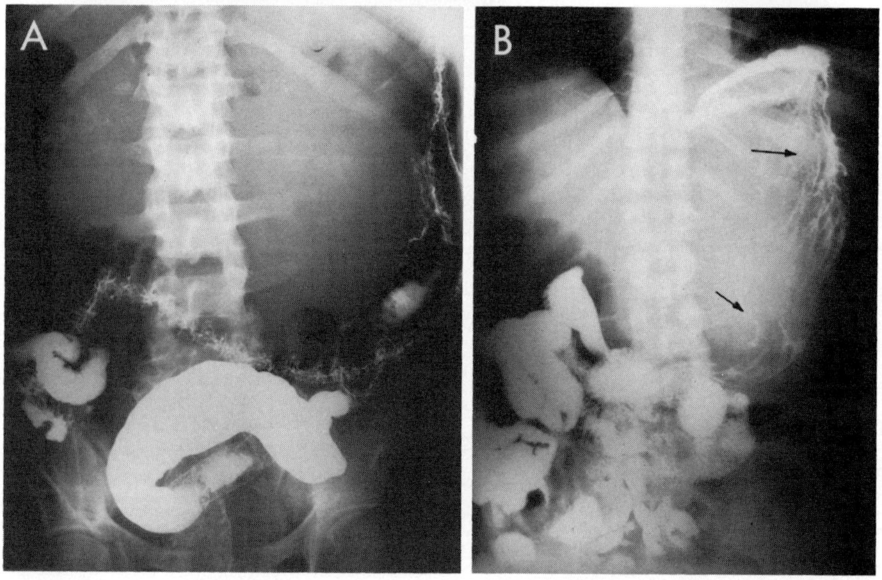

Fig 16–32 (top).—Colon cutoff sign, plain film finding suggestive, but not characteristic, of acute pancreatitis. As originally described, hepatic flexure was site of cutoff, with distention of right colon and collapsed colon distal to hepatic flexure. Actually, cutoff is more likely to occur at splenic flexure and is infrequently seen on plain abdominal films in patients with acute pancreatitis.[3, 7] **A,** sharp cutoff in distal transverse colon in patient with acute pancreatitis *(arrows).* **B,** "air lumenogram" of narrowing at splenic flexure (small arrow) without significant dilatation proximal to this point in patient with acute pancreatitis. Note encroachment on gas-outlined stomach by pancreatic mass *(arrows).*

Fig 16–33 (bottom).—Lesser sac pseudocyst. **A,** marked displacement of transverse colon by large lesser sac pancreatic pseudocyst. **B,** extrinsic compression of stomach (small arrows) and downward displacement of gastroduodenal junction. Lateral film showed mass to be retrogastric.

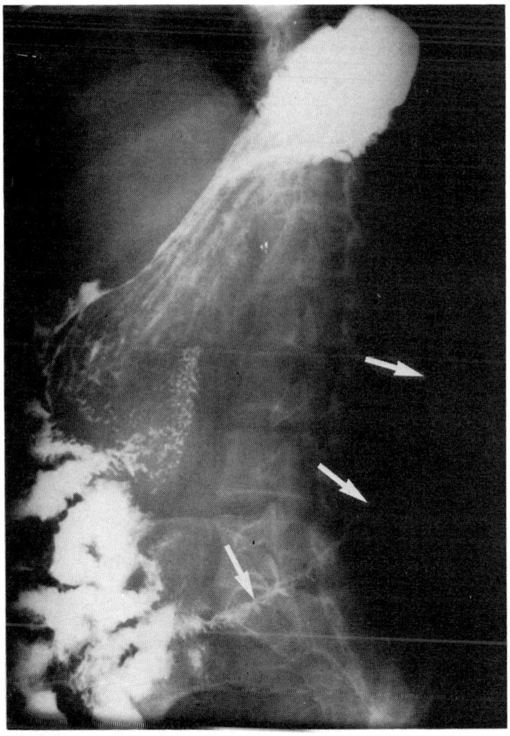

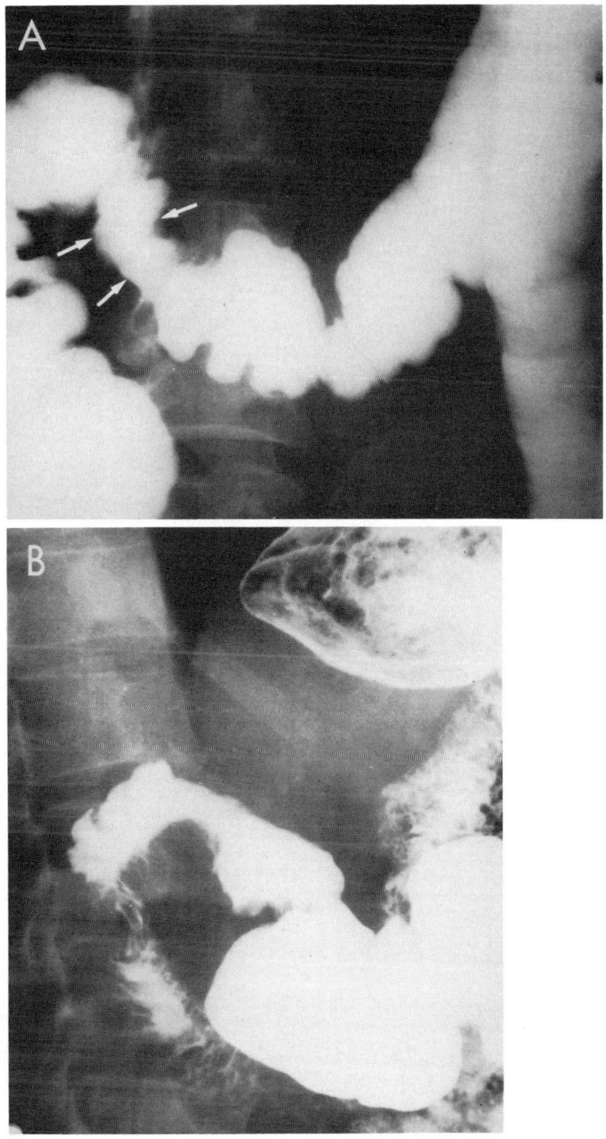

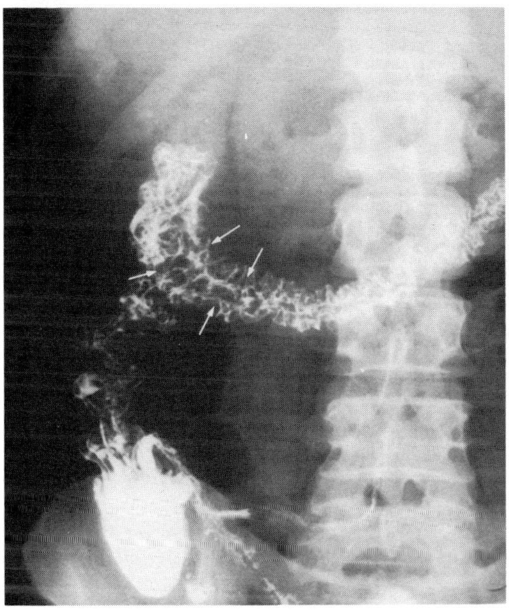

Fig 16–34 (top left).—Gastrocolic pseudocyst. Right posterior oblique gastrointestinal film immediately following barium enema, demonstrating large mass interposed between stomach and transverse colon *(arrows)*.

Fig 16–35 (right).—Pericolitis of proximal transverse colon associated with pancreatitis. **A,** narrowing and mucosal distortion in proximal transverse colon in patient with acute pancreatitis *(arrows)*. **B,** gastrointestinal study showing changes in proximal duodenal loop.

Fig 16–36 (bottom left).—Mucosal edema of proximal transverse colon secondary to acute pancreatitis. Postevacuation film demonstrating mucosal thickening *(arrows)* in proximal transverse colon in patient with acute pancreatitis.

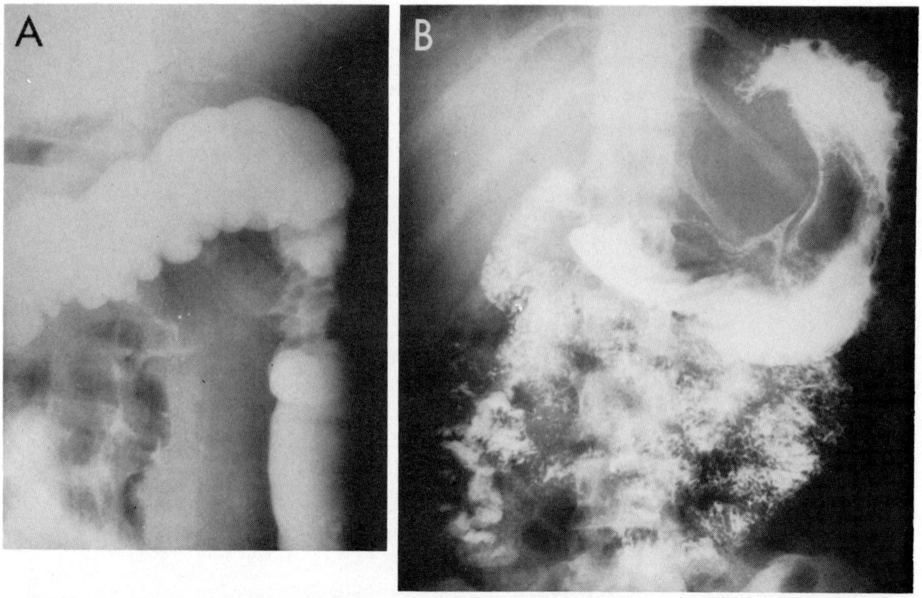

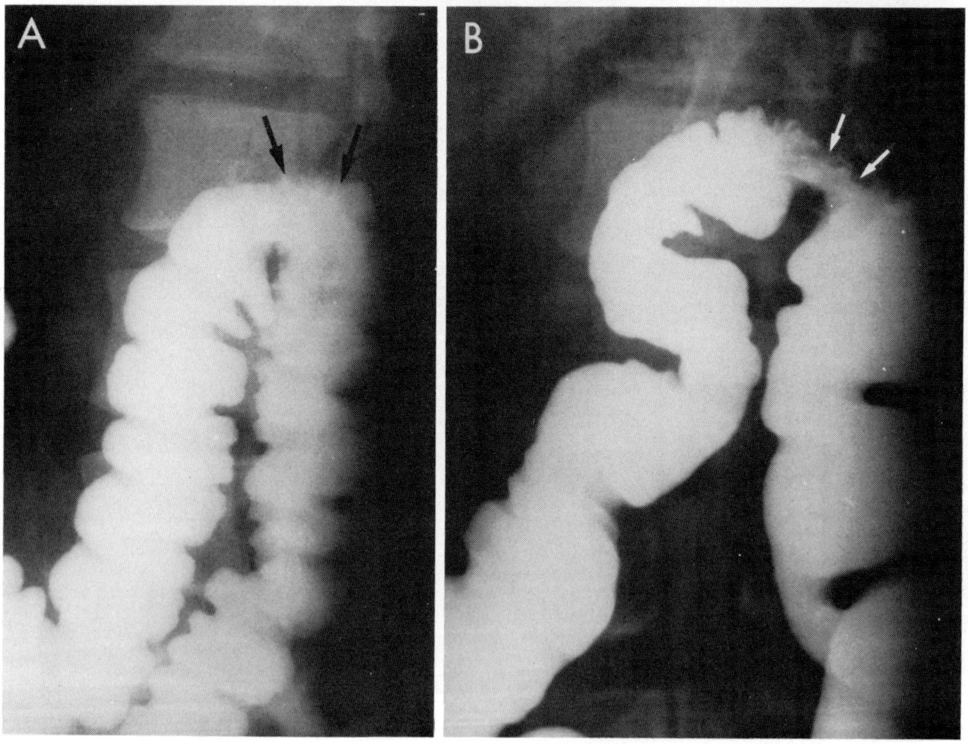

Fig 16–37 (top).—**A** and **B,** pancreatic pseudocyst with evidence of pericolitis involving proximal descending colon with narrowing and spiculation of mucosal pattern. **B,** barium contrast study in same patient demonstrates defect produced by large retrogastric pseudocyst.

Fig 16–38 (bottom).—Pericolitis involving splenic flexure. In patient with acute pancreatitis, **A** demonstrates minimal spiculation *(arrows)* of superior aspect of splenic flexure. **B,** in a different patient (with pancreatic pseudocyst), more marked changes in same area *(arrows),* with narrowing of lumen, are noted.

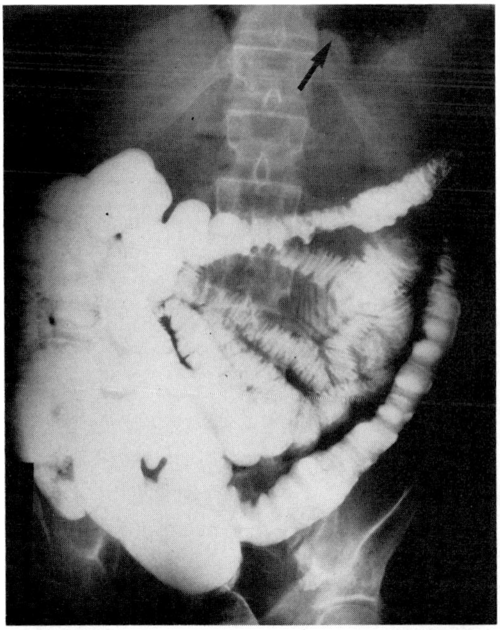

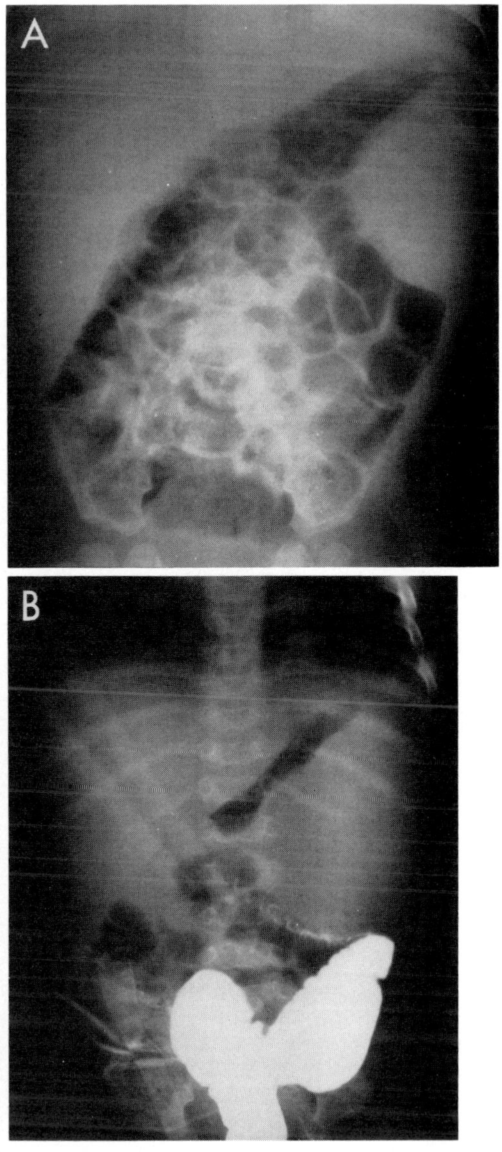

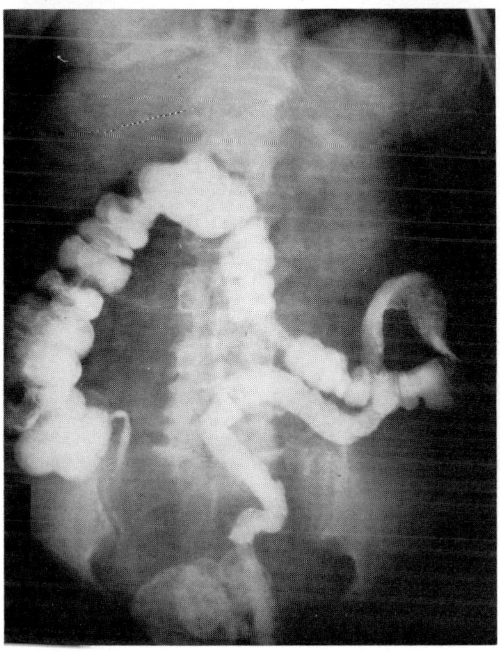

Fig 16–39 (top left).—Pericolitis of distal transverse colon and splenic flexure secondary to acute pancreatitis. There is narrowing of distal half of transverse colon and proximal descending colon at splenic flexure, which was nondistensible. Patient had acute pancreatitis. Note also distortion of gas-filled proximal stomach by extrinsic pancreatic mass *(arrow)*.

Fig 16–40 (right).—Infected pancreatic pseudocyst invading spleen and producing pericolitis at level of splenic flexure. An infant, age 2 years, had a pancreatic pseudocyst arising from tail of pancreas, apparently traumatic in origin. At surgery, pseudocyst had invaded the spleen. **A,** plain film demonstrating left upper quadrant mass. **B,** barium-filled colon study demonstrating marked pericolitis in region of splenic flexure with obstruction to retrograde flow of contrast material.

Fig 16–41 (bottom left).—Carcinoma of the pancreas encasing splenic flexure of colon. Filled barium enema film demonstrating downward displacement of distal transverse colon and splenic flexure, with encasement and stricture formation at level of splenic flexure. Entire colon distal to splenic flexure is distorted by diffuse peritoneal metastases and bilateral ovarian metastases from adenocarcinoma of pancreas.

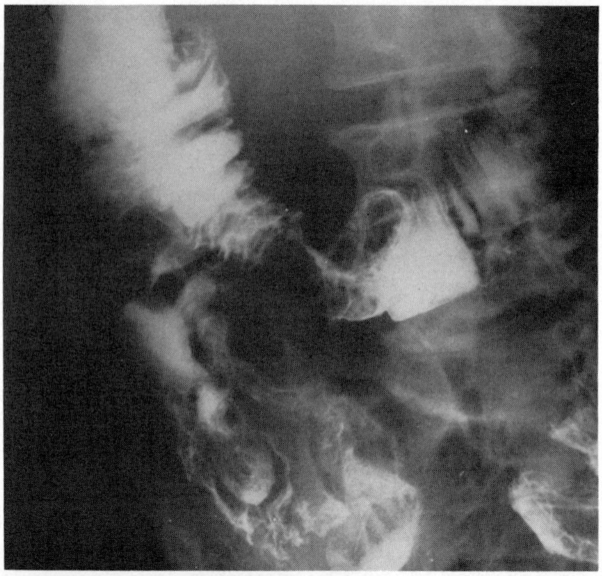

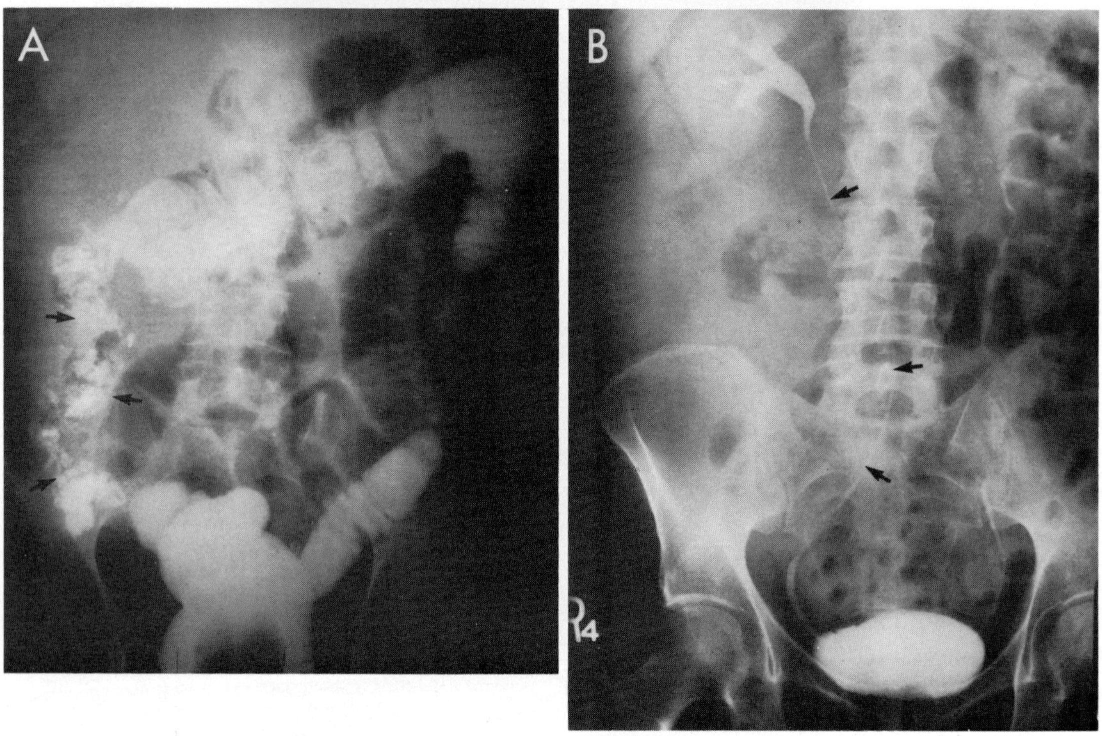

Fig 16–42 (top).—Carcinoma of pancreas invading transverse colon. Patient with carcinoma of head of pancreas with invasion and distortion of distal stomach and duodenal loop and contiguous constricting lesion of transverse colon, representing invasion of colon by pancreatic carcinoma. Note spiculation of mucosa of transverse colon proximal to stenotic lesion.

Fig 16–43 (bottom).—**A** and **B,** right lower quadrant pseudocyst. Filled barium enema film demonstrating narrowing and irregularity of cecum and ascending colon *(arrows)* secondary to pericolitis. **B,** intravenous pyelogram (same patient) shows displacement of right ureter to midline *(arrows)* by large right lower quadrant pseudocyst. (From Atkinson, et al., Clin. Radiol. 24:185, 1973, with permission.)

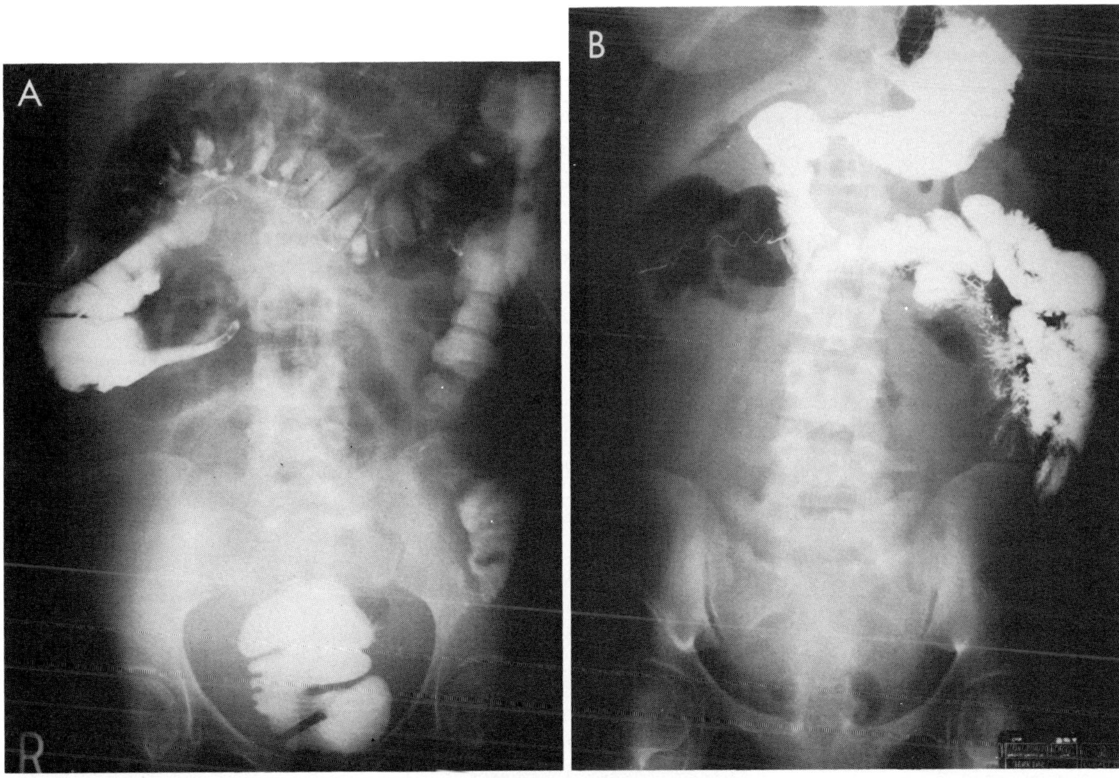

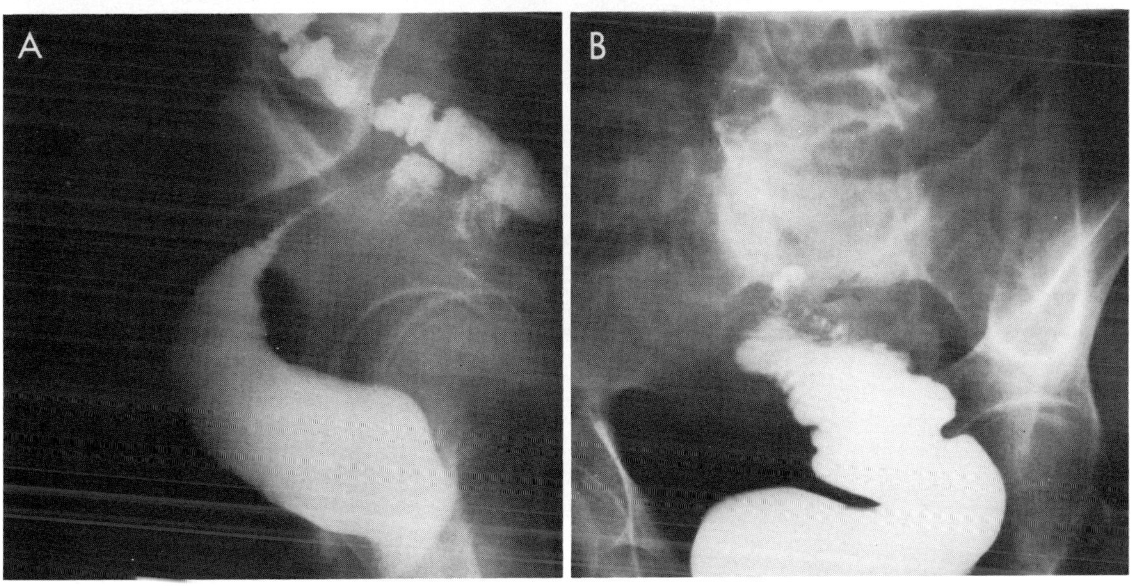

Fig 16–44 (top).—Massive right lower quadrant pseudocyst. **A,** elevation of cecum by this mass. **B,** small bowel examination demonstrating marked displacement of small intestinal loops from right lower quadrant.

Fig 16–45 (bottom).—**A** and **B,** pelvic pseudocyst. Patient with extension of pseudocyst retroperitoneally to pelvis with extrinsic compression and partial obstruction of distal sigmoid colon.

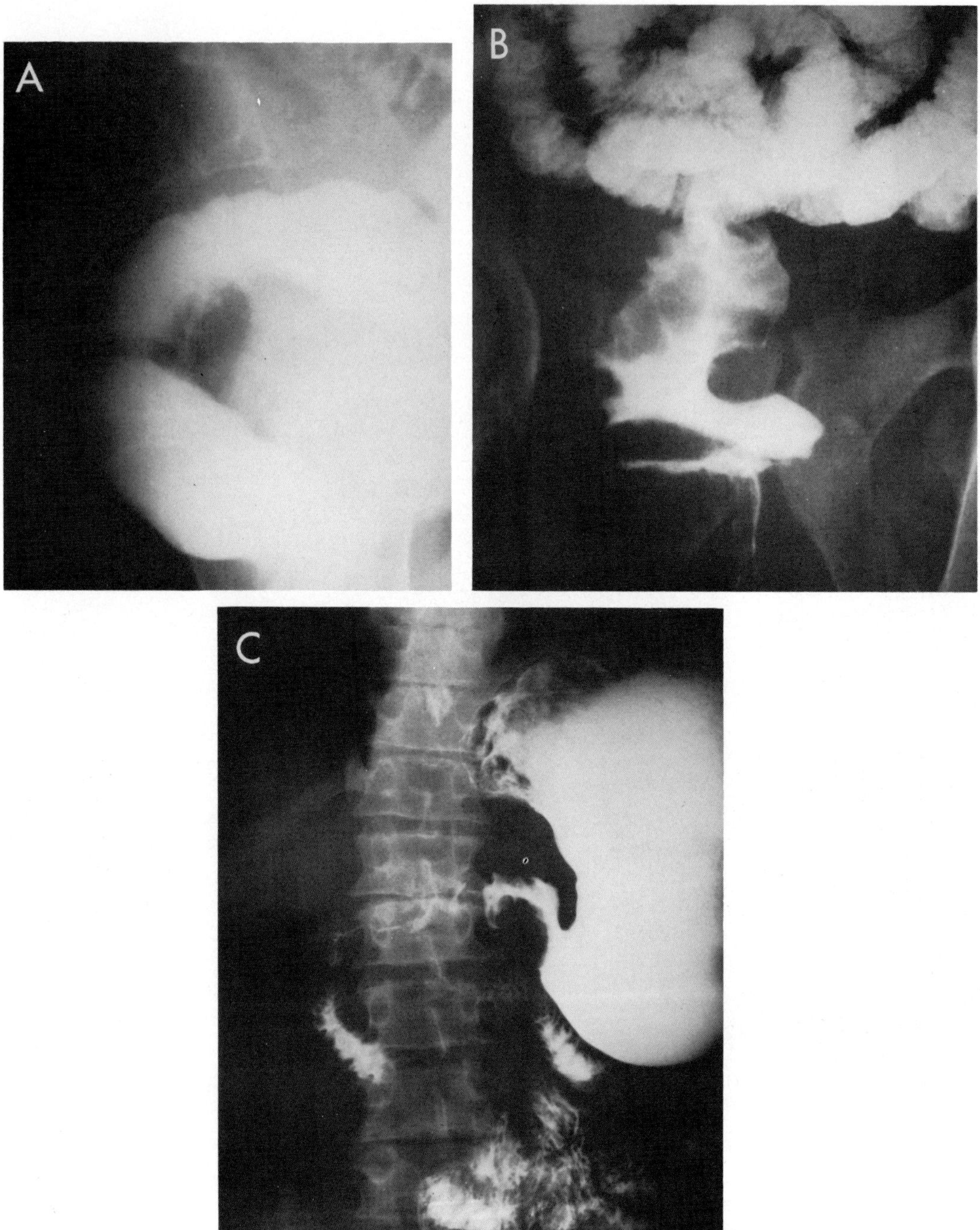

Fig 16–46.—Metastatic pancreatic carcinoma to pouch of Douglas. **A** and **B** demonstrate extrinsic mass encroaching on anterior aspect of rectosigmoid, distortion of mucosal folds being due to intraperitoneal spread of pancreatic carcinoma. Carcinoma of ovary is most common cause of this finding; however, spread of pancreatic, gastric and colonic carcinoma may produce the same appearance.[5, 6] **C,** upper gastrointestinal study on same patient demonstrating invasion of gastric antrum and duodenal loop by carcinoma of head of pancreas.

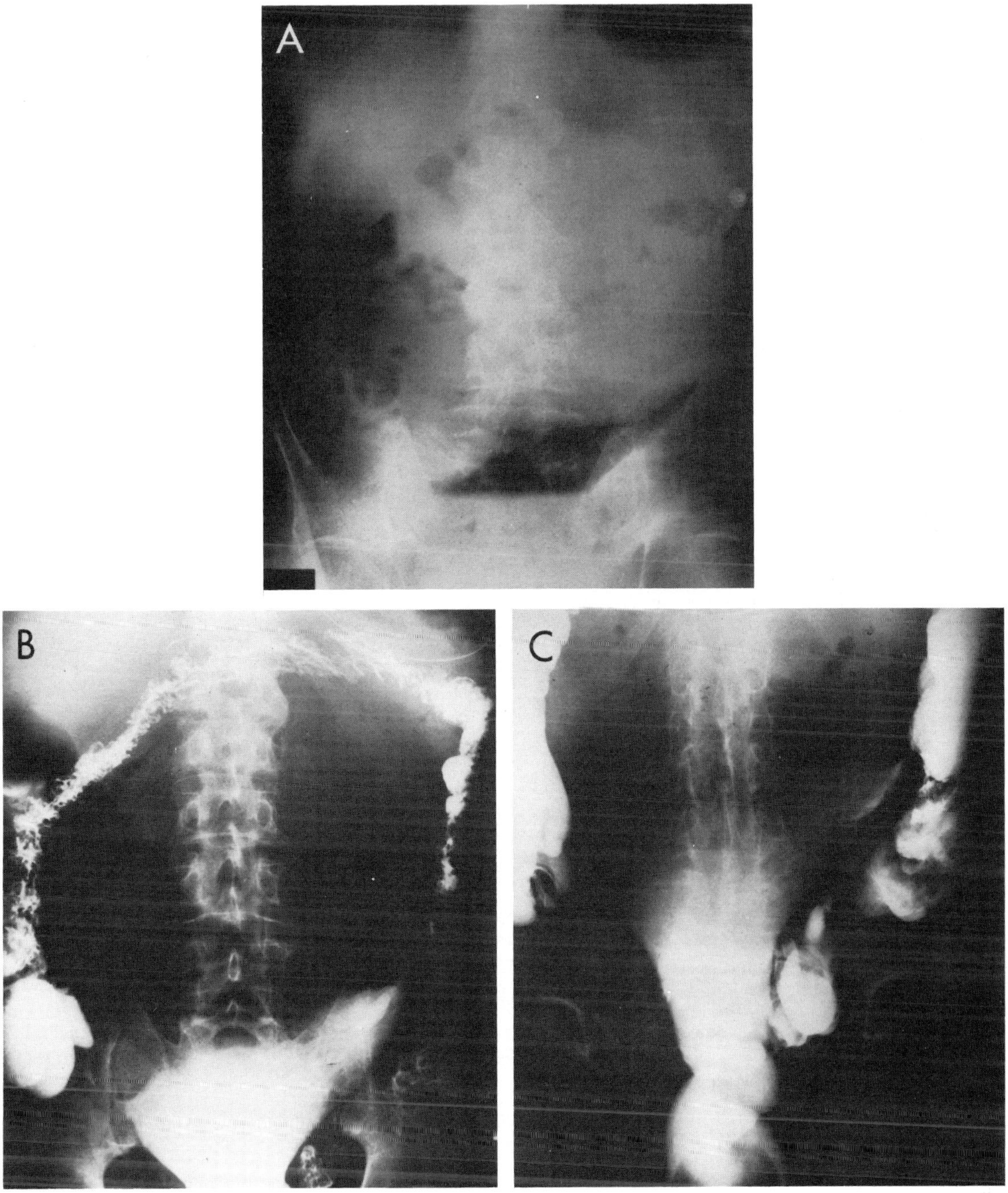

Fig 16–47. — Pelvic pseudocyst with spontaneous fistula formation to colon. **A,** erect plain film of abdomen showing extraluminal gas and fluid loculation in lower abdomen and pelvis. **B** and **C,** barium enema studies showing filling of large pelvic pseudocyst from fistula to proximal sigmoid colon. Pancreatic pseudocysts have been observed to form fistulas to the esophagus, stomach, duodenum and colon. Spontaneous fistulization occurs most commonly to the colon.[9] (From Shapiro et al., Film Interpretation sessions, RSNA November 1977, with permission.)

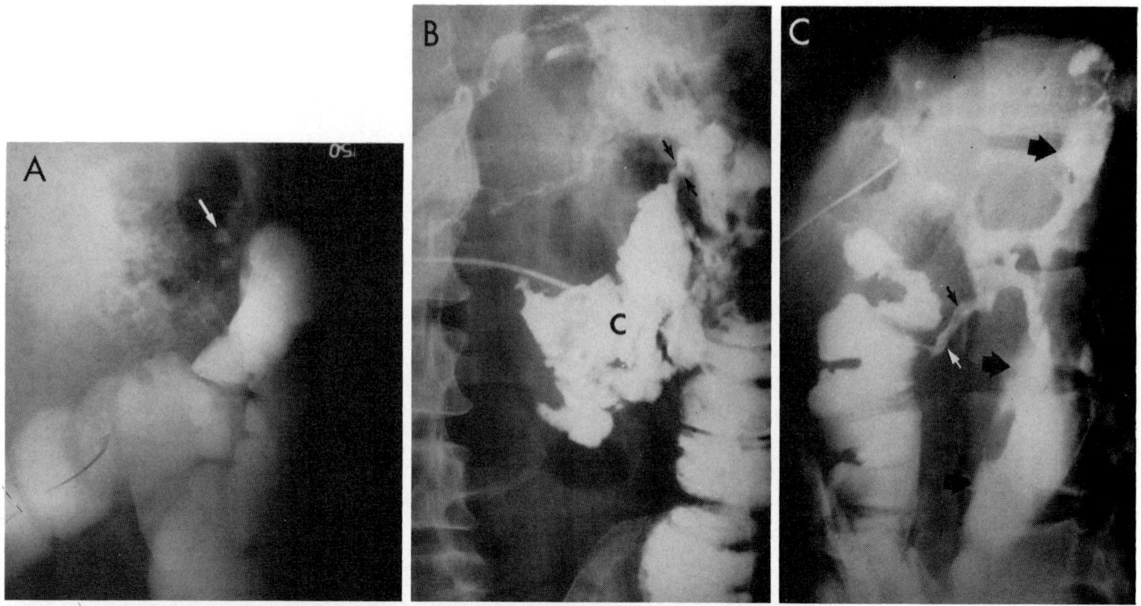

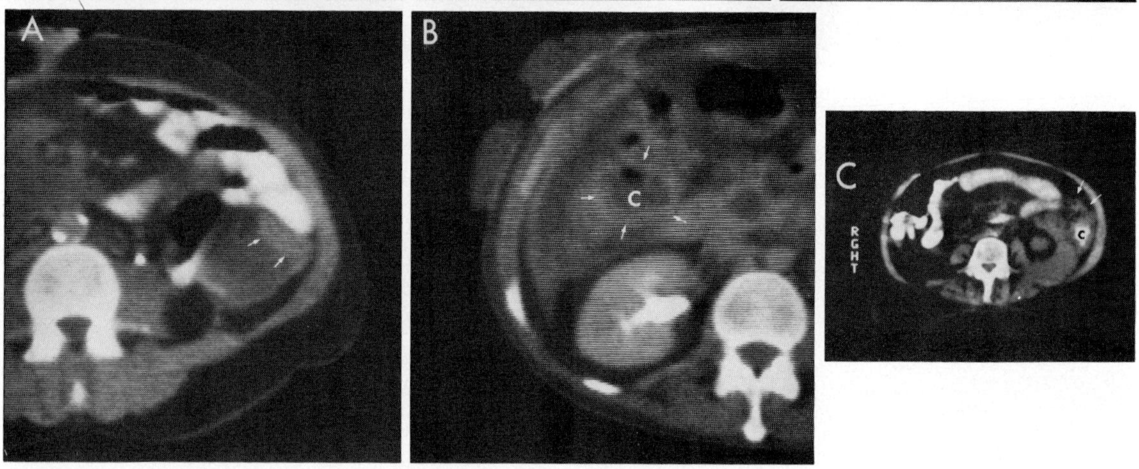

Fig 16–48 (top).—Pancreatic abscess with spontaneous fistula formation to colon. **A,** extraluminal gas loculation in left upper quadrant displacing splenic flexure of colon. Small amount of contrast material has extravasated into abscess *(arrow).* Pancreatic abscesses produce same colonic distortion as noninfected pseudocysts and pancreatitis. Presence of streaked or flocculent extraluminal gas shadows, as demonstrated here, indicates infected pseudocyst (gas-forming organisms). **B** and **C,** films from fistulogram performed after drainage of pancreatic abscess. **B,** frontal film demonstrating the irregular abscess outlined by contrast *(C)* material with the fistula *(large arrows)* extending to the colon. **C,** lateral view, again demonstrating the fistula *(small arrows)* and extent of retroperitoneal abscess in posterior paracolic gutter *(large arrows).* (**B** from Clements et al., Am. J. Roentgenol. 126:985, 1976, with permission.)

Fig 16–49 (bottom).—CT abdominal scans demonstrating retroperitoneal spread of pancreatic exudate in paracolic regions in three patients. **A,** in a patient with traumatic pancreatitis, retroperitoneal accumulation of pancreatic exudate in left paracolic region below plane of kidney. The colon is demonstrated to be collapsed and compressed anteriorly by exudate *(arrows).* **B,** in a patient with acute pancreatitis, right retroperitoneal exudate at plane of right kidney. Colon *(C)* is displaced medially and colonic wall demonstrates faint increase in density *(arrows).* **C,** left perirenal and paracolic infected pseudocyst. The scan is at level of upper pole of left kidney. Retroperitoneal exudation surrounds upper pole of left kidney and proximal descending colon *(C).* Gas secondary to infection by gas-forming organisms is demonstrated anterior to colon *(arrows).* (**A** and **B** courtesy of Drs. P. J. Sones and R. Steele, Atlanta.)

Chapter 17

Familial Colon Carcinoma in Nail-Patella Syndrome

LOUIS A. GILULA, M.D.

A FAMILY has been described with nail-patella syndrome, or onycho-osteodysplasia, and an increased incidence of colon carcinoma.[1] Major components of the syndrome consist of nail (Fig. 17 – 1) and patellar hypoplasia (Fig. 17 – 3), iliac horns (Fig. 17 – 2) and elbow dysplasia. There also is an increased incidence of renal abnormalities, with proteinuria and hematuria the main findings.[3, 4] Some members of this family also had increased lumbar lordosis and nonspecific arthralgias. A grandfather had rectal adenocarcinoma and a maternal aunt and mother had colon carcinoma.

The genes for nail-patella syndrome, adenylate kinase-1 (red cell A – K) enzyme, and the ABO blood groups are all located on the 9th chromosome.[5-8] Because of their close linkage, the genes cosegregate in families. The syndrome is passed as an autosomal dominant with complete penetrance and variable expressivity. There are occasional sporadic cases.[9]

Other reported families with the nail-patella syndrome did not indicate increased incidence of colon carcinoma. When compared with 3.5 cases of colon and rectal carcinoma per 100,000 population,[10] the three cases in this family represent an abnormally increased incidence.

REFERENCES

1. Gilula, L. A., and Kantor, O. K.: Familial colon carcinoma in nail-patella syndrome, Am. J. Roentgenol. 123:783, 1975.
2. Fong, E. E.: "Iliac Horns" (symmetrical bilateral central posterior iliac processes): Case report, Radiology 47:517, 1946.
3. Carbonara, P., and Alpert, M.: Hereditary osteo-onchyo-dysplasia (HOOD), Am. J. Med. Sci. 248: 37, 1964.
4. Morita, T., Laughlin, L. O., Kawano, K., et al.: Nail-patella syndrome: Light and electron microscopic studies of kidney, Arch. Intern. Med. 31: 271, 1973.
5. Elston, R. C., Lange, K., and Namboodiri, K. K.: Age trends in human chiasma frequencies and recombination fractions. II. Method for analyzing recombination fractions and applications to the ABO:Nail-patella linkage, Am. J. Hum. Genet. 28: 69, 1976.
6. Ferguson-Smith, M. A., Aitken, D. A., Turleau, C., et al.: Localisation of the human ABO:Np-1:AK-1 linkage group by regional assignment of AK-1 to 9q34, Hum. Genet. 34:35, 1976.
7. Pilling, D. W., and Levick, R. K.: Radiological abnormalities associated with anomalies of the ninth chromosome, Pediatr. Radiol. 6:215, 1978.
8. Westerveld, A., Jongsma, A. P. M., Khan, M. P., et al.: Assignment of the AK_1:Np:ABO linkage group to human chromosome 9, Proc. Natl. Acad. Sci. USA 73(3):895, 1976.
9. Duthie, R. B., and Hecht, F.: Inheritance and development of nail-patella syndrome, J. Bone Joint Surg. (Br) 45:259, 1964.
10. Burkett, D. P.: Epidemiology of cancer of colon and rectum, Cancer 28:3, 1971.

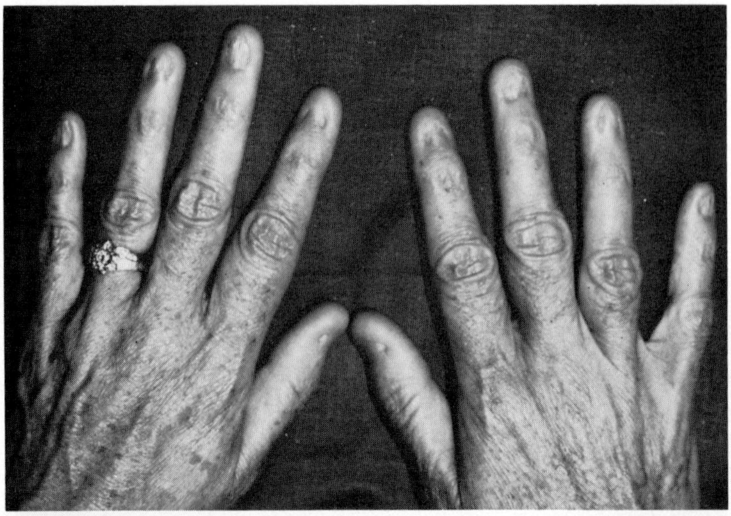

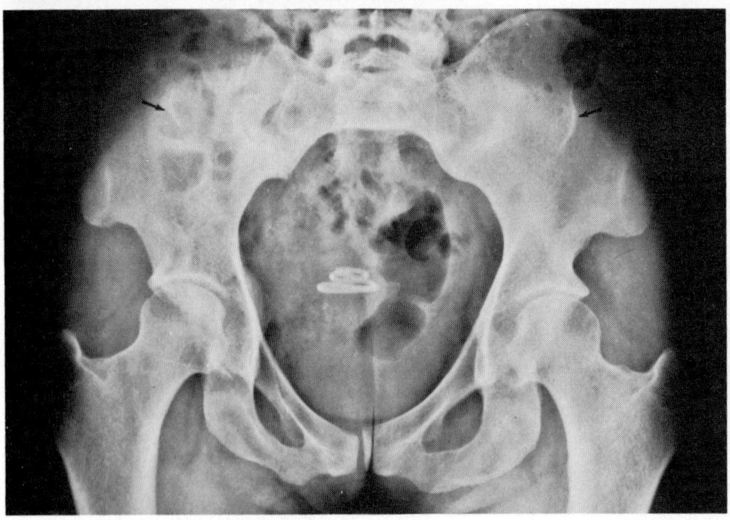

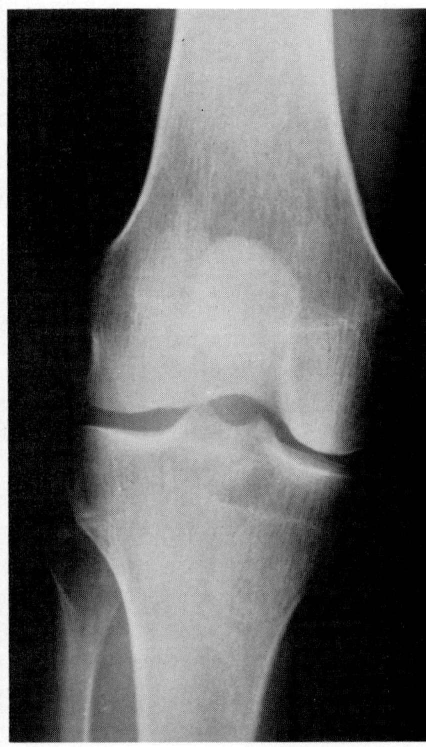

Fig 17–1 (top).—Nails are hypoplastic or aplastic. Characteristically, the findings are most marked on thumbs and are less prominent ulnarly.

Fig 17–2 (bottom left).—Exostoses *(arrows),* "iliac horns" or "Fong's horns,"[2] project off posterior surface of iliac crest.

Fig 17–3 (bottom right).—In this patient the patella is small. Medial aspect of patella usually is more prominently involved. In some patients the patella may be absent.

Chapter 18

Granulomatous Colitis

BARBARA M. KADELL, M.D.
MARVIN WEINER, M.D.

IN 1932 Crohn, Ginzberg and Oppenheimer[1] described the findings of regional ileitis or Crohn's disease. For many years this lesion was believed to involve the small intestine exclusively. In 1959 Lockhart-Mummery and Morson[2] described similar clinical and pathologic features involving the colon and, with their work and the description of the radiologic features by Wolf and Marshak,[3] granulomatous colitis became a distinct entity.

Clinical Features

The etiologic factors in granulomatous colitis are unknown. The disease appears to be increasing in frequency and, although genetic factors have been postulated, no definite proof of this link has been clearly established.[4] Granulomatous colitis is primarily a disease of young adults, the peak age range occurring between the late second and early third decades.[4, 5, 6]

Symptoms includes diarrhea, malaise, cramping abdominal pain and fever. Some rectal bleeding may occur, but gross bleeding is less commonly seen than in patients with ulcerative colitis. Perianal and perirectal fissures and fistulas frequently accompany these symptoms and may precede obvious bowel symptoms by months or years. Associated extracolonic manifestations are weight loss, anemia, arthritis and dermatitis, and occasionally these symptoms may be more disabling than the colonic manifestations.[2, 4, 6, 7]

Pathology

The colon is involved by a chronic granulomatous inflammatory process, characterized by edema, ulceration and fibrosis, which extends through the entire wall and may involve the mesentery.

In the early stage of the disease, hyperplasia of lymphoid tissue and lymphedema cause thickening of the bowel wall. Small ulcers may be seen scattered among patches of normal mucosa. With progression, the ulcers may coalesce and align themselves in a longitudinal and transverse direction. The surviving islands of mucosa among these interlacing ulcerations may give the appearance of cobblestones. When these islands are discrete, they have been called pseudopolyps. Excess fat adhering to the serosa is a prominent feature. In the late stages, fibrosis occurs and segments of the bowel may become stenotic.

Microscopically, numerous lymph follicles are found in the mucosa and submucosa. The principal diagnostic feature is noncaseating granulomas, which are located mainly in the submucosa and muscularis. These granulomas are found in a majority of cases,[4, 6, 7] but the diagnosis still can be made in their absence if the other features are present.

Partial colon involvement is more common than pancolitis. Pancolitis was reported in only 10–15% of cases in three large series.[4, 5, 7] The most typical distribution of the disease is involvement of the colon and terminal ileum, with sparing of the sigmoid and rectum. Exclusive involvement of the left colon is unusual. Rectal disease has been seen in 0–55% of patients in different series.[4, 7, 8] The terminal ileum is commonly involved and the reported incidence varies from 30 to 100%.[4, 6, 8, 9]

In early stages the disease is most commonly limited to the right colon but can spread rapidly, and a minimally involved colon may become severely diseased in a short time.[4, 6, 8] When the disease in the small bowel extends through the wall of the bowel, it may involve an adjacent portion of colon, usually the cecum or sigmoid. The phenomenon has been referred to as a "kissing" or secondary lesion in the colon.[3-6]

Radiology

Radiographically (Figs 18–1 to 18–32) the prominent features of granulomatous colitis are ulceration, which may be deep and penetrating; skip areas of disease; and colonic strictures. The earliest visible changes are demonstrated using a double contrast barium enema technique.[5, 8, 10-13] These are the presence of "aphthoid" ulcers, which are shallow 1–2 mm ulcers surrounded by a radiolucent halo of edema. Patches of normal mucosa may be seen. These tiny ulcers are only visible en face on air contrast examination. Punched-out ulcers, slightly larger and more irregular in outline, also may be seen in early colonic disease. These ulcers may be observed en face and in profile, giving the mucosal margin an irregular outline.

On full column or conventional barium enema, the earliest findings are small, irregular nodules along the contour of the bowel, with slight rigidity of the bowel, thickening of the haustra and eccentric loss of haustration in the area of involvement.[3, 4] Spasm and irritability may be prominent, and small ulcerations may be seen along the mucosal margin. The cecum may show a concave medial wall even without evidence of colonic disease elsewhere.[4, 8, 9] This finding may be due to thickened loops of adjacent inflamed ileum and indurated mesentery. Perianal disease, although common clinically, is not often well demonstrated radiographically.

As the disease progresses, the ulcers may become larger, deeper and elongated and may undermine the mucosa. These may resemble crosshatched streaks of barium interspersed with nonulcerated nodules of tissue or "cobblestones." As transverse ulcers invade the wall of the bowel, they may penetrate so deeply as to resemble spicules perpendicular to the long axis of the bowel. These spicules or fissures may join to form a tract parallel to the bowel[4] or may lead to the formation of abscesses and fistulas. Fistulas occur in as many as 10% of cases[9, 14] and may involve adjacent loops of bowel or the bladder, vagina or skin. Segments of the bowel may be spared, and asymmetric involvement is common, as is abrupt transition between diseased and normal bowel. Pseudodiverticula may be seen in an asymmetrically involved segment owing to distention of a relatively uninvolved zone in an area of fixed diseased bowel. When ileal involvement is present, the diseased segment is characterized by thickened mucosal folds, ulceration, nodularity, narrowing of the lumen and occasionally fistulas.

In late stages, strictures may occur due to fibrosis, and these may be variable in number, length and severity.[4, 15, 16] In early stages, areas of luminal narrowing may be reversible and are caused by spasm and submucosal thickening.

Reversibility of radiographic changes has been reported by many investigators[4, 5, 8, 17, 18, 19] and is most frequently seen in the early stages of the disease, especially in patients who have received medical therapy. When the disease has progressed to a stage showing extensive ulceration and cobblestoning, radiographic reversibility is unusual, even though clinical remissions may occur.

Complications

Complications are obstruction, fistulas, abscesses, free perforation, hemorrhage and intractable pain.[14] Toxic dilatation is being reported with greater frequency in patients with granulomatous colitis,[4, 7, 20] but the incidence is still not as high as that seen with ulcerative colitis. On pathologic examination of the colon of these patients, some localized perforations secondary to abscess formation were seen.

Carcinoma of the colon has been reported in association with granulomatous colitis, but the number of cases is still too small to make a valid statistical judgment as to the association.[21, 22]

A high recurrence rate after surgery has been reported by many authors.[4, 5, 6, 14] Recurrent disease may be seen on either side of an ileocolic anastomosis. Earliest findings are thickening and blunting of mucosal folds, which progress to ulceration, nodularity and stenosis.

Differential diagnosis includes ulcerative colitis, ischemic colitis, tuberculosis, amebiasis and other infectious colitides, diverticulitis, pseudomembranous enterocolitis, scirrhous carcinoma of the colon and lymphoma.

REFERENCES

1. Crohn, B. B., Ginzberg, L., and Oppenheimer, G. D.: Regional ileitis: Pathologic and clinical entity, J.A.M.A. 99:1323, 1932.
2. Lockhart-Mummery, H. E., and Morson, B. C.: Crohn's disease (regional enteritis) of the large intestine and its distinction from ulcerative colitis, Gut 1:87, 1960.
3. Wolf, B. S., and Marshak, R. H.: Granulomatous colitis (Crohn's disease of the colon). Roentgen features, Am. J. Roentgenol. 88:662, 1962.
4. Marshak, R. H.: Granulomatous disease of the intestinal tract (Crohn's disease), Radiology 114:3, 1975.
5. Hildell, J.: *Radiographic Patterns of Crohn's Disease.* A long-term study of pre- and postoperative findings in 195 patients, with special reference to recurrence of the disease (Thesis) (Malmo, Sweden: Department of Radiology University of Lund, Malmo General Hospital, 1978).
6. Reeves, B. R., Carlson, H. C., et al.: Segmental ulcerative colitis versus segmental Crohn's disease of the colon, Am. J. Roentgenol. 99:24, 1967.
7. Zetzel, L.: Granulomatous (ileo) colitis, New Engl. J. Med. 282:600, March 1976.
8. Brahme, F.: Granulomatous colitis, Roentgenologic appearance and course of the lesions, Am. J. Roentgenol. 99:35, 1967.
9. Kemp Harper, R. A.: The radiologic spectrum of Crohn's disease, Proc. Roy. Soc. Med. 64:1181, 1971.
10. Laufer, I.: Air contrast studies of the colon in inflammatory bowel disease, CRC Crit. Rev. Radiol. 9(4):421, 1977.
11. Fraser, G. M., and Findlay, J. M.: The double contrast enema in ulcerative and Crohn's colitis, Clin. Radiol. 27:103, 1976.
12. Laufer, I., and Hamilton, J.: The radiological differentiation between ulcerative and granulomatous colitis by double contrast radiology, Am. J. Gastroenterol. 66:259, 1976.
13. Laufer, I., Mullens, J. E., and Hamilton, J.: Correlation of endoscopy and double-contrast radiography in the early stages of ulcerative and granulomatous colitis, Radiology 118:1, 1976.
14. McGarity, W. C.: Crohn's disease, Mod. Med. 44: 78, 1976.
15. Simpkins, K. C., and Young, A. C.: The differential diagnosis of large bowel strictures, Clin. Radiol. 22: 449, 1971.
16. Marshak, R. H., Bloch, C., and Wolf, B. S.: The roentgen findings in strictures of the colon associated with ulcerative and granulomatous colitis, Am. J. Roentgenol. 90:709, 1963.
17. Marshak, R. H., and Lindner, A. E.: Reversibility in granulomatous colitis, Am. J. Gastroenterol. 57: 172, 1972.
18. Jones, J. H., Lennard-Jones, J. E., and Young, A. C.: Reversibility of radiologic appearances during clinical improvement in colonic Crohn's disease, Gut 10:738, 1969.
19. Goldstein, F., and Murdock, M. G.: Clinical and radiologic improvement of regional enteritis and enterocolitis after treatment with Salicylazosulfapyridine, Am. J. Dig. Dis. 16:421, 1971.
20. Javett, S. L., and Brooke, B. N.: Acute dilatation of colon in Crohn's disease, Lancet, 2:126, 1970.
21. Fielding, J. F., Prior, P., et al.: Malignancy in Crohn's disease, Scand. J. Gastroenterol. 7:3, 1972.
22. Darke, S. G., Parks, A. G., et al.: Adenocarcinoma and Crohn's disease, Br. J. Surg. 60:169, 1973.

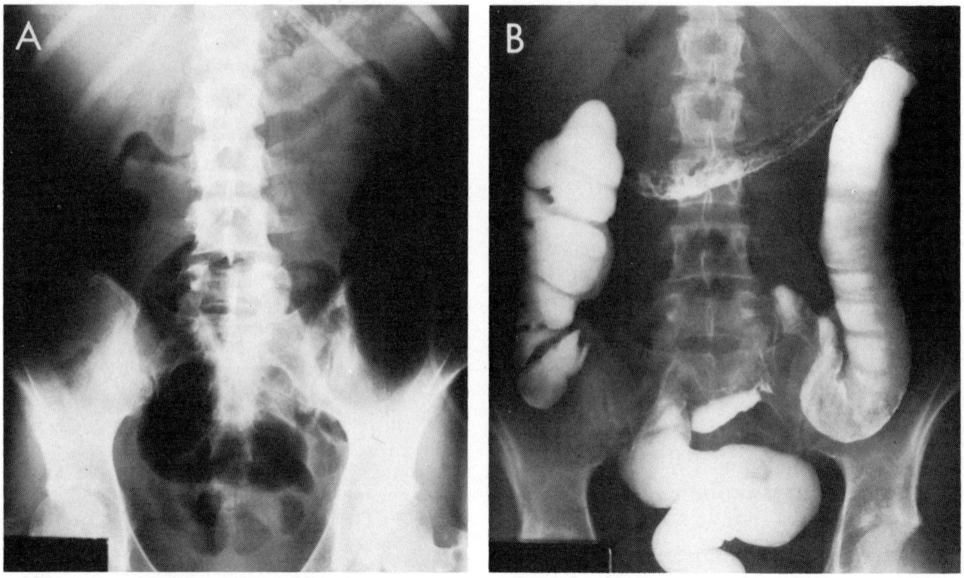

Fig 18–1. – **A,** plain film of abdomen in granulomatous colitis. Irregular narrowing and loss of haustration are seen in transverse colon. Ascending and descending colon appear normal. **B,** barium enema confirms involvement of transverse colon and shows additional disease in sigmoid colon. "Skip lesions" are typical of granulomatous colitis.

Fig 18–2 (left). – Plain film of abdomen in granulomatous colitis. Bowel has tubular appearance, with loss of haustration. Rectal air collection appears normal. *Arrows* point to thickened bowel wall in involved segments.

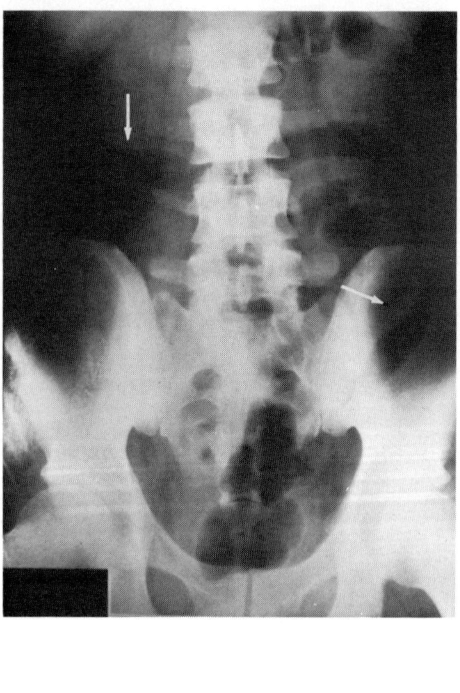

Fig 18–3 (right). – Granulomatous colitis, double contrast examination. Many shallow ulcerations are viewed en face in background of normal mucosa.

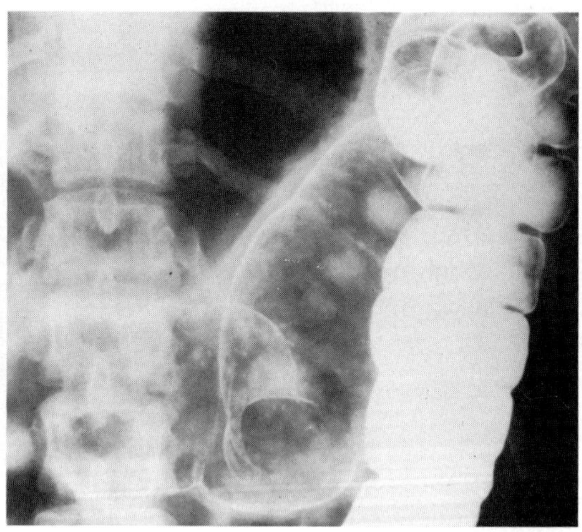

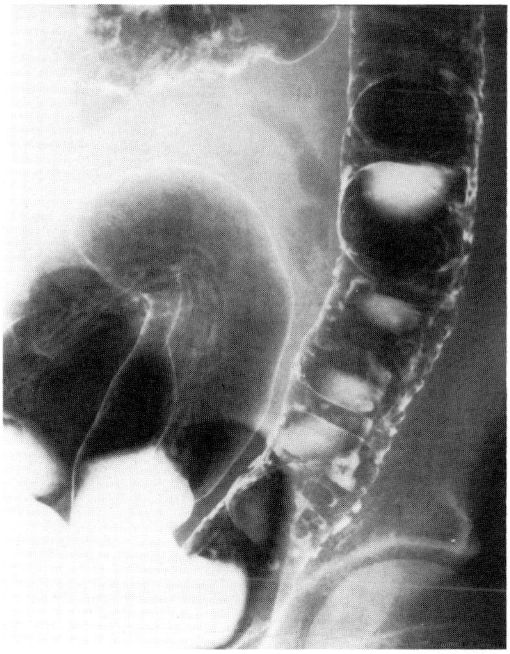

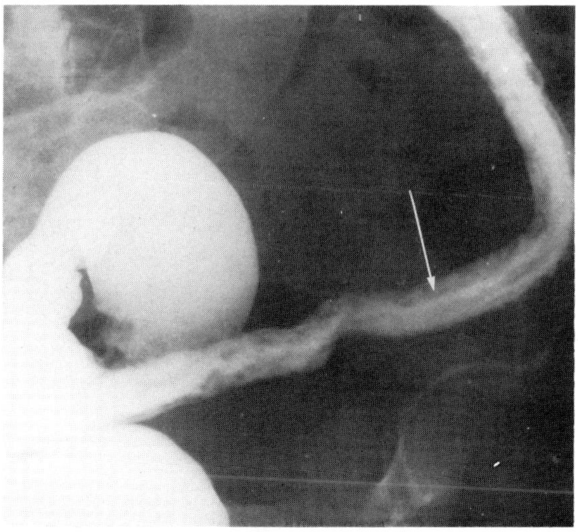

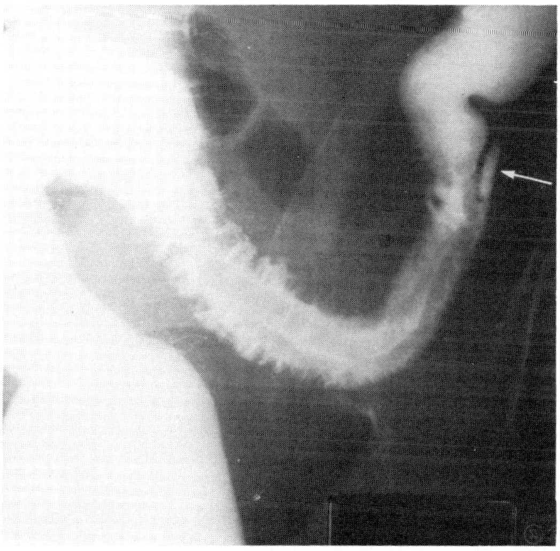

Fig 18–4 (top left).—Granulomatous colitis, double contrast examination. Descending colon is diseased and shows ulcers undermining mucosa. Involvement is asymmetric, with more extensive changes seen on lateral wall of descending colon. Note sigmoid sparing.

Fig 18–5 (top right).—Granulomatous colitis involving proximal sigmoid colon. *Arrow* points to extensive longitudinal ulceration. Rectum and distal sigmoid spared.

Fig 18–6 (bottom).—Granulomatous colitis involving sigmoid colon. Longitudinal and transverse ulcerations present in sigmoid colon. Lucencies between these ulcerations represent cobblestoning. *Arrow* points to tract extending into wall of bowel. Rectum is spared, and transition between normal and abnormal bowel is abrupt.

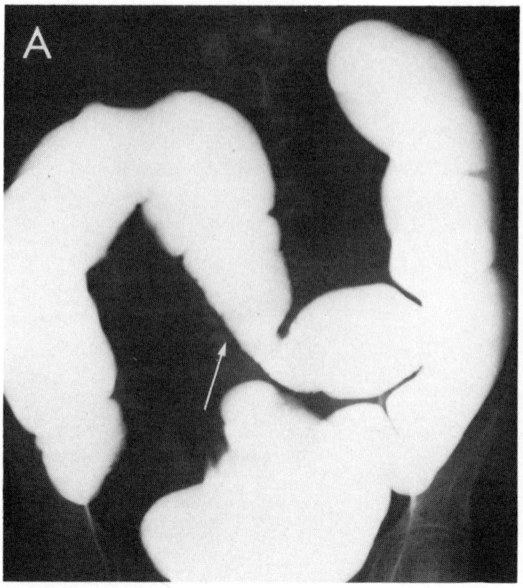

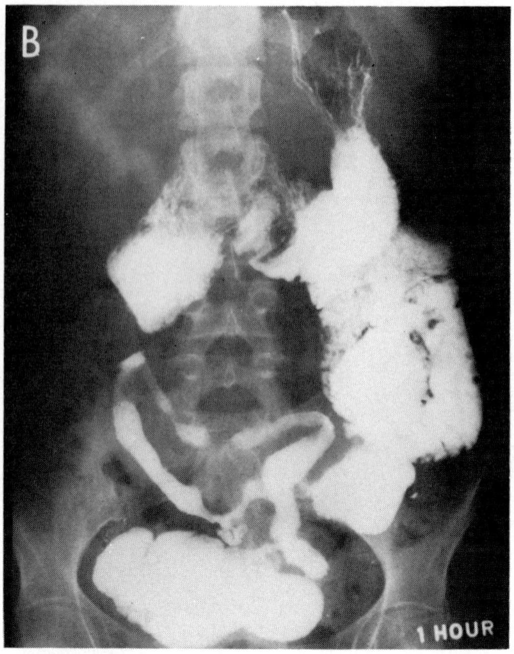

Fig 18–7.—**A,** granulomatous colitis with segmental colonic involvement *(arrow).* Nodularity and rigidity are demonstrated along inferior margin of proximal transverse colon. **B,** small bowel study (same patient). Extensive regional enteritis involves ileum.

Fig 18–8.—**A,** granulomatous colitis. *Arrows* point to skip areas of disease in descending and sigmoid colon. Involvement of bowel is asymmetric in diseased areas. **B,** small bowel study with extensive involvement of distal ileum. Loss of mucosal pattern, longitudinal ulceration, cobblestoning and markedly thickened bowel wall are present.

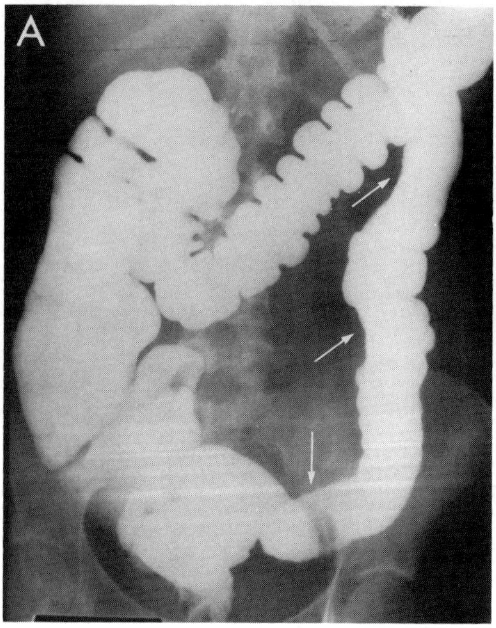

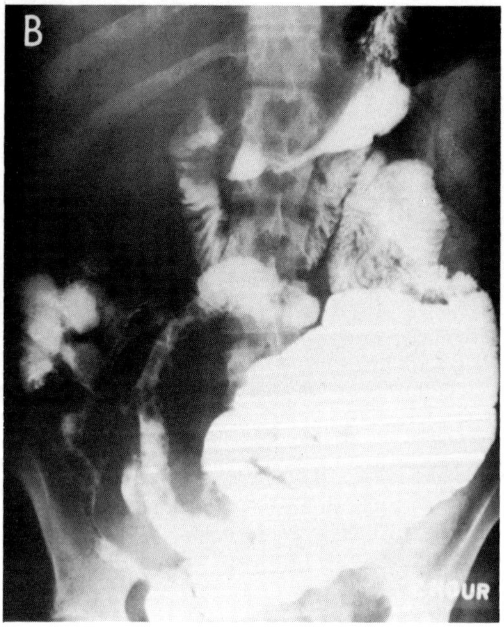

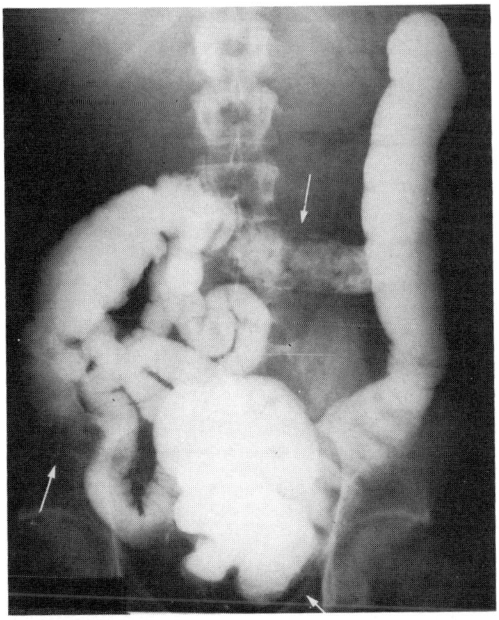

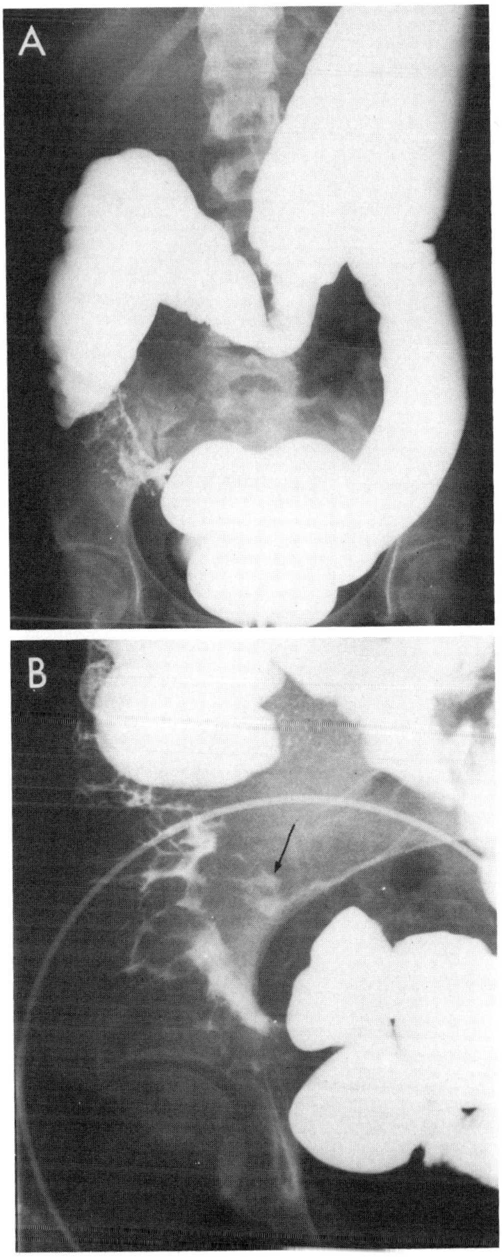

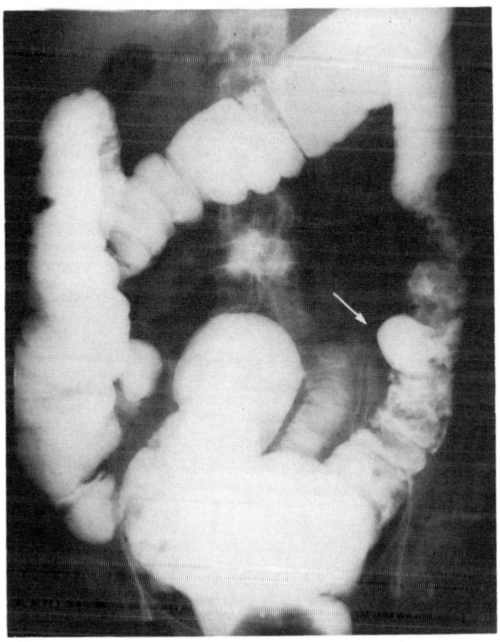

Fig 18–9 (top left).—Granulomatous colitis with skip areas of disease *(arrows)* in cecum, transverse colon and sigmoid.

Fig 18–10 (right).—**A,** granulomatous ileocolitis. Narrowing and deformity of cecum and midtransverse colon are present. **B,** pressure spot film shows multiple ileocolic fistulas *(arrow)*.

Fig 18–11 (bottom left).—Granulomatous colitis with skip lesions. Hepatic flexure, superior aspect of transverse colon and descending colon are involved. *Arrow* indicates island of normal bowel in extensively involved descending colon.

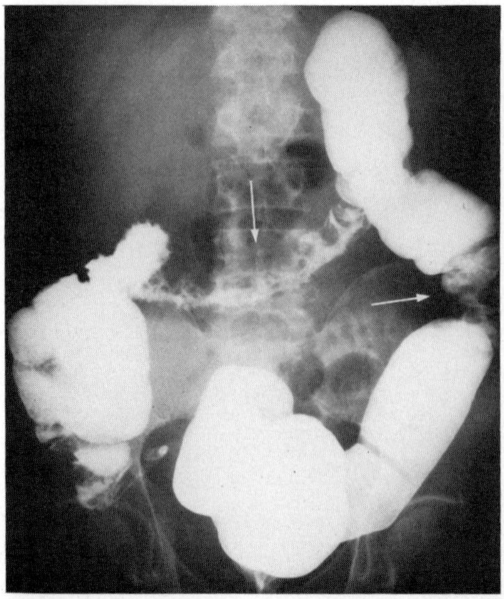

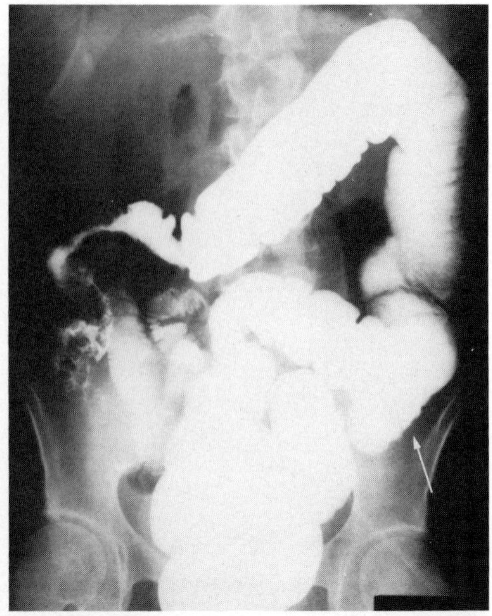

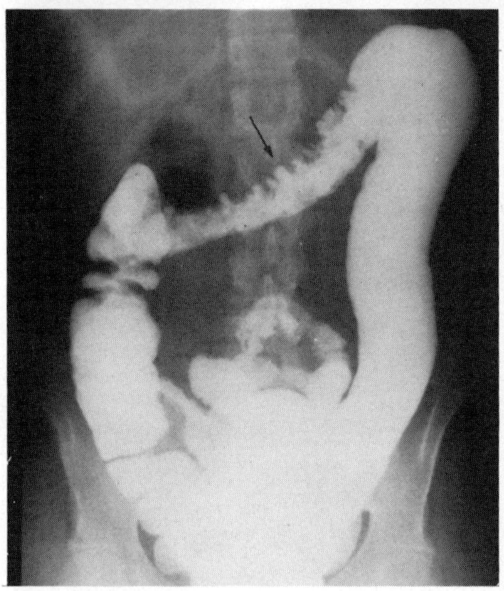

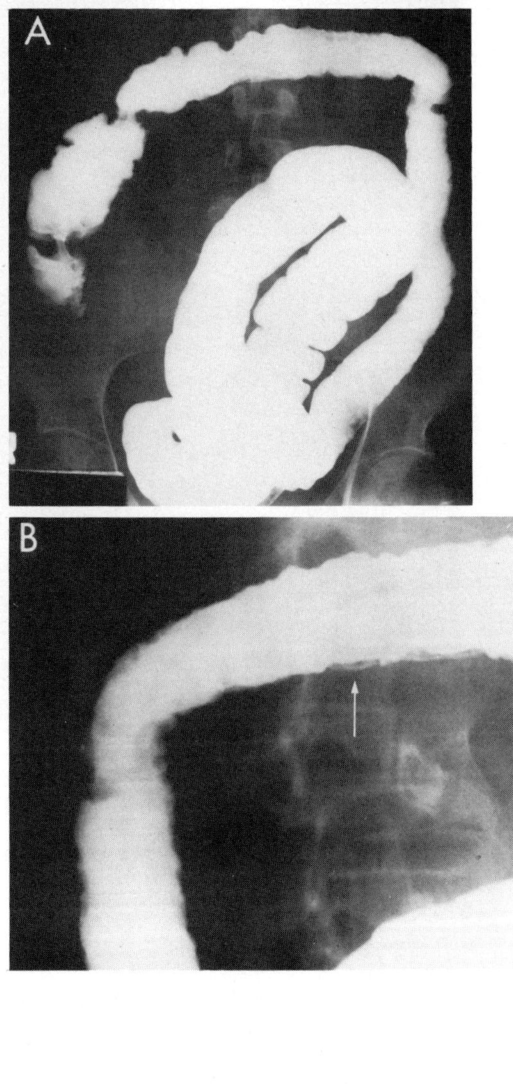

Fig 18–12 (top left).—Granulomatous colitis. Cecum and transverse and descending colon are diseased and show significant narrowing, loss of haustration and nodularity.

Fig 18–13 (bottom left).—Granulomatous ileocolitis. Distal ascending and transverse colon and terminal ileum are involved. Lumen is narrowed, and extensive ulceration is present. *Arrow* points to one of the multiple pseudo-diverticula seen in transverse colon.

Fig 18–14 (top right).—Granulomatous colitis with extensive involvement of ascending and proximal transverse colon. Skip area of disease in descending colon indicated by *arrow*. Marked narrowing of lumen as well as nodularity present in right side of colon.

Fig 18–15 (bottom right).—**A,** granulomatous colitis involving right and midcolon. Extensive nodularity and irregular narrowing present in diseased segments. **B,** long intramural tract is indicated by *arrow*.

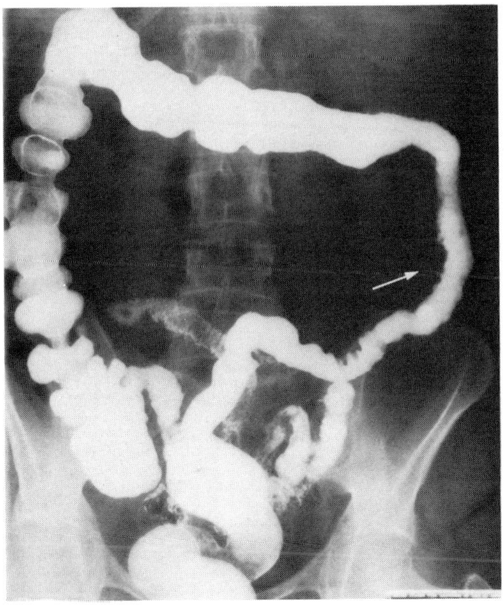

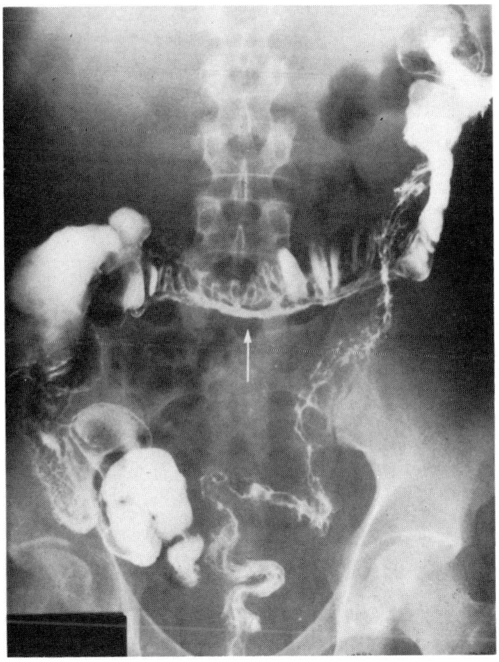

Fig 18–16 (left). – Granulomatous colitis (surgically proved). All of colon except rectum is involved. *Arrow* points to fistulous tract into wall of descending colon.

Fig 18–17 (right). – Granulomatous colitis, postevacuation contrast study. Long, longitudinal ulceration on inferior margin of transverse colon indicated by *arrow*.

Fig 18–18. – **A** and **B**, granulomatous colitis. Extensive involvement of colon, but rectum and distal sigmoid are spared. Marked narrowing, longitudinal and transverse ulcerations, and cobblestones are seen throughout transverse colon. *Arrows* point to tracts in wall of transverse colon. Discrete lucencies, representing pseudopolyps, are seen in ascending colon.

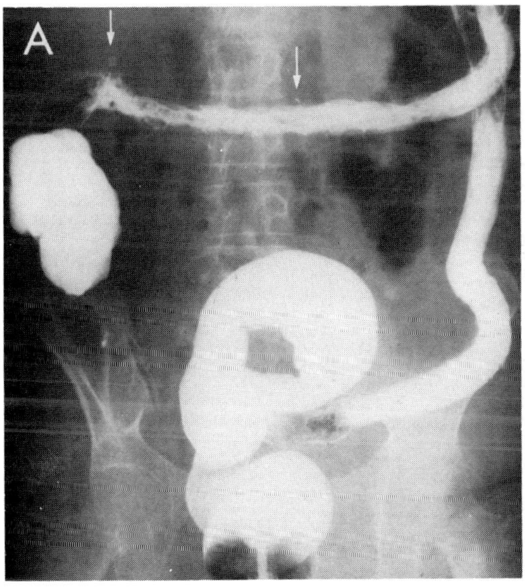

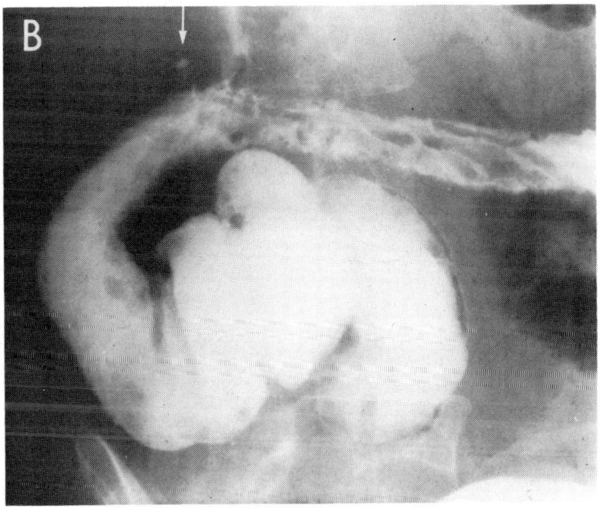

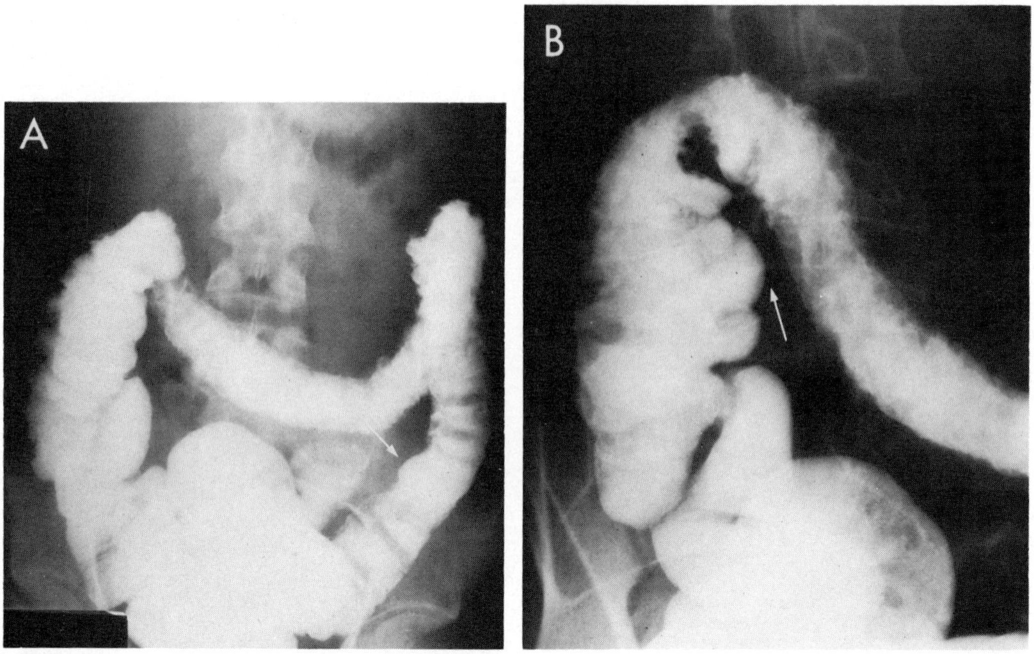

Fig 18–19.—**A** and **B,** granulomatous colitis with extensive colonic disease. Rectum and sigmoid are spared. Ascending and descending colons are asymmetrically involved. *Arrows* show localized spared areas.

Fig 18–20.—**A** and **B,** granulomatous colitis with extensive involvement. Long longitudinal ulcers present in splenic flexure and descending colon, as indicated by *arrows.*

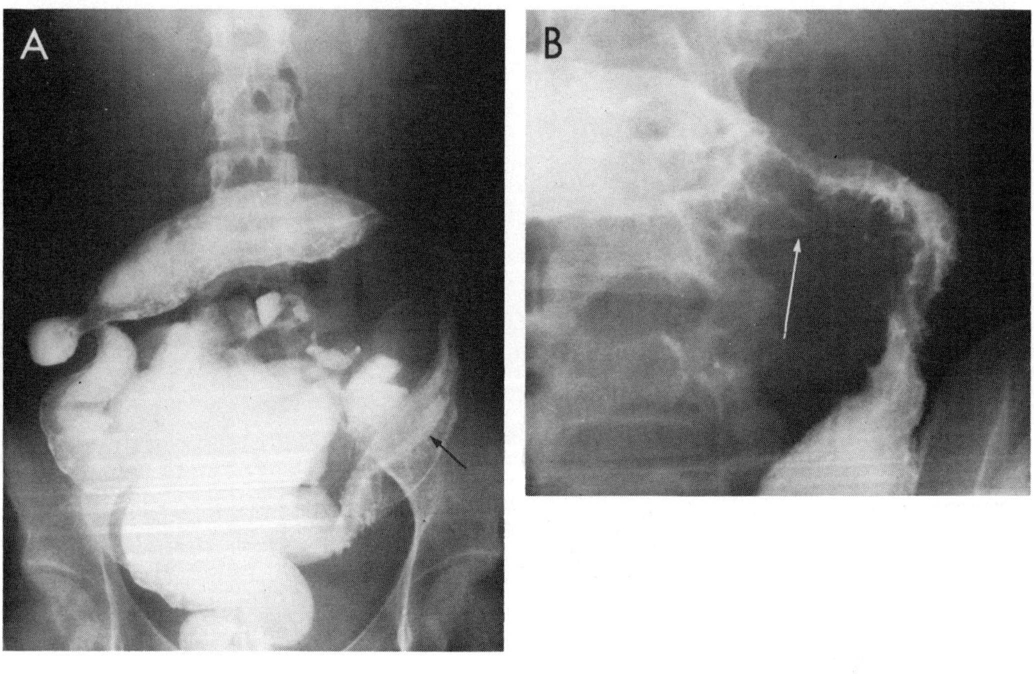

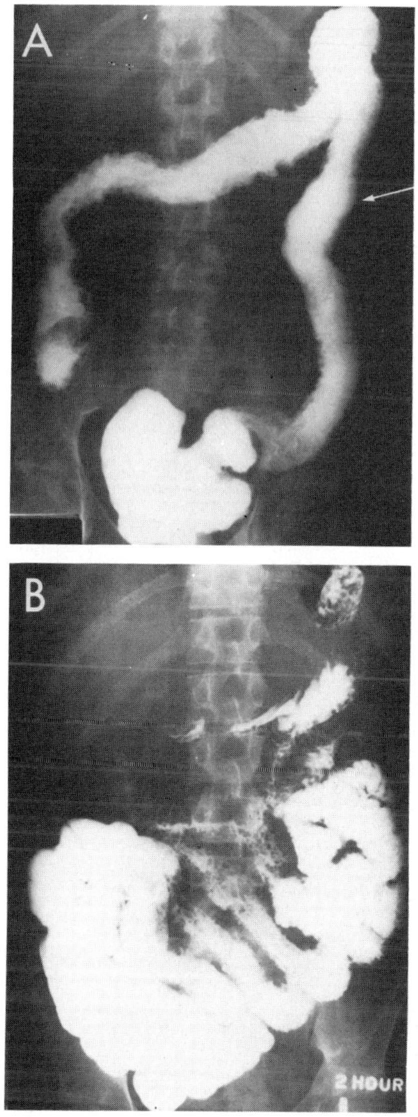

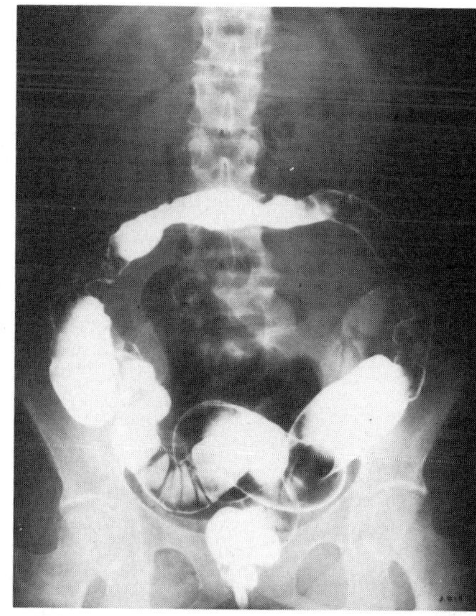

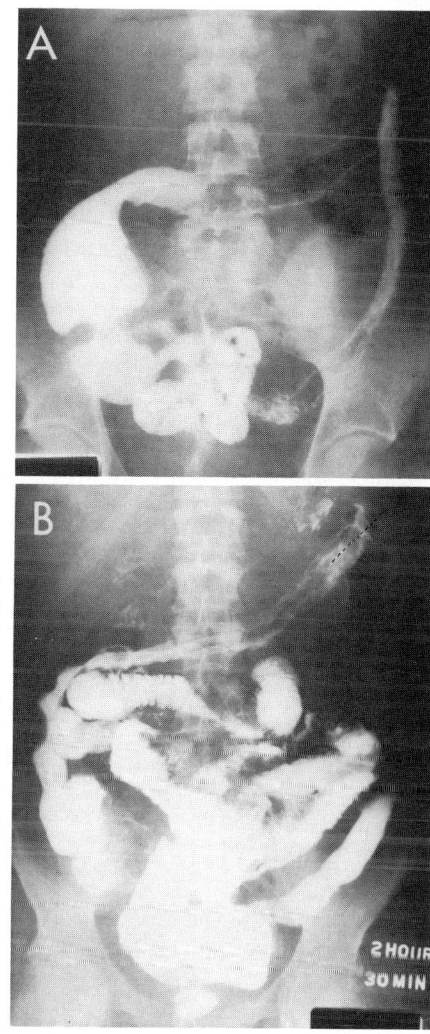

Fig 18–21 (left).—**A** and **B,** granulomatous colitis with extensive colonic involvement. Bowel is nondistensible, and extensive cobblestoning is present. *Arrow* in **A** shows area not involved in otherwise diseased descending colon. **B,** small bowel series shows Chron's disease in jejunem and proximal ileum.

Fig 18–22 (top right).—Granulomatous colitis with extensive colon involvement. Except for normal rectum and sigmoid, entire colon is narrowed and markedly shortened.

Fig 18–23 (bottom right).—**A** and **B,** granulomatous colitis with total colonic involvement. This appearance could easily be confused with that of ulcerative colitis were it not for extensive ileal disease, as demonstrated by small bowel study.

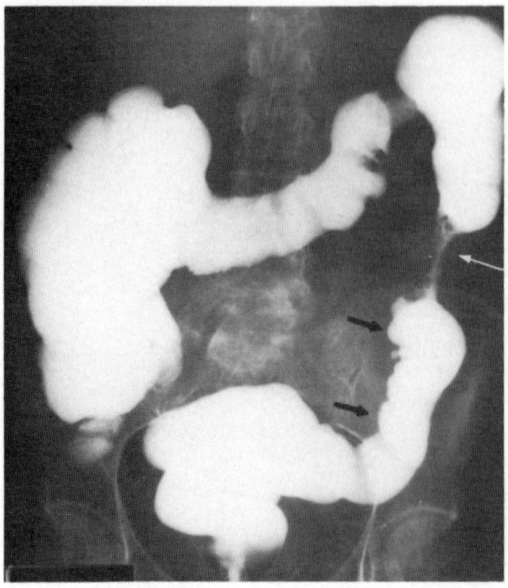

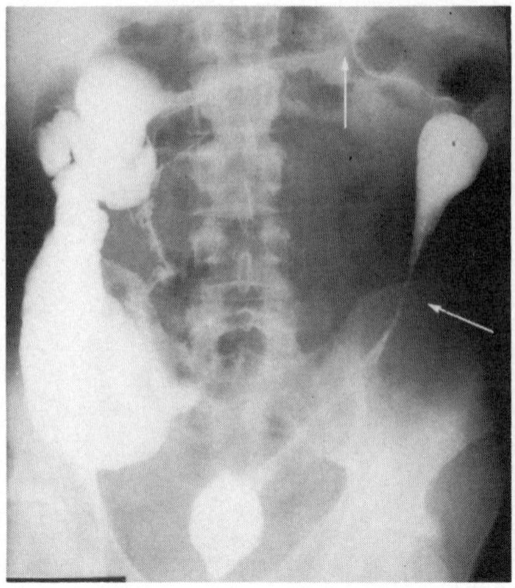

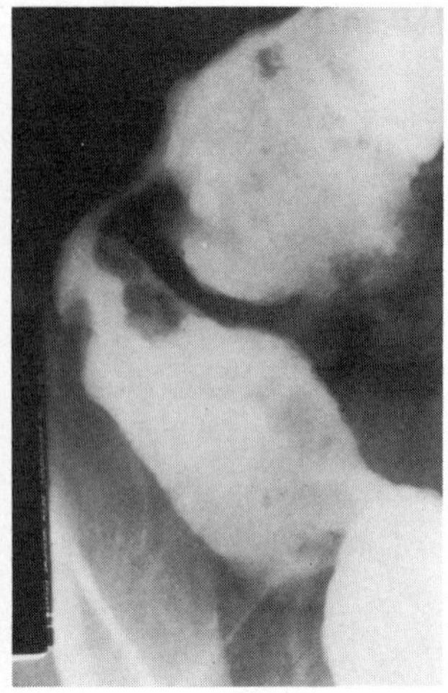

Fig 18–24 (left). – Granulomatous colitis. Transverse and descending colon is involved. Strictures are present in distal transverse and mid-descending colon, and pseudodiverticula *(black arrows)* are seen on inferior margin of distal descending colon. *White arrow* indicates tract into wall of bowel.

Fig 18–25 (center). – Granulomatous colitis (surgically proved) with total colonic involvement. Localized stricture *(upper arrow)* is seen in distal transverse colon. A long stricture involves most of descending colon. *Lower arrow* points to small tract in wall of descending colon.

Fig 18–26 (right). – Granulomatous colitis with benign stricture involving right colon (biopsy proved). Zone of fixed narrowing present at hepatic flexure, with large inflammatory pseudopolyps proximal to area of narrowing.

Fig 18–27. – **A,** regional enteritis with "kissing" lesion in sigmoid colon. An extrinsic mass effect, causing narrowing and distortion of sigmoid colon, is present. **B,** small bowel study demonstrates extensive Crohn's disease in adjacent ileal segment, with fistulous communication to sigmoid.

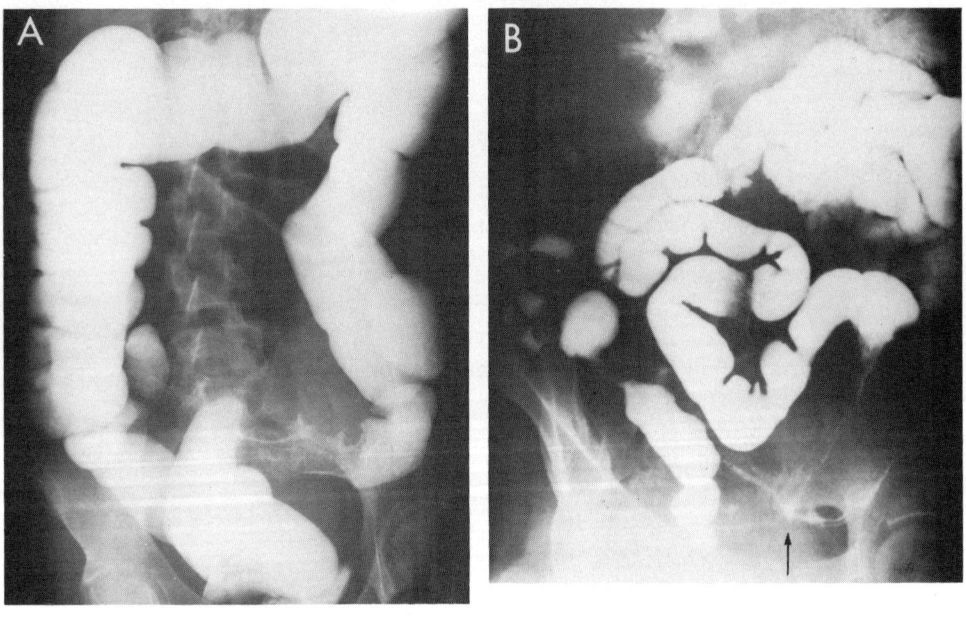

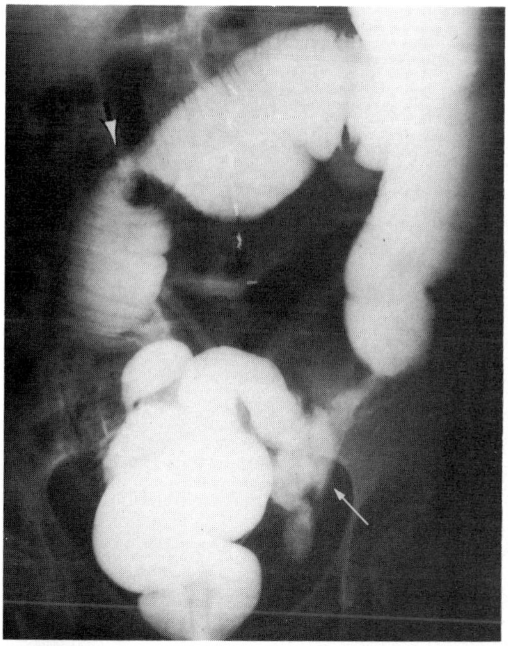

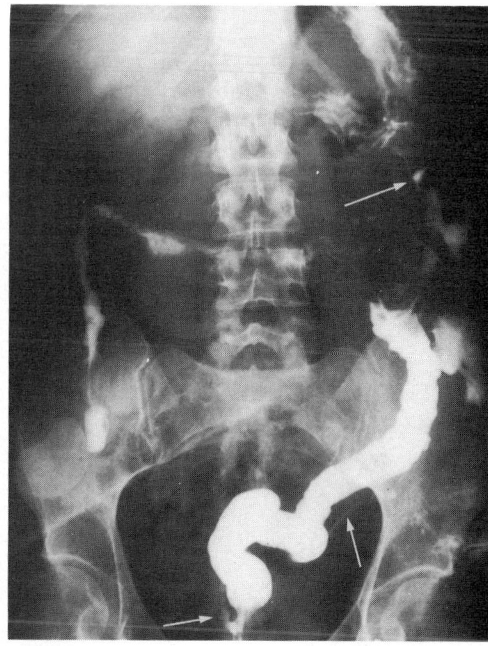

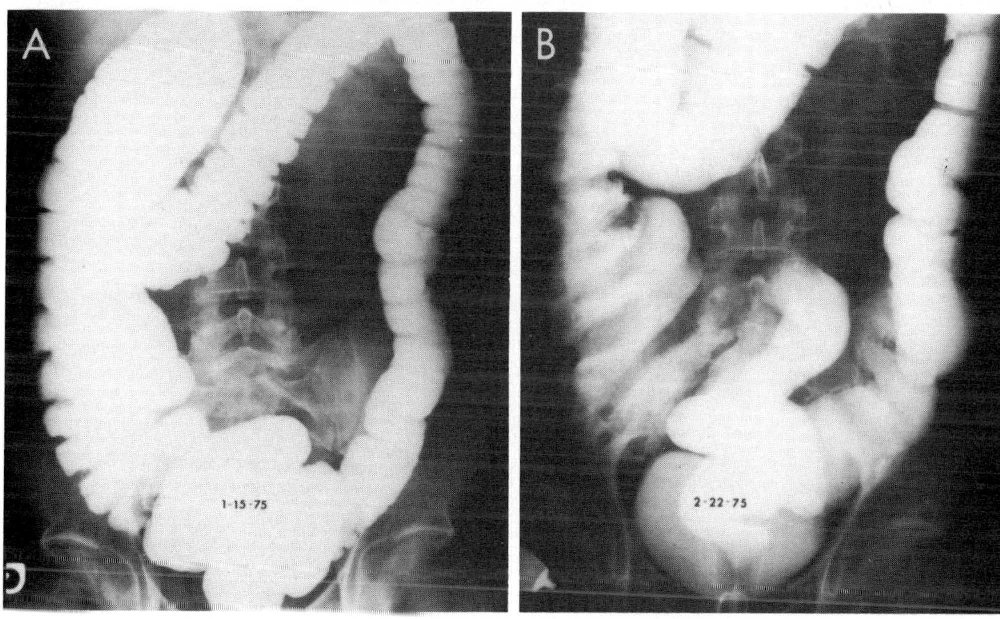

Fig 18–28 (top left).—Granulomatous ileocolitis with fistula from sigmoid to ileum. *White arrow* marks site at which small bowel communicates with diseased sigmoid colon.

Fig 18–29 (top right).—Granulomatous colitis with extensive involvement. Several fistulas arise from left colon *(arrows). Arrow* in left upper quadrant indicates gastrocolic fistula.

Fig 18–30 (bottom).—**A,** granulomatous colitis with rapid progression. Examination shows minimal widening of haustra in right colon. **B,** study 5 weeks later shows marked thickening of haustra in ascending colon. Nodularity and ulceration also seen in ascending, transverse and sigmoid colon.

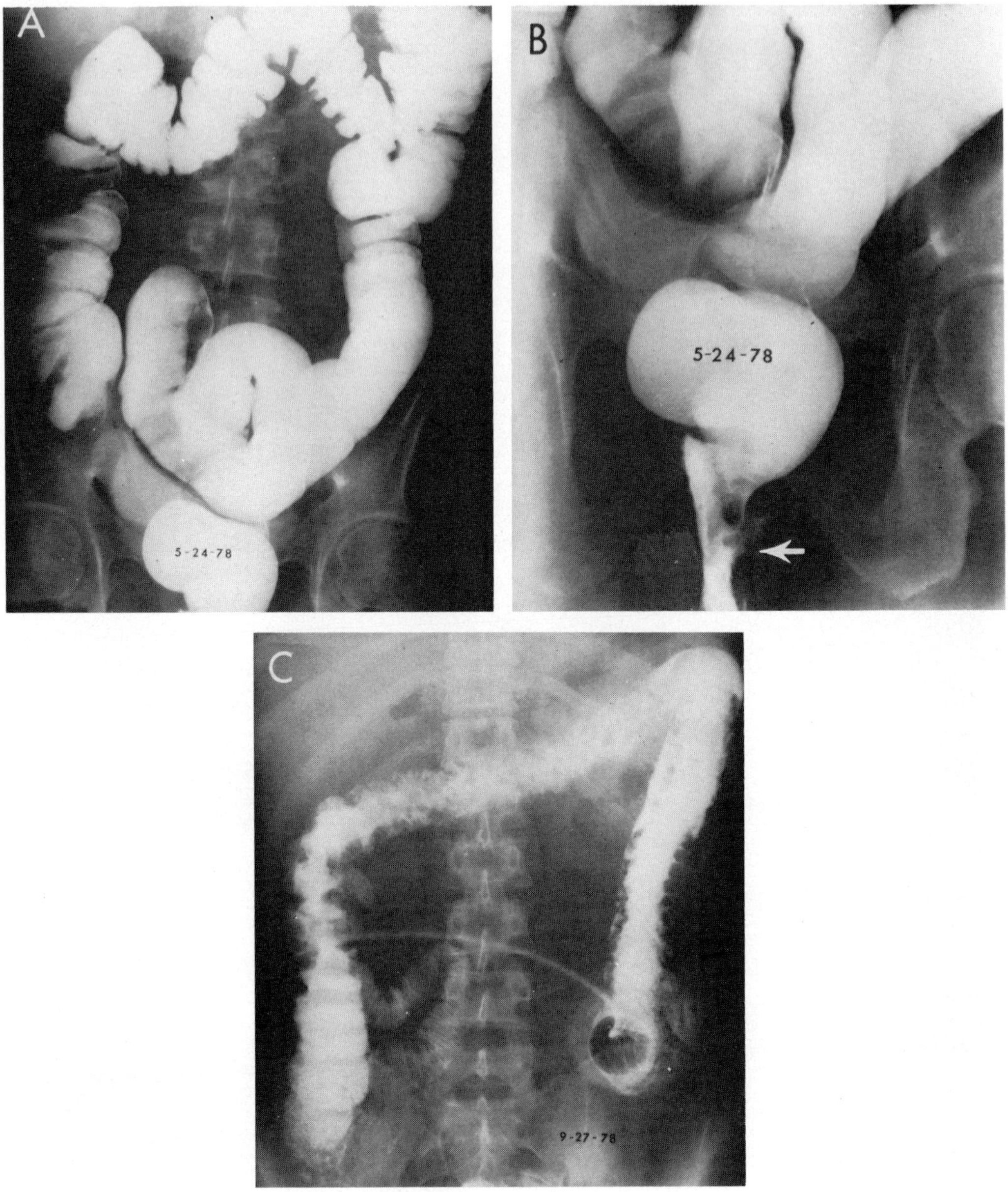

Fig 18–31.—Granulomatous colitis with rapid progression. **A,** study shows normally haustrated, distensible colon. **B,** *arrow* indicates large rectal ulceration on same examination. **C,** 4 months later, after a descending colostomy was performed, extensive ulceration and nodularity involve entire remaining colon.

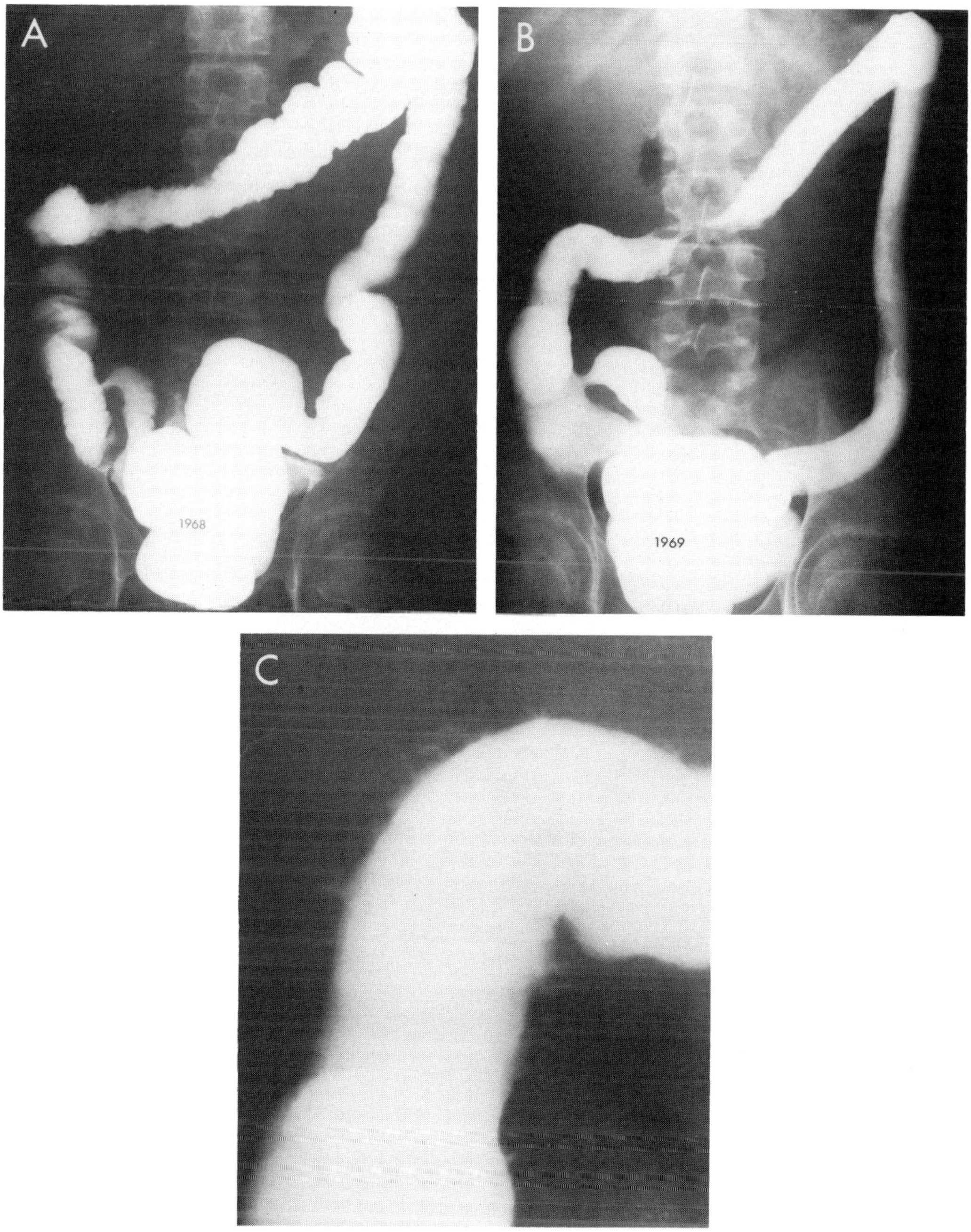

Fig 18–32. – **A,** granulomatous colitis with progression of disease. Barium enema reveals involvement of ascending and proximal transverse colon. **B,** examination 1 year later shows significant extension of disease. A stricture involving transverse colon is present. **C** (same examination), multiple deep spicules project into wall of hepatic flexure.

Chapter 19

Herniations of the Colon

GARY G. GHAHREMANI, M.D.
MORTON A. MEYERS, M.D.

ABDOMINAL HERNIAS occur in about 1.5% of the population and account for almost half a million operations per year in the United States.[1,2] Most of these hernias involve the groin and anterior abdominal wall, thus permitting a clinical diagnosis to be made based on inspection and palpation. Nevertheless, radiologic studies, including barium examination of the gastrointestinal tract, are often performed for preoperative delineation of the hernial content or when complications such as mechanical bowel obstruction are the presenting symptoms. Radiologic evaluation is crucial as the primary diagnostic means if the hernia is located within the abdominal cavity or extends through the diaphragm.[3]

It is important to note that the designation of various hernias is based on an anatomical location of the hernial orifice rather than on the type or ultimate position of the protruding viscera. Accordingly the following two general categories of hernias are commonly recognized.

1. *External abdominal hernias.*—The hernial opening or ring is located in the encompassing walls of the abdominal cavity so that the viscera protrude beyond their normal area of confinement.[1,2] Various types of diaphragmatic hernias and those involving the abdominal wall, groin and pelvic regions are included in this category.

2. *Internal abdominal hernias.*—An aperture is present in the mesentery or peritoneum, which permits protrusion and encapsulation of a viscus in another compartment of the abdominal cavity.[3] The hernial ring is usually a preexisting anatomical structure, e.g., foramen of Winslow, through which intestinal herniation into the lesser sac may occur. Less commonly, the internal hernial ring is formed by pathologic defects, either congenital or acquired.[2,3]

Most abdominal hernias include a peritoneal sac, which passes through the hernial orifice and receives the eventrated viscera. Usually the omentum and segments of the small intestine or colon constitute the content of the hernial sac, whereas other abdominal organs are only occasionally involved.[1-3] In this chapter, however, the emphasis will be placed primarily on those entities in which herniation of the colon alone or together with other viscera has been a recognizable feature.

External Abdominal Hernias

DIAPHRAGMATIC HERNIAS

Esophageal Hiatus Hernia

The esophageal hiatus is the most common site for development of diaphragmatic hernia in adults. The stomach is the only organ routinely involved in both the sliding and paraesophageal type of herniation. With progressive upward migration of the stomach and further dilation of the hiatus, however, the stomach can eventually assume an intrathoracic position and undergo organoaxial or mesenteroaxial torsion.[4] Because of the attachment of the greater curvature to the transverse colon by the gastrocolic ligament, the colon may be pulled upward into the chest (Fig 19–1). Patients may experience upper abdominal pain and obstructive symptoms owing to associated gastric torsion, but herniation of the colon itself remains an asymptomatic incidental finding.

Foramen of Bochdalek Hernia

The pleuroperitoneal canal, or foramen of Bochdalek, represents a congenital anomaly owing to failure in the formation of the posterolateral portion of the diaphragm. The resultant intrathoracic protrusion of the abdominal viscera through this defect is the most common type of diaphragmatic herniation in the pediatric age group. More (80–90%) of these hernias occur on the left side, primarily because the liver protects against a similar defect in the right hemidiaphragm.[5]

Small Bochdalek hernias are often first recognized on routine chest radiographs as a localized bulge on the posterolateral aspect of the diaphragm. The hernial content usually includes portions of the omentum and the transverse colon and occasionally the upper pole of the left kidney (Fig 19–2). Some initially small, clinically silent Bochdalek hernias become symptomatic later in adulthood when gradual enlargement of the diaphragmatic defect results in massive herniation of the abdominal viscera. In such cases, operative repair is required owing to potential for incarceration and strangulation of the intrathoracically displaced intestinal loops.[6]

In infants with large Bochdalek hernia, acute respiratory distress develops shortly after birth when the herniated intestinal loops fill with gas and food. The frequent absence of a confining hernial sac allows free communication between the abdominal and thoracic cavities. Therefore, the protruding intestinal loops can interfere with the maturation and function of the lungs.[7] Clinical manifestations are progressive dyspnea, cyanosis, absent respiratory sounds on the affected side and a scaphoid abdomen. Chest radiographs show the gas-filled loops of bowel in the pleural space, collapse of the ipsilateral lung and mediastinal shift to the opposite side. Partial or complete absence of the intestinal gas pattern also may be seen on abdominal radiographs.

Barium studies of the gastrointestinal tract are seldom necessary for the diagnosis of Bochdalek hernias. However, they provide useful information concerning preoperative delineation of the herniated segments and for differential diagnosis from cystic disease of the lungs and pneumatocele in infants.

Foramen of Morgagni Hernia

The foramina of Morgagni are triangular defects located just posterior to the sternum on either side of the midline. They represent embryologic defects in fusion of the sternal and costal portions of the diaphragm. The foramen on the left side is protected by the heart so that most Morgagni hernias develop on the right and account for nearly 10% of congenital diaphragmatic hernias.[5,7] The usual contents are portions of the omentum, liver or transverse colon. Massive herniation occurs rarely owing to the presence of a true membranous sac confining the protruding viscera.

The diagnosis usually is first made on a routine chest radiograph because of the characteristic appearance of a well-defined soft tissue mass or gas-containing loop in the right cardiophrenic angle (Fig 19–3). Barium enema, upper gastrointestinal series, liver scans and diagnostic pneumoperitoneum are all useful in establishing the nature and content of the hernia. In unusual instances, there may be an associated defect in the diaphragmatic portion of the pericardium.[8] As a result, the herniated viscera can enter the pericardial sac and be visible anterior to the cardiac shadow on lateral chest films. Such patients present with severe cardiorespiratory symptoms requiring prompt diagnosis and corrective surgery.

Traumatic Diaphragmatic Hernias

About 5% of diaphragmatic hernias are traumatic in origin. These develop through tears in the diaphragm caused by blunt abdominal trauma (automobile accidents or fall) and through direct penetrating injuries of the diaphragm (gunshot or stab wounds).[9] On rare occasions, dehiscence of diaphragmatic suture lines after transthoracic hiatus hernia repair or severe vomiting may be the causal factors.[10]

Traumatic hernias involve the central and/or posterior portions of the left hemidiaphragm in over 90% of cases.[9] Lacerations of the right hemidiaphragm rarely occur because of the liver, which dissipates the force of abdominal trauma.[10] The stomach, together with portions of the transverse colon and small intestine, makes up the usual contents of a traumatic hernia (Fig 19–4). Plain film features include (1) mediastinal shift by the gas- and fluid-filled intestinal loops in the pleural space and (2) the obliterated outline of the involved hemidiaphragm.

Differentiation between a large Bochdalek hernia and traumatic hernia is at times difficult. The association with fractures of the lower ribs or vertebrae, penetrating wounds of the upper abdomen and hemothorax are particularly suggestive of traumatic herniation in adults. In contrast, the Bochdalek hernias usually are recognized at an earlier age, and the defect involves the posterolateral portion of the diaphragm. Furthermore, the intrathoracic position of ascending or descending colon, kidney or duodenal loop suggests that the herniation had occurred prior to retroperitoneal fixation of these organs during fetal life. In such cases, it is not uncommon to find the stomach displaced inferiorly in the abdomen, whereas traumatic diaphragmatic hernias commonly contain the stomach and intraperitoneally mobile intestinal loops.[10]

INGUINAL HERNIAS

Nearly 75% of all abdominal hernias occur in the inguinal regions and predominantly affect males.[1,2] Because of the relative ease of clinical diagnosis, radiologic studies are performed mostly for evaluation of complications or when preoperative delineation of the herniated viscera appears desirable.

In *indirect inguinal hernia* the peritoneal sac (processus vaginalis) and the herniated viscera protrude at the internal inguinal ring and, in males, pass down the course of the inguinal canal anterior to the structures of the spermatic cord. They then emerge through the external inguinal ring and may actually extend into the scrotum. In females, the hernial sac follows the course of the round ligament of the uterus into the labium majus.[1]

The contents of indirect inguinal hernias usually are segments of the small bowel and omentum. However, barium enema examination may show herniation of the cecum, appendix or sigmoid (Figs 19–5 to 19–7). In rare instances, the protruding viscera have shown evidence of inflammation (appendicitis, diverticulitis) or involvement by primary or metastatic tumors.[2]

Indirect inguinal hernias (Fig 19–8) are a major cause of intestinal obstruction and strangulation.[1,2] Such complications also may be seen with other types of hernias and represent one of the 10 leading causes of mortality in the United States. The symptoms of strangulated inguinal hernias are those of mechanical bowel obstruction, together with a painful and tense swelling in the inguinal region or scrotum.

Radiologic diagnosis of strangulated hernia is based primarily on plain films of the abdomen and pelvis obtained in supine, upright and lateral decubitus positions. Typical findings are (1) visualization of distended loops converging toward the inguinal region; (2) gas-filled bowel overlying the obturator foramen and (3) bulging groin mass with air-fluid level. When the diagnosis is not clearly evident, barium enema examination should be attempted. In addition to visualizing the colon, reflux of contrast beyond the ileocecal valve can demonstrate the site of small bowel herniation and obstruction.

Sliding inguinal hernia is the term used to indicate that partially retroperitoneal structures, e.g., ascending or descending colon or the bladder, form a portion of the wall of the hernial sac (Fig 19–9).[1, 2] The preoperative diagnosis by barium enema and excretory urography is important because the blood vessels to the involved bowel lie behind the colon and are prone to injury if incorrect surgical approach is used.[1, 11]

Direct inguinal hernia is a protrusion of viscera directly through the posterior wall of the inguinal canal, medial to the inferior epigastric vessels. Direct hernias are very uncommon in children and women.[1, 2] Strangulation seldom is a complication because of the blunt, diffuse character of the protrusion. Radiographic differentiation between direct and indirect types of inguinal hernias may be difficult. However, the obliquely elongated tubular course of indirect hernia and the frequent extension into the scrotum are useful diagnostic features.

Combined inguinal hernia denotes the simultaneous presence of indirect and direct hernias in the same inguinal region. The inferior epigastric vessels separate the two hernial sacs and produce a bilocular appearance, accounting for the name *saddlebag* or *pantaloon hernia*.[2]

Femoral hernias occur primarily in women. The hernial content usually includes preperitoneal fat, omentum and short segments of the small bowel (Fig 19–10). The protruding viscera enter the femoral canal along the femoral vein and emerge through the fossa ovalis. The firm, unyielding margins of the femoral ring account for the frequency of strangulated hernia at this site. At times, only a portion of the antimesenteric wall of the bowel is incarcerated in the hernia even though the intestinal lumen remains patent. This uncommon condition is known as Richter's hernia.[1, 2]

ABDOMINAL WALL HERNIAS

Umbilical Hernia

The protrusion of viscera at the umbilical ring is relatively common in children prior to age 3 years but often remains asymptomatic and may disappear spontaneously. Clinically significant are the umbilical hernias in adults, which account for 4% of all hernias and usually affect middle-aged women.[1] Predisposing conditions are obesity, multiple pregnancies and ascites.

The contents of umbilical hernia, usually the omentum and portions of small or large intestine, are particularly prone to incarceration and strangulation (Fig 19–11). In such cases the radiographs of the abdomen may show the signs of mechanical bowel obstruction and a tumor-like density of the hernia. Barium enema and small bowel series may be used to further confirm the diagnosis by showing the narrowed loops as they enter the hernial sac and by dilatation proximally.

Ventral Hernia

This general term refers to all herniations of the viscera through the anterolateral abdominal wall except those involving umbilical and inguinal regions.[1, 2]

Midline ventral hernias emerge through the linea alba and usually contain omentum together with segments of the gastrointestinal tract. Most are located above the umbilicus and are also referred to as *epigastric hernias*.

Lateral ventral hernias, which appear through the semilunar line, also are known as *spigelian hernias.*[12, 13] The defect of the transversalis abdominis aponeurosis, which forms the hernial ring, usually is sharply defined and less than 5 cm in diameter. The organs commonly involved in this type of hernia include the small bowel and colon (Fig 19–12).

Lumbar hernias emerge through the potential areas of weakness in the loin known as the inferior lumbar space, or Petit's triangle, and the larger superior lumbar space, or Grynfelt's triangle.[1, 2] The hernia usually presents as a bulging mass in the lumbar region, particularly when intra-abdominal pressure is increased by coughing and straining. The hernial content may include retroperitoneal fat, omentum, kidneys and portions of the small or large intestine (Fig 19–13).

Incisional hernias are essentially a complication of accidental or surgical wounds of the abdominal wall and account for nearly 1.7% of all hernias.[2] About half of the cases develop after hysterectomy or appendectomy, usually within the first postoperative year.[14] Depending on the size and location of the incisional hernia, various portions of the small bowel or colon may protrude through the defect (Fig 19–14). Incarceration of the hernial content is reported to occur in one third of patients and may be further complicated by strangulation in 5%.[1, 2, 14]

Internal Abdominal Hernias

An internal hernia represents the protrusion of a viscera through either a normal peritoneal fossa or pathologic orifice within the confines of the otherwise intact abdominal cavity.[3] Most of these hernias are the result of congenital anomalies of intestinal rotation and peritoneal attachment. Although an autopsy incidence of 0.2–0.9% has been reported, most of the small reducible hernias remain asymptomatic during a lifetime.[15] The usual clinical presentation is, however, that of recurrent epigastric and periumbilical pain, nausea, vomiting and intermittent small bowel obstruction. In such patients a correct radiologic diagnosis may be reached if barium studies are performed during symptomatic periods and prior to spontaneous reduction of the hernia.[3, 16]

Figure 19–15 shows the susceptible site of occurrence and the relative incidence of various internal hernias based on a collective review of 467 cases.[17] The small intestine is the principal organ involved in the herniation, so that the small bowel series is crucial for radiographic diagnosis. It should be realized, however, that embryologic development of the colon with its subsequent mesenteric attachment is responsible for the formation of most internal hernias. Accordingly, the barium enema examination provides indirect but useful information toward diagnosis of many internal hernias, notably those involving the paraduodenal, pericecal and sigmoid regions. It is in this context that the following brief description of internal hernias is presented.

Paraduodenal Hernias

The most common type of internal hernias, accounting for half of the cases, occurs in the paraduodenal region. These hernias are basically congenital and essentially represent small bowel entrapment beneath the mesentery of the colon during embryologic rotation of the midgut.[3, 16]

Seventy-five percent of paraduodenal hernias occur on the left side of the abdomen within the fossa of Landzert. This is a peritoneal pocket lateral to the fourth portion of the duodenum and deep to the left colic branches of the inferior mesenteric vessels. A variable length of the small intestine herniates posteriorly and to the left to fill the paraduodenal fossa. Therefore, a more accurate designation would be "hernia into the descending and transverse mesocolon".[3] The typical radiographic finding is a circumscribed ovoid mass of intestinal loops, which appear encapsulated in the left upper quadrant immediately lateral to the ascending duodenum (Fig 19–16). The distal transverse colon usually is depressed, the posterior wall of the stomach indented or elevated. Stasis of barium in the herniated loops and duodenal dilatation are often visible.[15, 16]

The remaining 25% of paraduodenal hernias develop on the right side of the abdomen within the mesenterico-parietal fossa of Waldeyer.[3, 16] This peritoneal pocket of jejunal mesentery opens behind the superior mesenteric artery just inferior to the third portion of the duodenum. Small bowel loops protrude downward and to the right, actually representing a hernia into the ascending mesocolon (Fig 19–17).

Foramen of Winslow Hernias

The lesser omental bursa or sac is the space behind the lesser omentum partly limited by the medial aspect of the liver, the posterior wall of the stomach and the posterior abdominal wall. It communicates with the free peritoneal cavity through the epiploic foramen (foramen of Winslow). Excessive intestinal mobility due to long mesenteric attachment and an enlarged foramen of Winslow are among the predisposing conditions for herniation of the bowel loops into the lesser sac.[3] In such cases, plain films of the abdomen show evidence of small bowel obstruction, together with a collection of gas-filled loops within the lesser sac, medial and posterior to the stomach. On upper gastrointestinal series, the stomach is seen displaced to the left and anteriorly, and the proximal duodenum appears deviated to the left.[18] The small bowel series may further reveal the presence and cause of the intestinal obstruction by showing the exact site of obstruction to be at the anatomical location of the foramen of Winslow around the hilus of the liver (Fig 19–18).

In about 60% of cases the hernial content is the small intestine, usually the terminal ileum.[19] The cecum and ascending colon are involved in only 25% (Fig 19–19). In these patients the barium enema may disclose a tapered narrowing and obstruction of the colon near the hepatic flexure. Failure to visualize the cecum in its normal location on plain films and barium enema also has been mentioned as a sign of cecal herniation.[18, 19]

On rare occasions herniation into the lesser sac may not involve the foramen of Winslow but, rather, defects in the gastrocolic ligament or gastrohepatic omentum forming the anterior wall of the lesser sac.[3, 14] For example, in patients with partial gastrectomy and Billroth II procedure, the created surgical defect in the anterior wall of the lesser sac can serve as the hernial ring. A portion of the transverse colon may then protrude upward and posteriorly into the lesser sac and be visible on barium enema examination (Fig 19–20).

Transmesocolic Hernias and Related Conditions

Peritoneal pockets and areas of congenital or acquired weakness in the mesentery of the colon are potential sites for a variety of internal herniations. Radiologic diagnosis of these hernias may be suspected on small bowel series or barium enema examination in which reflux into the small intestine has been achieved.

Pericecal hernias usually are congenital and account for 13% of internal hernias.[17] They represent entrapment of the small bowel loops behind the mesentery of the cecum and terminal ileum. In addition to at least four peritoneal fossae in the ileocecal region, other pathologic defects in the mesentery of the cecum and appendix may form the hernial ring.[3] In most cases a portion of ileum protrudes through the cecal mesentery to occupy the right paracolic gutter (Fig 19–21).

Intersigmoid fossa is a peritoneal pouch formed between the two loops of sigmoid colon and its mesentery. This pocket is found in 65% of cadavers and represents a potential site of intersigmoid herniation of the small bowel (Fig 19–22).[3, 20] Similarly, the *transmesosigmoid hernia* is a rare condition in which a defect in both layers of the sigmoid mesentery serves as a hernial ring through which the small bowel loops protrude and occupy the left lower abdomen.[21]

Another entity that should be recognized for differential diagnosis and as a possible factor in development of internal hernia is the *persistent mesocolon*.[22] Normally the mobile and intraperitoneal portions of the colon are the cecum, transverse colon and sigmoid. These segments are attached to the posterior abdominal wall by their respective mesocolons. In contrast, the ascending and descending colon have a retroperitoneally fixed position because their mesocolons fuse with the posterior parietal peritoneum during fetal life. In probably 2–5% of individuals, however, this fusion fails to occur, producing an anomaly referred to as *persistent ascending mesocolon* and/or *descending mesocolon*.[3, 22] The first condition is more common and results in excessively mobile cecum and ascending colon. In patients with persistent descending mesocolon, the left side of the colon usually moves medially, thus enlarging the left paracolic gutter and ileac fossa. The small bowel loops may then occupy the free space and be visible lateral to the descending colon (Fig 19–23). Less commonly, an internal hernia may develop in the same location if the small bowel loops pass through defects in the descending mesocolon and become incarcerated within the left paracolic gutter.[22, 23] Therefore, it is important to appreciate the significance of variations in length and attachment of the mesocolon as potential predisposing elements, not only for volvulus but also for development of internal hernias.

REFERENCES

1. Nyhus, L. M., and Bombeck, C. T.: Hernias, in Sabiston, D. C., Jr. (ed.): *Davis Christopher Textbook of Surgery* (Philadelphia: W. B. Saunders Co., 1977), pp. 1335–1360.
2. Zimmerman, L. M., and Anson, B. J.: *Anatomy and Surgery of Hernia* (2d ed.; Baltimore: Williams & Wilkins Co., 1967).
3. Ghahremani, G. G., and Meyers, M. A.: Internal Abdominal Hernias, in Moseley, R. D. (ed.): *Current Problems in Radiology* (Chicago: Year Book Medical Publishers, Inc., 1975).
4. Gerson, D. E., and Lewicki, A. M.: Intrathoracic stomach: When does it obstruct?, Radiology 119: 257, 1976.
5. Reed, J. O., and Lang, E. F.: Diaphragmatic hernia in infancy, Am. J. Roentgenol. 82:437, 1959.
6. Keshishian, J. A., and Cox, P. A.: Diagnosis and management of strangulated diaphragmatic hernias, Surg. Gynecol. Obstet. 115:626, 1962.
7. Berdon, W. E., Baker, D. H., and Amoury, R.: The rule of pulmonary hypoplasia in the prognosis of newborn infants with diaphragmatic hernia and eventration, Am. J. Roentgenol. 103:413, 1968.
8. Smith, L., and Lippert, K. M.: Peritoneo-pericardial diaphragmatic hernia, Ann. Surg. 148:798, 1958.
9. Ebert, P. A., Gaetner, R. A., and Zuidema, G. D.: Traumatic diaphragmatic hernia, Surg. Gynecol. Obstet. 125:59, 1967.
10. Fraser, R. G., and Pare, J. A. P.: *Diagnosis of Diseases of the Chest,* Vol. 2 (1st ed.; Philadelphia: W. B. Saunders Co., 1970), pp. 1224–1232.
11. Liebeskind, A. L., Elkin, M., and Goldman, S. H.: Herniation of the bladder, Radiology 106:257, 1973.
12. Hunter, T. B., Freundlich, I. M., and Zukoski, C. F.: Preoperative radiographic diagnosis of a Spigelian hernia containing large and small bowel, Gastrointest. Radiol. 1:379, 1977.
13. Holder, L. E., and Schneider, H. J.: Spigelian hernias: Anatomy and roentgenographic manifestations, Radiology 112:309, 1974.
14. Akman, P. C.: A study of five hundred incisional hernias, J. Int. Coll. Surg. 37:125, 1962.
15. Williams, A. J.: Roentgen diagnosis of intra-abdominal hernia. An evaluation of the roentgen findings, Radiology 59:817, 1952.
16. Meyers, M. A.: Paraduodenal hernias. Radiologic and arteriographic diagnosis, Radiology 95:29, 1970.
17. Hansmann, G. H., and Morton, S. A.: Intra-abdominal hernia. Report of a case and review of the literature, Arch. Surg. 39:973, 1939.
18. Henisz, A., Matesanz, J., and Westcott, J. L.: Cecal herniation through the foramen of Winslow, Radiology 112:575, 1974.
19. Jones, T. W.: Paraduodenal Hernia and Hernias of the Foramen of Winslow, in Nyhus, L. M., and Harkins, H. N. (eds.): *Hernia* (Philadelphia: J. B. Lippincott Co., 1964), pp. 577–601.
20. Zimmermann, L. M., and Laufman, H.: Intra-abdominal hernias due to developmental and rotational anomalies, Ann. Surg. 138:82, 1953.
21. Bertelsen, S., and Christiansen, J.: Internal hernia through mesenteric and mesocolic defects. A review of the literature and report of two cases, Acta Chir. Scand. 133:426, 1967.
22. Popky, G. L., and Lapayowker, M. S.: Persistent descending mesocolon, Radiology 86:327, 1966.
23. Callander, C. L., Rusk, G. Y., and Nemir, A.: Mechanism, symptoms, and treatment of hernia into the descending mesocolon (left duodenal hernia): Plea for change in nomenclature, Surg. Gynecol. Obstet. 60:1052, 1935.

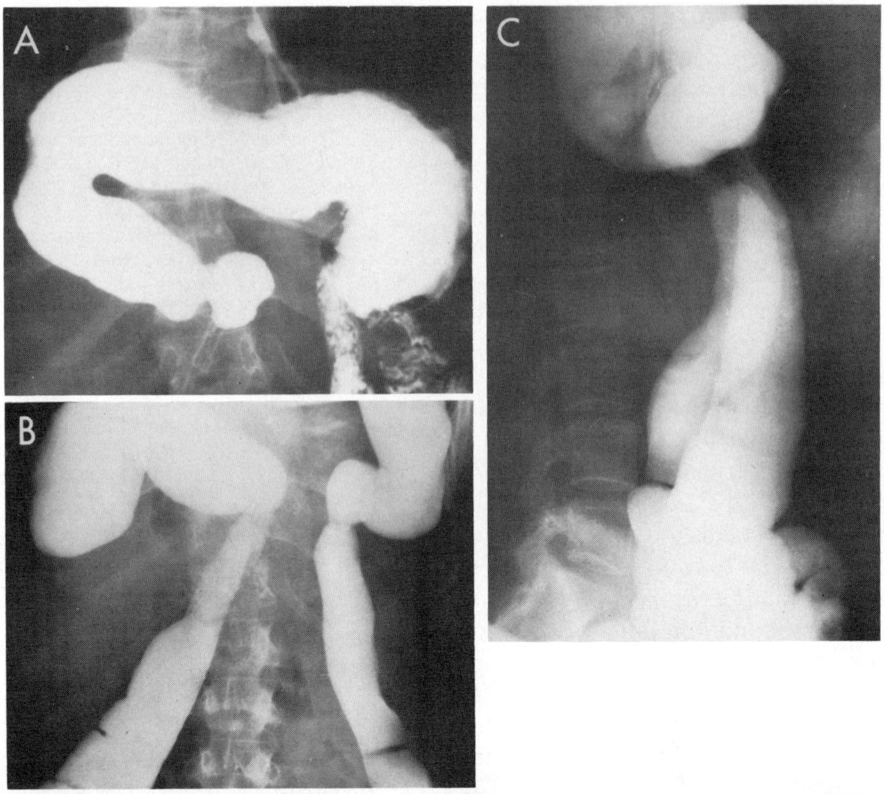

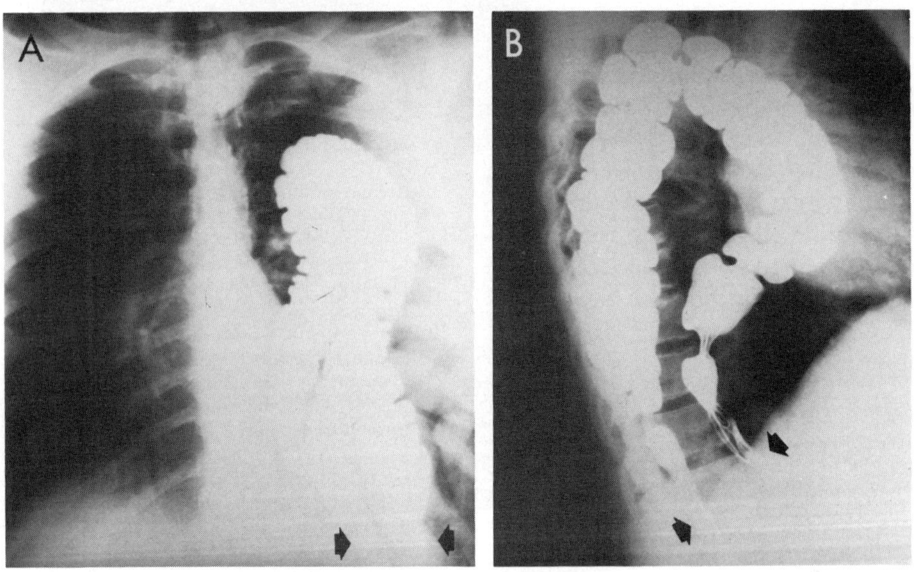

Fig 19–1 (top).—Sliding hiatal hernia with intrathoracic stomach and concomitant herniation of colon. **A,** 180-degree anterior organoaxial torsion of stomach so that its greater curvature now lies above lesser curvature. **B** and **C,** barium enema examination demonstrates associated herniation of transverse colon through enlarged esophageal hiatus.

Fig 19–2 (bottom).—Herniation of colon through foramen of Bochdalek. **A** and **B,** chest radiographs obtained during barium enema examination show colon within left pleural cavity. Note typical posterolateral location of diaphragmatic defect *(arrows).*

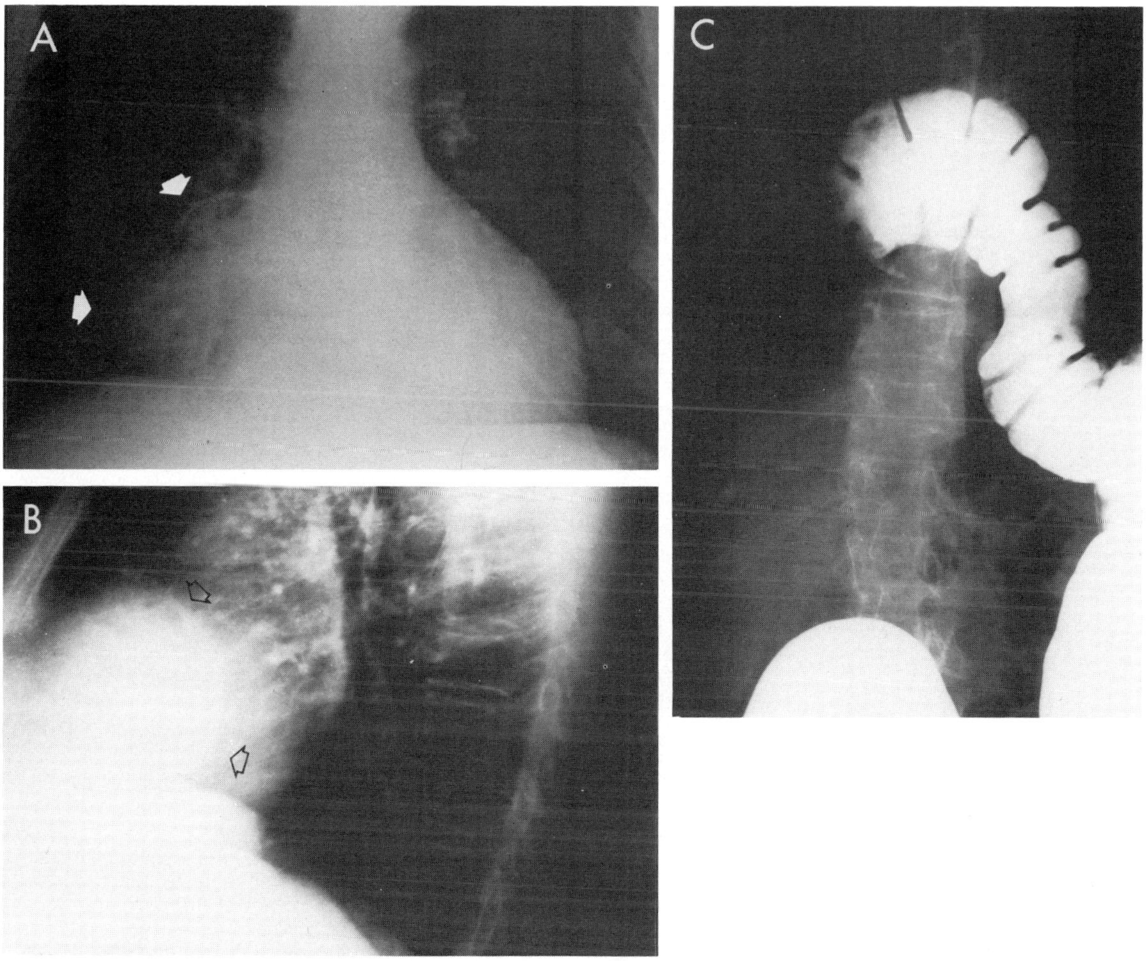

Fig 19–3. – Herniation of colon through foramen of Morgagni. **A** and **B**, chest radiographs show gas-containing soft tissue mass in right cardiophrenic angle *(arrows)*. **C**, barium enema examination confirms herniation of loop of transverse colon.

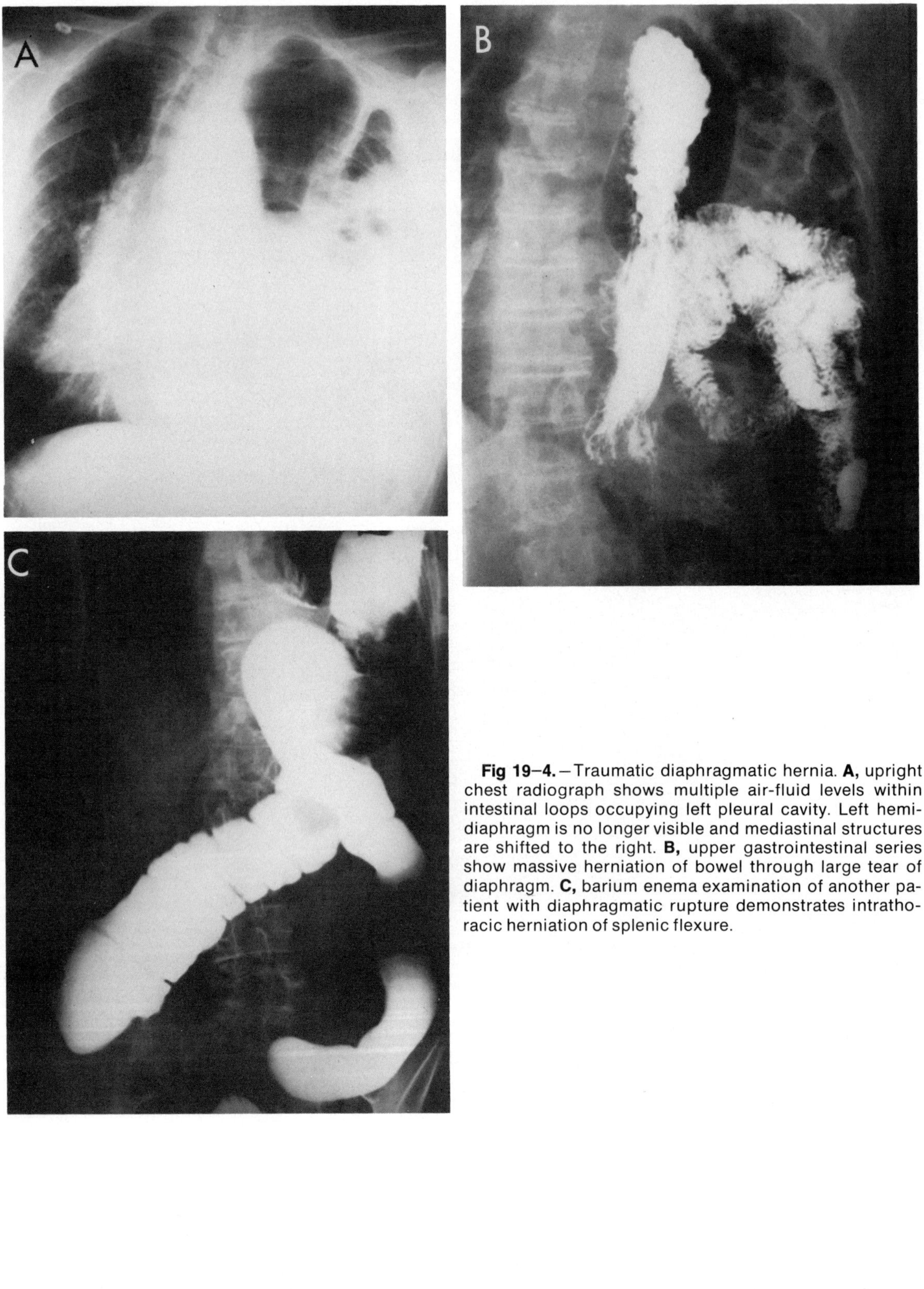

Fig 19–4.—Traumatic diaphragmatic hernia. **A,** upright chest radiograph shows multiple air-fluid levels within intestinal loops occupying left pleural cavity. Left hemidiaphragm is no longer visible and mediastinal structures are shifted to the right. **B,** upper gastrointestinal series show massive herniation of bowel through large tear of diaphragm. **C,** barium enema examination of another patient with diaphragmatic rupture demonstrates intrathoracic herniation of splenic flexure.

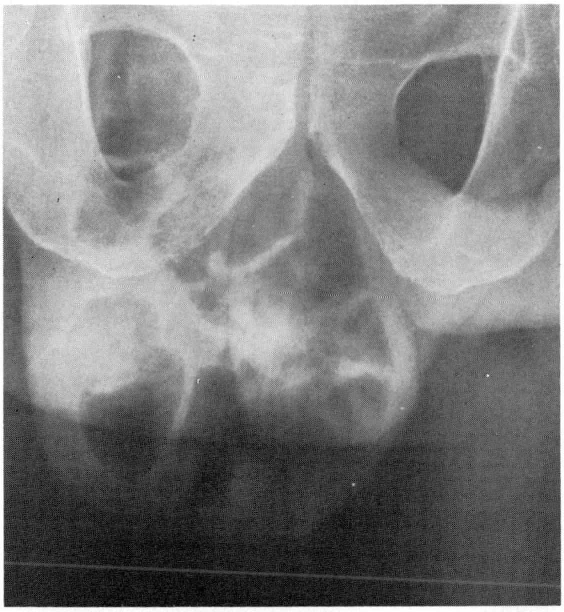

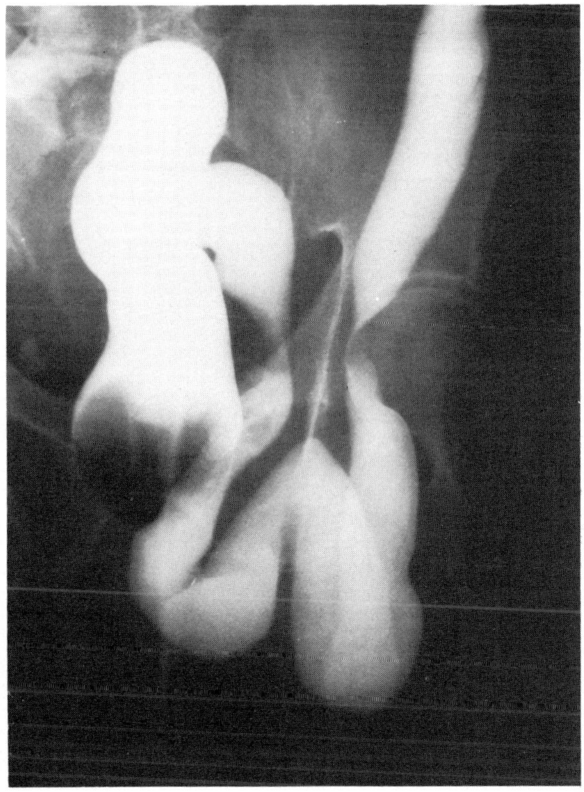

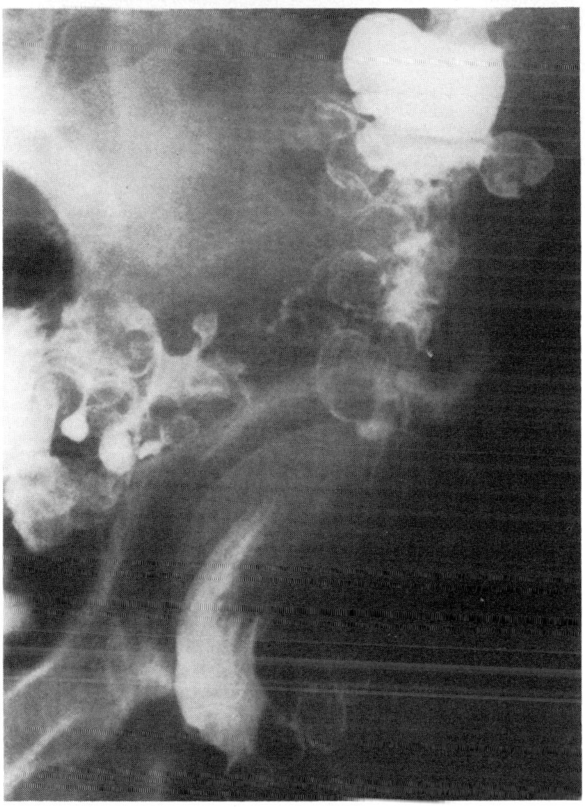

Fig 19–5 (top left).—Large indirect inguinal hernia. Haustral markings of herniated cecum and ascending colon are visible within scrotum and over right obturator foramen.

Fig 19–6 (right).—Left indirect inguinal hernia. Barium enema examination demonstrates narrowing of both sigmoid loops at hernial orifice.

Fig 19–7 (bottom left).—Barium enema examination shows diverticulosis of sigmoid loop within left inguinal hernia.

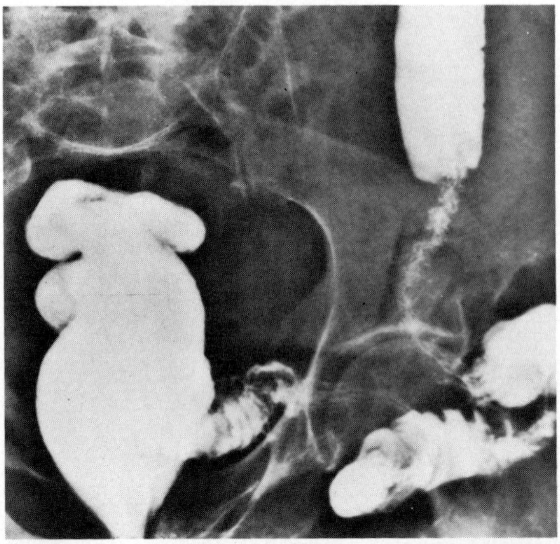

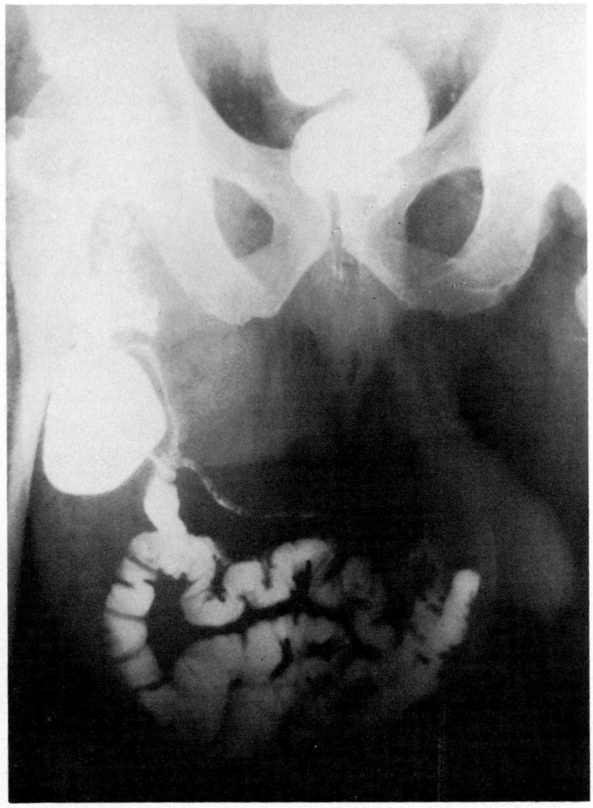

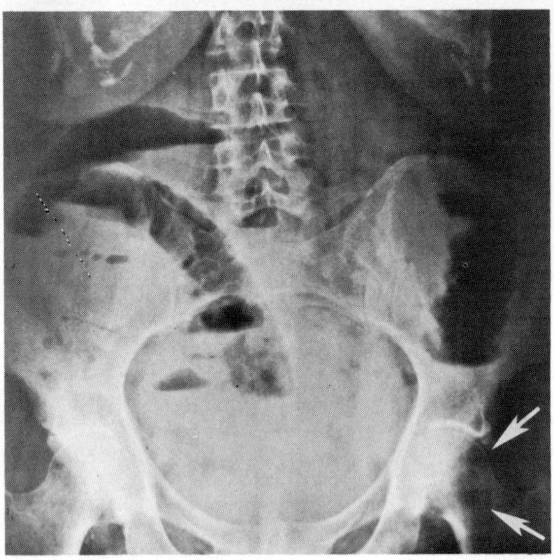

Fig 19–8 (top left). – Incarcerated left inguinal hernia. Note narrowed sigmoid loops entering hernial ring and edematous ischemic segment within hernial sac.

Fig 19–9 (right). – Sliding right inguinal hernia. In this patient, ascending colon constitutes lateral wall of hernial sac, whereas cecum, appendix and ileal loops are visible within scrotum.

Fig 19–10 (bottom left). – Strangulated left femoral hernia. Preoperative upright film of abdomen shows air-fluid containing bowel loops converging toward left lower quadrant. Two small gas collections over left femoral neck indicate site of strangulated hernia *(arrows)*.

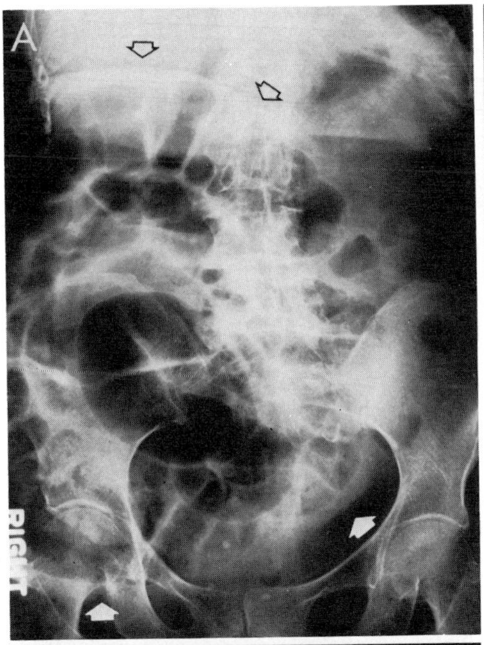

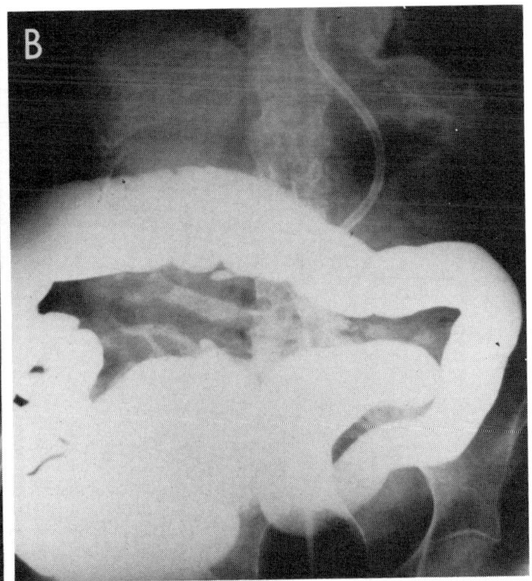

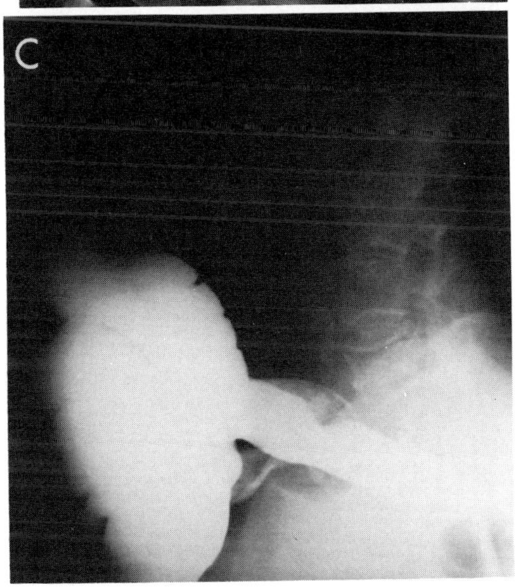

Fig 19–11 (top and above).—Large umbilical hernia. **A,** supine radiograph of abdomen shows gas-filled intestinal loops within large hernial sac *(arrows).* **B,** and **C,** barium enema study demonstrates that colon, with exception of rectosigmoid, has herniated anteriorly.

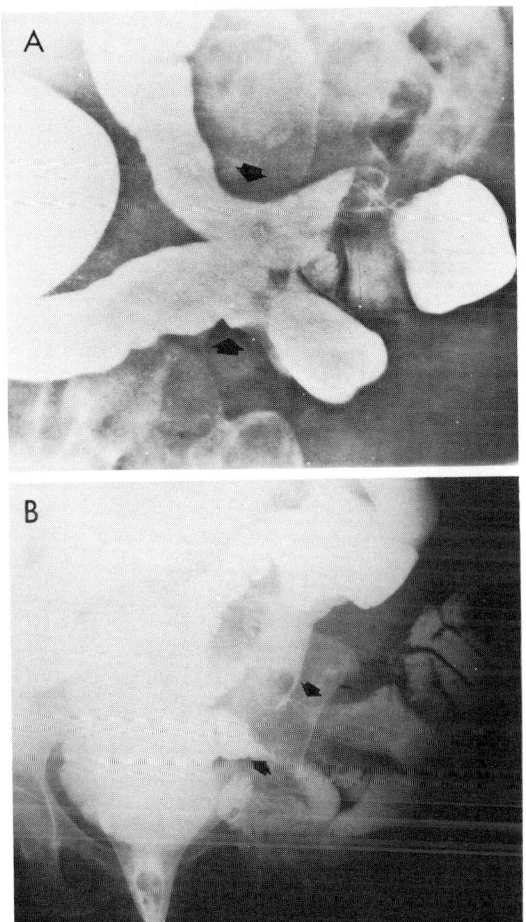

Fig 19–12 (right center and bottom).—Spigelian hernia. **A** and **B,** barium enema studies of two patients demonstrate sigmoid herniation *(arrows)* through left semilunar line. (**B** from Hunter et al., Gastrointest. Radiol. 1:379, 1977, with permission.)

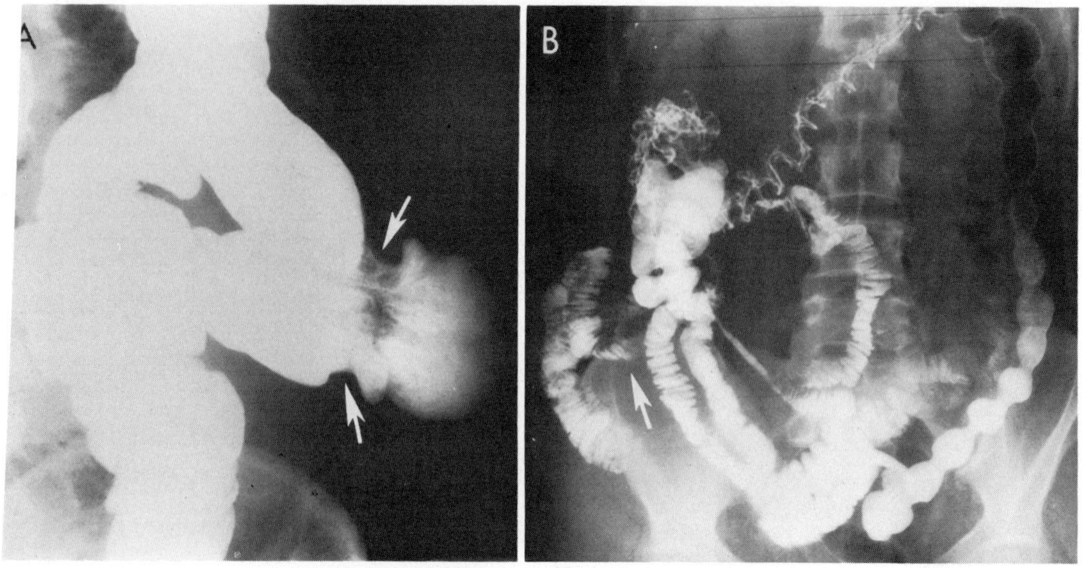

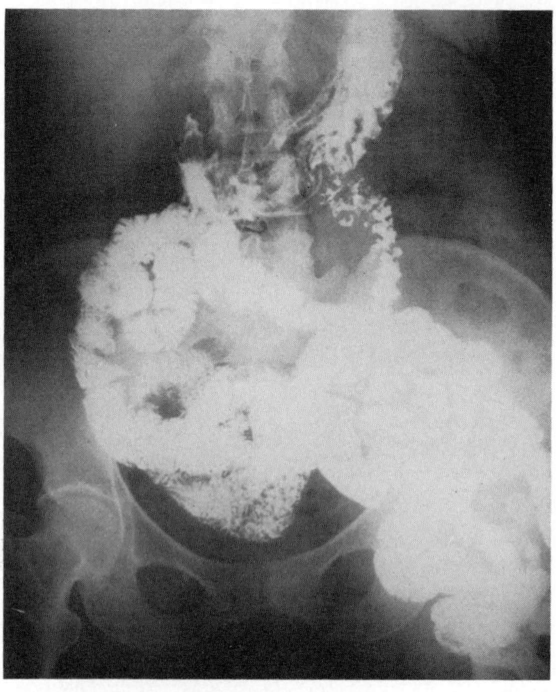

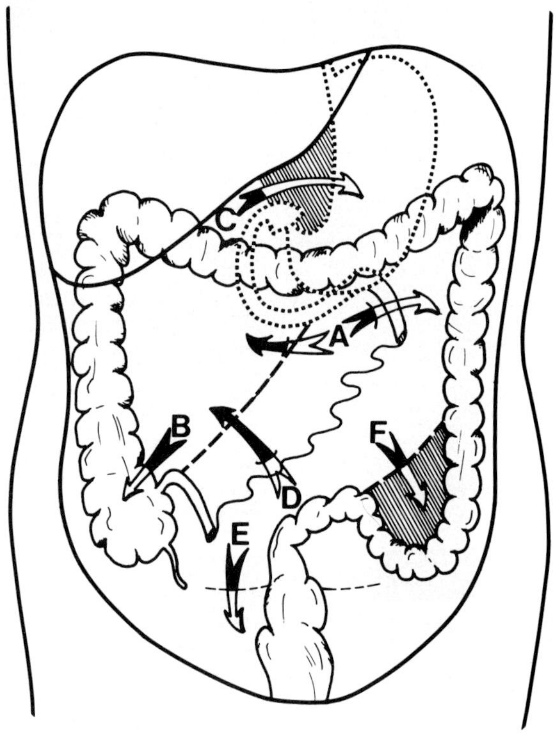

Fig 19–13 (top).—Lumbar hernia in two patients. **A,** barium enema examination shows short segment of redundant descending colon herniating through left lumbar space *(arrow)*. **B,** postevacuation film of barium enema study shows ileal loop protruding through right lumbar space *(arrows)*.

Fig 19–14 (bottom left).—Large incisional hernia complicating resection of sigmoid colon for carcinoma. Note protruding small bowel loops in left lower abdomen.

Fig 19–15 (bottom right).—Distribution and relative incidence of internal hernias based on 467 cases cited in Ref. 17. *A:* paraduodenal, 53%; *B:* pericecal, 13%; *C:* foramen of Winslow, 8%; *D:* transmesenteric, 8%; *E:* pelvic, 7%; and *F:* transmesosigmoid, 6%. (From Ghahremani and Meyers, Internal Abdominal Hernias, in Moseley, R. D. [ed.]: *Current Problems in Radiology,* Vol. V [Chicago: Year Book Medical Publishers, Inc., 1975], used by permission.)

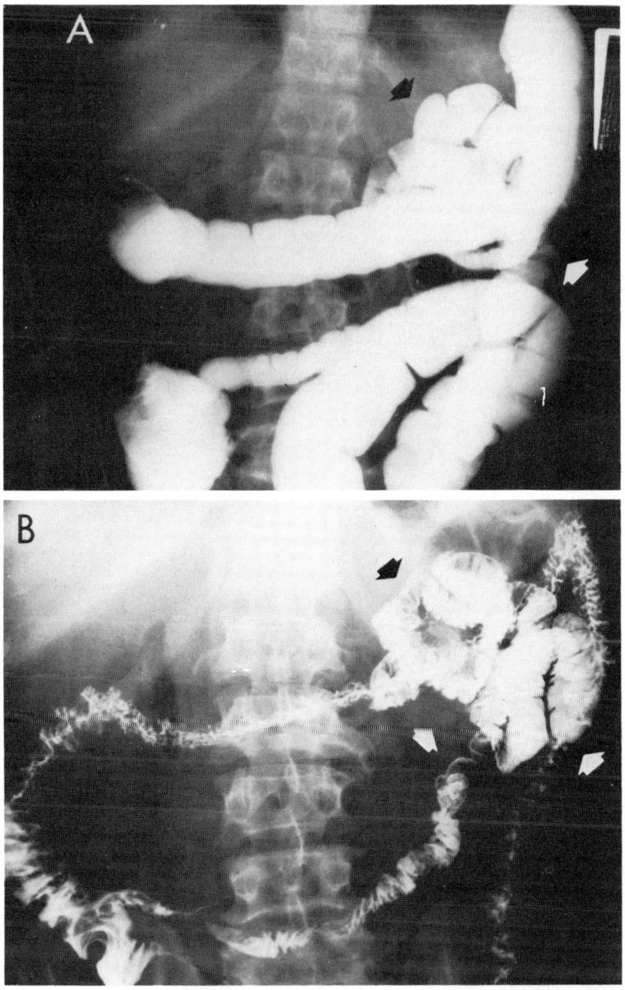

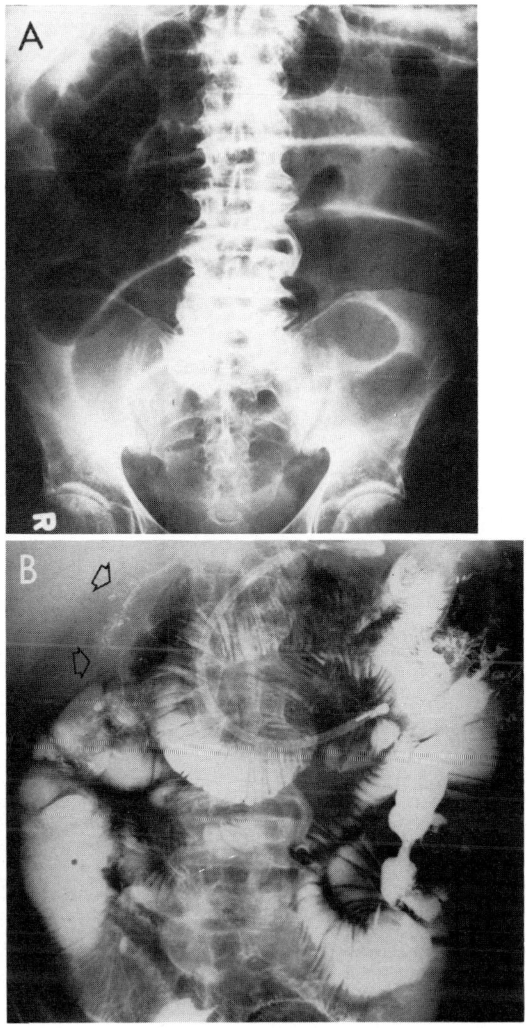

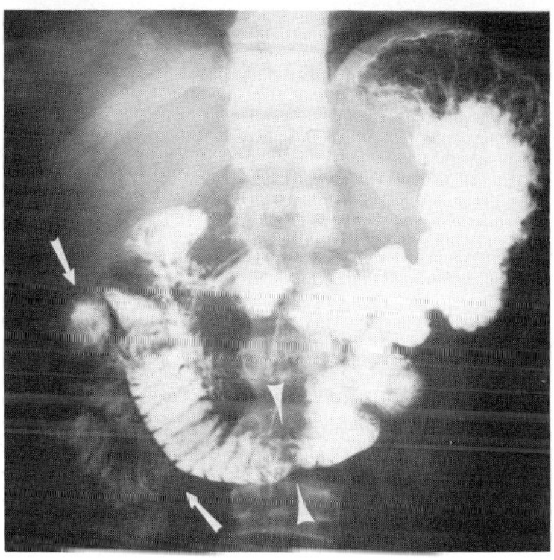

Fig 19–16 (top left).—Left paraduodenal hernia. **A** and **B,** filled view and postevacuation film of barium enema examination show unusual course of terminal ileum toward left upper abdomen. Proximal ileal loops form circumscribed ovoid mass within left paraduodenal fossa *(arrows).*

Fig 19–17 (bottom left).—Right paraduodenal hernia. Circumscribed grouping of proximal jejunal loops *(arrows)* represents herniation into right paraduodenal fossa and right portion of transverse mesocolon. Note that duodenal loop and ligamentum of Treitz are situated normally. However, afferent loop of jejunum shows localized narrowing *(arrowheads)* at hernial orifice as it passes behind superior mesenteric vessels.

Fig 19–18 (right).—Foramen of Winslow hernia. **A,** supine film of abdomen reveals marked dilatation of small bowel but no gas in colon. **B,** delayed radiograph of small bowel series shows narrowed terminal ileum *(arrows)* as it passes between liver and duodenal bulb toward foramen of Winslow.

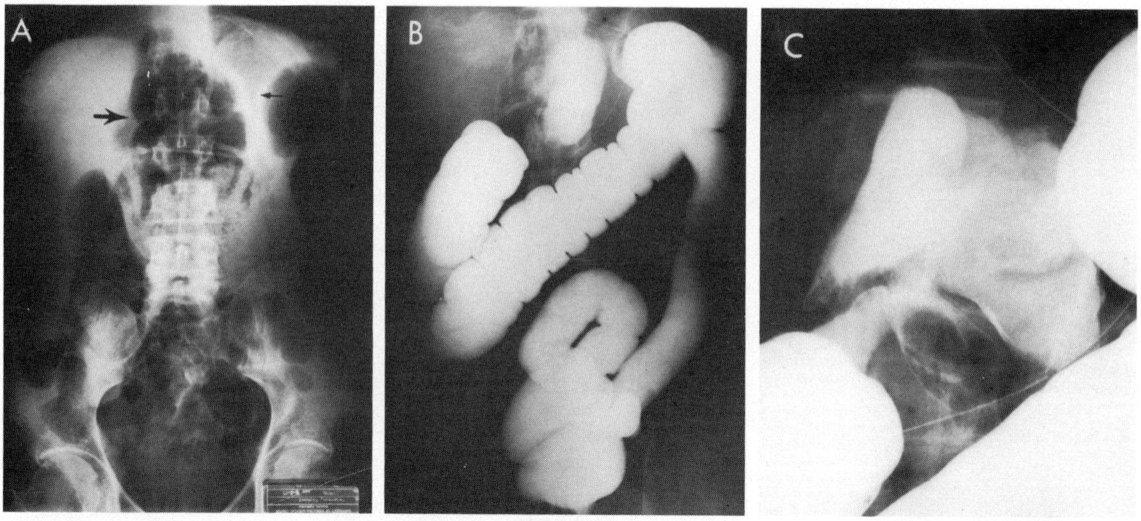

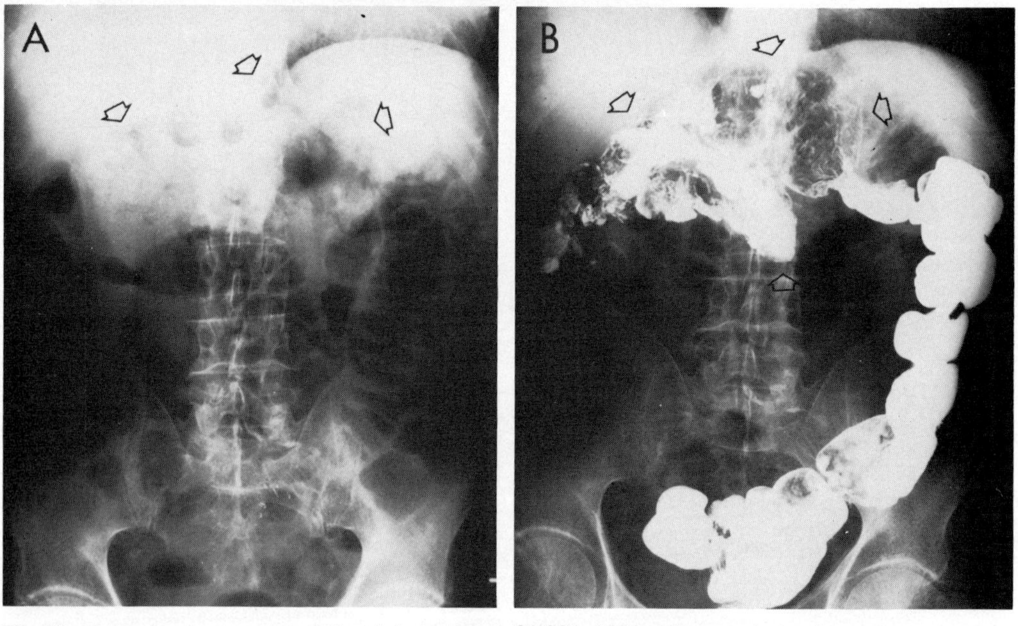

Fig 19–19 (top).—**A,** cecal herniation into lesser sac. Plain film shows cecum in epigastrium *(large arrow).* Stomach *(small arrow)* is compressed and displaced to left. **B,** barium enema shows displaced cecum within lesser peritoneal sac. On lateral view (not shown), cecum is posterior to stomach. **C,** cone view shows detail of tapered segment of ascending colon as it passes through foramen of Winslow. (From Harned, R.: Am J. Gastroenterol. 61:304, 1974, with permission.)

Fig 19–20 (bottom).—Herniation of colon into lesser sac. **A,** radiograph of abdomen in patient with previous Billroth II gastroenterostomy shows moderate distention of small bowel loops and gas-containing soft tissue mass *(arrows)* in region of lesser sac. **B,** barium enema examination demonstrates herniated loop of transverse colon within lesser sac *(arrows).*

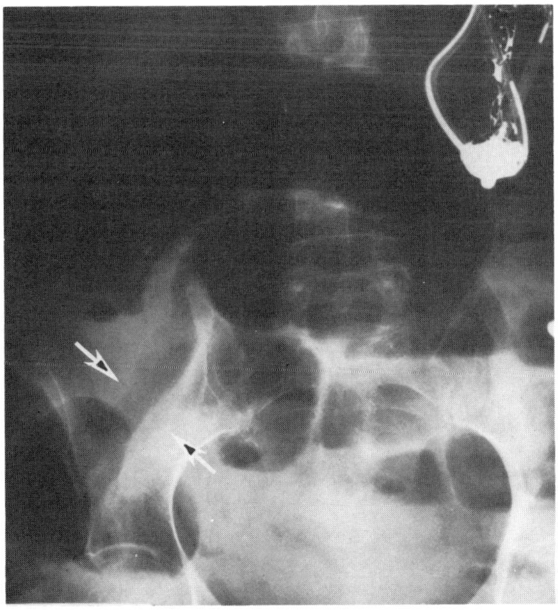

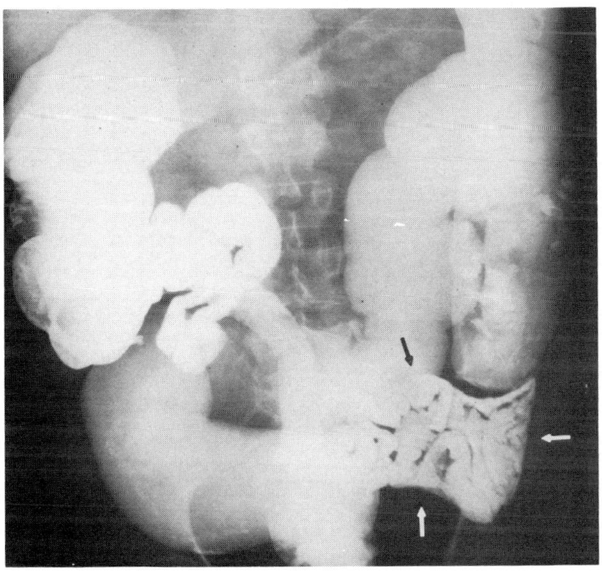

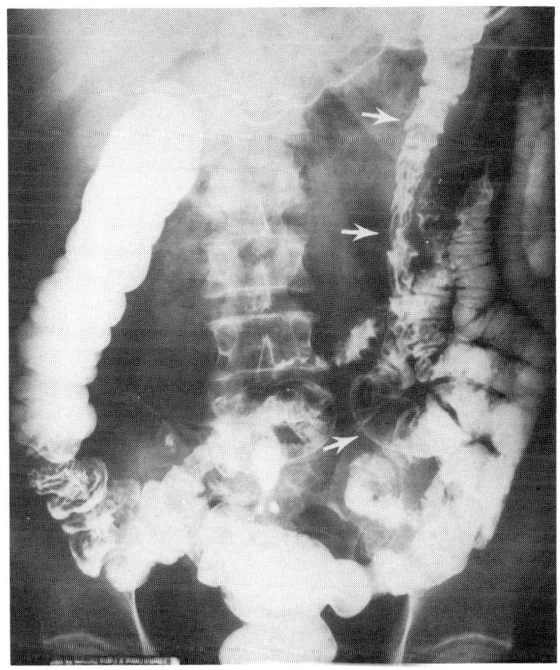

Fig 19–21 (top).—Pericecal herniation of ileal loop through defect in mesentery of cecum. Constriction and approximation of loops at hernial orifice *(arrows)* cause massive distention of more proximal small intestine. (From Ghahremani and Meyers, Internal Abdominal Hernias, in Moseley, R. D. (ed.): *Current Problems in Radiology,* Vol. V (Chicago: Year Book Medical Publishers, Inc., 1975, used by permission.)

Fig 19–22 (bottom left).—Intersigmoid hernia. Retrograde filling of small bowel during barium enema examination demonstrates encapsulation of several ileal loops *(arrows)* within intersigmoid fossa.

Fig 19–23 (bottom right).—Persistent descending mesocolon. Small bowel loops opacified by reflux during barium enema examination occupy left paracolic gutter. Descending colon *(arrows)* is displaced medially. (From Ghahremani and Meyers, Internal Abdominal Hernias, in Moseley, R. D. [ed.]: *Current Problems in Radiology,* Vol. V [Chicago: Year Book Medical Publishers, Inc., 1975], used by permission.)

Chapter 20

Herpetic Colitis

LESLIE S. MENUCK, M.D.

EXTRACUTANEOUS manifestations of herpes zoster have been described both in patients with an altered immune response and in patients who are otherwise healthy.[1-4] The presence of gastrointestinal tract involvement has been substantiated by the demonstration of intranuclear inclusion bodies of the virus itself within the ganglion cells of the myenteric plexus and in inflammatory and epithelial cells within the mucosa.[1]

The onset of colonic lesions may shortly precede, follow or coincide with the skin manifestations. Resolution of the colonic lesions may lag behind the skin changes, especially if there has been mucosal ulceration. The segment of involved colon may or may not correspond to the associated cutaneous dermatome.[1, 5]

The radiographic appearance of these lesions will depend on the stage of the disease at the time of barium enema. The small, discrete, polygonal filling defects with sharp angular margins correspond morphologically to the vesicular phase of the cutaneous lesions (Fig 20–1 and 20–2), whereas the presence of minute ulcerations in a short segment represents progression to the ulcerative phase[5, 6] (Fig 20–3). The presence of focal narrowing probably represents a stage of residual narrowing following the resolution of the small ulcerations.[5]

The differential diagnosis of the colonic herpetic lesions will depend on whether the vesicular or ulcerative phase is present. The sharp, angular, polygonal appearance of these vesicular lesions differs from the rounded margins of colonic polyps. This appearance and the focal segmental involvement should greatly help in differentiating colonic herpes from any lesions of the polyposis syndrome, inflammatory pseudopolyposis or lymphoma. The presence of a narrowed segment of colon with small ulcerations may be similar superficially to inflammatory or ischemic colitis. However, the rapid disappearance of these lesions, as well as their relationship in time to the typical cutaneous findings, will be helpful in making the diagnosis of colonic herpes.

REFERENCES

1. Lever, W. F., and Schaamburg, G.: *Histopathology of Skin* (5th ed.; Philadelphia: J. B. Lippincott Co., 1975).
2. Curtin, R. G.: Herpes zoster and its relation to internal inflammation and disease, especially of the serous membranes, Am. J. Med. Sci. 73:264, 1902.
3. Eisenbad, M.: Chickenpox with visceral involvement, Am. J. Med. 12:740, 1952.
4. Wyburn-Mason, R.: Visceral lesion in herpes zoster, Br. Med. J. 1:678, 1957.
5. Menuck, L., Brahme, F., Amberg, J., and Sherr, H.: Colonic changes of herpes zoster, Am. J. Roentgenol. 127:273, 1976.
6. Khilnani, M. T., and Keller, R. J.: Roentgen and pathological changes in the gastrointestinal tract in herpes zoster generalisata, Mt. Sinai J. Med. NY 38: 303, 1971.

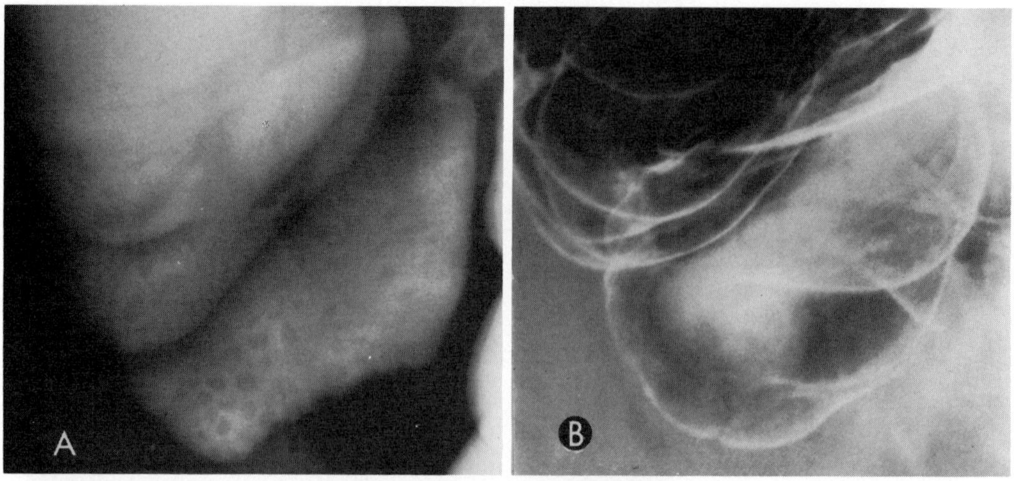

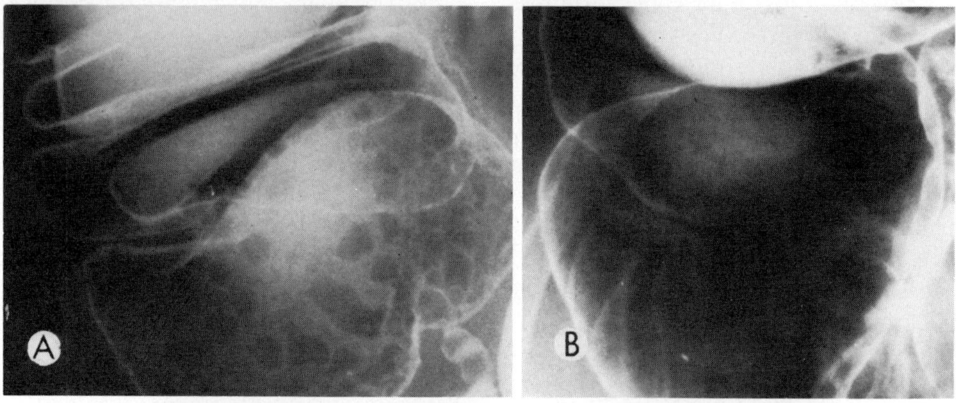

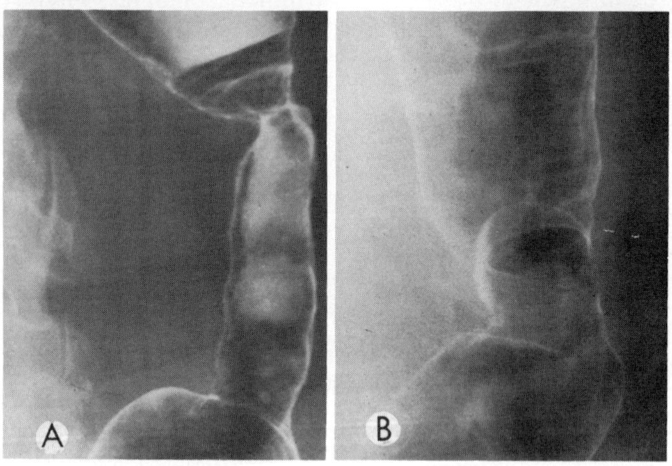

Fig 20–1 (top). – **A,** single contrast barium enema showing multiple polygonal filling defects within cecum. **B,** repeat examination 1 month later showing normal cecum.

Fig 20–2 (center). – **A,** double contrast barium enema showing sharply angular polygonal filling defects of cecum. **B,** repeat examination 3 weeks later showing total resolution of cecal filling defects.

Fig 20–3 (bottom). – **A,** double contrast barium enema showing short focal narrowing with mucosal irregularity in middescending colon. **B,** repeat examination 2 months later showing some residual narrowing of involved segment.

Chapter 21

Infectious Colitis

JEFFERSON O. JANES, M.D.

INFECTIOUS COLITIS caused by bacterial organisms has been reported with increasing frequency over the past few years.[1-7] This increased incidence is primarily due to social conditions related to mass production and transport of meat and food products, with the associated problems of exposure and inadequate refrigeration[8]; poor hygienic conditions related to the preparation of food[4, 7, 8]; the large number of household pets, many of which harbor and excrete toxic organisms[2]; and the increase in the incidence of colonic venereal infection.[5, 7] Concomitantly, the diagnosis of idiopathic inflammatory colitis (Crohn's versus ulcerative colitis) frequently cannot be made upon clinicoradiologic criteria alone,[9, 10] and the nonspecific inflammatory colitides have begun to be further categorized, allowing more specific diagnosis and treatment. The recent additions of Behçet's colitis,[11-12] evanescent colitis in the young adult,[13, 14] leukemic typhlitis in the adult,[15] uremic colitis[1] and postrenal transplant colitis[16-18]—along with clarification of the older colitides (drug-induced colitis[19-24] and ischemic colitis[25, 26])—has made the radiologic diagnosis of inflammatory colonic conditions more complicated. As a result, knowledge of the clinical and radiologic picture of infectious colitis has become increasingly important.

Bacillary Dysentery (Shigellosis)

Bacillary dysentery is an acute or chronic disease, caused by members of the genus Shigella, which produce a potent endotoxin accounting for epidemics as well as sporadic cases. The condition occurs almost exclusively in man and is spread by fomites contamination of polluted water supplies; infected food handlers; or transfer of the organism by flies, cockroaches or other insects.[27] A recent report also describes an increased incidence in male homosexuals.[7]

Clinically the history usually is that of an acute episode of diarrhea with abdominal cramps and vomiting, although chronic diarrhea of varying severity has been described. Swollen, diffusely inflamed colonic mucosa, often covered with mucus and pus and associated with irregular, shallow ulcerations, is seen at endoscopy. Pathologically, acute diffuse inflammation with hyperemia of the mucosa is followed by edema, hemorrhage and leukocytic infiltration, which often extends into the submucosa, causing marked thickening of the bowel wall. The distribution of the inflammation usually is not uniform throughout the colon but is often most severe distally.[1, 27] Chronic cases may show scarring and fibrosis with intermittent exacerbation and acute changes.[27]

The roentgen findings, as would be expected, correlate well with those seen by the endoscopist and pathologist and are influenced by the severity and stage of disease. As illustrated in Figure 21 – 1, mild disease shows only minimal mucosal edema with prominence of the interhaustral folds usually localized to the distal colon. Early ulceration may be suspected by the slightly irregular margins of the barium column and is best shown by the air contrast technique. Frequently these early changes are not recognized as abnormal. More advanced disease (Fig. 21 – 2) shows distinct shallow ulcerations that extend into the muscularis and are more common in the rectosigmoid.[27]

Severe disease (Fig. 21 – 3) may show increased involvement of the distal colon, with extension to the region of the right colon. Marked bowel wall thickening, spasticity and diffuse ulceration, which may be collar button in nature, is characteristic.[1, 27] Pneumatosis, which has been reported in other inflammatory bowel disease,[28] is illustrated in the splenic flexure area of Figures 21 – 3, (C and D). Such changes should strongly suggest bowel necrosis with consideration given to surgical intervention.

Roentgenographic differential diagnosis includes other forms of infectious as well as idiopathic inflammatory bowel disease. Final diagnosis must be confirmed by bacteriologic and clinical findings. Follow-up examination after appropriate antibiotic therapy usually is normal.

Salmonellosis

Salmonella colitis as a result of a contaminated food source may involve the entire colon rather than the ileocecal area, as is the usual case in typhoid fever. Although only one third of cases of classic typhoid fever involve the colon as well as the terminal ileum[27] (Fig. 21 – 4), patients who present with diarrheal symptoms are more likely to have barium enema as the primary radiologic examination. Details of the roentgenographic changes of typhoid fever are readily available.[14, 27]

Many species of salmonella organisms may be responsible for the explosive diarrheal syndrome associated with food poisoning. Such a condition is caused by thermostable endotoxin that irritates the entire gastrointestinal system. Differentiation from similar disease caused by enterotoxin-producing organisms such as staphylococci must be made. After a short incubation period, worsening symptoms usually appear, with a 1 – 2% mortality occurring from fulminant disease.[27]

Endoscopic[1] findings, as well as those at necropsy,[14, 27] demonstrate similar pathology: inflamed mucosa with associated exudate, small hemorrhages and superficial ulcerations similar to that seen in shigellosis and in idiopathic ulcerative colitis. Diffuse involvement with thickened edematous fold enlargement (giving a corrugated pattern on the radiograph) or a more segmental pattern may be seen. Usually distal colon involvement includes the rectum. These changes may be associated with deep "collar button" ulceration[1, 27] (see Fig 21 – 5). This type of deep ulceration is said to be more common in paratyphoid fevers.[27]

Radiographic differentiation from other inflammatory bowel disease can be difficult, and diagnosis remains principally clinical and bacteriologic. One recent report has noted coincident salmonella infections and acute ulcerative colitis.[29] One death occurred from sepsis caused by a usually noninvasive organism following institution of corticosteroid therapy for what was thought to be idiopathic ulcerative colitis. However, recovery in the noncompromised individual usually is complete after institution of appropriate antibiotic therapy and is associated with a normal follow-up barium enema examination.

Venereal Colitis

GONOCOCCAL PROCTOCOLITIS

Anorectal gonococcal infection is increasing in incidence. A recent review estimates that 44% of women who have gonorrhea have positive rectal cultures with 4% having anorectal disease alone. Proctocolitis infection in males is almost exclusively in homosexuals with an estimated prevalence of 45%.[5] Most patients complain of mucoid or purulent discharge, anal irritation, painful defecation, tenesmus or hematochezia. Endoscopically, erythema and edema are seen correlating with biopsy specimens, which show patchy disorganization and derangement of columnar epithelium with some areas of mucosal destruction and inflammatory cell infiltration.[5]

The radiographic findings (Figs 21-6 and 21-7) are those of proctitis manifested by spasticity, edematous mucosa, shallow ulcerations and loss of distensibility.[5, 6] Amebiasis or shigellosis may be associated with gonococcal infection in these patients.[7] Although most cases resolve completely after confirmed diagnosis from bacterial cultures and subsequent appropriate antibiotic therapy, untreated disease produces a 20% incidence of rectal stricture.[5]

LYMPHOGRANULOMA VENEREUM

Also known as lymphopathia venereum or lymphogranuloma inguinale, this venereal disease causing proctocolitis results from infection by a filterable organism larger than a virus of the psittacosis-lymphogranuloma group. A common disease among females in the tropics,[30] it has been recently reported to be increasing in male homosexuals.[7] Early symptoms include rectal bleeding and purulent discharge in the acute stage, with rectal stricture formation and associated symptoms of tenesmus, constipation and pain in the late stages. Rectovaginal fistulas may develop. Endoscopy in acute disease reveals proctitis with pseudomembrane formation. Biopsy may show granulomas with destructive changes and cellular infiltration. Late changes are fibrotic. The diagnosis is confirmed by the intradermal Frei test as well as complement fixation tests.[27]

Roentgenographic findings on barium enema depend on the phase and activity of the disease. Ulceration with irregular narrowing and spasm, fistulous tracts and perirectal abscesses have been described in the acute stages.[27, 30] Progression to fibrosis and stricture formation is then seen with extensive involvement reaching into the sigmoid and descending colon (Fig 21-8). Differential diagnosis in the chronic stricture stage includes long infiltrating scirrhous carcinomas of the rectosigmoid and the unusual occurrences of tuberculosis or schistosomiasis.[27] Although the Schistosoma is not a true bacterium, antibiotic therapy is effective in the early acute stages, with surgery required following development of chronic strictures.

Summary

The recent literature related to bacterial infectious colitis suggests several points, as summarized below.

Shigellosis

1. Common disease is common, and therefore shigellosis should be a serious consideration in any inflammatory colitis. The nonspecificity of the findings, including the common occurrence of ulceration, requires that this entity be looked for bacteriologically in the patient with acute colitis.
2. The high association of shigellosis and proctocolitis in homosexual men should be noted. The public health implica-

tions related to such patients who may be employed as food handlers, or in other roles where dissemination of the disease could occur, are noteworthy.

Salmonellosis

1. The fact that Salmonella infection occurs other than in the usual setting of typhoid fever with distal or diffuse colonic disease is a point of diagnostic interest as well as one having public health implications.
2. The possibility of concomitant infection associated with acute idiopathic ulcerative colitis raises the problem of high-dose steroid therapy in such patients.

Venereal Colitis

1. Although there are few reliable statistics regarding male homosexuality in the United States, most sources agree that its incidence is increasing. Since gonorrheal infection is now the most common communicable disease in the United States, the public health problem of anorectal gonorrhea is becoming increasingly important.
2. The clinical implications of inflammatory colitis in the homosexual male or in the female who has a history compatible with gonorrheal infection should be noted.
3. The incidence of lymphogranuloma venereum infection in homosexual patients with acute inflammatory colitis should be noted in radiographic differential diagnosis.

REFERENCES

1. Farman, J., Rabinowitz, J. G., and Meyers, M. A.: Roentgenology of infectious colitis, Am. J. Roentgenol. 119:375, 1973.
2. Bennett, I. L., Jr., and Hook, E. W.: Infectious diseases (some aspects of salmonellosis), Ann. Rev. Med. 10:1, 1959.
3. Lowenstein, M. S., Fox, M. D., and Martin, S. A.: Surveillance for Salmonella, J. Infect. Dis. 123: 332, 1971.
4. Vijil, C.: Epidemic of dysentery in Nicaragua, Lancet 2:471, 1970.
5. Klein, E. J., Fisher, L. S., Chow, A. W., and Guze, L. B.: Anorectal gonococcal infection, Ann. Intern. Med. 86:340, 1977.
6. Goodman, K. J.: Radiologic findings in anorectal gonorrhea, Gastrointest. Radiol. 3:223, 1978.
7. Sohn, N., and Robilotti, J. G.: The gay bowel syndrome, Am. J. Gastroenterol. 67:478, 1977.
8. Wilder, A. N., and MacCready, R. A.: Isolation of salmonella from poultry, poultry products and poultry processing plants in Massachusetts, New Engl. J. Med. 274:1453, 1966.
9. Lockhart-Mummery, H. E., and Morson, B. C.: Crohn's disease of the large intestine and its distinction from ulcerative colitis, Gut 1:87, 1960.
10. Margulis, A. R., Goldberg, H. I., Lawson, T. L., Montgomery, C. K., Rambo, O. N., Noonan., and Amberg, J. R.: The overlapping spectrum of ulcerative and granulomatous colitis: A roentgenographic-pathologic study, Am. J. Roentgenol. 113:325, 1971.
11. Stanley, R. J., Tedesco, F. J., Melson, G. L., Geisse, G., and Herold, S. L.: The colitis of Behçet's disease: A clinical-radiographic correlation, Radiology 114:603, 1975.
12. Smith, G. E., Kime, L. R., and Pitcher, J. L.: The colitis of Behçet's disease: A separate entity? Colonoscopic findings and literature review, Am. J. Dig. Dis. 18:987, 1973.
13. Miller, W. T., DePoto, D. W., Scholl, H. W., and Raffensperger, E. C.: Evanescent colitis in the young adult: A new entity?, Radiology 100:71, 1971.
14. Berk, R. N., and Lasser, E. C.: *Radiology of the Ileocecal Area* (Philadelphia: W. B. Saunders Co., 1975), pp. 228–230.
15. Archibald, R. B., and Nelson, J. A.: Necrotizing enterocolitis in acute leukemia: Radiographic findings, Gastrointest. Radiol. 3:63, 1978.
16. Peterson, R.: Gastrointestinal abnormalities in renal homotransplant patients, J. Can. Assoc. Radiol. 27:240, 1976.
17. Perloff, L. J., Chon, H., Petrella, E. J., Grossman, R. A., and Barker, C. F.: Acute colitis in the renal allograft recipient, Ann. Surg. 183:77, 1976.
18. Thompson, W. M., Meyers, W., Seigler, H. F., and Rice, R. P.: Gastrointestinal complications of renal transplantation, Semin. Roentgenol. 13:319, 1978.
19. Hyson, E. A., Burrell, M., and Toffler, R.: Drug-induced gastrointestinal disease, Gastrointest. Radiol. 2:183, 1977.
20. Stanley, R. J., and Tedesco, F. J.: Antibiotic-associated pseudomembranous colitis, CRC Crit. Rev. Clin. Radiol. Nucl. Med. 8:255, 1976.
21. Toffler, R. B., Pingoud, E. G., and Burrell, M. I.: Acute, transient antibiotic colitis: Ischemic colitis and bloody diarrhea related to penicillin and penicillin derivatives (Abst.), in Scientific Section, Proc. Soc. Gastrointest. Radiol., 1976.
22. Stein, H. B., and Urowitz, M. B.: Gold-induced enterocolitis: Case report and literature review, J. Rheumatol. 3:21, 1976.
23. Roe, M., Sears, A. D., and Arndt, J. H.: Gold reaction panenteritis, Radiology 104:59, 1972.

24. Kaplinsky, N., Pras, M., and Frankl, O.: Severe enterocolitis complicating chrysotherapy, Ann. Rheum. Dis. 32:574, 1973.
25. Wittenberg, J., Athanasoulis, C. A., Williams, L. F., Jr., Garedes, S., O'Sullivan, P., and Brown, B.: Ischemic colitis: Radiology and pathophysiology, Am. J. Roentgenol. 123:287, 1975.
26. Ghahremani, G. G., Meyers, M. A., Farman, J., and Port, R. B.: Ischemic disease of the small bowel and colon associated with oral contraceptives, Gastrointest. Radiol. 2:221, 1977.
27. Margulis, A. F., and Burhenne, H. J.: *Alimentary Tract Roentgenology* (2d ed.; St. Louis: C. V. Mosby Co., 1973), pp. 1579–1585; 1591–1595.
28. Meyers, M. A., Ghahremani, G. G., Clements, J. L., Jr., and Goodman, K.: Pneumatosis intestinalis, Gastrointest. Radiol. 2:91, 1977.
29. Dronfield, M. W., Fletcher, J., and Langman, M. J. S.: Salmonella infections and ulcerative colitis: Problems of recognition and management, Br. Med. J. 1:99, 1974.
30. Annamunthodo, H., and Marryatt, J.: Barium studies in intestinal lymphogranuloma venereum, Br. J. Radiol. 34:53, 1961.

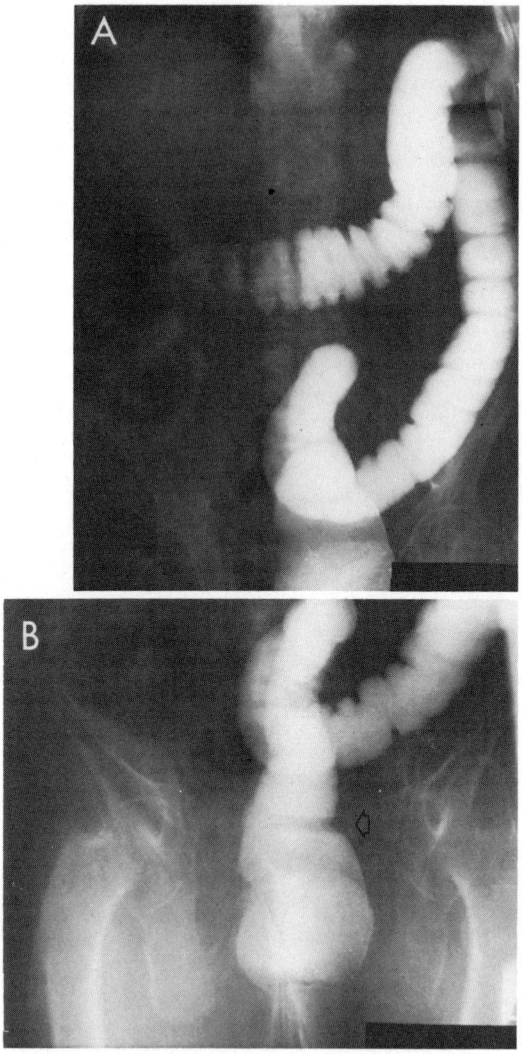

Fig 21–1 (above).—**A,** film from barium enema showing minimal mucosal edema with increased width of interhaustral folds, distal colon and rectum. Patient was young Mexican male with diarrhea and culture-proved shigellosis. **B,** close-up of rectum and sigmoid colon in same patient showing minimal irregularity of margins of rectum indicating shallow ulceration, which was seen at proctoscopy. Slight thickening of one of the valves of Houston *(arrow)* is also present.

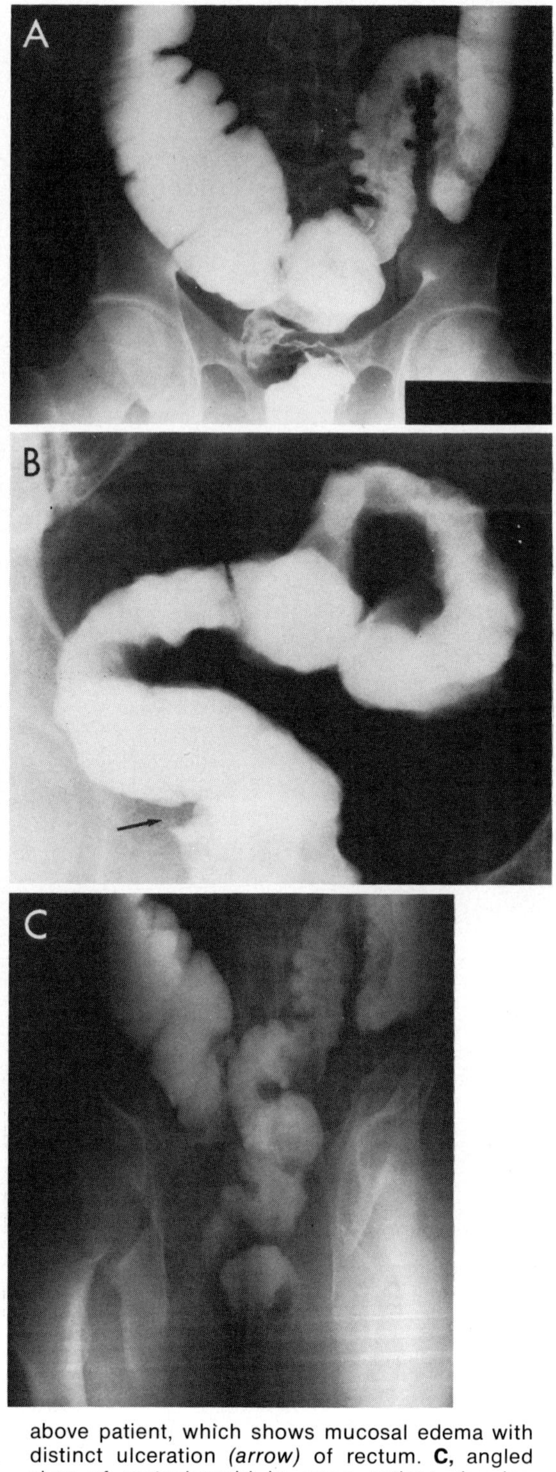

Fig 21–2 (right).—**A,** more advanced case than that in Figure 21–1 of culture-proved Shigella colitis with shallow ulcerations of rectum. **B,** fluoroscopic spot film of rectum and sigmoid colon in above patient, which shows mucosal edema with distinct ulceration *(arrow)* of rectum. **C,** angled view of rectosigmoid in same patient showing mucosal edema and shallow ulceration.

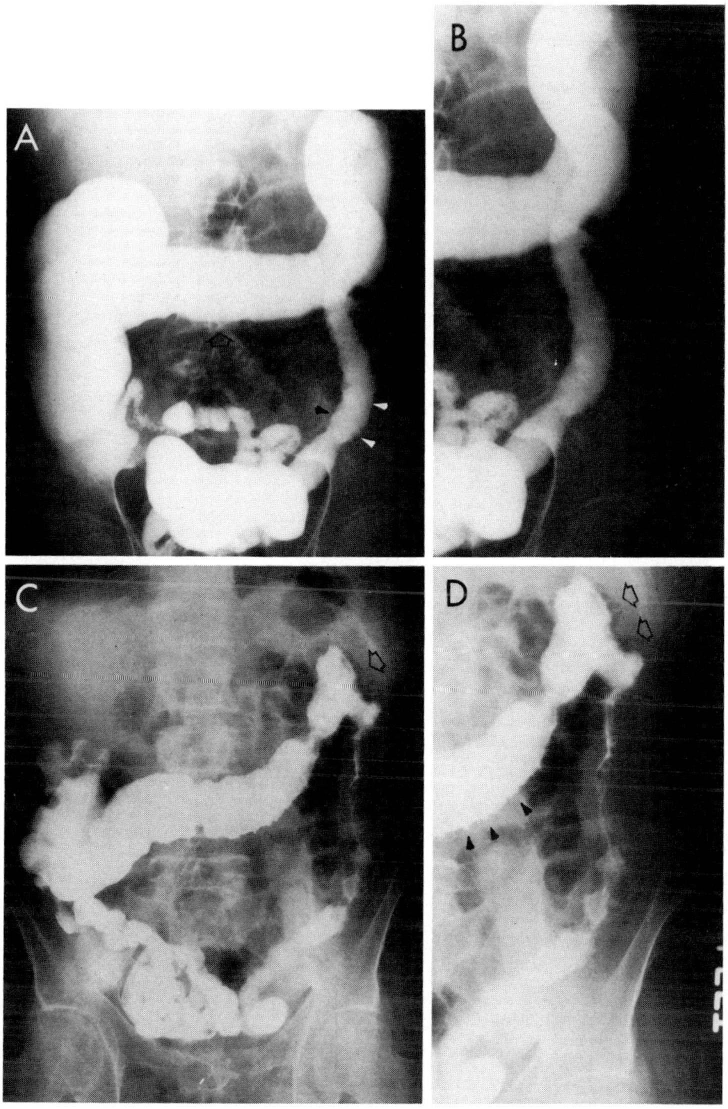

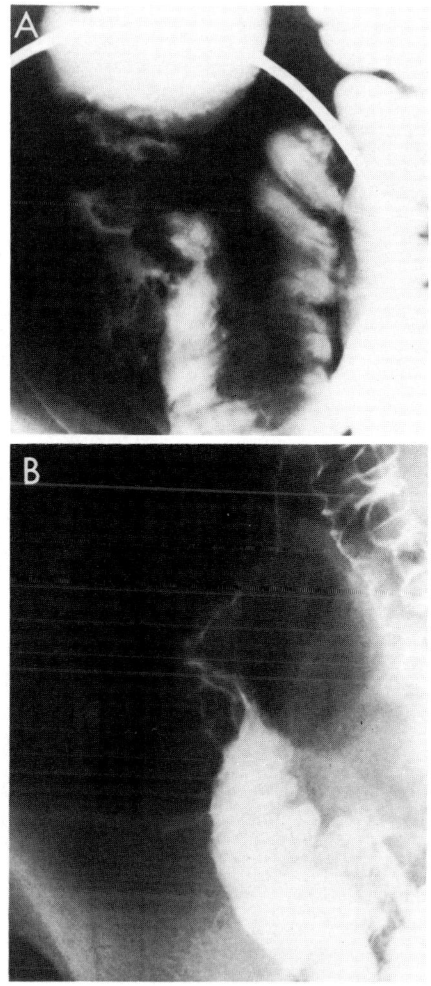

Fig 21–3 (left).—**A,** filled film in severe case of culture-proved shigellosis of colon. Bowel wall thickening can be appreciated in transverse colon *(arrows)*. Ulceration with rigidity of descending colon is also present *(arrowheads)*. **B,** close-up of descending colon in same patient showing ulcerations and lack of distensibility. **C,** postevacuation film in same patient with severe shigellosis showing shallow collar button ulcerations of transverse colon not noted on filled films, with pneumatosis *(arrow)* of splenic flexure secondary to necrosis of bowel wall. Splenic flexure was removed at surgery and proved to be necrotic. **D,** close up of distal transverse and descending colon in same patient. Collar button ulcerations *(arrowheads)* of distal transverse colon and pneumatosis *(arrows)* within wall of necrotic splenic flexure are shown.

Fig 21–4 (right).—**A,** compression spot film during barium enema of ileocecal area in patient with typhoid fever. Nodular mucosal pattern with constricted cecum and mucosal edema of terminal ileum is shown. Patient had history of exposure to contaminated water supply and a positive stool culture for *Salmonella typhi*. **B,** air contrast view of same patient with typhoid fever showing poor distensibility of cecum and nodular, spastic terminal ileum.

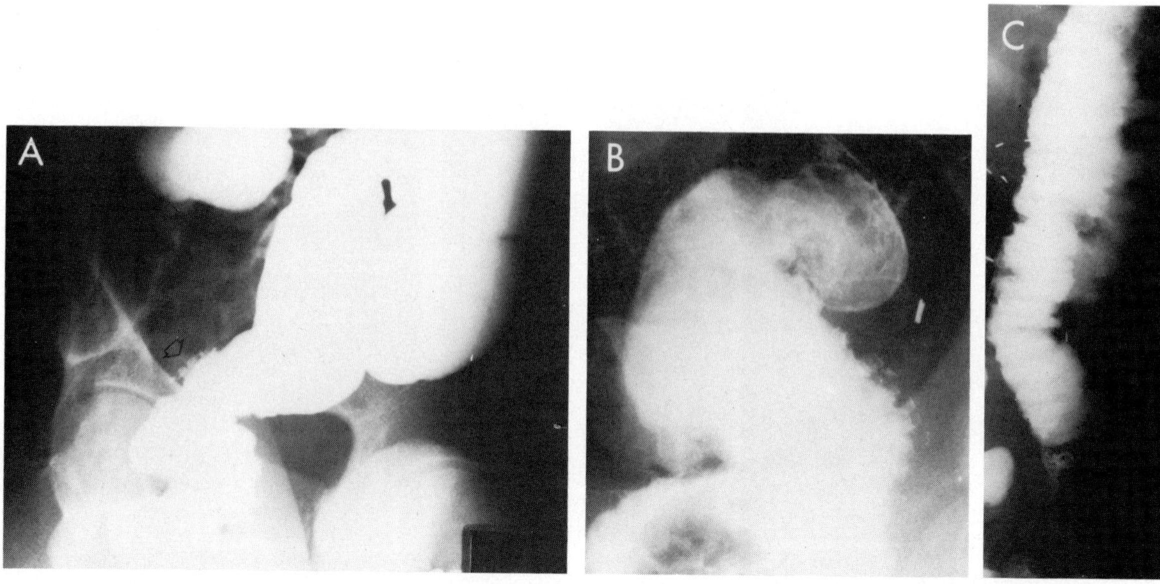

Fig 21–5. – **A,** oblique view of rectosigmoid in patient with culture-proved Salmonella colitis with deep collar button ulcerations *(arrow)* and mucosal edema. Terminal ileum was normal. **B,** close-up of rectum showing deep collar button ulcerations in same patient. **C,** close-up of descending colon, which shows diffuse mucosal edema, in same patient.

Fig 21–6. – **A,** prone PA view of colon during air contrast barium enema showing poor distensibility of rectum in known homosexual male with culture-proved gonococcal proctitis. **B,** lateral rectal view in same patient. Note lack of distensibility and suggestion of shallow ulceration seen at proctoscopy. Widened pre-sacral space is also seen.

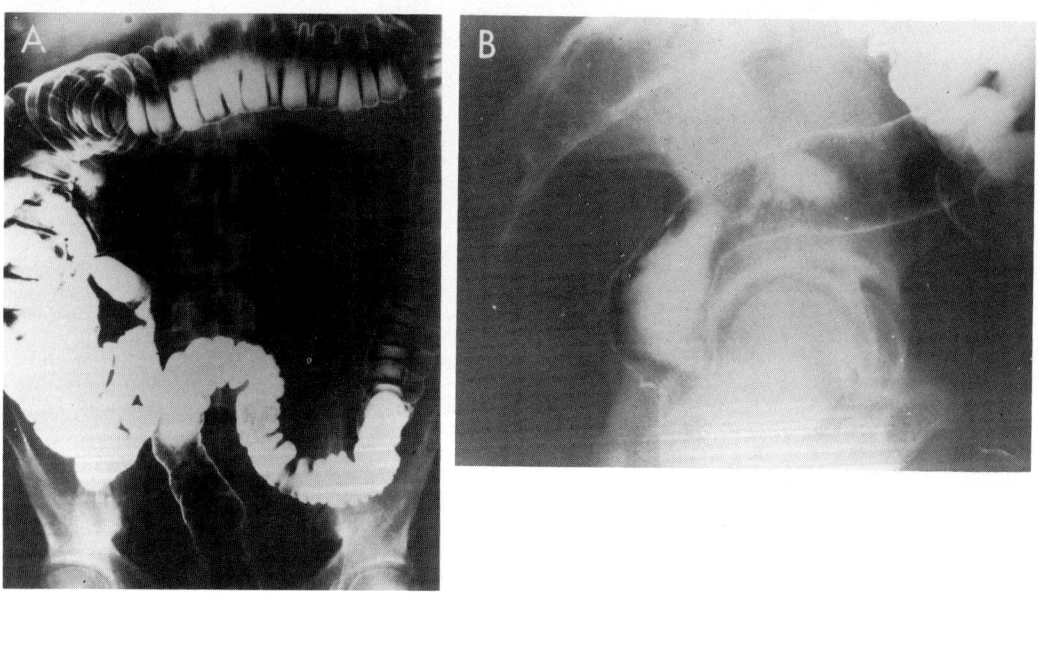

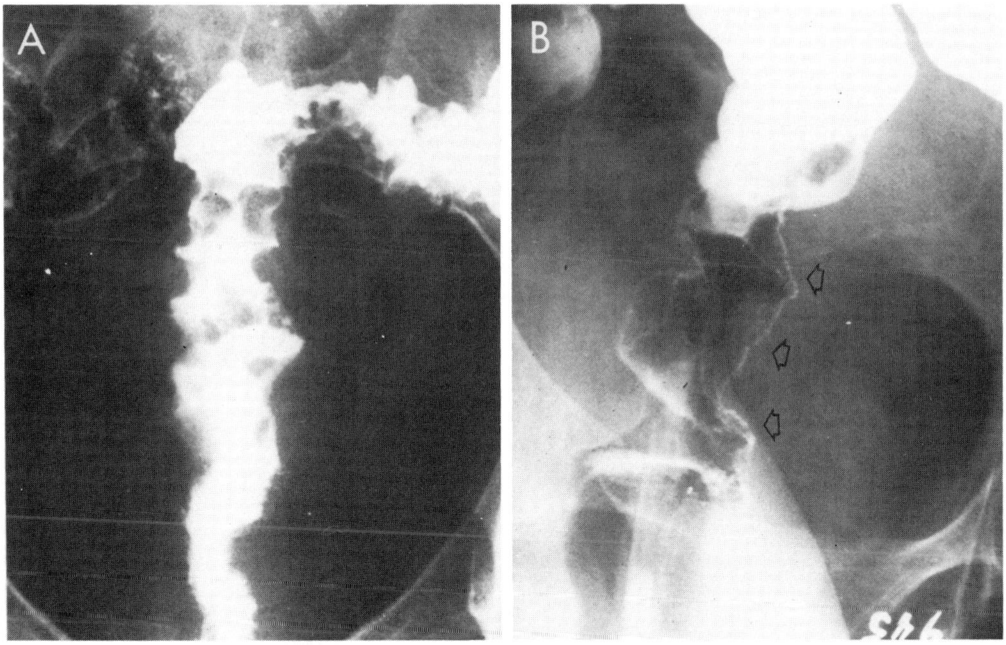

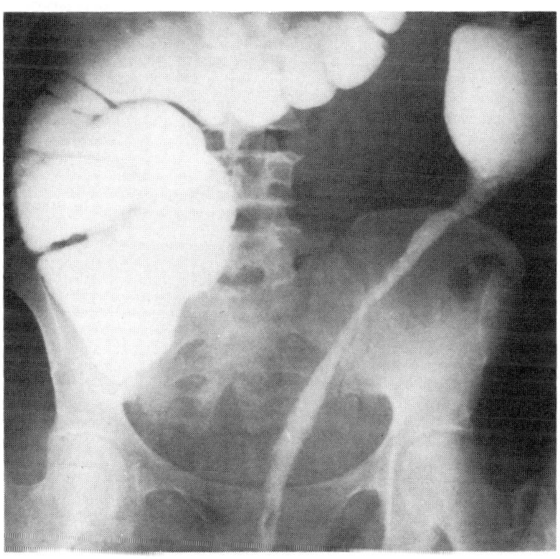

Fig 21–7 (top). — **A,** marked mucosal edema with diffuse ulceration of rectum in another homosexual male patient with proved gonococcal proctitis. **B,** air contrast view in same patient showing lack of distensibility and fine granular pattern along margins of rectum *(arrows)*, corresponding to shallow ulcerations seen at proctoscopy.

Fig 21–8 (bottom). — Long stricture of descending and sigmoid colon and rectum in woman with long-standing history of lymphogranuloma venereum infection of colon diagnosed by positive Frei skin test.

Chapter 22

Intussusception

LEO S. FIGIEL, M.D., F.A.C.R.
STEVEN J. FIGIEL, M.D., F.A.C.R.

ADULT FORMS of colocolic intussusception will generally be due to tumors of the right colon or proximal transverse colon, and obstruction due to intussusception will most frequently be encountered in the transverse colon. Occasionally, colocolic intussusception may be encountered in the descending or sigmoid colon. In such cases the underlying tumor usually will originate in either the transverse or sigmoid colon.

In our experience with 21 patients at the Harper-Grace Hospital, colocolic intussusception was always associated with a benign or malignant tumor. In all cases the tumors were large, measuring at least 4–6 cm in size. Benign tumors were found in eight instances: of these, five were lipomas and three were adenomas, two of the latter being villous. Of the lipomas, one was a lesion involving the ileocecal valve, which measured about 7 cm in diameter; two were located in the midascending colon; and two were located in the proximal sigmoid colon. Of the adenomas, two were located in the midascending colon and the third in the distal transverse colon. Polypoid or annular malignancies of the colon were present in the remaining 13 patients. With the exception of an annular carcinoma at the proximal sigmoid and an annular carcinoma at the apex of the splenic flexure, all of the malignant tumors were located in the right or proximal transverse colon.

It can be assumed that any lesion or pathologic process producing an impediment to normal peristaltic activity could result in intussusception. The presence of a neoplasm involving the mucosa and/or other elements of the intestinal wall that are subject to traction during peristaltic activity over a long period of time can theoretically result in an intussuscepting process. This will be the mechanism responsible for intussusception in colonic neoplasms. We are not aware of any instance in which an inflammatory process of the colon was associated with colocolic intussusception. Recently, Johnson and Caldwell[5] implicated "angioneurotic edema of the colon" as a cause of recurring colocolic intussusception. Submucosal tumefactive changes due to the presence of fluid in the bowel wall produced a localized disturbance in the bowel equivalent to a tumor mass.

Roentgenographic Findings (Figs 22–1 to 22–9)

Radiologists will recognize classic findings of intussusception when complete obstruction is encountered during barium enema study.[8] A convex, meniscus-shaped deformity associated with compacted mucosal folds, the "accordion pleating or concertina pattern," may be regarded as pathognomonic. Often the bowel lumen is expanded at the site of obstruction. In some instances, rather than a sharp convex defect, sausage-like intraluminal polypoid tumor-like defect may actually be shown extending into the bowel distal to the obstruction. The surface of this tumor-like defect often shows the compacted mucosal pattern typical of intussusception, especially in expulsion study.

Colocolic intussusception is frequently reducible during barium enema study. Substantial changes in position are possible, e.g., an obstruction can shift from the left colon into the transverse colon; from the splenic flexure to the area of the hepatic flexure; from the transverse colon to the right colon. Complete reduction will permit precise localization and identification of the underlying pathologic process. Such information will be invaluable to the surgeon in planning his operative procedure in terms of his incision and the type of resective procedure required.

Unfortunately in some instances when radiologists encounter shifting deformities, they assume that they are dealing with fecal matter. This may be the source of a substantial number of errors in the diagnosis of malignancies of the colon.[2] In reviewing our cases, we noted that radiologists had failed to diagnose the presence of neoplasm in four instances on previous examinations, often performed within a day to a few weeks before our examination. In one of our personal cases, a staff radiologist with substantial experience overlooked an intussuscepting polypoid tumor while preoccupied with a pedunculated polypoid lesion that he had discovered in the sigmoid. Failure to observe the head of the barium column as it filled the colon was probably the cause of his not having noted the shifting obstruction, which was completely reduced during his examination. Presence of the intussuscepting lesion was suspected on review of the expulsion study of the colon. On reexamination of this patient, an obstruction was encountered in the proximal transverse colon with gradual reduction of the intussusception, and finally demonstration of a 4-cm sessile tumor in the midascending colon was demonstrated. We must again emphasize that whenever the radiologist encounters a meniscus-shaped deformity associated with a temporary or high-grade obstruction, especially if there is a shifting deformity of this type, he must suspect colocolic intussusception and must investigate the proximal colon with great care. Advanced lesions may be readily overlooked, especially in the presence of fecal matter. It is a known fact that the incidence of error on the part of the radiologist in detection of colonic neoplasms increases as one reaches the right colon and is highest in the cecal region.[2]

We regard the expulsion study as probably the single most important film in the investigation of the colon. Many pathologic conditions become evident on study of the expulsion study, including many small polypoid lesions. An expanded bowel lumen at the site of an intussuscepted mass may be recognized as potentially significant when such expansion is associated with a compacted mucosal fold pattern at the surface of the mass, and when, in addition, the bowel proximal and distal to the expanded segment is in a collapsed state. Several examples of the bowel pattern in colocolic intussusception on the expulsion study are shown.

Diagnosis of colocolic intussusception is occasionally possible on scout studies of the abdomen. Whenever an elongated soft tissue mass presents its longest diameter in the longitudinal axis of the colon, this possibility should be suspected. The shifting nature of such defects on clinical examination and the conformance to the anatomical site of the colon provide a clue to the clinician. In some instances the intussusceptum may be partly outlined by a ring or sheathlike accumulation of gas, or the apex of the intussusceptum may be visible as a soft tissue density in the gas immediately distal to it. Comprehensive reports of this entity have been published by Laurell,[6] Schatzki,[7] Sussman,[9] Dick and

Green[1] and by the authors.[3] Otherwise most of the literature consists of single case reports.

Summary

In our experience with 21 adults with colocolic intussusception, the obstruction always was associated with an underlying carcinoma or polypoid tumor. Benign tumors were present in eight cases, of which five were lipomas and three adenomas. Polypoid or annular malignancies were present in the remaining 13 cases.

The presence of a cupula or meniscus-shaped deformity associated with a temporary or high-grade obstruction is the most reliable indication of colocolic intussusception. The bowel lumen is often expanded at the site of obstruction. Compaction of mucosal folds, the accordion pleating pattern, is frequently present at the site of deformity, and is often best seen on the expulsion study. In some instances an intraluminal sausage-like tumor mass will be present in the bowel distal to the obstruction.

Colocolic intussusception is frequently reducible during fluoroscopic study. A shifting defect of this type must be regarded as highly suspicious of a colocolic intussusception, and the bowel proximal to the obstruction must be studied with great care in order to avoid missing an underlying neoplasm. Complete reduction of colocolic intussusception with visualization of the underlying pathologic process permits precise localization and accurate identification of the underlying pathology. The prognosis in colocolic intussusception is good, since a high percentage of underlying tumors is benign.

REFERENCES

1. Dick, A., and Green, G. J.: Large bowel intussusception in adults, Br. J. Radiol. 34:769, 1961.
2. Figiel, L. S., Figiel, S. J., and Hennessey, A.: Carcinoma of the colon: Accuracy of roentgen diagnosis, Gastroenterology 40:487, 1963.
3. Figiel, L. S., and Figiel, S. J.: Colo-colic intussusception, Am. J. Dig. Dis. 8:1017, 1963.
4. Jackson, H.: A sign of intussusception, Br. J. Radiol. 26:323, 1953.
5. Johnson, T. H., and Caldwell, K. W.: Angioneurotic edema of the colon, Radiology 99:61, 1971.
6. Laurell, H.: Uber reine Coloninvagination vor allem von roentgenologischen Gesichtspunkt, Acta Radiol. 14:122, 1933.
7. Schatzki, R.: Intussuscepted tumors of the colon, Am. J. Roentgenol. 41:549, 1939.
8. Solis-Cohen, L., and Levine, S.: X-ray diagnosis of complete and partial acute intestinal obstruction, Radiology 31:8, 1938.
9. Sussman, M. L.: Roentgenologic aspect of subacute and chronic intestinal intussusception, Am. J. Roentgenol. 27:373, 1932.

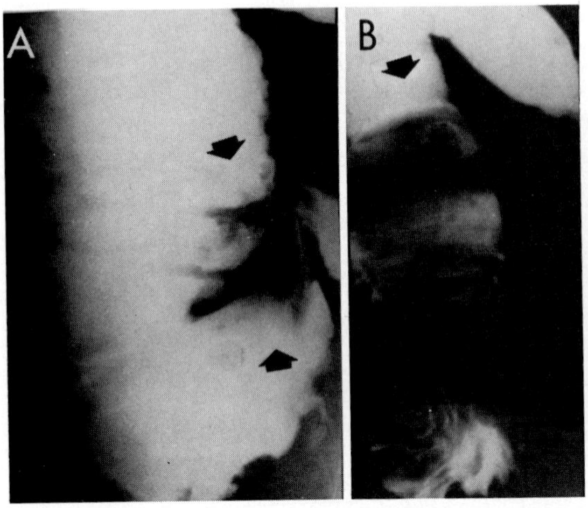

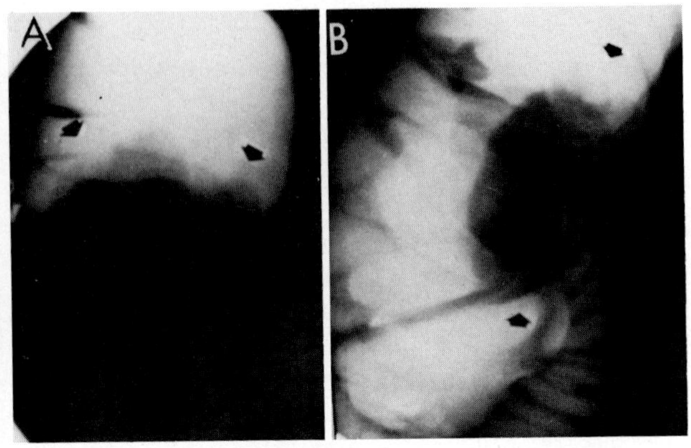

Fig 22–1 (left).—**A,** 7-cm lipoma of ileocecal valve with cecocolic intussusception *(arrows).* On expulsion study **(B)** note convex margin *(arrow)* of superior border of intussusceptum in midascending colon, expanded bowel lumen and compacted mucosal fold pattern.

Fig 22–2 (right).—Polypoid carcinoma of cecum and ascending colon with intussusception. **A,** note lobulated, convex margin *(arrows)* at site of obstruction in midascending colon. **B,** note complete reduction of intussusception *(arrows)* and demonstration of large polypoid tumor, which involves ileocecal valve and ascending colon.

Fig 22–3.—Note variations in appearance of colocolic intussusception secondary to 5-cm villous tumor of midascending colon. Obstruction was originally encountered at hepatic flexure. **A,** high-grade obstruction with convex, meniscus-shaped deformity and expanded bowel lumen and compacted mucosal fold pattern. **B,** polypoid mass *(arrows)* in midascending colon. **C,** complete reduction of intussusception with demonstration of large sessile tumor *(arrow)* in midascending colon.

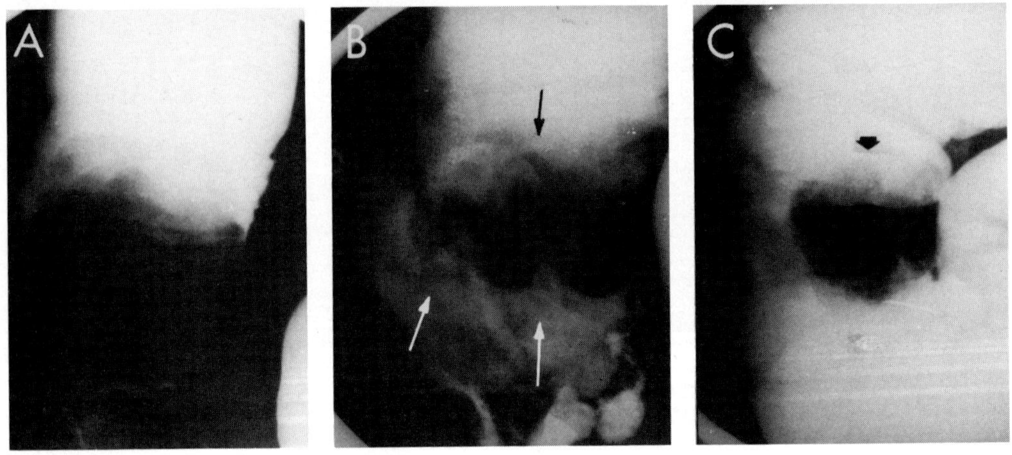

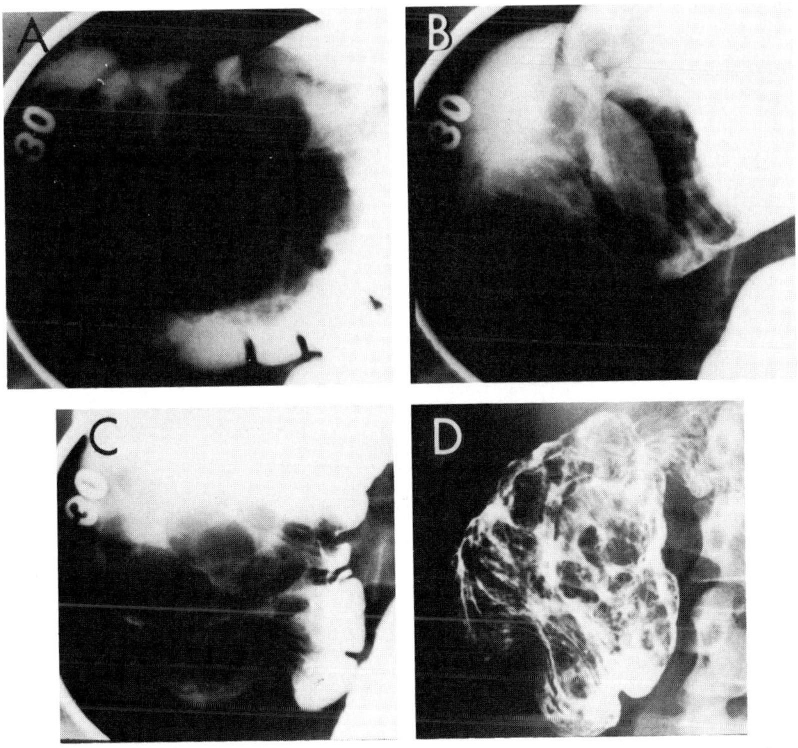

Fig 22–4. – Large polypoid carcinoma of ascending colon, with intussusception. **A,** large polypoid defect encountered in midtransverse colon. **B,** defect shifting to hepatic flexure. **C,** defect shifting to midascending colon. **D,** pattern of intussuscepting mass on expulsion study.

Fig 22–5. – **A,** radiographic study of abdomen showing large soft tissue mass *(arrow)* in right midflank conforming to intussuscepted mass in transverse colon. **B,** small bowel study demonstrating intussuscepted mass in transverse colon. Note expanded lumen at site of intussusception and compacted mucosal fold pattern, in addition to lobulated margin of distal extremity of intussuscepting mass due to presence of large polypoid neoplasm. The ileum is noted to enter intussuscepted colon and can be identified near leading edge of intussusceptum.

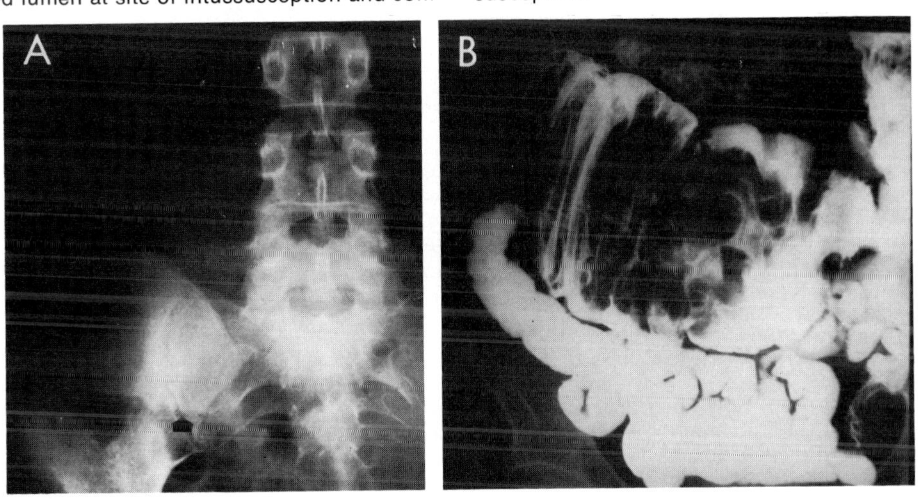

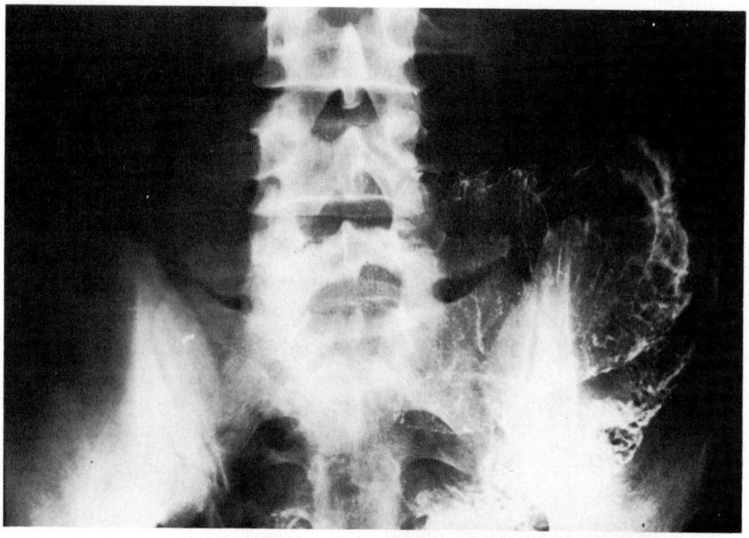

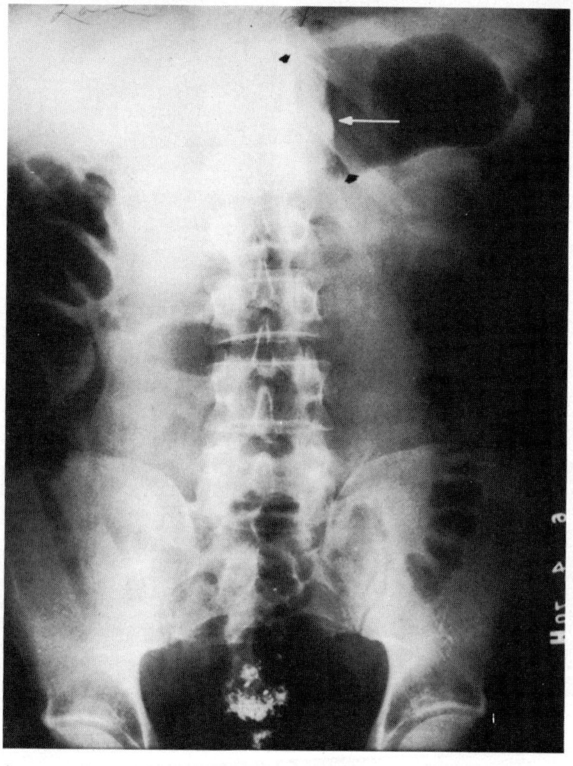

Fig 22–6 (top). – Annular carcinoma of hepatic flexure with intussusception: note long intraluminal, sausage-shaped mass in distal transverse colon, with apex of intussusceptum at splenic flexure of colon. Note also expanded bowel lumen and compacted mucosal fold pattern.

Fig 22–7 (bottom). – A 5-cm villous tumor of mid-ascending colon with colocolic intussusception. Note soft tissue mass in right upper and midabdomen with leading edge of colocolic intussusception identifiable in transverse colon *(arrows)*.

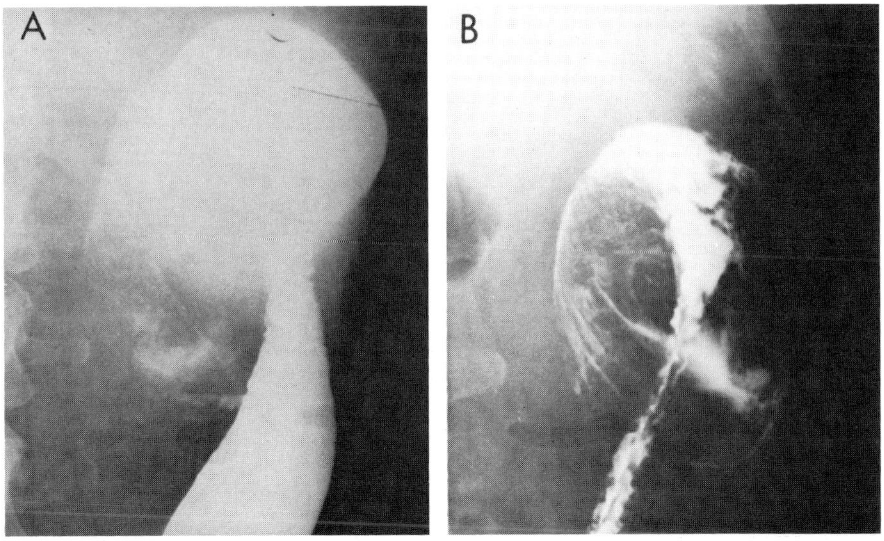

Fig 22–8.—Annular carcinoma of hepatic flexure with irreducible intussusception presenting at splenic flexure. **A,** classic features of sausage-shaped, intraluminal mass with distal convex margin, expanded bowel lumen and compacted mucosal fold pattern. **B,** characteristics of the mass and compacted mucosal fold pattern are more clearly seen on expulsion study.

Fig 22–9.—Sigmoidorectal intussusception due to annular carcinoma of proximal sigmoid. **A,** note intraluminal, sausage-shaped mass; expanded bowel; and mucosal fold pattern at margins of intraluminal mass. **B,** intussusceptum fills rectum. Note curvilinear mucosal fold pattern at surface of mass.

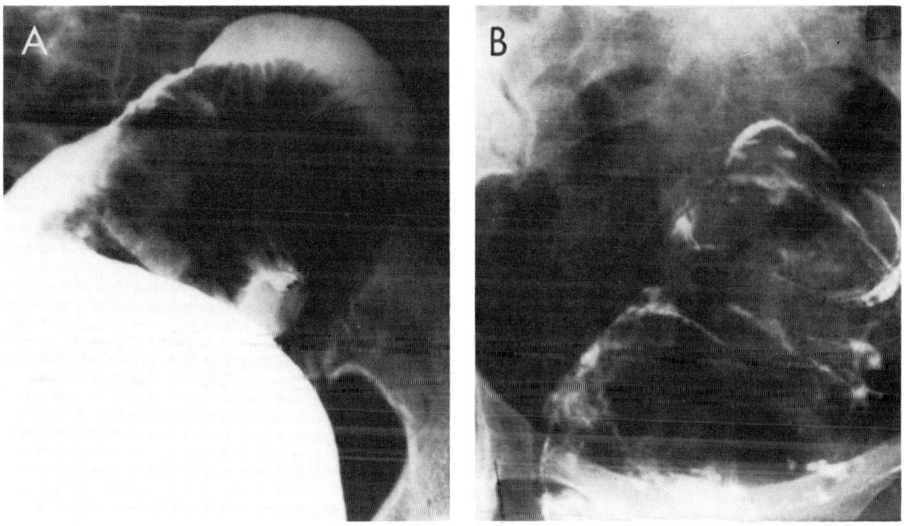

Chapter 23

Ischemic Colitis and Discrete Colonic Ulceration Secondary to Oral Contraception

THOMAS L. LAWSON, M.D.

SMALL OR LARGE BOWEL ischemic disease is rare in young patients in the absence of predisposing conditions such as heart disease, abdominal infections, systemic vasculitis, hypercoagulation states or secondary to some drugs, including those taken for oral contraception.[1-11] Ischemic colitis secondary to mesenteric venous or arterial thrombosis associated with various progesterone or estrogen compounds taken for oral contraceptives is an idiopathic disorder, the diagnosis depending on clinical suspicion and associated radiographic findings. Most commonly, these young women present with crampy abdominal pain; a change in bowel habits, which may progress to bloody diarrhea; and a history of taking oral contraceptive pills for a variable length of time. The drug-induced vascular occlusion may be mild, self-limited and reversible or severe, progressive and leading to extensive bowel necrosis.

The barium enema roentgen findings in the usual mild self-limited case are thickening of the bowel wall with narrowing and irregularity of the lumen and focal submucosal fluid collections (thumbprints) indenting the barium column (Fig 23 – 1). An expected feature is a return to health, with follow-up roentgen examinations demonstrating a slow resolution of the pathologic process and a return to normal. More severe ischemic changes in these young patients, leading to infarction with subsequent healing and stricture formation on follow-up barium examinations, have not been described, but theoretically they should exist. Rarely there may be severe progressive ischemic changes leading to bowel gangrene and subsequent patient death.[1, 7]

Rarely the ischemic changes may present as large, discrete colon ulcers (Fig 23 – 2). When this is the case, the diagnosis may be difficult, as the large, discrete ulcerations may be confused with ulcerating mural or submucosal tumors, delaying the correct diagnosis of ischemic ulcers. In such instances, colonoscopy may be helpful in making the correct diagnosis. Visceral angiography is of no value in these cases and is not indicated.

The etiologic factors in ischemic disease in patients taking oral contraceptives are obscure. Oral contraceptives are known to increase the platelet count, decrease partial thromboplastin time, accelerate thromboplastin regeneration and decrease antithrombin III levels. These findings have led to a "hypercoagulation state theory," which clinically has not been supported.[5, 12] A "low flow state" also has been postulated, as oral contraceptives are known to decrease venous return and venous distensibility in the extremities. Such a low flow state might cause ischemia in the splenic flexure area, where the blood supply is transitional, although this theory has not been proved.[13, 14]

The usual differential diagnosis of ischemic colitis in these young women would include inflammatory bowel disease, such as Crohn's disease, or ulcerative colitis and lymphoma. In ischemic colitis presenting as focal ulcerations, the differential diagnosis would include ulcerating mural tumors and solitary, nonspecific colon ulcer. The correct diagnosis may be difficult to reach and require follow-up or ancillary examinations; it does require clinical suspicion and a history of oral contraceptive pill ingestion. Inflammatory bowel disease may be differentiated from ischemic colitis in these young women by a slightly different distribution of ulcerations and an entirely different clinical course. Lymphoma may be differentiated by clinical and laboratory evaluation as well as by a dissimilar clinical course. Ulcerating mural tumors or solitary, nonspecific colon ulcer may be differentiated from focal ischemic colonic ulcers by clinical history, colonoscopy with biopsy and clinical follow up.

REFERENCES

1. Brennan, M. F., Clarke, A. M., and MacBeth, W. A.: Infarction of the midgut associated with oral contraceptives, N. Engl. J. Med. 279:1213, 1968.
2. Kilpatrick, Z., Silverman, J., Betancourt, E., Farman, J., and Lawson, J. T.: Vascular occlusion of the colon and oral contraceptives—possible relation, N. Engl. J. Med. 278:438, 1968.
3. Reed, D., and Coon, W.: Thromobembolism in patients receiving progestional drugs, N. Engl. J. Med. 269:622, 1963.
4. Cotton, P. B., and Thomas, M. L.: Ischemic colitis and the contraceptive pill, Br. Med. J. 3:27, 1971.
5. Hurwitz, R., Martin, A., Grossman, B., and Waddell, W.: Oral contraceptives and gastrointestinal disorders, Ann. Surg. 172:892, 1970.
6. Welin, G., and Persson, T.: Oral contraceptives and thrombosis of the celiac artery, Lancet 2:1348, 1968.
7. Civetta, J., and Kolodney, M.: Mesenteric venous thrombosis associated with oral contraceptives, Gastroenterology 58:713, 1970.
8. Gelfand, M.: Ischemic colitis with a depot synthetic progestogen, Am. J. Dig. Dis. 178:275, 1972.
9. Castelli, M. F., Qizilbash, A. H., Salem, S., and Fyshe, T. G.: Ischemic bowel disease, Can. Med. Assoc. J. 111:935, 1974.
10. Bernardino, M., and Lawson, T. L.: Discrete colonic ulcers associated with oral contraceptives, Am. J. Dig. Dis. 21:503, 1975.
11. McClennan, B. L.: Ischemic colitis secondary to premarin: Report of a case, Dis. Colon Rectum 19: 618, 1976.
12. Handin, R. I.: Thromboembolic complications of pregnancy and oral contraceptives, Prog. Cardiovasc. Dis. 16:395, 1974.
13. Goodrich, S. M., and Wood, J. E.: Effects of estradiol 17 beta on peripheral venous distensibility and velocity of venous flow, Am. J. Obstet. Gynecol. 76:407, 1966.
14. Goodrich, S. M., and Wood, J. E.: Peripheral venous distensibility and velocity of venous blood flow during pregnancy or oral contraceptives, Am. J. Obstet. Gynecol. 90:740, 1964.

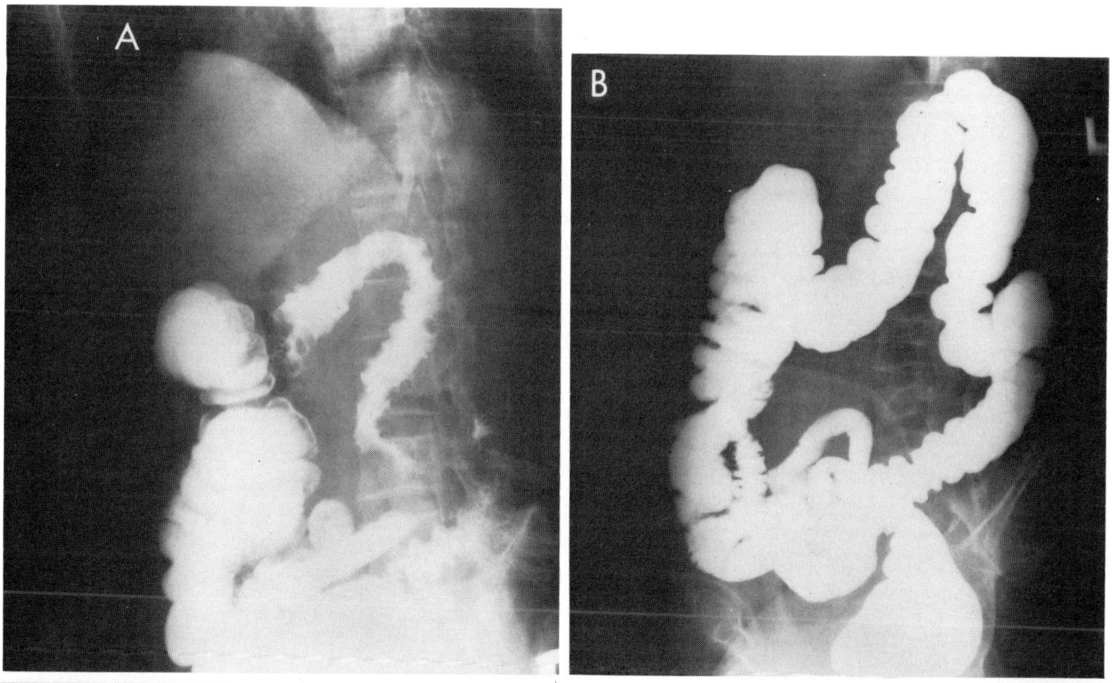

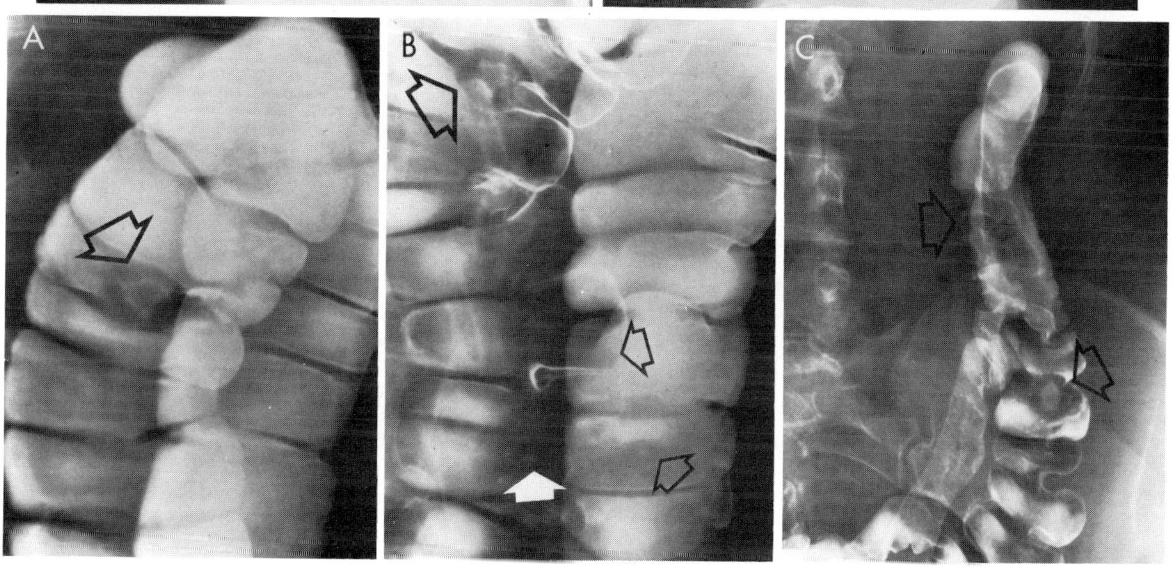

Fig 23–1 (top). – **A,** right posterior oblique roentgenogram obtained during initial barium enema examination demonstrates narrowing, irregularity and thumbprinting in splenic flexure region. **B,** follow-up right posterior oblique roentgenogram 8 weeks after initial examination demonstrates return to normal. (From McClennan, Dis. Colon Rectum 19:618, 1976, with permission.)

Fig 23–2 (bottom). – **A** and **B,** oblique roentgenogram of splenic flexure obtained during barium enema examination and **C,** postevacuation roentgenogram, demonstrate several large focal ulcers in distal transverse and proximal descending colon *(arrows).* Central ulceration is surrounded by mound of edema, which resembles a mural mass. (From McClennan, Am. J. Dig. Dis. 21:503, 1976, with permission.)

Chapter 24

Ischemic Disease of the Colon

DENIS C. ADLER, M.D.
HARVEY L. MEYERS, M.D.

RADIOLOGIC CHANGES accompanying ischemia of the colon have been widely recognized since 1963 when Boley et al,[1] reported five cases of what they called "reversible vascular occlusion of the colon." The characteristic radiologic finding emphasized in their report was the formation of pseudotumors described as thumbprinting.

The radiologic findings of severe vascular compromise, known variably as intestinal necrosis, mesenteric thrombosis and mesenteric infarction were the subject of many excellent earlier studies[2-5] and are for the most part nonspecific in nature. These reports were based most frequently on roentgen studies of the acute abdomen without administration of contrast material.

Before the report of Boley et al.,[1] Engelhardt and Jacobson[6] in 1956 reported a case of infarction of the colon for which a barium enema was performed shortly before the death of the patient. It showed a "narrowed, rigid segment of the splenic flexure with thickened, edematous mucosa."

Wang and Reeves[7] in 1960, in a thorough study of mesenteric vascular disease, reported a case of inferior mesenteric artery occlusion in which a barium enema showed superficial ulcerations and a narrowed segment, which could be distended to almost normal size. Repeat barium enema 3 days later demonstrated "multiple intraluminal defects which are due to severe mucosal swelling."

Since the report of Schwartz, Boley et al.,[8] Marston et al.,[9] Marshak and Linder[10] and Wittenberg et al.[11] have described the radiologic findings in more detail. It became obvious that ischemic disease of the colon is a spectrum from transient ischemic colitis, which heals without sequelae, to colonic infarction. The pathologic changes form a continuum from mucosal edema, submucosal hemorrhages and ulcerations to gangrene, and from a completely reversible to an irreversible process and massive necrosis.

The radiologic changes of colon ischemia had already been investigated and reproduced in animal experiments by Boley et al.[1] in 1963. On the basis of their experiments, they believed that the pseudotumor formation responsible for thumbprinting was caused by submucosal hemorrhage or by pericolic fat inflammation or both. More recently Matthews and Parks[12, 13] showed not only the effect of both gradual and sudden obstruction of the mesenteric vessels but also the role of hypovolemia. Diminished blood flow in experimental animals in the presence of previous arterial constriction or obstruction may lead to reduction of mesenteric perfusion and result in ischemia. Mucosal edema and swelling of the folds occurred early – 2 – 4 hours after occlusion. Thumbprinting occurred after 12 – 24 hours, and marked pseudotumor formation in 24–48 hours. Regression of these events occurred in 10–21 days. It also was noted that increase in intraluminal pressure resulted in a decrease in mesenteric blood flow, which returned to normal when the pressure was released. The pathologic and radiologic findings in these animals were similar to the clinical and radiologic observations in human beings.

Although there is universal acceptance of the premise that poor blood flow to the involved colonic wall is the causative factor in ischemic colitis in human beings, there has not yet been incontrovertible demonstration that ischemia is the chief cause of the clinical complex known in human patients as ischemic colitis.[14]

All the manifestations of colonic ischemia from infarction to transient changes without sequelae may occur in a number of pathologic conditions and may have numerous predisposing factors. Partial or complete occlusion of the mesenteric vessels may occur in arterial or venous thrombosis, embolic phenomena, vasculitis, incarceration by hernia or volvulus.[15] Proximal to obstructive lesions of the colon, e.g., cancer of the sigmoid,[16] severe ulcerating mucosal changes have been noted, presumably caused by ischemia.

Some of the diseases predisposing to thrombosis are atherosclerosis, polycythemia, leukemia, lymphoma and altered hemicoagulability. Beside the so-called nonocclusive ischemia secondary to hypovolemia, as seen in shock and congestive heart failure, there remain numerous cases in which a definite etiology could not be established. Several drugs that cause thromboembolic phenomena and ischemic disease of the colon have been recognized in the past decade. Among these, oral contraceptives are particularly important.[17] Ischemic colon disease also has been described in patients who received ergotamine[18] and in drug abusers, particularly users of amphetamines.[19] Some surgical procedures involving the abdominal aorta, such as aortic reconstruction, may result in the complication of colon ischemia.[20]

Pathologically and also radiologically, the effect of insufficient blood supply to the bowel may result in the following:

1. Vascular compromise with completely reversible changes. Complete healing occurs without a permanent lesion.

2. Vascular compromise with irreversible changes. The colonic blood supply is sufficiently intact to prevent complete necrosis of the colon wall, although not adequate to prevent mucosal sloughing. This produces fibrosis and stricture. It may involve only a very short segment. Longer segments of the colon may be involved, however, particularly in the region of the splenic flexure and descending colon. A subgroup may be recognized in this category where, beside the persistent narrowed segment, chronic nonhealing ulcerations occur. These cases may represent a chronic active disease with repeated episodes of bleeding.

3. Insufficiency of the blood supply to the bowel. This may result in gangrene of the colon, with necrosis of the entire thickness of the bowel wall and sloughing of the mucosa. Some patients may survive if early resection is carried out. Most, however, die from gangrene leading to perforation and generalized peritonitis.

It is important to note that the radiologic findings in ischemic disease of the colon are not specific and may be seen in other disease processes, especially inflammatory bowel disease. Only when combined with clinical findings can a reliable diagnosis of ischemia of the colon be established.

Also noteworthy is the limited value of angiography in establishing the diagnosis of colon ischemia. There may be no notable vascular changes present, or the changes may be indistinguishable from those of inflammatory disease. Additionally, there is overall poor correlation between the extent of vascular disease demonstrated angiographically and the severity of ischemic involvement of the colon.

Summary

1. The barium enema is the most sensitive and accurate radiographic method for detection of ischemic disease of the colon.

2. The combination of an appropriate clinical history and a barium enema with characteristic findings permits an accurate differential diagnosis between ischemic, inflammatory and neoplastic disease in the majority of cases.

3. Angiography is of limited value both in differential diagnosis of ischemic and inflammatory disease of the colon and in diagnosis of ischemic disease of the colon in general.[11, 14]

REFERENCES

1. Boley, S. J., Schwartz, S. S., Lash, J., and Sternhill, V.: reversible vascular occlusion of colon, Surg. Gynecol. Obstet. 116:53, 1963.
2. Rendich, R. A., and Harrington, L. A.: Roentgenologic observations in mesenteric thrombosis, Am. J. Roentgenol. 52:317, 1944.
3. Frimann-Dahl, J.: *Roentgen Examinations in Acute Abdominal Diseases* (2d ed.; Springfield, Ill. Charles C Thomas, 1960).
4. Nelson, S. W., and Eggleston, W.: Findings on plain roentgenograms of the abdomen associated with mesenteric vascular occlusion with a possible new sign of mesenteric venous thrombosis. Am. J. Roentgenol. 83:886, 1960.
5. Rigler, L. J., and Pogue, W. L.: Roentgen signs of intestinal necrosis, Am. J. Roentgenol. 94:402, 1965.
6. Engelhardt, J. E., and Jacobson, G.: Infarction of colon demonstrated by barium enema, Radiology 67:573, 1956.
7. Wang, C. G., and Reeves, J. D.: Mesenteric vascular disease, Am. J. Roentgenol. 83:895, 1960.
8. Schwartz, S. S., Boley, S. J., Robinson, K., Kreiger, H., Schultz, L., and Allen, A. C.: Roentgenologic features of vascular disorders of intestines, Radiol. Clin. North Am. 2:71, 1964.
9. Marston, A., Pheils, M. T., Lea, T. M., and Morson, B. C.: Ischemic colitis, Gut 7:1, 1966.
10. Marshak, R. H., and Linder, A.: Ischemia of colon, Semin. Roentgenol. 3:81, 1968.
11. Wittenberg, J., Athanasoulis, C. A., Williams, L. F., Jr., Paredes, S., O'Sullivan, P., and Brown, B.: Ischemic colitis, Am. J. Roentgenol. 123:287, 1975.
12. Matthews, J. G. W., and Parks, T. G.: Ischemic colitis in the experimental animal. I. Comparison of the effects of acute and subacute vascular occlusion, Gut 17:671, 1976.
13. Matthews, J. G. W., and Parks, T. G.: Ischemic colitis in the experimental animal, II. Role of hypovolemia in the production of the disease, Gut 17:677, 1976.
14. Williams, L. F., and Wittenberg, J.: Ischemic colitis: A useful clinical diagnosis, but is it ischemic?, Ann. Surg. 182:439, 1975.
15. Meyers, M. A., Gharemaini, G. G., and Govoni, A. F.: Ischemic colitis associated with sigmoid volvulus: New observations, Am. J. Roentgenol. 128: 591, 1977.
16. Schwartz, S., and Boley, S. J.: Ischemic origin of ulcerative colitis associated with potentially obstructing lesions of the colon, Radiology 102:249, 1972.
17. Cotton, P. M., and Thomas, M.: Ischemic colitis and the contraceptive pill, Br. Med. J. 3:27, 1971.
18. Stillman, A. E., Weinberg, M., Mast, W. C., and Palpant, S.: Ischemic bowel disease attributable to ergot, Gastroenterology 72:1336, 1977.
19. Citron, B. P.: Personal communication.
20. Ernst, C. B., Hagihara, P. F., Dougherty, M. E., Sachatello, C. R., and Griffen, W. O.: Ischemic colitis incidence following abdominal aortic reconstruction. A prospective study, Surgery 80:417, 1976.

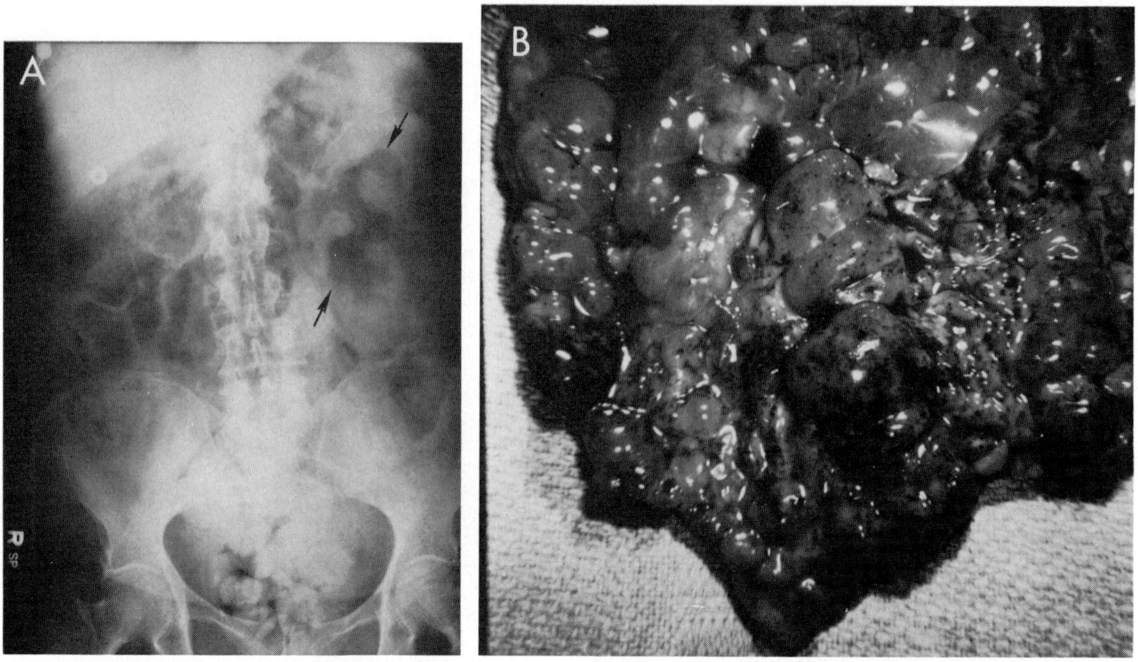

Fig 24–1. – **A,** woman, age 54, with heart disease and diabetes who presented with sudden onset of crampy abdominal pain and tenderness and watery diarrhea, strongly positive for occult blood. Sigmoidoscopy revealed wet gangrene of sigmoid. Abdominal film shows abnormal gas luminogram of distal transverse colon, with coarse thumbprinting *(arrows)* caused by edematous hemorrhagic masses of necrotic mucosa. **B,** photograph of surgical specimen gives vivid demonstration of gangrene of colonic mucosa with edema, hemorrhage, bleb and blue cyst formation, responsible for changes seen in plain film of abdomen.

Fig 24–2. – Male alcoholic, age 62, who had sudden onset of abdominal pain and bloody diarrhea. **A,** plain film, left lateral decubitus, shows straightening and narrowing of lower descending and sigmoid colon. **B,** barium enema 3 days later shows irregular narrowing of entire descending colon, mucosal edema and occasional thumbprinting.

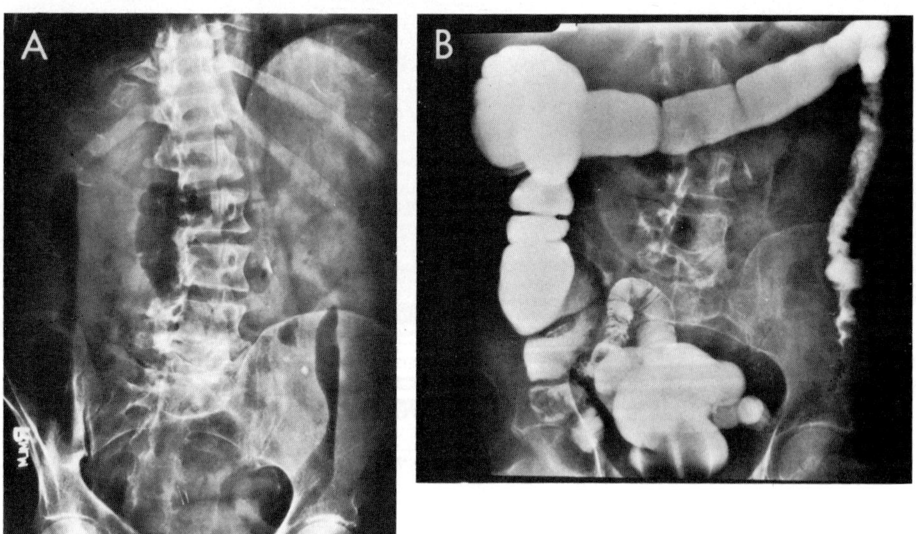

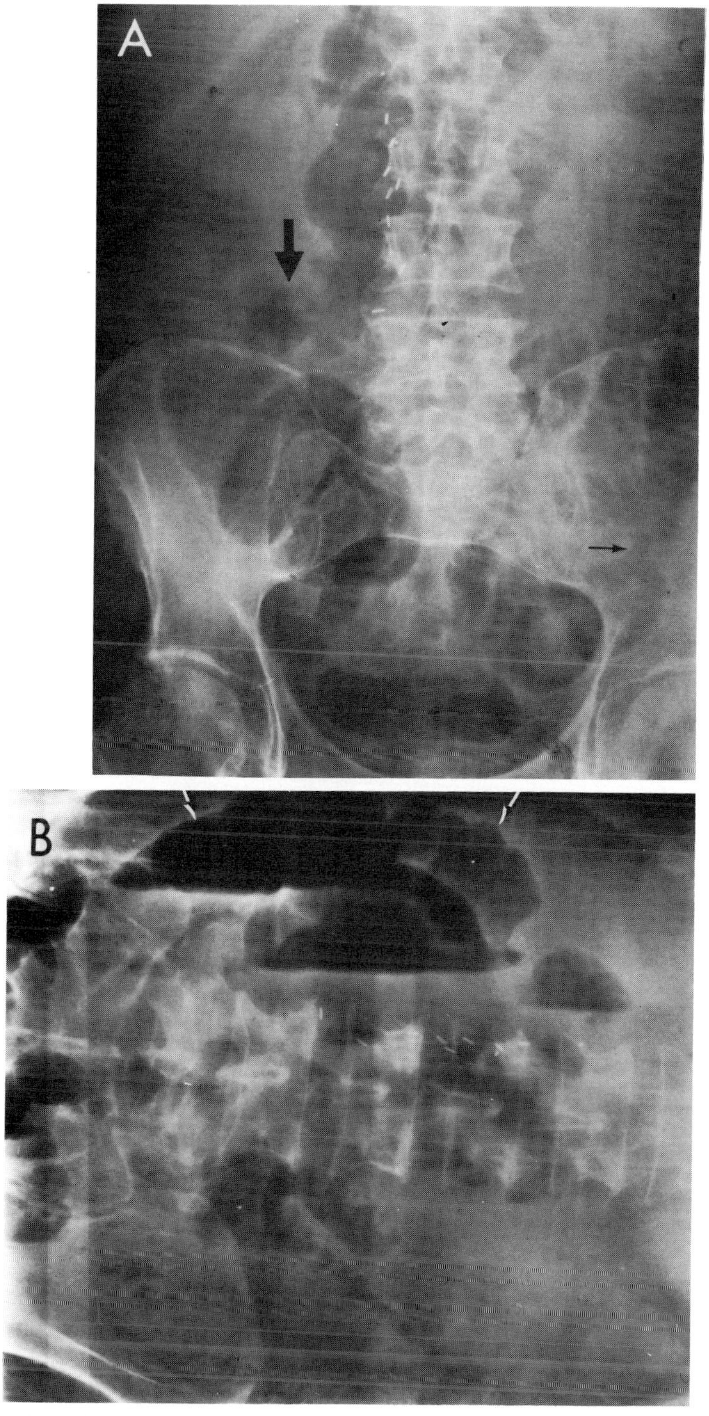

Fig 24–3. – Male alcoholic, age 64, with history of pneumonectomy for bronchogenic carcinoma followed by thrombosis of femoral artery for which a sympathectomy was performed. Presenting complaint was passage of blood from rectum and severe abdominal pain. Paracentesis yielded feculent material. Immediate exploration revealed gangrene of colon from cecum to sigmoid with multiple perforations and peritonitis. Patient did not survive. **A,** areas of dilatation and narrowing *(small arrow)* of colon as well as thumbprinting *(large arrow)*. **B,** left lateral decubitus film shows large amount of intraluminal fluid and mucosal irregularity in gas luminogram *(arrows)*.

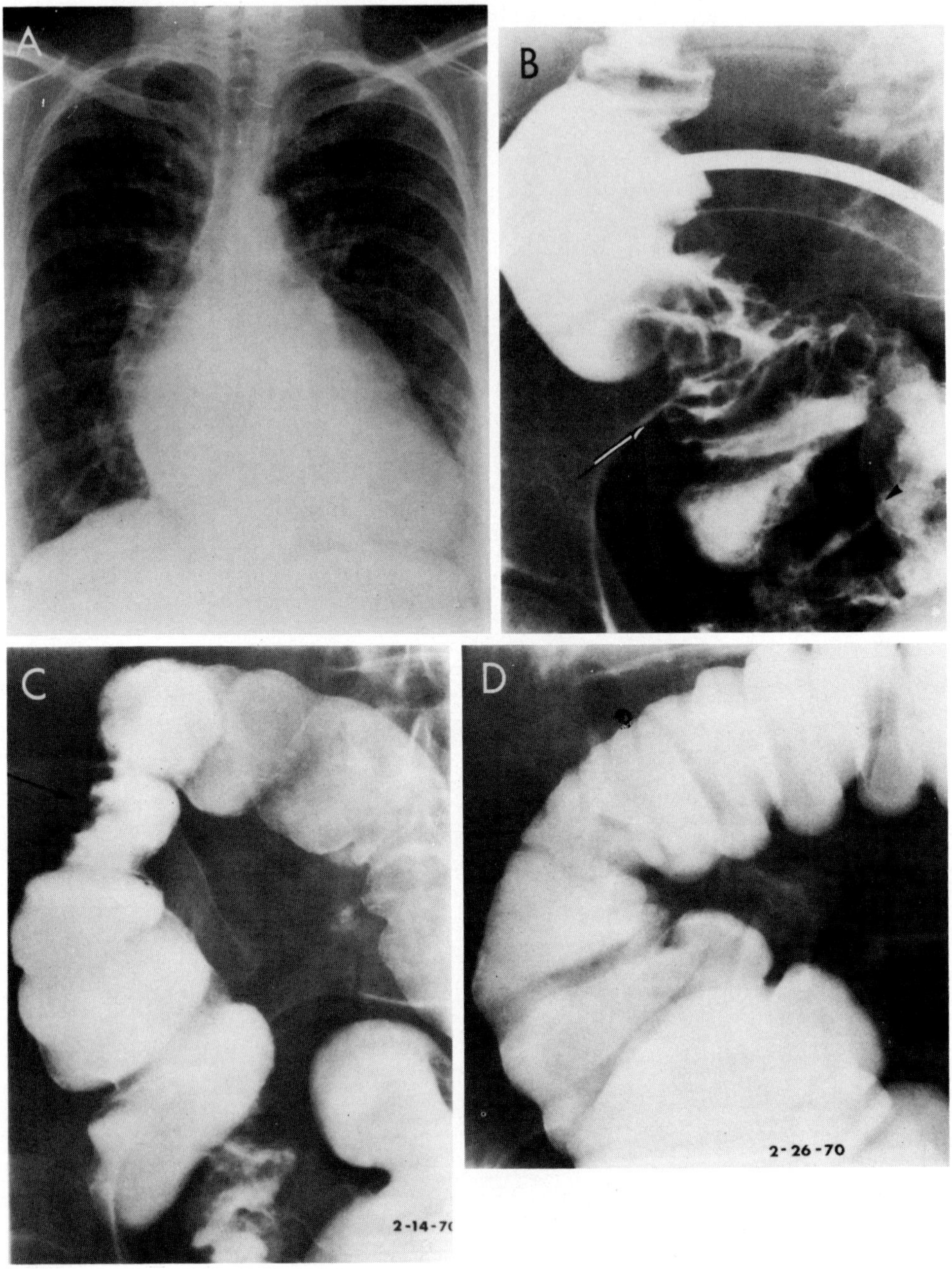

Fig 24–4.—Woman, age 44, with long history of rheumatic heart disease with mitral stenosis and insufficiency, and recent development of atrial fibrillation. **A,** chest film shows typical mitral configuration. Onset of diarrhea and melena occurred 2 days before barium enema was performed. **B,** severe spasm of ascending colon *(arrow)* and edema of ileocecal valve *(arrowhead)*. **C,** *arrow* points to area of thumbprinting and narrowing near hepatic flexure. Bleeding stopped 2 days after barium enema and patient became asymptomatic. **D,** repeat barium enema 12 days later shows reversion to normal. (Courtesy of Dr. Richard Fortin, Fontana, California.)

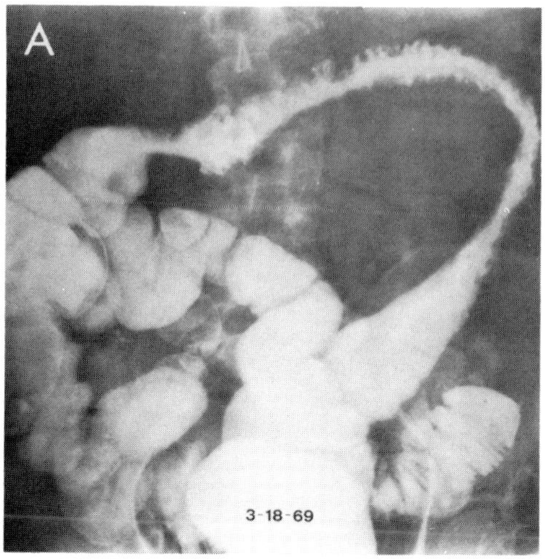

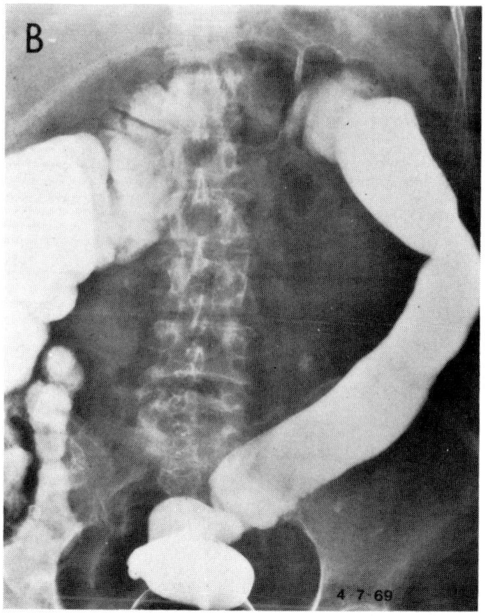

Fig 24–5.—Woman, age 64, with history of resection of sigmoid colon for adenocarcinoma 2 years previously. Patient developed gross rectal bleeding and lower abdominal pain. **A,** barium enema reveals narrowing, thumbprinting, rigidity and ulceration of much of left colon. **B,** repeat barium enema 3 weeks later reveals normal colon with foreshortening from previous surgery.

Fig 24–6.—Man, age 63, who had had resection of a gastric carcinoma 2 years previously. Bloody diarrhea and suprapubic pain developed. **A,** barium enema shows ulcerations, thumbprinting and mucosal edema. **B,** 2 months later colon has returned to normal.

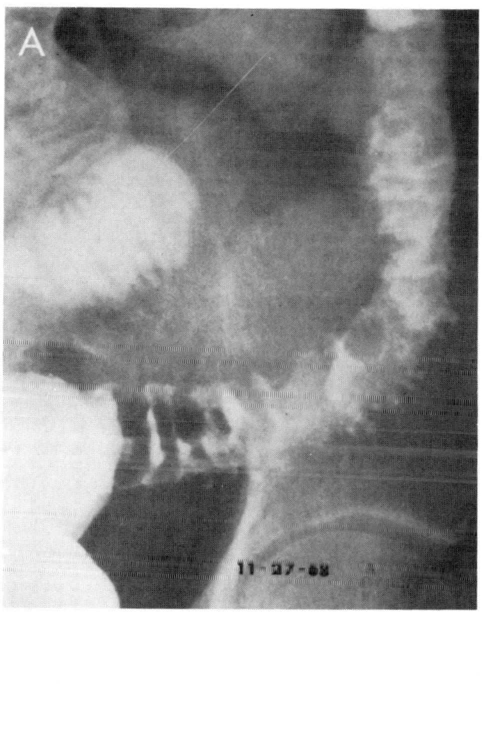

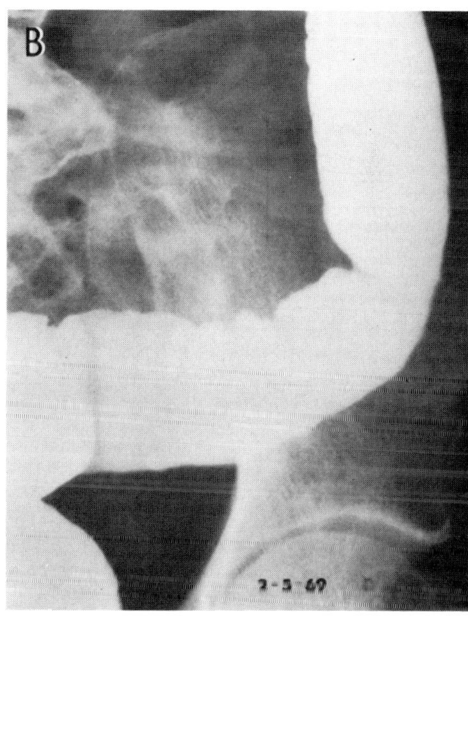

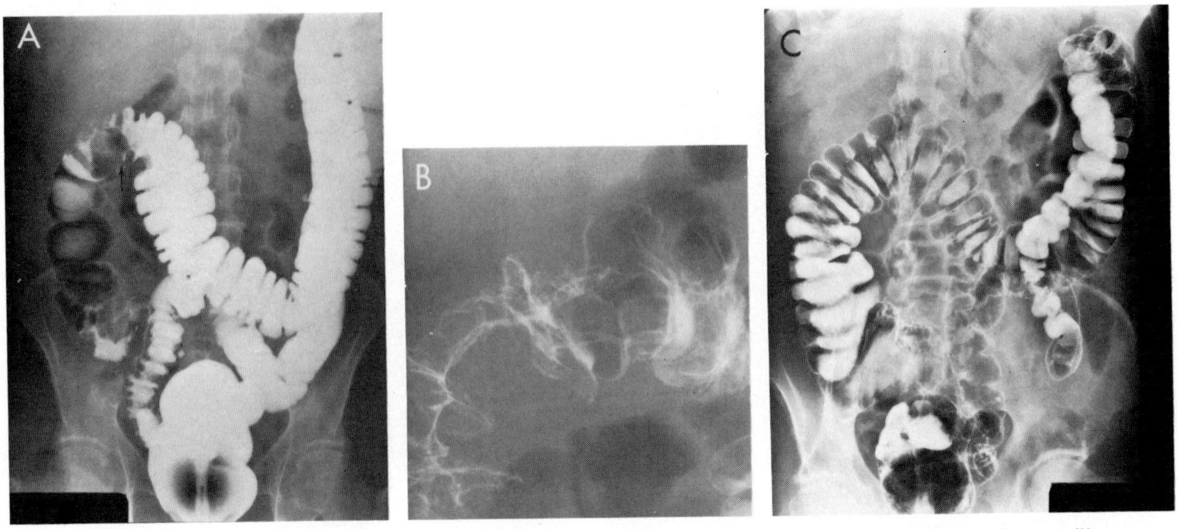

Fig 24–7.—In a man, age 63, with long-standing chronic obstructive airway disease, severe cramping abdominal pain and bloody diarrhea developed, with localized tenderness in right upper and lower quadrants. **A,** barium enema showing large polypoid filling defect in hepatic flexure *(arrow)* and deformity of cecum and ileocecal valve. **B,** spot film of hepatic flexure showing marginal filling defects and mucosal deformity simulating neoplasm. **C,** 3 weeks later barium enema shows complete return to normal. Patient asymptomatic.

Fig 24–8.—In a young woman who had been taking birth control pills for several years, bloody diarrhea developed. **A,** note spasm, thumbprinting *(arrow)* and deformity of cecum. **B,** 4 months later, colon has returned to normal. (Courtesy of Dr. I. J. Pincus, Beverly Hills, California.)

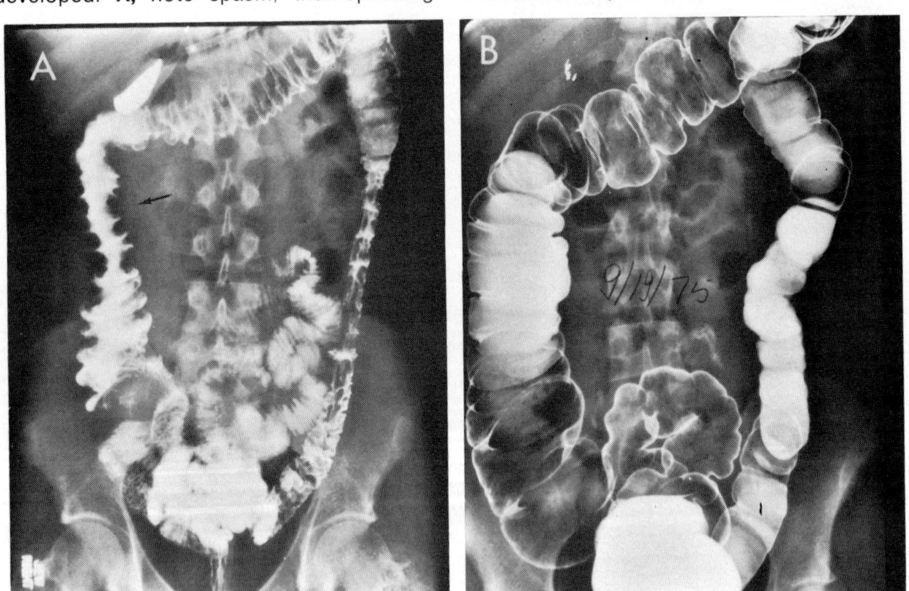

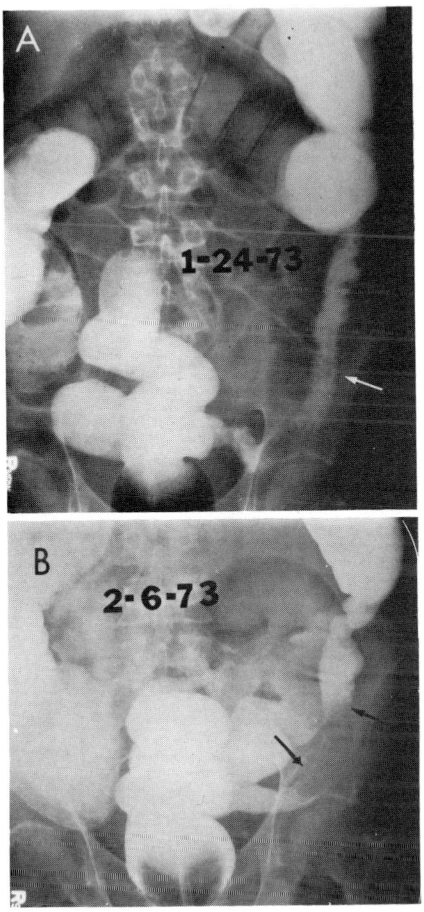

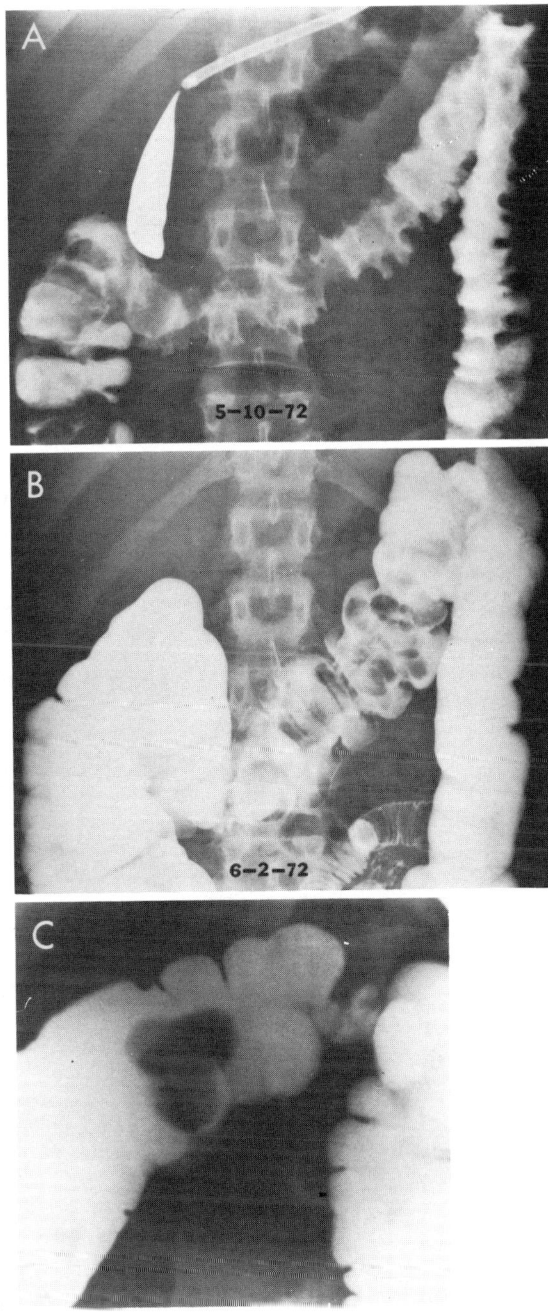

Fig 24–9 (left). – Man, age 55, with sudden onset of painful, bloody diarrhea. **A,** initial barium enema reveals multiple ulcerations, marked mucosal irregularity and irregular narrowing of distal descending and sigmoid colon *(arrow)*. **B,** 2 weeks later all that remains is diminished distensibility *(arrows)* of involved area.

Fig 24–10 (right). – A woman, age 26, an amphetamine user undergoing steroid therapy for sarcoidosis, admitted with rectal bleeding. **A,** marked thumbprinting with ulcerations and narrowing are noted in transverse and descending colon. **B,** 3 weeks later colon has returned nearly to normal. **C,** spot film of splenic flexure reveals area of localized narrowing and pseudodiverticulum formation. Lobulated filling defect is caused by fecal material.

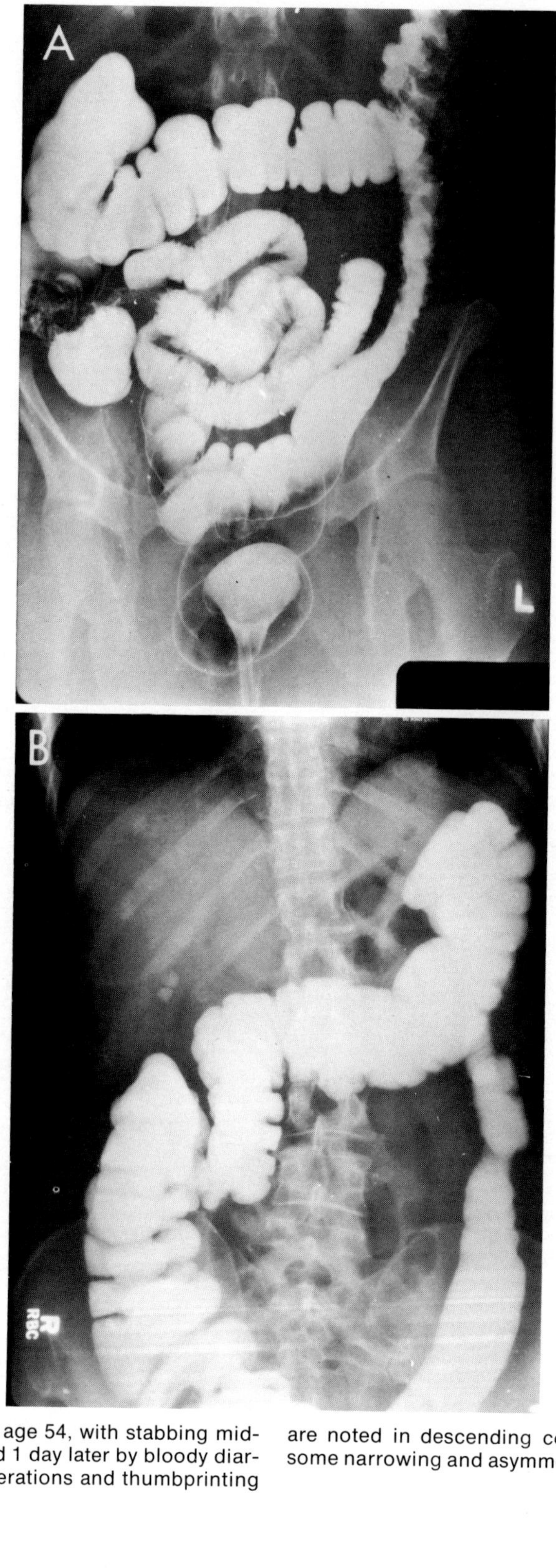

Fig 24–11.—Woman, age 54, with stabbing midepigastric pain followed 1 day later by bloody diarrhea. **A,** narrowing, ulcerations and thumbprinting are noted in descending colon. **B,** 12 days later, some narrowing and asymmetric deformity persist.

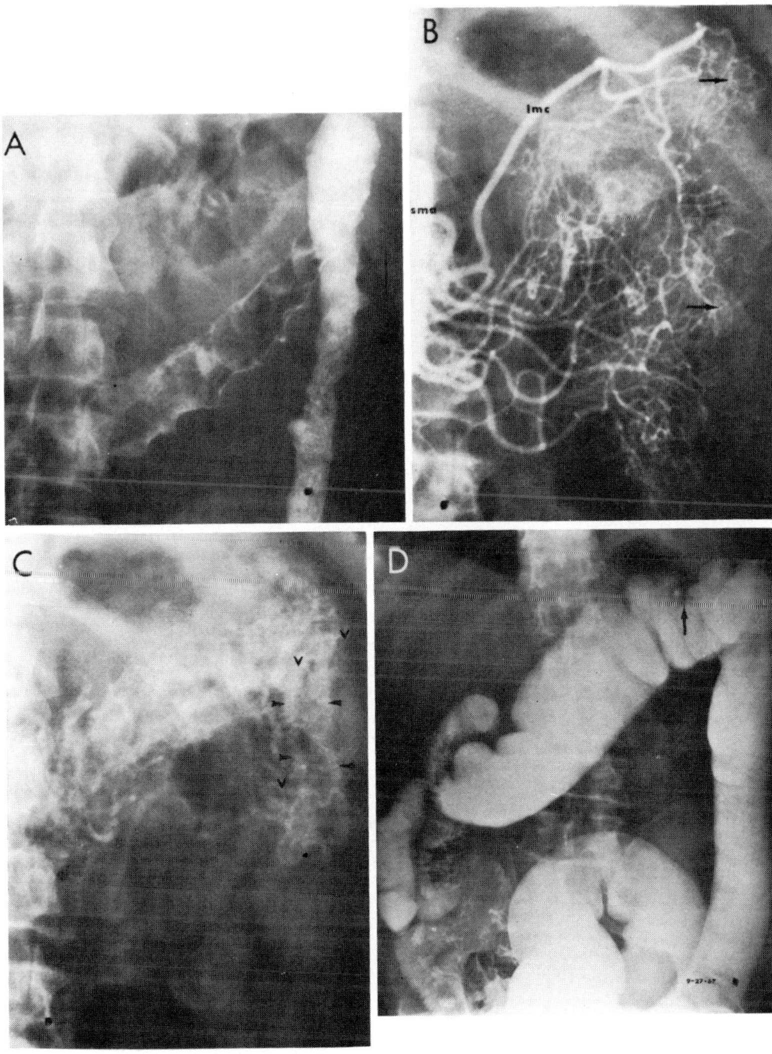

Fig 24–12. — Man, age 62, with several-day history of crampy abdominal pain and melena. **A,** extensive thumbprinting in transverse colon, narrowing and ulceration in descending colon. **B,** arterial phase of arteriogram shows slightly dilated left middle colic artery *(lmc)* and tortuous end arteries *(arrows)*. **C,** venous phase shows thickening of bowel wall *(arrowheads)* and tortuous, ectatic small draining veins *(v)*. **D,** 2 years later the only residual is localized narrowing with pseudodiverticulum in splenic flexure *(arrow)*.

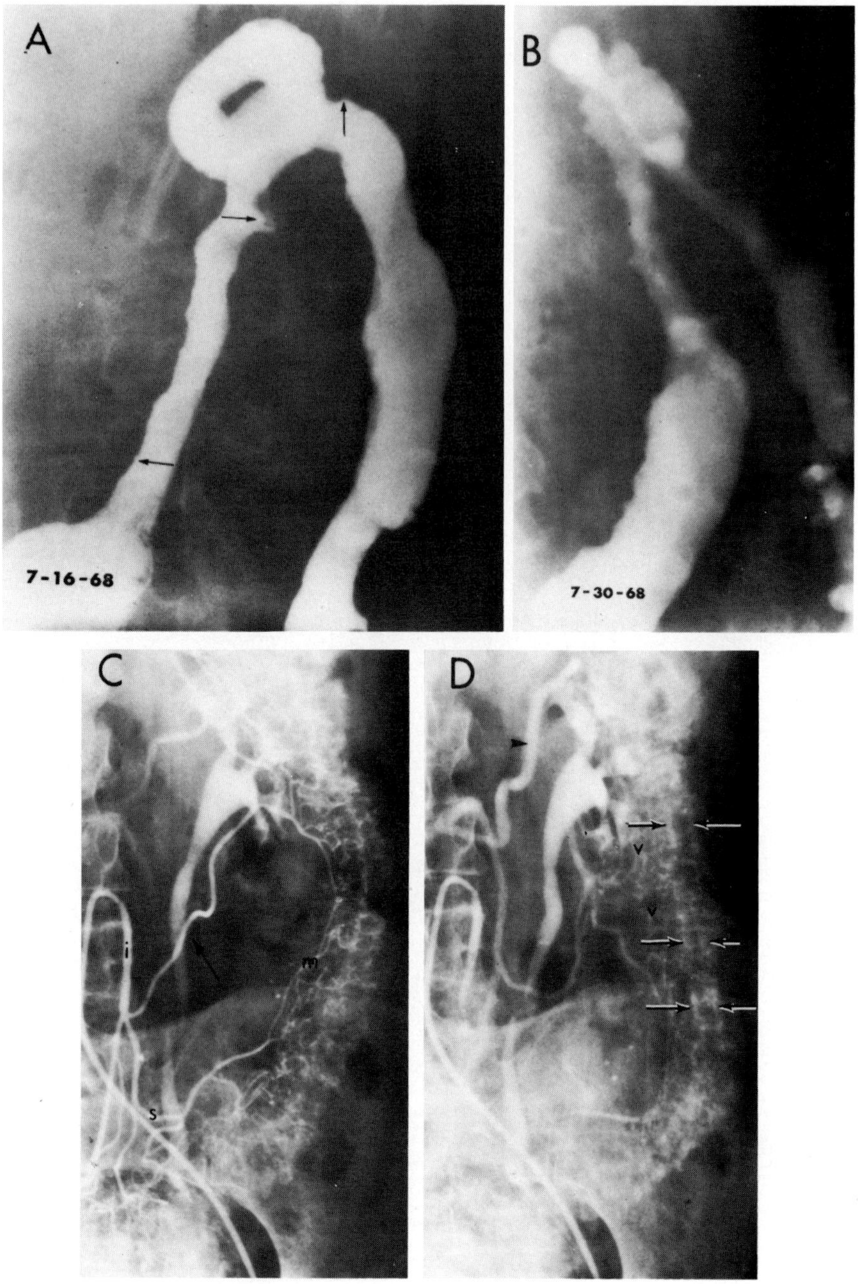

Fig 24–13. – Man, age 80, who had been experiencing left abdominal pain and intermittent melena for a year. Symptoms subsided 2 days before examination. **A,** splenic flexure shows irregular narrowing, ulcerations and pseudodiverticula *(arrows).* **B,** 2 weeks later pseudodiverticula are more strikingly seen and narrowing is more marked. **C,** normal major arteries are seen in angiogram. (*i* = inferior mesenteric artery; *m* = marginal artery of Drummond; *s* = sigmoidal artery; *arrow* = ascending left colic artery.) Slight tortuosity of end-arteries is noted. **D,** in venous phase small veins *(v)* are slightly irregular. Thickening of bowel wall is indicated by *arrows.* Increased density of middle colic vein indicated by *arrowhead.*

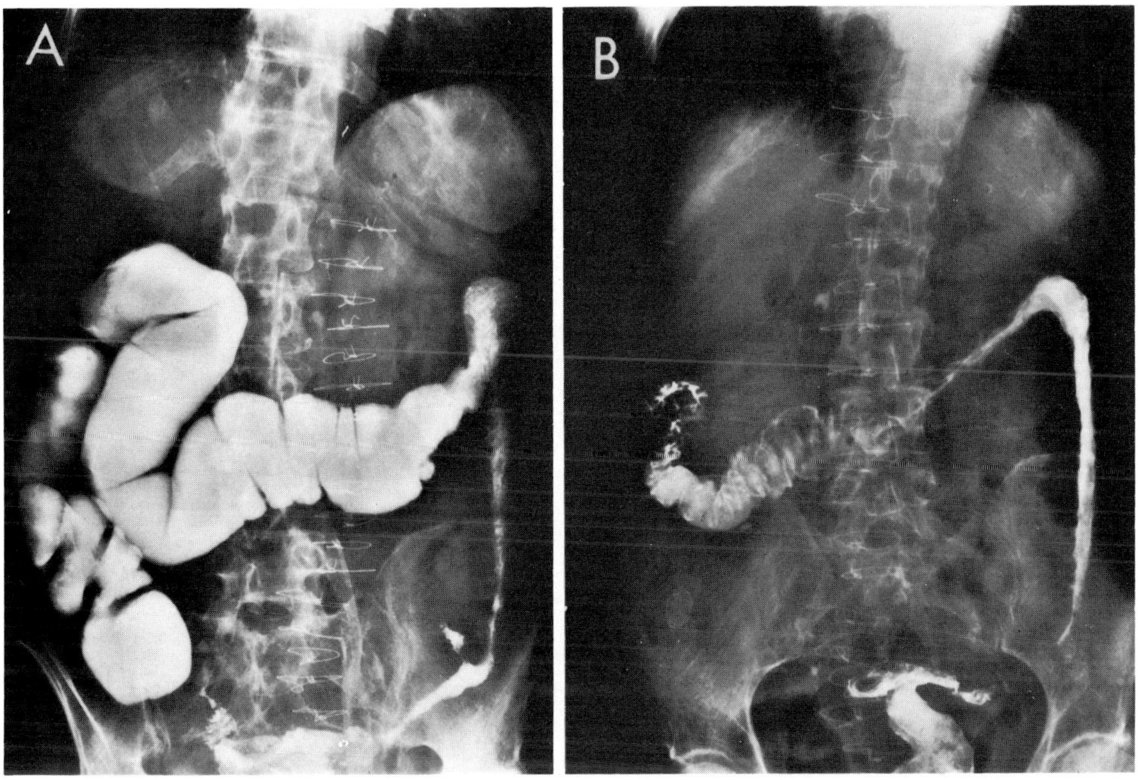

Fig 24–14.—Woman, age 66, who was followed for many years with chronic colon complaints for which many normal barium enemas were performed. After iliofemoral bypass graft for peripheral arterial disease, diarrhea and bleeding developed. **A,** barium enema 1 month following aortic surgery shows marked narrowing of descending and sigmoid colon, ulcerations and fistulous tract. **B,** 4 months later fistulous tract has healed, but ulceration and narrowing have extended to include left transverse colon. Ulcerations were confirmed by endoscopic biopsy. (Courtesy of B. Philip Citron, Glendale, California.)

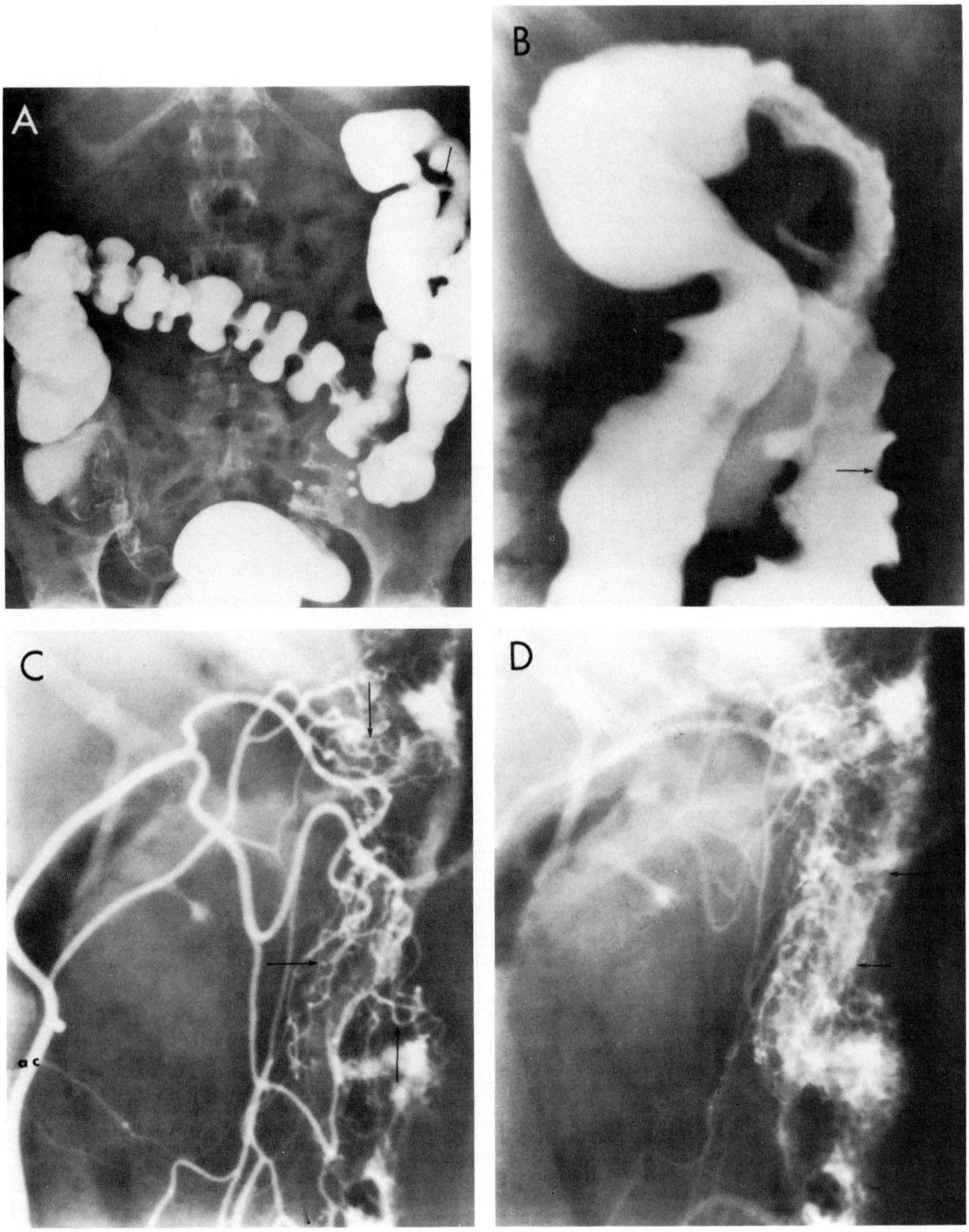

Fig 24–15.—Woman, age 53, with 2-year history of intermittent diarrhea, left upper quadrant pain and bloody stools. **A,** barium enema shows narrowing of splenic flexure with pseudodiverticulum *(arrow)*. **B,** spot film shows additional finding of thumbprinting *(arrow)*. **C,** arteriogram shows tortuosity and mild ectasia of end-arteries *(arrow)*. **D,** later phase shows no venous abnormalities. Thickened bowel wall is visible *(arrows)*. Note: Patient was operated on, with preoperative surgical diagnosis of diverticulitis. Pathologic diagnosis was ulcerative colitis. This points out the difficulty of arriving at an accurate diagnosis of ischemic colon disease by clinical or pathologic findings alone.

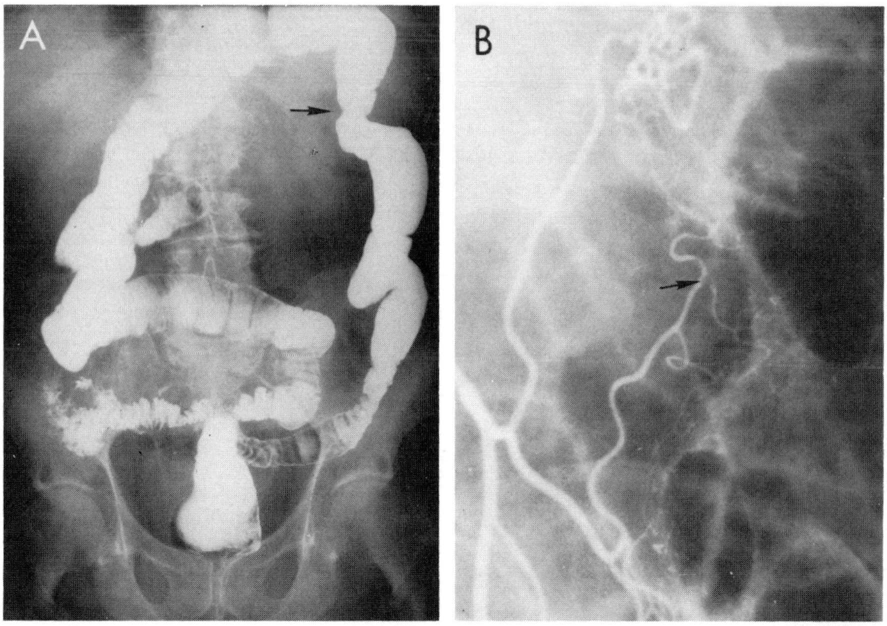

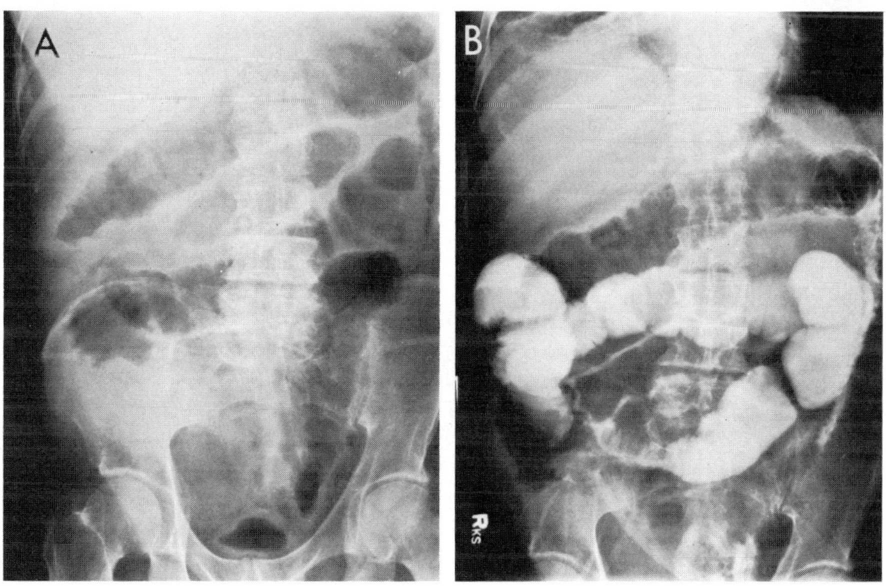

Fig 24–16 (top).—Man, age 74, who previously had had a partial small bowel resection for multiple small intestinal infarcts. He complained of rectal bleeding and diarrhea for several months. **A,** barium enema shows only a small area of narrowing in upper descending colon *(arrow)*. **B,** arteriogram shows thrombus at branch of marginal artery *(arrow)*. At surgery, a stricture with mucosal scarring was found. A small ulcer with underlying necrosis and organized thrombus in end artery was also noted.

Fig 24–17 (bottom).—Man, age 78, who complained of diarrhea and abdominal pain. No gross bleeding but stools were positive for occult blood. **A,** abdominal film shows thumbprinting of right colon, abnormal haustration of transverse colon and narrowing of descending colon. **B,** water-soluble contrast enema confirms findings above and shows numerous ulcerations of descending colon. Colon was resected. Specimen revealed numerous ulcerations, thickening of bowel wall and sealed perforation at splenic flexure. Large arteries were patent.

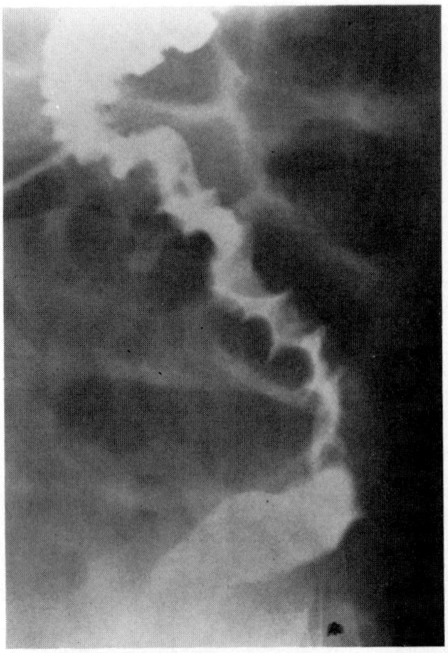

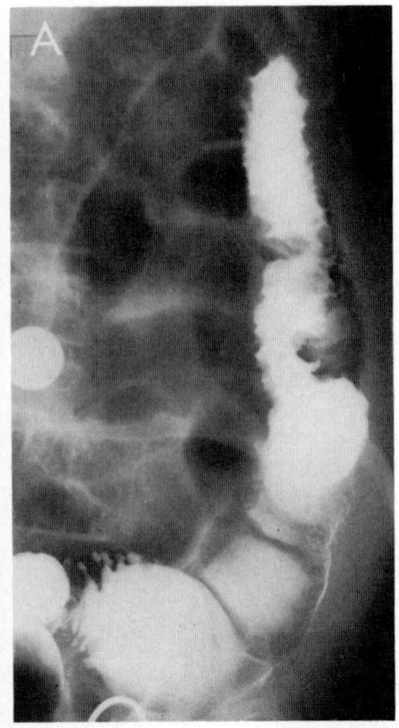

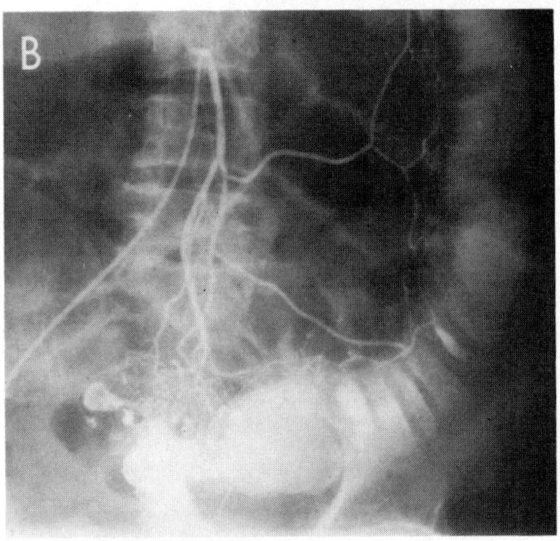

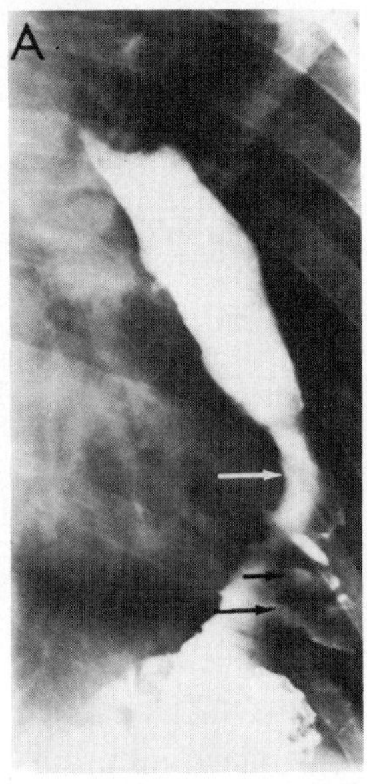

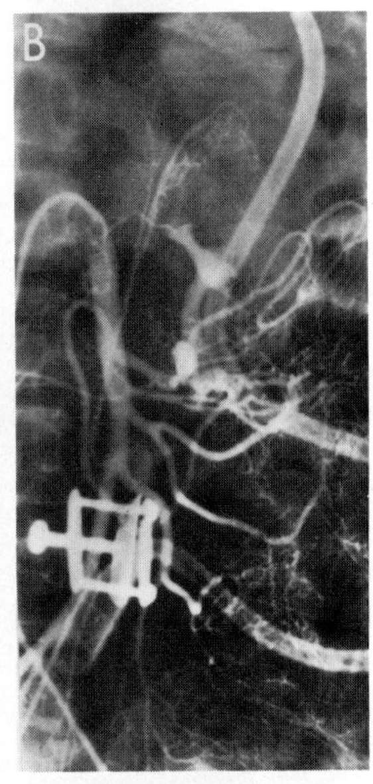

Fig 24–18 (top left).—Man, age 38, initially believed to have acute pancreatitis. When his pain became localized in left lower quadrant, a barium enema was performed. Marked thumbprinting and narrowing were noted in distal descending colon. Ulcerations were also noted in sigmoid. At surgery, gangrene of sigmoid colon with thrombosis of inferior mesenteric artery and vein was found. Subsequently the patient incurred multiple thromboembolic episodes. Hematologic studies revealed a severe hypercoagulation state.

Fig 24–19 (top right and bottom left).—Woman, age 84, with crampy abdominal pain for 6 days. Abdomen was distended and tender. Sigmoidoscopy showed inflamed mucosa. **A,** barium enema showed extensive ulcerations and thumbprinting in descending colon and sigmoid diverticula. **B,** angiography performed immediately after barium enema showed no significant vascular changes. Immediate operation showed thickened left colon, dusky with poor venous return. A colostomy was performed, but patient did not survive.

Fig 24–20 (bottom right).—Man, age 49, with carcinoma of esophagus treated with right colon interposition. **A,** follow-up barium study revealed unusually large pseudodiverticulum *(black arrows),* narrowing *(white arrow)* and ulcerations. **B,** superior mesenteric arteriogram showed complete interruption of blood supply to interposed colon segment.

Chapter 25

Lesions of the Ileocecal Valve

BRUCE D. SMITH, M.D.
WELLAND F. SHORT, M.D.

TO DISTINGUISH the prominent or unusual ileocecal valve from one that is involved with inflammatory or neoplastic disease may be difficult. Familiarity with the anatomy of the valve and with the circumstances that may lead to confusion frequently allows the radiologist to make a confident differentiation (Fig 25 – 1).

Radiologic Procedure

The ileocecal valve can be identified in the great majority of barium enema examinations.[1] During fluoroscopy, localization of the valve confirms cecal filling, enabling the examiner to avoid excessive reflux of barium into the ileum. With accurate identification of the valve, an intraluminal cecal filling defect can be properly identified and the normalcy of the valve itself assessed.

Prior to examination, thorough bowel preparation to eliminate fecal material and excess mucus is essential. Following catharsis, a high cleansing enema on the morning of the examination is recommended.

A low density (about 12% w/v), well-suspended barium, in our experience, is optimal for evaluation of the ileocecal region and the valve. Using an intermittent flow of barium allows the barium column to equilibrate throughout the colon and helps to avoid unwanted flooding of the ileum. Nonvisualization of the ileocecal valve, appendix or terminal ileum usually results from spasm before the cecum has filled. On occasion, if the cecum is filled with air or fluid, tilting the table partially erect or palpating the cecum may be necessary. If cecal filling cannot be confirmed, differentiation between spasm and organic obstruction by parenteral administration of an antispasmodic (e.g., glucagon[2] or propantheline bromide[3]) may be helpful.

If disease in the ileocecal region is suspected or the ileocecal valve is unusually prominent, visualization of the terminal ileum is essential. When no reflux occurs with the barium enema, orally administered barium should be followed to the ileocecal region and spot films obtained. Evaluation of the ileocecal valve is improved if concomitant air insufflation of the colon or barium enema is used.[4, 5]

To completely evaluate the ileocecal valve by barium enema, it should be viewed in more than one projection during varying degrees of external compression and evaluated on both filled and postevacuation films. Although the double contrast barium enema may give more detail of the valve, it is more difficult and time consuming, and we use it as

This chapter was adapted from Short, W. F., Smith, B. D., and Hoy, R. J.: Roentgenologic evaluation of the prominent or unusual ileocecal valve, Med. Radiogr. and Photogr. 52:2, 1976.

the initial study only in patients with gastrointestinal blood loss, unexplained anemia or symptoms suggestive of a colon polyp or malignancy.

Normal Valve

The ileocecal valve is located at the junction of the cecum and ascending colon, marked by the first complete haustral fold above the cecal tip (Fig 25–2). With the appendix filled,[6] the valve is noted in 90% of adults to be on the same side of the colon as the appendix (Figs 25–3 and 25–4). The valve is medial or posteromedial in 90% of instances, 7–8% being posterior, 1% posterolateral or lateral and the remainder anterior (Fig 25–5).[1,7] The position of the valve may vary somewhat with changes in cecal filling or patient position.[8]

The ileocecal valve may be papillary or bilabial in appearance. The papillary shape has a mound with a central orifice seen more often with incomplete colonic distention, whereas the bilabial shape is seen with complete colon distention (Fig 25–6).

Radiologically the valve shape is determined by both the degree of distention and the projection in which it is viewed (Figs 25–1 to 25–9). En face, it appears as a papillary structure with mucosal folds radiating from a central ostium, a "rosette" (Fig 25–7), or it may have a spindle shape with a central orifice (Fig 25–8).

The profile view, in which the valve usually is viewed, has various shapes based on the shape, thickness and length of the lips, to which terms such as spindle, funnel, shark mouth, ampullary and polypoid rosette have been applied.[1] The valve lips are smoothly marginated, club-shaped structures, which may be multilobular in shape, the upper lip generally being slightly longer than the lower (Fig 25–11). Occasionally there may be underdevelopment or absence of the lower lip (Fig 25–10), and rarely of both lips, resulting in loss of functional valve competence.

The valve labia consist of muscular, submucosal and mucosal layers. The muscularis is primarily from the ileum, with colonic mucosa on its outer surface and ileal mucosa on the inner surface, with the transition at the free margin of the valve. Some fat is present normally in the submucosa of the valve in an adult. The normal labial thickness and shape are variable (Fig 25–12). This, in addition to the effect of radiographic magnification, external compression and cecocolonic distention, make valve size alone unreliable as a criterion of abnormality (Figs 25–1, 25–9, 25–12 to 25–15).

Two crescentic folds or frenula, one on each side of the valve, are noted where the lips coalesce; these extend partially around the cecocolonic junction, with the colon distended or the specimen fixed in formalin. At the valve the frenula divide into arches to both the upper and lower lips. The transverse diameter of the frenula of the upper lip is shorter, and with colonic distention it tenses first, so that the lower lip rests against it as a flap valve. If the upper lip is too lax, the lower lip may have inadequate contact with its undersurface, and incompetence and reflux may then occur. Extreme laxity of the upper lip, resulting in retrograde prolapse of the lower lip into the terminal ileum, was reported by Rigler and Lasser.[9] Owing to the variability and frequent incomplete development of both the frenula and valve labia, valve function of the ileocecal junction is seldom completely competent.

The ileocecal valve functions both as a valve and as a sphincter. The sphincteric function has become important to an understanding of the physiologic role of the ileocecal valve in regulating passage of ileal contents to the colon. The valvular function serves to prevent bacterial contamination of the ileum by colon content.

Although true valvular function exists only with the colon distended and the valvular labia tensed, the fact that reflux of barium to the ileum during a barium enema occurs does not necessarily indicate physiologic incompetence of the ileocecal valve. Absolute competence occurs in only 5% of patients during a barium enema. With large bowel obstruction, physiologic competence of the valve from elevated intracolonic pressure and bowel distention creates the potential for cecal perforation,[10] although this is infrequent.[11] When complete incompetence exists without appreciable colonic distention, the possibility of inflammatory disease or chronic laxative abuse affecting the valve should be considered.

Conditions Simulating Disease of the Valve

LIPOMATOSIS

Prominence of the ileocecal valve usually is the result of a large accumulation of unencapsulated fat in the submucosa of the labia, which may simulate inflammatory or neoplastic disease. This condition, termed lipomatosis, is not well defined and is not considered pathologic. Its incidence is unknown, but Zettergren[12] found large amounts of subcutaneous fat in five of 43 adult cadavers, suggesting that it is relatively more common than some surgical reports suggest.[13, 14] Lipomatosis appears to affect women twice as often as men[12, 14] and is most common after age 40,[13] increasing with age,[16] and there is some correlation with the amount of retroperitoneal and subserosal fat present.[12]

The cause of accumulation of a large amount of fat in the ileocecal valves of otherwise normal, nonobese persons is unclear. If prolapse of ileal mucosa is present, lipomatosis could be the result of relative ischemia with fat deposition.[17, 18]

The clinical importance of lipomatosis of the ileocecal valve is uncertain. An association of a prominent valve with bloating and colicky pain with tenderness over the valve has been described.[13-15,18-23] Stark[16], however, believes that the symptoms could be attributed to other causes, and the presence of edema, congestion, low-grade inflammation and occasional superficial mucosal ulceration in resected specimens with lipomatosis suggests that it may cause symptoms. Castleman[24] thought that intermittent ileocecal intussusception, and Berk et al.[25] that narrowing of the valve orifice, could cause partial obstruction.

Although an association between massive hemorrhage and mucosal erosion of a lipomatous ileocecal valve has been reported,[12, 18, 21, 22] Corry et al.,[26] in reporting five cases of massive gastrointestinal hemorrhage attributed to cecal erosion, noted involvement of the ileocecal valve in one, without apparent valve enlargement or mucosal prolapse noted.

Although vascular dysplasia with mucosal erosion is an important cause of chronic hemorrhage in the cecum and ascending colon,[27] no definite dysplasias specifically involving the ileocecal valve have been described. Selective mesenteric angiography should precede exploratory surgery, if a prominent ileocecal valve is considered a potential bleeding site, to exclude a vascular dysplasia.

Concern over differentiation of a prominent normal ileocecal valve and an ileocecal tumor has led to numerous surgical explorations, and to resection of the valve in some cases.[13, 18, 28] Strauch et al.[29] diagnosed lipomatosis of the valve by colonoscopy with biopsy and believed that radiologic differentiation of a benign and malignant tumor of the ileocecal valve cannot be made radiologically. However, if a prominent but otherwise normal-appearing ileocecal valve is properly studied by radiologic means, we believe that further evaluation is rarely necessary.[15, 25]

Radiologic determination of whether an ileocecal valve is to be considered abnormal should not be based on size alone as measured on the radiograph, as this varies on radiographs and spot films, as well as with compression and colonic distention. The valve also may appear large in double contrast radiographs or those made with low density barium, as it is seen in its entirety.

A papillary-shaped valve, particularly if located posteriorly, may be mistaken for a mass unless the valve ostium, rosette pattern or terminal ileum is identified. Rarely a tumor within the lumen could cause the valve to appear prominent and yet normal. The borders of a normal valve may be lobulated, but the mucosal surface should be smooth. Rarely the valve surface may have multiple grapelike nodules, which require surgery for diagnosis.[25] The valve lips normally may be unequal in size (see Fig 25–14), but localized enlargement of the labia is a suspicious finding. Changeability of a prominent valve, with compression and colonic filling, will help to confirm that the valve is normal.

PROLAPSE

Prolapse of ileal mucosa alone can cause the ileocecal valve to appear prominent and it is frequently associated with lipomatosis of the valve. Although its incidence as a sole cause of a prominent ileocecal valve appears infrequent, several such cases have been reported.[1, 7, 30] Fleischner and Bernstein[7] found several ileocecal valves with the transition of ileal to colonic mucosa on the colonic portion of the labia and not at the free margin.

When pronounced, prolapse of ileal mucosa, like lipomatosis, may be confused with a tumor,[10] but marked change in size or volume not attributable to differences in compression or bowel distention is noted with prolapse (see Fig 25–15). In fact, valve size was thought by Nagasako and Takemoto[31] to reflect muscular activity in the terminal ileum. It is difficult and rarely important to distinguish lipomatosis from mucosal prolapse. Mucosal prolapse alone does not appear to lead to intussusception in an adult. If the presence of a tumor cannot be excluded, endoscopy or surgery may be necessary for diagnosis.

The rosette-fold pattern, viewed en face, was thought by Fleischner and Bernstein[7] to indicate mucosal prolapse, but this appearance is common in normal papillary-shaped valves, indicating valve pliability and intact mucosa.

Retrograde prolapse of the valvular mucosa, noted on occasion, may be due to increased hydrostatic pressure during a barium enema examination[32] (Fig 25–17). More unusual is retrograde prolapse of the lower lip of the valve, which should not be confused with an ileal tumor.[9]

EDEMA

In most cases edema of the ileocecal valve is associated with lipomatosis,[17] a recently reduced intussusception or inflammatory disease of the large intestines. Edema of unknown origin is an unusual cause of a prominent ileocecal valve, although Debray et al.[33] reported two cases associated with recurrent diarrhea and weight loss.

Benign Tumors

LIPOMAS

Lipomas are true encapsulated tumors, distinct from lipomatosis, which has no true capsule. They are common in the large intestines, especially the cecum, and are the most common tumor of the ileocecal valve.[25] Their peak incidence is in the sixth and seventh decades with no notable sex preference. Most are asymptomatic, but they may cause obstruction, intussusception or bleeding.

Radiologically they may appear similar to other types of tumors. Being encapsulated, they are confined to only one portion of the valve and appear smooth and pliable (Fig 25–18). In the colon they frequently are multiple and usually are pedunculated, occasionally arising from the valve itself (Fig 25–19). Use of a water enema following the barium enema, as suggested by Margulis and Jovanovich,[37] may identify the high fat content characteristic of a lipoma. Generally, however, when a localized enlargement or pedunculated lesion of the ileocecal valve is present on radiographs, evaluation with endoscopy or surgery is required.

OTHER BENIGN TUMORS

Benign adenomatous tumors of the ileocecal valve are unusual[10, 34, 38, 39] (Fig 25–20). Tumors arising from the valve may be of clinical importance as a cause of intussusception or obstruction. Radiologic differentiation of a benign adenomatous tumor, malignant tumor or lipoma may be impossible, although the lipoma is the most common and tends to be smooth, whereas an adenoma or polypoid carcinoma usually will have a rougher surface.

Fibromas arising from the ileocecal valve are rare.[34, 40, 41] These lesions are of intramural origin, with no distinctive radiologic appearance, in this location. The presence of a smooth, sessile, polypoid mass localized to one portion of the valve would be expected.

One case of ganglioneuroma of the ileocecal valve has been reported by Haff and San Diego.[42] The lesion was poorly defined, with an ulcerated nodular surface, suggestive of malignancy, although all reported intestinal gangliomas have been benign.[42]

Malignant Tumors

CARCINOMA

Adenocarcinoma is the most common malignant tumor of the large intestine, as well as of the ileocecal valve. The incidence of carcinoma of the valve differs with the definition of an ileocecal tumor. Most authorities include carcinoma arising in the cecum and ascending colon affecting the valve, as the exact site of origin usually is difficult to ascertain (Figs 25–21 and 25–22). Careful studies by Wapshaw[43] and Berk et al.[44] indicate that 6.5–15% of carcinomas in the ascending colon and hepatic flexure arise on the ileocecal valve. In Wapshaw's series, about 1.5% of all malignancies of the large intestine were ileocecal lesions.[43]

Early symptoms often are vague and vary from digestive upset to severe abdominal pain. Anemia, rectal bleeding and weight loss usually occur.[43, 45] A palpable mass in the right lower abdomen most often will be present. Obstruction is a frequent complication, which usually occurs late in the course of carcinoma of the ileocecal valve, as the ileal contents are fluid.

Ileocecal carcinomas are classified by gross and histologic type: columnar adenocarcinoma, either polypoid or annular stenosing; and colloid, a bulky fungating type, the least common type.[46] Classification of ileocecal valve carcinoma is also made according to the area of involvement: (1) cecovalvular or colovalvular (most common), (2) ileovalvular and (3) valvular (least common). Spread of tumor to the terminal ileum is infrequent, probably due to the absence of lymphatic channels between the colonic and ileal side of the valve, noted by Bargen et al.[47] (see Fig 25–21).

Carcinoma of the cecal region frequently is misdiagnosed with barium enema studies[48] (Figs 25–23 and 25–24). In a series of 708 cases of colonic malignancy, McSwain et al.[49] noted radiographic accuracy of 75% in cecal lesions, compared with 90% accuracy from the ascending colon to the rectosigmoid junction. Allcock[50] in 123 cases found that 14 (11%) of colon cancers were overlooked or misdiagnosed, and nine of these were in the cecal area. Several factors may contribute to the difficulty in diagnosing cecal and ileocecal valve tumors. Among these are (1) incomplete filling of the cecum with barium;

(2) presence of fecal residue, mucus or gas; (3) failure to penetrate the cecum with x-rays owing to the large diameter of the colon, insufficient kilovoltage, excessive barium density or absence of compression; (4) confusion of a tumor with the ileocecal valve; and (5) uncertainty caused by nonneoplastic lesions (e.g., chronic appendiceal abscess) and postoperative changes (e.g., as inverted appendiceal stump)[42] (see Fig 25–4).

Carcinoma of the ileocecal valve, in the reported cases reviewed and in our cases, did not appear as a prominent but otherwise normal valve. Signs of malignancy included (1) destruction or marked irregularity of the mucosal pattern with or without ulceration (see Fig 25–21), (2) a filling defect (see Fig 25–23, A), (3) a mass with overhanging edges (see Fig 25–22), (4) an annular growth or stricture (see Fig 25–24) and (5) a valve with a nodular surface (Fig 25–25). Berk et al.,[25] however, noted that in infrequent instances lipomatosis may be nodular, but never shaggy or moth-eaten. The tumor rarely remains confined to the valve but spreads to the adjacent cecum, ascending colon or both—rarely to the terminal ileum (Fig 25–26). Visualizing the ileum is necessary to confirm tumor location and to detect ileal involvement.

CARCINOID TUMOR

Carcinoid tumors frequently arise in the ileocecal region and on occasion in the ileocecal valve itself.[52-58] Metastasis of this chromaffin cell tumor may occur from the gastrointestinal tract, although rarely from the appendix.[58-60] When metastasis to the liver is present, the carcinoid syndrome may occur as a result of secretion of serotonin by the tumor. Most lesions appear after the fifth decade,[61] and long-term survival is not uncommon, even with distant spread.[58]

In reported cases of carcinoid of the ileocecal valve, the valve varies radiologically from a prominent but otherwise normal valve[10, 54] to being indistinguishable from that with primary carcinoma.[57] The terminal ileum is a common site of carcinoids. In at least one reported case, a carcinoid of the ileum was completely contained within the lumen of the valve,[52] which may explain the prominent but otherwise normal appearance of the valve (Fig 25–27).[54] Since a carcinoid tumor may be contained in the ileocecal valve lumen, it is important to evaluate the terminal ileum if a prominent ileocecal valve is noted (Fig 25–28). Also, with suspicion of ileocecal carcinoid, the remaining small bowel should be evaluated by barium meal, as the small bowel is a common site of metastasis. If clinical or radiographic findings are suggestive of a carcinoid tumor, abdominal angiography should be considered to help confirm the diagnosis of these highly vascular tumors and reveal other areas of involvement, including hepatic metastasis.[62]

LYMPHOMA AND LYMPHOSARCOMA

Lymphosarcoma involving the cecum and ileoceal valve is not uncommon (Fig 25–29). In contrast to carcinoma, the terminal ileum usually is also involved,[25] the ileal involvement being less localized than with either carcinoma or carcinoid (Fig 25–30). Its appearance is of diffuse infiltration, multiple nodules, discrete polypoid lesions and ulcerating masses.[63] On occasion, differentiation from other primary and metastatic tumors or inflammatory disease, particularly regional enteritis, may be difficult (Fig 25–31).

Because lymphosarcoma is a medullary tumor, it may become large before symptoms of obstruction are present. However, lymphoma or lymphosarcoma involving the terminal ileum occasionally acts as a lead point and causes ileocolic intussusception earlier in its course (Fig 25–32).[40] Hemorrhage, perforation, fistula formation and malabsorption also may occur.

Inflammatory Disease

Radiologic changes in the ileocecal valve associated with inflammatory disease of the intestines alone are not diagnostic but are important when considered as a part of the total radiologic and clinical picture.

REGIONAL ENTERITIS (CROHN'S DISEASE)

Golden[64] in 1943 described "edema" of the ileocecal valve on a barium enema in a patient with regional enteritis with terminal ileitis. The cause of the enlargement was not recognized owing to the competent valve and nonvisualization of the ileum. Golden recommended, and it is still relevant, that the terminal ileum be evaluated if a prominent ileocecal valve on barium enema is noted.

The radiologic appearance of the ileocecal valve in Crohn's disease depends on the extent of involvement and duration of the disease. Early in the course of granulomatous colitis, ileocolitis or disease restricted to the terminal ileum, the valve may appear normal. Later the valve enlarges, often as the result of fatty hypertrophy (Fig 25–33). Sinus tracts may develop and traverse the valve[65, 66] (Fig 25–34). Later the lips may atrophy, with gaping of the valve ostium (Fig 25–35).

ULCERATIVE COLITIS

Radiologically the ileocecal valve in ulcerative colitis may be normal, atrophic or (least often) enlarged (Fig 25–36). The valve in regional enteritis by comparison tends to be enlarged, with a narrowed ostium. A gaping incompetent valve, with or without atrophy of the labia, is frequent in ulcerative colitis[65] (see Fig 25–36). With backwash ileitis, valvular incompetence usually is present. The valve in ulcerative colitis rarely contains sinus tracts, as in granulomatous disease[65] (Fig 25–37).

AMEBIASIS

A contracted, cone-shaped cecum and skip lesions of the colon, sparing the terminal ileum, are well-known features of amebiasis (Figs 25–38 and 25–39). The frequency of involvement of the ileocecal valve in this disease recently has been emphasized. In five of eight cases reported by Kolawole and Lewis,[67] and in all seven cases reported by Balikian et al.,[68] the cecum was coned and the valve was gaping and incompetent, resembling ulcerative colitis (see Fig 25–39). Mucosal necrosis and ulceration may occur, and amebomas and fistula formation in the cecum may be present. The appearance may suggest either tumor or Crohn's disease of the colon, if terminal ileal changes are not demonstrated.

TUBERCULOSIS

The ileocecal valve area is that most affected in intestinal tuberculosis with involvement of both colon and ileum. Initially the valve is usually competent owing to spasm. The inflammation causes irregularity of the valvular mucosa and thickening of the labia, which later become distorted and eroded, resulting in a gaping orifice. The ileum develops mucosal ulceration and nodularity, as well as rigidity or narrowing of the terminal ileum, and fistulas may be present.[69] With distortion of the valve and narrowing of the terminal ileum, the "inverted umbrella" appearance of the valve, described by Fleischner,[7] develops (Fig 25–40). This appearance was considered specific for ileocecal tuberculosis but may result from other granulomatous diseases (Fig 25–41); Crohn's disease should be included in the differential diagnosis, with involvement of the terminal ileum and proximal colon.[71] A chest x-ray may be helpful, as gastrointestinal tuberculosis, at least in the United States, usually follows pulmonary tuberculosis.[72]

OTHER INFLAMMATORY DISEASES

The ileocecal valve may be affected by a variety of inflammatory diseases. Fungal diseases (e.g., histoplasmosis,[73] blastomycosis[74]) may resemble tuberculosis (see Fig 25–41). Other diseases, e.g., typhoid fever,[75] ascariasis (infestation with roundworms),[76] and schistosomiasis,[77] may in some instances resemble those of more common diseases (e.g., Crohn's disease) radiologically.

Cathartic colon, a result of chronic laxative abuse, may resemble chronic burned-out ulcerative colitis, although the cecum generally is more distended than in ulcerative colitis, with loss of haustrations and atrophy. Atrophy and incompetence of the ileocecal valve result,[78] and narrowing, with loss of a normal mucosal pattern in the terminal ileum, may occur (Fig 25–42).

An appendiceal abscess with compression of the cecum, nonfilling of the appendix, distortion of the ileocecal valve and displacement of the terminal ileum may be evident on barium enema[79] (Fig 25–43). Endometriosis also may involve the appendix and cecum and, if symptomatic, may suggest appendicitis.[28]

Summary and Conclusions

A prominent ileocecal valve visualized during a barium enema examination usually is the result of lipomatosis or occasionally of mucosal prolapse of the valve. On rare occasions a prominent valve may be caused by a tumor. It would be most unusual for a carcinoma of the ileocecal valve to appear prominent but be otherwise normal, although a tumor of the lumen of the valve that arises from the ileal mucosa (e.g., a carcinoid) may have this appearance.

Tumors other than carcinoma arising from the colonic side of the valve always cause localized enlargement of the valve and marked asymmetry of the valvular labia, or give rise to polypoid lesions.

Enlargement of the valve can be secondary to inflammatory disease, particularly Crohn's disease. Because of this, and to exclude the rare tumor arising in the lumen of the valve, it is essential that the terminal ileum be evaluated whenever an unusually prominent ileocecal valve is encountered with a barium enema, which may necessitate oral administration of barium.

Although a prominent ileocecal valve visualized during a barium enema infrequently requires endoscopy or surgery to confirm the radiologic impression that the valve is normal, familiarity with the normal and pathologic appearance, as well as careful performance of appropriate examinations, is necessary to avoid misdiagnosis of ileocecal tumors.

REFERENCES

1. Hinkel, C. L.: Roentgenological examination and evaluation of the ileocecal valve, Am. J. Roentgenol. 68:171, 1952.
2. Miller, R. E., et al.: Hypotonic roentgenography with glucagon, Am. J. Roentgenol. 121:264, 1974.
3. Ferrucci, J. T., Jr.: Hypotonic barium enema examination, Am. J. Roentgenol. 116:304, 1972.
4. Kellett, M. J., Zboralske, F. F., and Margulis, A. R.: Per oral pneumocolon examination of the ileocecal region, Gastrointest. Radiol. 1:361, 1977.
5. Heitzman, E. R., and Berne, A. S.: Roentgen examination of the cecum and proximal ascending colon with ingested barium, Radiology 76:415, 1961.
6. Sakover, R. P., and Del Fava, R. L.: Frequency of visualization of the normal appendix with the barium enema examination, Am. J. Roentgenol. 121: 312, 1974.
7. Fleischner, F. G., and Bernstein, C.: Roentgen-anatomic studies of the normal ileocecal valve, Radiology 54:43, 1950.
8. Gottlieb, C., Berenbaum, S. L., and Dorfman, M.: Roentgen features of non-malignant periappendiceal and ileocecal lesions, Am. J. Dig. Dis. 18:79, 1951.
9. Rigler, L. G., and Lasser, E.: Prolapse of the lower lip of the ileocecal valve into the terminal ileum, Am. J. Roentgenol. 65:878, 1951.
10. Berk, R. N., and Lasser, E. C.: Radiology of the Ileocecal Area (Philadelphia: W. B. Saunders Co., 1975), pp. 15–62.
11. Gazet, J.-C.: The surgical significance of the ileo-

caecal junction, Ann. R. Coll. Surg. Engl. 43:19, 1968.
12. Zettergren, L.: Lipohyperplasia of the ileocolic valve, Acta Soc. Med. Upsal. 59:61, 1953.
13. Boquist, L., Bergdahl, L., and Andersson, A.: Lipomatosis of the ileocecal valve, Cancer 29:136, 1972.
14. Bennert, H. W., Jr., Andrews, R. P., and Porter, J. E.: Lipomatosis of the ileo-cecal valve. A problem in diagnosis and treatment, J. Maine Med. Assoc. 58:196, 1967.
15. Lasser, E. C., and Rigler, L. G.: Ileocecal valve syndrome, Gastroenterology 28:1, 1955.
16. Stark, S.: Diagnostic implications of the ileocecal valve, Gastroenterology 35:485, 1958.
17. Cabaud, P. G., and Harris, L. T.: Lipomatosis of the ileocecal valve, Ann. Surg. 150:1092, 1959.
18. Hulten, J.: Lipomatosis of the ileocaecal valve, Acta Chir. Scand. 129:104, 1965.
19. Grayson, C. E.: Enlargement of the ileocecal valve, Am. J. Roentgenol. 79:823, 1958.
20. Kelby, G. M.: Submucous lipomas of the ileocecal valve, J. Lancet 68:301, 1948.
21. Marsh, A. P.: The enlarged ileocecal valve. Report of cases, Dis. Colon Rectum 3:407, 1960.
22. Seabrook, D. B., et al.: Lipomatosis of the ileocecal region, Am. J. Surg. 92:214.
23. Weiner, M. F., and Polayes, S. H.: Benign tumors of the ileocecal region, with survey of the literature, Am. J. Surg. 40:538, 1938.
24. Castleman, B.: Case records of the Massachusetts General Hospital (case 29502), N. Engl. J. Med. 229:950, 1943.
25. Berk, R. N.: Davis, G. B., and Cholhassey, E. B.: Lipomatosis of the ileocecal valve, Am. J. Roentgenol. 119:323, 1973.
26. Corry, R. J.: Bartlett, M. K., and Cohen, R. B.: Erosions of the cecum; A cause of massive hemorrhage, Am. J. Surg. 119:106, 1970.
27. Baum, S., et al.: Angiodysplasias of the right colon: A cause of gastrointestinal bleeding, Am. J. Roentgenol. 129:789, 1977.
28. Felson, B., and Wiot, J. F.: Some interesting right lower quadrant entities. Myxoglobulosis of the appendix, ileal prolapse, diverticulitis, lymphoma, endometriosis, Radiol. Clin. North Am. 7:83, 1969.
29. Strauch, M., Remmele, W., and Ottenjann, R.: Endoscopic-bioptic diagnosis of lipomatosis of the ileocecal valve, Acta Hepatogastroenterol. (Stuttg.) 19:408, 1972.
30. Hawley, C., and Mithoefer, J.: Ileal prolapse, Radiology 54:380, 1950.
31. Nagasako, K., and Takemoto, T.: Endoscopy of the ileocecal area, Gastroenterology 65:403, 1973.
32. Rubin, S., et al.: Retrograde prolapse of the ileocecal valve, Am. J. Roentgenol. 87:706, 1962.
33. Debray, C., et al.: La bauhinite oedemateuse: Oedeme inflammatoire pseudo-tumoral de la valvule de Bauhin, Arch. Fr. Mal. Appar. Dig. 42:163, 1953.
34. River, L., Silverstein, J., and Tope, J. W.: Collective review: Benign neoplasms of the small intestine; a critical comprehensive review with reports of 20 new cases, Int. Abstr. Surg. 102:1956, in Surg. Gynecol. Obstet. 1956.
35. Mayo, C. W.: Pagtalunan, R. J. G., and Brown, D. J.: Lipoma of the alimentary tract, Surgery 53: 598, 1963.
36. Castro, E. B., and Stearns, M. W.: Lipoma of the large intestines. A review of 45 cases, Dis. Colon Rectum 15:441, 1972.
37. Margulis, A. R., and Jovanovich, A.: The Roentgen diagnosis of submucous lipomas of the colon, Am. J. Roentgenol. 84:1114, 1960.
38. Knechtges, T. C., and Carrasquilla, C.: Piggy-back adenopapillomas over lipomatosis of the ileocecal valve, Dis. Colon Rectum 13:255, 1970.
39. Tandon, R., Buhac, I., and Rodgers, J. B., Jr.: Obstruction of the ileocecal valve by an adenomatous polyp mimicking regional enteritis, Am. J. Dig. Dis. 17:929, 1972.
40. Sherwood, W. A.: Neoplasms of the ileocecal valve. Report of 3 cases complicated by intussusception, Surg. Clin. North Am. 7:1057, 1927.
41. Jefferson, J. C.: Fibroma of the ileo-caecal valve, Br. Med. J. 2:819, 1920.
42. Haff, R. C., and San Diego, A. G.: Ganglioneuroma of the ileocecal valve. Review of the literature, Arch. Pathol. 93:549, 1972.
43. Wapshaw, H.: Carcinoma of the ileo-caecal valve. Report of 3 cases and statistical survey, Glasgow Med. J. 129:280, 1938.
44. Berk, R. N., Sadowsky, N. L., and Levenson, S. S.: Carcinoma of the cecum and ascending colon. An analysis of ninety-one cases, Am. J. Surg. 104:27, 1962.
45. Ng, A. C., and Margulis, A. R.: Roentgenographic findings of primary carcinoma of the illeocecal valve, Surgery 54:861, 1963.
46. Glasser, S. T., and Mersheimer, W.: Carcinoma of the ileocecal valve, Am. J. Surg. 56:650, 1942.
47. Bargen, J. A., Wesson, H. R., and Jackman, R. J.: Studies on the ileocecal junction (ileocecus), Surg. Gynecol. Obstet. 71:33, 1940.
48. Cooley, R. N., Agnew, C. H., and Rios, G.: Diagnostic accuracy of the barium enema study in carcinoma of the colon and rectum, Am. J. Roentgenol. 84:316, 1960.
49. McSwain, B., Sadler, R. N., and Main, F. B.: Carcinoma of colon, rectum and anus, Ann. Surg. 155: 782, 1962.
50. Allcock, J. M.: An assessment of the accuracy of the clinical and radiological diagnosis of carcinoma of the colon, Br. J. Radiol. 31:272, 1958.
51. Myllarniemi, H., Perttala, Y., and Peltokallio, P.: Tumor-like lesions of the cecum following inversion of the appendix, Am. J. Dig. Dis. 19:547, 1974.
52. Whiting, J. A., Wallace, F. T., and Wilson, R. S.: Chronic intussuscepting carcinoid of the ileocecal valve and cecum. A case report, Am. Surg. 19: 1180, 1953.

54. Calenoff, L.: Rare ileocecal lesions, Am. J. Roentgenol. 110:343, 1970.
55. Shulman, H., and Giustra, P.: Invasive carcinoids of the colon, Radiology 98:139, 1971.
56. Pearson, C. M., and Fitzgerald, P. J.: Carcinoid tumors. A reemphasis of their malignant nature: Review of 140 cases, Cancer 2:1005, 1949.
57. Hudson, H. L., and Margulis, A. R.: The roentgen findings of carcinoid tumors of the gastrointestinal tract. A report of 12 recent cases, Am. J. Roentgenol. 91:833, 1964.
58. Horn, R. C., Jr.: Carcinoid tumors of the colon and rectum, Cancer 2:819, 1949.
59. Richie, A. C.: Carcinoid tumors, Am. J. Med. Sci. 232:311, 1956.
60. Ponka, J. L.: Carcinoid tumors of the appendix. Report of 35 cases, Am. J. Surg. 126:77, 1973.
61. Rosato, F. E., and Rosato, E. F.: Carcinoid tumors of the large bowel, Cancer 20:352, 1970.
62. Goldstein, H. M., and Miller, M.: Angiographic evaluation of carcinoid tumors of the small intestine: Value of epinephrine, Radiology 115:23, 1975.
63. Messinger, N. H., Bobroff, L. M., and Beneventano, T. C.: Lymphosarcoma of the colon, Am. J. Roentgenol. 117:281, 1975.
64. Golden, R.: Enlargement of the ileocecal valve, Am. J. Roentgenol. 50:19, 1943.
65. Margulis, A. R., et al.: The overlapping spectrum of ulcerative and granulomatous colitis: A roentgenographic-pathologic study, Am. J. Roentgenol. 113: 325, 1971.
66. Marshak, R. H., and Lindner, A. E.: Ulcerative and Granulomatous Colitis, in Margulis, A. R., and Burhenne, R. J. (eds.): Alimentary Tract Roentgenology, vol. 2 (2d ed.; St. Louis: C. V. Mosby Co., 1973), p. 991.
67. Kolawole, T. M., and Lewis, E. A.: Radiologic observations on intestinal amebiasis, Am. J. Roentgenol. 122:257, 1974.
68. Balikian, J. P., Uthman, S. M., and Khouri, N. F.: Intestinal amebiasis. A roentgen analysis of 19 cases including 2 case reports, Am. J. Roentgenol. 122:245, 1974.
69. Gershon-Cohen, J., and Kremens, V.: X-ray studies of the ileocecal valve in ileocecal tuberculosis, Radiology 62:251, 1954.
70. Fleischner, F.: Die Darmtuberkulose im Röntgenbild, Ergeb. Med. Strahlenforsch. 3:359, 1928.
71. Marshak, R. H.: Granulomatous disease of the intestinal tract (Crohn's disease), Radiology 114:3, 1975.
72. Mitchell, R. S., and Bristol, L. J.: Intestinal tuberculosis. An analysis of 346 cases diagnosed by routine intestinal radiography on 5,529 admissions for pulmonary tuberculosis, 1924–49, Am. J. Med. Sci. 227:241, 1954.
73. Dietz, M. W.: Ileocecal histoplasmosis, Radiology 91:285, 1968.
74. Auritchir, Y., and Perroni, A. A.: Radiologic manifestations of small intestinal South American blastomycosis, Radiology 127:607, 1978.
75. Francis, R. S., and Berk, R. N.: Typhoid fever, Radiology 112:583, 1974.
76. Richman, R. H., and Lewicki, A. M.: Right ileocolitis secondary to anisakiasis, Am. J. Roentgenol. 119:329, 1973.
77. Medina, J. T., et al.: The roentgen appearance of schistosomiasis mansoni involving the colon, Radiology 85:682, 1965.
78. Uroso, F. P., Uroso, M. J., and Lee, C. H.: The cathartic colon: Pathological findings and radiological/pathological correlation, Radiology 116:557, 1975.
79. Beneventano, T. C., et al.: The roentgen aspects of some appendiceal abnormalities, Am. J. Roentgenol. 96:344, 1966.

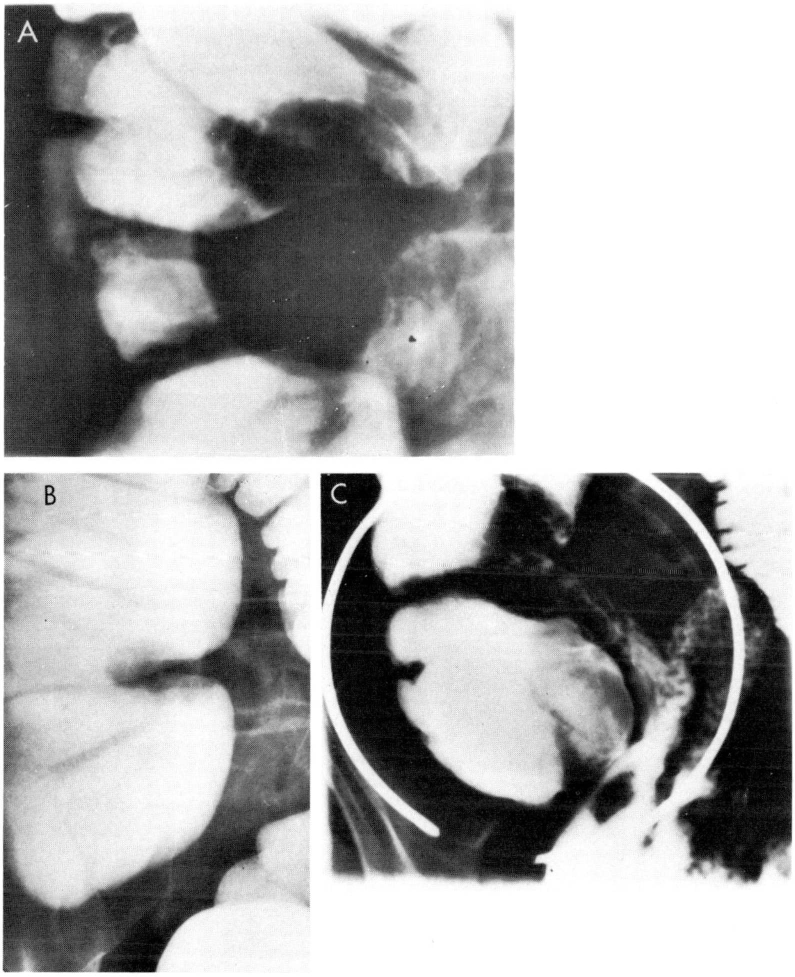

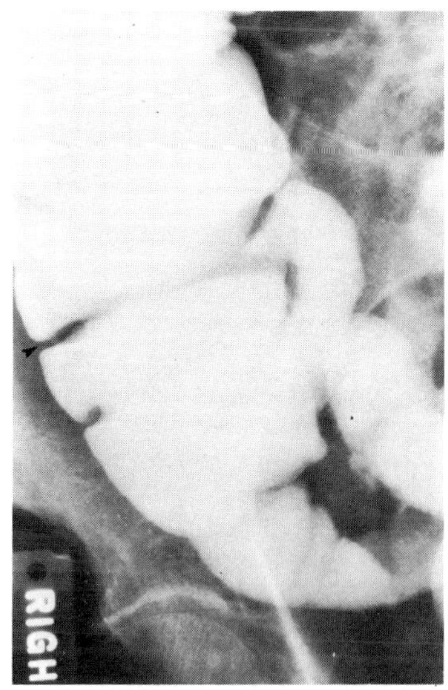

Fig 25–1 (left).—Possible cecal mass. **A,** compression spot film obtained during barium enema shows smooth spherical filling defect measuring 5 cm in diameter in region of ileocecal valve. **B,** radiograph during same study. Valve measures 2.3 cm vertically in same location. This papillary shape is that of an ileocecal valve, with the colon incompletely distended with barium. **C,** spot film during small bowel examination shows terminal ileum entering center of ileocecal valve, which at surgery was normal.

Fig 25–2 (right).—Normal ileocecal valve. Valve is at junction of cecum and ascending colon, almost always at first complete haustral fold *(arrowhead)* above cecal tip and usually either medial or posteromedial.

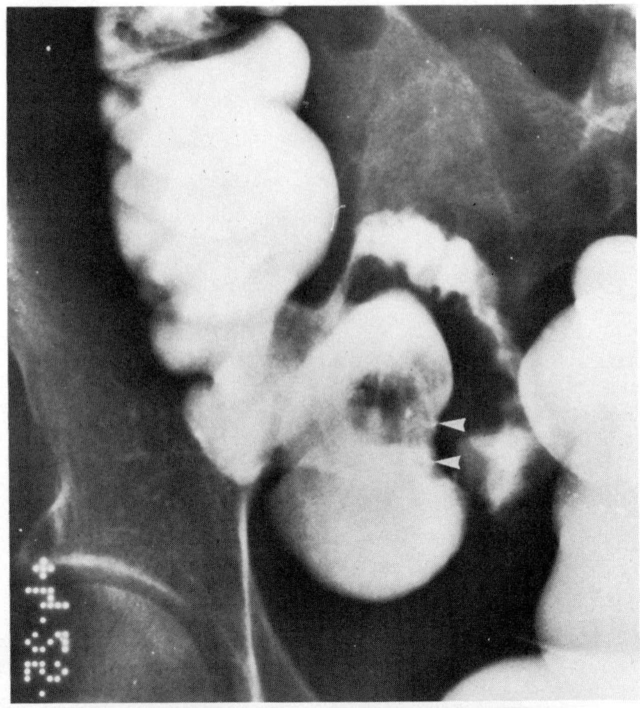

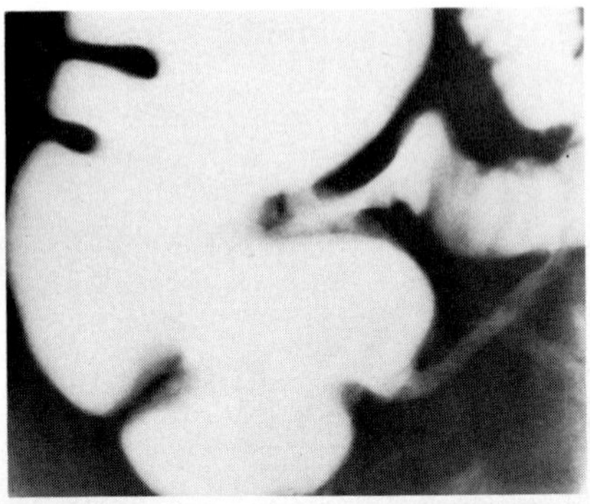

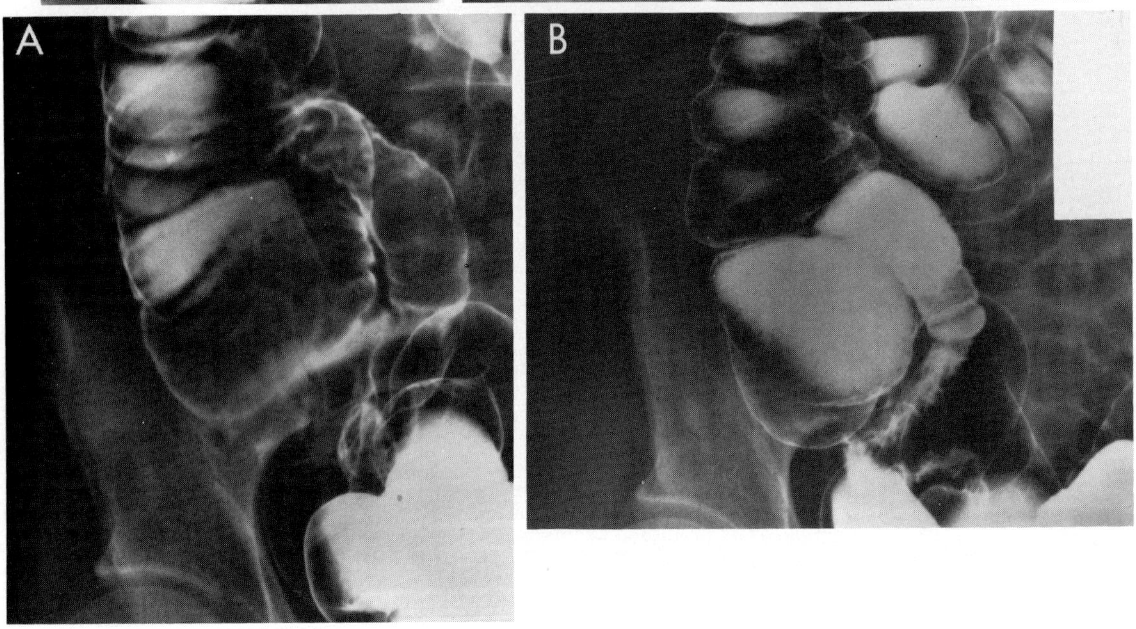

Fig 25–3 (top left). – Normal ileocecal valve. Profile view shows ileocecal valve on same side of colon as appendix in 90% of adults in whom appendix arises from cecal tip.

Fig 25–4 (top right). – Inverted appendiceal stump. By relating appendix to position of ileocecal valve, filling defect is noted to be in expected location of appendix. Note fine wire sutures *(arrowheads)*. Note also normal configuration of ileocecal valve in profile. Upper lip normally is larger.

Fig 25–5 (bottom). – Posteromedial ileocecal valve. **A,** air contrast study shows valve outline with small amount of barium in its ostium. **B,** a few minutes later barium refluxed through valve, obscuring it and opacifying terminal ileum.

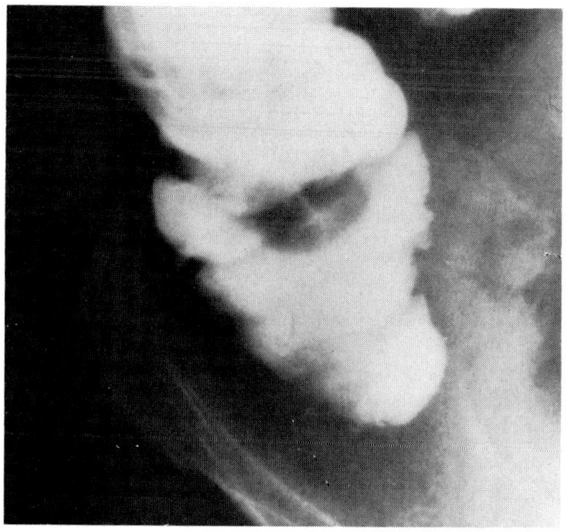

Fig 25–6.—Normal papillary-shaped ileocecal valve. Note rosette-fold pattern, which identifies valve and indicates pliability. Normal valve outline may be lobular, but its mucosal surface always is smooth.

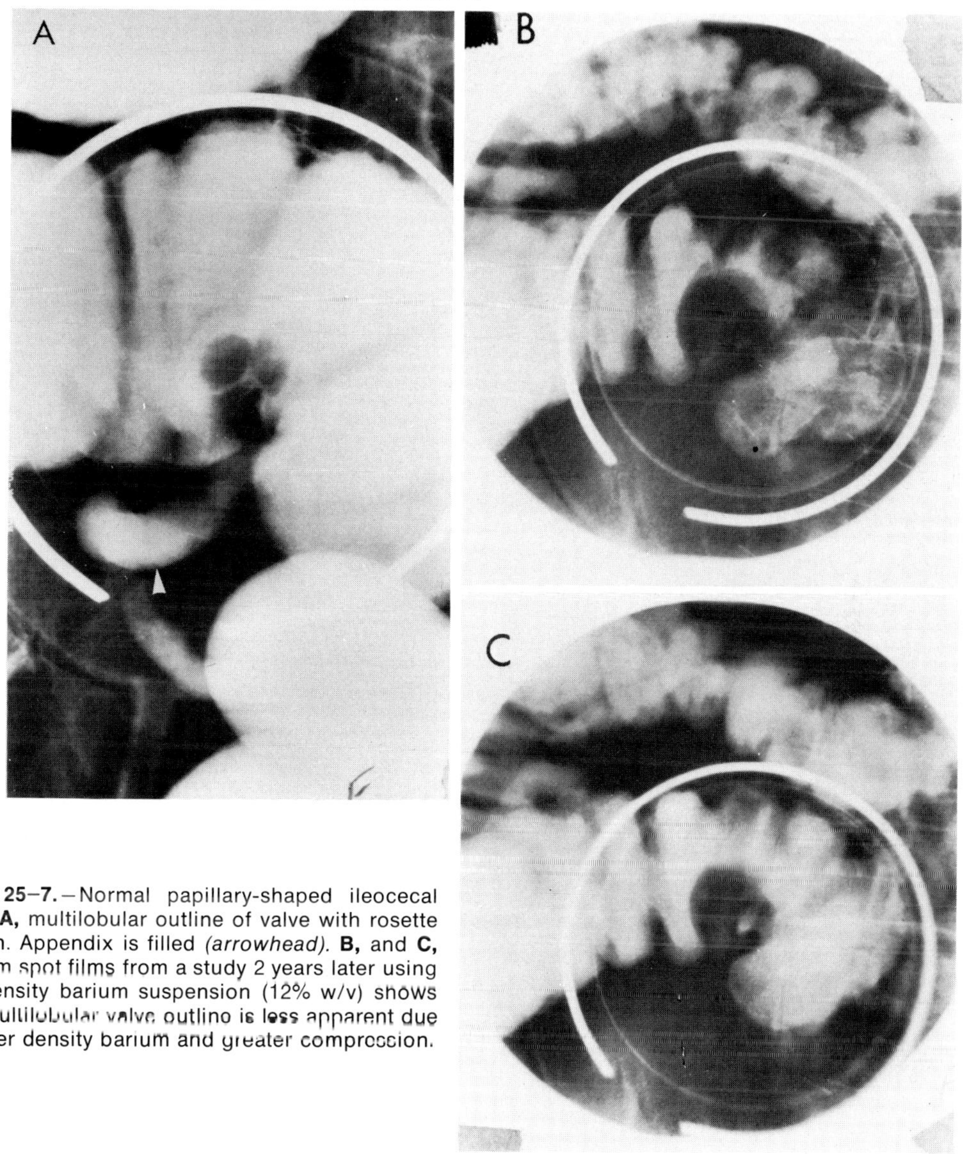

Fig 25–7.—Normal papillary-shaped ileocecal valve. **A,** multilobular outline of valve with rosette pattern. Appendix is filled *(arrowhead).* **B,** and **C,** 105 mm spot films from a study 2 years later using low density barium suspension (12% w/v) shows that multilobular valve outline is less apparent due to lower density barium and greater compression.

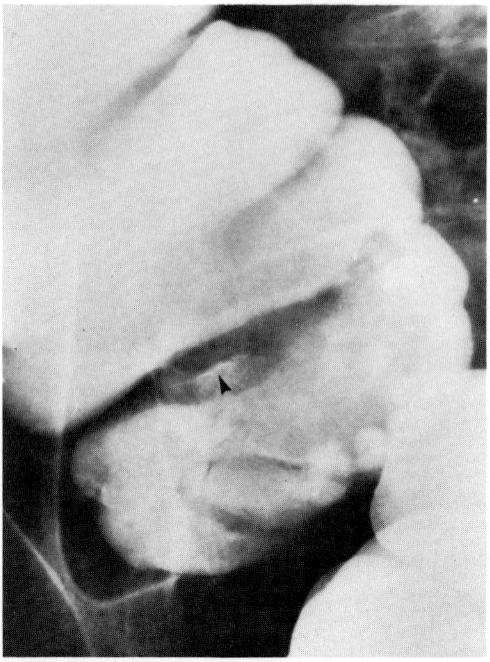

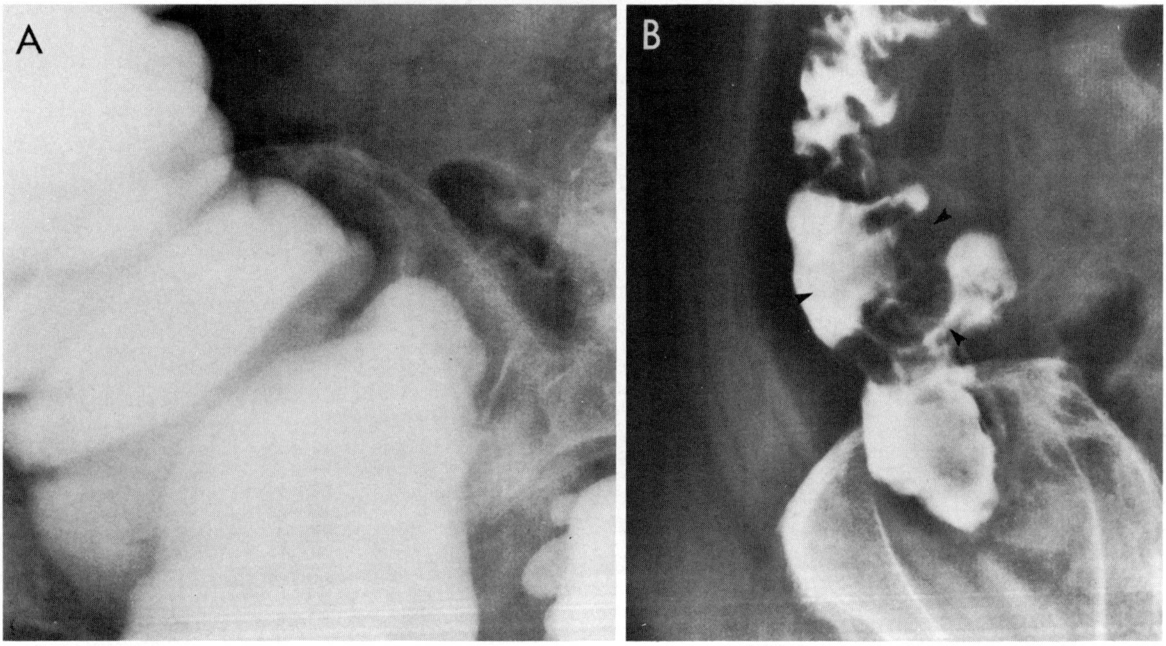

Fig 25–8 (top). – Normal spindle-shaped ileocecal valve. Valve is posterior. Central ostium *(arrow)* and frenula are evident.

Fig 25–9 (bottom). – Variation in shape of ileocecal valve. Shape varies with degree of distention. **A,** with colonic distention, bilabial shape of valve occurs due to frenula pull from medial and lateral valve margins. **B,** after evacuation frenula pull has relaxed and valve *(arrowheads)* has become papillary shaped.

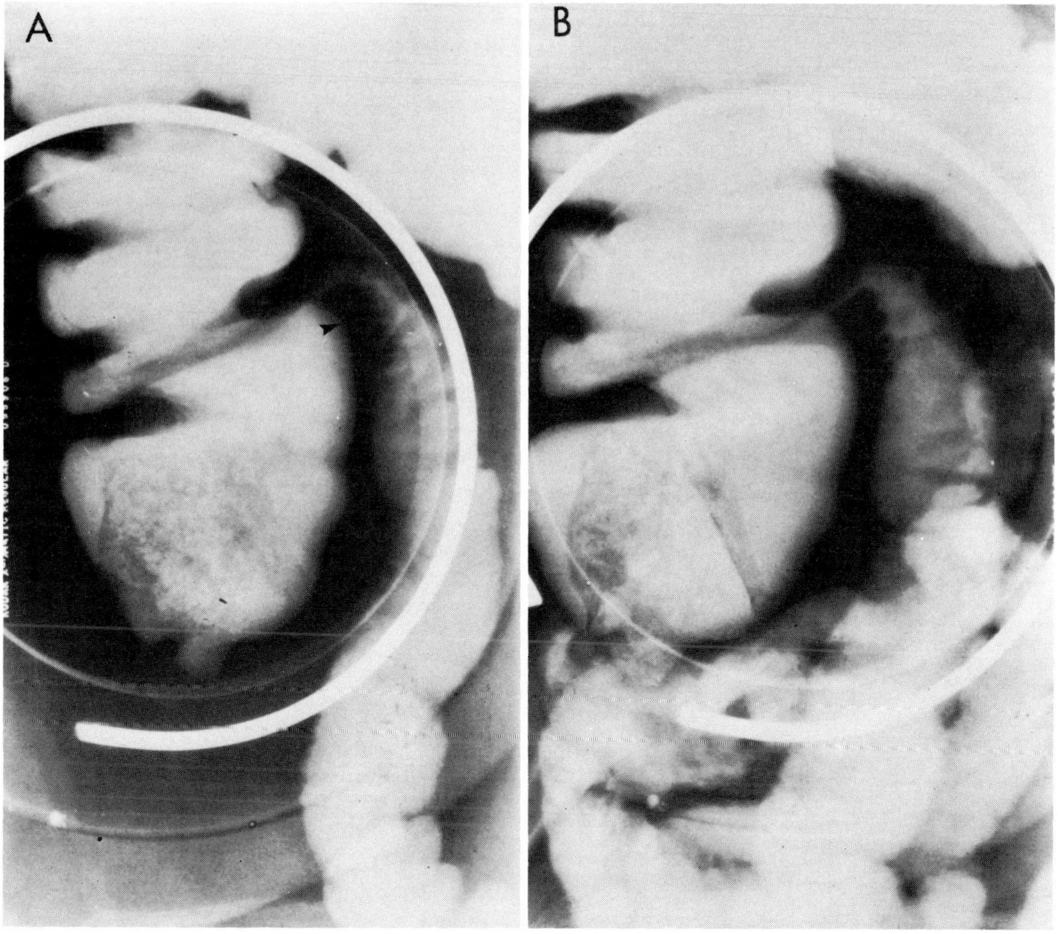

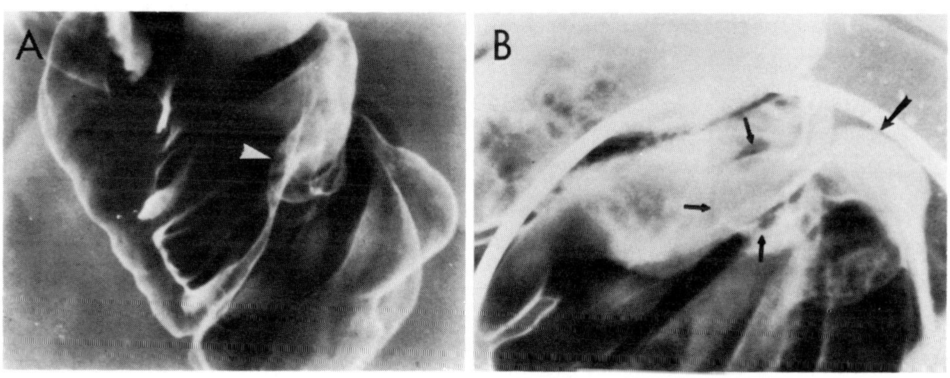

Fig 25–10 (top). – Underdeveloped lower lip of ileocecal valve. **A,** lower lip of ileocecal valve *(arrowhead)* has prolapsed into ileum, an appearance that could be mistaken for ileal tumor. **B,** a minute later, prolapse has disappeared. Incompetence of normal valve during barium enema may be due to underdevelopment of labia or frenula of valve.

Fig 25–11 (bottom). – Multilobular ileocecal valve. **A,** spot film during air contrast barium enema shows filling defect, which suggests a polyp *(arrowhead).* **B,** spot film obtained after oral administration of barium and air insufflation of colon by way of rectum identifies filling defect in **A** as ileocecal valve by visualizing both the valve *(left small arrows)* and the terminal ileum *(right large arrow)*. The greater cecocolonic distention in **B** has caused valve to appear less multilobular.

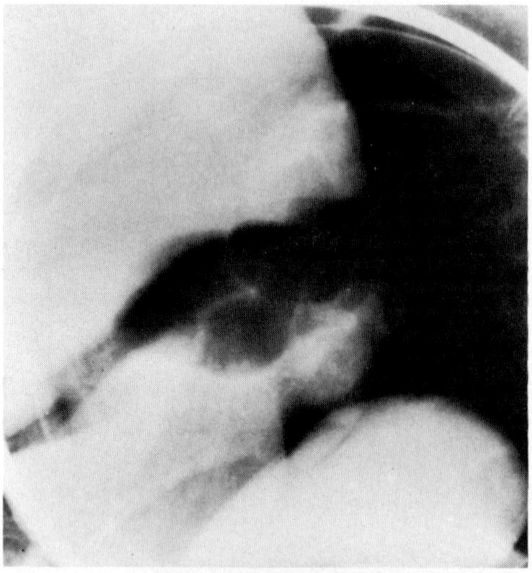

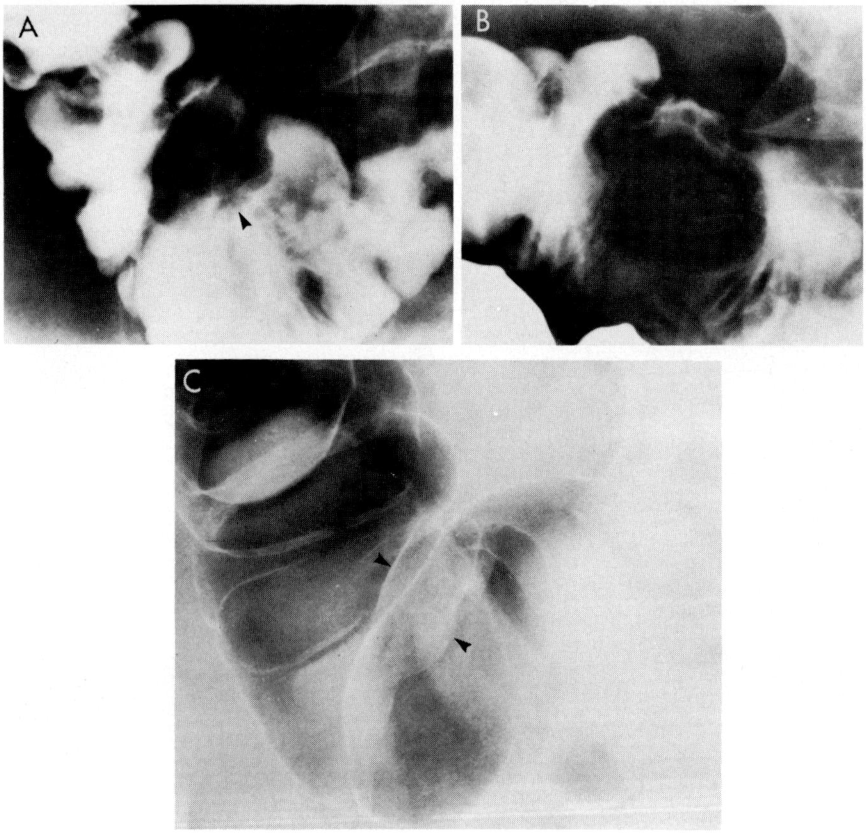

Fig 25–12 (top).—Normal ileocecal valve. Standard spot film shows ileocecal valve measuring 3 cm in height. Few normal valves exceed 3 cm in diameter, but size alone is not a criterion of abnormality. Rosette-fold pattern converging on valve ostium is evident.

Fig 25–13 (bottom).—Variation in size of ileocecal valve. Valve size varies with colonic distention and with external compression. **A,** spot film shows valve diameter is 3 cm without complete colonic distention and without compression *(arrowheads).* **B,** spot film with compression a few seconds later shows that valve now measures 5 cm. **C,** spot film with good colonic distention, valve diameter measuring 1.7 cm *(arrowheads).*

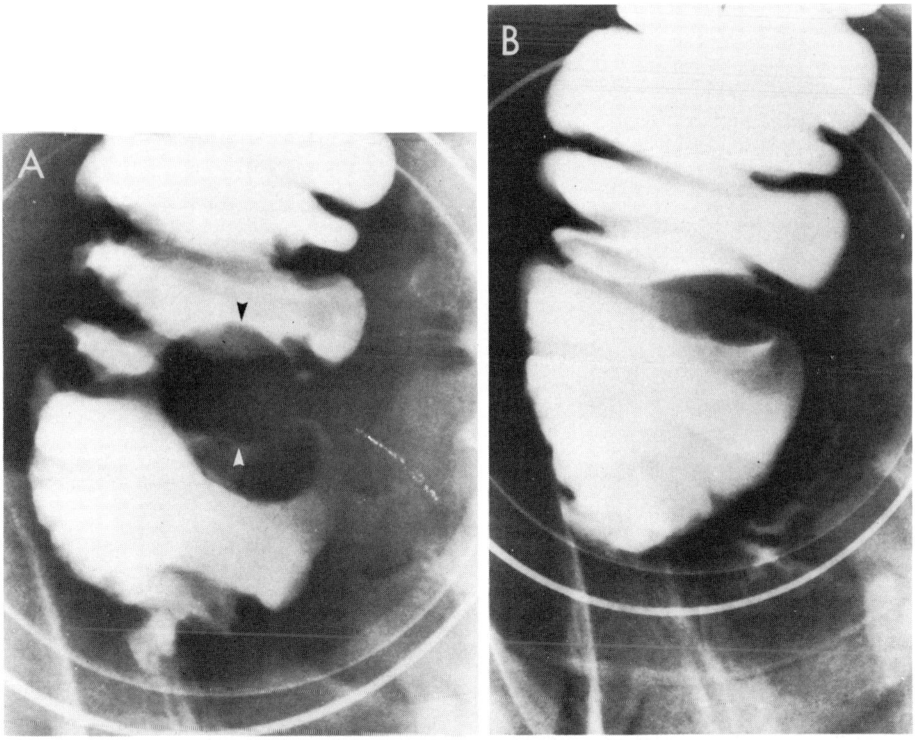

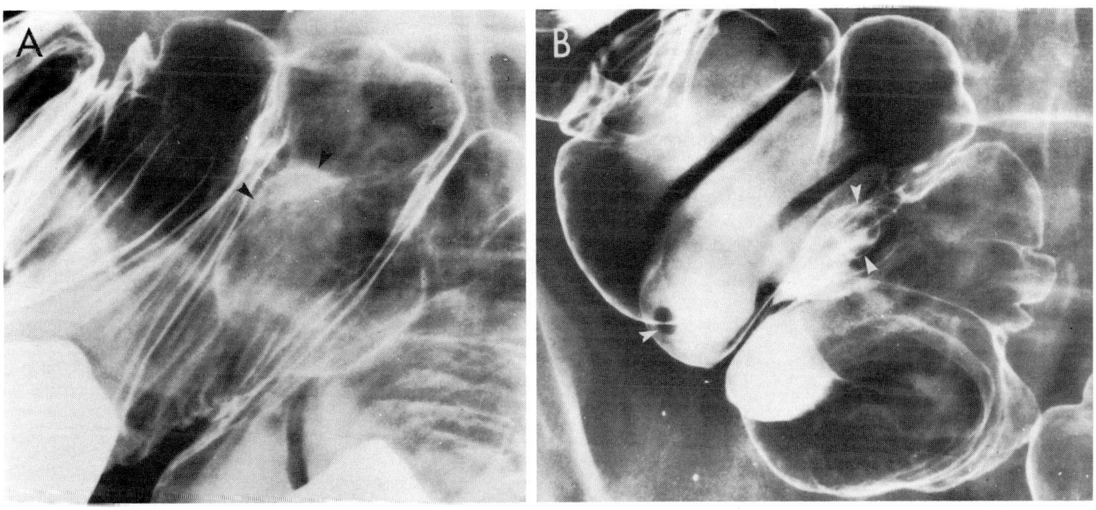

Fig 25–14 (top). – Normal ileocecal valve. **A,** spot film with marked prominence of upper lip *(arrowheads)* of valve. Lips of normal valve are not necessarily equal in size. **B,** a few minutes later with better colonic distention, valve configuration changed from papillary to funnel shape. Valve is pliable without localized enlargement of upper lip, indicating that it is normal.

Fig 25–15 (bottom). – Probable prolapse of ileocecal valve. **A,** spot film shows large papillary-shaped valve. There is smooth, polypoid lobulation of upper lip *(arrowheads).* **B,** a few minutes later spot film shows valve to be much smaller, with a spindle shape. Change in volume of valve, not attributable to differences in compression or colonic distention, suggests prolapse. Smooth, polypoid lobulation of upper lip *(right arrowheads)* is localized; this appearance may suggest a tumor, particularly a lipoma. Small polyp *(left arrowhead)* noted in ascending colon. Over the next 2 years, follow-up studies showed no change in ileocecal valve.

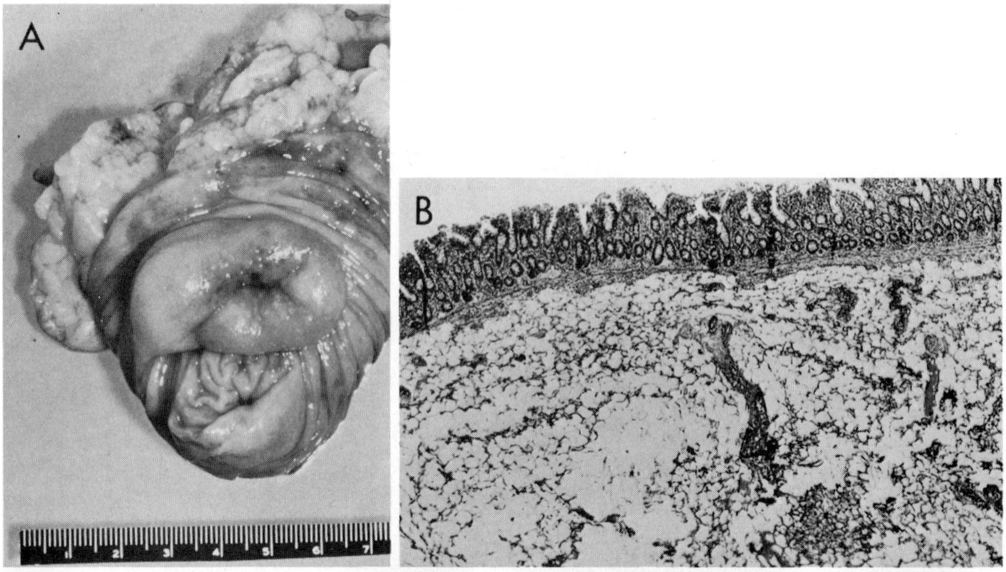

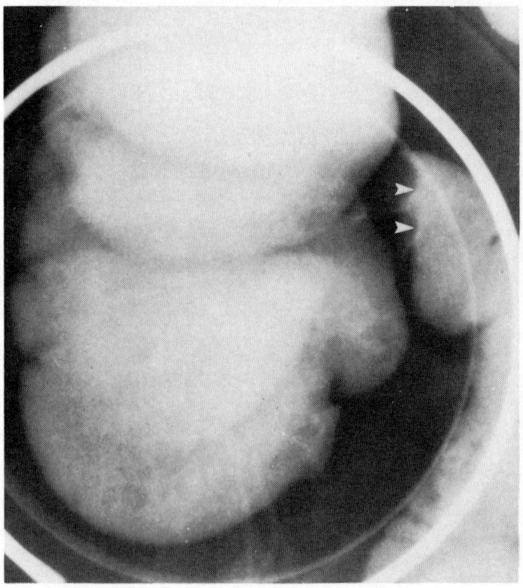

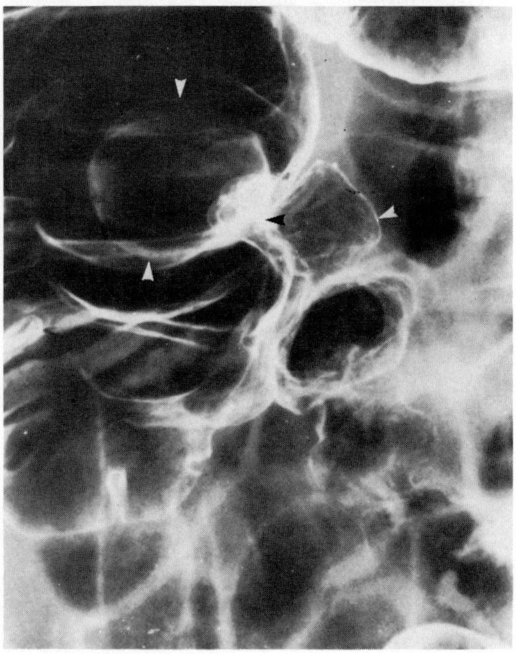

Fig 25–16 (top). – Lipomatosis of ileocecal valve. **A,** surgically resected valve of patient with vague complaints referable to lower abdomen. Valve is smooth, although prominent. **B,** histologic section of portion of one lip of same valve with marked submucosal fat in otherwise unremarkable valve.

Fig 25–17 (bottom left). – Retrograde prolapse of valvular mucosa. Mucosal prolapse *(arrowheads)* is seen occasionally during barium enemas but has no known significance.

Fig 25–18 (bottom right). – Lipoma of ileocecal valve. Lipoma *(left arrowheads)* arises from upper lip of small ileocecal valve *(black arrowhead)*. Note terminal ileum *(right arrowhead)*.

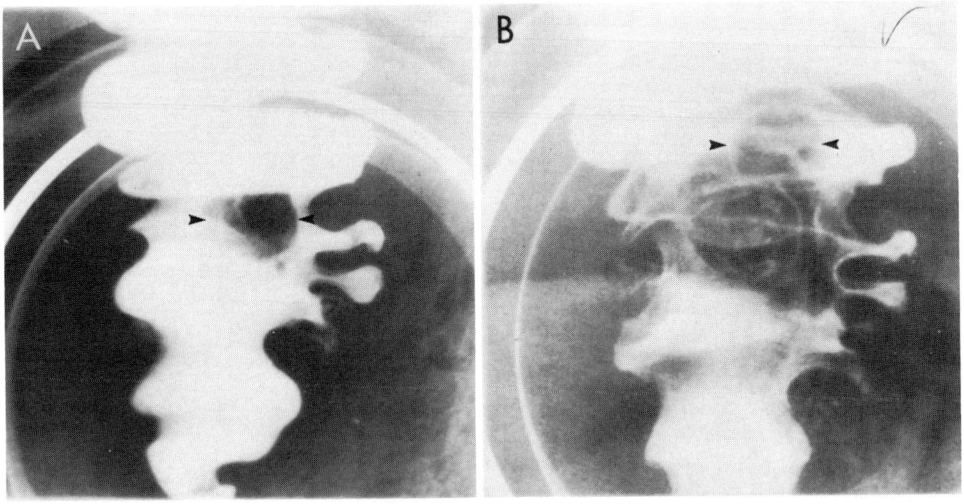

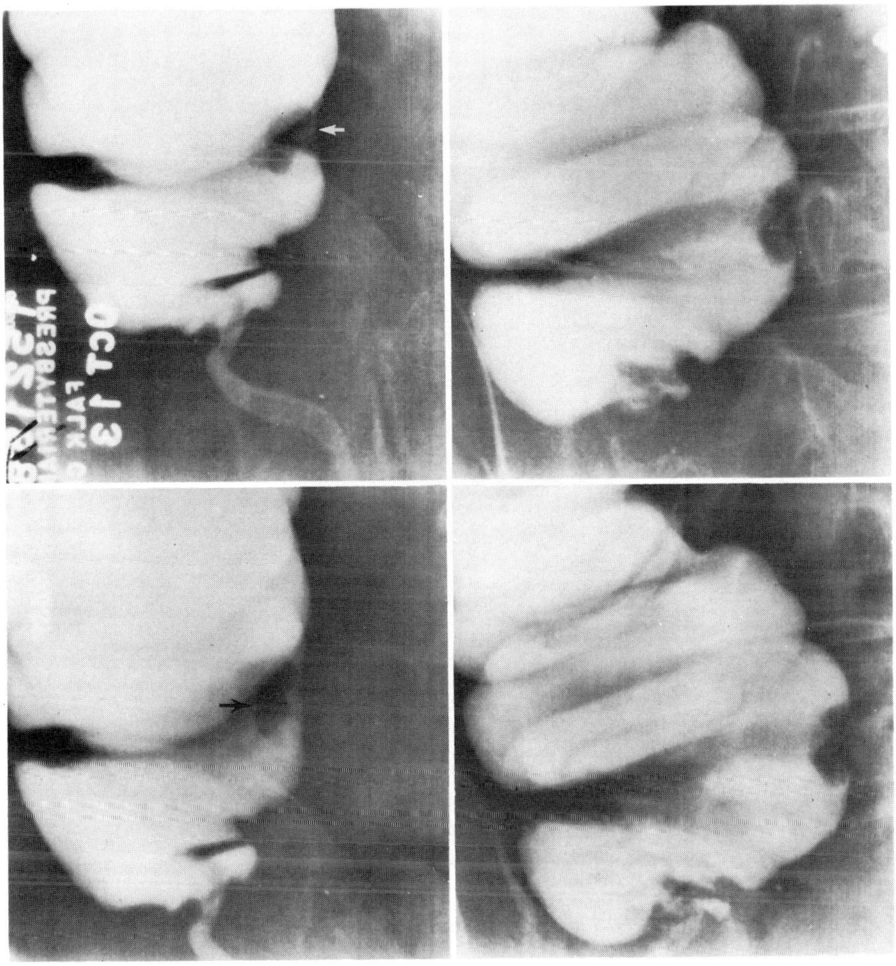

Fig 25–19 (top). – Pedunculated lipoma of ileocecal valve. **A,** lipoma *(arrowheads)* is noted before application of external compression. **B,** after external compression, lipoma has been displaced 1.5 cm cephalad *(arrowheads),* indicating that it is pedunculated.

Fig 25–20 (center and bottom). – Adenoma of upper lip of ileocecal valve. Slightly nodular and creased surface of polyp *(arrow)* is suggestive of either adenoma or polypoid carcinoma, rather than lipoma.

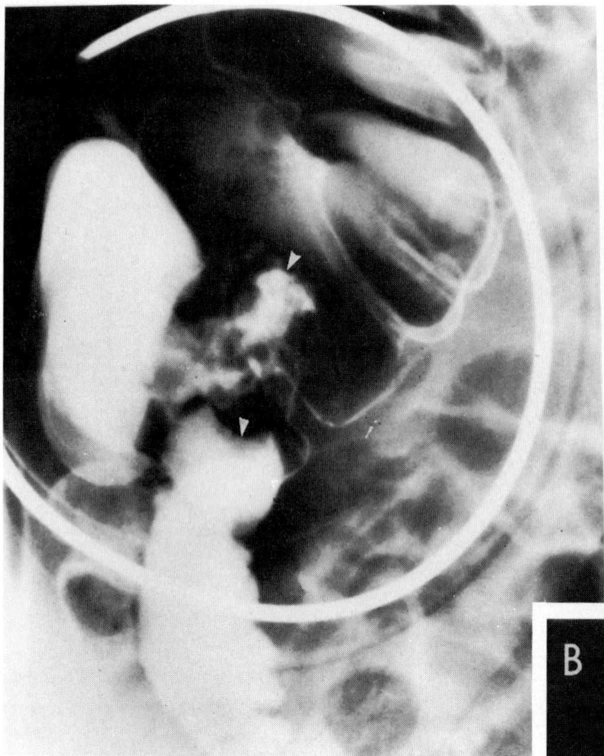

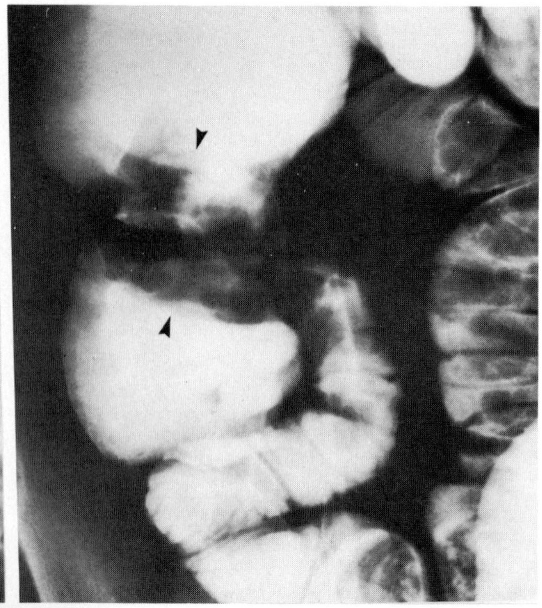

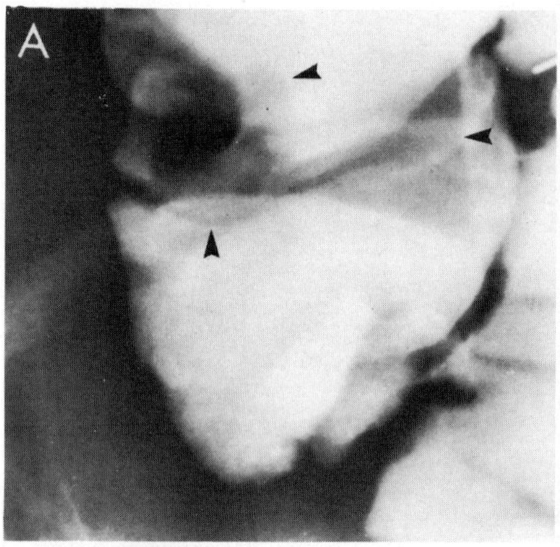

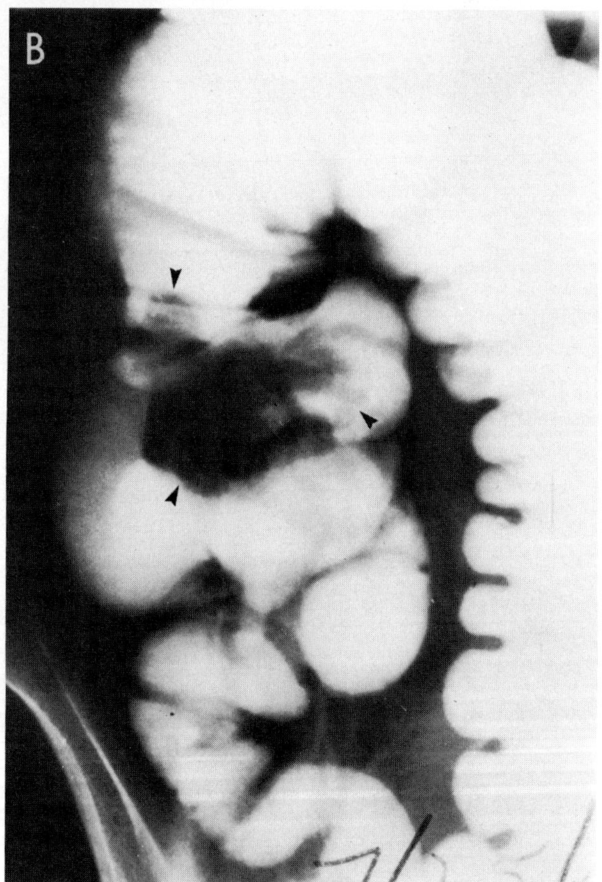

Fig 25–21 (top left).—Carcinoma of ileocecal valve. Carcinoma *(upper arrowhead)* has markedly irregular, ulcerated surface, with spread to terminal ileum *(lower arrowhead),* cecum and ascending colon. Invasion of terminal ileum with carcinoma is usually more limited than with either lymphosarcoma or carcinoid.

Fig 25–22 (top right).—Large ileocecal carcinoma. Annular growth of tumor *(arrowheads)* with overhanging edges involves valve as well as surrounding structures so that point of origin is difficult to determine.

Fig 25–23 (bottom).—Carcinoma apparently mistaken for ileocecal valve. **A,** radiograph shows carcinoma *(left arrowheads)* and ileocecal valve *(right arrowhead).* **B,** radiograph 11 months later shows that tumor *(arrowheads)* has grown to involve ileocecal valve.

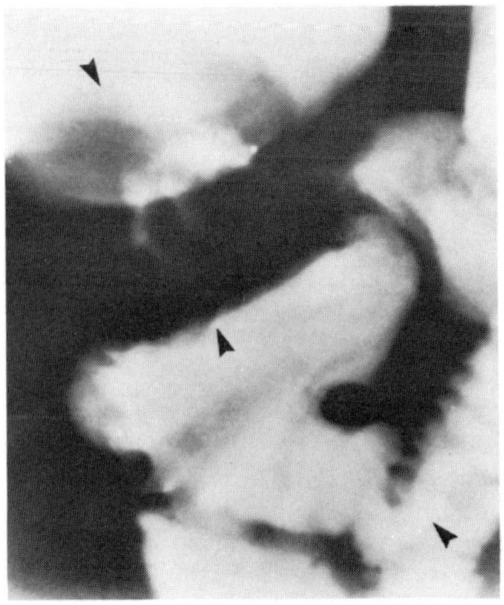

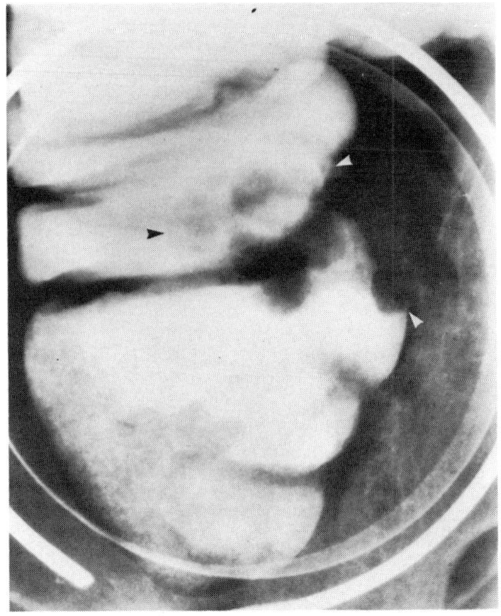

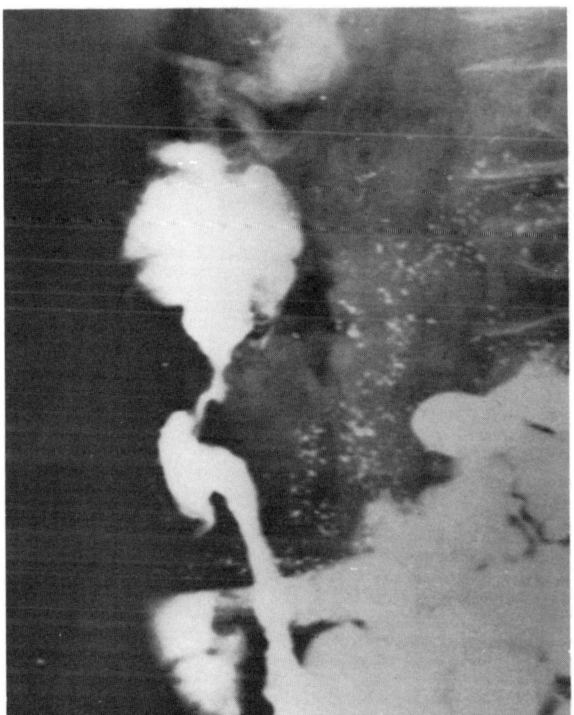

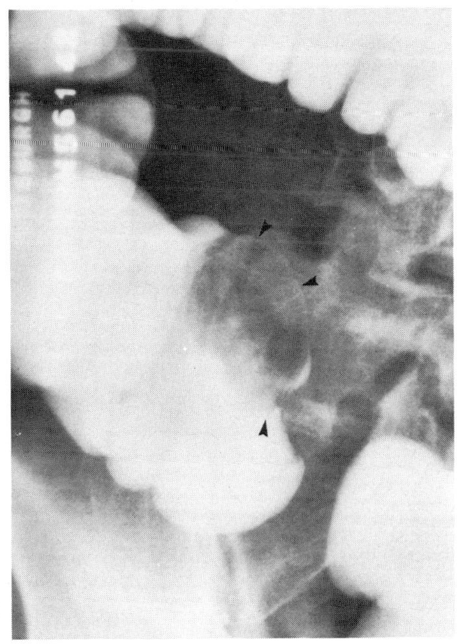

Fig 25–24 (top left). – Annular ileocecal carcinoma tumor *(upper and middle arrowheads)* may cause obstruction. Spasm may obscure cecal filling and a lesion missed if care is not taken to identify ileocecal valve, terminal ileum or appendix. Note fetal-shaped cecum with centrally placed appendix *(lower arrowhead)*, which would not help to localize ileocecal valve.

Fig 25–25 (top right). – Carcinoma almost confined to ileocecal valve. Valve has an irregular, nodular surface *(arrowheads)*.

Fig 25–26 (bottom left). – Linitis plastica of cecum. Diffuse involvement has infiltrated bowel wall, narrowing it and destroying ileocecal valve, with free reflux to ileum. This type of tumor usually occurs in patients with preexisting ulcerative colitis. (Courtesy of Dr. Robert Armstrong, Audie Murphy V. A. Hospital, San Antonio, Texas.)

Fig 25–27 (bottom right). – Carcinoid of ileocecal valve. Prominence of ileocecal valve noted during barium enema examination was due to malignant carcinoid arising in terminal ileum *(arrowheads)*. (Courtesy of Dr. David Bryk, Jewish Hospital and Medical Center of Brooklyn, Brooklyn, N. Y., and of Armed Forces Institute of Pathology, Washington, D. C.)

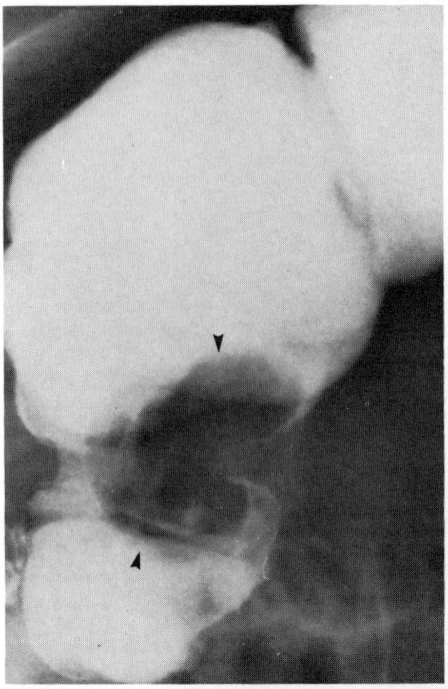

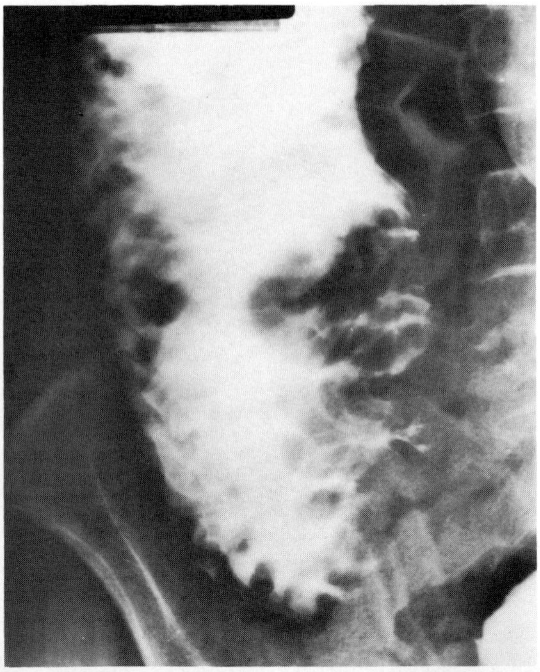

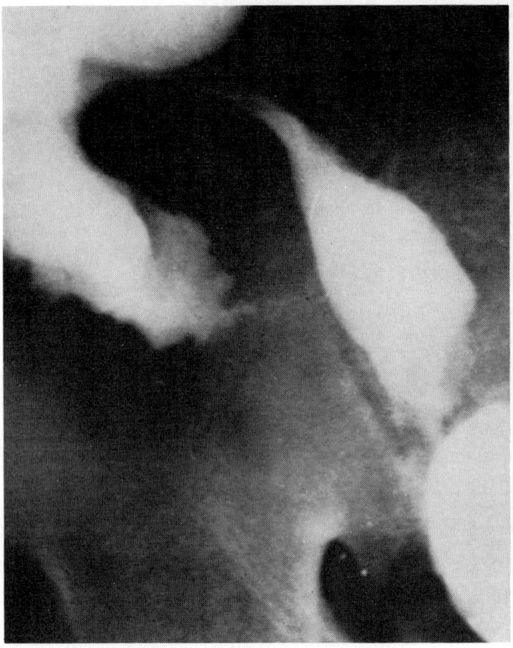

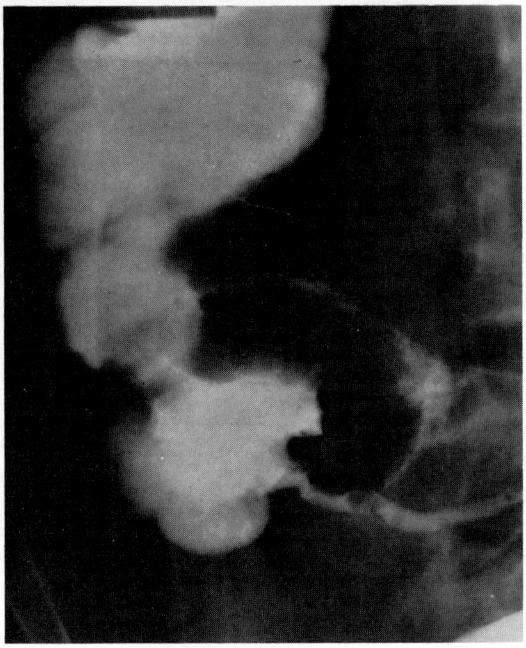

Fig 25–28 (top left).—Carcinoid of ileocecal valve *(arrowheads)*. Tumor, measuring 5 cm in diameter, was contained within valve lumen. Some small nodules on colonic surface of valve are not visualized. A carcinoid tumor may appear as smooth, symmetric enlargement of valve, so it is important to visualize terminal ileum if prominent, nonpliable valve is present.

Fig 25–29 (top right).—Lymphosarcoma involving ileocecal valve, ascending colon, cecum and terminal ileum. Irregular nodularity and diffuse involvement visualized are common features of lymphosarcoma.

Fig 25–30 (bottom left).—Reticulum cell sarcoma of terminal ileum. Marked narrowing of terminal ileum crossing ileocecal valve to cecum is noted, with infiltration of cecum causing narrowing. This appearance may simulate that of regional enteritis. (Courtesy of Dr. Robert Armstrong, Audie Murphy Veterans Administration Hospital, San Antonio, Texas.)

Fig 25–31 (bottom right).—Non-Hodgkins lymphoma. Infiltrating variety with more than usual narrowing of terminal ileum and invasion of ileocecal valve and cecum. Appearance would be difficult to definitely differentiate from regional enteritis. (Courtesy of Dr. Harvey Goldstein, Methodist Hospital, San Antonio, Texas.)

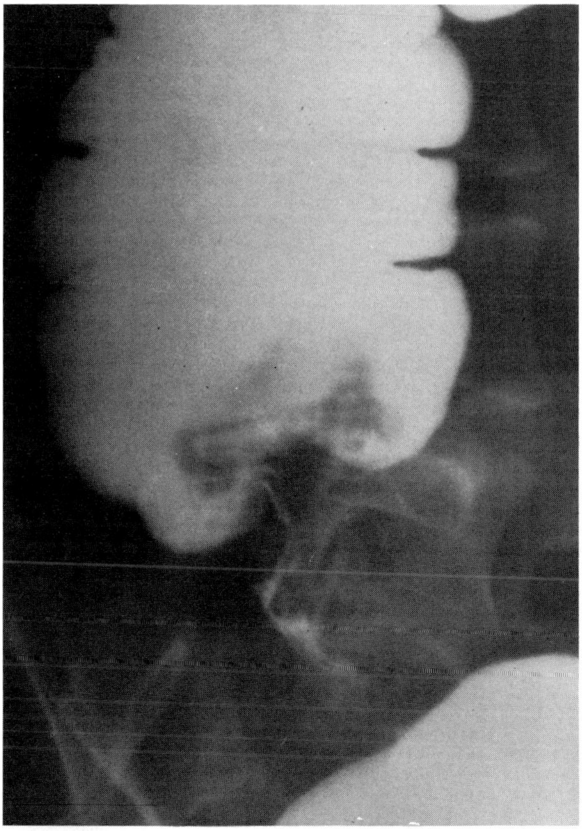

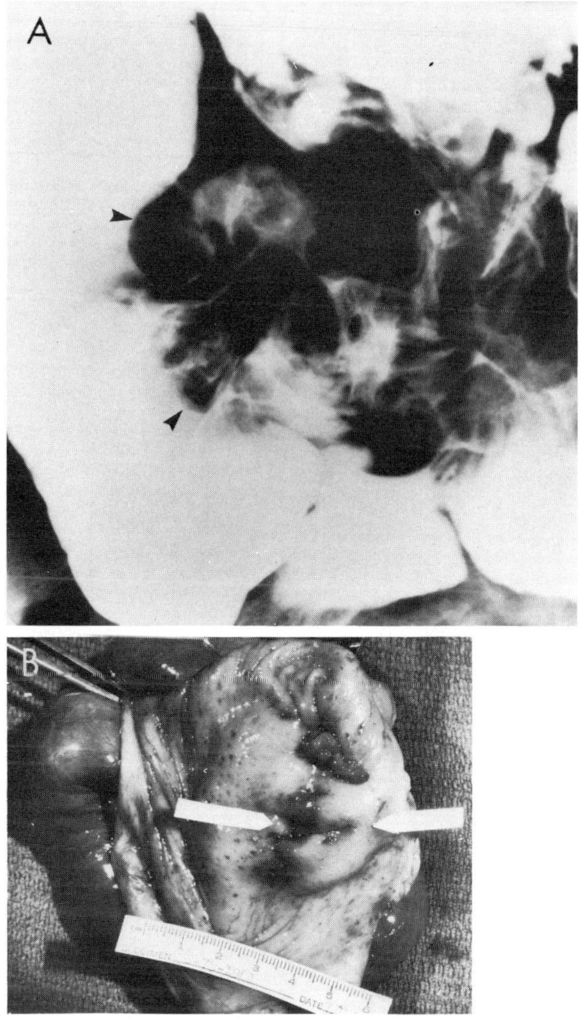

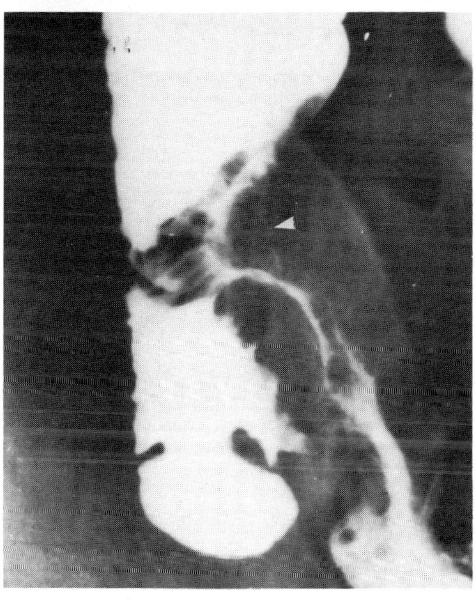

Fig 25–32 (top left). – Lymphoma of terminal ileum with intussusception. Polypoid lymphoma of terminal ileum is a relatively common cause of ileocolic intussusception, although carcinoid tumors or other benign or malignant masses of ileum or ileocecal valve may act as lead point. (Courtesy of Dr. Harvey Goldstein, Methodist Hosp., San Antonio, Texas.)

Fig 25–33 (right). – Lipomatosis of ileocecal valve in granulomatous enterocolitis. **A,** spot film made during examination of small intestines of man, age 10, shows thickened labia *(arrowheads)* of ileocecal valve. **B,** resected valve of same patient shows prominent labia caused by deposition of fat. Multiple small ulcers are noted surrounding valve ostium *(arrows)*.

Fig 25–34 (bottom left). – Granulomatous enterocolitis. Fistula *(arrowhead)* traverses thickened upper lip of ileocecal valve.

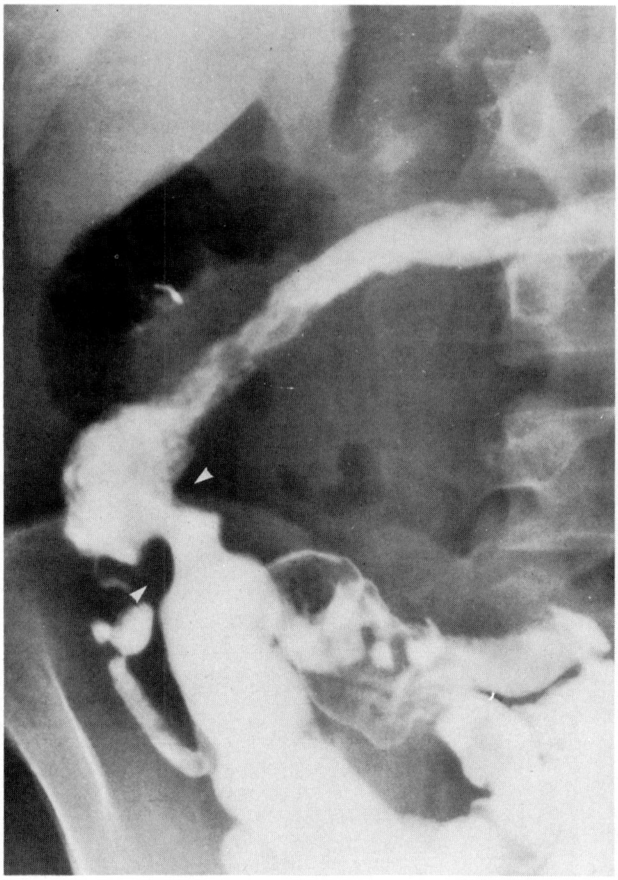

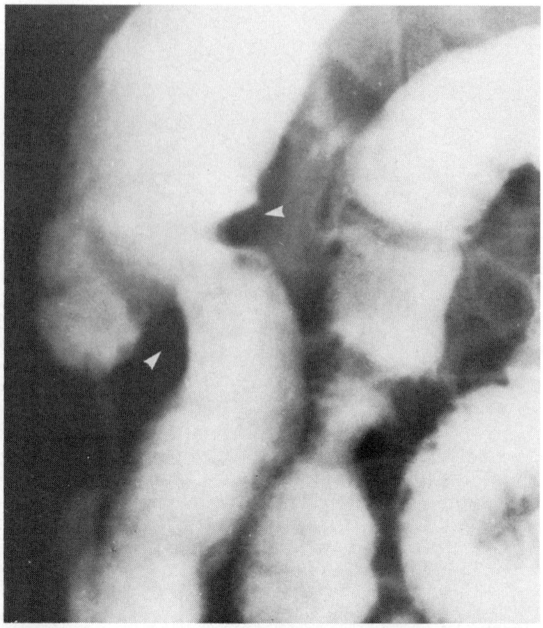

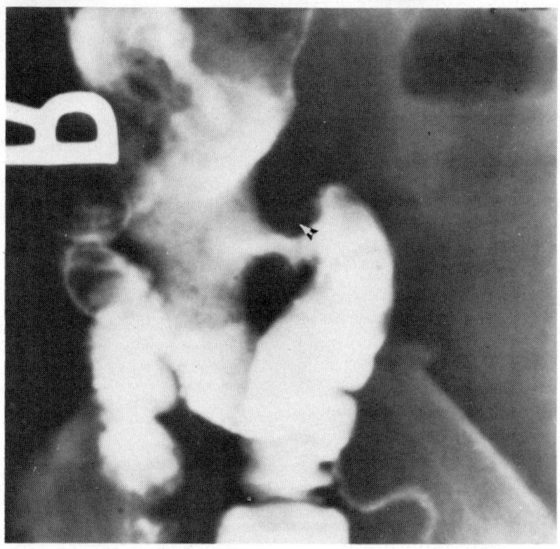

Fig 25–35 (top left). – Granulomatous colitis with atrophy of ileocecal valve. Note gaping valve due to atrophy of lips *(arrowheads),* with smooth and slightly dilated terminal ileum.

Fig 25–36 (top right). – Late changes of ulcerative colitis. Atrophic, gaping ileocecal valve *(arrowheads)* and backwash ileitis are usually associated with ulcerative colitis but may be seen with other inflammatory bowel diseases, including Crohn's disease, tuberculosis and amebiasis.

Fig 25–37 (bottom right). – Ulcerative colitis with thickened ileocecal valve. Valve involved with inflammation becomes thickened. Fistula *(arrowhead)* traversing upper lip of valve is noted. Fistulas across valve are a more common result of Crohn's disease.

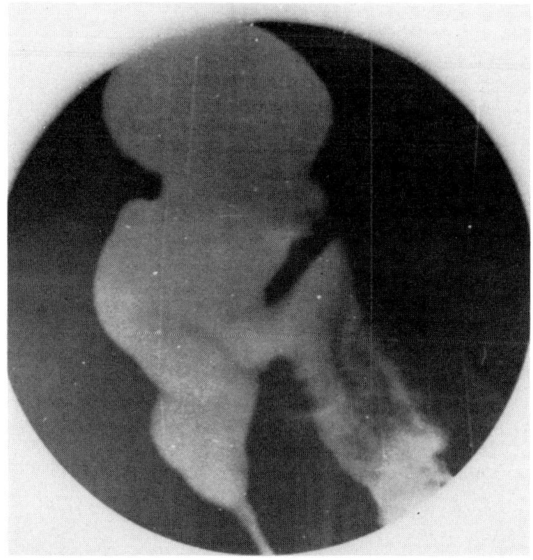

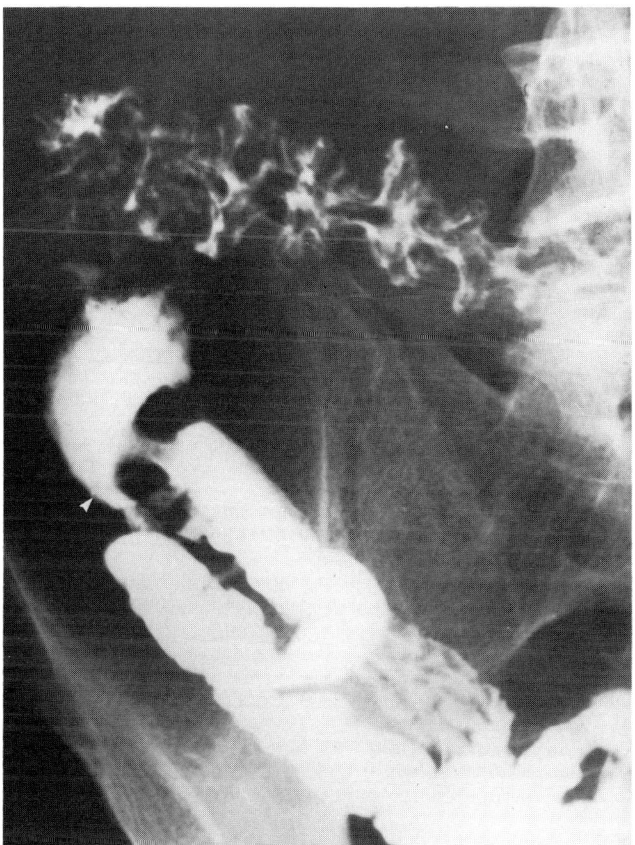

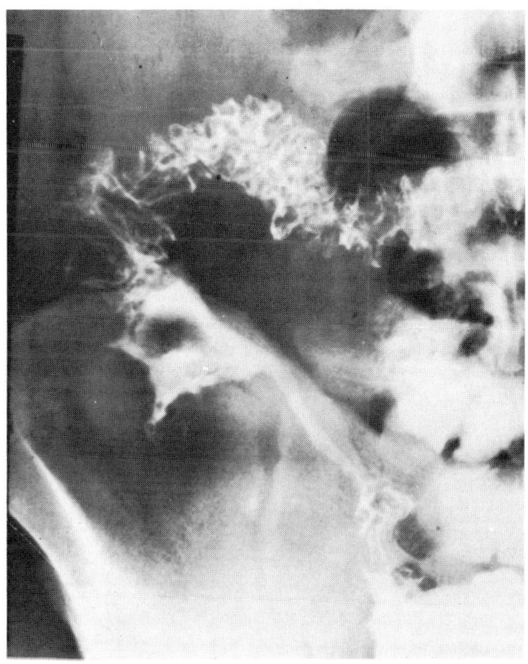

Fig 25–38 (top right). Amebiasis involving ileocecal region. There is conical narrowing of cecum with atrophy of ileocecal valve. Note relatively normal appearance of terminal ileum. (Courtesy of Dr. Robert Armstrong, Audie Murphy Veterans Administration Hospital, San Antonio, Texas.)

Fig 25–39 (left). —Amebiasis of ileocecal region. Entire right side of colon is foreshortened, cecum conical *(arrowhead),* with hypertrophy and rigidity of ileocecal valve, permitting easy coloileal reflux during barium enema. (Courtesy of Dr. Maurice M. Reeder, University of Hawaii at Manoa, Honolulu, Hawaii.)

Fig 25–40 (bottom right). —Ileocecal tuberculosis. Severe distortion of ileocecal valve and narrowing of terminal ileum have produced "inverted umbrella" appearance of valve, which had been thought a specific sign of this disease. Advanced changes of ileocecal tuberculosis cannot be confidently distinguished radiographically from Crohn's disease involving distal ileum and proximal colon.

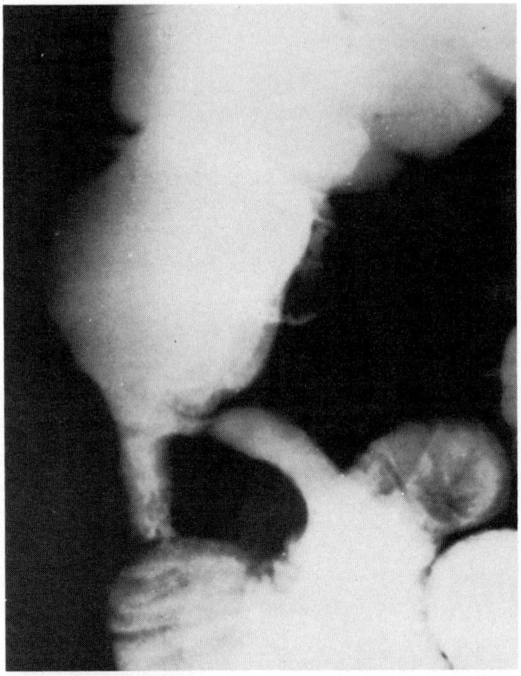

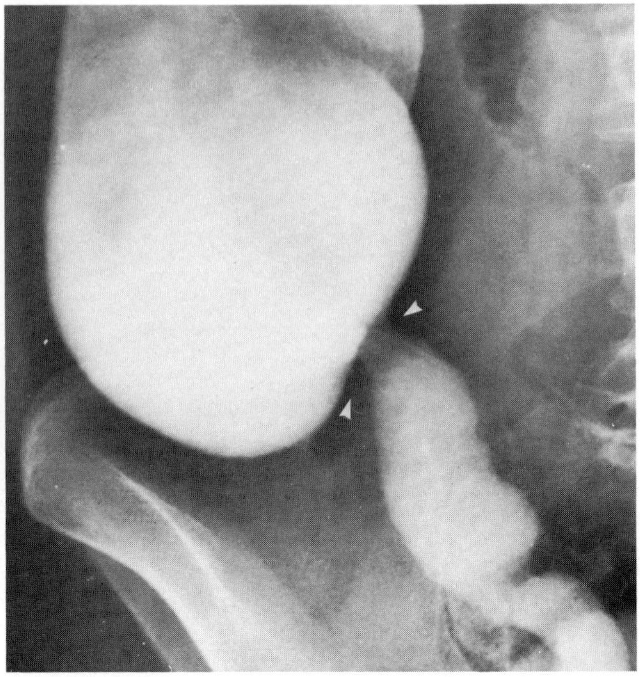

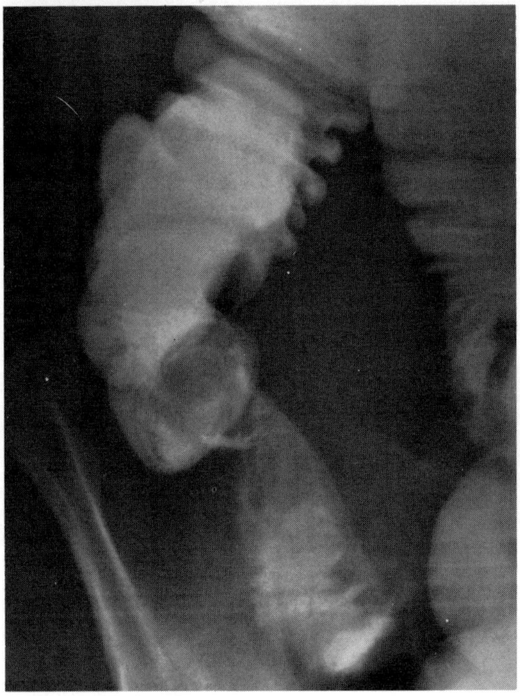

Fig 25–41 (top left).—Ileocecal blastomycosis. Conical appearance of cecum is present with atrophy primarily of lower lip of ileocecal valve with some involvement of terminal ileum. The findings are similar to those of other inflammatory diseases of ileocecal area, particularly tuberculosis. (Courtesy of Dr. Y. Auritchir, Sao Paulo, Brazil.)

Fig 25–42 (top right).—Cathartic colon. Gaping, atrophic ileocecal valve *(arrowheads),* associated with tubular shortening of colon, and an appropriate clinical history of laxative abuse are characteristic.

Fig 25–43 (bottom left).—Appendiceal abscess. A large extrinsic lesion has distorted cecum, ileocecal valve and terminal ileum. Appendix is not filled. This appearance, with an appropriate clinical history, is highly suggestive of this entity. Rarely other inflammatory or neoplastic disease involving the appendix could have this appearance. (Courtesy of Dr. Harvey Goldstein, Methodist Hospital, San Antonio, Texas.)

Chapter 26

Lipomas of the Colon

LAWRENCE W. BASSETT, M.D.
MARVIN WEINER, M.D.

LIPOMAS ARE THE SECOND most common benign tumor of the large intestine, exceeded only by adenomatous polyps. According to autopsy data, they are found in 0.25% of the population.[1] They occur somewhat more frequently in females and are rarely diagnosed before middle age.[2] They usually are solitary lesions averaging 3 cm in size,[2] but larger lesions measuring up to 30 cm in diameter have been reported.[3] They may occur in any part of the large intestine but are more frequently located on the right side of the colon. Most lipomas are submucosal, a few originating in the subserosa. Submucosal lipomas usually are covered by an intact mucosa, although ulceration may occur.[4]

The most common symptoms associated with lipomas are diarrhea, constipation and bleeding.[5] Pedunculated lipomas may cause intussusception, and complete colonic obstruction has been reported with larger tumors.[6] However, lipomas even moderate in size may produce no symptoms, being discovered at the time of barium examination for unrelated reasons.

Submucosal lipomas produce characteristic findings on barium enema examinations. Like other submucosal tumors, they are sharply marginated and smooth in contour (Fig 26–1). Changes in their configuration occur with peristalsis or external compression (Fig 26–2). This feature has been termed the "squeeze sign" and, in combination with a smooth contour, is diagnostic of submucosal lipomas[7, 8] (Fig 26–3). This inherent pliability also accounts for their frequent sausage-shaped or elongated appearance (Fig 26–4).

Larger lipomas frequently are pedunculated and pear shaped, lacking the sharp demarcation between stalk and body seen in adenomatous polyps (Fig 26–5).

Owing to their fatty composition, one might expect these tumors to appear more radiolucent than other neoplasms. In fact, this finding is not of sufficient reliability to be helpful in most cases.

Table 26–1 is useful in differentiating lipomas from other colonic neoplasms.

TABLE 26–1.—DIFFERENTIATION OF LIPOMAS AND OTHER NEOPLASMS

NEOPLASM	SMOOTH CONTOUR	PLIABILITY
Lipoma	+	+
Carcinoma; large adenoma	−	
Small adenoma	+	−
Villous adenoma	−	+
Other nonepithelial tumors (e.g., Leiomyoma, neurofibroma)	+	−

REFERENCES

1. Helwig, E. B.: Benign Tumors of the Large Intestine, Surg. Gynecol. Obstet. 76:419, 1943.
2. Castro, E. B., and Stearns, M. W.: Lipoma of the large intestine: A review of 45 cases, Dis. Colon Rectum:441, 1972.
3. Weinberg, T., and Feldman, M.: Lipomas of the gastrointestinal tract, Am. J. Clin. Pathol. 25:272, 1955.
4. Berk, R. N., and Werner, L. G.: The radiology corner—Lipoma of the colon, Am. J. Gastroenterol. 61: 145, 1974.
5. Pemberton, J. D., and McCormack, C. J.: Submucous lipomas of colon and rectum, Am. J. Surg. 37(2): 205, 1937.
6. Pemberton, L. B., and Manax, W. G.: Complete obstruction of the colon by lipoma, Surgery 69(1):139, 1971.
7. Hurwitz, M. M., Redleaf, P. D., Williams, H. J., and Edwards, J. E.: Lipomas of the gastrointestinal tract: An analysis of seventy-two tumors, Am. J. Roentgenol. 99(1):84, 1967.
8. Wolf, B. S., Melamed, M., and Khilnani, M. T.: Lipoma of the colon, Mt. Sinai J. Med. NY 21:80, 1954–1955.

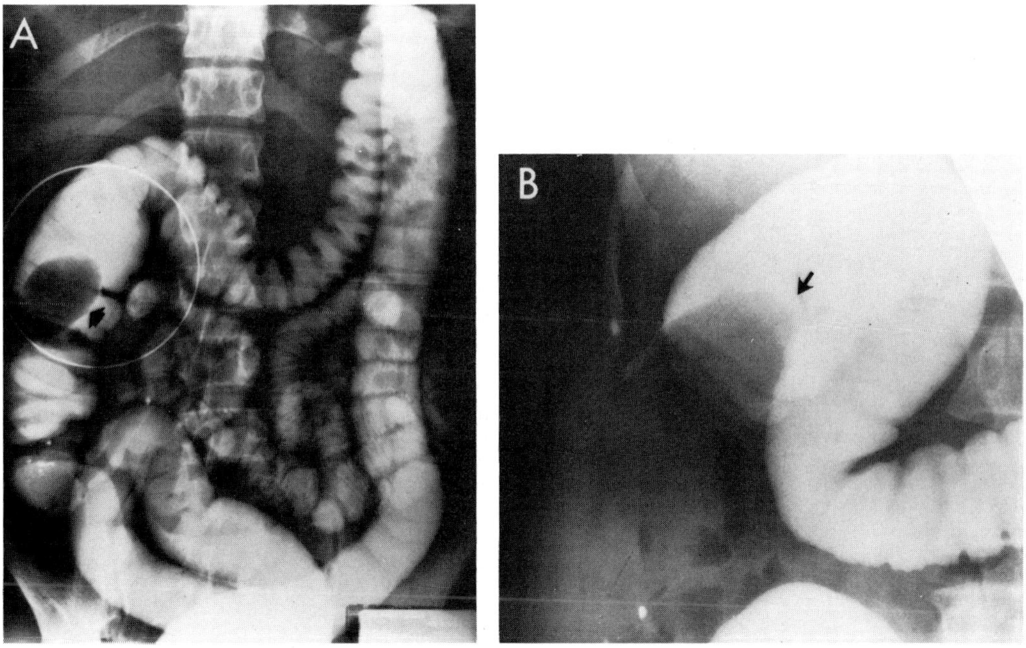

Fig 26–1. – **A,** oval, sharply marginated, smoothly contoured appearance of this lipoma *(arrows)* of ascending colon is typical. **B,** patient presented with obstructive symptoms secondary to intussusception of lipoma. (Courtesy of Drs. Edward I. Greenbaum and Milton Lerner.)

Fig 26–2. – **A** and **B,** broad-based submucosal lipoma of descending colon demonstrates changes in contour and position observed during barium examination.

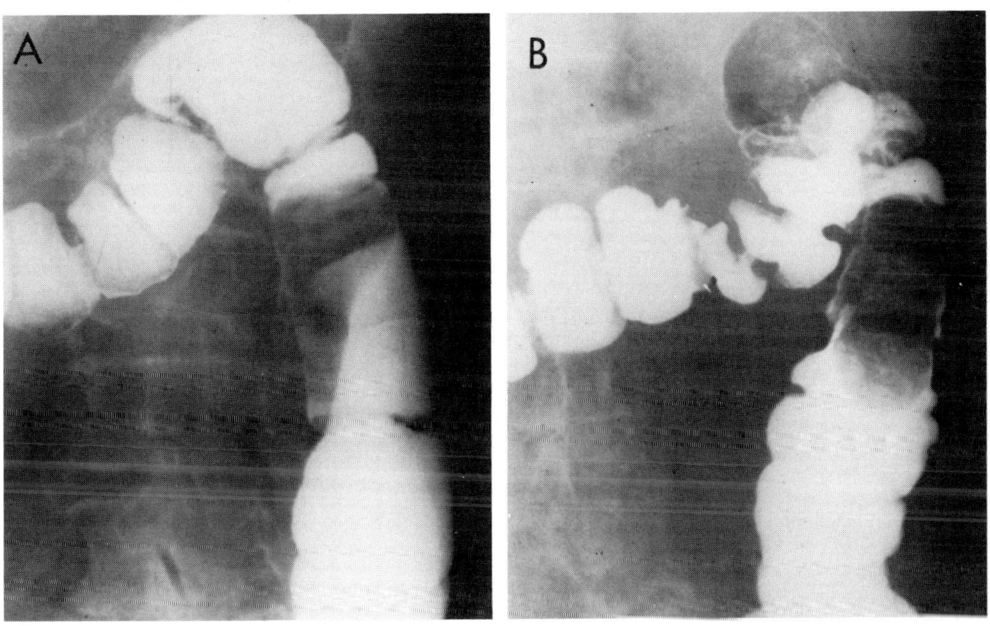

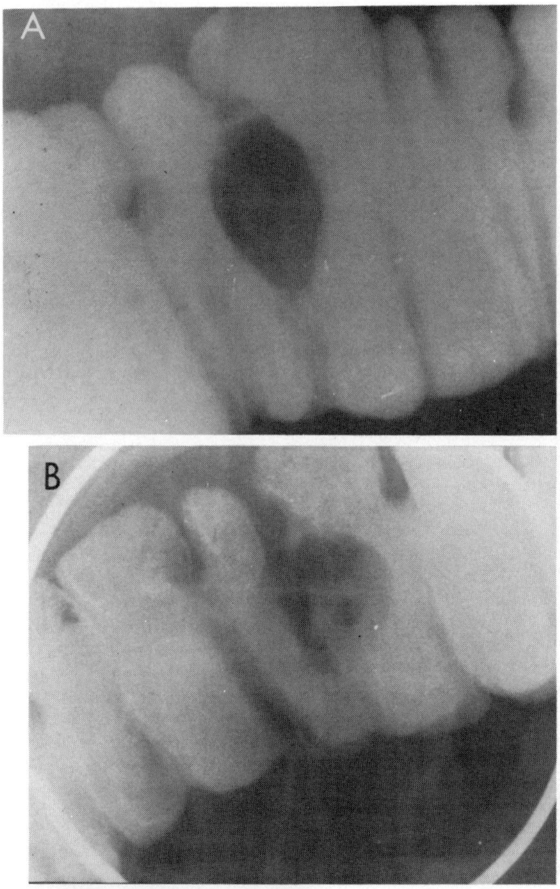

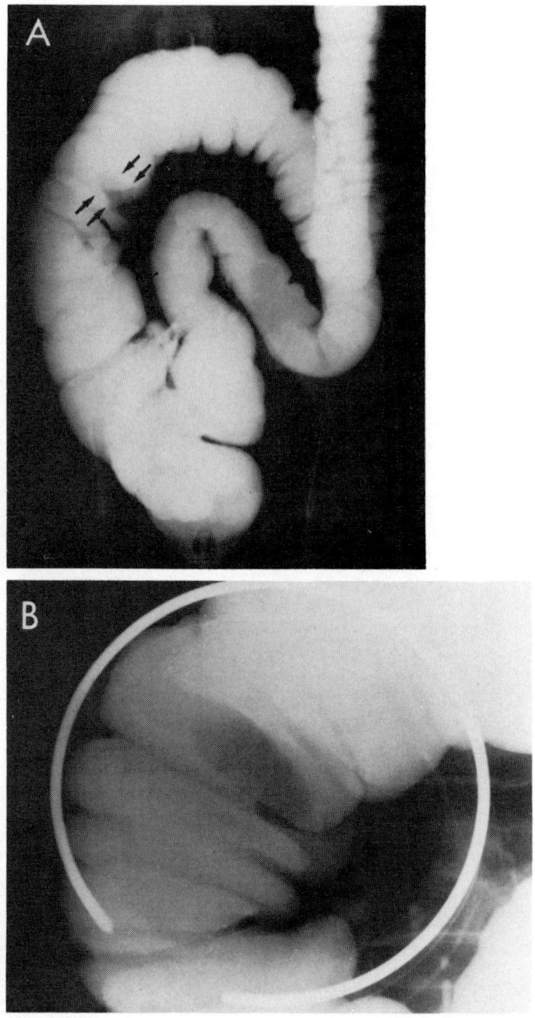

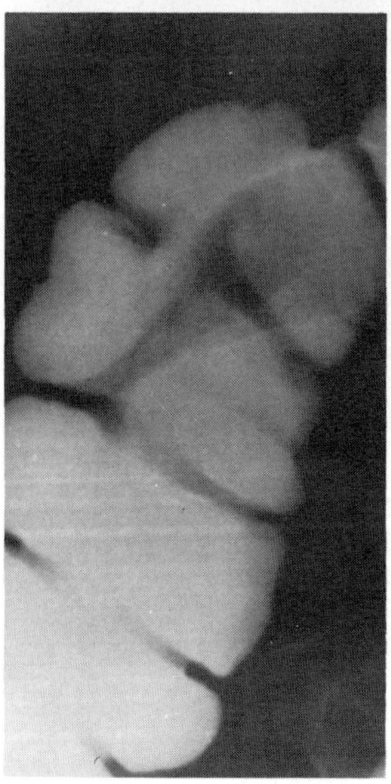

Fig 26–3 (top left).—**A** and **B,** ovoid-shaped lipoma of transverse colon shows characteristic changes in contour and configuration with external compression ("squeeze sign").

Fig 26–4 (top right).—**A** and **B,** lipoma *(arrows)* near hepatic flexure demonstrated smooth, sausage-shaped appearance frequently encountered.

Fig 26–5 (bottom).—Pedunculated lipoma of hepatic flexure exhibiting pear-shaped appearance with lack of demarcation between head and stalk.

Chapter 27

Lymphomas of the Large Intestine

JAMES M. HALLS, M.B., F.R.C.P.(C)

LYMPHOMATOUS INVOLVEMENT of the gastrointestinal tract is not common. Warren and Lulensky[1] report an 0.9% incidence in a total of 3,132 gastrointestinal tumors. In about one half of the 362 cases in Berg's series[2] the stomach was involved, one-third showed disease in the small intestine and in one-sixth there was sole or predominant involvement of the colon. Lewin et al.[3] report similar ratios in their study of 117 cases presenting with gastrointestinal disease. Warren and Lulensky[1] also described an 0.3% incidence of lymphoma of the large bowel in a series of 2,510 cases of colonic and rectal cancers.

The most common site of involvement is the ileocecal region and, less frequently, the rectosigmoid,[4] reflecting the fact that there is normally more lymphoid tissue in these two areas than in any other part of the colon. However, lymphoma may occur in other areas of the large bowel, including the appendix.

Frequently, multiple lesions are seen, usually confined to one anatomical segment of the intestine, but other sites may be concurrently involved. In the latter instances, the lesions are often accompanied by massive mesenteric and retroperitoneal involvement.

Lesions usually occur in the fifth to seventh decades, but occasionally the disease is seen in patients under age 16. There is no racial bias, but a significant sex difference exists in lymphomas located in the ileocecal region, where the male/female ratio is 3.3:1.

Diffuse histiocytic lymphoma is the most common histologic type, characteristic of extranodal lymphoma, and Hodgkin's disease is the rarest.

Earlier reports stated that gastrointestinal lymphoma was invariably fatal, but more recent studies have documented survival rates varying between 30% and 45%. Prognosis does not appear to be significantly affected by cell type but is seriously influenced by extension into regional lymph nodes. Dissemination beyond the regional lymph nodes also is of great prognostic significance, and none of the patients in the Lewin et al.[3] series, in whom this had occurred, were alive more than 2 years from the time of diagnosis. Ileocecal lymphoma appears to have a slightly better prognosis than lymphoma of the rectum.

Patients with lymphoma of the colon may present with anemia from chronic blood loss, malaise, weight loss and abdominal pain. Occasionally the presentation may be acute, resulting from intestinal obstruction, either simple or complicating an intussusception, or it may be a catastrophic illness precipitated by perforation. Rectal lesions most often manifest themselves by bright red rectal bleeding of varying degree.

Radiologic Considerations

Lymphoma of the colon may present in two forms: (1) localized—infiltrative or polypoid, and (2) diffuse—infiltrative, often extending over long segments.

LOCALIZED DISEASE

This form of lymphoma may present with nonspecific features of an irregular intraluminal lesion (Fig. 27–1) and mimic other forms of colonic disease. Differentiation from carcinoma may be impossible, and even the surgeon may be surprised that the histologic diagnosis of the resected specimen is lymphoma. On the other hand, segmental lymphomatous infiltration is sometimes more suggestive of inflammatory disease than of neoplasia (Fig. 27–2).

Some radiologic presentations, however, strongly suggest lymphoma.

PRESENCE OF BULKY EXTRACOLONIC COMPONENT: Figure 27–3 illustrates such a case, a man age 45, who presented with abdominal pain and increasing malaise. A smooth filling defect was demonstrated in the pole of the cecum (see Fig. 27–3, A), covered by normal mucosa and thought initially to be an appendiceal abscess. After a downhill course of 2 months, the study was repeated, at which time a huge extracolonic component was demonstrated, together with irregular narrowing of the lumen and destruction of the mucosa (see Fig. 27–3, B). The radiographic appearances and the rapid growth rate were strongly suggestive of lymphoma.

CONCENTRIC DILATATION OF THE LUMEN OF THE COLON: This dilatation, secondary to destruction of full thickness of the bowel wall, also is suggestive of lymphoma. As there is no accompanying desmoplastic reaction, aneurysmal dilatation may be similar to that seen in small bowel lymphoma. Owing to the lack of a fibrous response, it is not surprising that perforation of some of the lesions may occur. Two patients recently at our medical center presented with acute abdominal pain and rigidity after a short history of chronic ill health and were found to have perforated cecal lesions (Fig. 27–4).

NONSPECIFIC COLONIC LESION ACCOMPANYING RADIOGRAPHICALLY DIAGNOSABLE LESIONS ELSEWHERE IN GASTROINTESTINAL TRACT: Figure 27–5, A, shows an irregular cecal filling defect in a patient who had a diffuse infiltrative process in the stomach (see Fig. 27–5, B), the radiographic characteristics of which suggest lymphoma.

POLYPOID FILLING DEFECTS APPEARING IN PROXIMAL COLON: Such defects, when they result from disease of the ileocecal valve and distal ileum (Fig. 27–6), suggest lymphoma. The size of the filling defects may be exaggerated by partial intussusception.

DIFFUSE DISEASE

This form of disease is characterized by extensive submucosal thickening secondary to cellular infiltration. Long segments of colon may be involved, often in a continuous fashion, but variation in the degree of infiltration may give rise to discontinuous radiographic appearances mimicking skip lesions (Fig. 27–7).

Wolfe and Marshak[5] described examples of diffuse lymphomatous infiltration appearing as hugely thickened mucosal folds and finger-like indentation along the contour of the colon. Increased distensibility and retention of the haustral fold pattern also were features of the cases described in their series.

In early involvement, "tethering" of intact mucosa, similar to that seen in metastatic carcinoma, may be present (see Fig. 27–7, A), and differentiation may be impossible. At a later stage, the mucosa becomes serrated over long segments (Fig. 27–8), the irregularity being due to formation of innumerable sessile protrusions into bowel lumen. Numerous flat-based projections of barium suggest ulceration, but most of these merely represent pools of contrast medium lying between the polypoid projections, since histologic ulceration usually is not marked.

Differentiation from familial polyposis and pseudopolyposis associated with inflammatory bowel disease may be difficult. Careful analysis of the lesions, as demonstrated by air contrast enema, may give important clues, since the polyps seen in familial polyposis often are both sessile and pedunculated with great variation in size, and the polyps seen in healed inflammatory bowel disease are filiform and may even be branched.

The association of adenocarcinoma with chronic ulcerative colitis is well known, but this chronic inflammatory disease is rarely complicated by lymphoma.[6] Whether lymphoma develops as a complication of longstanding ulcerative colitis or whether lymphoma masquerades from the outset as ulcerative colitis has not been established.

REFERENCES

1. Warren, S., and Lulensky, C. R.: Primary solitary lymphoid tumors of the gastrointestinal tract, Ann. Surg. 115:1, 1942.
2. Berg, J. W.: Primary lymphoma of the human gastrointestinal tract, Natl. Cancer Inst. Monogr. 32: 211, 1969.
3. Lewin, K. J., Ranchod, M., and Dorfman, R. F.: Lymphoma of the gastrointestinal tract, Cancer 42: 693, 1978.
4. Morson, B. C., and Dawson, I. M. P.: *Gastrointestinal Pathology* (Oxford: Blackwell Scientific Publications, 1972).
5. Wolf, B. S., and Marshak, R. H.: Roentgen features of diffuse lymphosarcoma of the colon, Radiology 75:733, 1960.
6. Friedman, H. B., Silver, G. M., and Brown, C. H.: Lymphoma of the colon simulating ulcerative colitis, Am. J. Dig. Dis. 13:910, 1968.

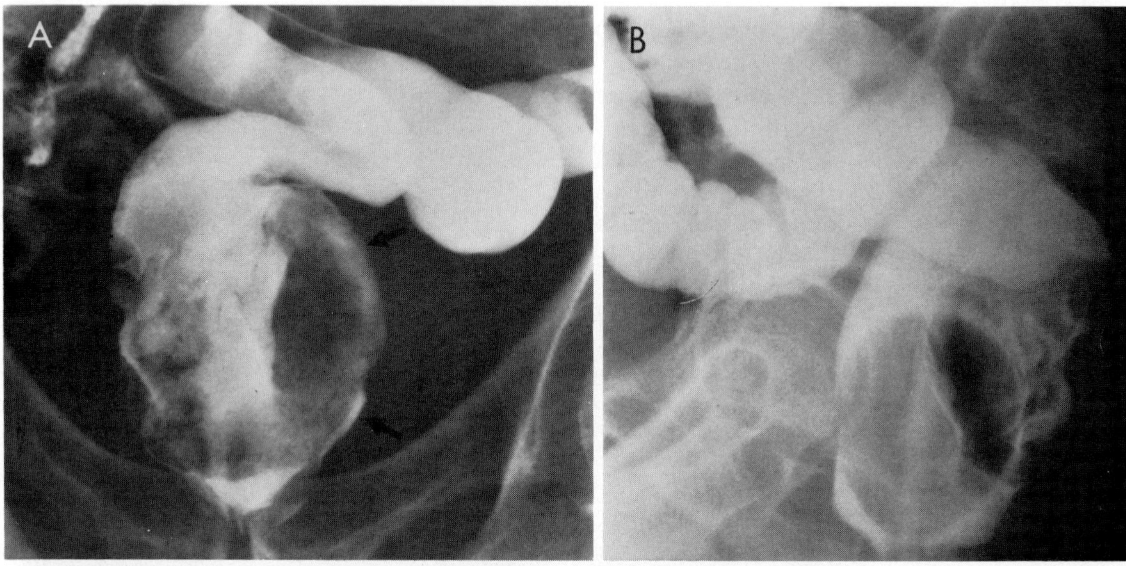

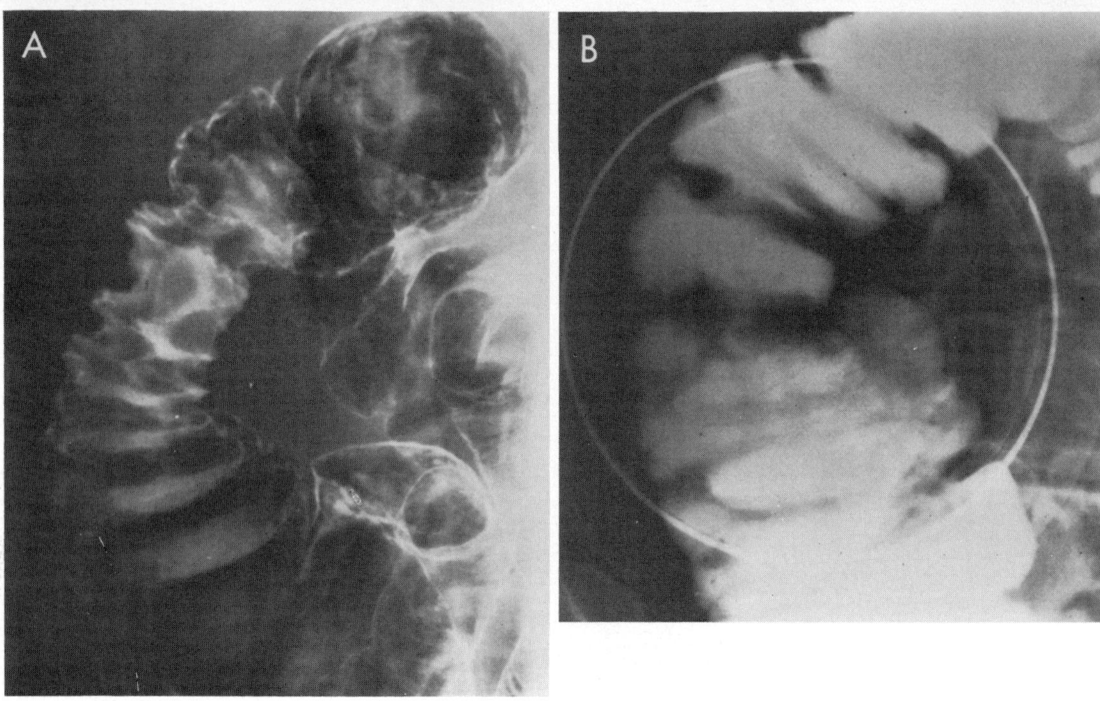

Fig 27–1 (top). – **A,** supine view. Large irregular filling defects *(arrows)* in rectum mimicking carcinoma. **B,** lateral view. Histologic diagnosis: lymphoma.

Fig 27–2 (bottom). – **A,** short segment of irregular narrowing in ascending colon. Note cobblestone appearance of mucosa. The appearances suggested Crohn's disease of colon. **B,** after radiation therapy. Histologic diagnosis: lymphoma.

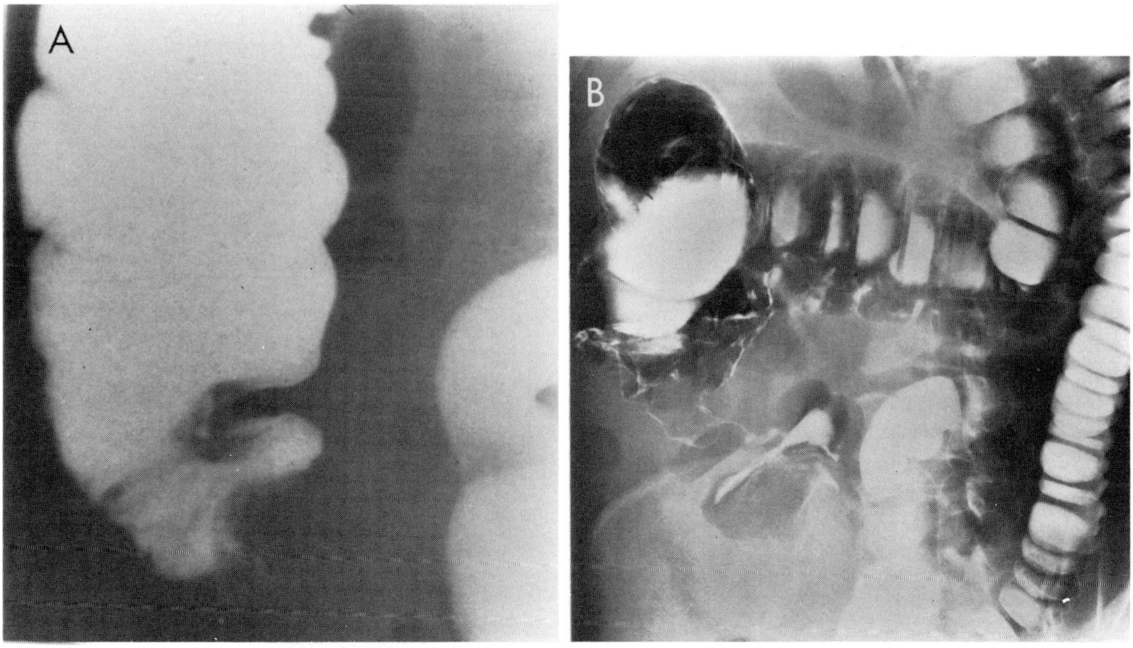

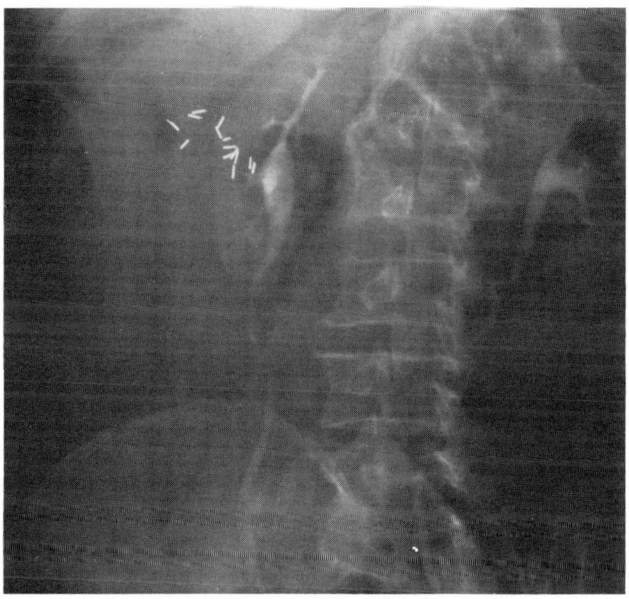

Fig 27–3 (top). – **A,** filling defect in pole of cecum with normal mucosa. Abnormality was diagnosed as an appendix abscess. **B,** 2 months later, long segment of irregular narrowing was demonstrated in ascending colon accompanied by bulky extracolonic component. Irregular mucosal destruction also was noted. Histologic diagnosis: lymphoma.

Fig 27–4 (bottom). – Extracolonic gas from perforation of cecal lesion. Histologic diagnosis: lymphoma.

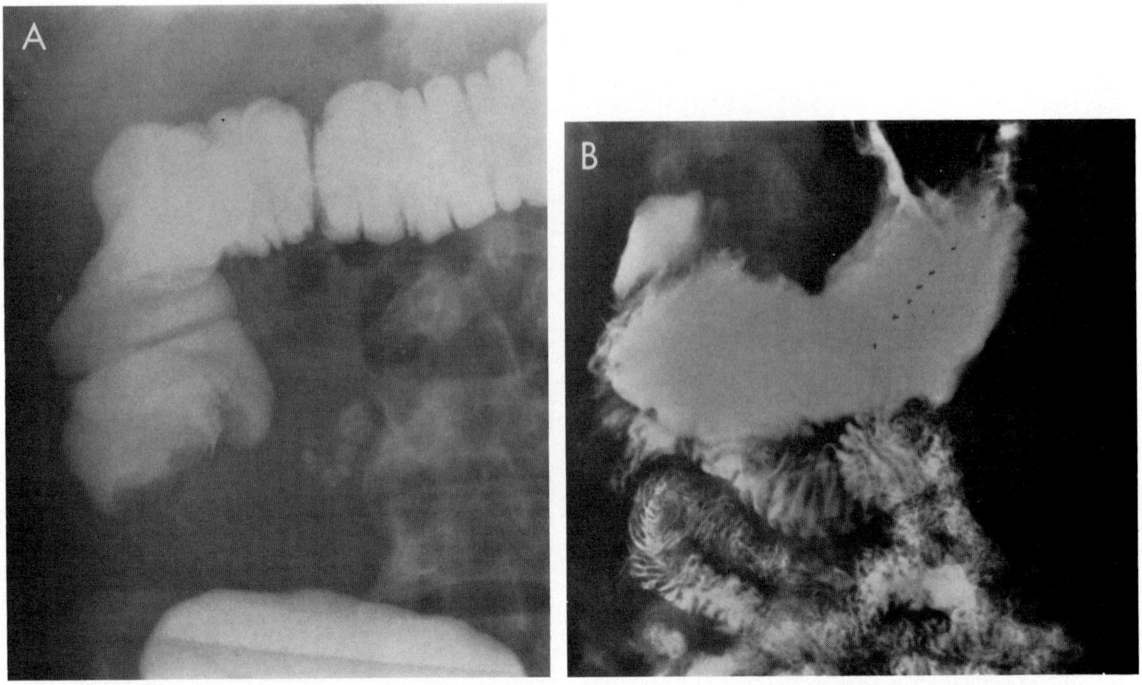

Fig 27–5. – **A,** lesion of cecum mimicking carcinoma. **B,** patient also had diffuse infiltration of stomach. Histologic diagnosis: lymphoma.

Fig 27–6. – **A,** patient presenting with small bowel obstruction. **B,** partially intussuscepted mass in ileocecal region demonstrated by barium enema. Histologic diagnosis: lymphoma.

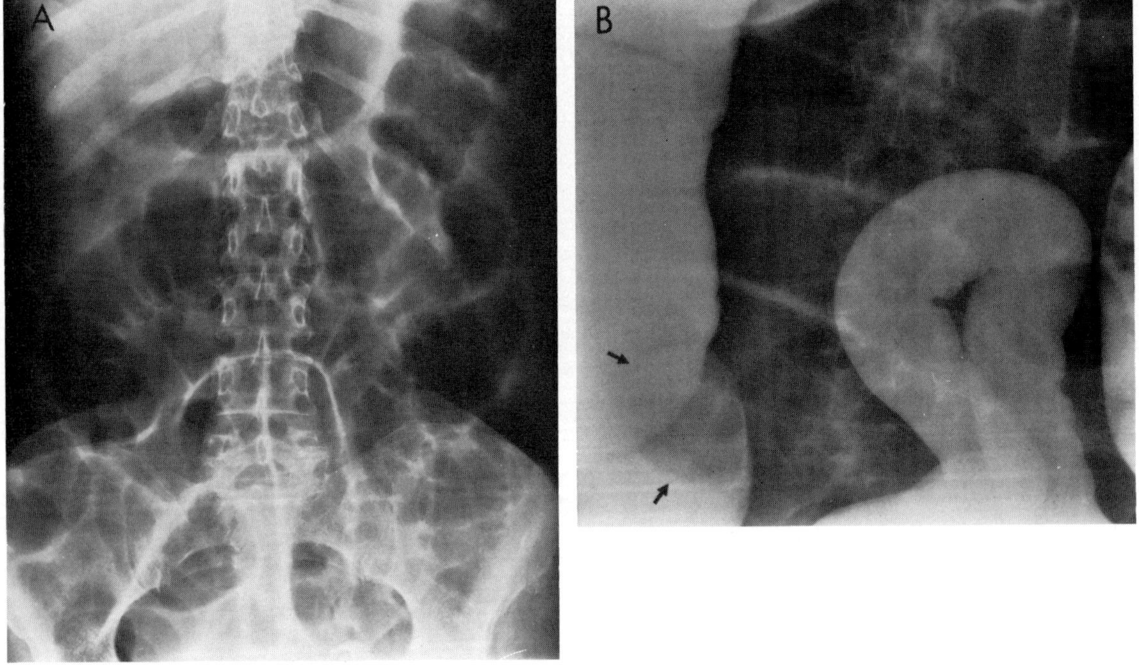

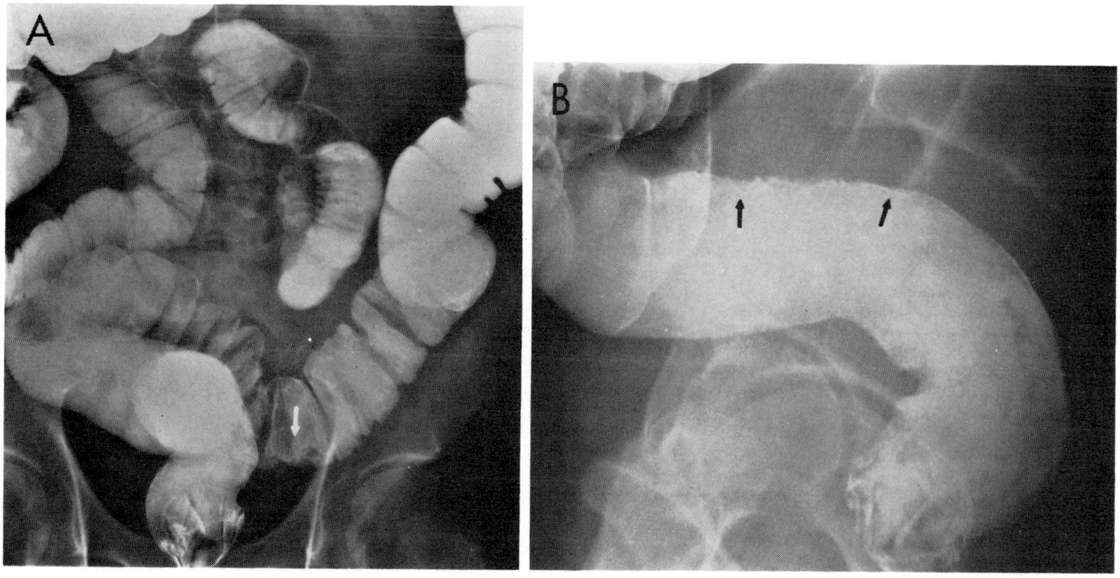

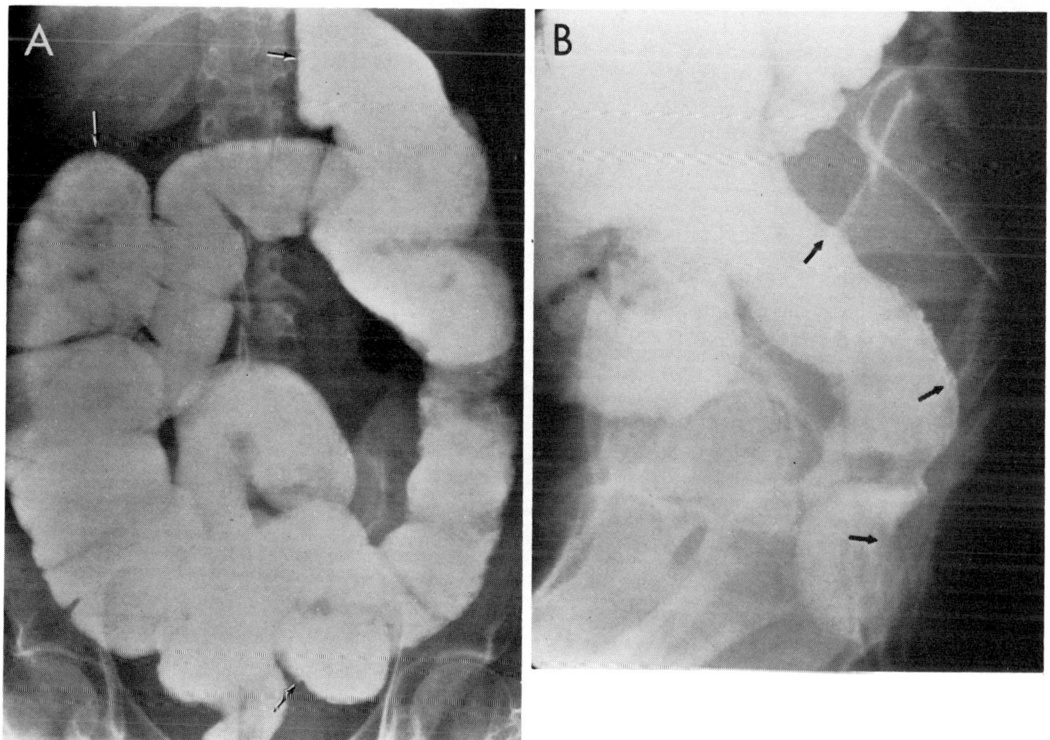

Fig 27–7 (top). – **A,** barium enema showing patchy small, nodular asymmetric lesions in left side of colon *(arrow)*. **B,** lateral view of section showing irregularity of posterior-superior aspect of rectosigmoid *(arrows)*. Histologic diagnosis: lymphoma.

Fig 27–8 (bottom). – **A,** extensive involvement of colon and rectum. Numerous sessile projections into lumen have been demonstrated, as well as flat-based projections beyond lumen *(arrows)* mimicking ulceration. **B,** irregularity of outline of rectum with some loss of distensibility *(arrows)*. Histologic diagnosis: lymphoma.

Chapter 28

Miscellaneous Lesions of the Colon

EDWARD I. GREENBAUM, M.D.

BIBLIOGRAPHY

1. Bargen, J. A.: Chronic ulcerative colitis: Diagnostic and therapeutic problems – A lifetime study, Am. J. Roentgenol. 99:5, 1967.
2. Stein, G. N., Roy, R., and Finkelstein, A. K.: Roentgen changes in ulcerative colitis, Semin. Roentgenol. 3:3, 1968.
3. Dodds, W., and McGlaughlin, P.: Intestinal intussusception in adults, Am. J. Gastroenterol. 55:284, 1971.
4. Briggs, D., Carpathios, J., and Zollinger, R.: Intussusception in adults, Am. J. Surg. 101:109, 1961.
5. Maroun, W. J., Nelson, S., Zimmer, J., and Reeder, M. M.: RPC of the Month from the AFIP, Radiology 96:649, 1970.
6. Cavanagh, R. C., Buchignani, J. S., and Rulon, D. B.: RPC of the Month from the AFIP, Radiology 101: 195, 1971.
7. Tellum, G.: *Special Tumors of the Ovary and Testes – Krukenberg Tumor* (Philadelphia: J. B. Lippincott Co., 1971), p. 260.
8. Smith, T. R., Freedman, S. N., and Adler, H.: Streptococcus bovis septicemia as a clue to colon neoplasms in two cases, Am. J. Roentgenol. 131:887, 1978.
9. Fainsinger, M. H.: Unusual foreign bodies in the bowel, J.A.M.A. 2225, 1977.

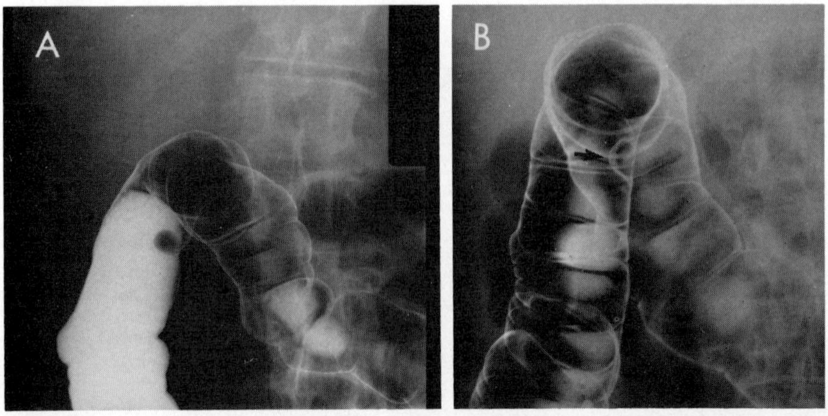

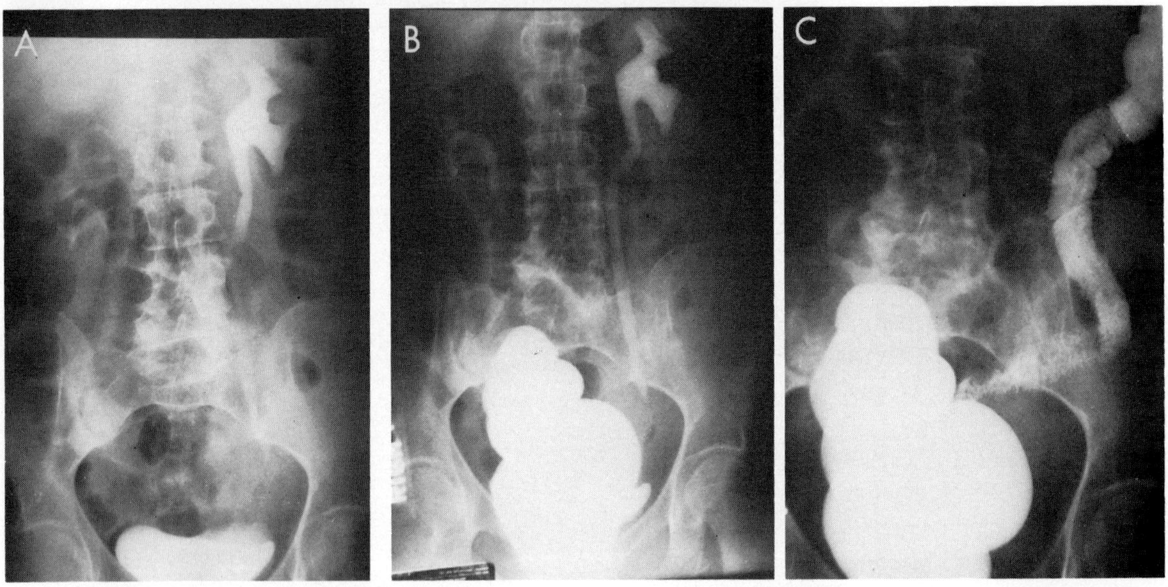

Fig 28–1 (top). – Leiomyoma of hepatic flexure of colon. **A,** smooth, sharply demarcated mass, which in **B** is clearly intramural. Margin of tumor forms 90-degree angle with adjacent colon wall. (Courtesy Drs. Angelo Dagradi and Jane McMillan, Long Beach VA Hosp., Long Beach, Cal.)

Fig 28–2 (bottom). – Tubo-ovarian abscess simulating diverticulitis. **A** soft tissue mass in left hemipelvis with obstruction of pelvic ureter and secondary hydroureter and hydronephrosis on left. **B,** initial barium examination was incomplete due to spasm and inability to fill colon. **C,** 2 days later barium enema was repeated with aid of glucagon. A long, narrowed segment of sigmoid colon is seen, with mucosa preserved. Several diverticula are seen in vicinity. At surgery this was thought to be a "diverticulic mass"; however, at pathology it was found to be a tubo-ovarian abscess. (Courtesy Drs. Herbert Roedling and Wolfgang Hallauer.)

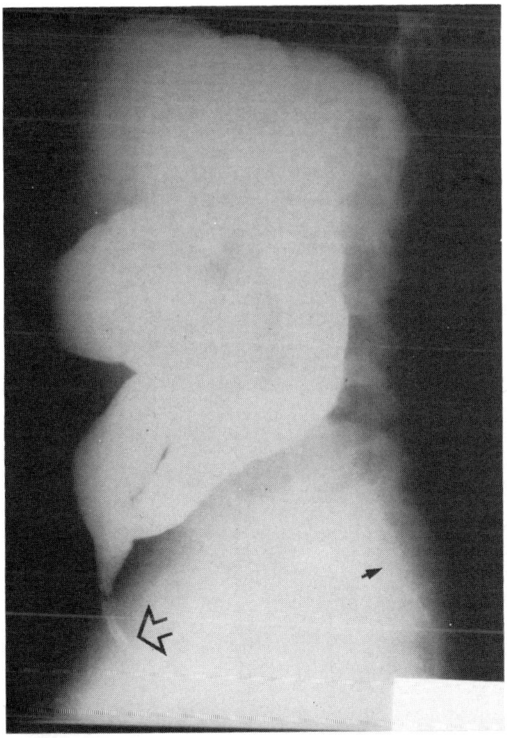

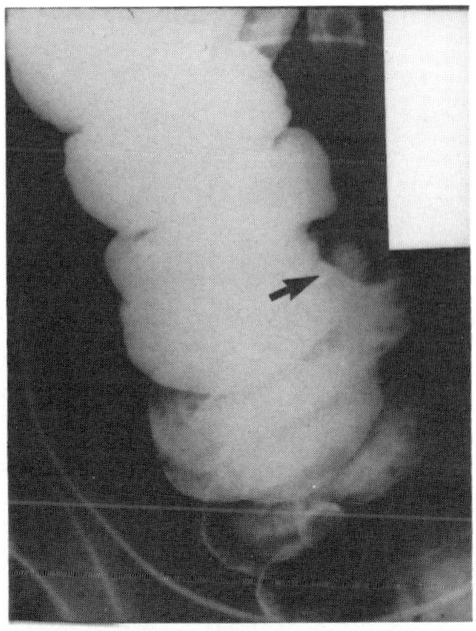

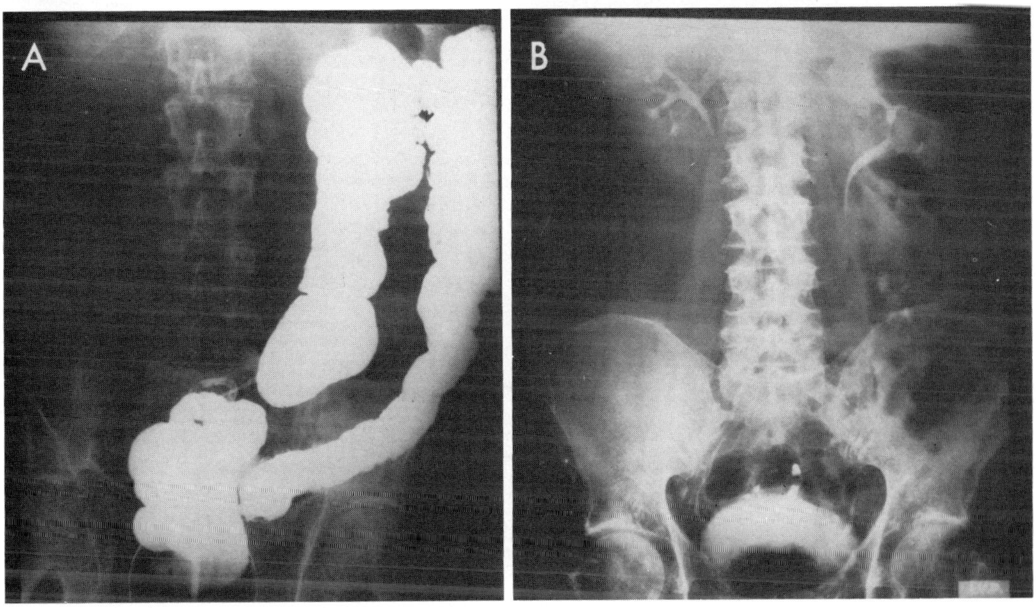

Fig 28–3 (top left).—Rectal duplication cyst. Lateral rectal view shows huge presacral mass with marked anterior displacement of rectum (see *open arrow* on lateral view; *small arrow* denotes anterior margin of sacrum).

Fig 28–4 (top right).—Metastatic melanoma with metastases to cecum *(arrow)*. Metastatic nodule has central collection of barium creating "bulls-eye" appearance.

Fig 28–5 (bottom).—**A,** huge retroperitoneal liposarcoma causing displacement of right hemicolon across midline. Radiolucency is seen in right retroperitoneal area due to fat density of this tumor. **B,** superior displacement of right kidney.

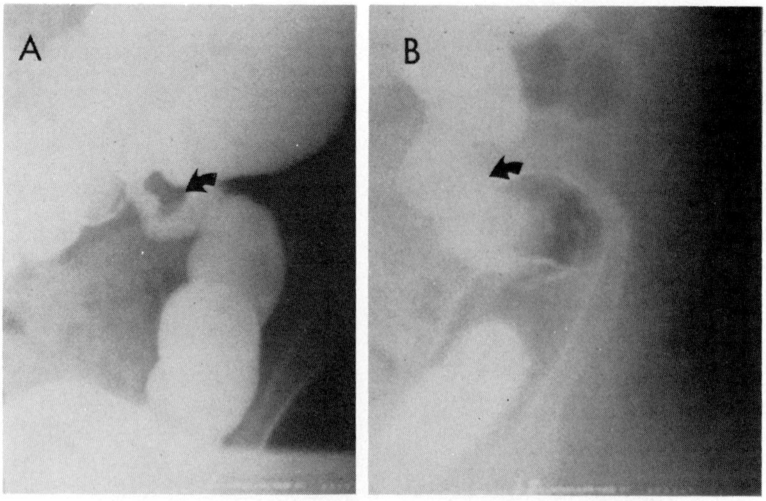

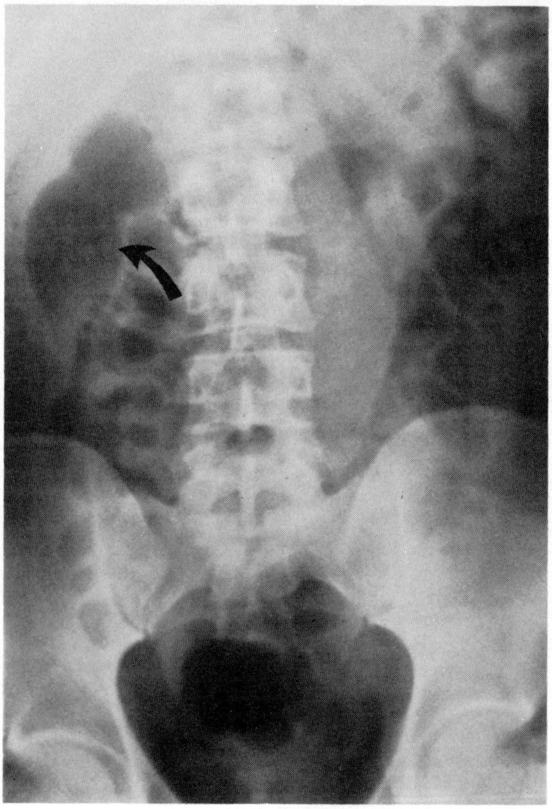

Fig 28–6 (top). – Small carcinoma of colon originally misdiagnosed as a spasm. **A,** filled column showed narrowed segment in midportion of descending colon *(arrow),* which on air contrast examination **B,** appeared to distend. Note, however, persistent fixation and rigidity at lateral margin of this lesion. Also, luminal diameter is diminished due to fixation of lateral wall *(arrow).* At surgery small, dime-sized, ulcerating, flat carcinoma of colon was seen that occupied about one fifth of total circumference of colon in this area.

Fig 28–7 (bottom). – Colon duplication. Air-filled sacular structure *(arrow)* is seen in right upper quadrant, which on barium enema (not shown) was seen to lie lateral to ascending colon and communicated with ileocecal region.

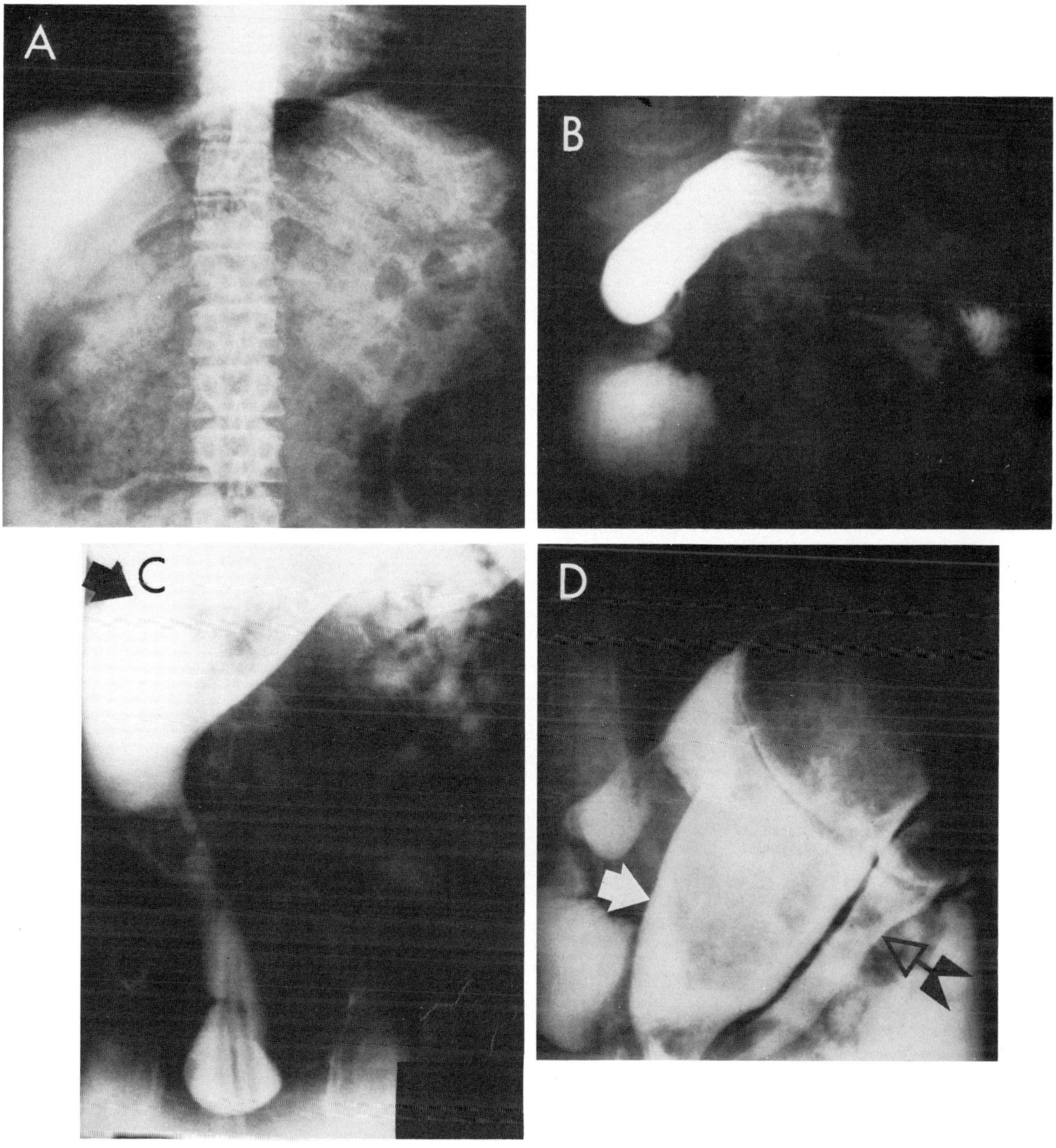

Fig 28–8.—Megasigmoid causing duodenal obstruction. **A,** fecal-filled mass occupying entire upper abdomen. **B,** Gastrografin (diatrizoate) upper gastrointestinal examination shows an extrinsic lesion obstructing duodenum at its third portion. **C,** Gastrografin enema shows megasigmoid with its ascending limb *(arrow)* extending toward duodenum. **D,** Gastrografin-filled megasigmoid is seen crossing third portion of duodenum and extending to level of left diaphragm; *(white arrow* marks ascending limb of megasigmoid colon at point just superior to crossing of third portion of duodenum); descending limb *(open arrow)* also is noted. (Courtesy of Dr. Mary Oda, Serra Memorial Hospital, Sun Valley, Calif.)

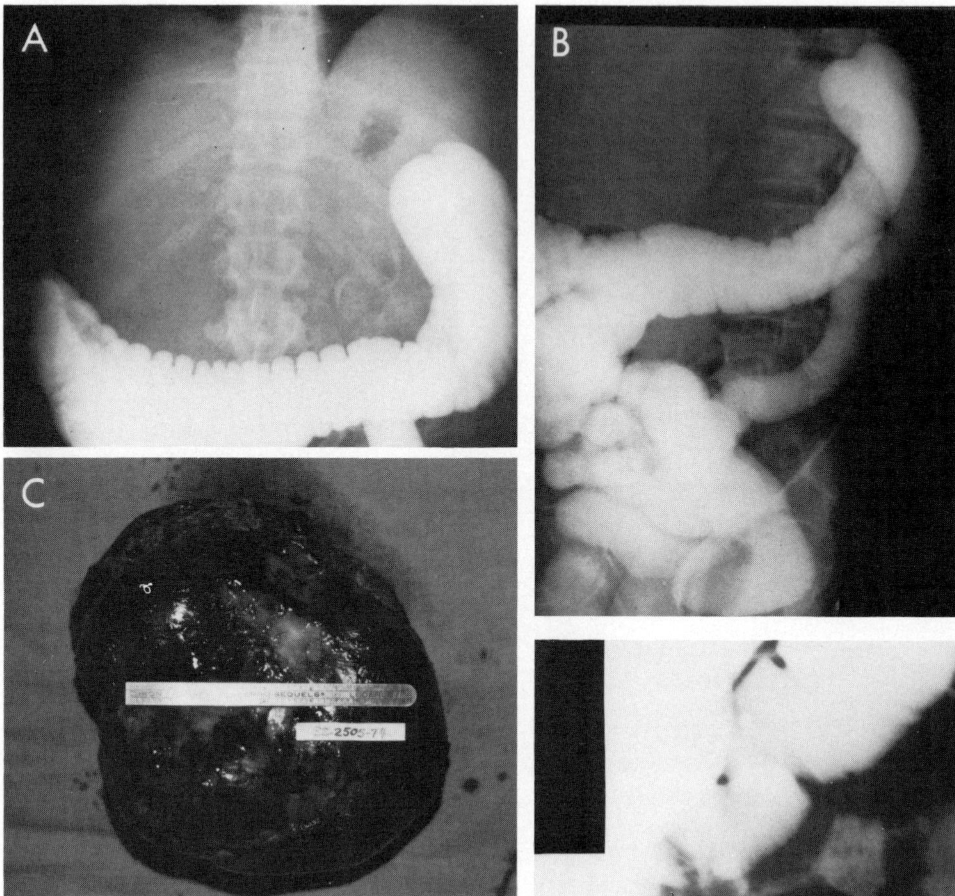

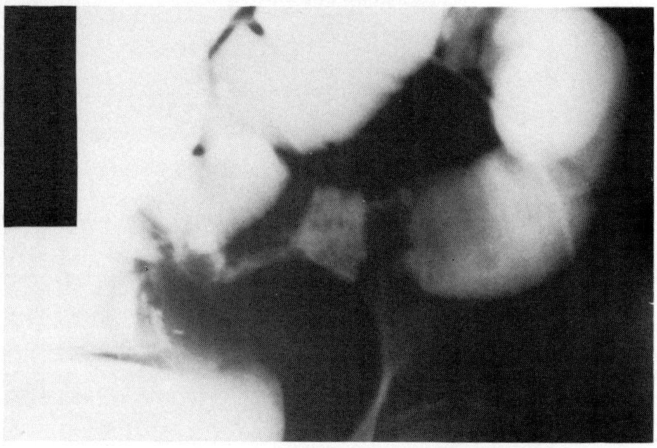

Fig 28–9 (top and left).—Large calcified adrenal carcinoma, causing **(A)** extrinsic compression of hepatic flexure. **B,** right posterior oblique view of barium examination of colon shows adrenal carcinoma causing extrinsic compression at hepatic flexure. **C,** adrenal carcinoma—gross specimen. (Gross specimen courtesy of Dr. Otto Klinger, Newhall, Calif.)

Fig 28–10 (bottom right).—Pelvic inflammatory disease (PID) with colon involvement. Irregular narrowing of midsigmoid colon is seen secondary to chronic PID.

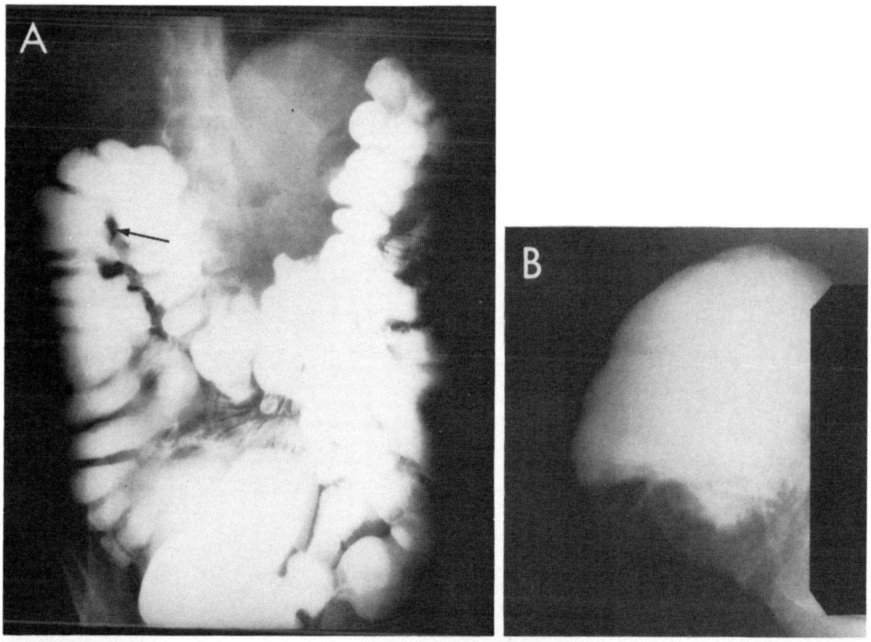

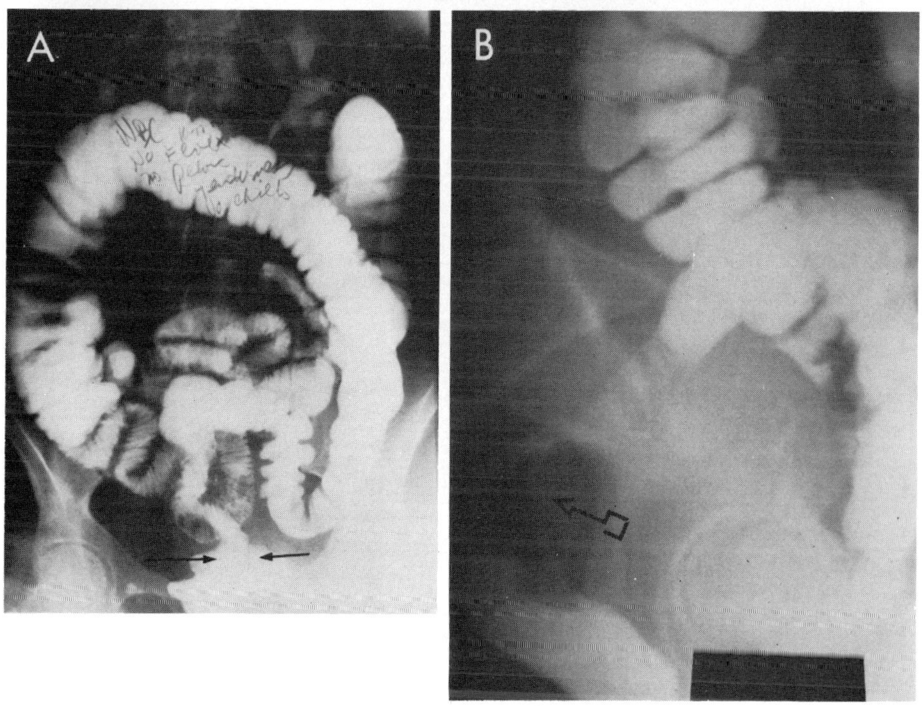

Fig 28–11 (top).—Carcinoma of colon in ulcerative colitis. **A,** small, flat, nonpliable segment of medial wall of ascending colon in region of hepatic flexure *(arrow)*. In ulcerative colitis, early infiltrating lesion may be extremely difficult to diagnose radiographically, and any flattening or loss of normal contours with rigidity and/or loss of pliability should be viewed with suspicion. **B,** 1 year later, obstructing annular carcinoma was noted.

Fig 28–12 (bottom).—Pelvic abscess secondary to pelvic inflammatory disease with rectal involvement. **A,** elongation, narrowing and distortion of rectum. **B,** lateral rectal view shows extrinsic mass compressing anterior wall of rectum.

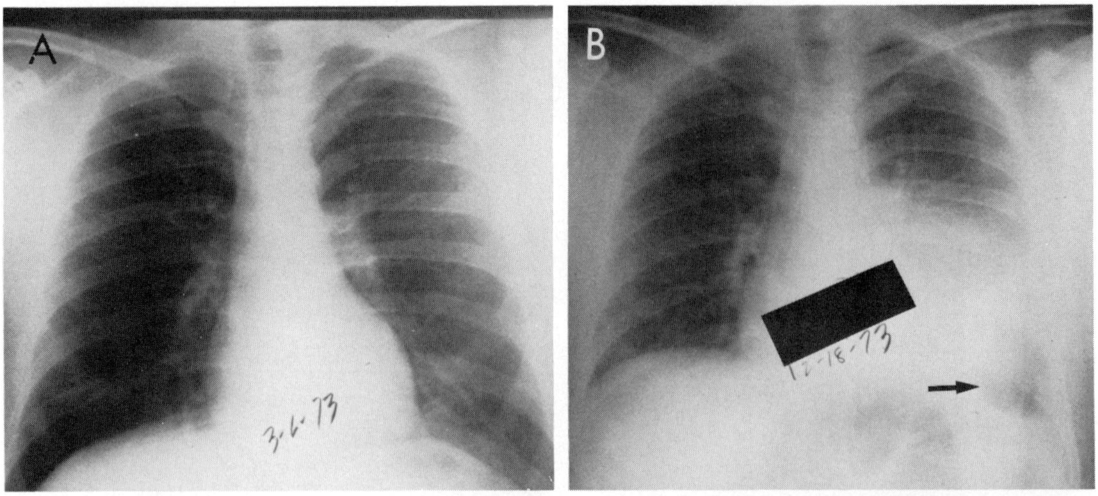

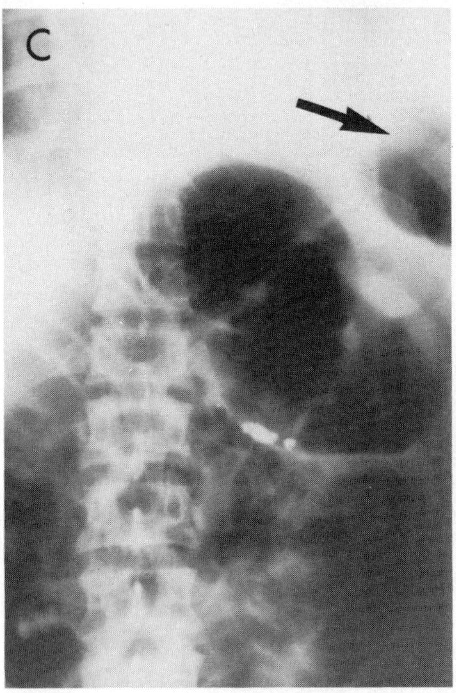

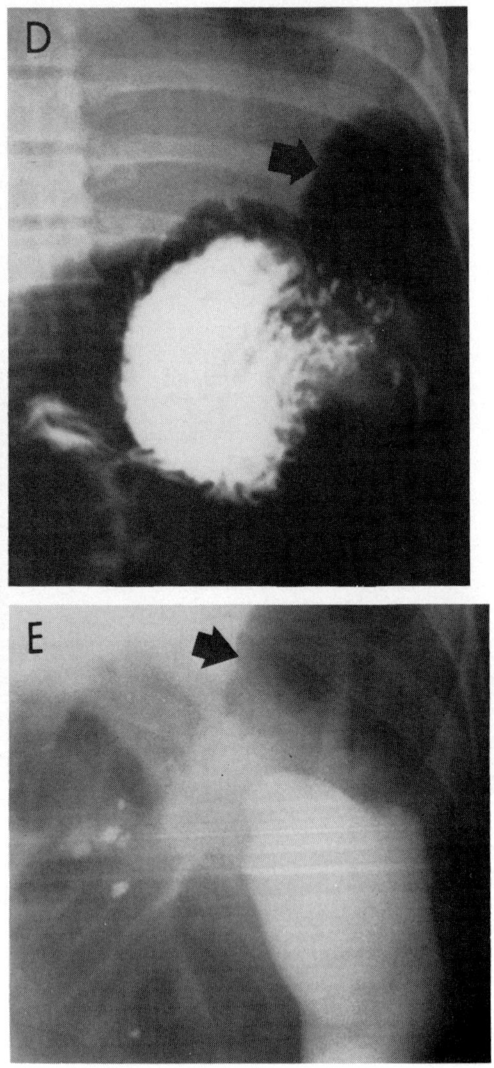

Fig 28–13. – **A,** traumatic left-sided diaphragmatic hernia. Patient presented originally with chest injury and evidence of haziness in left chest. No evidence of diaphragmatic rupture noted at this time. **B,** 9 months later patient returned and a left pleural effusion was seen with a knuckle of gas noted in region of left costophrenic angle *(arrow)*. **C,** KUB done at that time revealed a colon obstruction with dilatation of colon to level of splenic flexure *(arrow)*. **D,** Gastrografin was given by mouth to outline stomach and once again knuckle of splenic flexure *(arrow)* is seen at left base. **E,** barium enema examination showed total obstruction to flow of barium in region of splenic flexure. Knuckle of colon *(arrow)* is within chest secondary to herniation through diaphragm.

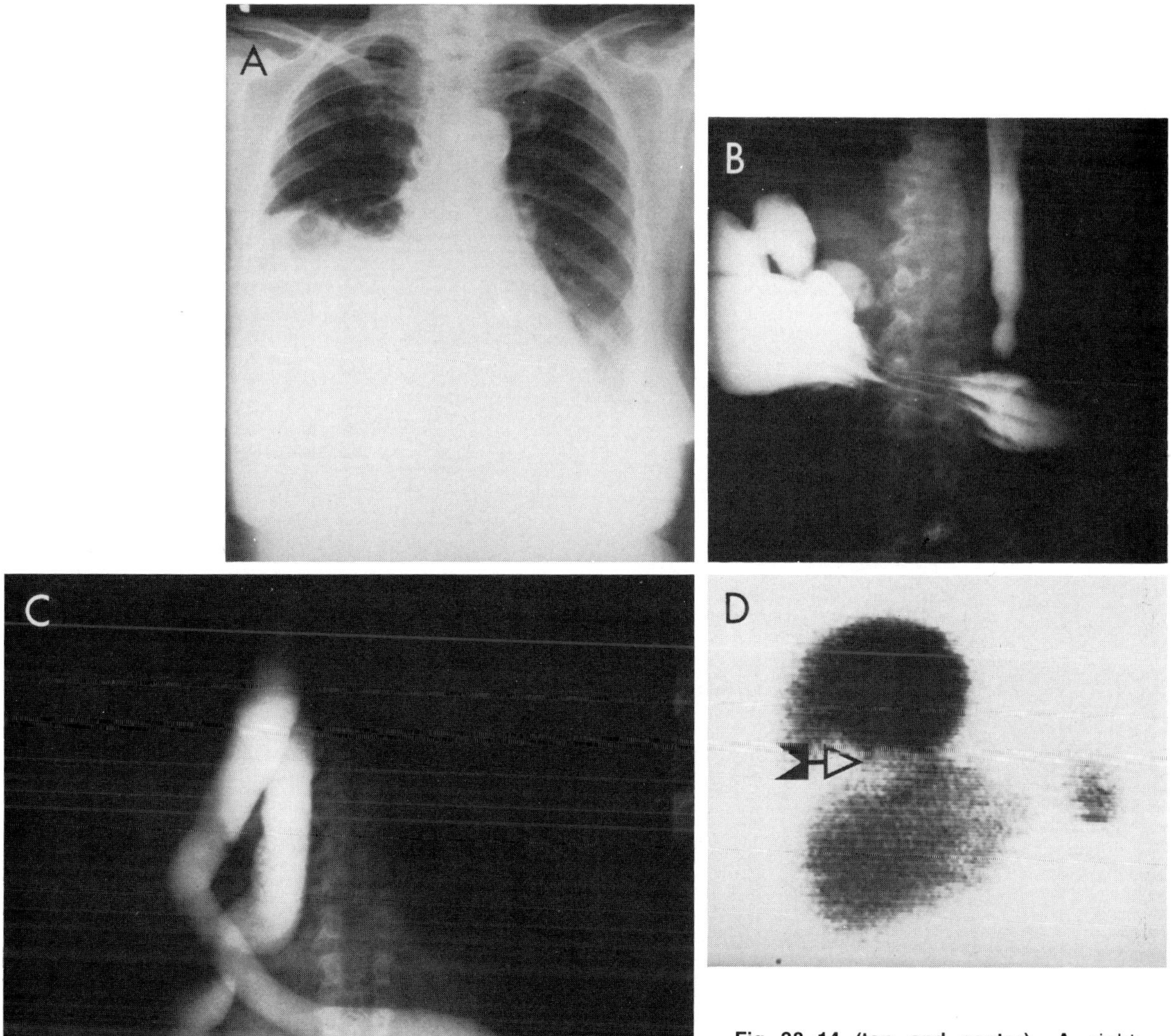

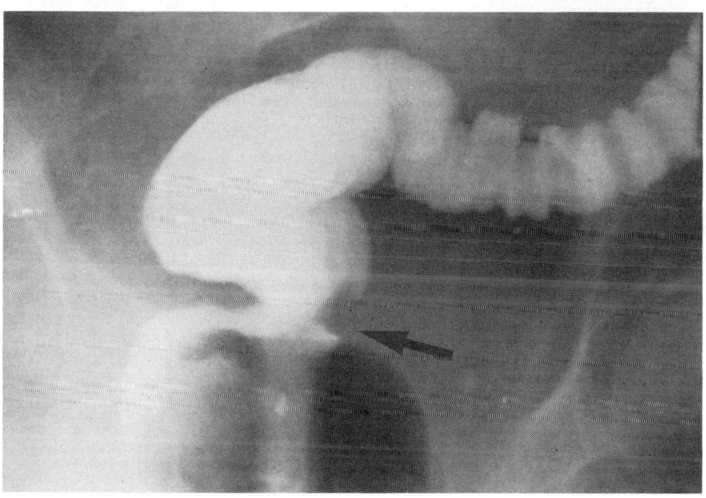

Fig 28–14 (top and center).—**A,** right-sided diaphragmatic hernia. Chest film reveals small gas collection and "elevated right hemidiaphragm." **B,** upper gastrointestinal examination reveals stomach and duodenum as well as gallbladder to be located in right upper quadrant. **C,** colon examination shows transverse colon to be superiorly displaced into right hemithorax. **D,** liver scan reveals 90-degree axial rotation of liver with large portion noted in right hemithorax.

Fig 28–15 (bottom).—Rectal stricture of 15-years' duration. Colonoscopy revealed benign-appearing stricture with several superficial erosions. Biopsy was performed; pathologist found colitis cystica profunda. (Courtesy of Dr Theodore Coutsoftides, Chief, Dept. Colorectal Surgery, Long Beach VA Hosp., Long Beach, Calif.)

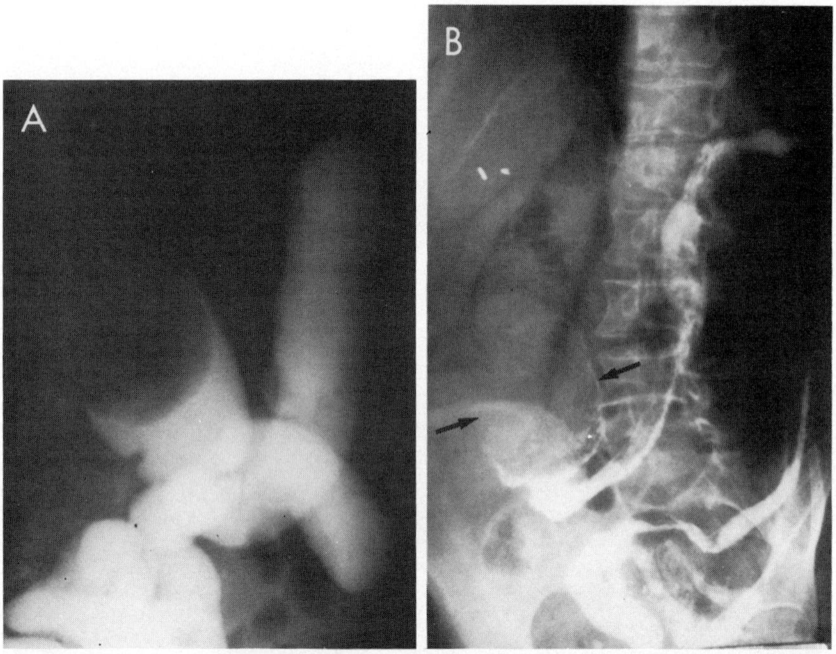

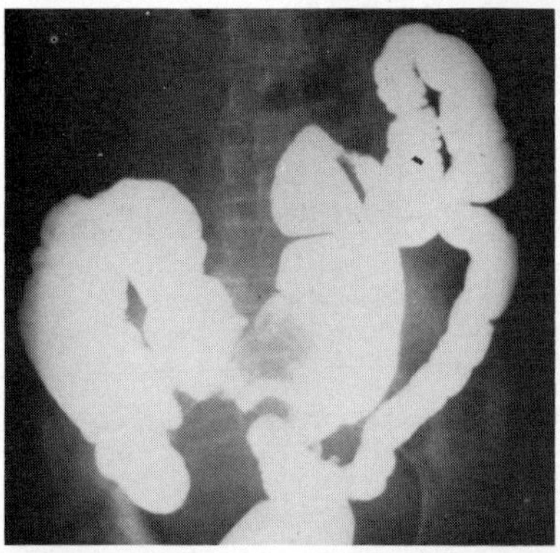

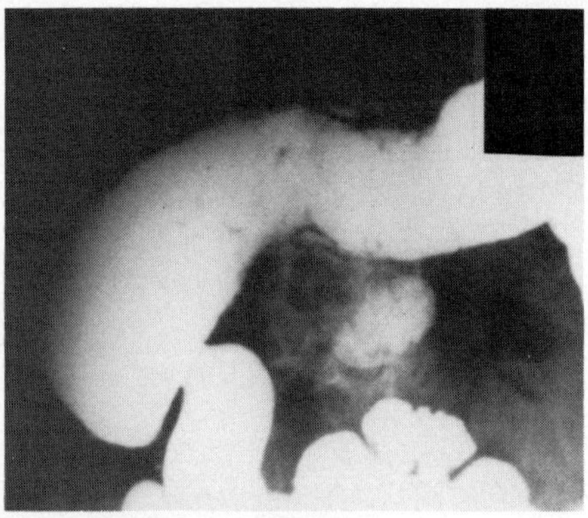

Fig 28–16 (top). – **A** and **B,** carcinoma of colon with colocolic intussusception.

Fig 28–17 (center left). – Krukenberg tumor of ovaries secondary to carcinoma of midtransverse colon. Although, classically, Krukenberg tumors of ovary are associated with drop-metastases of stomach, this lesion may occur secondary to peritoneal seeding from any gastrointestinal source.

Fig 28–18 (center right). – Cathartic colon with loss of haustration and marked shortening of right colon.

Fig 28–19 (bottom). – Carcinoma in ulcerative colitis. **A,** typical changes of ulcerative colitis with loss of haustration, narrowing, shortening and tubulation. **B,** lateral rectal view shows flattening, induration and plaque-like lesion of posterior rectal wall with widening of presacral space secondary to carcinoma in this region.

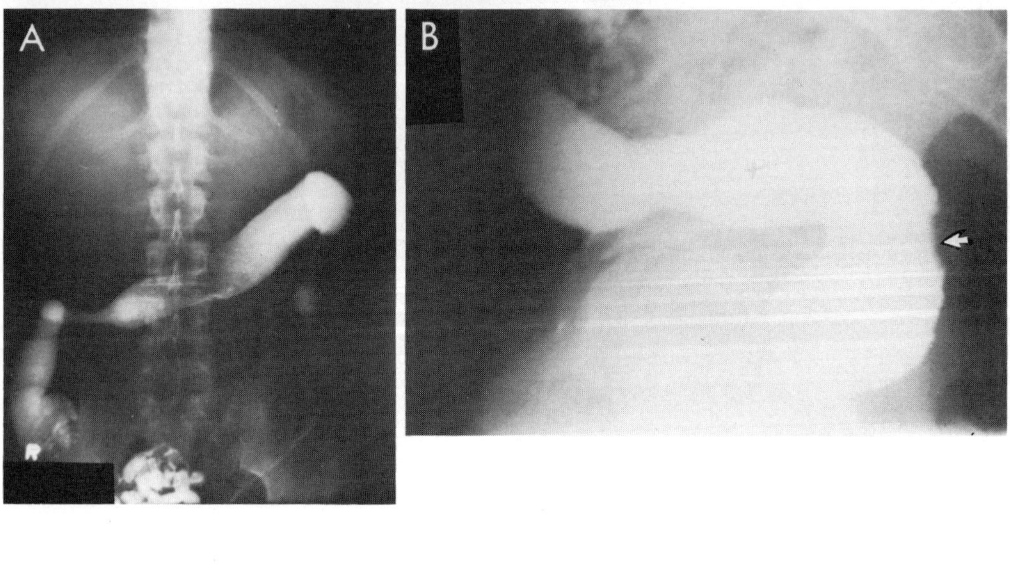

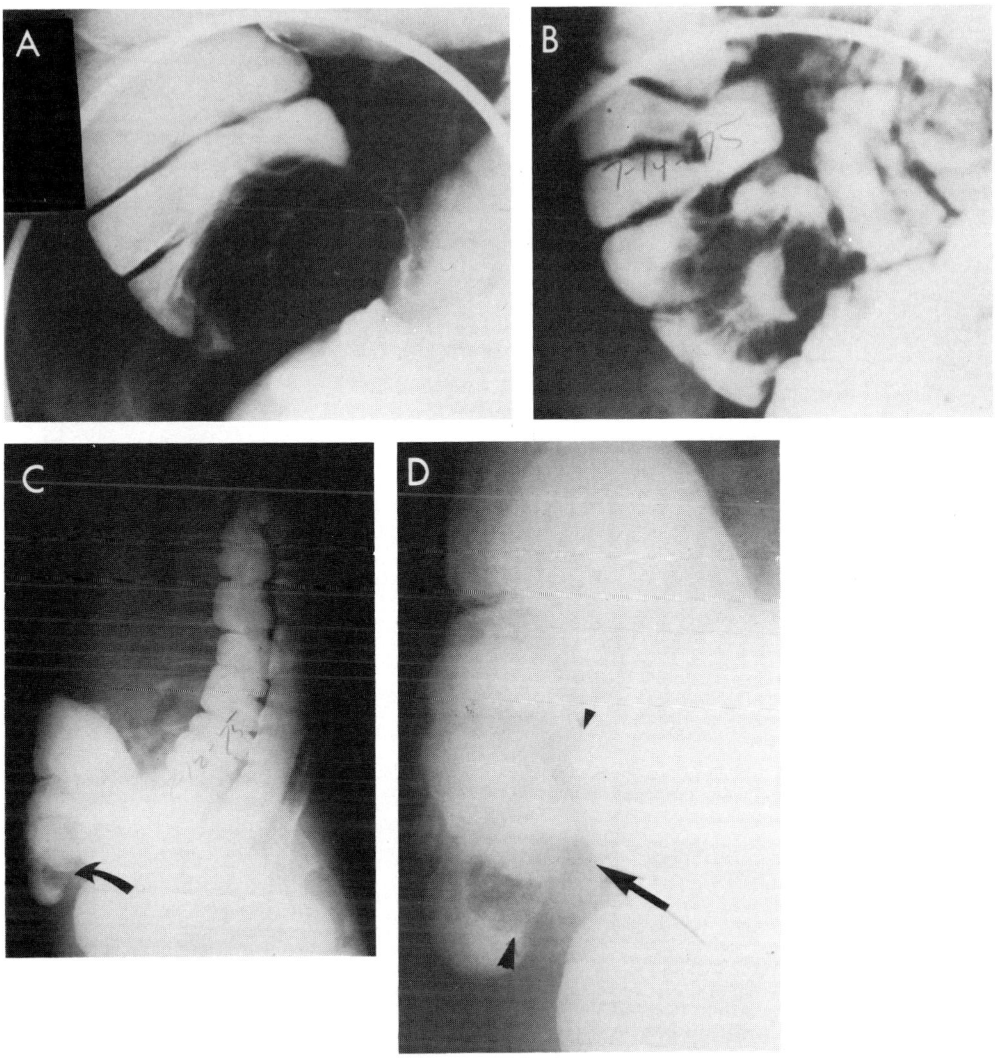

Fig 28–20. – Carcinoma of cecum simulating an extrinsic lesion. **A,** mass at inferomedial aspect of cecum. This originally was thought to represent a mucocele or other extrinsic mass. **B,** several days later a small bowel follow-through revealed central collection of barium within this mass. It was believed that this barium might be within terminal ileum viewed en face; possibility of prolapse of ileocecal valve also was considered. **C,** right posterior oblique view of barium enema. The lesion *(arrow)* was shown to reside in medial aspect of cecum. **D,** close-up view of above. Arrowheads delineate mass. Arrow points to central ulcer.

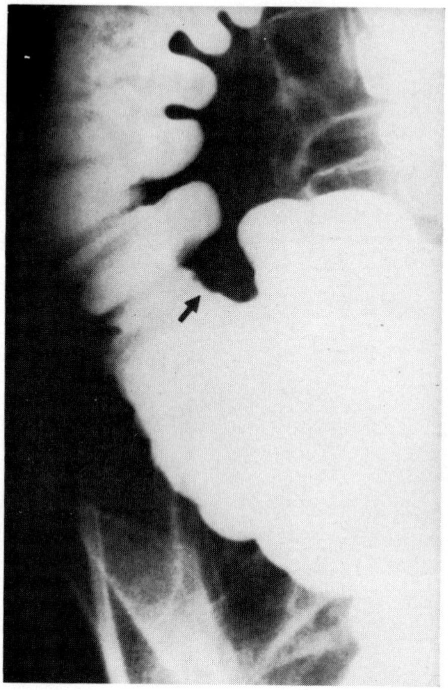

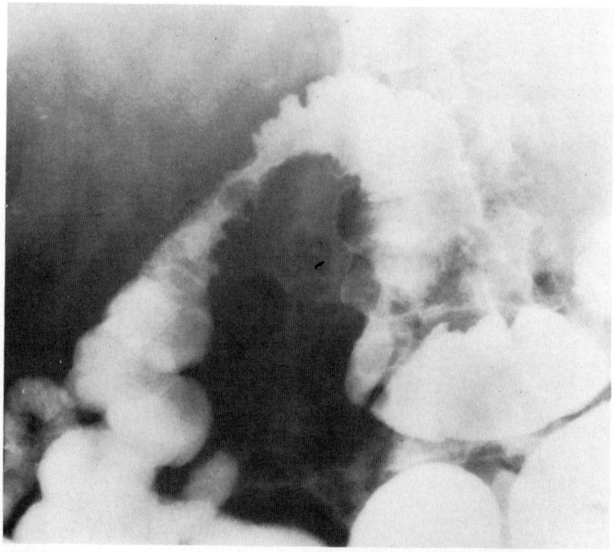

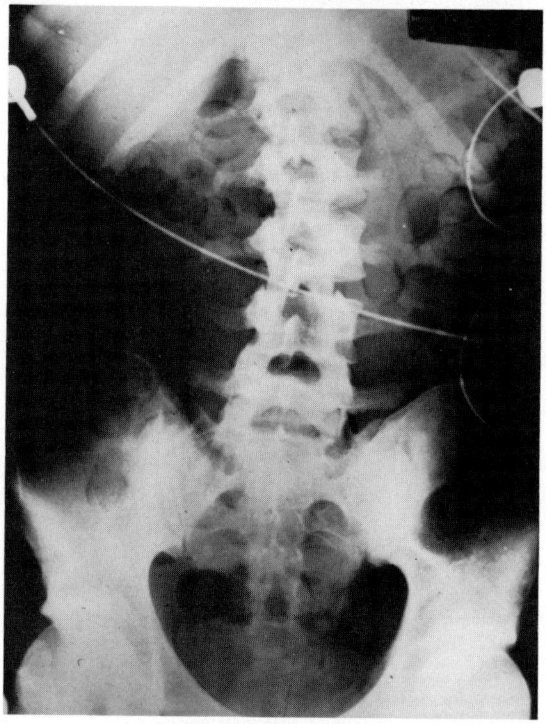

Fig 28–21 (top left).—Early carcinoma of right colon. This lesion presented as irregular plaque-like lesion infiltrating medial wall of ascending colon *(arrow)*. Wall at this site was infiltrated, rigid and nonpliable at fluoroscopy.

Fig 28–22 (top right).—Carcinoma of breast metastatic to hepatic flexure. Long segmental area of narrowed colon is seen in region of hepatic flexure with irregular plicated folds, narrowed lumen and rigid indurated contours. Patient had far-advanced carcinomatoses.

Fig 28–23 (bottom).—Ingested narcotic seen in multiple latex condoms within colon. In wrapping the narcotic, air is trapped, producing multiple radiolucent ring shadows, interspersed throughout colon on above KUB film. If condom ruptures, patient may present with signs of narcotic overdose. (Courtesy of Fainsinger, M. H.: J.A.M.A. 237: 2225–2226, 1977; copyright 1977, American Medical Association.)

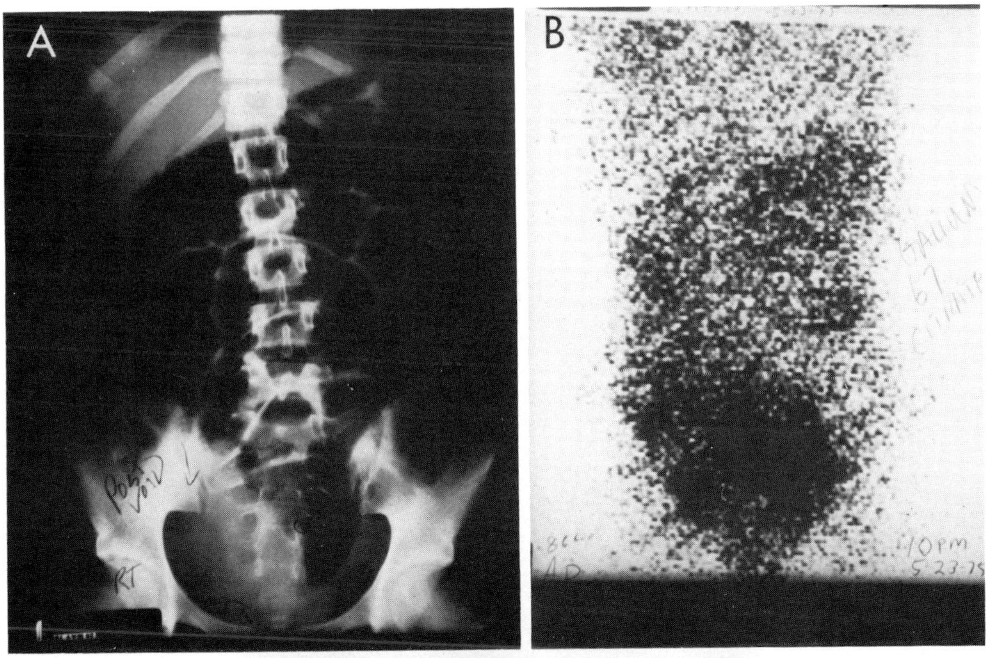

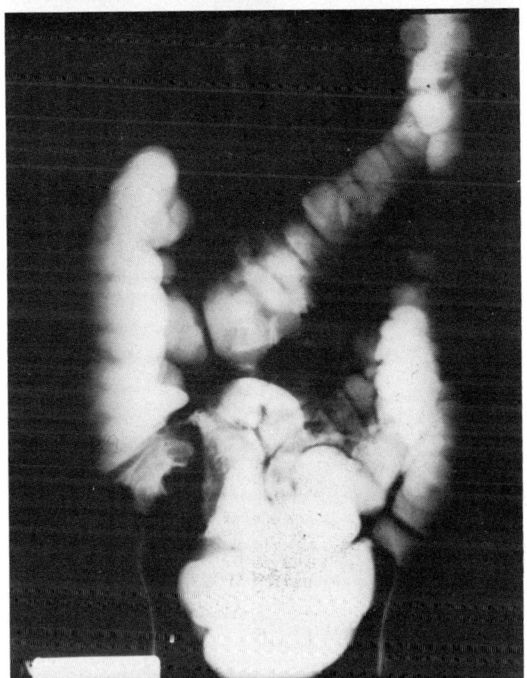

Fig 28–24 (top). – **A,** postoperative pelvic abscess 2 weeks following appendectomy for perforated appendicitis. Patient had a mass palpable in right lower quadrant. KUB film done in postvoiding state showed soft tissue mass involving right lower quadrant and right pelvis. **B,** Galium scan at 24 hours shows marked increased activity in area of above soft tissue mass. About 700–800 cc of pus was drained from this region at laparotomy.

Fig 28–25 (bottom). – Appendicitis with involvement of cecum. Barium enema shows irregular thickoned edematous folds at inferomedial aspect of cecum secondary to appendicitis.

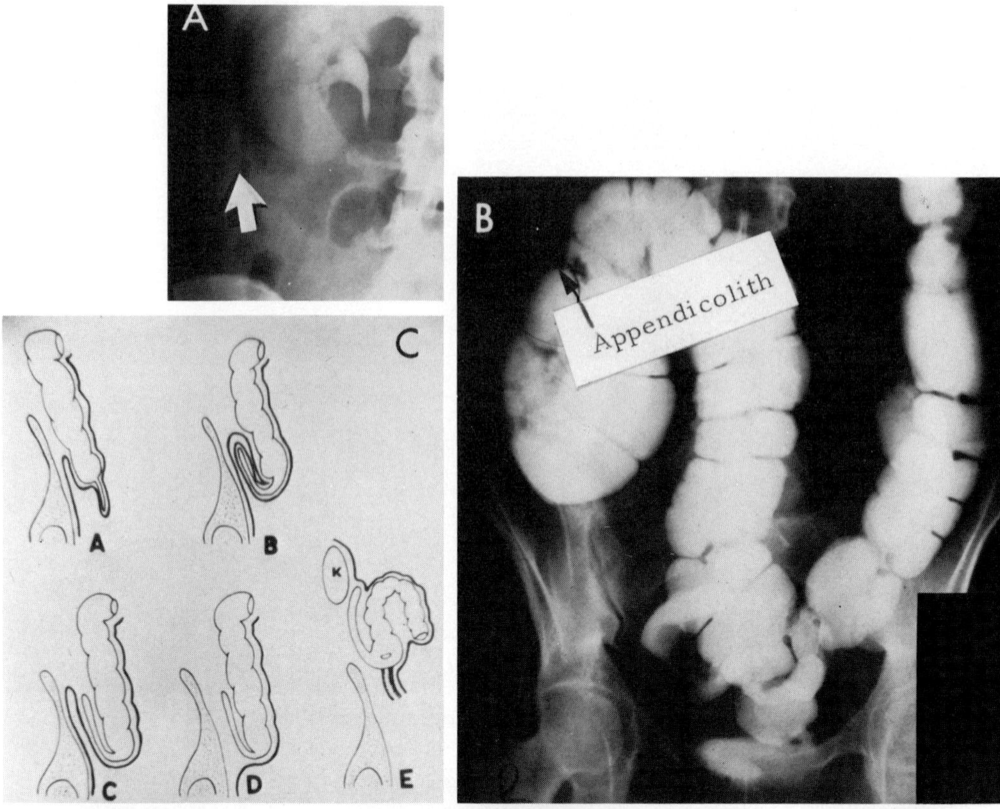

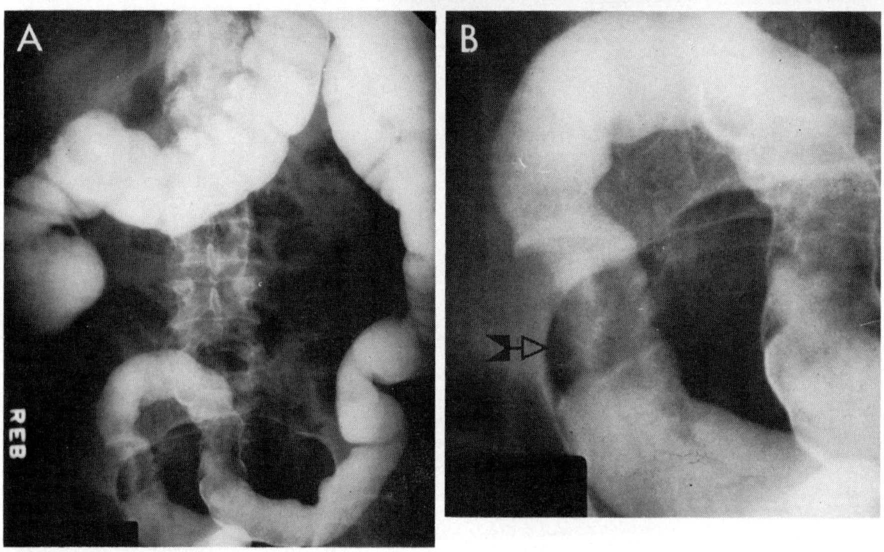

Fig 28–26 (top).—Appendicitis presenting with pain in right upper quadrant. **A,** intravenous pyelogram shows an appendicolith at inferolateral margin of right kidney *(arrow)*. **B,** barium enema shows malrotated cecum with cecal tip inverted and presenting in right upper quadrant. By bright-lighting the original film, appendicolith was seen at tip of cecum. **C,** normal variations in position and peritoneal fixation of appendix: *(a)* intraperitoneal, pointing over brim of pelvis; *(b)* intraperitoneal, ascending retrocecal, within fossa; *(c)* extraperitoneal, ascending retrocecal—paracecal fossa present; *(d)* extraperitoneal, ascending retrocecal—no paracecal fossa; *(e)* extraperitoneal, ascending retrocecal, lying anterior to right kidney *(k)* deep to liver, associated with undescended subhepatic cecum—terminal ileum, also extraperitoneal, enters cecum from behind.

Fig 28–27 (bottom).—**A** and **B,** streptococcus bovis septicemia associated with colon carcinoma. Cases of streptococcus bovis endocarditis and septicemia have been reported not only with colonic carcinoma but also with villous adenoma. Carcinoma sigmoid colon best seen on close up view *(arrow)*. (Courtesy of Dr. Keith Burnett, UCI-LB VA Hospitals.)

Chapter 29

Neoplasia of the Colon Over a Long Segment

EDWARD I. GREENBAUM, M.D.

NEOPLASTIC LESIONS may involve a long segment of the colon, producing areas of narrowing that may be confused with inflammatory processes such as diverticulitis and granulomatous colitis or vascular processes such as ischemic colitis.

Whereas adenocarcinoma of the colon ordinarily presents with a polypoid mass or a "napkin ring" lesion, tumors differing in cell type (carcinoid, lymphoma, scirrhous carcinoma) or in growth pattern (e.g., extensive submucosal and/or extracolonic extension or early vascular necrosis) present a different and less recognizable roentgen pattern. This may occur similarly when the colon is invaded from without by a contiguous mass or hematogenous metastasis. Finally, the nature of the "soil" in which the carcinoma takes root may cause an additional variable, as exemplified by carcinoma arising in ulcerative colitis.

Frequently in these instances a long segment of colon is involved, and the sharp demarcations seen with more typical adenocarcinomas of the colon are absent.

Diffusely Infiltrating Adenocarcinoma

In Figure 29-1, a long segmental zone of narrowing was produced by a poorly differentiated anaplastic carcinoma infiltrating the colon wall, with extensive extracolonic extension. The mucosal folds are thick and somewhat nodular appearing but the mucosal pattern is relatively preserved. A similar case was found in a case record of the Massachusetts General Hospital.[1] There the barium enema showed a 12 cm area of narrowing in the sigmoid, with tapered margins and markedly thickened mucosal folds. This case was shown pathologically to represent a mucin-producing colloid adenocarcinoma, which extended in an intramural and extramural manner, resulting in elevation and distortion of the overlying mucosa.[1]

This type of diffuse involvement may easily simulate granulomatous colitis, and colonoscopy may be necessary to make this differential diagnosis.

Perforating Carcinoma of the Colon

In Figures 29-2 to 29-7, the long segment involvement of the sigmoid is the result of a perforated carcinoma with extracolonic extension. The extracolonic component may be secondary to tumor extension, infected neoplasm or abscess formation. Differentiation between this entity and diverticulitis may be extremely difficult, but inasmuch as resection of the diverticular mass is connected with a high operative mortality and is indicated in comparatively rare instances, the necessity of making the correct diagnosis before opening the abdomen is obvious. Clinical data in regard to age, weight loss, pain, stool habits, temperature and blood picture usually are not decisive in making this distinction. In both conditions a tender left lower quadrant mass may be palpable. The presence of blood in the stool strongly favors carcinoma in questionable cases.[2]

Diverticulitis usually presents as a long zone of narrowing with preserved mucosa and tapered margins. Scattered diverticula usually are seen in the immediate vicinity. Occasionally, fistulas, sinus tracts and/or extravasation of barium into an extracolonic abscess may be present. In these cases the radiologic diagnosis is relatively clear-cut, but this entity frequently overlaps perforated carcinoma, and this latter possibility must always be kept in mind. Perforation obscures the more usual criteria for radiographic diagnosis of carcinoma of the colon (1) by opening avenues of infection into the pericolic tissues, producing what may be called infected neoplasm; and (2) by permitting rapid, gross extension of the neoplastic process, producing a lesion much larger and over a longer segment than would be seen without this complication.[3]

Carcinoma Mimicking Ischemic Colitis

In Figure 29-8 the tumor eroded a vessel early in its course, and there was resultant intramural hemorrhage over a long segment in the transverse colon. Radiographically thumbprinting was seen, which taken together with the history of acute onset of epigastric pain, was initially thought to represent ischemic colitis. Because of the radiographic configuration, other possibilities, including a spontaneous bleed due to Coumadin overdose or an inflammatory process (e.g., granulomatous colitis) were entertained but clinically excluded. The possibility of neoplasm with this initial roentgen presentation was not considered and, to our knowledge, has not been previously reported as a presenting feature of primary carcinoma of the colon. It was only later that the clinical course and radiographic picture pointed to the correct diagnosis.

Carcinoma in Ulcerative Colitis (Fig 29–9)

In patients with ulcerative colitis, carcinoma may present as a long strictured area. In adults with a history of ulcerative colitis longer than 10 years, carcinoma occurs about 20 times more often than in the corresponding age group in the general population. Marshak et al.[4] noted carcinoma arising as a complication of ulcerative colitis in about 6% of 1,700 cases. He states that in 18 cases the carcinoma presented as a filiform stricture with none of the usual roentgen characteristics associated with carcinoma. The roentgen findings consisted of a narrowed segment measuring up to 6 cm in length with an eccentric lumen, irregular contours and mucosa with flattened, rigid, tapered margins. Pathologic studies of these cases revealed deep layers of fibrous tissue to be infiltrated by scirrhous carcinoma.

Metastatic Carcinoma (Figs 29–10 to 29–12)

Metastatic carcinoma may involve the colon from direct extension from an adjacent viscus or via hematogenous or peritoneal seeding. The study of 30 cases by Wigh and Tapley[5] showed that 19 patients had a single site of involvement. In some of these patients, there were long areas of narrowing with incomplete distensibility and a normal mucosal pattern. The margins of the lesion were conical and tapered. The authors attributed this to tumor encapsulation of the affected portion of the colon. Khilnani et al.[6]

noted that with metastases to the colon there often is involvement over a long segment with narrowing of the lumen and limited distensibility. With mural extension, the mucosal folds are "stretched, fixed, transversely arranged and oriented towards the extra-colonic mass." Only in the later stages does the mucosa become involved, and in this instance the transverse folds are replaced by nodular defects; finally there is a rigid tube-like segment with no recognizable mucosa.

Primary Scirrhous Carcinoma (Figs 29–13 to 29–15)

Primary scirrhous carcinoma of the colon may present as a long area of segmental narrowing. About one third of reported cases arise as a complication of long-standing ulcerative colitis. The lesion may be simulated exactly by metastatic scirrhous carcinoma of the stomach or breast.[7] The tumor is a diffusely infiltrating anaplastic carcinoma, which produces marked fibrosis, with segmental thickening and rigidity of a relatively long segment of colon, throughout its entire circumference. The mucosal folds are flattened and obliterated, but ulceration is minimal, superficial or absent. The margins are often tapered in appearance. According to Wolf and Marshak,[8] this lesion may be considered "when the involved area appears rigid or irregularly scalloped with eccentric flat defects along the borders and fixed tapered margins on barium examination."

Carcinoid Tumors (Fig 29–16)

Carcinoid tumors of the colon ordinarily are found in the rectum or appendix and usually present as small polypoid masses less than 2 cm in diameter, which rarely show microscopic invasion. Schulman and Giustra[9] in reviewing 116 carcinoids of the colon found 15 cases that presented as bulky, invasive lesions with large extracolonic components. Once through the serosa and mesentery, the resultant desmoplastic reaction and extraluminal tumor resulted in masses several times larger than the primary lesion. Roentgenographically an apple core lesion was seen infrequently. When the extramural component was visualized, a long segment of colon involvement was noted, with a radiographic appearance similar to that seen with a perforated adenocarcinoma. The carcinoid syndrome with colonic carcinoids is a rare finding.

Lymphoma of the Colon (Figs 29–17 and 29–18)

Last in differential diagnosis of neoplasia over a long segment is lymphoma of the colon, a rare entity occurring about 0.05% as frequently as adenocarcinoma in the same region. The several histologic forms of malignant lymphoma of the colon are similar in roentgen appearance The annular configuration typical of adenocarcinoma was seen in only 6% of a series reviewed by Woodruff and Skorneck.[10] These authors state that "lymphosarcomas tend to be longer, more distensible, less sharply demarcated and more frequently polypoid than adenocarcinomas in the same location." Wolf et al.[11] state that differentiation of the discrete variety of lymphosarcoma from carcinoma is difficult, but it is suggested when there is dilatation of the lumen of the bowel in a concentric fashion at the site of the lesion. This aneurysmal dilatation is associated with infiltration of the bowel wall and destruction of the mucosa. Lymphosarcoma also may present as a bulky intramural mass with extensive extracolonic involvement. Another discrete type is the endo-exocolonic or dumbbell variety, in which the bulk of the lesion is located in the serosa or mesentry.

REFERENCES

1. Castleman, B., and McNeely, B.: Case records of the Massachusetts General Hospital, N. Engl. J. Med. 277:1141, 1967.
2. Schatzki, R.: The roentgenologic differential diag-

nosis between cancer and diverticulitis of the colon, Radiology 34:651, 1940.
3. Stevenson, C. A., and Sommer, A. W.: Differential diagnosis of chronic perforating carcinoma of the colon, Radiology 60:485, 1953.
4. Marshak, R. H., Block, C., and Wolf, B. S.: The roentgen findings in strictures of the colon associated with ulcerative and granulomatous colitis, Am. J. Roentgenol. 90:709, 1963.
5. Wigh, R., and du V. Tapley, N.: Metastatic lesions to the large intestine, Radiology 70:222, 1958.
6. Khilnani, M., Marshak, R. H., Eliasoph, J., and Wolf, B.: Roentgen features of metastases to the colon, Radiology 96:302, 1966.
7. McQueeney, A. J., Olson, R. W., and Medwid, A.: Primary scirrhous carcinoma of colon, Am. J. Roentgenol. 101:306, 1967.
8. Wolf, B. S., and Marshak, R. H.: Linitis plastica or diffusely infiltrating type of carcinoma of the colon, Radiology 81:502, 1963.
9. Schulman, H., and Giustra, P.: Invasive carcinoids of the colon, Radiology 98:139, 1971.
10. Woodruff, J. H., and Skorneck, A. B.: Malignant lymphoma of the colon and rectum, Calif. Med. 96:181, 1962.
11. Wolf, B. S., and Marshak, R. H.: Roentgen features of diffuse lymphosarcoma of the colon, Radiology 75:733, 1960.

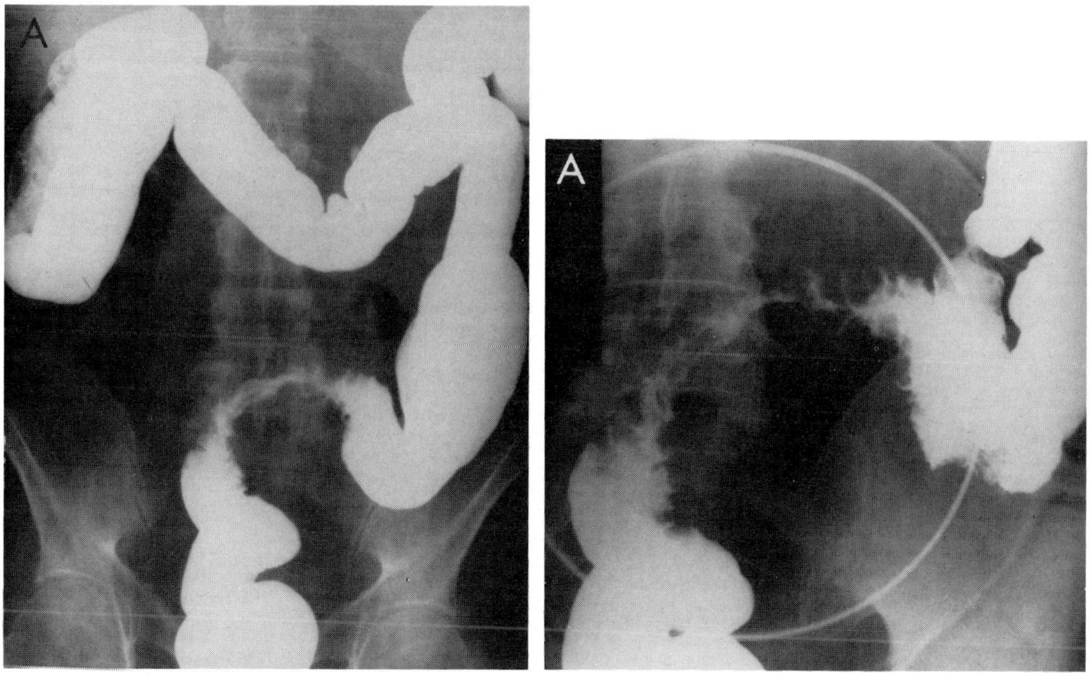

Fig 29–1. – **A,** deeply infiltrating adenocarcinoma, which extends through colon wall to serosal surface. Thickened colonic wall compromises lumen, causing long segmental zone of narrowing with tapered margins. **B,** with compression, mucosal folds are thickened and irregular and in some areas have fixed, nodular configuration. (From Clin. Radiol. 24:416, 1973, with permission.)

Fig 29–2. – **A,** perforated adenocarcinoma with extracolonic abscess. Sigmoid is narrowed over long segment and, although the mucosa appears coarsened, it is preserved. Note large soft tissue density *(arrows)* representing extracolonic abscess. No annular lesion is seen. **B,** Gastrografin enema done 3 months later through colostomy shows carcinoma *(small arrows)* as a smooth denuded short segment with fixed contours. Extracolonic extension is present with extrinsic compression of more proximal sigmoid. Mucosa in this area is preserved *(large white arrow).*

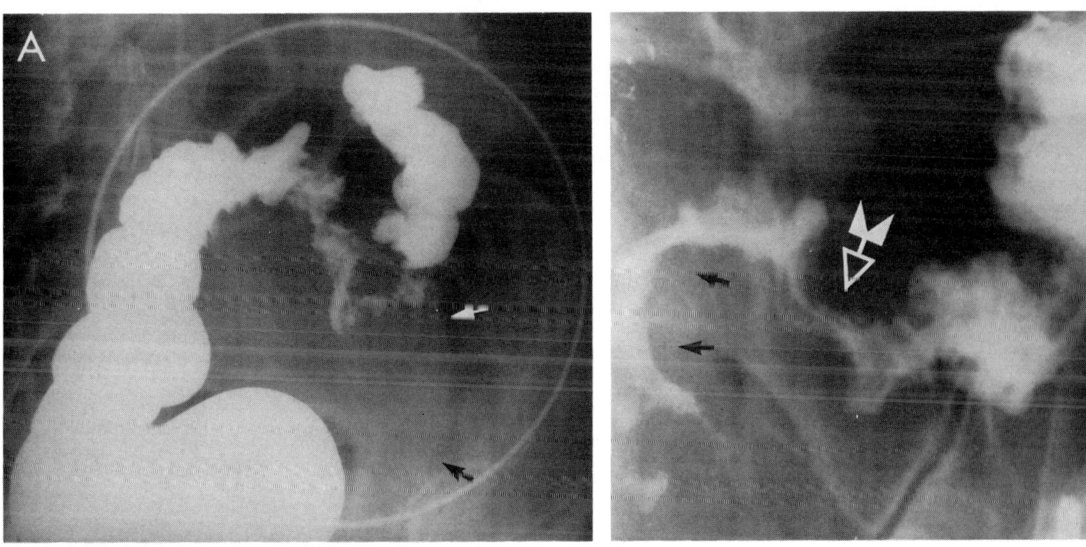

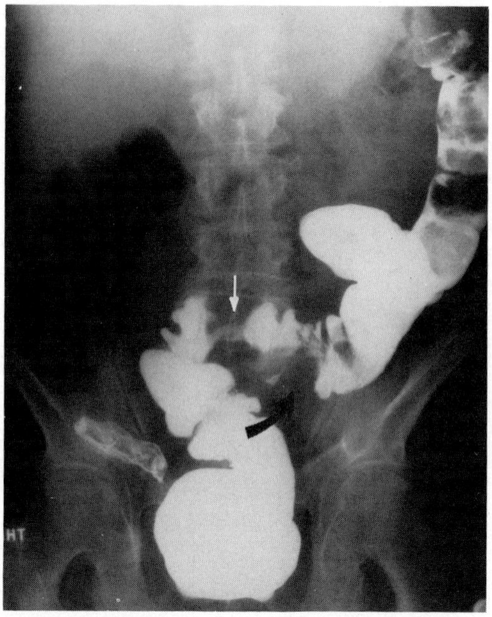

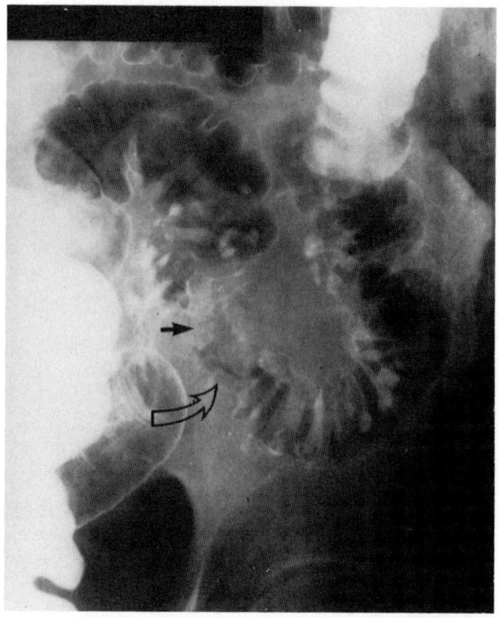

Fig 29–3 (left).—Perforating carcinoma. Long segmental zone of narrowing has two components. At distal aspect of lesion, annular carcinoma is seen *(small arrow)*. More proximally, large extracolonic mass *(large arrow)* is seen causing extrinsic pressure along inferior border, with eccentric narrowing of lumen and preservation of mucosa in this area. Fistulous tract is seen extending into extracolonic mass.

Fig 29–4 (right).—Perforated adenocarcinoma with typical apple core component seen at distal aspect of lesion *(closed arrow)*. Large extracolonic mass composed of infected neoplasm narrows adjacent sigmoid *(open arrow)*.

Fig 29–5 (left).—**A,** perforating adenocarcinoma with large bulky extracolonic mass involving long segment of splenic flexure. **B** and **C,** air contrast barium examination showing the above in greater detail.

Fig 29–6 (right).—Line drawing showing perforated adenocarcinoma with large bulky extracolonic mass extending proximally to involve a long segment of colon. (From Stevenson and Sommer, Radiology 34:651, 1953, with permission.)

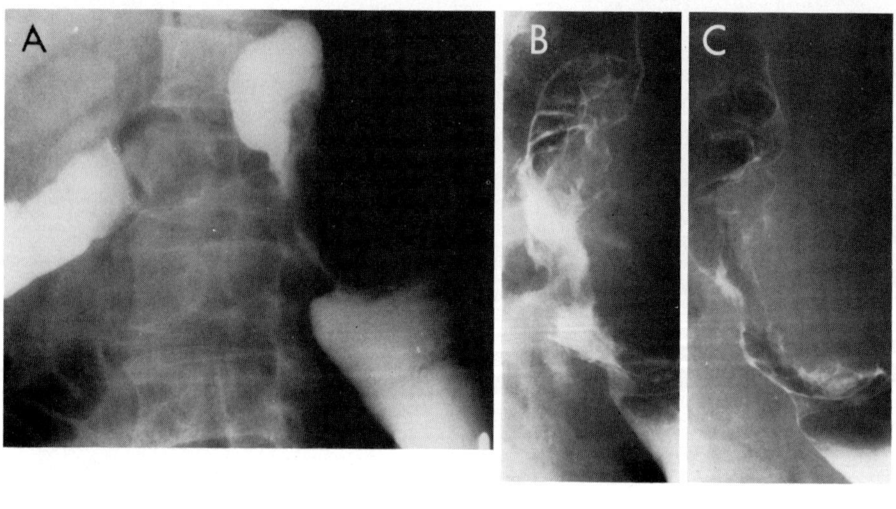

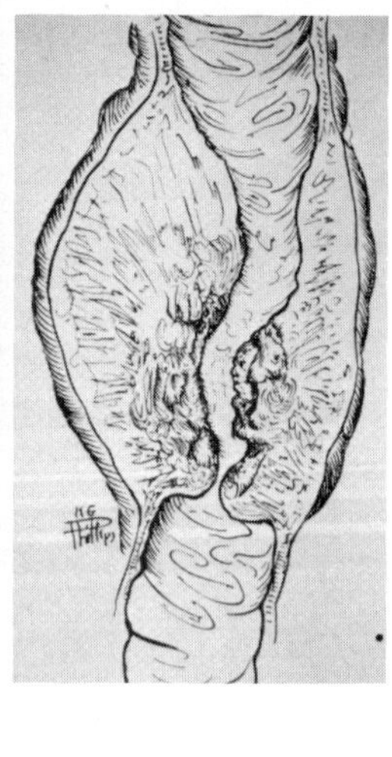

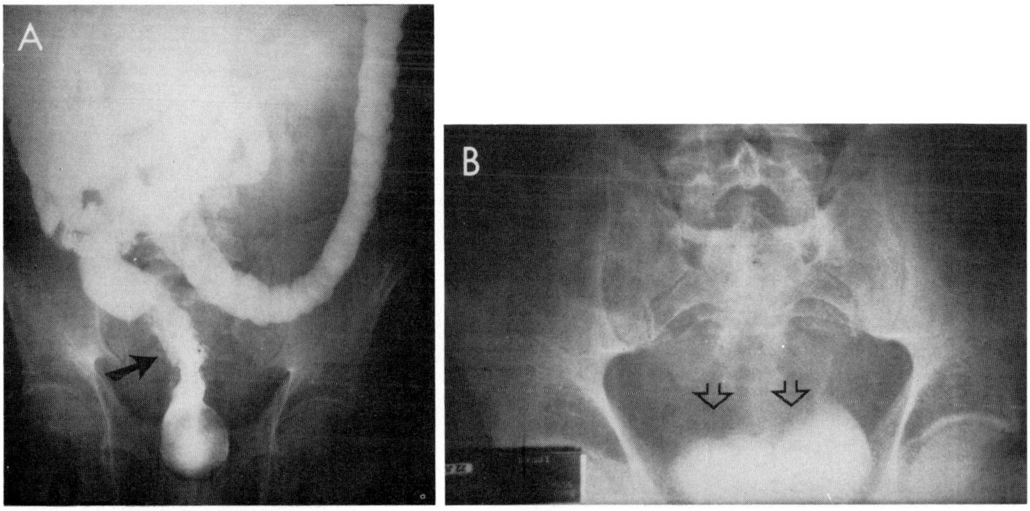

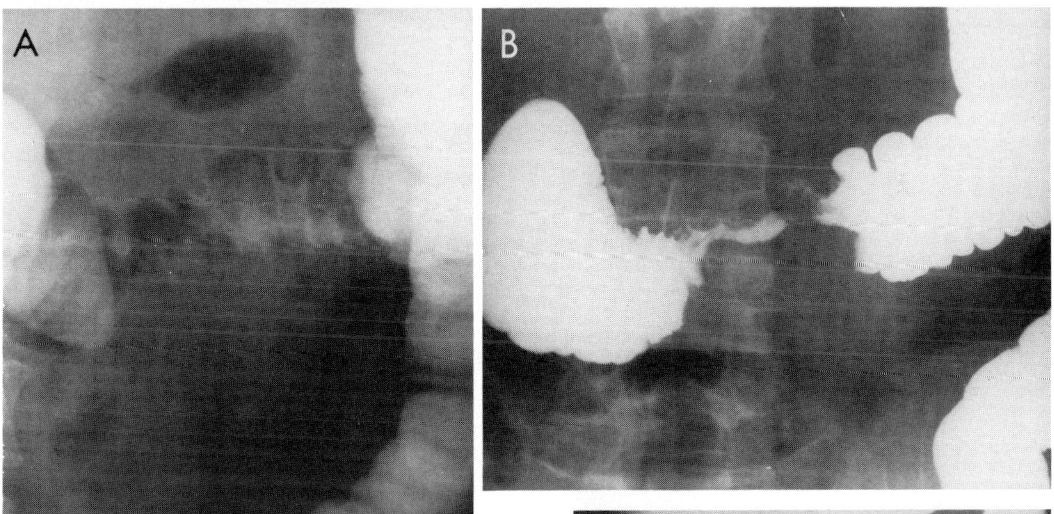

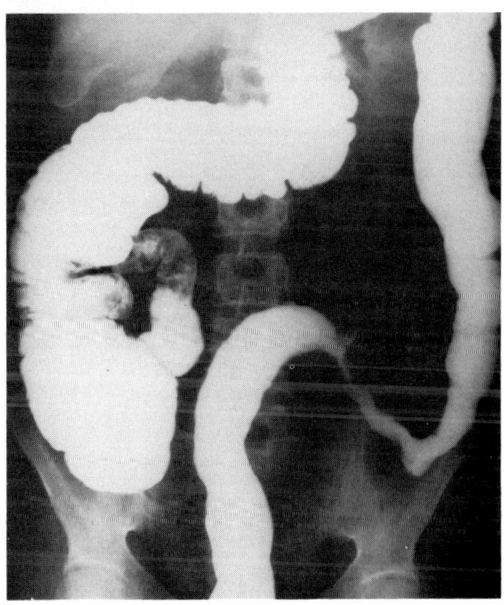

Fig 29–7 (top). – **A,** carcinoma of colon with large extracolonic component *(arrow)*. **B,** On intravenous pyelogram there is evidence of an extrinsic mass effect with scalloping and irregularity at dome of bladder *(arrows)*.

Fig 29–8 (center). – **A,** carcinoma of colon with early vascular invasion and intramural hemorrhage. There is long narrowed segment of midtransverse colon with thumbprinting at superior and inferior margins. Mucosa otherwise preserved with no frank intraluminal mass. **B,** barium enema 8 months later reveals annular adenocarcinoma with typical overhang edges and denuded mucosa.

Fig 29–9 (bottom). – Carcinoma complicating ulcerative colitis. Rectum is narrowed in transverse diameter and resembles burnt-out ulcerative colitis. In sigmoid, long carcinomatous structure is seen with irregular margins, which were rigid and nonpliable throughout examination.

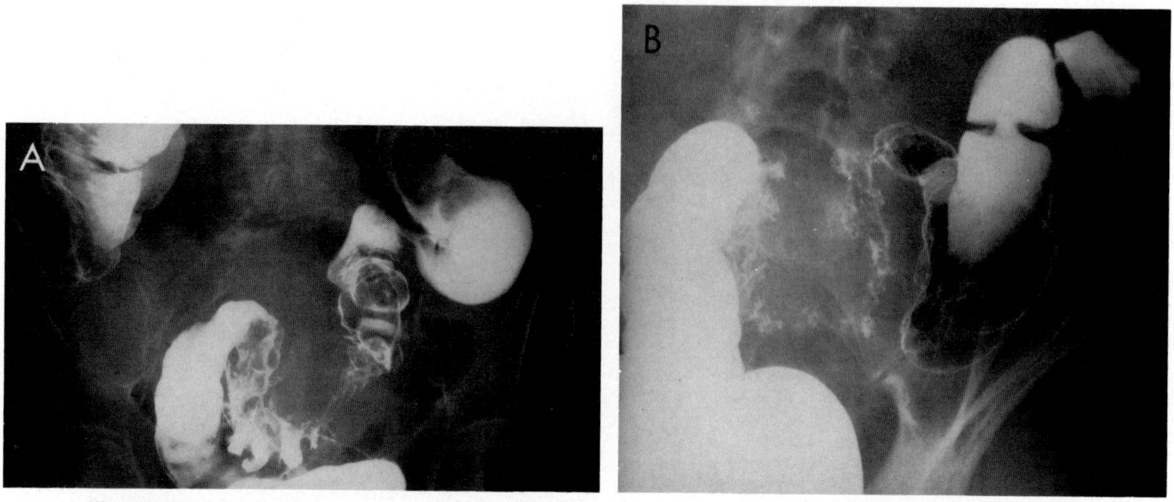

Fig 29–10.—**A** and **B,** ovarian carcinoma with involvement of sigmoid. A large pelvic mass is seen surrounding sigmoid colon. There is encapsulation with narrowing of lumen and incomplete distensibility. Mucosa is preserved and margins are tapered in appearance.

Fig 29–11.—**A** and **B,** metastatic carcinoma of breast to rectosigmoid. Long area of narrowing with incomplete distensibility and mural extension with mucosal folds noted to be "stretched, fixed, transversely arranged and oriented towards the extracolonic mass."[6] An additional mass is seen involving inferior medial aspect of cecum.

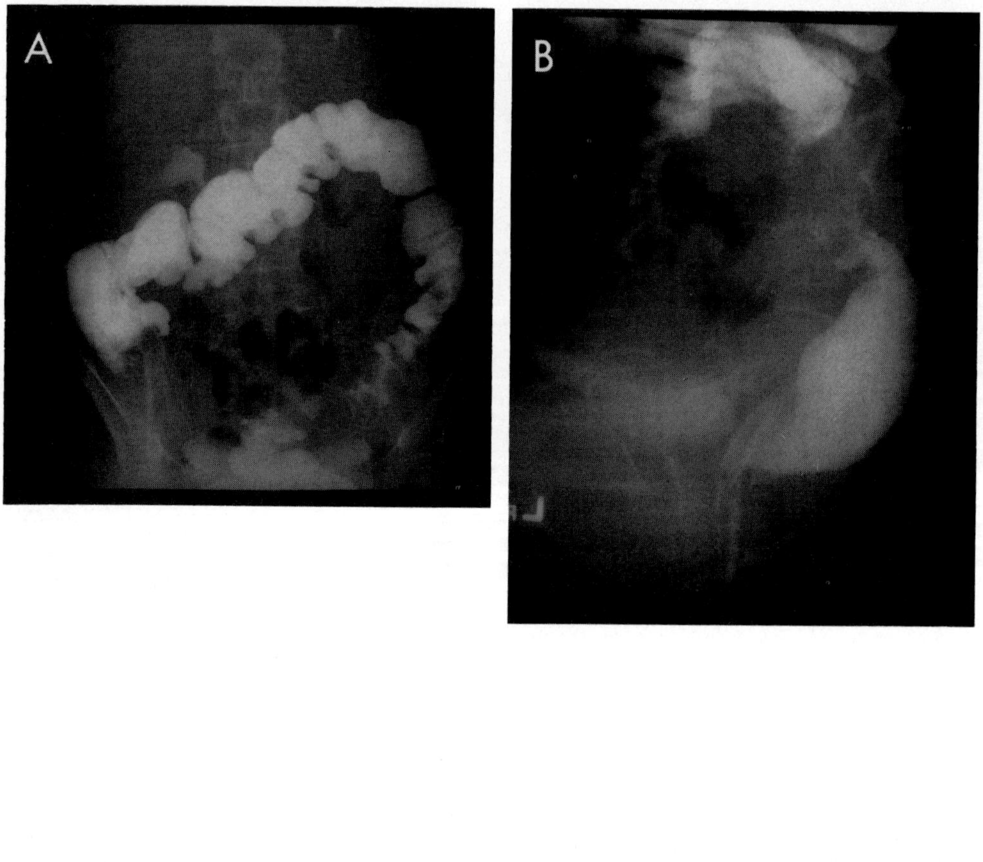

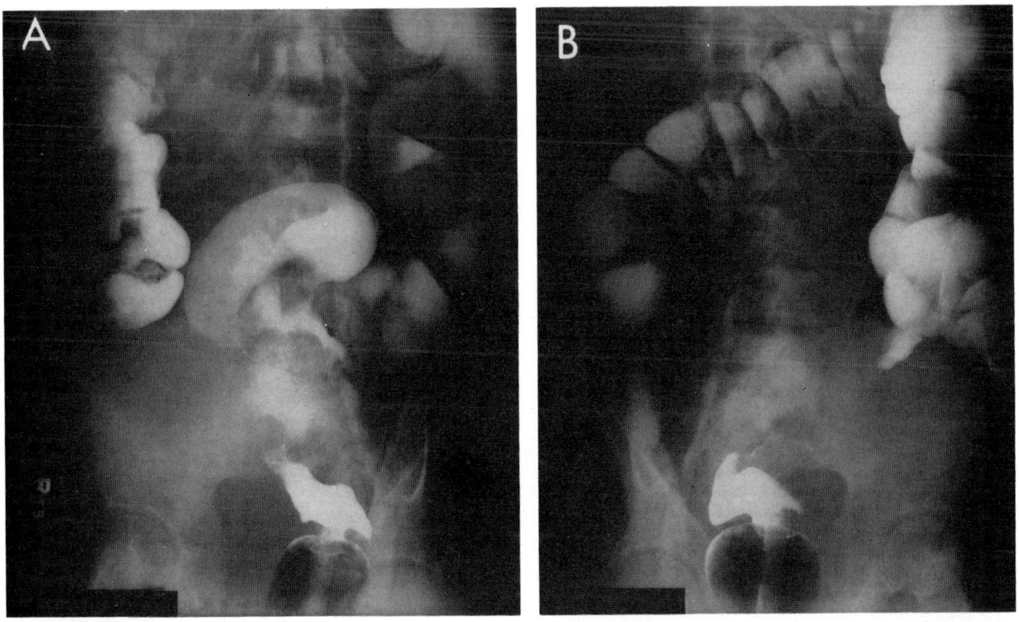

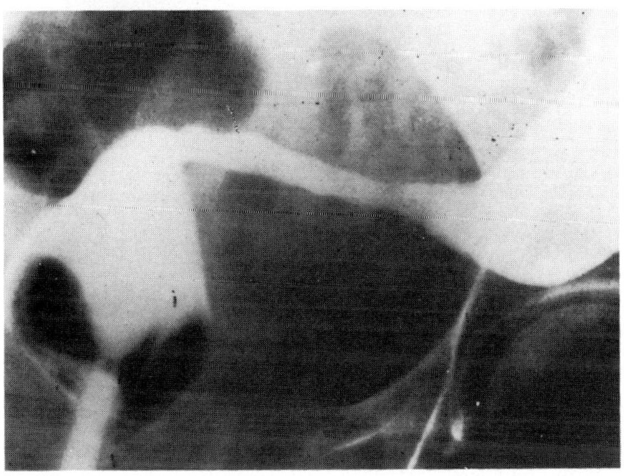

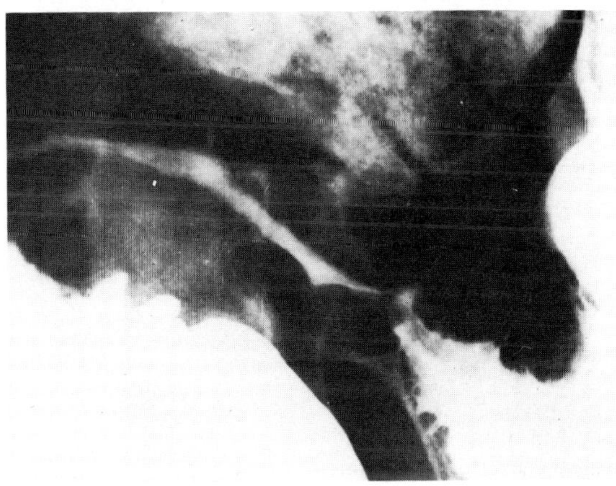

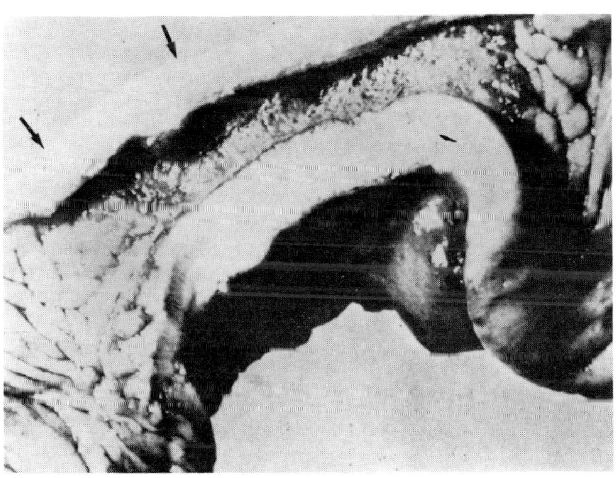

Fig 29–12 (top).—**A** and **B,** advanced carcinoma of prostrate with rectal and sigmoid involvement. Osteoblastic bony metastases are noted. Rectosigmoid shows long strictured segment with nodular defects and rigid tube-like segment with no recognizable mucosa. This is the end state in evolution of metastatic disease to colon.

Fig 29–13 (center left).—Scirrhous carcinoma presenting as long segmental zone of narrowing. Rectosigmoid was rigid in appearance and had tapered margins, the mucosa flattened and smooth in appearance.

Fig 29–14 (center right).—Scirrhous carcinoma presenting as long filiform narrowing of sigmoid with fixed tapered margins and obliteration of mucosa. Lesion is fixed and rigid in appearance.

Fig 29–15 (bottom).—Gross pathologic specimen showing scirrhous carcinoma with marked infiltration and thickening of colonic wall *(arrows)*.

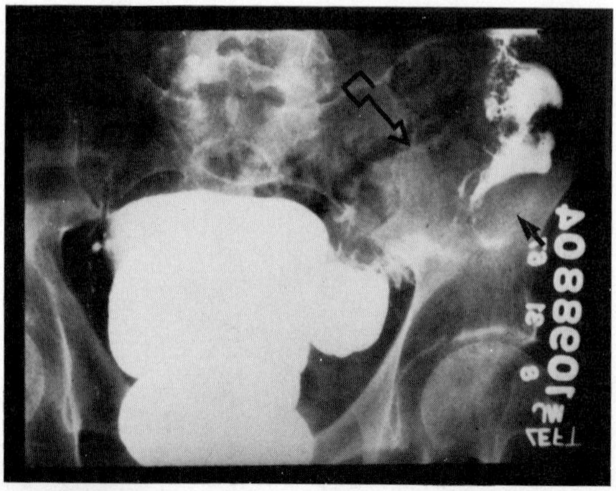

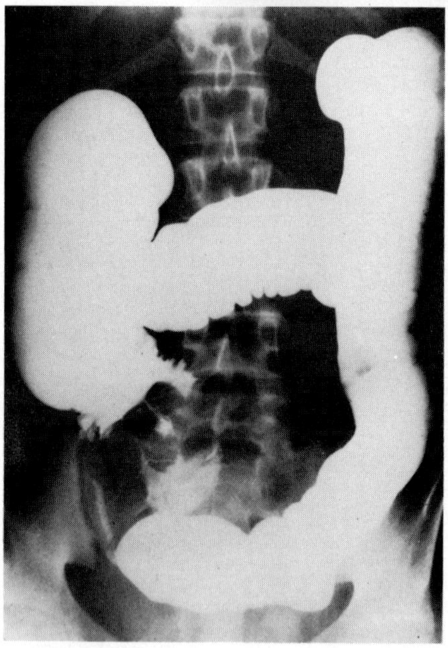

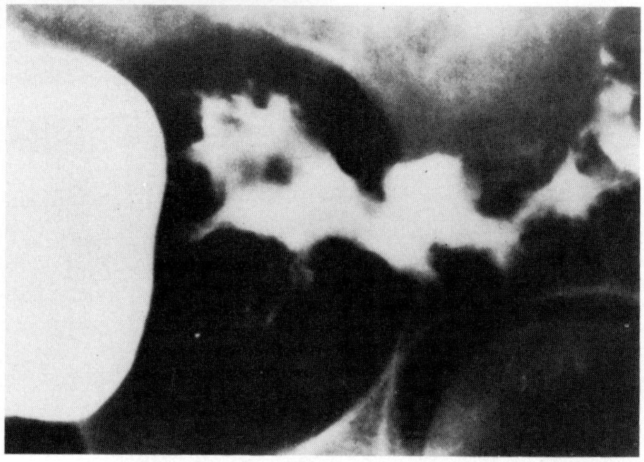

Fig 29–16 (top).—Invasive carcinoid of colon. Poorly delineated 5-cm mass in distal descending colon *(small arrow).* Large extraluminal mass displaces small bowel *(large arrow)* and extrinsically compresses adjacent sigmoid colon. Carcinoid tumor with mesenteric abdominal nodes and liver metastasis was found at surgery.

Fig 29–17 (left).—Lymphoma of colon. Girl, age 16, with large intramural lymphomatous mass in right posterior lateral wall of cecum extending into adjacent cecum. Mucosa is intact and no extracolonic extension was noted at surgery.

Fig 29–18 (right).—Man, age 77, with severe diarrhea and 40-pound weight loss. Long segment of sigmoid is irregularly narrowed with only gradual transition to normal bowel. Lumen was ragged in appearance secondary to ulceration. Multiple nodular lesion defects produced a contour very much resembling thumbprinting. Lesion was resected and found to be a polymorphous lymphoma, probably reticulum cell sarcoma.

Chapter 30

The Pediatric Colon

FRED A. LEE, M.D.

THE NORMAL COLON in the newborn and young infant differs significantly in appearance from that of an older child or adult. At birth the colon is relatively elongated with redundant flexures. The sigmoid projects high into the midabdomen and frequently to the right lower quadrant. The hepatic flexure is slightly low, owing to the relatively large size of the liver. The cecum normally may be high and even slightly medially directed or retroverted and may preserve a fetal conical configuration.

Haustral markings are poorly developed. Identification of the colon on plain radiograms is difficult and rests primarily on its position and its larger caliber rather than on mucosal characteristics.[1] With growth of the child, the haustrations become distinct and the length and course of the colon more like the adult configuration.

The colonic lymphoid follicles in infants and children often are quite prominent and hyperplastic, and on air contrast studies these may appear as a myriad of small nodular filling defects with tiny umbilicated centers filled with retained barium (Fig 30–1). They are usually found in patients presenting with lower gastrointestinal bleeding, but this association probably is coincidental rather than causal, since air contrast studies are seldom performed except in children with rectal bleeding to exclude polyps. These prominent lymphoid follicles are normal and of no clinical significance.[2-4]

Radiologic examination of the colon in infants and children should be an individualized procedure tailored to answer specific questions prompted by the patient's symptoms and clinical findings. There should be no single, set routine examination for all patients. Each institution should develop its own methodology; no one method is necessarily the best. The methods of examination for various abnormalities to be discussed reflect our own personal philosophy and experience. Our basic goal is to arrive at a correct conclusion with the least discomfort to the patient and the least expenditure of radiation to patient and staff.

Some general comments, however, are pertinent. The patient's physical well-being is of paramount importance. In young infants particularly, maintenance of hydration and prevention of heat loss should supersede any diagnostic manipulations. Fluoroscopic time should be kept at a minimum and the field of fluoroscopy should be restricted to the area of immediate interest. Unlike in the adult patient, there is no concern over an occult malignancy. The colon is not routinely prepared, and numerous spot films of all the flexures are unnecessary.

We do not use Foley or Bardex catheters because of the risk of rectal laceration and the possibility (albeit theoretical) of obscuring a transitional zone in infants with Hirschsprung's disease. In neonates the colon examination is performed with a no. 8 or 10 French disposable soft rubber radiopaque catheter and a 50 ml syringe filled with barium. The tip of the catheter is inserted into the rectal ampulla and fixed in place by a single strip of adhesive tape. The buttocks are then taped tightly together with two wide strips of tape. Barium spillage is uncommon unless the baby has been subjected to numerous recent digital rectal examinations. In this circumstance, the baby's buttocks also may have to be pinched tightly together with the leaded gloved hand during the study. Barium is injected manually without excessive pressure and the flow of barium observed fluoroscopically.

In older children any of the commercially available disposable enema tube and bag setups may be used, and barium is introduced by gravity flow. The tip of the catheter is usually taped to the buttocks, more for the patient's reassurance than to prevent incontinence, which is seldom a problem in children.

Barium is the contrast medium of choice in most cases. Meglumine diatrizoate (Gastrografin) is used when there is suspected meconium blockage in neonates or fear of a possible perforation in infants or older children. Single contrast studies generally suffice. Air contrast is used only when there is a question of polyps. We do not routinely prepare the colon in children, but obviously the colon must be well cleansed if air contrast is to be used. Cleansing enemas are administered in the evening before and on the morning of the examination. The patient is placed on a clear liquid diet on the preceding day, and a laxative in appropriate dosage for the patient's size is given on the evening before the study. Unfortunately, the initial barium enema will frequently demonstrate residual fecal debris, but it can serve as a final purge before a satisfactory air contrast study is obtained.

Congenital Malformations

ANORECTAL MALFORMATIONS

Anorectal malformations occur in about one in every 5,000 births. A wide spectrum of abnormalities may be encountered, ranging from mild distal anal strictures or cutaneous covering of the anus to high atresias with or without fistulous communications and other associated anomalies. A full discussion of the embryology and clinical presentations of these lesions is presented by Stevens and Smith[5] and Louw.[6]

The simplest classification is that of Ladd and Gross,[7] which divides these malformations into four major types:

Type I: Stenosis of the patent lower anal canal.

Type II: Complete obliteration of the distal anal opening by a thin septum.

Type III: Imperforate anus with atretic rectum. This is further divided according to whether the rectum ends blindly below (IIIa) or above (IIIb) the puborectalis sling.

Type IV: The anus and distal rectum are normal and separated from the upper atretic rectum.

Type III accounts for 90% of all cases. Over half of these will have fistulas into either the perineum or genitourinary system.

Table 30–1 shows the more comprehensive and descriptive International Classification, which categorizes the various possible abnormalities according to the patient's sex and the level of rectal atresia.[8]

From a practical point of view, the most important differentiation to be made is whether the rectal atresia is high or low, i.e., whether the atresia is above or below the levator ani muscle. This differentiation is vital, as it determines the type of surgical procedure needed. A low lesion can be treated by anoplasty or dilatation of the fistula, whereas a high lesion will require a colostomy and a future abdominal perineal approach for definitive repair. This differentiation fre-

TABLE 30-1.—SUGGESTED INTERNATIONAL CLASSIFICATION OF ANORECTAL ANOMALIES

MALE	FEMALE
A. Low (translevator)	
1. At normal anal site	1. Same
a. Anal stenosis	a. Same
b. Covered anus—complete	b. Same
2. At perineal site	2. Same
a. Anocutaneous fistula (covered anus—incomplete)	a. Same
b. Anterior perineal anus	b. Same
	3. At vulvar site
	a. Anovulvar fistula
	b. Anovestibular fistula
	c. Vestibular anus
B. Intermediate	
1. Anal agenesis	1. Same
a. Without fistula	a. Without fistula
b. With fistula	b. With fistula
1) Rectobulbar	1) Rectovestibular
	2) Rectovaginal—low
2. Anorectal stenosis	2. Same
C. High (supralevator)	
1. Anorectal agenesis	1. Same
a. Without fistula	a. Without fistula
b. With fistula	b. With fistula
1) Rectourethral	1) Rectovaginal—high
2) Rectovesical	2) Rectocloacal
	3) Rectovesical
2. Rectal atresia	2. Same
D. Miscellaneous	
1. Imperforate anal membrane	
2. Cloacal exstrophy	
3. Others	

From Santulli et al., J. Pediatr. Surg. 5:281, 1970, with permission.

quently can be determined by careful clinical inspection of the perineum. Detection of a perineal fistula always indicates a low lesion. The presence of "perineal pearls"—a median bar of slightly lobulated tissue—or corrugations at the extrinsic sphincter always indicate a low lesion. In girls a separate orifice for the urethra and the vagina with an intact hymen would suggest a low lesion. In contrast, boys with a smooth perineum and no perineal opening, and girls with a single perineal opening (cloacal anomaly) and with no visible hymen, most likely will have a high lesion.[9]

The radiographic landmark indicating the level of the levator ani muscle is the pubococcygeal (PC) line, a line drawn from the middle of the pubis to the sacrococcygeal junction. Traditionally this line is used in conjunction with the Wangensteen-Rice inverted lateral projection of the neonate pelvis. This view was initially devised to determine the actual distance separating the distalmost air filled rectum from the anal dimple. Its primary usefulness now is to determine the presence of gas in the bladder or vagina, and hence the presence of a fistula. Less importantly, the distal air-filled rectum is evaluated to see whether it terminates above or below the PC line. To correctly use this maneuver, at least 12 hours must pass after birth to allow sufficient time for swallowed intestinal gas to reach the distal rectum. The baby is then inverted (Cremin[10] urges inverting the neonate for at least 7 minutes to assure that gas will reach the distalmost portion of the rectum) and a lateral radiogram exposed with the beam centered at the hips. As reported by Berdon and colleagues,[11] this maneuver is fraught with potential inaccuracies apart from those purely technical in nature. The gas may in fact never reach the distalmost portion of the rectum, which may be impacted with meconium, and this would lead to a false assumption of a high lesion (Fig 30–2). A straining or crying baby may momentarily project a high rectal obstruction downward below the PC line. For these reasons, we do not routinely and seldom ever use this procedure for investigation of newborn infants with imperforate anus.

Other radiographic studies, however, are useful to define the type of malformation present. In rectal stenosis, studies by contrast injection into the rectum would permit assessment of the length and degree of stenosis present. Further, contrast injection into the rectum would exclude presacral masses, which may cause distal rectal stenosis.[12]

The covered anus is usually recognized by detection of meconium behind the thin anal membrane. Wagner et al,[13] have injected water-soluble contrast medium directly through these thin membranes, and also percutaneously in other types of rectal atresias, in order to visualize the distal rectal segment and demonstrate fistulas from the rectal pouch.

Plain abdominal radiograms in neonates with rectal atresia and imperforate anus will show evidence of distal bowel obstruction. Rarely pneumoperitoneum from bowel perforation may be present. Intraluminal calcified meconium pellets may be seen in the colon in both boys and girls with rectovesical fistulas or cloacal anomalies[14, 15] (Fig 30–3). Presumably the calcification occurs as a result of the admixture of urine and meconium within the colon. Air in the bladder, urethra or vagina indicates a fistula between the rectal pouch and these structures, as does presence of meconium in the vagina or urine.

Obstruction to retrograde passage of a catheter and separation of the proximal air-filled rectum from the catheter are diagnostic radiographic features (Fig 30–4) of type IV (Ladd-Gross classification) anorectal malformation.

Over half the cases of rectal atresia with imperforate anus will have fistulas to the perineum or contiguous structures. Some authors consider these fistulas to be ectopic anal openings, but histologically they differ from the normal anal canal. Fistulas are especially common in supralevator rectal atresia and involve the upper vagina in girls and the bladder or urethra in boys. Urethral communication usually occurs at the cavernous or membranous urethra and only rarely in the bulbar urethra.[16] In low lesions, fistulas to the perineum (Fig 30–5)—the low vagina in girls (Fig 30–5) and the urethra in boys—are not uncommon (Fig 30–6). Retrograde filling of these structures with water-soluble contrast injections may demonstrate the communication with the atretic rectum. Following a diverting colostomy for obviously high lesions, water-soluble contrast study of the distal colostomy segment can demonstrate both the presence of a fistula and the level and configuration of the distal rectal pouch. Anterior tapering of the distal rectum by the puborectalis sling would indicate an intermediate position of the atresia.

Radiography also plays an important role in evaluating the multitude of associated anomalies that may occur with imperforate anus. Anomalies of the lumbosacral spine are common in both sexes in low and especially in high lesions.[17, 18] Renal anomalies are also common and must be evaluated by routine excretory urography. Esophageal or duodenal atresias and sometimes both may occur concomitantly (Fig 30–7). Hand and forearm anomalies and cardiac lesions may also be present. These anomalies may occur singly or in any combination. A useful mnemonic device for the different organs and structures that may be involved is the acronym, VATER association, which stands for V = vertebral/vascular, A = anal, T = tracheal, E = esophageal; R = renal/rectal/radial.[19]

COLON ATRESIA

Atresia of the large bowel other than in the anorectal region is uncommon. It occurs in about one per 40,000 live births, presumably as a result of an intrauterine vascular accident. Louw[20] classifies colon atresias as three separate types:

Type I: Complete obstruction of the lumen by a diaphragm.

Type II: Blind proximal and distal ends connected by an atretic cordlike remnant of bowel.

Type III: Complete separation of proximal and distal blind ends with a V-shaped defect of the adjacent mesentery.

The clinical presentation of colon atresia is similar to any other cause of low intestinal obstruction.

Plain abdominal radiograms will depict evidence of distal bowel obstruction. The colon just proximal to the atresia, particularly with type I atresia, may be remarkably distended. With type I atresia, the flow of barium may demonstrate a localized expansion and retrograde invagination of the stretched obstructing diaphragm and produce a "windsock" or "club" appearance at the obstruction[21, 22] (Fig 30–8). Contrast study of the distal colon will demonstrate abrupt nondistorted obstruction at a type II atresia.

Selke and Jona[23] described a "hook" appearance to the mobile proximal portion of the distal colonic segment in type III atresias. The recoil movement responsible for the hook occurs by virtue of the V shaped mesenteric defect present.

Congenital colon strictures are uncommon. We have seen one child with a congenital band, causing stenosis in the proximal descending colon (Fig 30–9).

MALROTATION AND VOLVULUS

Symptoms of midgut malrotation generally appear early owing to obstruction of the duodenum by peritoneal or Ladd's bands. These residual embryonic peritoneal folds extend from the malplaced colon across the duodenum to the lateral abdominal wall and can be responsible for midgut volvulus. Bilious vomiting and radiographic demonstration of gaseous distention of the stomach and duodenum (double bubble sign), with relative paucity of gas in distal bowel loops, clearly indicate duodenal obstruction and the necessity for prompt surgical intervention. Whether the duodenal obstruction is caused by malrotation with bands or by other abnormalities, e.g., congenital stenosis, annular pancreas or a preduodenal portal vein, is academic at this point and further diagnostic studies are seldom helpful. Occasionally a surgeon may wish to temporize, if he can be reassured that there is no risk of intestinal volvulus, and a barium study may be requested for this reason.

Traditionally a barium enema is the study of choice but, in fact, there are equally sound reasons for doing either an upper gastrointestinal series or a barium enema.[24] Malrotation may be diagnosed by either method if carefully performed. On barium enema, malrotation is demonstrated by malposition of the proximal colon. The proximal colon may be grossly displaced to the mid or left side of the abdomen, or the displacement may be relatively subtle. An upper gastrointestinal study may be needed to differentiate this subtle finding of malrotation from a normal cecum, which may be high and slightly medial in position in some neonates (Fig 30–10). Barium usually fills the neonatal colon rapidly and also refluxes freely into terminal small bowel; the exact position of the cecum and the ileocecal valve may be observed. In addition partial malrotation of the proximal small bowel may be present even when the cecum is normally placed. For these reasons we prefer to study the upper gastrointestinal tract if duodenal obstruction is not complete and the infant is not critically ill. The upper gastrointestinal study will more easily and accurately demonstrate the level of obstruction and presence of duodenojejunal malrotation. A twisted or spiral appearance of the proximal displaced small bowel loops will indicate the presence of volvulus and need for immediate surgery (Fig 30–11). However, in a critically ill neonate who has passed bloody stools, an enema study is the preferred route if any barium study is to be performed at all. Obstruction to retrograde flow of barium in the region of Canon's point indicates complete midgut volvulus (Fig 30–12). Colon malrotation may be one part of a complex of abdominal anomalies such as the asplenia complex, gastroschisis, omphalocele and "Christmas tree" (or apple peel) deformity of the mesentery[25] (Fig 30–13).

Localized volvulus of the cecum or sigmoid colon is extremely uncommon in children, in contrast to its relative frequency in older adults. These types of volvulus occur presumably because the local mesocolon is congenitally long and is fixed to a narrow base. The only significant series of sigmoid volvulus in children is that reported by Parker and Nordstrom.[26] Unlike classic adult sigmoid volvulus, which is characterized by closed loop obstruction, marked distention of the sigmoid loop and obstruction to retrograde flow of barium at the distal limb of the obstruction, the children studied had normal abdominal films and only partial obstruction, with a slightly twisted, pointed configuration at the proximal limb of the volvulus. The volvulus was reduced hydrostatically, and this may account for the paucity of reported cases in children, since these cases may go unrecognized.[27, 28]

Other localized volvulus of the colon is extremely rare. We have seen one 5-year-old boy with localized volvulus of the transverse colon present in conjunction with a normal cecum and malrotation of the proximal small bowel (Fig 30–14).

DUPLICATIONS

Colon duplications are found twice as frequently in girls as in boys and are less common than small bowel duplications. They may be either spherical or tubular masses and generally occur on the mesenteric side of the colon or posterior to the rectum. They may be completely isolated from or communicate with the colon lumen. The isolated spherical lesion causes symptoms by its mass effect and occasionally because of bleeding (Fig 30–15). Long tubular duplications may represent an abortive attempt at twinning and may occur in conjunction with other severe anomalies of the spine and pelvis and duplication of kidneys and other pelvic organs (Fig 30–16).

Meconium and Stool Blockage Problems

The normal neonate usually passes meconium within the first 24 hours after birth. Failure of a newborn infant to pass meconium 24–48 hours after birth should alert the clinician to the possibility of an anatomical or functional abnormality of the colon.

Congenital Aganglionosis of the Colon (Hirschsprung's Disease)

This represents a functional obstruction of the colon caused by congenital absence of the ganglion cells in Auerbach's and Meissner's plexus in the submucosa and intermuscular layers of the rectum and adjacent colon. This aganglionosis occurs in about one in 5,000 births. Absent or faulty peristalsis in the aganglionic segment results in inspissation of stool in the progressively dilated normal bowel proximal to the involved segment. In 80% of cases, only the rectum and sigmoid are aganglionic. A striking (4 to 1) predominance of males is present in this classic "short segment" Hirschsprung's disease. In about 10–15% of cases, the entire colon and parts of the distal small bowel are aganglionic. Rarely the entire gut from the duodenum distally is aganglionic, and this would be incompatible with life. The male predominance is less striking in long segment disease. Familial occurrence has been reported and is usually but not exclusively of the long segment variety. In the other 5–10% of patients with Hirschsprung's disease, varying lengths of the colon proximal to the sigmoid are involved. For practical consideration, separate regions of aganglionosis with intervening normally innervated areas, i.e., skipped areas of aganglionosis, do not occur.[29]

Hirschsprung's disease is almost never found in the prematurely born. The vast majority of full-term neonates with aganglionosis become symptomatic in the early weeks of life but others may escape detection for years. Death from Hirschsprung's disease in the neonatal period nearly always results from fulminating enterocolitis (Fig 30–17). Enterocolitis developed in 25% of Tank's series of 50 patients and accounted for 50% of the deaths in his series.[30] The cause of the supervening enterocolitis is unknown, but a prompt colostomy in the normally innervated segment is mandatory to prevent its occurrence.

Clinically, neonatal Hirschsprung's disease presents with abdominal distention, vomiting, constipation and failure to thrive. Plain abdominal films show varying degrees of intestinal distention with air-fluid levels. Diagnosis can usually be made on barium enema study, although conclusive diagnosis can only be made histologically.

No cleansing enema should be given prior to the barium study. The stool impaction is useful in accentuating and facilitating detection of the transition zone. A straight catheter tip should be used and, once aganglionosis is detected or excluded by the appearance of the barium-filled rectum and sigmoid colon, the study should be stopped without filling the entire colon. Barium mixed with saline rather than water has been advocated to avoid the risk of water intoxication from retention of the enema, but as long as the colon is not routinely filled and the patient is satisfactorily hydrated, this risk is more theoretical than real.

The patient should be studied initially in lateral projection, as this allows an unobstructed view of the rectum and sigmoid junction. The findings on barium enema in neonates are not as pronounced as in older children but are nonetheless diagnostic in most cases.[31] Abnormal peristaltic activity of the aganglionic segment may be present and produce a sawtoothed configuration to the rectum.[32] The aganglionic segment is normal or only slightly diminished in caliber and is frequently empty of stool. There is usually a detectable transition as barium flows into the normally innervated, more dilated proximal colon. The dilatation is a secondary effect caused by piling up of stool that cannot be propelled past the aganglionic segment. Hence the transition zone becomes more obvious with passage of time. This transition zone, however, may be quite prominent in some neonates (Fig 30–18). Rarely a fecaloma may be tightly impacted at or near the transition zone and prevent retrograde flow of barium (Fig 30–19). The fecaloma may become calcified in older children.[33]

Overhead films in AP and lateral projection before and following evacuation are routinely obtained after the fluoroscopic study. If the diagnosis is not apparent, 24- and 48-hour follow-up films have been advocated by most authors. If there is significant retention of barium and stool on these delayed films, the concern for Hirschsprung's disease is heightened. In our opinion, the usefulness of these delayed films is overrated. What constitutes a significant retention has never been quantitated. Obviously, it is abnormal if the entire barium bolus remains after 48 hours, but the significance of retention of a half or even a third of the barium bolus is debatable. Furthermore, neonates with aganglionosis and enterocolitis will usually evacuate completely. Rather than risk an unnecessary delay of 24–48 hours when enterocolitis may develop, it is our approach to recommend suction mucosal biopsy of the rectum to exclude Hirschsprung's disease, if the enema study is not diagnostic and if there is strong clinical suspicion of Hirschsprung's disease.

In older children with aganglionosis, the diagnosis nearly always can be made on barium enema study. The transition zone is more clearly defined and frequently can be suspected even on plain abdominal radiograms (Fig 30–20). Lateral projections are more valuable than frontal views, as the fecal-filled dilated sigmoid can project over and obscure the low transitional zone (Fig 30–21).

Total colon Hirschsprung's disease is more difficult to recognize radiographically.[34] The most important factor in diagnosis is to consider its possibility in any infant who acts obstructed but in whom no obstructing lesion can be demonstrated on barium enema study. Abnormal peristaltic activity of the colon; relative dilatation of the ileal compared to colonic caliber; unusually free reflux into proximal small bowel; prolonged retention of barium in small bowel; and apparent shortening of the colon, with rounding of the usually redundant flexures, are some nonspecific signs that should suggest the diagnosis of total colon Hirschsprung's[35] (Fig 30–22). Rarely intraluminal calcifications in the terminal ileum may be present.[36] Prompt rectal suction mucosal biopsy should be performed if the diagnosis is suspected.

Associated anomalies are uncommon with congenital aganglionosis, except for a higher incidence in Down's syndrome. In the series reported by Kilcoyne and Taybi,[37] 5 of 31 children with Hirschsprung's disease had Down's syndrome. One of our cases had Ivemark syndrome (asplenia complex) (Fig 30–23). An infant with asplenia, total colon aganglionosis and congenital microgastria was also reported by Shackelford et al.[38] Aganglionosis has been reported with imperforate anus, but absence of ganglion cells in these patients may be secondary to surgery. Urinary problems are secondary to pressure effects from the fecal masses in the rectum and sigmoid rather than to "aganglionosis" of the bladder or ureters[39] (Fig 30–24).

MECONIUM ILEUS

Distal small bowel obstruction caused by inspissation of abnormally viscid and tenacious meconium may be the initial clinical and radiographic manifestation of cystic fibrosis. Whereas 10–20% of patients with cystic fibrosis present with meconium ileus, all cases of meconium ileus have cystic fibrosis. Failure to pass meconium, abdominal distention and vomiting are the principal clinical features.

Classic plain film findings in uncomplicated meconium ileus include presence of a bubbly mass in the right lower quadrant and generally absence of air-fluid levels on the erect films. The bubbly appearance represents admixture of meconium and gas in the distal small bowel, and the thick meconium in the small bowel loops prevent air and fluid accumulation. Contrast study of the colon will demonstrate a microcolon and numerous retained pellets of meconium in the proximal colon and distal small bowel (Fig 30–25). A microcolon indicates a colon that has not been distended by passage of meconium and it is not an intrinsic developmental abnormality. It is not diagnostic of cystic fibrosis. Berdon et al.[40] suggest that microcolon can occur only with distal small bowel obstruction, but we have observed it in proximal (i.e., duodenal) as well as distal small bowel atresias and do not consider it a reliable indicator of the level of atresia or obstruction.

Uncomplicated meconium ileus may be treated by meglumine diatrizoate enema.[41, 42] The hypertonic solution draws fluid into the lumen of the ileum, which loosens the meconium mass and allows it to pass spontaneously. The primary effective agent in Gastrografin, however, may be Tween-80, a wetting agent.[43, 44] Several repeated enemas may be necessary before the obstruction is relieved (Fig 30–26). This treatment must not be undertaken lightly. The baby must be carefully observed to prevent fluid and electrolyte imbalance. A surgeon's cooperation and permission should be obtained and his help available in case the procedure is unsuccessful or if perforation occurs (Fig 30–27).

Nearly half of the patients with meconium ileus have fetal complications of volvulus, intestinal atresia, perforation, pseudocyst formation and meconium peritonitis. In utero, intestinal perforation results in spillage of meconium into the peritoneal cavity, which produces a sterile chemical peritonitis. The meconium spreads widely throughout the peritoneal cavity and may also pass through the patent processus vaginalis into the scrotum. Calcification of the meconium occurs rapidly. Meconium peritonitis develops secondary to intestinal perforation from whatever cause. Although meconium ileus is a common cause (about 33%) of meconium peritonitis, not all patients with meconium peritonitis have cystic fibrosis. Nonetheless, the diagnosis of cystic fibrosis must be excluded in all neonates with meconium peritonitis.

If perforation occurs shortly before birth, air-fluid levels within the peritoneal cavity may be noted shortly after birth. The initially sterile peritonitis may become secondarily contaminated very quickly in the neonatal period. Intrauterine intestinal volvulus caused by meconium ileus may lead to subsequent intestinal atresias or development of inflammatory pseudocyst

About a third of the cases of complicated meconium ileus will have essentially normal abdominal radiograms.[45] The presence of numerous air-fluid levels in a neonate with meconium ileus should alert the clinician to possible associated complications. Meconium peritonitis is heralded by presence of calcifications scattered throughout the abdomen. These frequently are thin, plaque-like calcifications around the periphery of the peritoneal cavity and liver (Fig 30–28). Rarely, meconium calcifications in the scrotum may be present and may cause concern for a possible testicular tumor. Intramural calcifications with intestinal atresias and circumferential curvilinear calcifications around pseudocysts rarely occur.

The generalized abnormality of the exocrine glands in cystic fibrosis results in obstruction and enlargement of the intestinal glands, which produce a coarsened, cobblestone mucosal pattern throughout the colon[46] (Fig 30–29). These changes are distinct and may provide the first clue to the diagnosis of cystic fibrosis in children with mild pulmonary problems. Impaction of persistently abnormally sticky stools in the distal small bowel or colon in older children with cystic fibrosis is equivalent to meconium ileus in the newborn infant (Fig 30–30). Meconium ileus equivalent can also be treated successfully with Gastrografin enemas. The fecal mass may act as a lead point for colocolic intussusception. An adherent fecalith may produce a mass lesion in the appendiceal region. Pneumatosis cystoides intestinalis is a rare complication of cystic fibrosis.

MECONIUM PLUG SYNDROME

Infrequently some newborn babies are unable to evacuate meconium, although there is no apparent abnormality of the meconium or of the anatomy of the gut. These babies act obstructed, but the obstruction is self-limited and promptly relieved following passage of the initial meconium mass. Although generally benign, a few cases of intestinal perforation have been reported.[47] This may occur in normal full-term babies but tends to occur more frequently with premature babies or infants of diabetic or prediabetic mothers.

The cause is unknown. Various etiologic theories are reflected in the plethora of names that have been applied to this condition, i.e., functional intestinal obstruction in premature infants,[48] functional immaturity of the large bowel,[49, 50] meconium plug,[51] meconium blockage[52] and small left colon syndrome.

Evacuation of a large meconium impaction may follow digital or thermometer manipulation of the rectum, or a contrast enema examination, particularly when diatrizoate is the medium used (Fig 30–31). The meconium mass may fill and dilate the entire colon (Fig 30–32) or only the terminal ileum and proximal colon. Davis et al.[53] reported a series of infants of diabetic mothers with impaction of meconium proximal to the descending colon and a remarkably small left colon and rectum (Fig 30–33). Many of these impactions were detected in infants who were asymptomatic.[54] The growing consensus is that these different patterns represent the same functional abnormality[55] (Fig 30–34).

The diagnosis of meconium plug syndrome should be a tentative one and the baby closely observed. If stooling difficulties persist, appropriate tests must be undertaken to rule out cystic fibrosis and congenital aganglionosis. Both may present initially with meconium blockage followed by a transient asymptomatic period.[56]

FUNCTIONAL (PSYCHOGENIC) MEGACOLON

In some preschool children, severe constipation may develop associated with overflow incontinence and fecal soiling (encopresis). Their previous general health and bowel habits have been normal and no anatomical abnormality is detected. Periodically they are capable of a voluminous bowel movement, which may plug up the plumbing. The cause for this is conjectural, but it is thought to be a reaction to coercive bowel training.

On physical examination, large fecal masses can be palpated through the abdominal wall. The perineum, especially in boys, is soiled and the rectal ampulla is markedly dilated and impacted with stool. On barium enema the capacious rectum is filled with stool down to the anal verge, and no distal transition zone is detected (Fig 30–35). The proximal colon is relatively less distended than the rectum. The radiographic distinction from Hirschsprung's disease is usually clear-cut, but rectal mucosal biopsy should be performed if there is any equivocation.

OTHER CAUSES OF CONSTIPATION

Many causes of constipation are clearly related to obvious medical problems, such as acute infections and electrolyte imbalance, or are secondary to medical treatment (Fig 30–36). Congenital cretinism may mimic neonatal Hirschsprung's disease (Fig 30–37). The megacystis–microcolon–intestinal hypoperistalsis syndrome[57] and the chronic idiopathic pseudo-obstruction syndrome[58, 59] are uncommon causes of functional intestinal obstruction of unknown cause.

Colon Masses

INTUSSUSCEPTION

Invagination of a bowel loop into the lumen of an adjacent segment of bowel may occur at any point in the small or large intestines. Ileoileal and colocolic intussusceptions account for less than 10% of all cases and usually result from a lead point such as a polyp, Meckel's diverticulum or a small duplication. The vast majority occurs in the ileocecal region, with invagination of the ileum into the colon. These occur over half the time in the first year of life, principally in boys. It is rare in the immediate postnatal period, when its occurrence usually is caused by a small benign mass acting as a lead point.[60] Similarly a lead point will commonly be found if intussusception develops after 3 years of age. Most ileocolic intussusceptions will occur between these two periods, and only 5% of these cases will have a lead point. The cause in most of these cases is unknown but is generally believed to be related to the increased peristaltic activity of the bowel at this age and to the presence of prominent lymphoid follicles (Peyer's patch) in the terminal ileum.

Clinically these infants are well nourished and healthy and present with recurrent bouts of sudden crampy abdominal pain with intervening asymptomatic periods. The bouts of pain increase in frequency and duration and may be accompanied by vomiting and drawing up of the legs. Listlessness, pallor, diaphoresis and dehydration may develop. The vascularity of the intussuscepted bowel becomes compromised, and stool admixed with blood and mucus (currant jelly stools) are passed. A soft tubular or round abdominal mass may be felt in the right upper quadrant or epigastric region. Plain abdominal films may show the head of the intussusceptum projecting into the air-filled distal transverse colon. A vague suggestion of a soft tissue mass in the right side of the abdomen and absence of gas in the right lower quadrant, associated with varying degrees of small bowel distention, are also commonly present. The diagnosis is confirmed on barium enema by demonstrating an intraluminal concave filling defect with a "coiled spring" appearance in the barium column as the barium encounters the distal intussusceptum and passes slightly around its periphery (Fig 30–38).

Hydrostatic reduction of ileocolic intussusception is gratifying and safe and easy to accomplish if performed according to strict guidelines. The ease by which intussusception is reduced in most cases should not lull the clinician and radiologist into forgetting the basic fact that ileocolic intussusception is a *surgical* disease with a potentially lethal outcome. Ideally the patient will have been examined by the surgeon, who is then immediately available to operate should hydrostatic reduction fail or if intestinal perforation occurs. The latter should happen rarely if the criteria for patient selection and performance of hydrostatic reduction are strictly adhered to. Two absolute contraindications to hydrostatic reduction in our judgment are clinical evidence of peritonitis and radiographic evidence of frank small bowel obstruction. On the other hand, we would not hesitate to do a *diagnostic* barium enema under these circumstances (Fig 30–39). In small bowel obstruction, the concern is not one of causing perforation of the distal viable colon but of reducing a segment of already ischemic bowel.

Duration of symptoms per se has not been an important consideration. We have demonstrated and easily reduced intussusception in children who have had complaints for several days and, conversely, have been unsuccessful in treating children seen within a few hours of onset of complaints.

A Bardex catheter is probably useful to insure a tight hydraulic system but it is not necessary and we do not use it. The patient should be normally hydrated and clinically stable. The barium reservoir should be kept no higher then 3–3.5 feet above table top. The patient should be adequately restrained, and his knees should be held down by a compression band or sandbag so that he cannot draw up his knees to evacuate. There should be no manipulation of the patient or the barium enema bag or tube once the enema is started. The head of the barium column is carefully watched fluoroscopically. Usually there will be momentary delay of the barium flow when the intussusceptum is initially encountered and intermittently as it is being reduced. The holdup may appear interminable in the area of the ileocecal valve. Reduction is achieved when barium suddenly flows freely through the ileocecal valve well back into proximal small bowel. Frequently at this point the patient, who has been fretful before and throughout the procedure, will fall off into a peaceful sleep. If an ileoileal intussusception is demonstrated after reduction back through the ileocecal valve, the examination should be stopped, as there will usually be an anatomical cause, which requires surgical removal.

The concomitant use of sedation and bowel relaxants has been advocated and theoretically should increase the success rate of hydrostatic reduction, but we have no experience with this. Repeated attempts at hydrostatic reduction have also been advocated. Our philosophy is to try only once and, if we are unsuccessful, to allow the surgeons to take over. Morbidity from anesthesia and surgery for this procedure is now so low that it is foolhardy to invite disaster by repeated vigorous attempts at hydrostatic reduction.

We do not hesitate to try hydrostatic reduction of an intussusception in children over 2 or 3 years of age, knowing full well the higher likelihood of a causative lesion, but the examination is quickly stopped if an abnormal lesion is demonstrated.

POLYPS

The various polyposis syndromes are presented fully elsewhere in this volume and only those that occur in the pediatric age range with some frequency will be discussed here.

1. Familial polyposis is transmitted as an autosomal dominant trait, although 50% of cases occur as a result of spontaneous mutation. Innumerable small adenomatous polyps develop throughout the rectum and colon. These carry a nearly universal risk of eventual malignant degeneration in late adulthood, and prophylactic total colectomy has been advised. The normal lymphoid hyperplasia of the pediatric colon must not be mistaken for familial polyposis, which usually does not present until adolescence at the earliest.

2. The Peutz-Jeghers syndrome is transmitted as an autosomal dominant trait. These patients present with cutaneous and mucous membrane melanosis, most conspicuously on the face, in and about the mouth. Hamartomatous polyps develop anywhere from the stomach to the rectum and carry a very small (2–3%) risk of later malignant degeneration. Symptoms are caused by bleeding and intussusception (Fig 30–40). Treatment is by local resection as symptoms develop.

3. Juvenile polyps are the most common form of colon polyps in childhood. These originate presumably as a retention cyst following obstruction of a colon mucous gland and are universally regarded as a benign lesion with no malignant potential. They are rare under 1 year of age and uncommon after age 10. The majority occurs as an isolated pedunculated lesion in the rectal and sigmoid region. Most of them slough and are passed spontaneously. Symptoms are related primarily to bleeding, but pain from traction, intussusception and rectal prolapse also may occur. Open surgery is indicated only if bleeding is severe and persistent. These polyps rarely appear in massive numbers (juvenile polyposis of the colon) and cause pain, bleeding and protein loss.

Diagnosis is made on air-barium contrast enema study. The colon must be meticulously cleared of retained stool. The polyp can be detected either as a filling defect in the barium column, as a barium-coated mass projecting into the air-filled colon or as an outstanding mass in the collapsed colon following evacuation (Fig 30–41). A solitary polyp that is beyond the reach of a sigmoidoscope in a child is presumed to be a juvenile polyp, and surgical intervention is not indicated. Coexistence of a juvenile polyp and an adenomatous polyp has not been reported.[61]

Other types of polyps in children are uncommon and usually are benign.[62] These include lymphoid polyps, inflammatory polyps and rarely neurofibromas and hemangiomas.

MALIGNANT TUMORS

Carcinomas of the intestinal tract in children are extremely rare but most commonly involve the colon. They are principally mucus-producing colloid adenocarcinomas and usually are found in the 2d decade of life in the rectum and sigmoid colon[63] (Fig 30–42).

Lymphomas, the most common malignant lesions of the colon in children, are primarily lymphosarcoma, Burkitt's lymphoma or reticulum cell sarcoma. American Burkitt's lymphoma differs from African Burkitt's in its higher frequency of abdominal and lower incidence of jaw involvement[64, 65] (see Fig 30–44).

Most cases of colon lymphomas occur in boys of preschool and early school age. The cecal region and right colon are usually involved, in contrast to adults, in whom the stomach and proximal intestinal tract are the more usual sites (Fig 30–43). Abdominal pain, vomiting and malaise are the chief complaints. A hard, nontender mass in the right side of the abdomen and iron deficiency anemia are the principal clinical findings. Prognosis is generally extremely grim.[66]

Abdominal films may show evidence of a soft tissue mass in the right side of the abdomen, with varying degrees of small bowel distention. The tumor mass and its involvement of the colon and small bowel may be demonstrated on either barium enema or upper gastrointestinal follow-through studies. Differentiation from Crohn's disease is important and usually easily accomplished. Intussusception is a common complication, and lymphosarcoma must be a major consideration as cause of intussusception in an older child.

Inflammatory Diseases

ACUTE APPENDICITIS

This is responsible for more abdominal surgery in children than any other condition. It is uncommon before age 2 years, possibly because the wide, funnel-shaped infant cecum and broad-based appendix insure good drainage of the appendix. In younger children, acute appendicitis presents with more nonspecific symptoms, a more rapid progression to appendiceal perforation and a wider spread of infection throughout the abdomen.[67] The classic clinical findings are abdominal pain and tenderness in the right lower quadrant, vomiting, fever and leukocytosis. Detection of a calcified appendicolith is presumptive evidence of acute appendicitis in a child with abdominal pain. Usually round or oval and laminated, appendicoliths are found in the right lower quadrant or pelvic area. They may be multiple (Fig 30–45) and can be quite large (Fig 30–46). Air outlining the appendix is not by itself an abnormal finding[68] (Fig 30–47). Pneumoperitoneum is uncommon, as the inflammatory reaction usually seals off the area of perforation (Fig 30–48). Other signs of localized inflammation in the right lower quadrant include the presence of an indistinct soft tissue mass in the right lower quadrant due to inflammatory thickening and absence of gas in the cecum; mild paralytic ileus of adjacent bowel loops (sentinel loops); partial distal small bowel obstruction; loss of psoas and lateral properitoneal lines; and presence of multiple small bubbles of gas in the abscess cavity.

Barium enema is considered to be safe and has been used increasingly in the diagnosis of appendicitis.[69-71] Normally the appendix is easily filled on barium enema in 90% of cases. If the appendix is filled, the likelihood of appendicitis is minimal. However, whether the entire appendix is filled cannot always be clearly determined, and in some cases there will be nearly complete filling but inflammation at the distal tip. Failure to fill the appendix and deformity of the cecum and contiguous terminal ileum are reliable signs of acute appendicitis in the proper clinical setting (Fig 30-49). There is a minimal risk of spill of barium into the peritoneal cavity (Fig 30-50).

Necrotizing colitis of the cecum (typhlitis) may be a terminal event in children with acute lymphocytic leukemia or aplastic anemia.[72, 73] These children present with high, spiking fevers and severe abdominal pain that is not restricted to the right lower quadrant. Generalized tenderness but absence of rigidity may be noted. Plain abdominal radiograms may show mild small bowel distention and relative absence of gas in the right lower quadrant. Thickening of the wall of the cecum and proximal colon may be appreciated (Fig 30-51). Differentiation from acute appendicitis is not possible. Surgical intervention in these terminal patients has not been rewarding in the experience of our surgeons.[74]

NEONATAL NECROTIZING ENTEROCOLITIS

Necrotizing enterocolitis occurs predominantly but not exclusively in low birth weight prematures. The exact cause has not been established, but bowel ischemia may be part of a generalized hypoxia or may result from preferential shunting of the splanchnic circulation to more vital organs (diving reflex), or from local factors, e.g., bowel wall injury, infection or presence of umbilical vascular catheters.[75-77]

Clinically these babies present with abdominal distention, vomiting, lethargy, temperature instability, gastric retention and gross or occult bloody stools. If unattended, the disease progresses rapidly, with development of disseminated intravascular coagulopathy, intestinal perforation, sepsis, shock and death.

The classic radiographic findings of air in the bowel wall and the portal venous system are late findings[78-80] (Figs 30-52 and 30-53). Survival depends on early recognition of the disease. Consistent but not pathognomonic radiographic findings of early necrotizing enterocolitis are selective dilatation of small bowel with little or no air in the colon; dilatation and elongation (sausage shape) of bowel loops; loss of bowel wall definition; and presence of a disorganized atonic pattern of intestinal gas.[81, 82] In addition to supine abdominal films, films either in cross-bed lateral or decubitus projections should be obtained to detect early pneumoperitoneum or portal venous air. Contrast studies are usually not indicated but, in selected cases, can demonstrate pneumatosis intestinalis and areas of bowel stenosis[83] (Fig 30-54). These areas of stricture may eventually spontaneously resolve.[84]

Treatment is directed toward total gut rest, maintenance of nutrition by parenteral hyperalimentation, antibiotics and prompt surgery if perforation occurs.

GRANULOMATOUS AND ULCERATIVE COLITIS

These entities are discussed fully in Chapters 18 and 45. They involve primarily young adults, but children and rarely even infants may be affected.[85]

Granulomatous colitis (Crohn's disease of the colon) (see Fig 30-58) represents a focal idiopathic full thickness granulomatous inflammation of the bowel wall and is limited to the small intestine 50% of the time, to the colon 10% of the time, and simultaneously to the colon and small bowel 40% of the time. About 25-50% of patients with granulomatous colitis have onset before age 16.[86]

Ulcerative colitis is an idiopathic diffuse superficial inflammation of the colon mucosa and submucosa, although transmural involvement may occur. About one seventh of cases of ulcerative colitis occur in children under age 16.[87]

Both diseases may be insidious in onset and present with malaise, failure to thrive, fever and mild diarrhea. Abdominal pain, occasionally a soft tissue mass in the right lower quadrant, and mild to moderate diarrhea, usually without blood, are the clinical hallmarks of granulomatous colitis. Ulcerative colitis generally presents with a more severe, persistent diarrhea, which is frequently bloody.[88]

Radiographic studies are important in diagnosis and determination of the extent of disease. However, because of overlapping features, accurate differentiation between the two is not possible in about a third of cases.[89] Plain radiograms can show the presence of pneumoperitoneum, toxic megacolon, absence of haustra (lead pipe colon) and bowel wall thickening (see Fig 30–57). Calcium oxylate stones develop with increased incidence in Crohn's disease when the terminal ileum also is involved and may be seen in the kidneys or ureters.[90] Excretory urogram may show ureteral obstruction from either a stone or the adjacent inflammatory bowel process (Fig 30–55). Double air-barium contrast studies have recently been advocated for evaluation of early mucosal changes such as aphthoid ulcers, which are now thought to be diagnostic of Crohn's disease.[91, 92] Our experience is limited to single contrast barium studies of the colon with reflux of barium into the terminal ileum. Progressive radiographic alterations in both conditions may occur with alarming speed (Fig 30–56). The major radiographic findings of differential value in each condition are shown in Table 30–2.[93]

TABLE 30–2.—RADIOGRAPHIC FINDINGS IN ULCERATIVE AND GRANULOMATOUS COLITIS

Ulcerative colitis
Rectal involvement
Left colon or total colon involvement (Fig 30–57)
Shallow superficial ulcers
Pseudopolypoid mucosal filling defects
Symmetric involvement of colon wall
Patulous ileocecal junction with dilated terminal ileum (backwash ileitis)
Granulomatous colitis
Rectum usually not involved
Predominantly right colon
Multiple skipped areas of involvement
Deep ulcers (over 3 mm)
Cobblestone mucosal pattern (Fig 30–58)
Asymmetric involvement of colon wall
Multiple fistulas (rectal, enterocolic, duodenocolic)
Narrowed ileocecal valve with stenotic, thickened, nodular terminal ileum

MISCELLANEOUS INFLAMMATORY PROCESSES

Infectious colitides from amebiasis and tuberculosis may resemble either granulomatous or ulcerative colitis and are discussed in Chapters 2 and 43. Both usually involve the proximal colon and cause deformity of the cecum. The terminal ileum is seldom involved with amebiasis in contrast to tuberculous ileocolitis (Fig 30–59). Amebiasis, however, may involve the entire colon[94, 95] (Fig 30–60). Differentiation of these infectious colitides from Crohn's colitis or ulcerative colitis is important, since appropriate antibiotic treatment can lead to a successful cure.

The hemolytic uremic syndrome occurs in infants and young children with a prodrome of flulike illness and gastroenteritis, followed by hemolytic anemia and uremia.[96] Massive lower gastrointestinal bleeding may occur, and on barium enema the colon shows changes of colitis and submucosal hemorrhage and may mimic ulcerative colitis[97, 98] (Fig 30–61).

Pseudomembranous colitis usually develops as a side effect of antibiotic usage. The highest incidence appears to be with clindamycin, which produces diarrhea in about 20% of patients and pseudomembranous colitis in 1–10%.[99] Other incriminated antibiotics include lincomycin HCl monohydrate, chloramphenicol, ampicillin and penicillin G. The cause is now thought to be the toxigenic organism *Clostridium difficile*.[99, 100] Barium enema shows irregularity of the colon contour without ulcerations. The mucosa of the entire colon appears to be covered by flat plaque-like lesions 2–8 mm in size[101] (Fig 30–62).

REFERENCES

1. Kleinman, P. K., Winchester, P., Meyer, M. A., et al.: The neonatal colon: An anatomic approach to plain films, Am. J. Roentgenol. 128:61, 1977.
2. Capitanio, M. A., and Kirkpatrick, J. A.: Lymphoid hyperplasia of the colon in children, Radiology 94:323, 1970.
3. Franken, E. A., Jr.: Lymphoid hyperplasia of the colon, Radiology 94:329, 1970.
4. Laufer, I., and deSa, D.: Lymphoid follicular pattern: A normal feature of the pediatric colon, Am. J. Roentgenol. 130:51, 1978.
5. Stephens, F. D., and Smith, E. D.: *Ano-rectal Malformations in Children* (Chicago: Year Book Medical Publishers, Inc., 1971).
6. Louw, J. H.: *Congenital Abnormalities of the Rectum and Anus*. Current Problems in Surgery (Chicago: Year Book Medical Publishers, Inc., 1965).
7. Ladd, W. E., and Gross, R. E.: Congenital malformations of the anus and rectum: Report of 162 cases, Am. J. Surg. 23:167, 1934.
8. Santulli, T. V., Kiesewetter, W. B., and Bill, A. H., Jr.: Anorectal anomalies: A suggested international classification, J. Pediatr. Surg. 5:281, 1970.
9. Seibert, J. J., and Golladay, E. S.: Clinical evaluation of imperforate anus: Clue to a type of anal-rectal anomaly, Am. J. Roentgenol. 133:289, 1979.
10. Cremin, B. J.: The radiological assessment of anorectal anomalies, Clin. Radiol. 22:239, 1971.
11. Berdon, W. E., Baker, D. H., Santulli, T. V., et al.: The radiologic evaluation of imperforate anus. An approach correlated with current surgical concepts, Radiology 90:466, 1968.
12. Malangoni, M. A., Grosfeld, J. L., Ballantine, T. V. N., et al.: Congenital rectal stenosis: A sign a presacral pathologic condition, Pediatrics 62: 584, 1978.
13. Wagner, M. L., Harberg, F. J., Kumar, A. P. M., et al.: The evaluation of imperforate anus utilizing percutaneous injection of water soluble iodide contrast material, Pediatr. Radiol. 1:34, 1973.
14. Berdon, W. E., Baker, D. H., Wigger, H. J., et al.: Calcified intraluminal meconium in newborn males with imperforate anus—enterolithiasis in the newborn, Am. J. Roentgenol. 125:449, 1975.
15. Selke, A. C., Jr., and Cowley, C. E.: Calcified intraluminal meconium in a female infant with imperforate anus, Am. J. Roentgenol. 130:786, 1978.
16. Currarino, G., Votteler, T. P., and Kirks, D. R.: Anal agenesis with rectobulbar fistula, Radiology 126:457, 1978.
17. Berdon, W. E., Hochberg, B., Baker, D. H., et al.: The association of lumbosacral spine and genitourinary anomalies with imperforate anus, Am. J. Roentgenol. 98:181, 1966.
18. Thompson, W., and Grossman, H.: The association of spinal and genitourinary abnormalities with low anorectal anomalies (imperforate anus) in female infants, Radiology 113:693, 1974.
19. Barnes, J. C., and Smith, W. L.: The VATER association, Radiology 126:445, 1978.
20. Louw, J. H.: Congenital intestinal atresia and stenosis in the newborn: Observations on its pathogenesis and treatment, Ann. R. Coll. Surg. Engl. 25:209, 1959.
21. Blank, E., Afshani, E., Girdany, B. R., et al.: "Windsock sign" of congenital membranous atresia of the colon, Am. J. Roentgenol. 120:330, 1974.
22. Bley, W. R., and Franken, E. A., Jr.: Roentgenology of colon atresia, Pediatr. Radiol. 1:105, 1973.
23. Selke, A. C., Jr., and Jona, J. Z.: The hook sign in type 3 congenital colonic atresia, Am. J. Roentgenol. 131:350, 1978.
24. Berdon, W. E., Baker, D. H., Bull, S., et al.: Midgut malrotation and volvulus. Which films are most helpful?, Radiology 96:375, 1970.
25. Leonidas, J. C., Amoury, R. A., Ashcroft, K. W., et al.: Duodenojejunal atresias with "apple peel" small bowel, Radiology 118:661, 1976.
26. Allen, R. P., and Nordstrom, J. E.: Volvulus of sigmoid in children, Am. J. Roentgenol. 91:690, 1964.
27. Hunter, J. G., Jr., and Keats, T. E.: Sigmoid volvulus in children. A case report, Am. J. Roentgenol. 108:621, 1970.
28. Wilk, P. J., Ross, M., and Leonidas, J.: Sigmoid volvulus in an 11-year-old girl, Am. J. Dis. Child. 127:400, 1974.
29. Ehrenpreis, T.: *Hirschsprung's Disease* (Chicago: Year Book Medical Publishers, Inc., 1970).
30. Tank, E. S.: Pitfalls in the diagnosis and treatment of Hirschsprung's disease, Arch. Surg. 102:332, 1971.
31. Cremin, B. J.: The early diagnosis of Hirschsprung's disease, Pediatr. Radiol. 2:23, 1974.
32. Hope, J. W., Borns, P. F., and Berg, P. K.: Roentgenological manifestations of Hirschsprung's disease in infancy, Am. J. Roentgenol. 95:217, 1965.
33. Campbell, J. B., and Robinson, A. E.: Hirschsprung's disease presenting as calcified fecaloma, Pediatr. Radiol. 1:161, 1973.
34. Sane, S. M., and Girdany, B. R.: Total aganglionosis coli, Radiology 107:397, 1973.
35. Cremin, B. J., and Golding, R. L.: Congenital aganglionosis of the entire colon in neonates, Br. J. Radiol. 49:27, 1976.
36. Fletcher, B. D., and Yulish, B. S.: Intraluminal calcifications in the small bowel of newborn infants with total colonic aganglionosis, Radiology 126:451, 1978.
37. Kilcoyne, R. F., and Taybi, H.: Conditions associated with congenital megacolon, Am. J. Roentgenol. 108:615, 1970.
38. Shackelford, G. D., McAlister, W. H., Brodeur,

A. E., et al.: Congenital microgastria, Am. J. Roentgenol. 118:72, 1973.
39. Shopfner, C. E.: Urinary tract pathology associated with constipation, Radiology 90:865, 1968.
40. Berdon, W. E., Baker, D. H., Santulli, T. V., et al.: Microcolon in newborn infants with intestinal obstruction. Its correlation with the level and time of onset of obstruction, Radiology 90:878, 1968.
41. Frech, R. S., and McAllister, W. H.: Meconium ileus relieved by 40% water soluble contrast enemas, Radiology 94:341, 1970.
42. Lillie, J. G., and Crispin, A. R.: Investigation and management of neonatal obstruction by Gastrografin enema, Ann. Radiol. (Paris) 15:237, 1972.
43. Wood, B. P., and Katzberg, R. W.: Tween 80/diatrizoate enemas in bowel obstruction, Am. J. Roentgenol. 130:747, 1978.
44. Wood, B. P., Katzberg, R. W., Ryan, D. H., et al.: Diatrizoate enemas: Facts and fallacies of colonic toxicity, Radiology 126:441, 1978.
45. Leonidas, J. D., Berdon, W. E., Baker, D. H., et al.: Meconium ileus and its complications, Am. J. Roentgenol. 108:598, 1970.
46. Berk, R. N., and Lee, F. A.: The late gastrointestinal manifestations of cystic fibrosis of the pancreas, Radiology 106:377, 1973.
47. Nixon, G. W., Condon, V. R., and Stewart, D. R.: Intestinal perforation as a complication of the neonatal small left colon syndrome, Am. J. Roentgenol. 125:75, 1975.
48. Cremin, B. J.: Functional intestinal obstruction in premature infants, Pediatr. Radiol. 1:109, 1973.
49. LeQuesne, G. W., and Reilly, B. J.: Functional immaturity of the large bowel in the newborn infant, Radiol. Clin. North Am. 13:331, 1975.
50. Vanhoutte, J. J.: Roentgenographic manifestations of immaturity of the intestinal neural plexus in premature infants, Radiology 106:368, 1973.
51. Swischuk, L.: Meconium plug syndrome, Am. J. Roentgenol. 103:339, 1968.
52. Mikity, V. G., Hodgman, J. E., and Paciulli, J.: Meconium blockage syndrome, Radiology 88:740, 1967.
53. Davis, W. S., Allen, R. P., Favara, B. E., et al.: The neonatal small left colon syndrome, Am. J. Roentgenol. 120:322, 1974.
54. Davis, W. S., and Campbell, J. B.: Neonatal small left colon syndrome: Occurrence in asymptomatic infants of diabetic mothers, Am. J. Dis. Child. 129:1024, 1975.
55. Berdon, W. E., Slovis, T. L., Campbell, J. B., et al.: Neonatal small left colon syndrome: Its relationship to aganglionosis and meconium plug syndrome, Radiology 125:457, 1977.
56. Rosenstein, B. J.: Cystic fibrosis presenting with the meconium plug syndrome, Am. J. Dis. Child 132:167, 1978.
57. Berdon, W. E., Baker, D. H., Blanc, W. A., et al.: Megacystis-microcolon-intestinal hypoperistalsis syndrome: A new cause of intestinal obstruction in the newborn, Am. J. Roentgenol. 126:957, 1976.
58. Byrne, W. J., Cipel, L., Euler, A. R., et al.: Chronic idiopathic intestinal pseudo-obstruction syndrome in children—clinical characteristics and prognosis, J. Pediatr. 90:585, 1977.
59. Schuffler, M. D., Rohrmann, C. A., Jr., and Templeton, F. E.: The radiologic manifestations of idiopathic intestinal pseudo-obstruction, Am. J. Roentgenol. 127:729, 1976.
60. Patriquin, H. B., Afshani, E., Effman, E., et al.: Neonatal intussusception. Report of 12 cases, Radiology 125:463, 1977.
61. Holgersen, L. O., Miller, R. E., and Zintel, H. A.: Juvenile polyps of the colon, Surgery 69:288, 1971.
62. Cremin, B. J., and Louw, J. H.: Polyps in the large bowel in children, Clin. Radiol. 21:195, 1970.
63. Pemberton, M.: Carcinoma of the large intestine with survival in a child of nine and in his father. A study of carcinoma of the colon with particular reference to children, Br. J. Surg. 57:841, 1970.
64. Smedresman, P., and Finegold, M. J.: Fulminant right lower quandrant mass in a child, J. Pediatr. 90:312, 1977.
65. Dunnick, N. R., Reaman, G. H., Head, G. L., et al.: Radiographic manifestations of Burkitt's lymphoma in American patients, Am. J. Roentgenol. 132:1, 1979.
66. Bartram, C., and Chrispin, A. R.: Primary lymphosarcoma of the ileum and caecum, Pediatr. Radiol. 1:28, 1973.
67. Wilkinson, R. H., Bartlett, R. H., and Eraklis, A. J.: Diagnosis of appendicitis in infancy. The value of abdominal radiographs, Am. J. Dis. Child. 118: 687, 1969.
68. Lim, M. S.: Gas-filled appendix: Lack of diagnostic specificity, Am. J. Roentgenol. 128:209, 1977.
69. Jona, J. Z., Belin, R. P., and Selke, A. C.: Barium enema as a diagnostic aid in children with abdominal pain, Surg. Gynecol. Obstet. 144:351, 1977.
70. Schey, W. L.: Use of barium in the diagnosis of appendicitis in children, Am. J. Roentgenol. 118: 95, 1973.
71. Shimkin, P. M.: Radiology of acute appendicitis, Am. J. Roentgenol. 130:1001, 1978.
72. Sherman, N. J., and Woolley, M. M.: The ileocecal syndrome in acute childhood leukemia, Arch. Surg. 107:39, 1973.
73. Wagner, M. L., Rosenberg, H. S., Fernbach, D. J., et al.: Typhlitis: A complication of leukemia in childhood, Am. J. Roentgenol. 109:341, 1970.
74. Sherman, N. J., Williams, K., and Woolley, M. W.: Surgical complications in the patient with leukemia, J. Pediatr. Surg. 8:235, 1973.
75. Lehmiller, D. J., and Kanto, W. P., Jr.: Relationship of mesenteric thromboembolism, oral feeding, and necrotizing enterocolitis, J. Pediatr. 92:96, 1978.
76. Santulli, T. V., Schullinger, J. N., Heird, W. C., et al.: Acute necrotizing enterocolitis in infancy. A review of 64 cases, Pediatrics 55:376, 1975.
77. Brown, E. G., and Sweet, A. Y.: Preventing necrotizing enterocolitis in neonates, J.A.M.A. 240: 2452, 1978.
78. Bell, R. S., Graham, C. B., and Stevenson, J. K.: Roentgenologic and clinical manifestations of nec-

rotizing enterocolitis, Am. J. Roentgenol. 112: 123, 1971.

79. Berdon, W. E., Grossman, H., Baker, D. H., et al.: Necrotizing enterocolitis in the premature infant, Radiology 83:879, 1964.
80. Holt, S. A., and Friedland, G. W.: Neonatal necrotizing enterocolitis. Clinical and radiological features, West. J. Med. 120:110, 1974.
81. Kogutt, M. S.: Necrotizing enterocolitis of infancy. Early roentgen pattern as a guide to prompt diagnosis, Radiology 130:367, 1979.
82. Siegle, R. L., Robinowitz, J. G., Korones, S. B., et al.: Early diagnosis of necrotizing enterocolitis, Am. J. Roentgenol. 127:629, 1976.
83. Lloyd, D. A., and Cywes, S.: Intestinal stenosis and enterocyst formation as late complications of neonatal necrotizing enterocolitis, J. Pediatr. Surg. 8:479, 1973.
84. Tonkin, I. L. D., Bjelland, J. C., Hunter, T. B., et al.: Spontaneous resolution of colonic strictures caused by necrotizing enterocolitis: Therapeutic implications, Am. J. Roentgenol. 130:1077, 1978.
85. Berger, L. A., and Wilkinson, D.: The investigation of colitis in infancy, Pediatr. Radiol. 2:145, 1974.
86. Zetzel, L.: Granulomatous (ileo) colitis, N. Engl. J. Med. 282:600, 1970.
87. Friedland, G. W., Gray, G. M., Oberhelman, H. A., Jr., et al.: Inflammatory bowel disease—a symposium. Calif. Med. 119:14, 1973.
88. Glotzer, D. J., Gardner, R. C., Goldman, H., et al.: Comparative features and course of ulcerative and granulomatous colitis, N. Engl. J. Med. 282: 582, 1970.
89. Margulis, A. R., Goldberg, H. I., Lawson, T. L., et al.: The overlapping spectrum of ulcerative and granulomatous colitis: A roentgenographic-pathologic study, Am. J. Roentgenol. 113:316, 1971.
90. Gelzayd, E. A., Breuer, R. I., and Kirsner, J. B.: Nephrolithiasis in inflammatory bowel disease, Am. J. Dig. Dis. 13:1027, 1968.
91. Kelvin, F. M., Oddson, T. A., Rice, R. P., et al.: Double contrast barium enema in Crohn's disease and ulcerative colitis, Am. J. Roentgenol. 131: 207, 1978.
92. Laufer, I., and Costopoulos, L.: Early lesions of Crohn's disease, Am. J. Roentgenol. 130:307, 1978.
93. Stanley, P., Fry, I. K., Dawson, A. M., et al.: Radiological signs of ulcerative colitis and Crohn's disease of the colon, Clin. Radiol. 22:434, 1971.
94. Cardoso, J. M., Kimura, K., Stoopen, M., et al.: Radiology of invasive amebiasis of the colon, Am. J. Roentgenol. 128:935, 1977.
95. Hill, M. C., and Goldberg, H. I.: Roentgen diagnosis of intestinal amebiasis, Am. J. Roentgenol. 99: 77, 1967.
96. Lieberman, E.: Hemolytic-uremic syndrome, J. Pediatr. 80:1, 1972.
97. Bar-Ziv, J., Ayoub, J. I. G., and Fletcher, B. D.: Hemolytic uremic syndrome: A case presenting with acute colitis, Pediatr. Radiol. 2:203, 1974.
98. Beuman, W., Jr.: The hemolytic-uremic syndrome: Initial clinical presentation mimicking ulcerative colitis, J. Pediatr. 81:275, 1972.
99. Check, W.: Colitis following antibiotic therapy due to Clostridium difficile, J.A.M.A. 239:2101, 1978.
100. Bartlett, J. G., Chang, T. W., Gurwith, M., et al.: Antibiotic-associated pseudomembranous colitis due to toxin-producing clostridia, N. Engl. J. Med. 298:531, 1978.
101. Tedesco, F. J., Stanley, R. J., and Alpers, D. H.: Diagnostic features of clindamycin-associated pseudomembranous colitis, N. Engl. J. Med. 290: 841, 1974.

GENERAL REFERENCES

Caffey, J.: *Pediatric X-Ray Diagnosis* (7th ed.; Chicago: Year Book Medical Publishers, Inc., 1978).

Cremen, B. J., Cywes, S., and Louw, J. H.: *Radiological Diagnosis of Digestive Tract Disorders in the Newborn* (London: Butterworth & Co. 1973).

Franken, E. A., Jr.: *Gastrointestinal Radiology in Pediatrics* (Hagerstown: Harper & Row, 1975).

Schapiro, R. L.: *Clinical Radiology of the Pediatric Abdomen and Gastrointestinal Tract* (Baltimore: University Park Press, 1976).

Singleton, E. B., Wagner, M. L., and Dutton, R. V.: *Radiology of the Alimentary Tract in Infants and Children* (2d ed.; Philadelphia: W. B. Saunders Co., 1977).

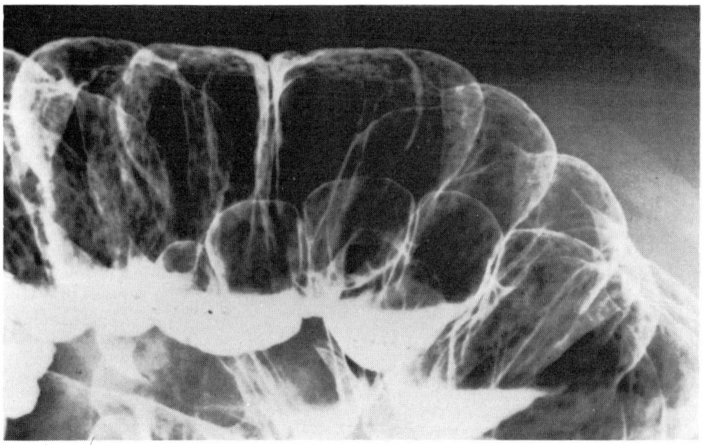

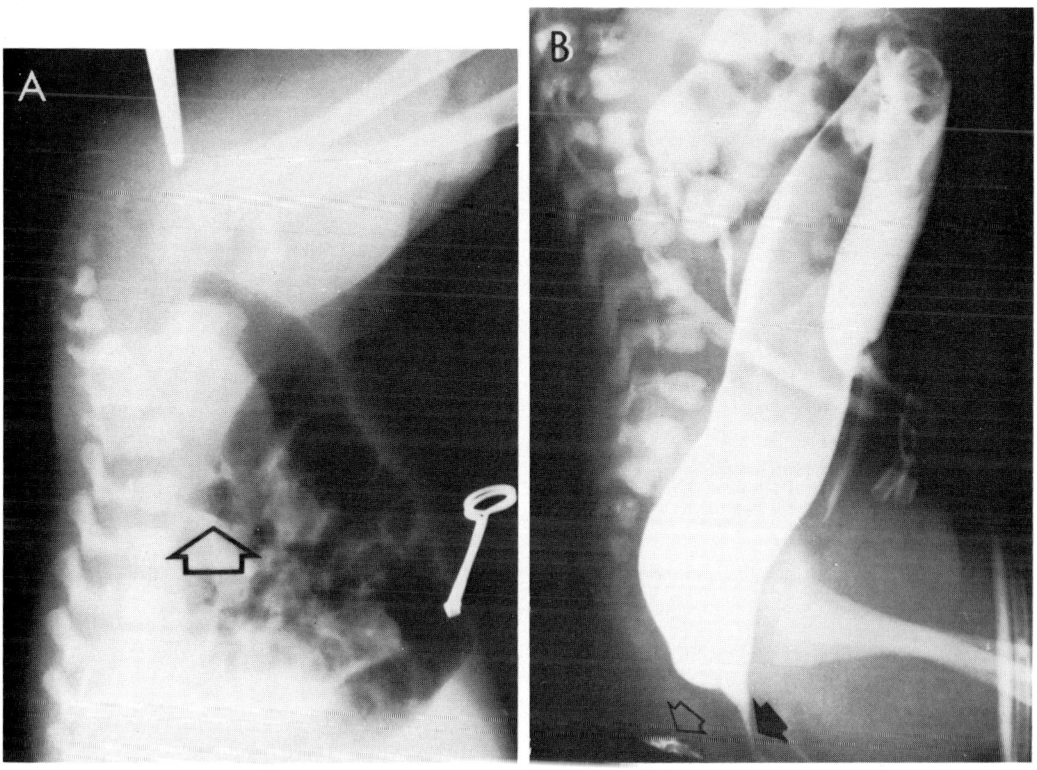

Fig 30–1 (top).—Hyperplastic lymphoid follicles demonstrated in wall of colon on air contrast study as numerous small round filling defects, which may have tiny umbilications that may retain barium.

Fig 30–2 (bottom).—**A,** Wangensteen-Rice inverted lateral view of pelvis shows distalmost air-filled loop of bowel *(arrow)* to lie above pubococcygeal line. **B,** following colostomy, water-soluble contrast study of distal colostomy shows ectopic anus with perineal fistula *(closed arrow)*. *Open arrow* points to area of anal dimple. On initial film, air never got down to distal rectum, which was filled with meconium.

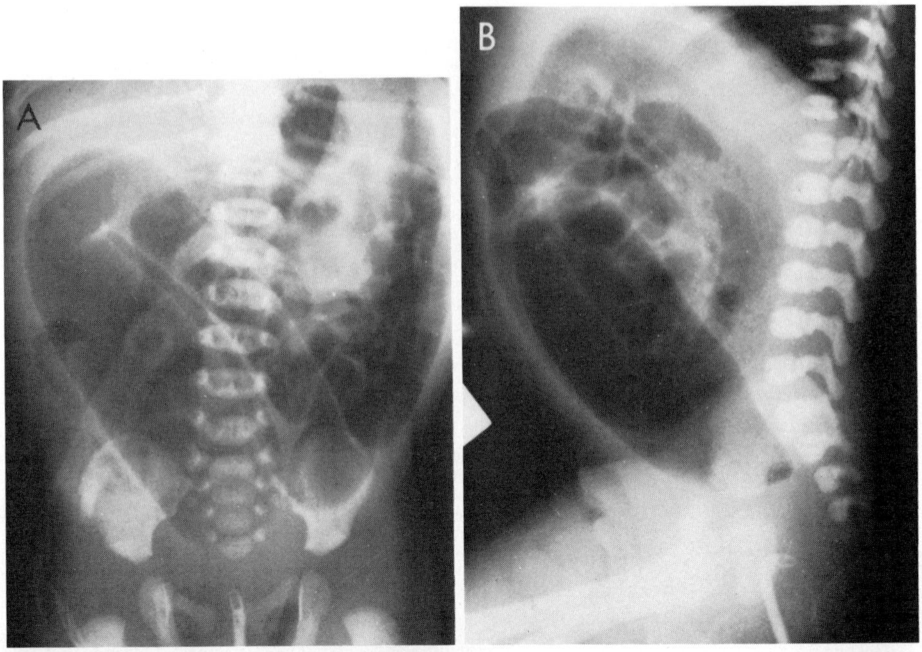

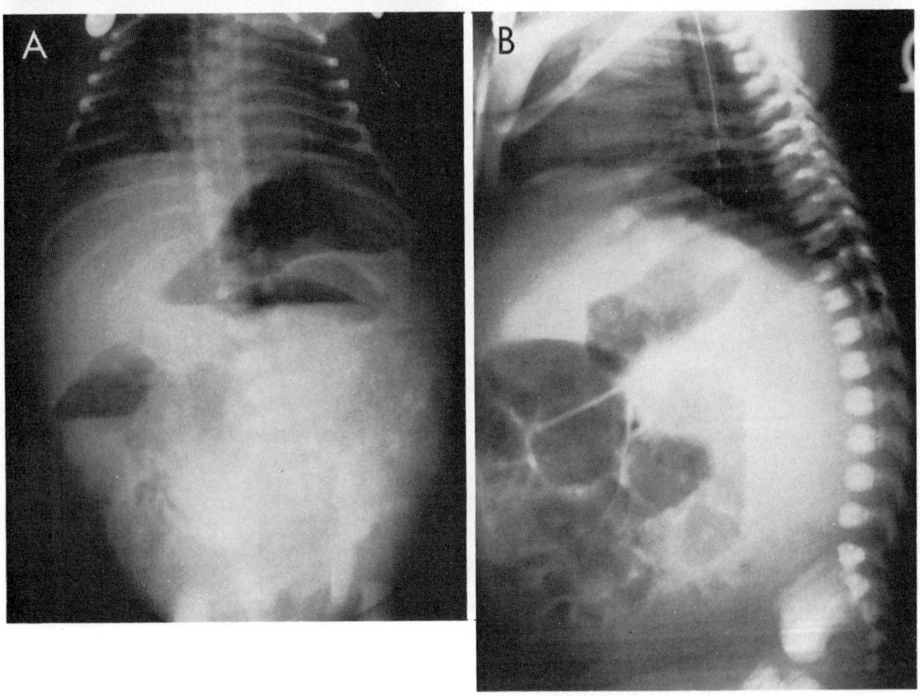

Fig 30–3 (top).– **A** and **B,** type IV rectal atresia in girl, age 3 days. Air in distal dilated rectum is separated from rectal tube by thick area of atresia.

Fig 30–4 (bottom).–Frontal **(A)** and lateral **(B)** abdominal films in newborn girl with markedly distended abdomen. Numerous calcified meconium liths present throughout colon. Imperforate anus and cloacal orifice were noted on physical inspection.

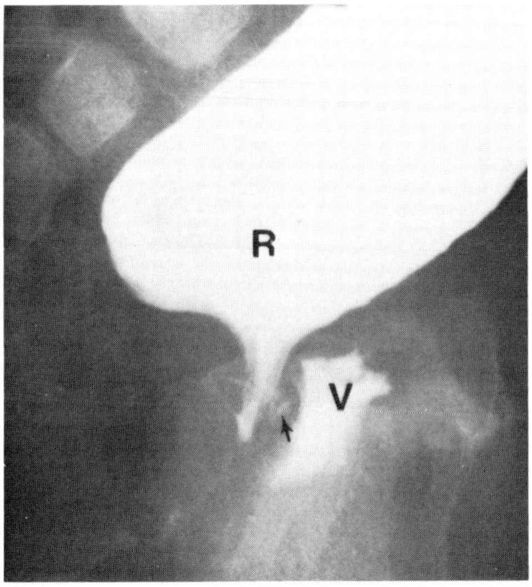

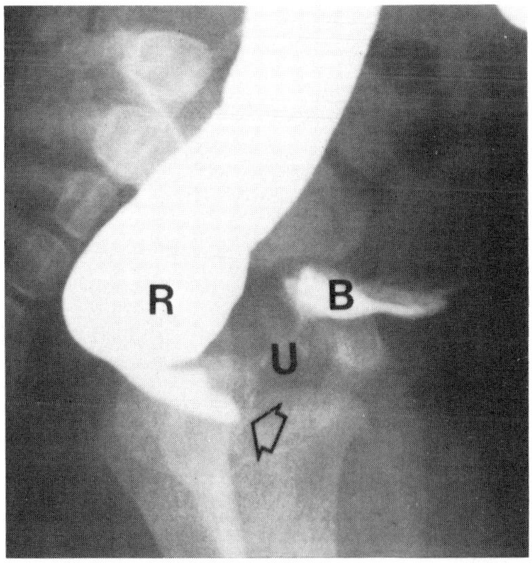

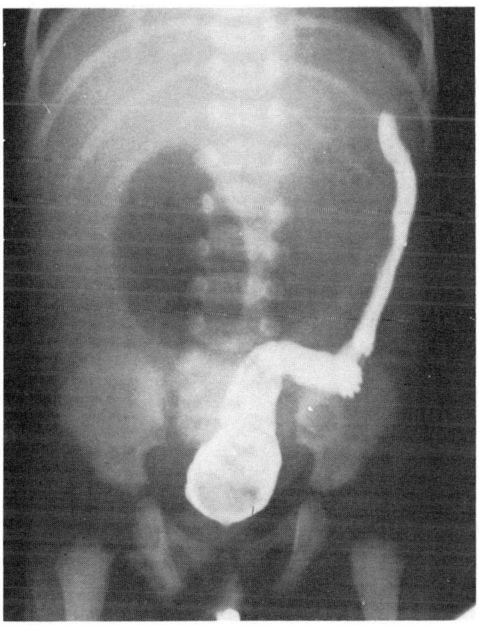

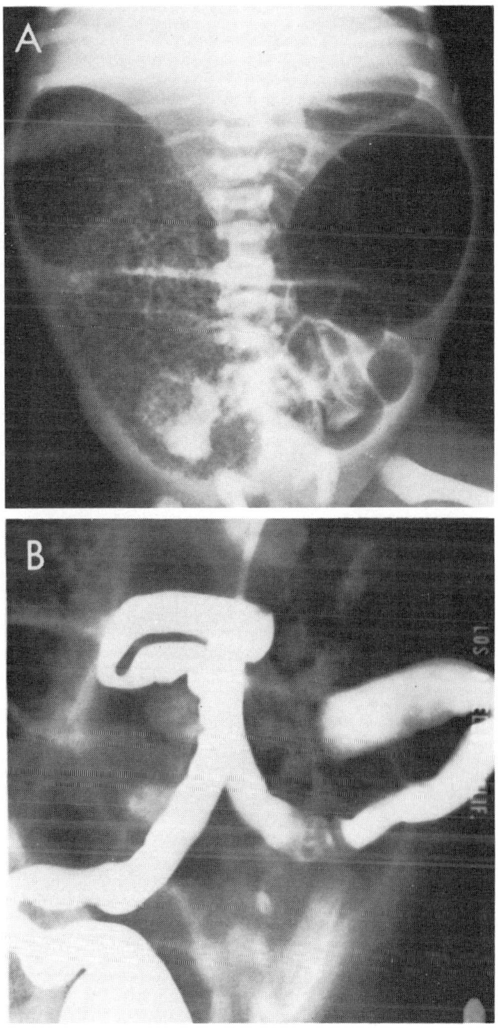

Fig 30–5 (top left). – Distal colostomy contrast study in girl, age 6 months, demonstrates perineal fistula and fistula to vagina *(v) (arrow)*. *R* = rectum.

Fig 30–6 (top right). – Boy, age 3 months, with rectourethral fistula *(arrow)* and reflux filling of bladder *(B)*. *R* = rectum; *U* = urethra

Fig 30–7 (bottom left). – Double bubble sign indicates presence of duodenal atresia in newborn infant who also had distal rectal atresia. Water-soluble contrast medium was injected percutaneously into distal rectal pouch.

Fig 30–8 (bottom right) – Membranous atresia of proximal descending colon. **A,** plain abdominal film shows marked dilatation of colon proximal to obstruction. **B,** barium enema shows slight clubbed appearance of proximal end of distal colon.

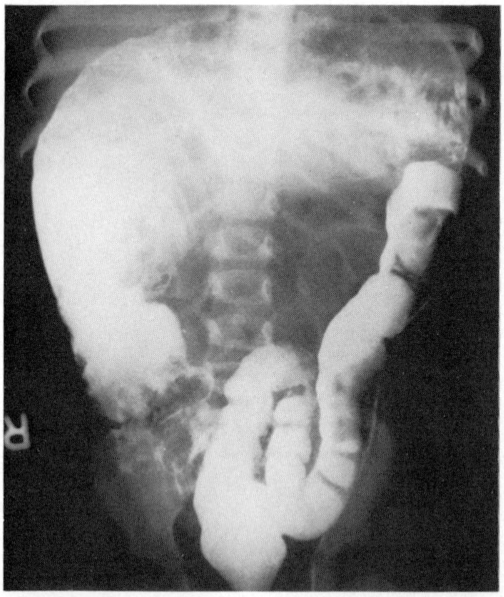

Fig 30–9 (top left).—Congenital stenosis of proximal descending colon due to congenital band found in child at surgery.

Fig 30–10 (center).—Boy age 1 year with bilious vomiting. **A,** malrotation demonstrated by high and medial position of cecum on barium enema. **B,** upper gastrointestinal series shows obstruction and distention of duodenum secondary to Ladd's band.

Fig 30–11 (bottom).—**(A),** on barium enema, rapid reflux of barium into ileum obscured position of cecum and ileocecal valve. **(B),** upper gastrointestinal series shows dilatation of duodenum and point of partial obstruction in descending duodenal loop with slight twist *(arrow)* of malpositioned duodenum, indicating presence of volvulus.

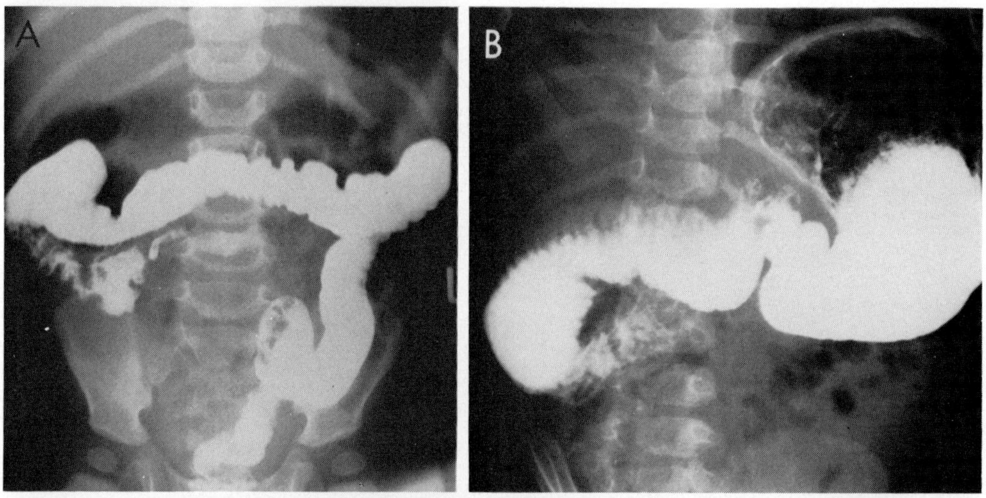

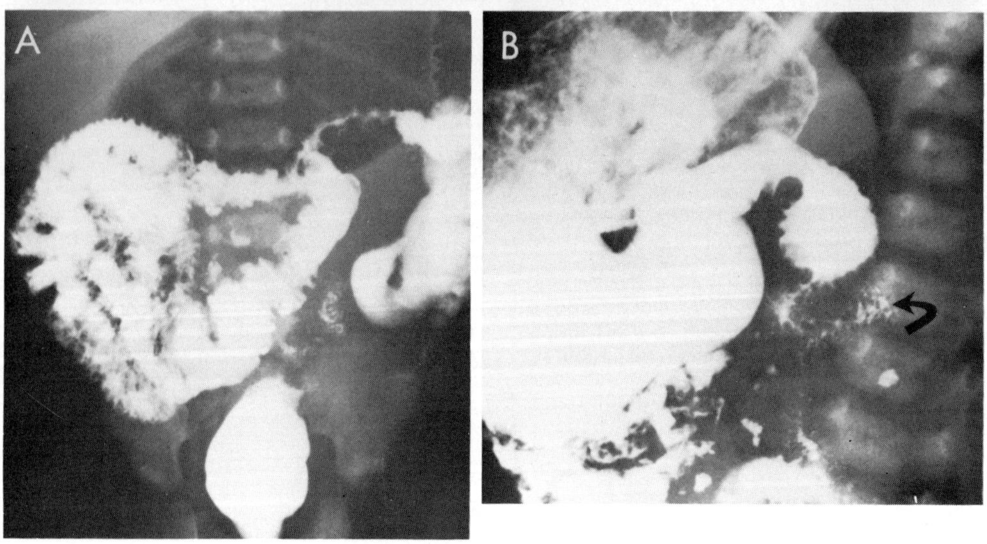

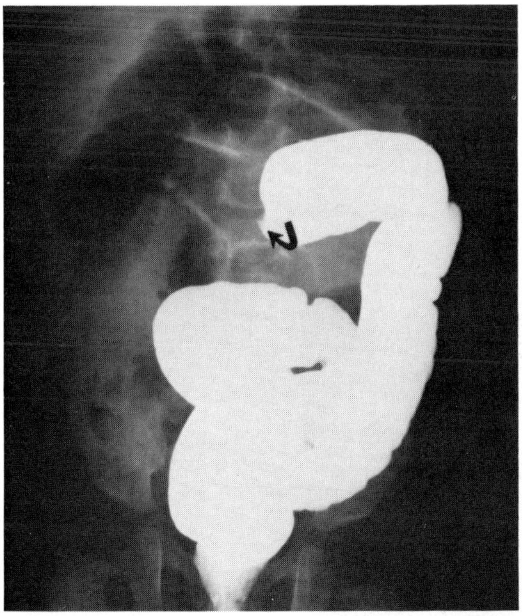

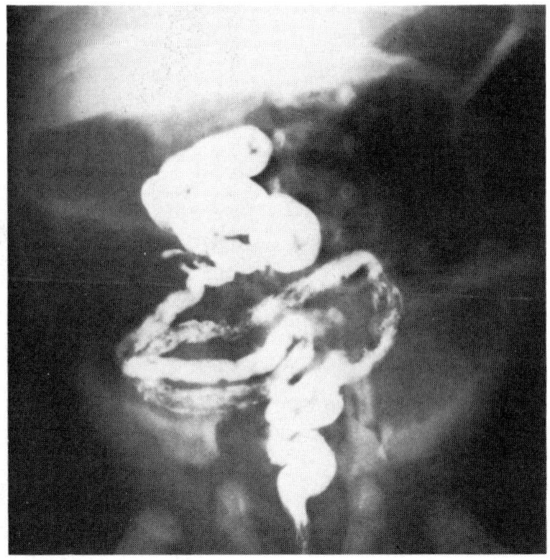

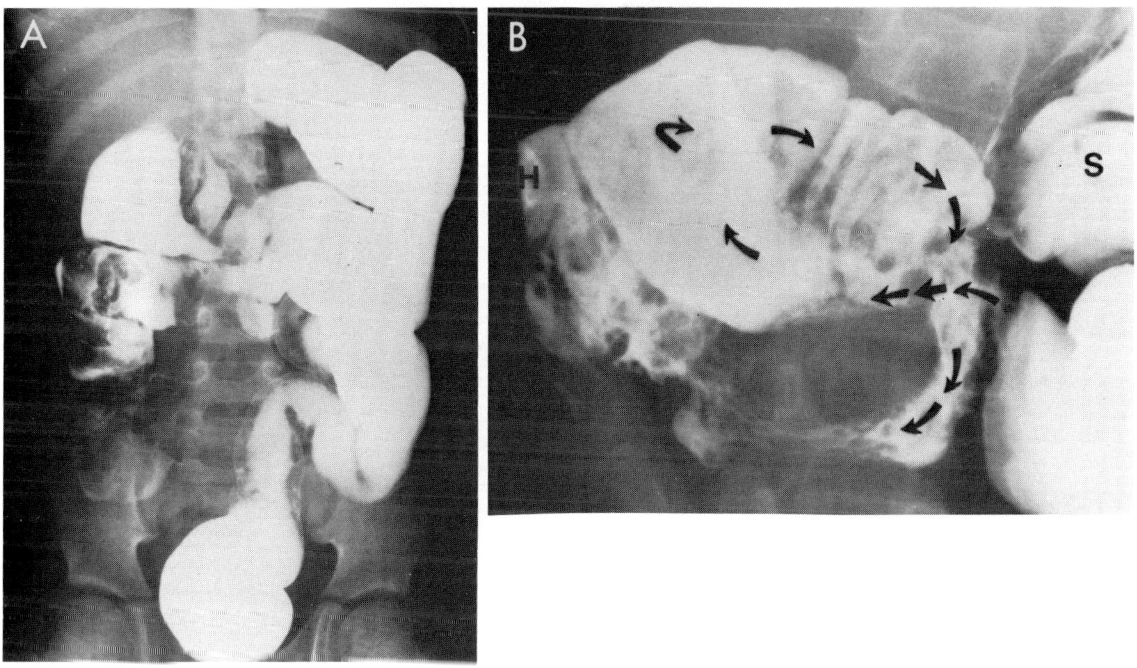

Fig 30–12 (top left).—Boy age 5 months with abdominal distention and hematochezia. Retrograde barium flow completely obstructed in mid-transverse colon, where mild beak deformity (*arrow*) is noted. This represents distal obstruction of complete midgut volvulus.

Fig 30–13 (top right).—Severe malrotation of colon and markedly dilated proximal small bowel loops in newborn girl with apple peel mesentery defect and jejunal atresia.

Fig 30–14 (bottom).—**A,** unusual partial volvulus of transverse colon in boy age 5 is demonstrated on barium enema. Cecum was normal in position but duodenum was malrotated. **B,** localized view shows dilatation of partly obstructed, volvulized transverse colon (*arrows*). S = splenic flexure; H = hepatic flexure.

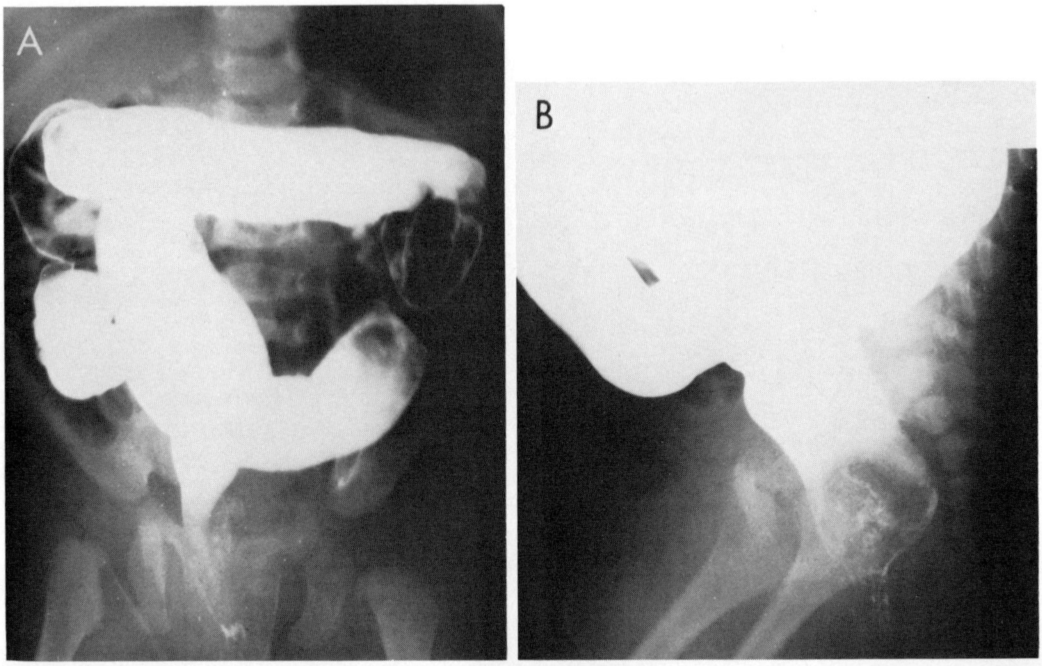

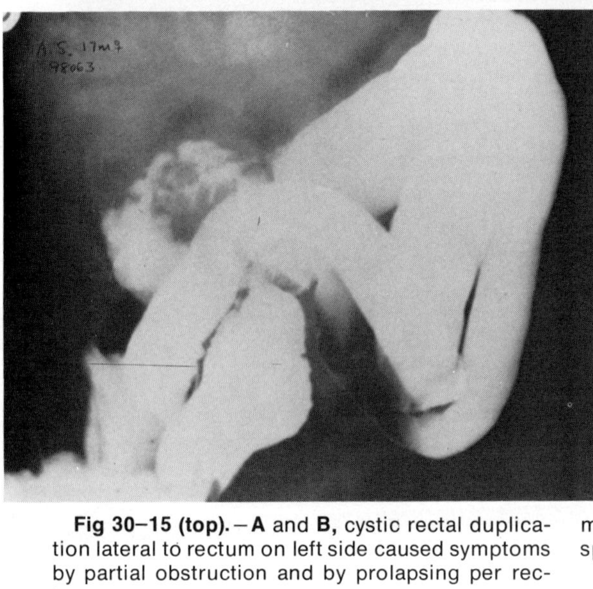

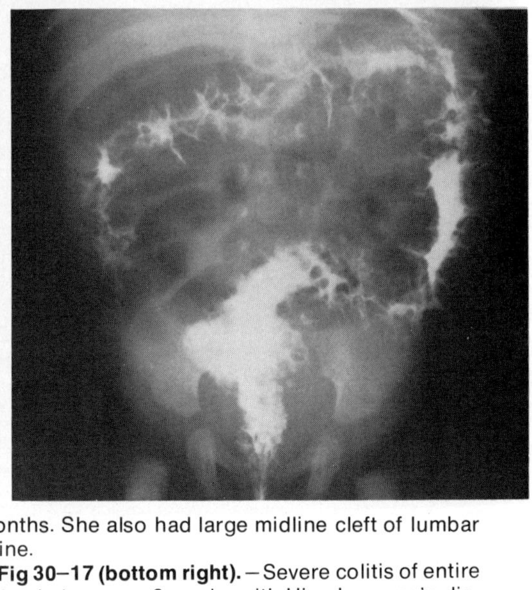

Fig 30–15 (top).—**A** and **B,** cystic rectal duplication lateral to rectum on left side caused symptoms by partial obstruction and by prolapsing per rectum.

Fig 30–16 (bottom left).—Complete duplication of colon from rectum to cecum in girl, age 17 months. She also had large midline cleft of lumbar spine.

Fig 30–17 (bottom right).—Severe colitis of entire colon in boy, age 3 weeks with Hirschsprung's disease.

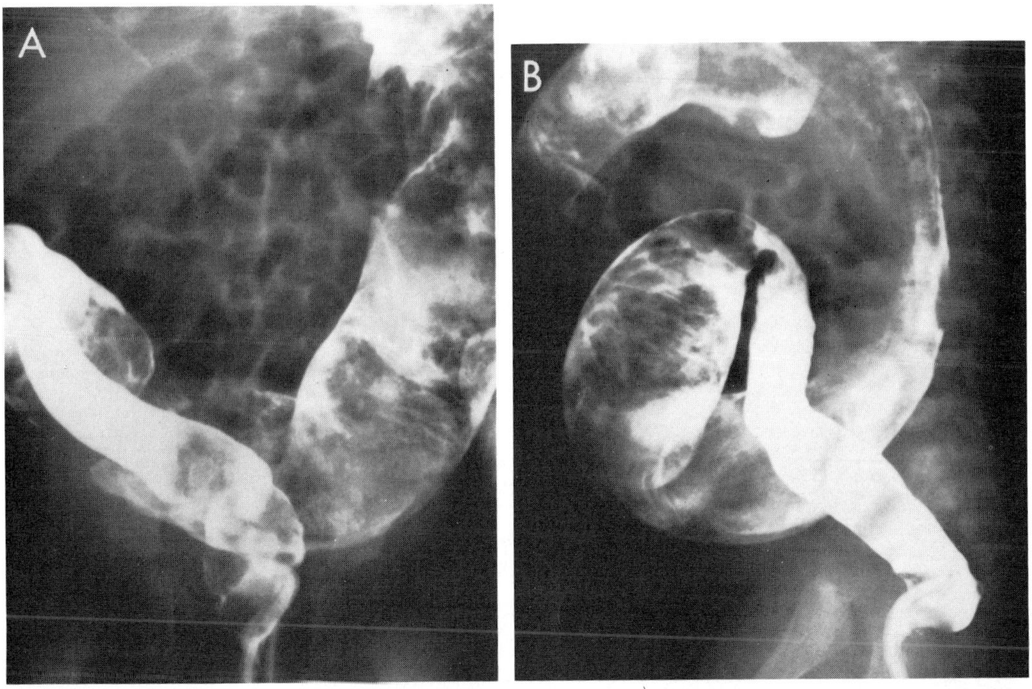

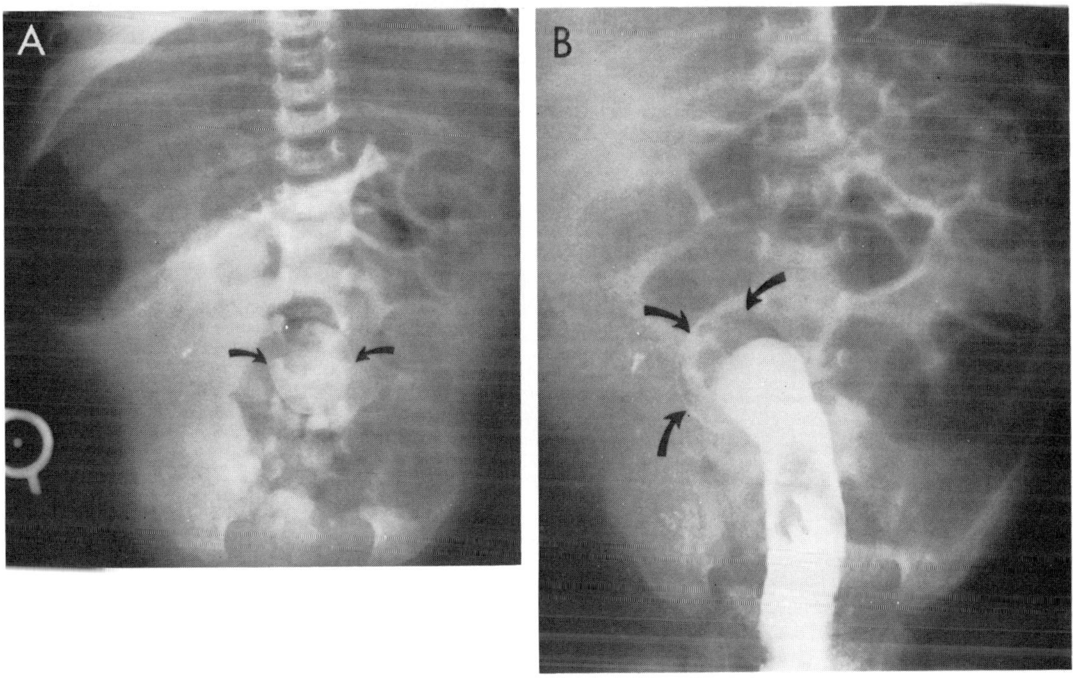

Fig 30–10 (top). Clearly defined transition zone on both AP **(A)** and lateral **(B)** views in girl, age 5 weeks, with typical short segment Hirschsprung's disease.

Fig 30–19 (bottom).—Girl, age 7 weeks, with Hirschsprung's disease. **A,** plain film shows marked gaseous distention of transverse colon and impacted fecaloma *(arrows)* in sigmoid region. **B,** fecaloma *(arrows)* obstructs retrograde flow of barium on enema study.

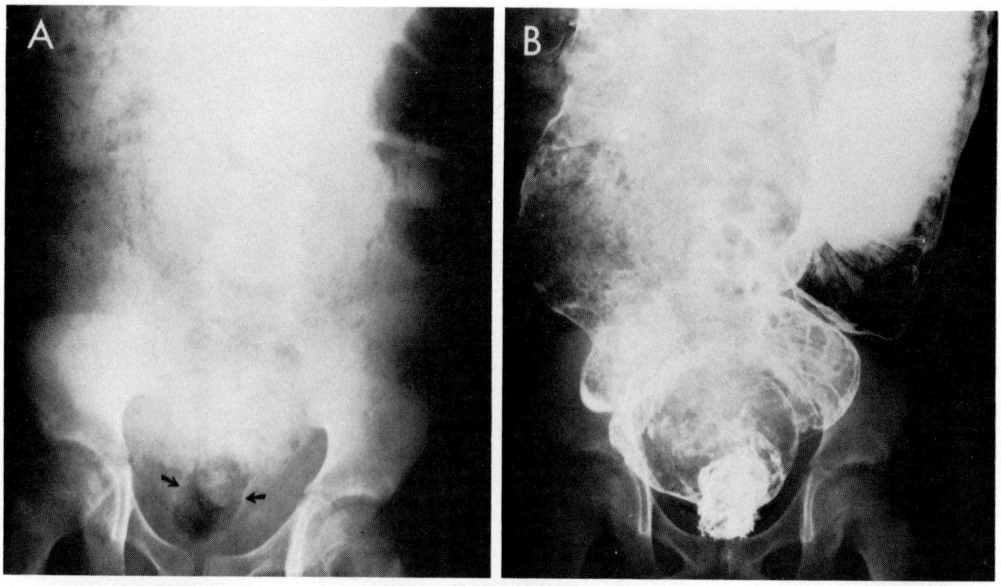

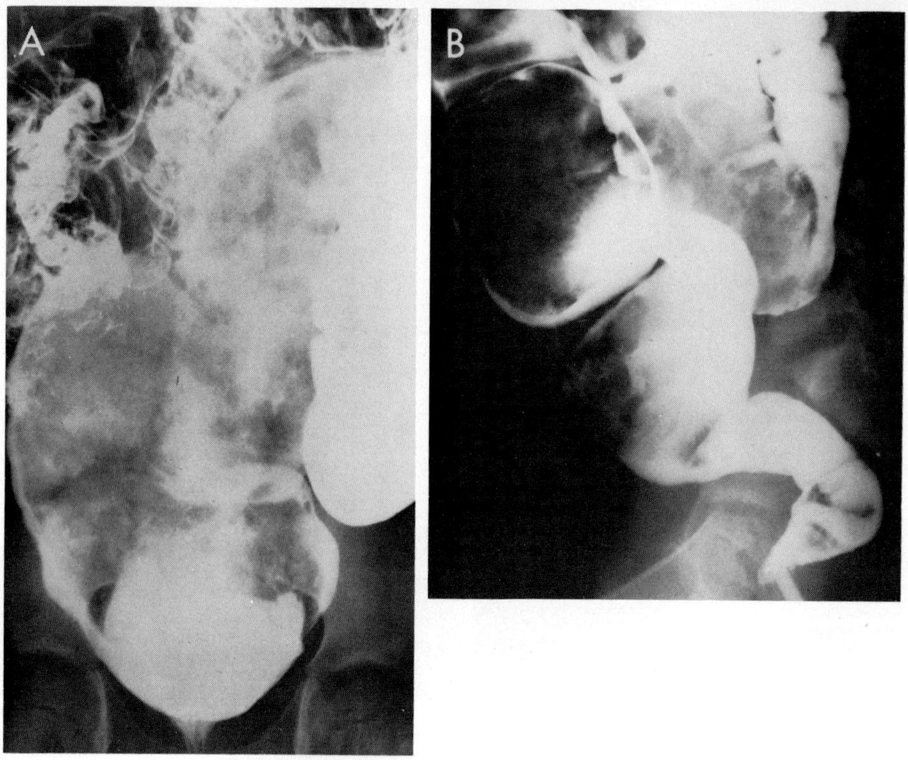

Fig 30–20 (top).—Girl, age 9, with short segment Hirschsprung's disease. **A,** plain film shows huge fecal mass in sigmoid colon. (*Arrows* point to empty rectum of obviously smaller caliber.) **B,** barium enema confirms small rectal caliber and gross dilatation of sigmoid.

Fig 30–21 (bottom).—Girl, age 5, with Hirschsprung's disease. **A,** on AP view, dilated sigmoid projects over and obscures transition zone. **B,** on lateral view difference in size of rectum and sigmoid is clearly demonstrated.

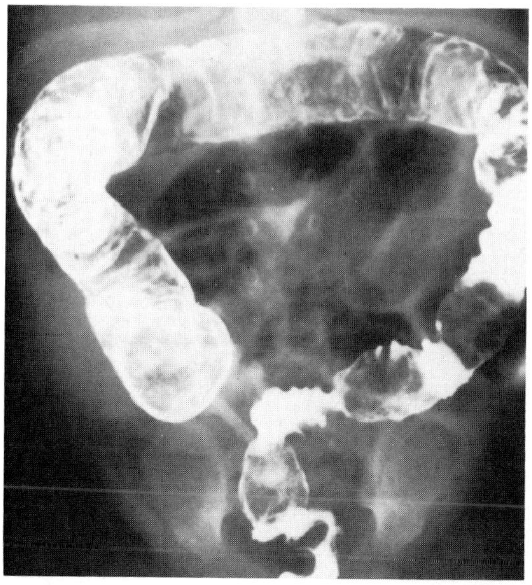

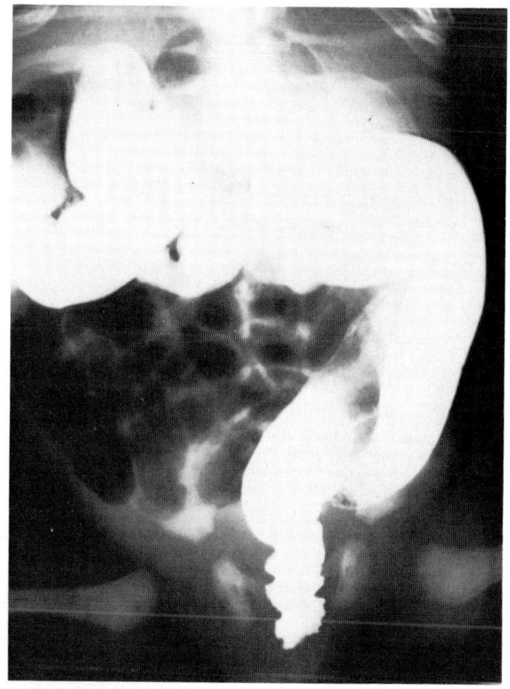

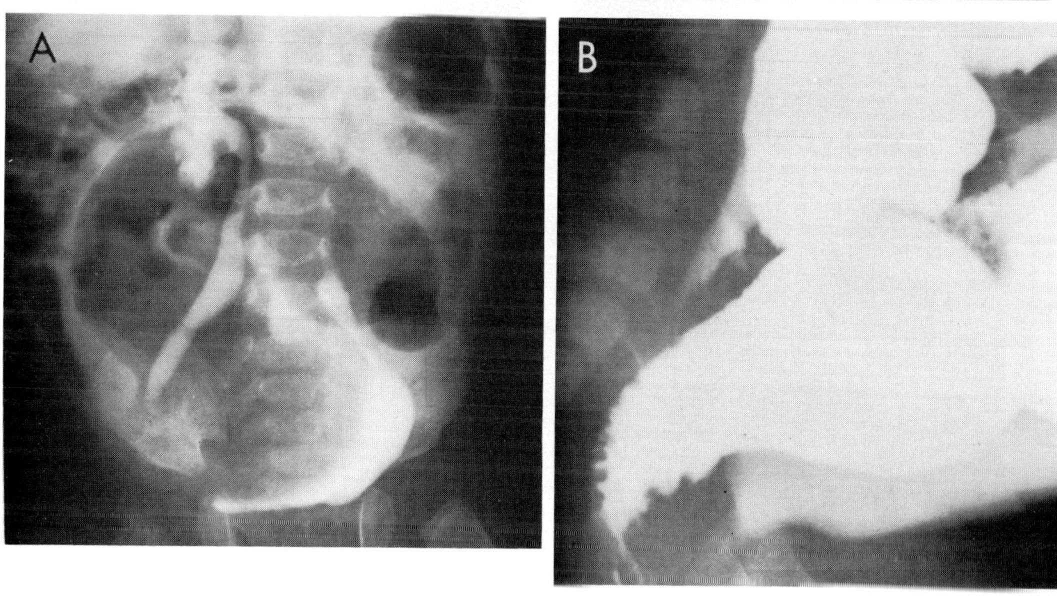

Fig 30–22 (top left). – Girl, age 1 month, with total colon aganglionosis. The 24-hour delayed film shows retention of barium throughout colon, which appears shortened, with rounded flexures. Spasm of relatively empty sigmoid and rectum also present.

Fig 30–23 (top right). – Sawtoothed configuration of slightly narrowed rectum and malrotation of proximal colon is demonstrated in newborn male. Patient also had asplenia (Ivemark) syndrome. Note horizontal liver in upper abdomen.

Fig 30–24 (bottom). – **A,** partial ureteral obstruction and bladder deformity may result secondarily from pressure by dilated fecal-filled rectum and sigmoid colon. **B,** spasm of rectum and dilatation of sigmoid with pressure effect on bladder are demonstrated in lateral view of barium enema in boy, age 3 months, with aganglionosis.

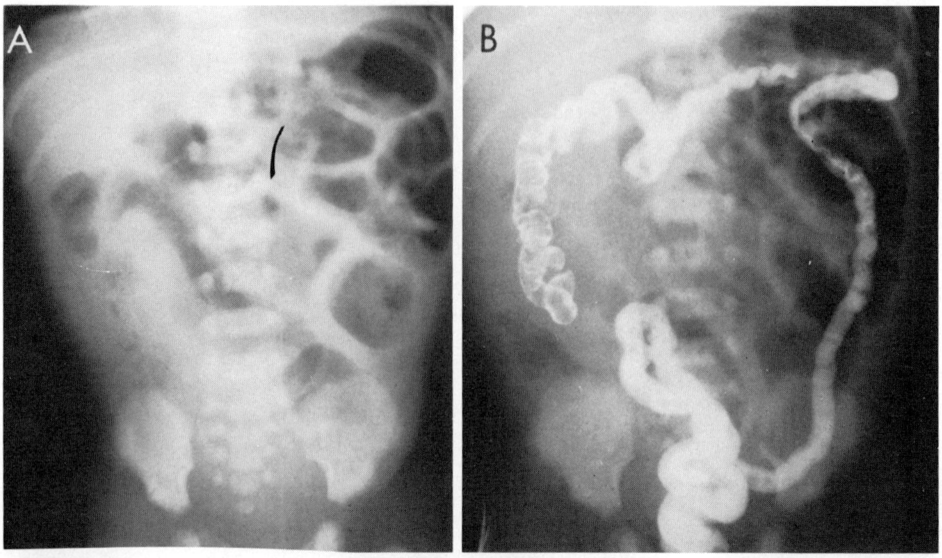

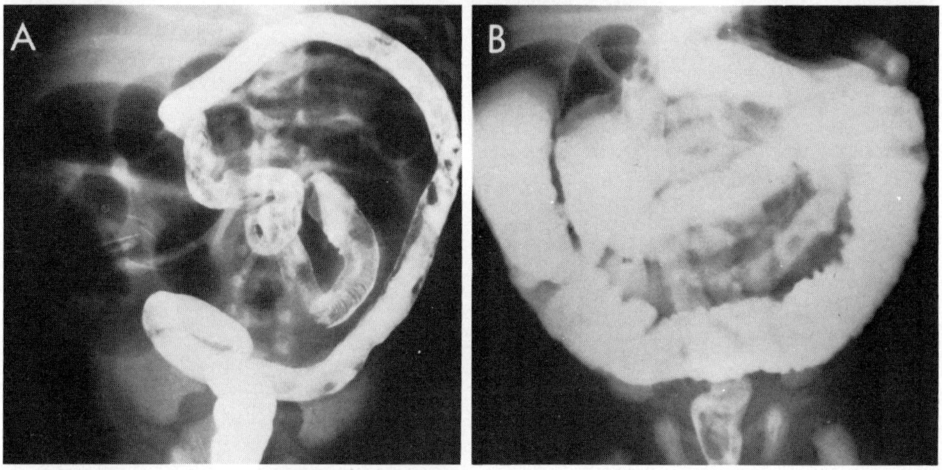

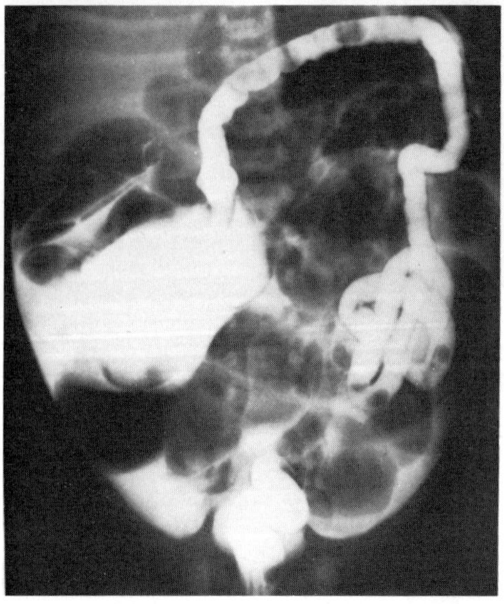

Fig 30–25 (top).—**A,** plain film of newborn girl with uncomplicated meconium ileus shows mild gaseous distention of small bowel loops and large bubbly mass in right lateral and lower abdomen. **B,** barium enema reveals microcolon with multiple impacted meconium pellets in proximal colon.

Fig 30–26 (center).—Repeated attempts may be needed to maneuver Gastrografin around meconium masses. **A,** initial enema shows malrotated meconium-filled proximal colon loops and obstruction to further retrograde flow of contrast medium. **B,** repeat study the following day shows good reflux filling of distal dilated small bowel loops.

Fig 30–27 (bottom).—Therapeutic Gastrografin enemas carry risk of causing fluid and electrolyte imbalance and bowel perforation, which has occurred in this boy, age 2 days, during second enema. The procedure must be performed with approval of surgeon available to intervene.

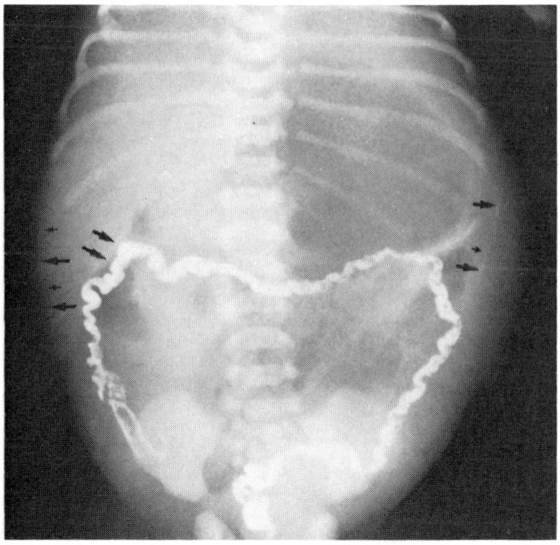

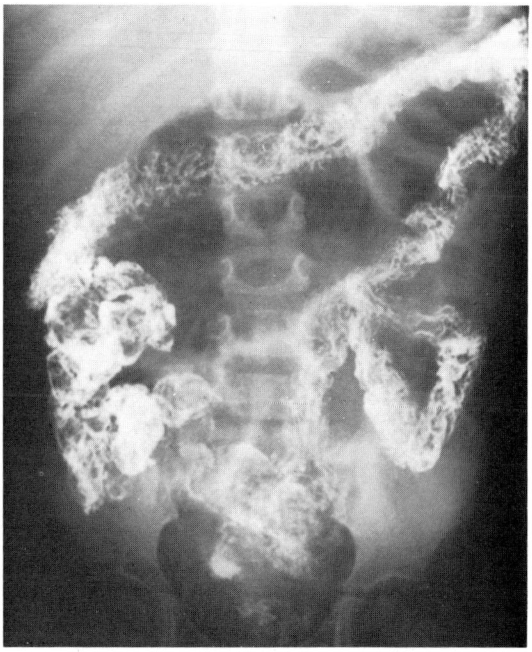

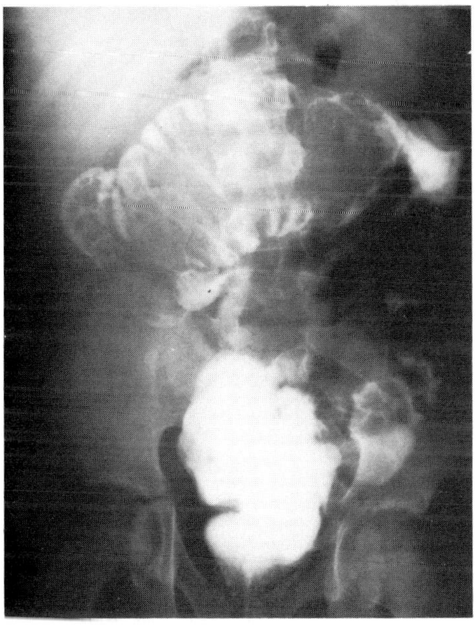

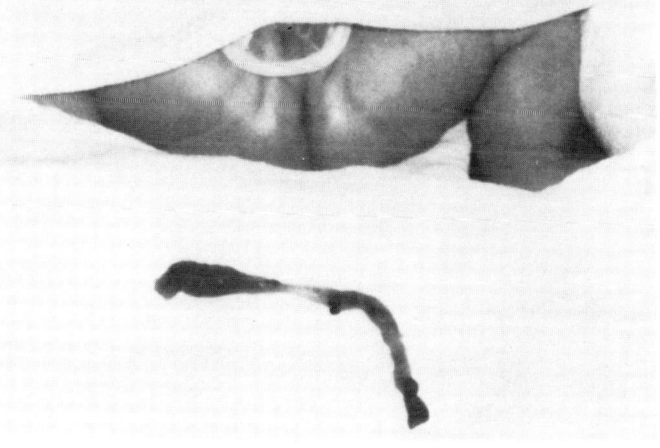

Fig 30–28 (top left).—Newborn male with meconium ileus and meconium peritonitis. Enema study shows abdominal distention and microcolon, with retained meconium in narrow distal ileum. Thin streaks of intraperitoneal calcifications *(arrows)* are noted peripherally and on undersurface of liver.

Fig 30–29 (top right).—Typical cobblestone mucosal pattern of colon in cystic fibrosis is caused by thickened mucosal mucous glands and is well demonstrated on postevacuation film in girl, age 2 years.

Fig 30–30 (bottom left).—Meconium ileus equivalent in boy, age 13 years, with cystic fibrosis. Gastrografin enema shows huge fecal impaction in distal transverse colon.

Fig 30–31 (bottom right).—Functional obstruction in meconium plug syndrome is usually promptly relieved following passage of long meconium mass.

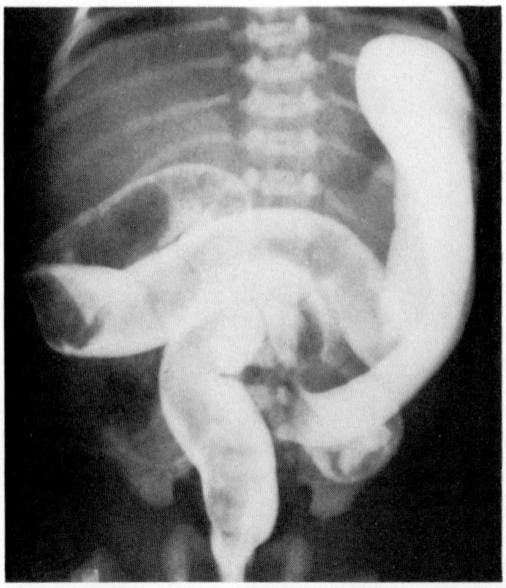

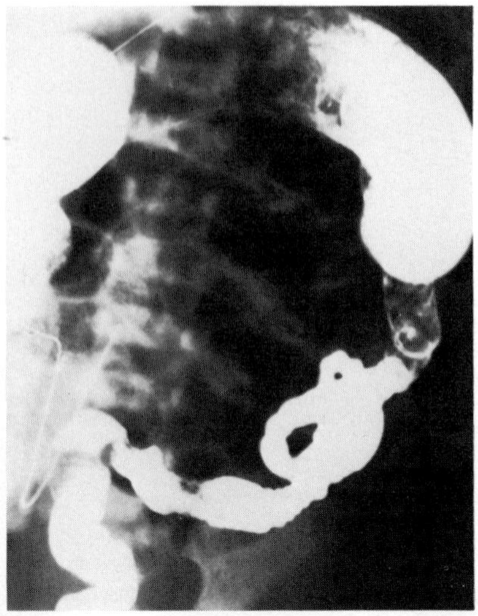

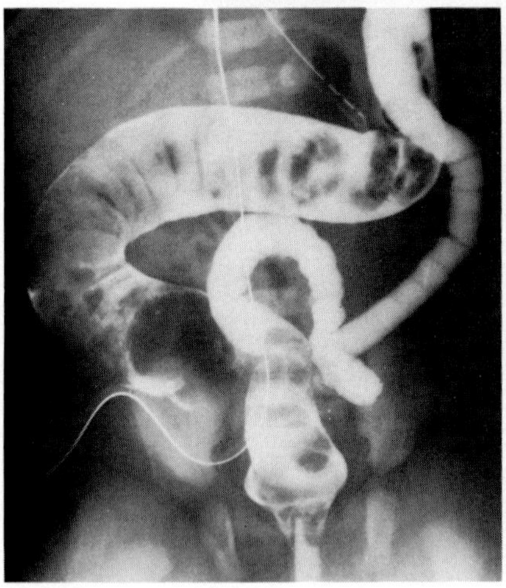

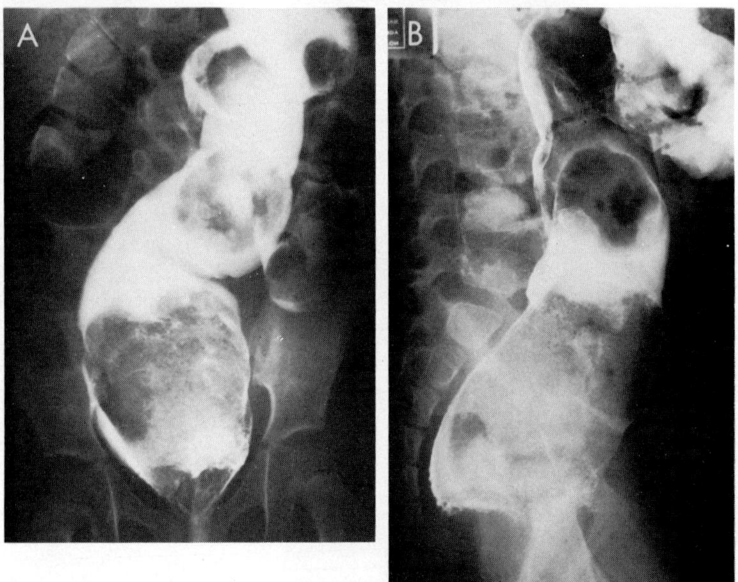

Fig 30–32 (top left).—Boy, age 2 days, with meconium plug syndrome shows large meconium masses causing moderate dilatation of colon.

Fig 30–33 (top right).—Small left colon syndrome is characterized by abruptly diminished caliber of distal colon from splenic flexure to rectum.

Fig 30–34 (bottom left).—Girl, age 2 days, with meconium plug syndrome demonstrates overlapping features of small left colon but with dilated rectum. Meconium plug syndrome and small left colon syndrome are probably similar with different radiographic manifestations.

Fig 30–35 (bottom right).—**A** and **B,** girl, age 4 years, with psychogenic megacolon. Rectal ampulla is impacted and dilated with large fecal mass down to anal verge. No distal transition is seen.

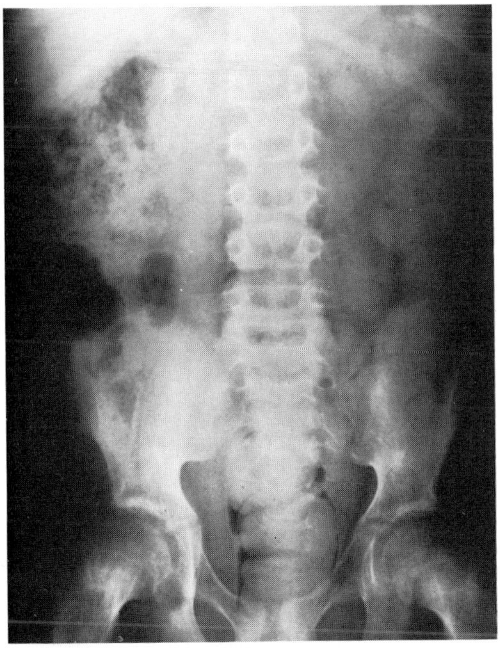

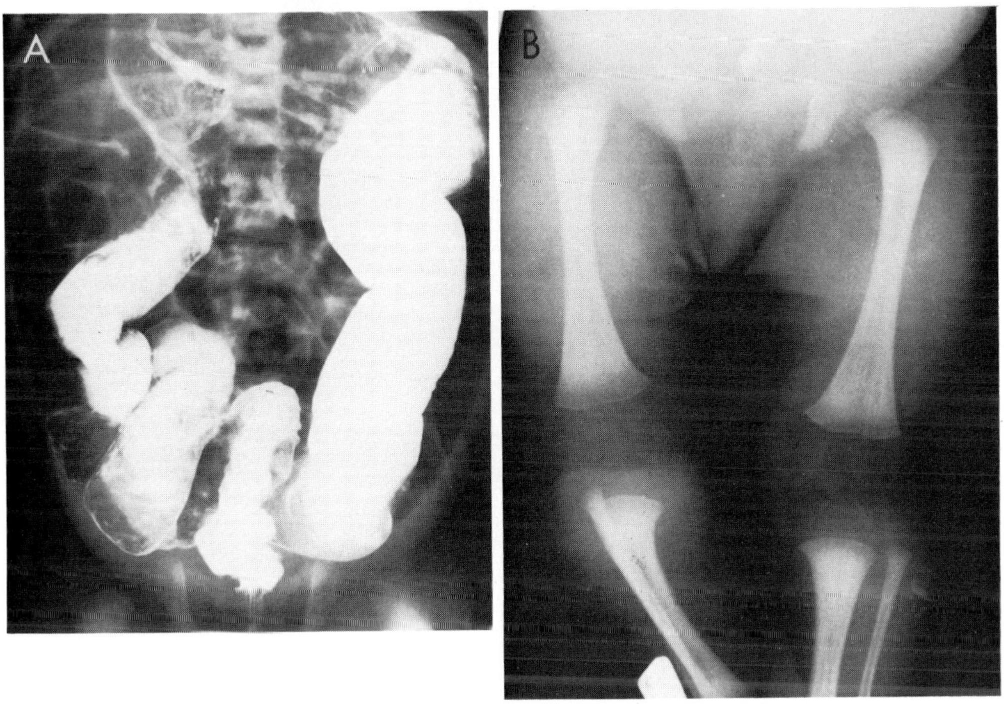

Fig 30–36 (top).—Many medications produce bowel inertia. Boy, age 11 years, with acute lymphocytic leukemia was being treated with vincristine, which can cause significant functional constipation.

Fig 30–37 (bottom).—Girl, age 3 months, with unrecognized congenital cretinism presented with abdominal distention and constipation. **A,** barium enema shows changes in distal rectum and sigmoid that mimic Hirschsprung's disease. **B,** absent ossification centers at knees reflect severely retarded skeletal maturation.

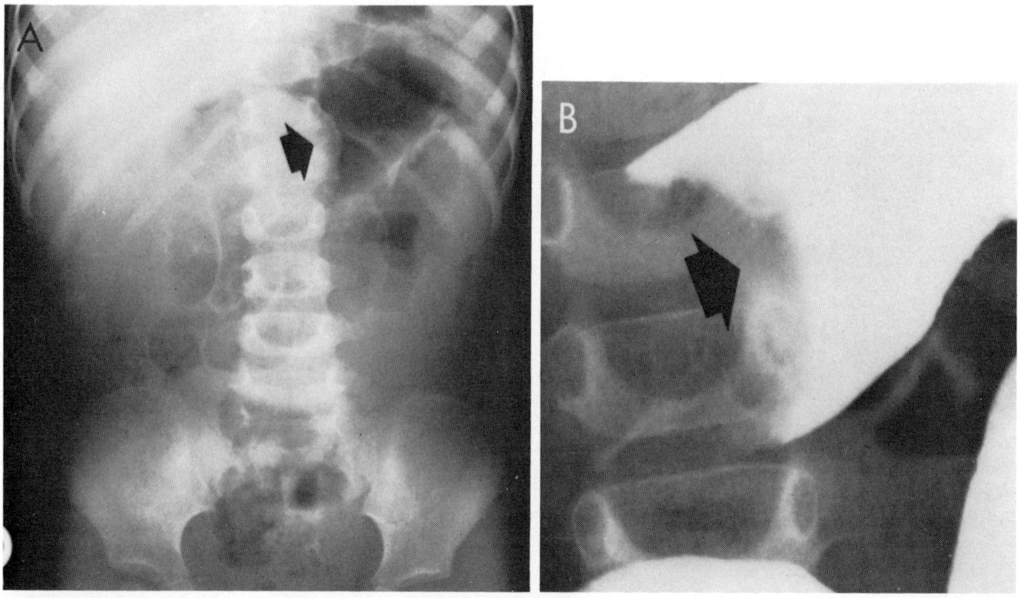

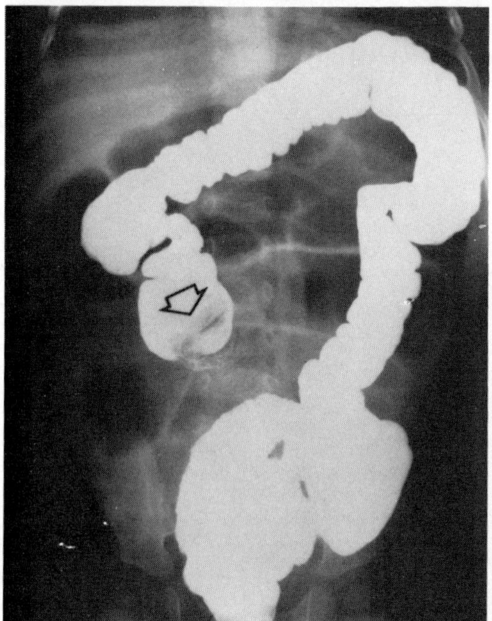

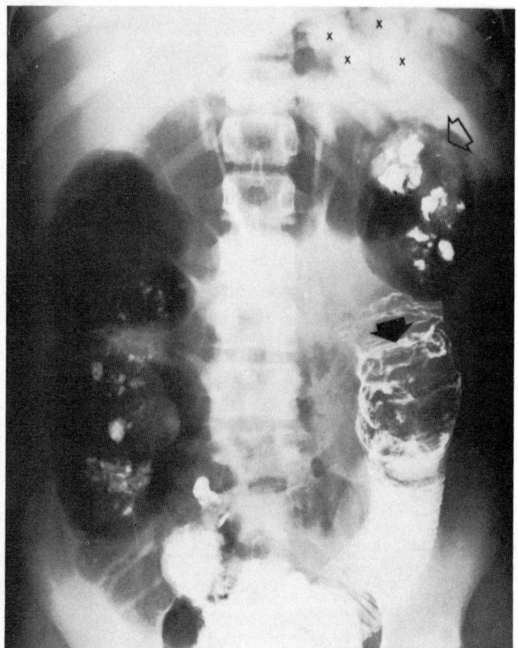

Fig 30–38 (top).—Ileocolic intussusception can be demonstrated occasionally on plain abdominal film **(A),** with intussusceptum *(arrow)* projecting into air-filled distal transverse colon. **B,** on barium enema, intussusception is diagnosed by demonstrating obstructing concave filling defect *(arrow)* in head of advancing barium column.

Fig 30–39 (bottom left).—No vigorous attempt was made to reduce this ileocolic intussusception *(arrow)* in presence of small bowel obstruction gas pattern on preliminary film.

Fig 30–40 (bottom right).—Girl, age 12 years, with Peutz-Jeghers syndrome. Plain abdominal film shows multiple gastric polyps (*X*'s) and large cluster of colonic polyps in splenic flexure *(open arrow). Closed arrow* points to colocolic intussusception.

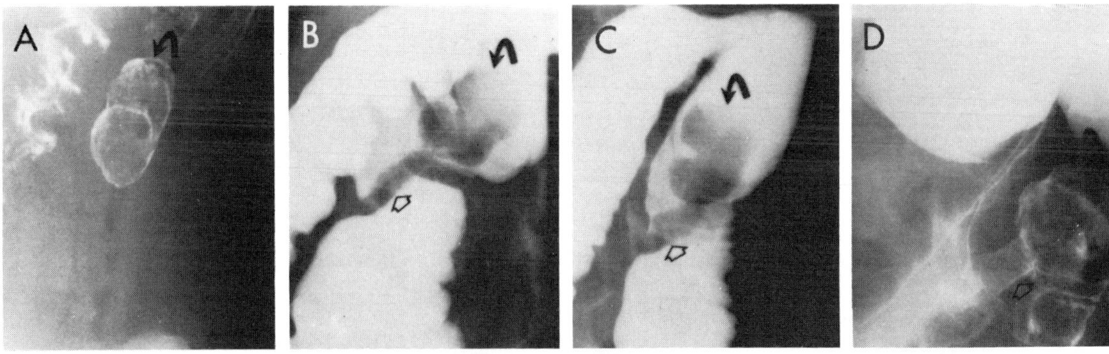

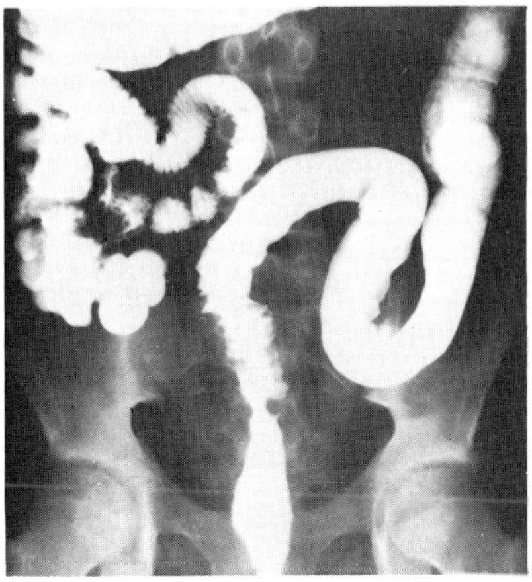

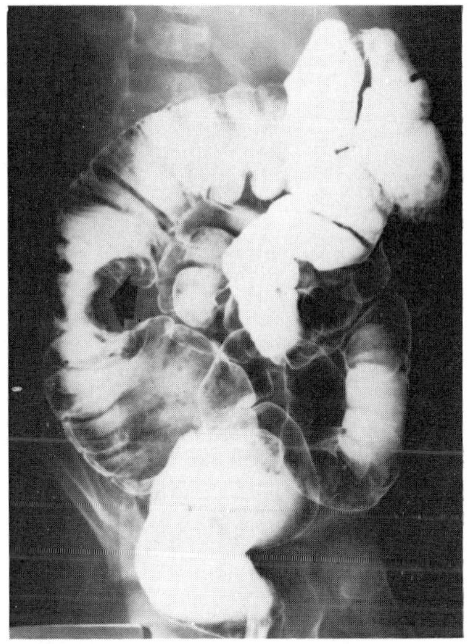

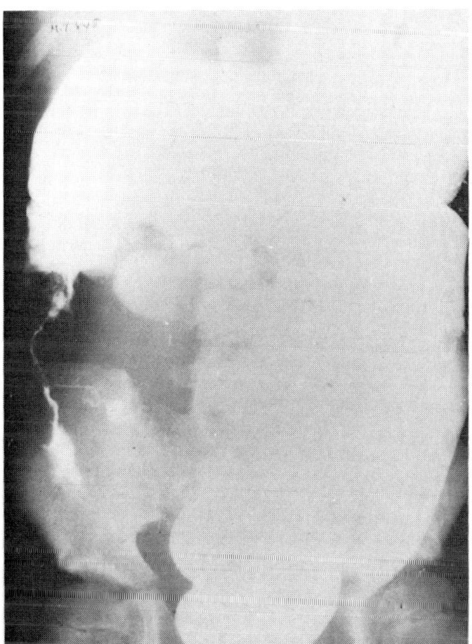

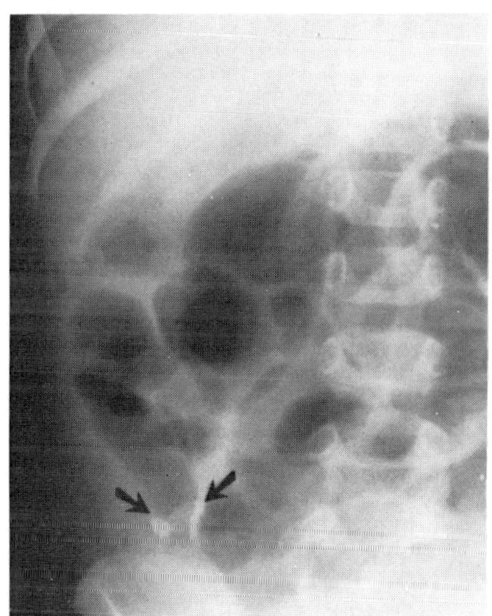

Fig 30–41 (top).—Pedunculated juvenile polyp can be demonstrated many ways, as on this four-on-one spot film. Polyp may present as **A,** barium-coated mass in decompressed postevacuation colon, **B** and **C,** as filling defect in barium-filled colon; or **D,** as mass coated with barium in air-distended lumen.

Fig 30–42 (center left).—Adenocarcinoma of rectosigmoid presenting as irregular annular infiltrating lesion in boy, age 12 years. (Courtesy of Dr. Morley Sloat, Los Angeles.)

Fig 30–43 (center right).—Napkin ring lesion of lymphosarcoma of midascending colon in boy, age 6 years. This had caused intermittent colocolic intussusception.

Fig 30–44 (bottom left).—Large Burkitt's lymphoma in right lower quadrant in boy, age 8 years. Terminal ileum and ascending colon markedly narrowed and deformed.

Fig 30–45 (bottom right).—Double appendicoliths in boy, age 1 year, with acute appendicitis.

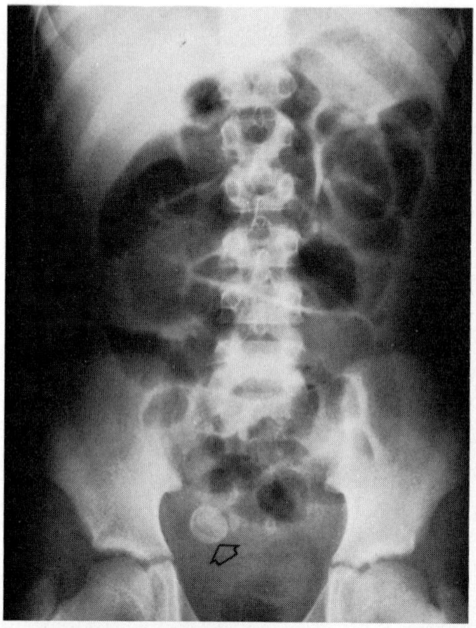

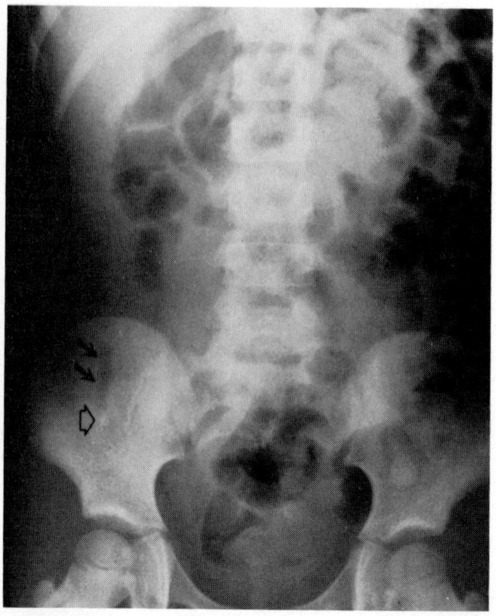

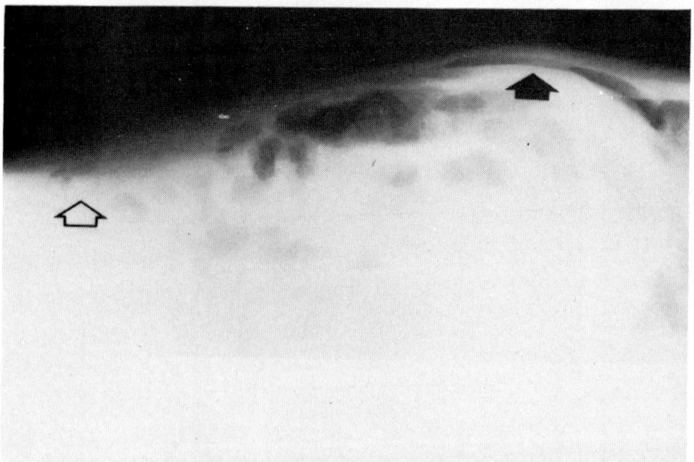

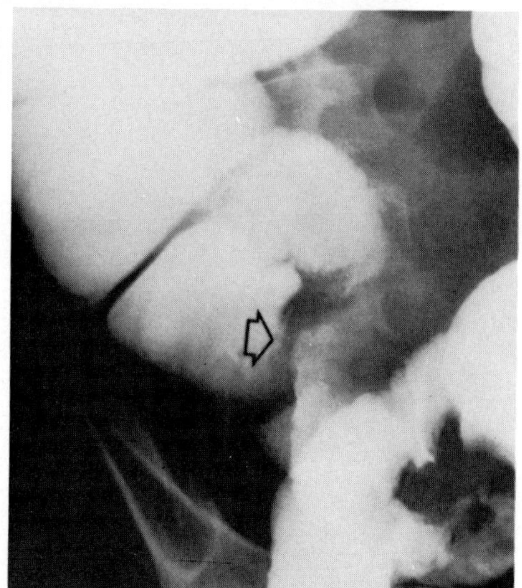

Fig 30–46 (top left).—Large laminated round appendicolith, with partial small bowel obstruction and absence of gas in right lower quadrant, seen on plain film in child with appendicitis.

Fig 30–47 (top right).—Air may normally be seen in appendix, but a girl, age 5, also had appendicolith *(open arrow)* at tip of air-filled appendix *(closed arrows)*.

Fig 30–48 (bottom left).—Cross-table lateral abdominal film in boy, age 14, with acute appendicitis shows small pneumoperitoneum *(closed arrow)* and small appendicolith *(open arrow)*.

Fig 30–49 (bottom right).—Film in boy, age 6 years, with acute appendicitis shows typical concave deformity of cecum *(arrow)* with nonfilling of appendix and inflammatory changes of adjacent terminal ileum.

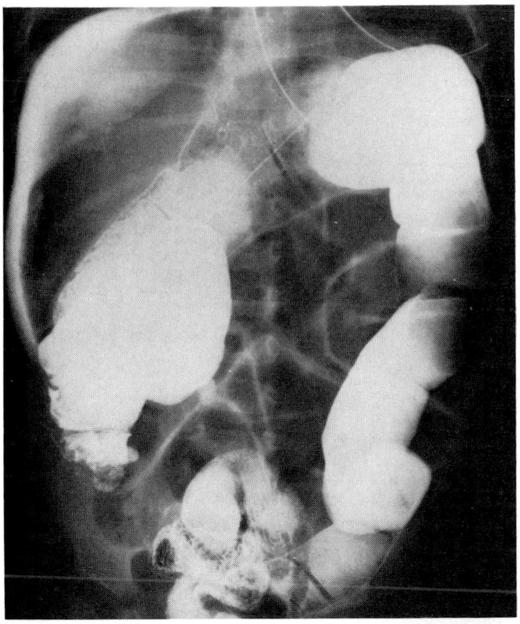

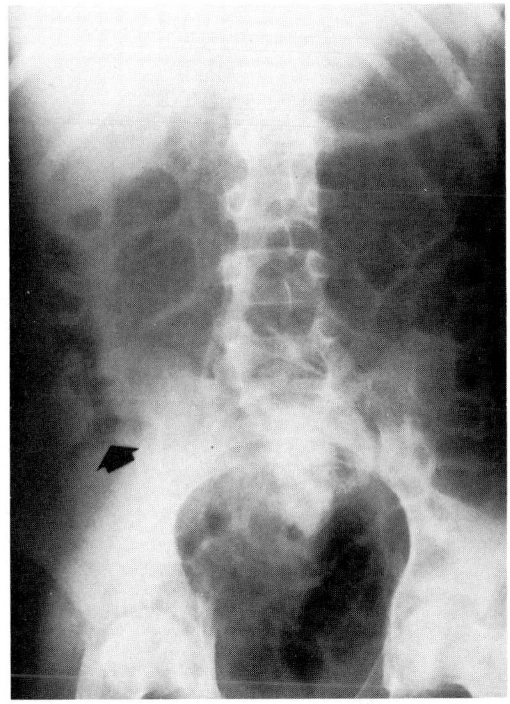

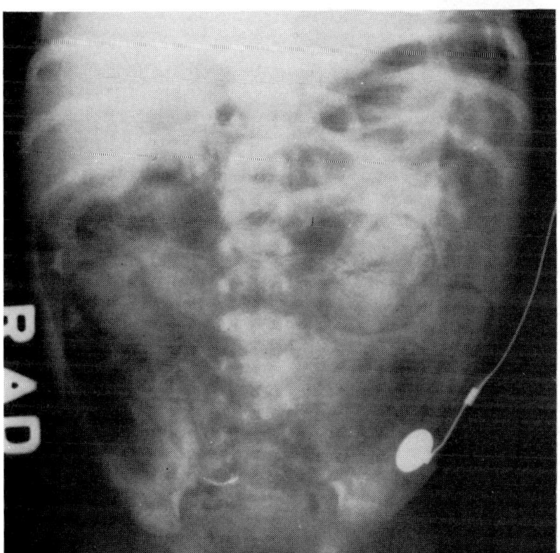

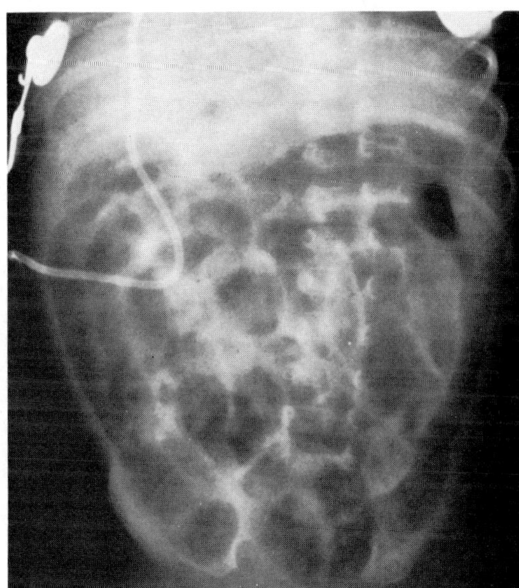

Fig 30–50 (top left).—Acute perforated appendicitis demonstrated on barium enema in boy, age 1 year. Barium has leaked through perforation into right upper quadrant of peritoneal cavity. No evidence of pneumoperitoneum on scout film.

Fig 30–51 (top right).—Girl, age 11, with acute lymphocytic leukemia complained of fever, abdominal pain, vomiting and bloody diarrhea. Film shows thickening of ascending colon wall and soft tissue mass deforming cecum. Acute typhlitis was confirmed at autopsy.

Fig 30–52 (bottom left).—Extensive pneumatosis intestinalis demonstrated in boy, age 1 month, with necrotizing enterocolitis.

Fig 30–53 (bottom right).—Extensive portal venous gas and moderate generalized gaseous distention of bowel loops seen on abdominal film of premature girl, age 1 month, with necrotizing enterocolitis.

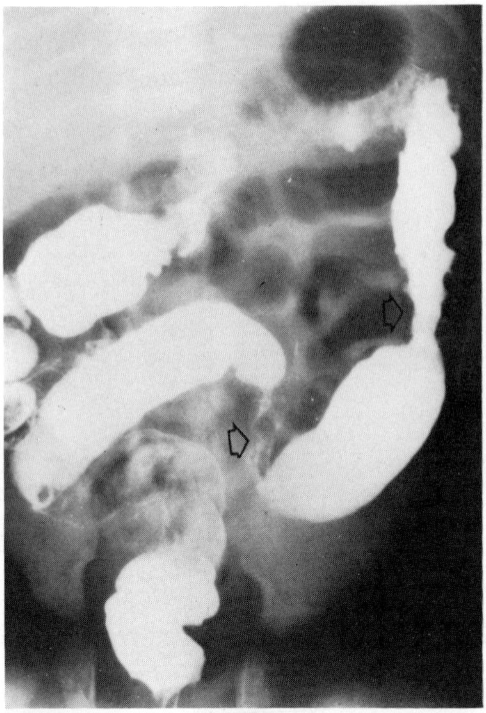

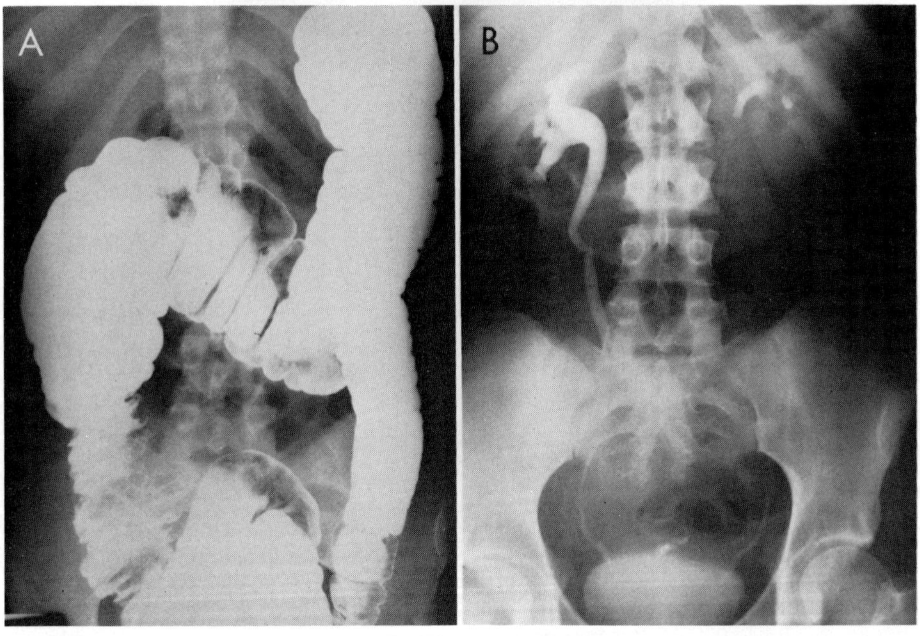

Fig 30–54 (top).—Several areas of irregular stenosis *(arrows)* of colon demonstrated on enema study in girl, age 3 days, with necrotizing enterocolitis.

Fig 30–55 (bottom).—Crohn's disease of cecum and ascending colon in teen-age girl. **A,** thickening and irregularity of involved area are seen on barium enema. **B,** right lower quadrant inflammatory process has caused slight obstruction of right ureter, demonstrated on excretory urography.

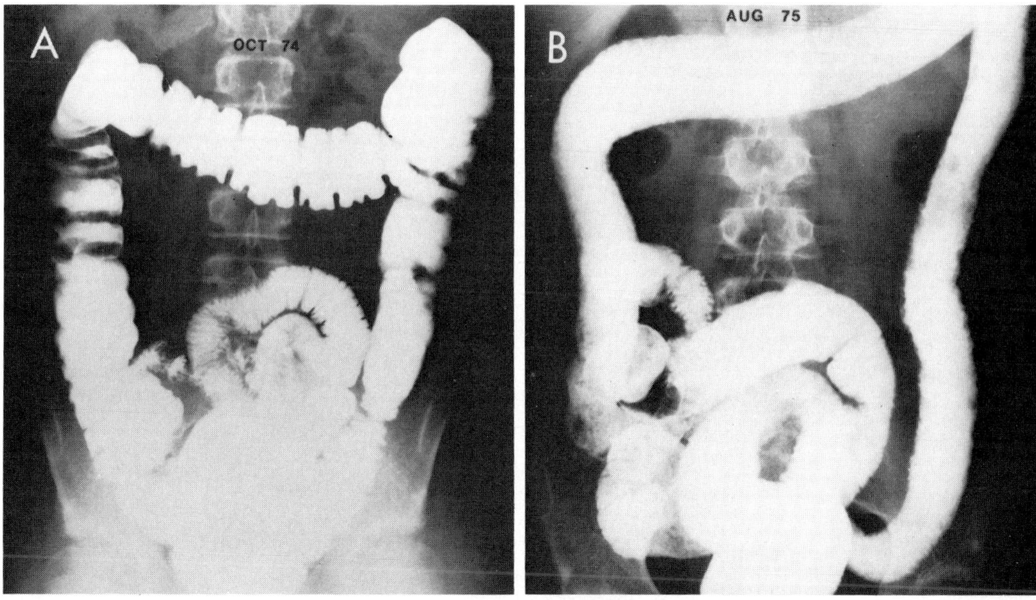

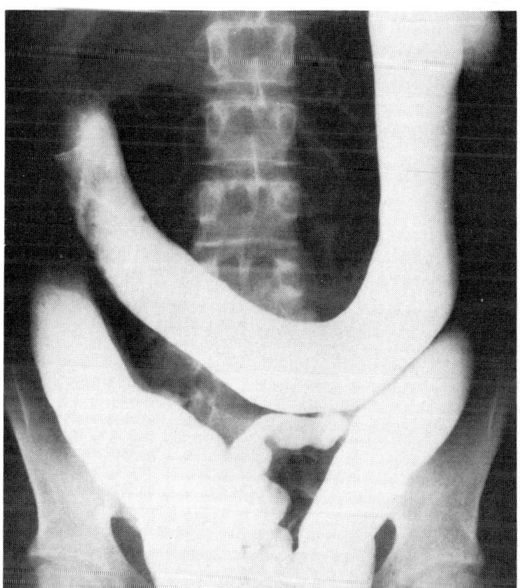

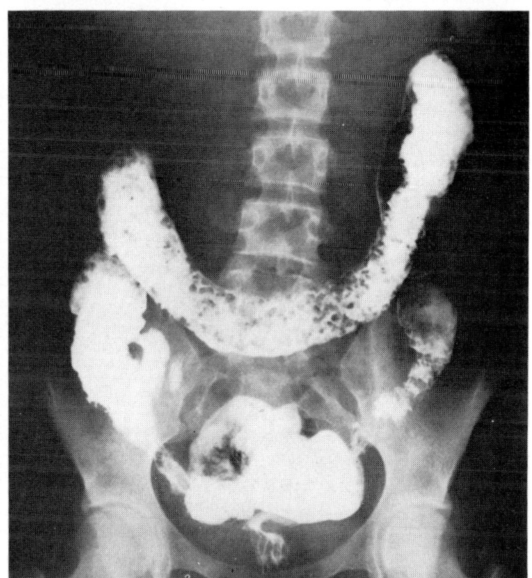

Fig 30–56 (top).—Rapid deterioration of colon in boy age 12 years with acute ulcerative colitis. **A,** initial enema shows only slight absence of haustration of descending colon. **B,** repeat study 10 months later shows progressive involvement of entire colon, with diffuse mucosal ulcerations throughout.

Fig 30–57 (bottom left).—Lead pipe configuration of entire colon in girl, age 14 years, with chronic ulcerative colitis.

Fig 30–58 (bottom right).—Extensive granulomatous ileocolitis in girl, age 16 years, with cobblestone mucosal pattern of colon and terminal ileum. Note fistula in region of terminal ileum.

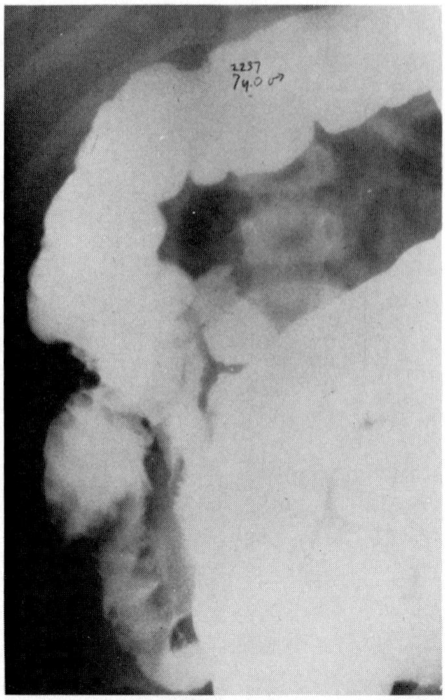

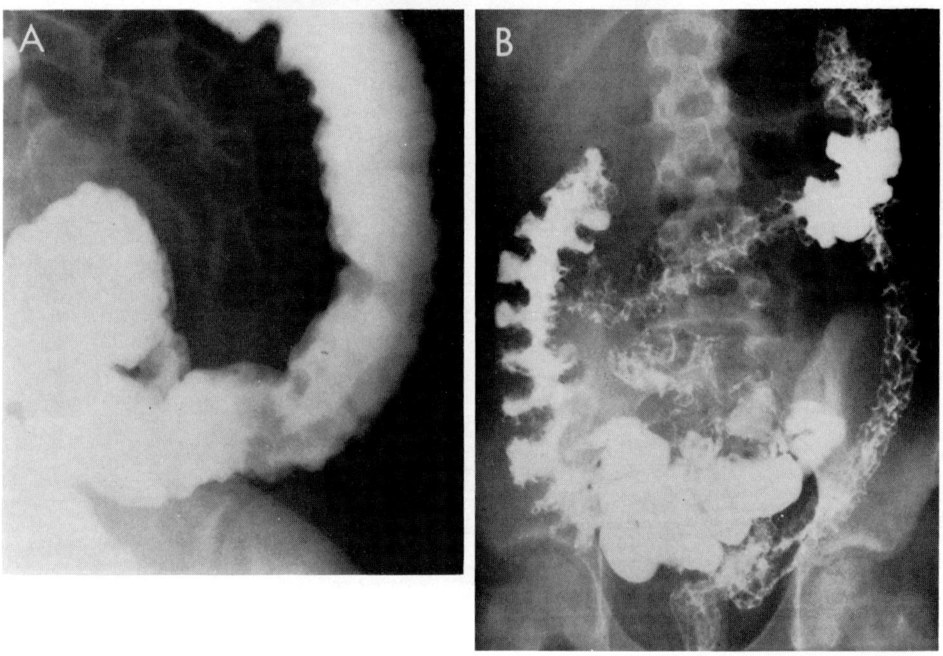

Fig 30–59 (top).—Tuberculous ileocolitis in boy, age 7 years, with marked inflammatory thickening and deformity of terminal ileum and cecum.

Fig 30–60 (bottom).—Girl, age 11 years, with diffuse amebic colitis. **A,** swollen nodular mucosal pattern demonstrated during barium filling of sigmoid and descending colon. **B,** extensive involvement of entire colon clearly seen on postevacuation film.

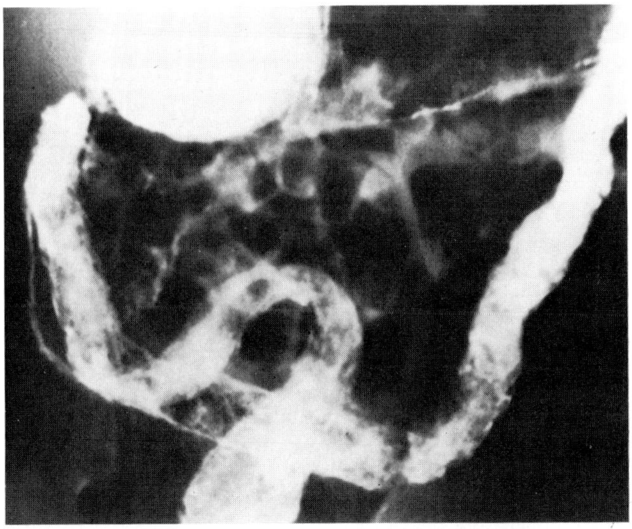

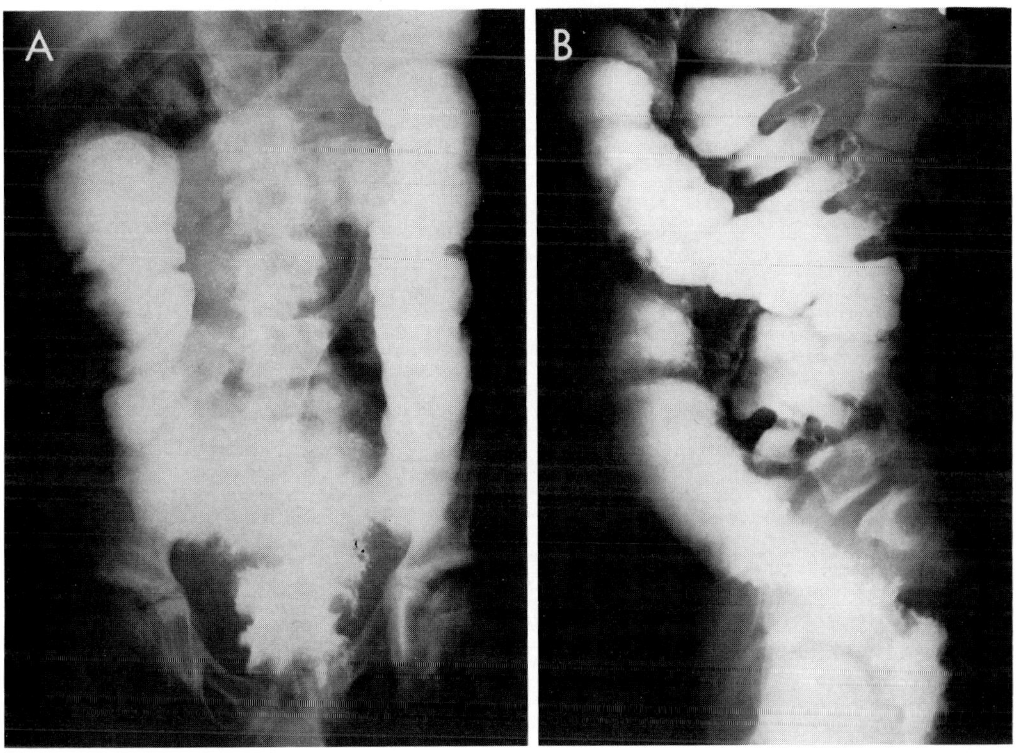

Fig 30–61 (top).—Inflammatory-like changes and narrowing of descending and rectosigmoid colon in young child with hemolytic uremic syndrome.

Fig 30–62 (bottom).—**A** and **B,** boy, age 14 years, with complex multiple system complaints, who had been treated extensively with numerous antibiotics, including lincomycin, shows extensive changes of pseudomembranous colitis of distal colon and rectum.

Chapter 31

Pelvic Lipomatosis

L. B. MORETTIN, M.D.

IN 1968 Fogg and Smyth[4] introduced the term "pelvic lipomatosis" to define a clinicoradiologic entity, originally described by Engels,[3] consisting of an unusual elevation and symmetric compression of the urinary bladder and rectum caused by an excessive deposition (proliferation) of fibroadipose tissue in the pelvis. The term pelvic lipomatosis aptly describes the anatomical and pathologic essence of this entity. With few exceptions,[7] the great majority of reported cases have been in males.

The radiologist may be the first to suspect this abnormality in an otherwise asymptomatic patient and, by recognizing its benign nature, could help to avoid other unnecessary diagnostic or therapeutic procedures.

Most individuals present with symptoms of chronic or recurrent nonspecific cystitis. Prostatic enlargement, described in most of the patients, is probably related to age. Subjective or objective signs of a suprapubic mass or fullness have been noted in less than half of the patients. Bladder neck obstruction and/or ureteral obstruction is rare and probably unrelated to the abnormality. Constipation has not occurred with more frequency than expected for the normal population of the same age group. Bowel obstruction has never been reported.

Cystoscopy can be very difficult and affords only incomplete visualization of the bladder. Sigmoidoscopy is consistently negative.

In some cases dense fibrosis of the diffuse lipomatosis infiltrating the pelvis is present. It does not seem justifiable to attribute the fibrosis to lower urinary tract infection. Rather, we believe that the fibrous connective tissue is an integral part of the abnormality. Urinary infection is either coincidental or secondary to chronic prostatic hypertrophy. It seems very unlikely that the accumulation of pelvic fat could be related to an increase in the patient's weight. If pelvic lipomatosis were related to obesity, one would expect to encounter this abnormality frequently.

Diffuse or localized deposition of an unusual amount of adipose tissue is known to occur in other clinical circumstances, e.g., Cushing's syndrome, hypothalamic lesions, islet cell adenomas and as a result of prolonged corticosteroid therapy. It is interesting that a hormonal disturbance is the common denominator of all these abnormalities. The roentgenographically demonstrable deposition of fat in several areas of the body in patients undergoing steroid therapy for a long period has received attention in recent publications.[9, 10] The most common location is the anterior and superior mediastinum. Other areas involved are the supraclavicular regions and presacral space.[10] In the latter location, anterior displacement of the rectum has been demonstrated, but diffuse fatty infiltration and the roentgenographic findings consistent with pelvic lipomatosis have not been described.

Radiographic Findings

Plain film examinations of the abdomen reveal an unusual radiolucency of the pelvis, which allows visualization of the muscular planes and better definition of the bony detail of the sacrum[8] (Fig 31–1). The roentgenographic appearance of the opacified rectum and urinary bladder is characteristic[8] (Figs 31–2 and 31–3). The rectum is narrowed. stretched and elongated. The sigmoid is elevated. The deformity is concentric and fixes the rectum and rectosigmoid in the midline.

The urinary bladder also is elongated in its vertical dimension. Its shape often resembles that of a pear or, as in the case referred to in Figure 31–3, that of an inverted teardrop with its narrow end at the base.[8] Emptying of the urinary bladder and rectum is normal and the walls are not rigid. Their mucosal patterns are not disturbed.

Differential Diagnosis

Because of its somewhat characteristic roentgenographic appearance, pelvic lipomatosis can be easily differentiated from other extrinsic abnormalities that may deform the rectum and bladder.

Computerized tomography (CT) clearly defining the abundant fat deposits, is very valuable in problem cases. Other conditions may similarly deform the rectum, bladder or both.

HEMATOMAS

When large, hematomas may surround the bladder and rectum, causing considerable narrowing. They are most common in extensive pelvic fractures (Fig 31–4) but may develop with moderate trauma in patients receiving anticoagulants or in those with bleeding disorders. When associated with extraperitoneal rupture of the bladder, the accumulation of blood and urine could produce an even more severe deformity as well as elevation of the bladder and rectum.

VENOUS OBSTRUCTION

Thrombosis with obstruction of the inferior vena cava can produce extensive collateral circulation in the pelvis. The engorged, tortuous veins compress and narrow the bladder and rectum. The ureters are displaced medially and may be notched. Similar findings may be present following caval ligation or in congenital interruption of the inferior vena cava (Fig 31–5).

LYMPHOMA

Extensive nodal involvement owing to lymphoma (Fig 31–6) or leukemia may cause a similar symmetric narrowing of the bladder. Metastatic nodes are generally smaller and rarely deform the pelvic organs.

One should keep in mind that pelvic lipomatosis may be an incidental unrelated finding in a patient with other reasons for deformities of the bladder and rectum. The patient illustrated in Figure 31–7 had had asymptomatic pelvic lipomatosis for many years and developed a carcinoma of the prostate, with extensive spread to the pelvic floor and obstruction of pelvic veins—three reasons for deformity of the rectum and bladder. Pelvic lipomatosis has also been reported in association with cystitis glandularis.[11]

LYMPHOCYSTS

Following extensive pelvic surgery, lymphocysts, when large and bilateral, may similarly deform the bladder. The rectum is not usually involved; ultrasonography, demonstrating the fluid-filled cysts, is diagnostic in most cases. Lymphangiography also is useful, demonstrating extravasation and pooling of contrast material in the cysts (Fig 31–8).

HYPERTROPHY OF PSOAS MUSCLES

Elongation and a gourdlike deformity of the bladder also may be caused by hypertrophy of the psoas muscles (Fig 31–9). CT allows clear differentiation between muscle and fat. This entity, which is probably more common than previously thought, should be suspected when a narrow bladder is found in a young, muscular or athletic individual.[2]

Pseudostenosis of the sigmoid colon also may be produced by a grossly distended bladder owing to urinary retention.[5]

ABSCESSES

Abscesses of the pelvic cavity or floor invariably produce some degree of asymmetric displacement of either the rectum or bladder.

METASTATIC TUMORS

Tumors that metastasize to the pelvic peritoneal cavity cause lobulated indentations in the rectum, and occasionally in the bladder, but usually do not produce significant elevation or elongation of these organs.

LYMPHOGRANULOMA VENEREUM

This systemic infectious disease transmitted by sexual contact is characterized by genital ulcerations followed by suppuration of regional lymph nodes. This may lead to fibrotic changes in the genital tract and rectum, the latter particularly found in homosexual men. The rectum in the latter stages may be considerably narrowed (Fig 31–10), but its walls are ragged and deformed by healed ulceration and fibrosis.

REFERENCES

1. Ambos, M. A., Bosniak, M. A., Lefleur, R. S., and Madayag, M. A.: The pear-shaped Bladder, Radiology 122:85, 1977.
2. Chang, S. F.: Pear-shaped bladder caused by large iliopsoas muscles, Radiology 128:349, 1978.
3. Engels, E. P.: Sigmoid colon and urinary bladder in high fixation: Roentgen changes simulating pelvic tumor, Radiology 72:419, 1959.
4. Fogg, L. B., and Smyth, W. J.: Pelvic lipomatosis: Condition simulating pelvic neoplasm, Radiology 90:558, 1968.
5. Kleinhaus, U., and Kaftori, J.: Rectosigmoid pseudostenosis due to urinary retention, Radiology 127:645, 1978.
6. Leuzinger, D. E., Bahr, R. D., Miller, C. D., and Shipman, G. A.: Case report of high fixation of bladder and sigmoid colon, J. Urol. 85:163, 1961.
7. Malter, I. J., and Omell, G. H.: Pelvic lipomatosis in a woman. A case report, Obstet. Gynecol. 37:63, 1971.
8. Morettin, L. B., and Wilson, M. C.: Pelvic lipomatosis, Am. J. Roentgenol. 43:181, 1971.
9. Price, J. E., Jr., and Rigler, L. G.: Widening of mediastinum resulting from fat accumulation, Radiology 96:497, 1970.
10. Teates, C. D.: Steroid-induced mediastinal lipomatosis, Radiology 96:501, 1970.
11. Yalla, S. V., Ivker, M., Burros, H. M., and Dorey, F.: Cystitis glandularis with perivesical lipomatosis, Urology 5:383, 1975.

Fig 31–1 (below).—Pelvic lipomatosis. Plain roentgenogram of abdomen showing diffuse increased radiolucency of pelvis. Shadows of obturator muscles are well seen bilaterally, outlined by radiolucent fat *(arrows).* (From Morettin and Wilson, Am. J. Roentgenol. 43:181, 1971, with permission.)

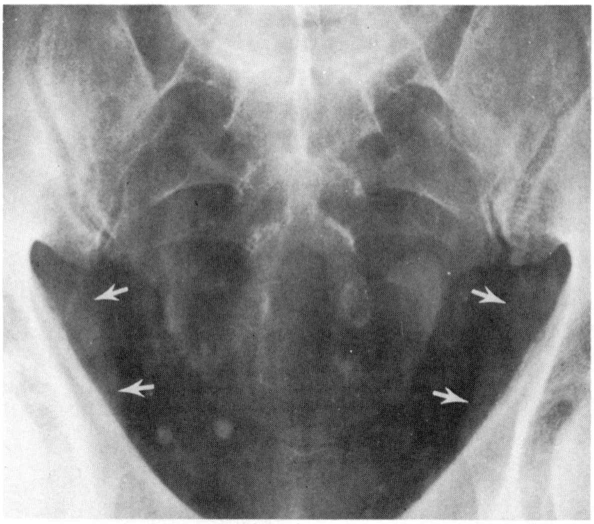

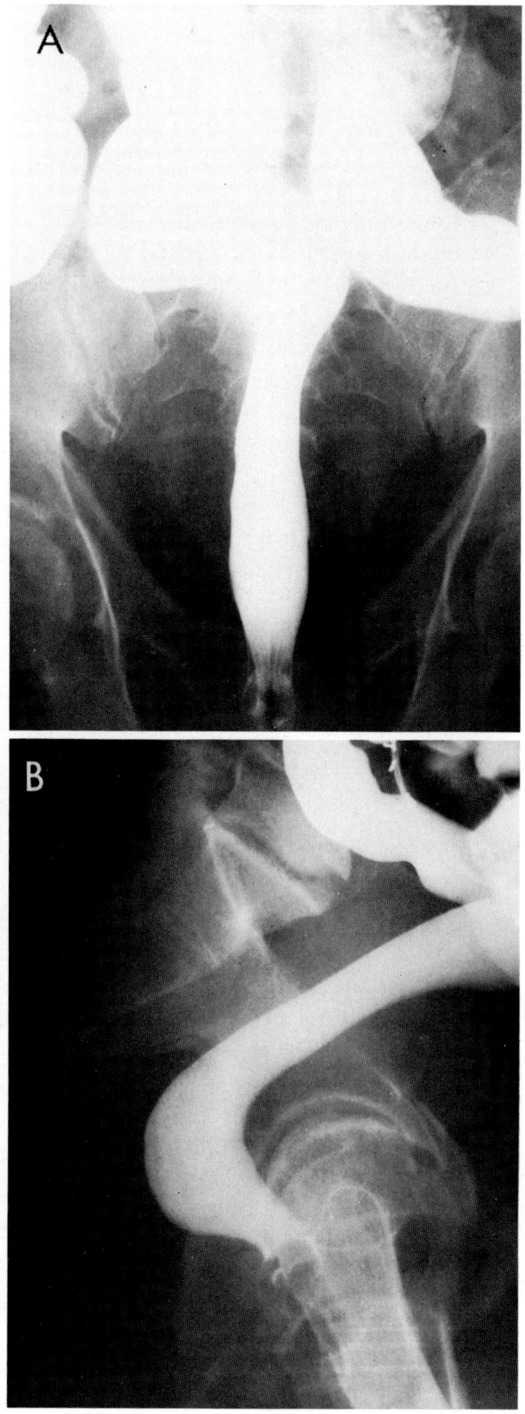

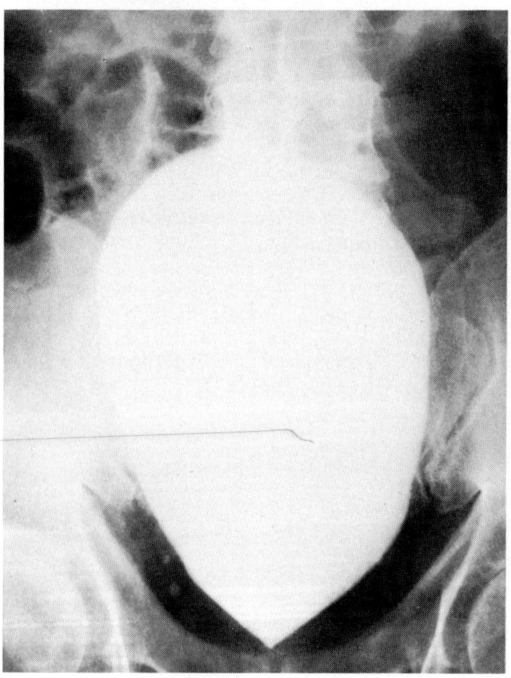

Fig 31–2. (right top and **bottom).**—Pelvic lipomatosis. Barium enema examination showing **(A),** anteroposterior view and **(B),** lateral view. Rectum is elongated and narrowed but remains in midline. Sigmoid is displaced outside of pelvis. (From Morettin and Wilson, Am. J. Roentgenol. 43:181, 1971, with permission.)

Fig 31–3 (bottom left).—Pelvic lipomatosis. Cystogram showing urinary bladder to be elongated in its vertical dimension and its base narrowed, assuming configuration of inverted teardrop. (From Morettin and Wilson, Am. J. Roentgenol. 43:181, 1971, with permission.)

Fig 31–4 (below).—Hematoma of pelvic floor and perivesical space caused by pelvic fractures. Bladder is elevated and symmetrically narrowed.

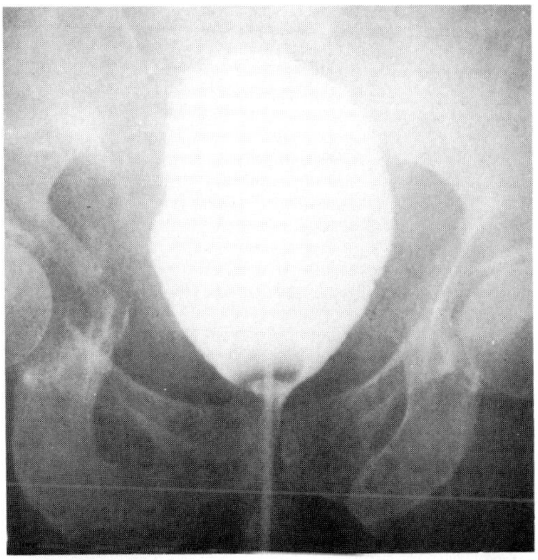

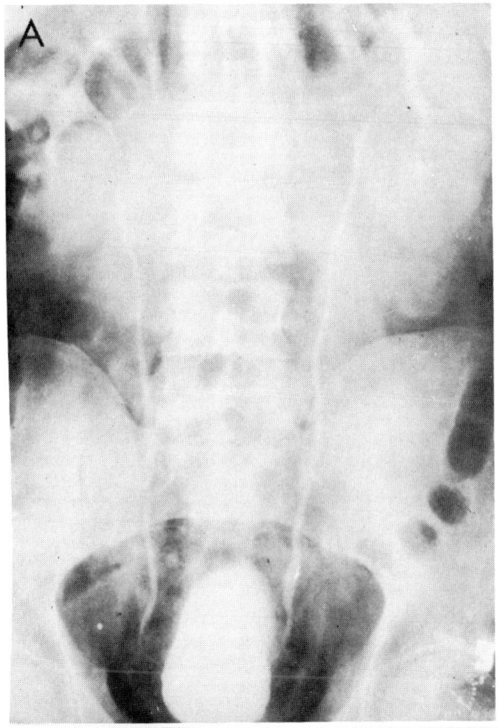

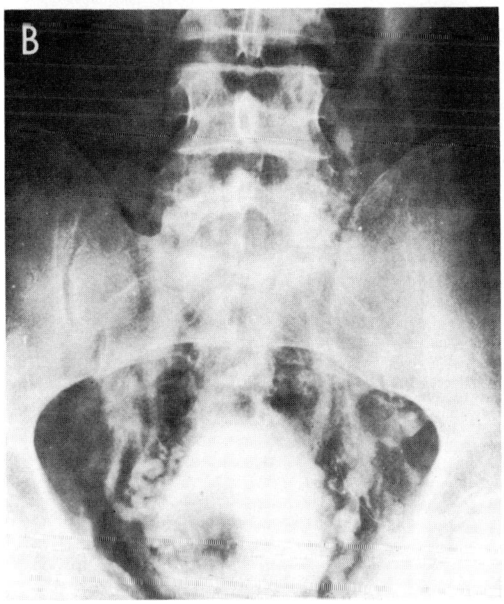

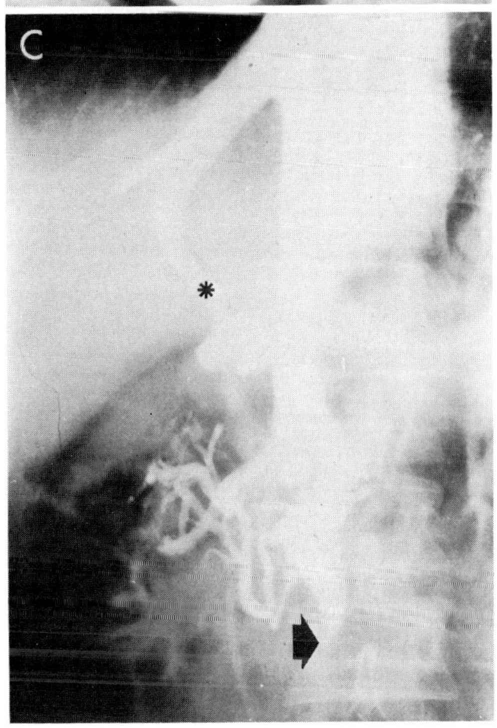

Fig 31–5 (top right and bottom).—Inferior vena cava obstruction (congenital). **A,** intravenous pyelogram shows bladder to be symmetrically narrowed and elongated. Both ureters are medially displaced but not obstructed. **B,** bilateral lower extremity venogram showing large, tortuous veins that surround and deform urinary bladder. **C,** inferior vena cavagram performed via brachial vein shows tapered complete obstruction below right renal vein *(arrow).* Patient had extensive venous systemic-portal communications, with persistent patent ductus venosum *(asterisk).*

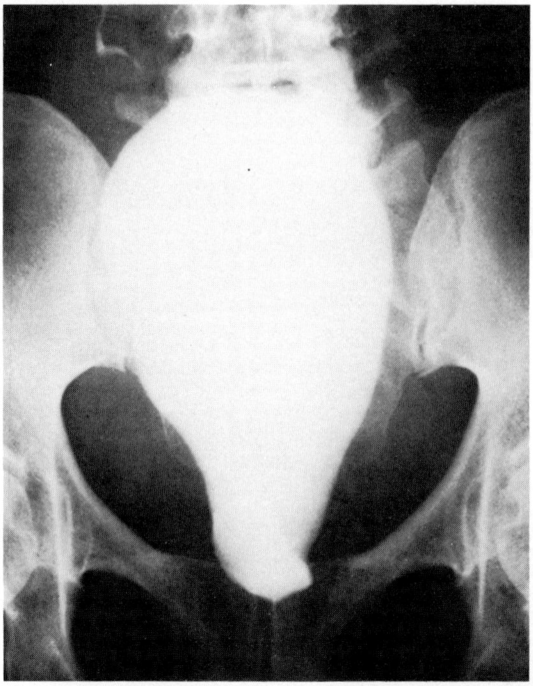

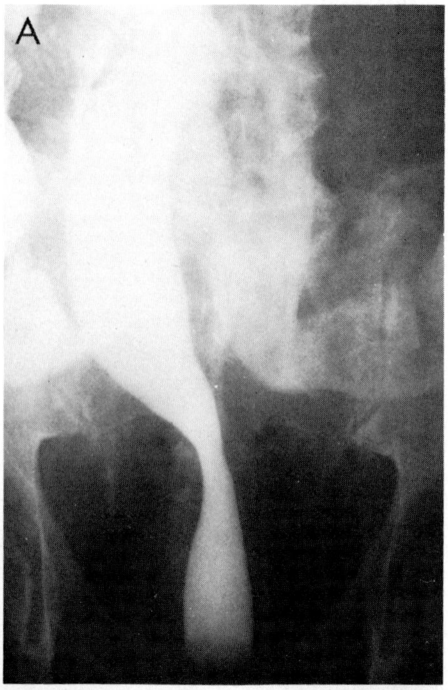

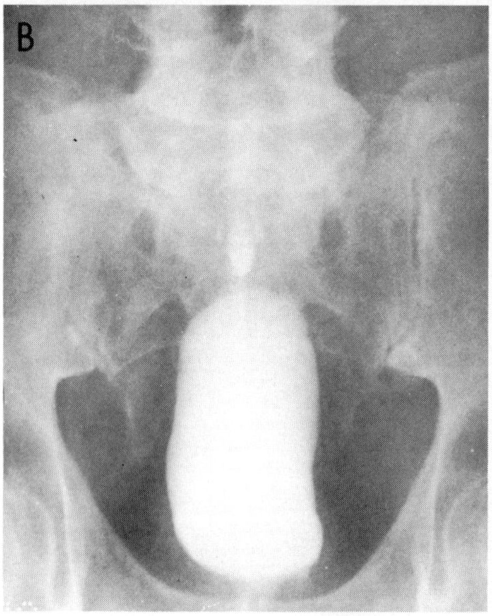

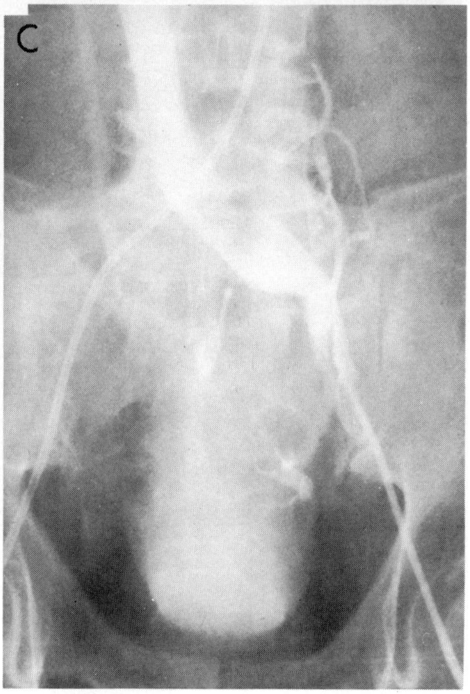

Fig 31–6 (top left). – Lymphoma. In a woman, age 25, intravenous urogram shows extensive lymphadenopathy compressing and elevating floor of bladder.[1] (From Ambos, Bosniak, Lefleur and Madayag, Radiology 122:85, 1977, with permission.)

Fig 31–7 (top right and **bottom).** – Man, age 67, with some narrowing of bladder and rectum present for many years caused by pelvic lipomatosis. He later developed prostatic carcinoma with extensive involvement of pelvic floor and pelvic nodes. **A,** barium enema examination shows narrowing and stretching of rectum. **B,** intravenous pyelogram shows elongation of urinary bladder. **C,** venogram shows irregular narrowing and compression of left iliac vein. At operation, in addition to abundant amounts of fat, extensive metastasis with enlarged nodes and venous engorgement was found.

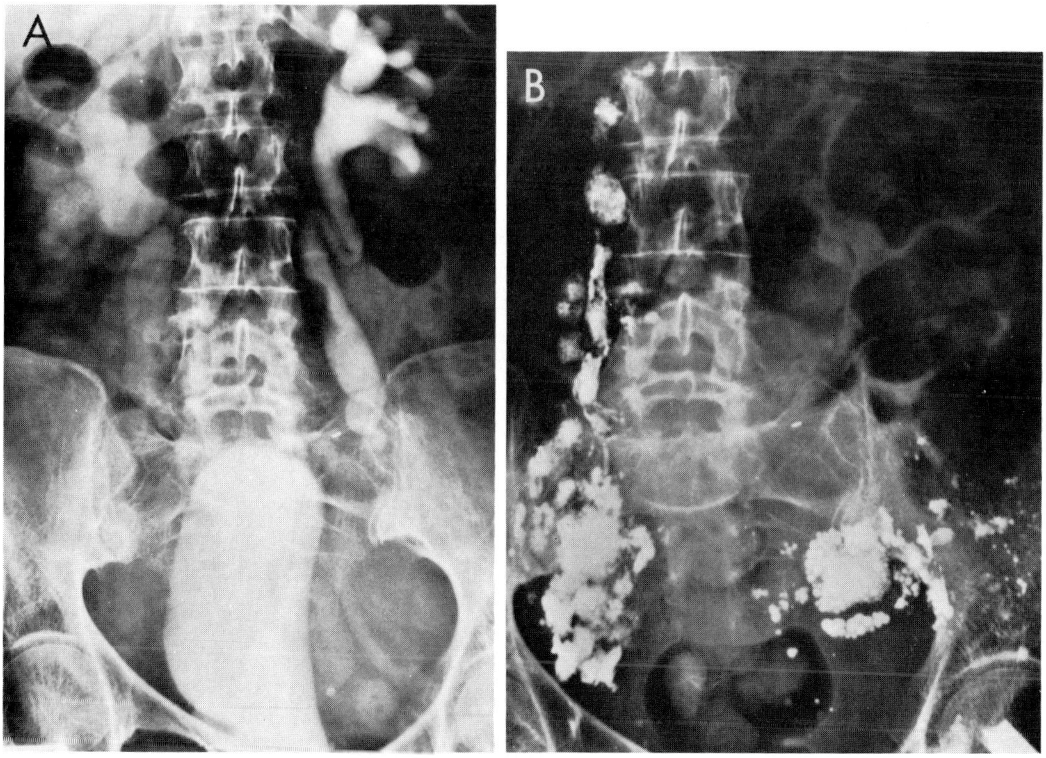

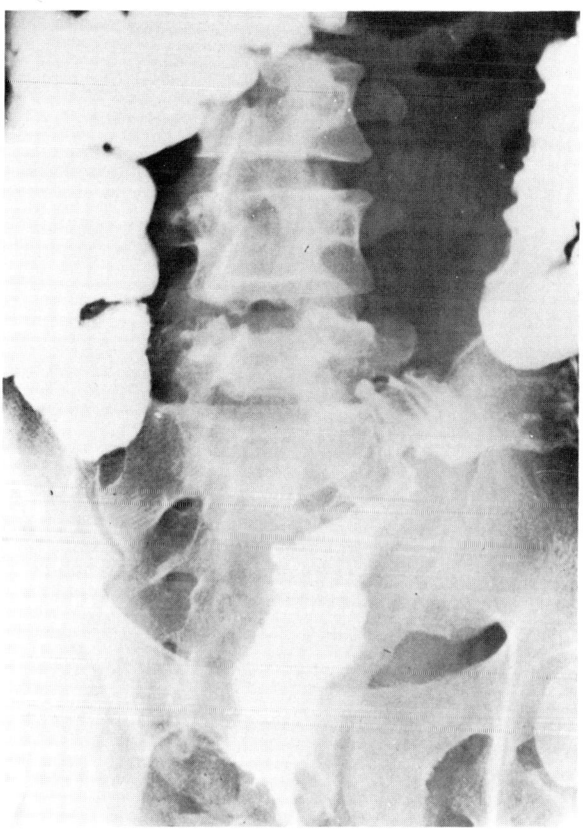

Fig 31–8 (top).—Postoperative lymphocysts.[1] Woman, age 65, had recurrent urinary tract infections several months after hysterectomy and extensive lymph node dissection. **A,** intravenous urogram shows bilaterally compressed bladder with increased density in pelvis. Bilateral hydronephrosis, more severe on the right, is secondary to compression of distal ureters. (Metallic clip from previous surgery is seen.) **B,** lymphangiogram demonstrates pooling of contrast medium in large bilateral lymphocysts. (From Ambos, Bosniak, Lefleur and Madayag, Radiology 122:85, 1977, with permission.)

Fig 31–9.—See page 382.

Fig 31–10 (left).—Lymphogranuloma venereum. Marked irregular narrowing of rectum and sigmoid with considerable mucosal distortion caused by extensive fibrosis.

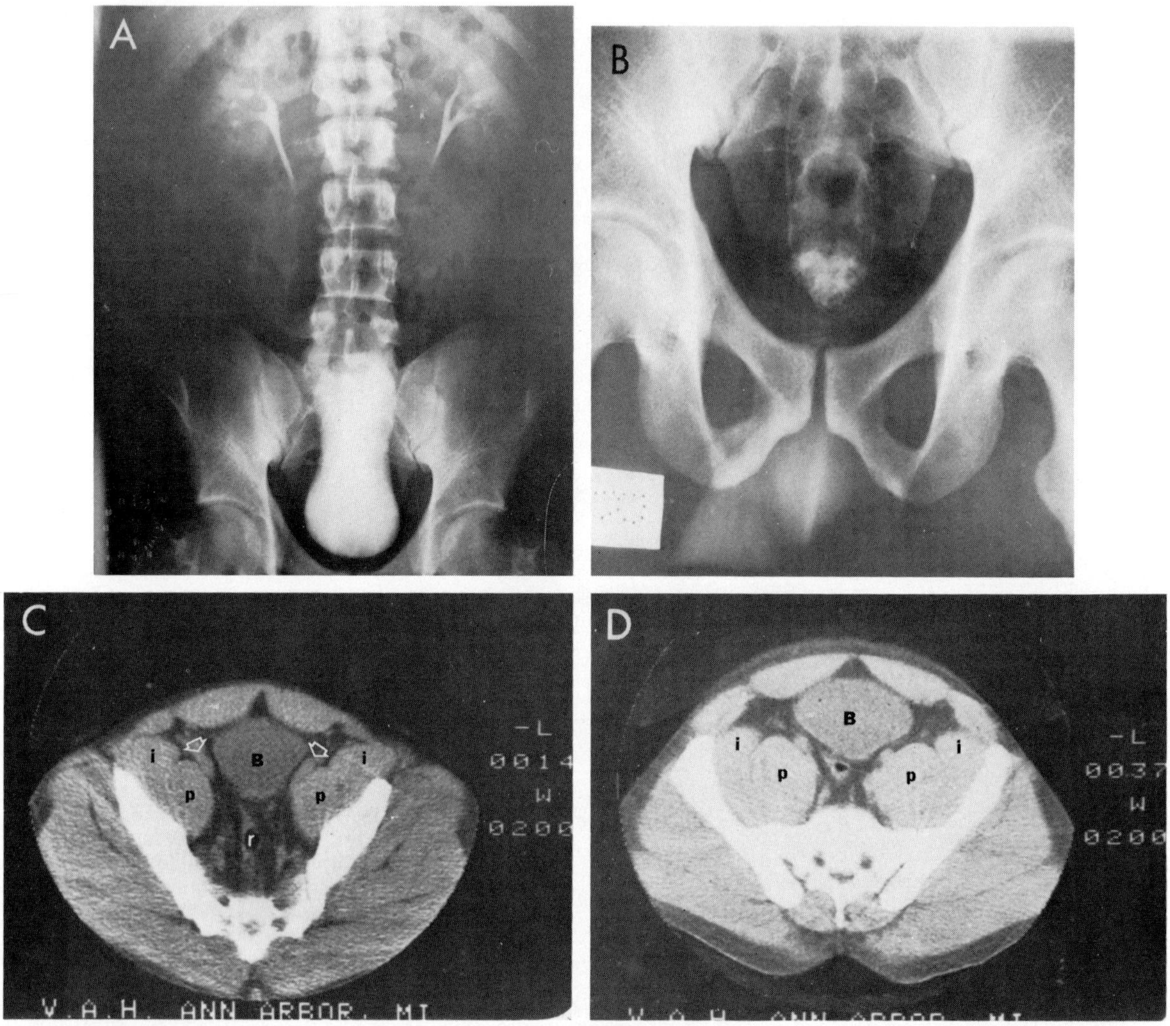

Fig 31–9. – **A,** excretory urogram showing bulging psoas muscles and pear-shaped bladder. Note narrow pelvis. Plain film did not show excessive lucency in pelvis. Lateral film showed smooth posterior draping of bladder. **B,** postvoid film showing symmetric, medial deviation of ureters. **C,** CT at 7 cm above pubic symphysis (level of S3). Bladder *(B)* is indented by iliacus *(i)* and psoas *(P)*. *Arrows* point to pelvic blood vessels. *r* = rectum. **D,** CT at 10 cm above pubic symphysis (level of L5–S1). Note that bladder is wider than in **C** at this higher level, consistent with its pear shape. (From Chang, Radiology 128:349, 1978, with permission.)

Chapter 32

Pneumatic Compression Paddle in Colonic Roentgenography

JOSEPH F. LINSMAN, M.D., F.A.C.R., F.A.C.P.

COMPRESSION TECHNIQUES in gastrointestinal radiology are well known and accepted maneuvers for disclosing and delineating the details of gastrointestinal lesions beginning with those in the stomach and continuing through the length of the colon. Manual manipulation with the lead-protected gloved hand is the most commonly used method. Spot filming devices with built-in compression cones are most useful. Localized pads of nonopaque material and balsa wood hemispheres have been utilized, but they do not permit *grading* of the compression. Palparium spoons work well in detecting and detailing lesions. In studying the colon, the pneumatic compression paddle (Fig 32–1) rates above all other methods as an aid in eduction of abnormalities involving this portion of the gastrointestinal tract.[1] Use of the paddle reflects the diligence and vigor on the part of the examiner in eliciting colonic lesions (notwithstanding the use of air contrast and multiple view types of examinations).

The pneumatic compression device* shown in Figure 32–1 produces graded compression and is most adaptable to study of the colon. It consists of a banjo-like frame made of five-ply plexiglass with a round housing and sturdy handle. An inflatable rubber bladder (balloon) is partially encased in the round housing. An inflation control bulb at the end of the handle permits both inflation and deflation of the balloon. The handle is notched and thus provides a nonslip grip. A circle of lead is embedded in the round plexiglass housing and surrounds the inflatable balloon, thus defining sharply under the fluoroscope the region under compression. The inflation control bulb permits graded compression. The back of the paddle has a rubberized cork facing so that it will not slip on the roentgenographic table once it is in position.

The best application of the paddle is made with the patient prone. However, it may also be used with the patient supine; it is then placed between the locked fluoroscopic screen and the patient.

When the paddle is positioned during fluoroscopy and spot filming, the device should be grasped close to its neck, since this permits more accurate initial placement. Minor adjustments, once the paddle is in place, may be made thereafter by manipulation with the notched handle. The balloon should be deflated during both positioning and adjustment

*Manufactured by Pennsylvania X-Ray Corporation, Ft. Washington, Pa. 19034; marketed as Smith Pneumatic Compression Paddle, U.S. Patent 2,619,599.

so as not to inadvertently force it from its housing container. The balloon should be deflated during paddle removal for the same reason. Rotation or movement of the patient to an optimal position may be accomplished with the paddle in place and the balloon deflated. The bladder should be overinflated initially, and then, with gradual deflation or reinflation, the proper amount of graded compression to demonstrate a lesion can be attained.

Grading the compression is very important and cannot be overemphasized. Spot films are made in the optimum phase of respiration, which best portrays the object being imaged. If desired, the patient may be left centered in position on the table with the paddle in place for over-table roentgenography.

The paddle is most useful in the pelvic colon, where it separates and compresses redundant loops. In the cecal region, it helps to depict the area of the ileocecal valve and ileum and appendix (if filled with contrast). Though useful anywhere along the course of the colon, it is of particular value in the area of both flexures. In these areas, deep inspiration is a distinct aid in displacing the flexures to a lower level, since this permits compression where it might not otherwise be attainable. Visual clarity is enhanced by the contrasting air in the rubber bladder.

If used with care, the pneumatic compression paddle is not discomforting to the patient. Jackson[2] recently issued a word of caution after a patient with osteopenia incurred a rib fracture when the bladder was inflated over the right lower rib cage.

The compression paddle thins the portion of the bowel beneath it, effectively displaces and separates overlapping intestinal loops and immobilizes moving lesions (e.g., pedunculated polyps). The air in the balloon enhances contrast of the demonstrated lesion, which is precisely and exquisitely documented. The procedure altogether is simple, rapid and safe.

The value of the pneumatic compression paddle in demonstrating lesions not otherwise shown, or not shown to an optimum degree, is depicted in Figures 32–2 to 32–10.

REFERENCES

1. Linsman, J. F.: The pneumatic compression paddle in colonic roentgenography, Am. J. Roentgenol. 91: 846, 1964.
2. Jackson, D. M.: Correspondence. (Letters to the Editor), N. Engl. J. Med. 298:856, 1978.

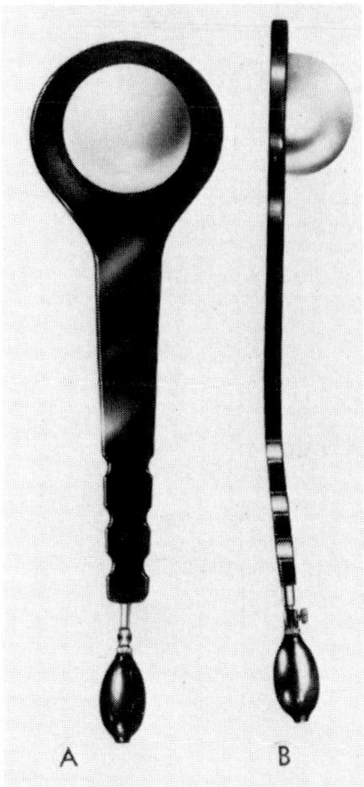

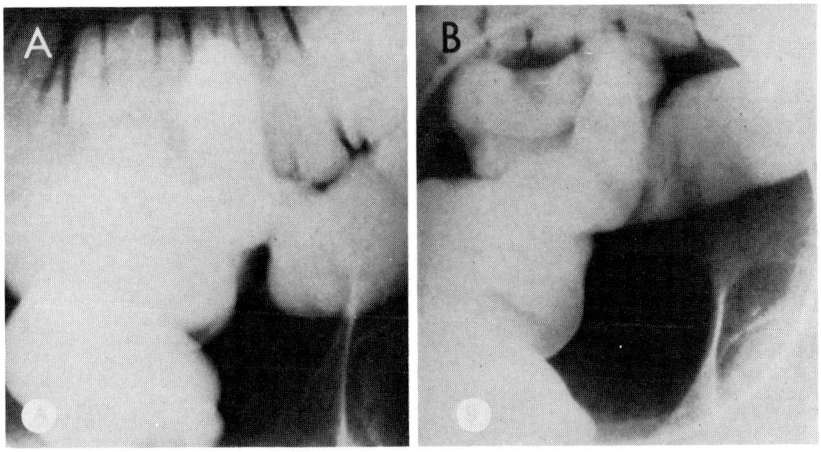

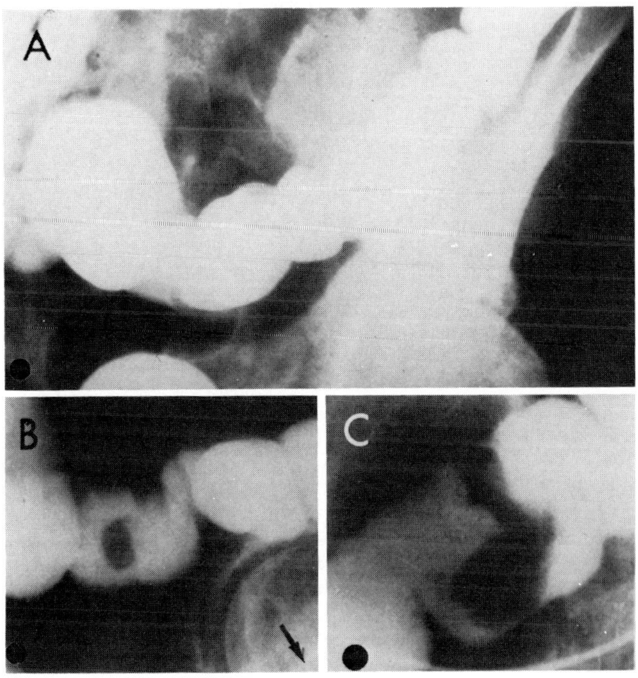

Fig 32–1 (left).—Pneumatic compression paddle with partial inflation of its rubber bladder shown in frontal **(A)** and profile **(B)** projections. Air is introduced by compressing rubber bulb and is released by turning thumb screw. (From Linsman, Am. J. Roentgenol. 91:846, 1964, with permission.)

Fig 32–2 (top right).—**A,** sigmoid colon is redundant and overlapping, and the transverse colon, because of its low position, is superimposed on it. **B,** compression paddle parts and thins these loops for better visualization and diagnosis. (From Linsman, Am. J. Roentgenol. 91:846, 1964, with permission.)

Fig 32–3 (bottom right).—**A,** both sigmoid and iliac portions of pelvic colon harbor pedunculated polypoid lesions, not demonstrable without benefit of graded compression. (**B** and **C**), with graded compression by paddle, areas of interest are immobilized and thinned so that pedunculated lesions are defined and documented. *Arrow* in **B** points to lead circle in housing of paddle, useful in fluoroscopic placement. (From Linsman, Am. J. Roentgenol. 91:846, 1964, with permission.)

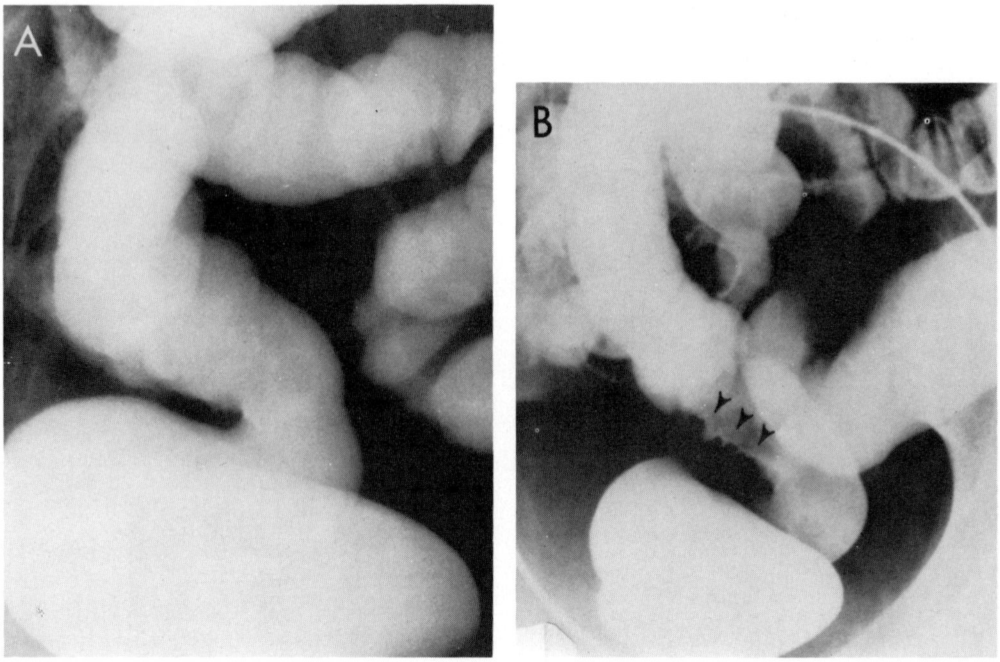

Fig 32–4. – **A,** sigmoid loop without compression is normal in appearance. **B,** with graded compression using the paddle, margin of distal sigmoid colon reveals pleating *(arrows)* due to serosal attachment of fairly large endometrioma.

Fig 32–5. – **A,** supine spot film of sigmoid colon without compression and with superimposed loops. **B,** prone spot film with paddle placed and properly inflated thins loops and separates them so as to delineate large villous adenoma *(arrows).*

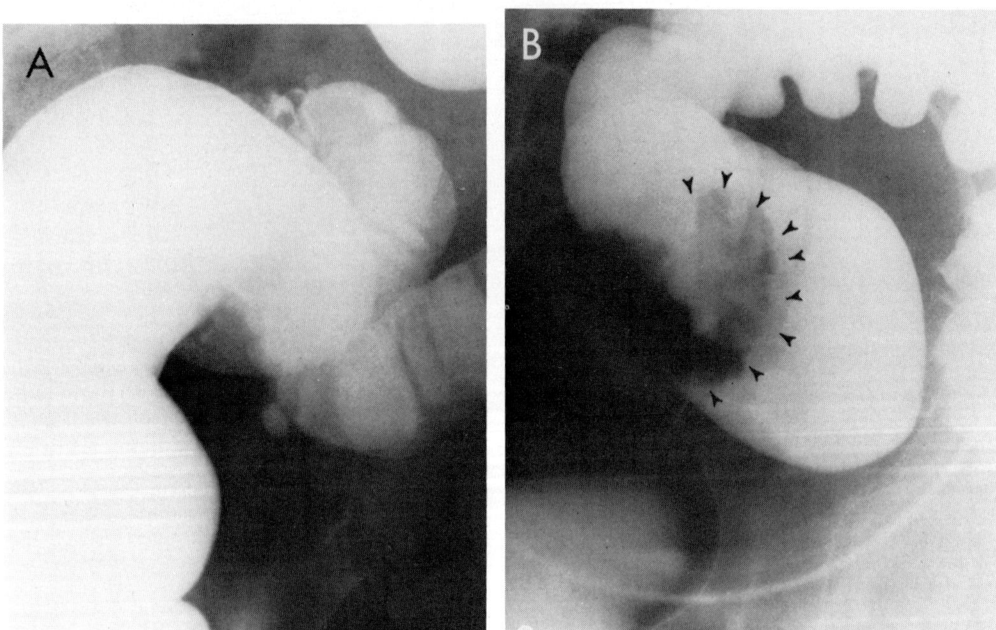

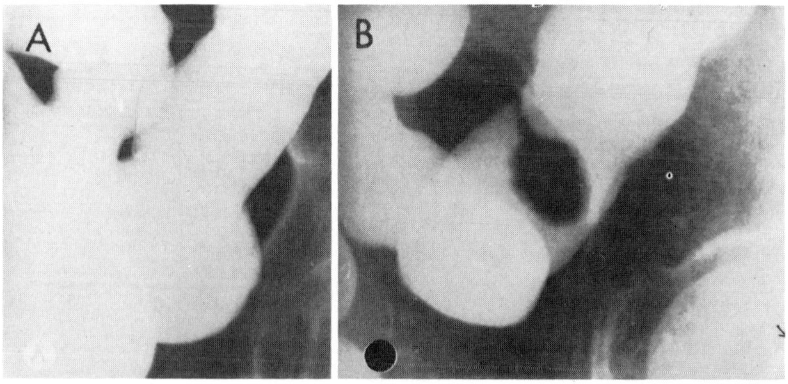

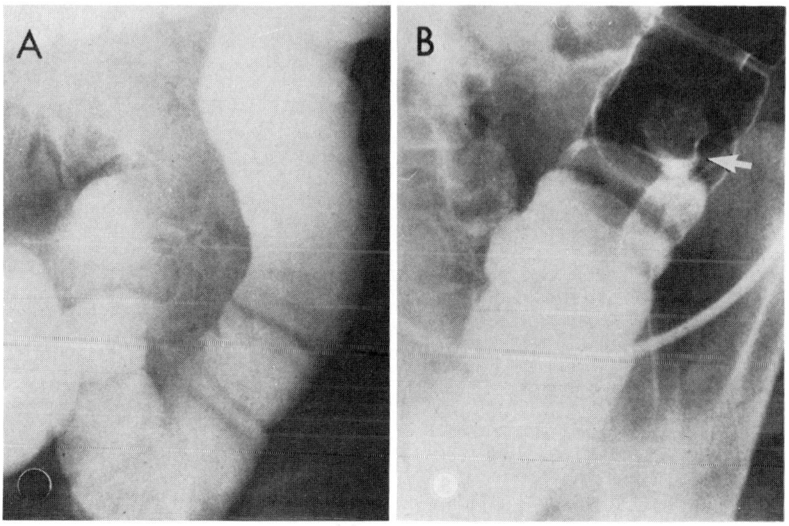

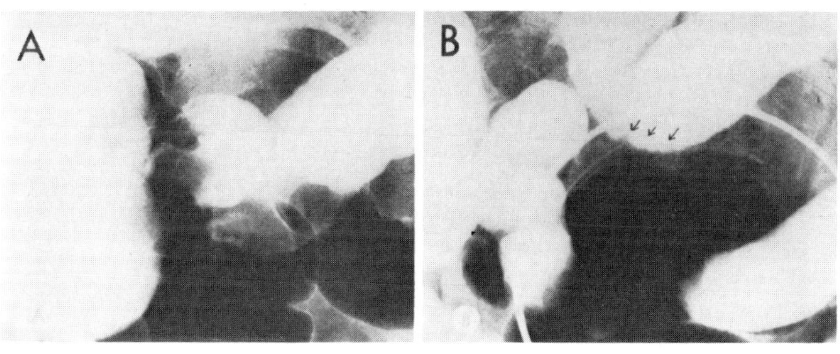

Fig 32–6 (top). – **A,** at brim of pelvis, colon appears normal with high kilovoltage technique. **B,** pedunculated, rather large polypoid lesion in this region now stands out sharply, not only because part is thinned but because lesion is fixed by compression paddle. *Arrow* points to lead ring embedded in paddle that houses balloon of compression paddle. (From Linsman, Am. J. Roentgenol. 91:846, 1964, with permission.)

Fig 32–7 (center). – Pneumocolon spot film of proximal iliac colon **(A)** contains stalked, free-floating polypoid lesion, which, with graded compression by paddle, becomes easily demonstrable *(arrow)* in **(B)**, since the part is thinned and stabilized. (From Linsman, Am. J. Roentgenol. 91:846, 1964, with permission.)

Fig 32–8 (bottom). – **A,** pneumocolon spot roentgenogram reveals low-lying midtransverse colon with inferior margin obscured by overlapping of sigmoid colon. **B,** pneumatic compression paddle has displaced transverse colon cephalad, separat ing it from pelvic colon and showing flat villous adenoma *(arrows)* on lower margin of transverse colon. (From Linsman, Am. J. Roentgenol. 91:846, 1964, with permission.)

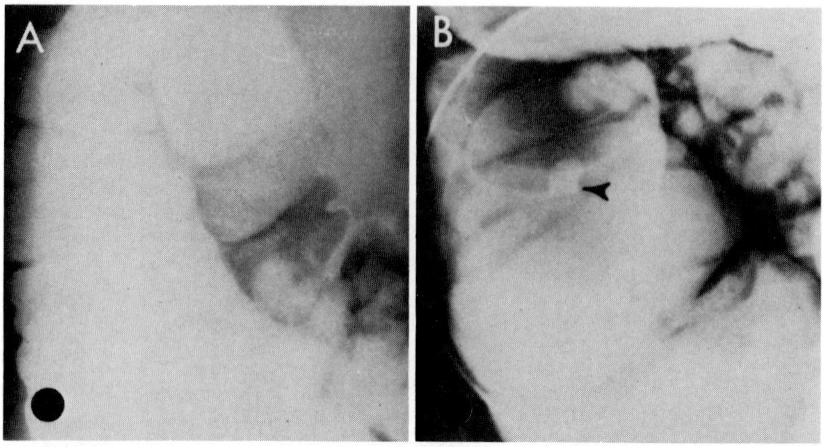

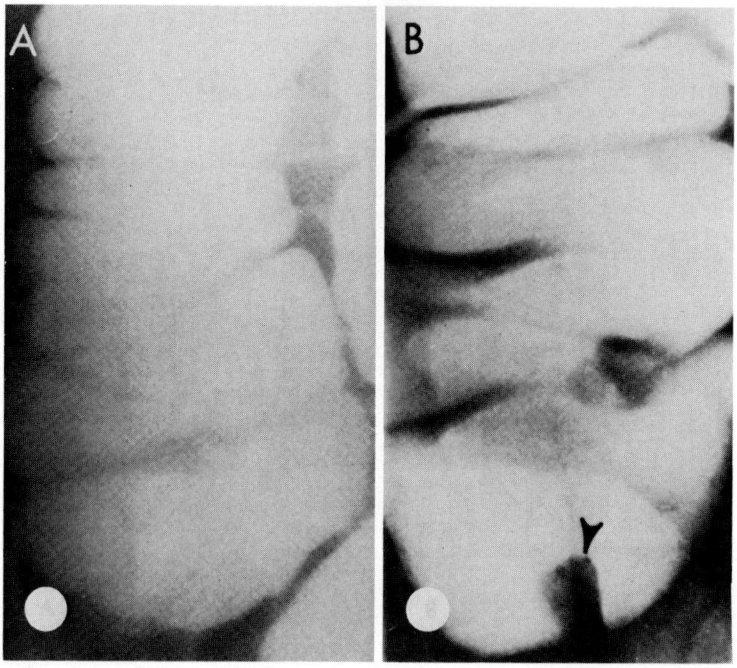

Fig 32–9 (top). – **A,** polypoid lesion is not demonstrable in ascending colon spot film. **B,** with pneumatic compression paddle in proper position and with graded compression, which stabilizes and thins the part, lesion *(arrowhead)* is nicely delineated. (From Linsman, Am. J. of Roentgenol. 91:846, 1964, with permission.)

Fig 32–10 (bottom). – **A,** cecum without compression shows neither inverted appendiceal stump nor ileocecal valve lips. **B,** with pneumatic compression paddle, both granulomatous inverted stump of appendix *(arrowhead),* which was ulcerating and a source of anemia, and ileocecal valve lips are clearly visualized. (From Linsman, Am. J. of Roentgenol. 91:846, 1964, with permission.)

Chapter 33

Pneumatosis Coli

MORTON A. MEYERS, M.D.
GARY G. GHAHREMANI, M.D.

CONCEPTS OF THE ETIOLOGY, pattern and significance of pneumatosis intestinalis (or coli) have undergone considerable change since the extensive classic review of the world literature in 1952 by Koss.[1]

Pneumatosis cystoides coli is a relatively uncommon condition characterized by multiple gas-containing cysts in the wall of the bowel. Historically, it has been held that this condition—also referred to as bullous emphysema or gas cysts of the intestine—is best classified as (1) a primary or idiopathic form (15%), which is encountered in adults and involves particularly the colon or (2) a secondary form, associated with many preexisting conditions and diseases. Subsequent reviews have subscribed to this type of classification.[2] Koss's review of the older literature found that severe pyloric stenosis was the single most common underlying disease, leading to pneumatosis cystoides of the small bowel. More recent studies strikingly differ concerning location and report a definite increased incidence of pneumatosis cystoides intestinalis involving the left colon.[3-7]

The term pneumatosis intestinalis includes not only the cystic form but other conditions of intramural gas that are typically linear in distribution and submucosal in location. Pneumatosis of the small intestine in premature infants is nearly always associated with an underlying necrotizing enterocolitis. Linear intramural pneumatosis of the colon has been increasingly recognized as associated with a variety of conditions—in the adult as well as in the child. Furthermore, pneumatosis cystoides coli may be encountered in several unique clinical situations. The spectrum of intra-abdominal entities predisposing to pneumatosis coli is listed in Table 33-1.

TABLE 33-1. —MAJOR INTRA-ABDOMINAL CAUSES OF PNEUMATOSIS COLI

Peptic ulcers
Intestinal obstruction
Abdominal trauma
Endoscopy
Acute necrotizing enterocolitis
Mesenteric vascular occlusion
Ischemic colitis
Inflammatory bowel disease
Postsurgical bowel anastomosis
Steroid therapy
Collagen disorders
Intestinal parasites

Modified from Meyers et al.[8]

Classic Pneumatosis Cystoides Coli

Classic pneumatosis cystoides coli is a readily recognizable entity. The peak of occurrence is between 30 and 60 years of age.[1] The thin-walled; noncommunicating, gas-containing cysts, which may measure up to several centimeters, are found predominantly in the serosa and subserosa and perhaps the submucosa. They appear to be composed primarily of nitrogen, presumably the residue after other gaseous components have been reabsorbed.[8] Colonoscopic and radiographic findings are characteristic, based on the presence and compressibility of intramural gas cysts and loss of pliability of the bowel wall[5, 7, 9] (Figs 33–1 and 33–2). The cysts may remain stationary, may increase in size and extension,[10] or may disappear either spontaneously,[1, 2, 10] with or without reappearance, or after treatment of any underlying gastrointestinal condition. A sterile and often asymptomatic pneumoperitoneum may be the consequence of spontaneous rupture of the cysts. Pneumatosis cystoides coli is generally a benign condition. Surgery is reserved for the rare patient with hemorrhage, obstruction or perforation. Recently oxygen administered by face mask to yield 70–75% oxygen and an arterial Po_2 of 300 mm Hg[11] has been used effectively to decompress cysts in patients with severe pneumatosis cystoides coli. By oxygen breathing, the balance of diffusion of gases between the cysts and venous blood is altered in favor of absorption of gases in the cyst, resulting in decompression. At present, it is recommended that therapy be continued for 48 hours after complete radiologic disappearance of all cysts,[12] since some instances of recurrence may be secondary to inadequate initial treatment.

Pneumatosis Coli Secondary to Pyloric Stenosis, with Chilaiditi's Syndrome

Interposition of the right colon between the liver and the diaphragm is known classically as Chilaiditi's syndrome.[13] It may be seen as an isolated phenomenon, which is often asymptomatic, but it implies failure of fusion to the posterior abdominal wall and unusually lax mesenteries. Its occasional association with pneumatosis cystoides intestinalis has been confirmed.[1, 8, 14] It has been postulated that intestine pneumatically changed by multiple gas cysts simply levitates to the upper abdomen, but the exact mechanism is unclear.

Figure 33–3 illustrates a striking triad of findings. The older literature has established the association of pneumatosis cystoides intestinalis, particularly of the jejunum, with pyloric stenosis. This case further documents that the gas cysts are within the colon interposed between liver and diaphragm.

Pneumatosis Coli Accompanying Ischemic Colitis

In 1965 Rigler and Pogue[15] reported cases of mesenteric arterial or venous thrombosis associated with crescentic linear gas collections in the wall of the infarcted bowel loops. The authors emphasized that simultaneous occurrence of gas in the portal veins is a reliable sign of intestinal necrosis. It has since been recognized that patients with *reversible* ischemic disease of the colon may present roentgen features characteristic of pneumatosis intestinalis[8] (Figs 33–4 and 33–5).

It is assumed that peripheral occlusion of mesenteric vascular branches, resulting in a transient ischemic break in the integrity of colonic mucosa, is responsible for intramural extension of bowel gas. These patients, however, do not exhibit the usual severe peritoneal irritation symptoms of intestinal necrosis or evidence of intravascular gas, and their pneumatosis typically disappears on improvement of blood circulation to the colon. The pneumatosis coli is typically localized to the area of ischemic colitis.[8] It is known that ischemic colitis may complicate reconstructive surgery of the cardiac valves or the aorta[16] or be produced by an aneurysm of the abdominal aorta.[17] In such instances careful evaluation of clinical and radiographic features is crucially important for differentiation of pneumatosis coli accompanying reversible ischemic bowel disease from that of frank intestinal gangrene.

Pneumatosis Coli Secondary to Endoscopy

Pneumatosis coli is an uncommon complication of endoscopy. Distention of the colon by gas insufflation facilitates negotiation of the colonoscope and visualization of the mucosa. However, the resultant increase in intraluminal pressure occasionally may cause a rupture of the colon in an area of anatomical weakness such as a diverticulum. Furthermore, a break in integrity of the colonic mucosa owing to ulceration or a biopsy site can permit dissection of intraluminally introduced gas into the wall of the colon, resulting in localized or generalized pneumatosis intestinalis[8] (Figs 33–6 and 33–7). Marshak and associates[18, 19] have reported several such patients in whom pneumatosis of the left side of the colon developed following sigmoidoscopy, with and without a mucosal biopsy. Although most such patients have an underlying gastrointestinal disorder, the pneumatosis coli itself can usually be managed successfully with medical treatment.

Pneumatosis Coli Secondary to Inflammatory Bowel Disease

In the toxic megacolon phase of acute ulcerative colitis, gaseous subserosal streaks are the consequence of an abnormally permeable bowel wall, perhaps further caused by gas-forming organisms, and indicate impending colonic perforation. The fulminant course of the disease and the characteristic radiographic features (Fig 33–8) clearly provide the diagnosis and prognosis of this grave condition.

In Crohn's disease, mucosal ulcerations, fistulas and stenotic segments lead to increased intraluminal pressure, which may predispose to development of pneumatosis coli. Ghahremani and co-workers[20] have noted this phenomenon (Fig 33–9).

Pneumatosis Coli in Collagen Diseases

The classic gastrointestinal changes in scleroderma consist of a dilated, atonic esophagus with decreased peristalsis in the lower two-thirds, delayed gastric emptying; decreased motility and dilatation of the small intestine; and colonic atony with sacculation or pseudodiverticulum formation. Pneumatosis may occur with sclerodermatous involvement of the bowel,[21] generally of the small intestine but rarely of the colon as well[8] (Fig 33–10), which usually has a long, progressive course. Occasionally this may be associated with a pneumoperitoneum, that is nearly always asymptomatic in itself. Although bacterial flora and electrolyte disturbances consequent to the stasis and malabsorption may play a role, the underlying mechanism for the development of the pneumatosis is probably related to the chronic intestinal distension and luminal pressures.

In contrast to the extensive fibrosis in scleroderma, the basic pathologic feature in systemic lupus erythematosus and polyarteritis nodosa is vasculitis. This involves small and medium-sized arteries and arterioles with acute and chronic perivascular cellular infiltrates. The vasculitis causes mucosal ischemia, which may lead to ulceration, infarction and perforation. With loss of mucosal integrity, gas and enteric organisms gain access to the bowel wall, and necrotizing enterocolitis ensues[22] (Fig 33–11). Intestinal vasculitis, however, was not evident clinically in benign transient pneumatosis of the colon in association with systemic lupus erythematosus; the intramural gas may have occurred secondary to structural changes in the connective tissue support in the bowel wall in the absence of intestinal ischemia.[23]

Pneumatosis Coli Secondary to Intestinal Anastomoses and to the Jejuno-Ileal Bypass Procedure

Mucosal defects at an anastomotic site may rarely permit the development of intramural cystic collections of gas, directed particularly distal to the anastomosis[8] (Fig 33–12).

Pneumatosis coli, however, is being increasingly recognized as a complication of the jejunoileal bypass procedure for morbid obesity[24-27] (Figs 33–13 and 33–14). The procedure involves an end-to-end anastomosis of the defunctionalized small bowel with the sigmoid colon. The pneumatosis has been identified from 2 weeks to 30 months after surgery and most commonly is confined to the colon, primarily the right colon, but may involve the defunctionalized small bowel or rarely both. Most observations indicate a mechanical origin of the pneumatosis through the anastomosis related to high intraluminal pressures.[24, 26] Since intraluminal pressures in the sigmoid colon often exceed 90 cm H_20 and average ileal intraluminal pressure is about 20 cm H_20, the gradient may allow dissection of gas. Some authors have suggested an inflammatory basis for the pneumatosis, involving the bypassed small bowel segment secondary to bacterial overgrowth, particularly anaerobic organisms.[25]

Pneumatosis Coli Secondary to Steroid Therapy

Steroid therapy has come to be considered a cause of pneumatosis coli (Fig 33–15), but this may not be warranted. Several case reports have appeared of patients receiving steroids who developed pneumatosis intestinalis.[28, 29] Borns and Johnston[28] postulated that steroid therapy results in severe submucosal lymphoid depletion, which then functions as a rent to allow intraluminal gas to dissect intramurally. Although this is an attractive theory, it understates the common denominator that the children receiving steroids are being treated for debilitating diseases that in themselves may account for or contribute to the development of pneumatosis.[8]

Pneumatosis Intestinalis Secondary to Hirschsprung's Disease

Robinson et al.[30] have described the association of pneumatosis intestinalis in children with obstructive lesions of the colon such as imperforate anus, Hirschsprung's disease (Fig 33–16) and meconium plug syndrome. It is believed that mucosal tears of a massively distended colon permit the intestinal gas to dissect into the submucosal and subserosal layers of the bowel wall. A contributing factor might be the mucosal ischemia resulting from diminished perfusion of the overdistended colon. Irrespective of the possible mechanisms, however, spontaneous regression of pneumatosis coli may be expected once the obstruction is relieved.[30]

Unifying Concept of Pathogenesis of Pneumatosis Coli

In pneumatosis cystoides limited to the colon, there is often associated asthma or pulmonary emphysema.[31] In 1961 Keyting et al.[32] proposed the concept that alveolar rupture may result in dissection of air along vascular channels not only to the mediastinum, as originally shown by Macklin,[33] but thereafter to the retroperitoneum and along the mesenteric attachments into the bowel wall. However, many objections exist to this explanation of the mechanism of pneumatosis cystoides coli.

In most instances of pneumatosis intestinalis, two basic mechanical factors—loss of mucosal integrity and increased intraluminal pressure—can be implicated. Kay-Butler[34] showed that cystic intramural collections of gas could be produced by inflating an excised cecum after small mucosal incisions had been made. These mechanical factors account for the pneumatosis intestinalis secondary to obstructive lesions such as pyloric stenosis and following endoscopy and intestinal anastomoses. These mechanical factors also probably account for those cases secondary to jejunoileal bypass procedure.

Infectious, ischemic or traumatic damage to the mucosa, with bacterial invasion, accounts for the pneumatosis coli in cases of necrotizing enterocolitis of infants and adults, ischemic enteritis and mesenteric infarction. The pneumatosis associated with collagen vascular disease appears to be mechanical in origin with chronic intestinal distention and increased intraluminal pressure associated with scleroderma, whereas pneumatosis associated with systemic lupus erythematosus and periarteritis nodosa appears to have an ischemic basis secondary to the vasculitis. The pneumatosis associated with cortisone therapy may be secondary to loss of mucosal integrity owing to many factors, including perhaps lymphoid depletion of Peyer's patches as well as the underlying debilitating disease.

Radiologic identification of pneumatosis intestinalis may be crucial in indicating the underlying condition, appropriate therapy and prognosis.

REFERENCES

1. Koss, L. G.: Abdominal gas cysts (pneumatosis cystoides intestinorum hominis). An analysis with a report of a case and a critical review of the literature, Arch. Pathol. 53:523, 1952.
2. Colquhoun, J.: Intramural gas in hollow viscera, Clin. Radiol. 16:71, 1965.
3. Ecker, J. A., Williams, R. G., and Clay, K. L.: Pneumatosis cystoides intestinalis – Bullous emphysema of the intestine. A review of the literature, Am. J. Gastroenterol. 56:125, 1971.
4. Olmsted, W. W., and Madewell, J. E.: Pneumatosis cystoides intestinalis, Gastrointest. Radiol. 1:177, 1976.
5. Varano, V., and Bonanno, C.: Colonoscopic findings in pneumatosis cystoides intestinalis, Am. J. Gastroenterol. 59:353, 1973.
6. Shallal, J., van Heerdon, J., Bartholomew, L., and Cain, J.: Pneumatosis cystoides intestinalis, Mayo Clin. Proc. 49:180, 1974.
7. Marshak, R. H., Lindner, A. E., and Maklansky, D.: Pneumatosis cystoides coli, Gastrointest. Radiol. 2:85, 1977.
8. Meyers, M. A., Ghahremani, G. G., Clements, J. L., Jr., and Goodman, K.: Pneumatosis intestinalis, Gastrointest. Radiol. 2:91, 1977.
9. Smith, W. G., Anderson, M. J., Jr., and Pemerton, H. W.: Pneumatosis cystoides intestinalis involving left portion of colon. Report of four cases diagnosed at sigmoidoscopy, Gastroenterology 35:528, 1958.
10. Bloch, C.: The natural history of pneumatosis coli, Radiology 123:311, 1977.
11. Gruenberg, J. C., Batra, S. K., and Prigst, R. J.: Treatment of pneumatosis cystoides intestinalis with oxygen, Arch. Surg. 112:62, 1977.
12. Simon, N., Nyman, K., Divertie, M., Rovelstad, R., and King, J.: Pneumatosis cystoides intestinalis: Treatment with oxygen via close fitting mask, J.A.M.A. 321:1354, 1975.
13. Chilaiditi, D.: Zur Frage der Hepatoptose and Ptose im Allemeinen im Anschluss and drei Fälle von temporärer partieller Leberverlagerung, Fortschr. Geb. Roentgenstr. 16:173, 1910–1911.
14. Kenney, J. G.: Pneumatosis intestinalis, Clin. Radiol. 14:70, 1963.
15. Rigler, L. O., and Pogue, W. L.: Roentgen signs of intestinal necrosis, Am. J. Roentgenol. 94:402, 1965.
16. Johnson, W. C., and Nasbeth, D. C.: Visceral infarction following aortic surgery, Ann. Surg. 180:312, 1974.
17. McKain, Jr., and Shumacker, H. B., Jr.: Ischemia of the left colon associated with abdominal aortic aneurysms and their treatment, Arch. Surg. 76:355, 1958.
18. Marshak, R. H., Lipsay, J. J., and Friedman, A. I.: Pneumatosis of the colon, J.A.M.A. 148:1416, 1952.
19. Marshak, R. H., Lindner, A. E., and Milano, A. M.: Pneumatosis coli, Am. J. Gastroenterol. 56:68, 1971.
20. Ghahremani, G. G., Port, R. B., and Beachley, M. D.: Pneumatosis coli in Crohn's disease, Am. J. Dig. Dis. 19:315, 1974.
21. Gompels, B. M.: Pneumatosis cystoides intestinalis associated with progressive systemic sarcoidosis, Br. J. Radiol. 42:701, 1969.
22. Kleinman, P., Meyers, M. A., Abbott, G., and Kazam, E.: Necrotizing enterocolitis with pneumatosis intestinalis in systemic lupus erythematosus and polyarteritis, Radiology 121:595, 1976.
23. Freiman, D., Chon, H., and Bilaniuk, L.: Pneumatosis intestinalis in systemic lupus erythematosus, Radiology 116:563, 1975.
24. Martyak, S., and Curtis, L.: Pneumatosis intestinalis a complication of jejunoileal bypass, J.A.M.A. 235:1038, 1976.
25. Passaro, E., Drenick, E., and Wilson, S.: Bypass enteritis, Am. J. Surg. 131:169, 1976.
26. Feinberg, S. B., Schwartz, M. Z., Clifford, S., Buchwald, H., and Varco, R. L.: Significance of pneumatosis cystoides intestinalis after jejunoileal bypass, Am. J. Surg. 133:149, 1977.

27. Clements, J. L., Jr.: Intestinal pneumatosis—A complication of the jejunoileal bypass procedure, Gastrointest. Radiol. 2:267, 1977.
28. Borns, P. F., and Johnston, T. A.: Indolent pneumatosis of bowel wall associated with immune suppressive therapy, Ann. Radiol. 16:163, 1973.
29. Keats, T. E., and Smith, T. H.: Benign pneumatosis intestinalis in childhood leukemia, Am. J. Roentgenol. 122:150, 1974.
30. Robinson, A. E., Grossman, H., and Brumley, G. W.: Pneumatosis intestinalis in the neonate, Am. J. Roentgenol. 120:333, 1974.
31. Doub, H. P., and Shea, J. J.: Pneumatosis cystoides intestinalis, J.A.M.A. 172:1238, 1960.
32. Keyting, W. S., McCarver, R. R., Kovarik, J. L., and Daywitt, A. L.: Pneumatosis intestinalis: A new concept, Radiology 76:733, 1961.
33. Macklin, C. C.: Transport of air along sheaths of pulmonic blood vessels from alveoli to mediastinum: Clinical implications, Arch. Intern. Med. 64: 913, 1939.
34. Kay-Butler, J. J.: Interstitial emphysema of the cecum, Gut 3:267, 1962.

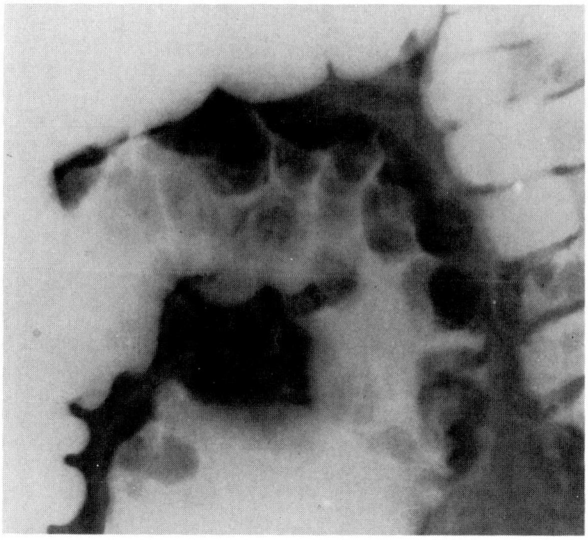

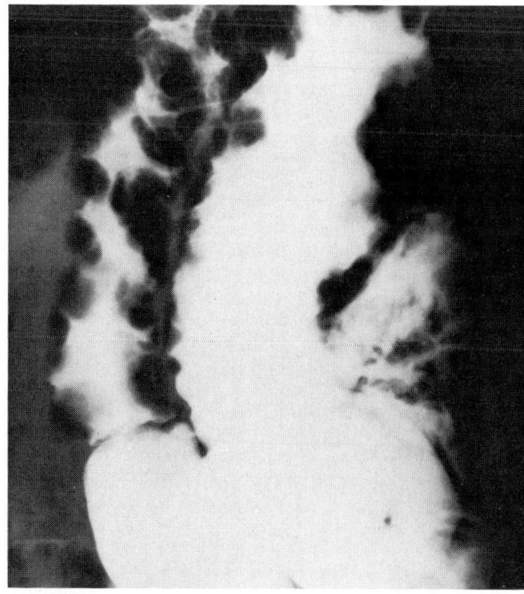

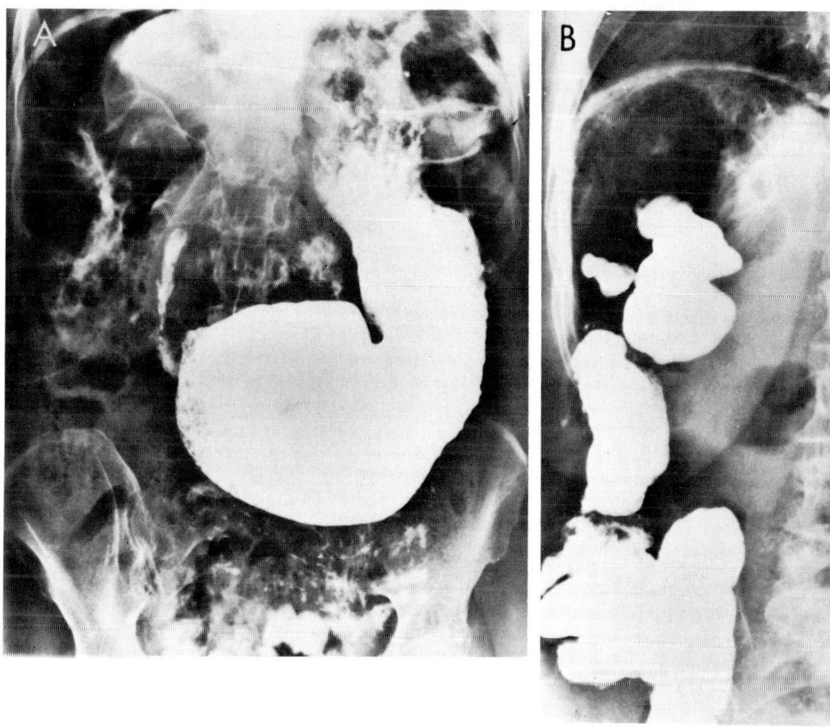

Fig 33–1 (top left).—Pneumatosis cystoides coli. Multiple intramural gas cysts along course of sigmoid colon produce nodular impressions on contrast-filled lumen and clearly extend as radiolucent collections.

Fig 33–2 (top right).—Pneumatosis cystoides coli. Sigmoid colon, which extends high into left upper quadrant, demonstrates indentations on bowel contour by numerous gas cysts. Outer margins of radiolucent cysts are well delineated.

Fig 33–3 (bottom).—Chilaiditi's syndrome with pneumatosis coli accompanying pyloric stenosis. **A,** upper gastrointestinal series demonstrates gastric outlet obstruction from markedly narrowed pyloroduodenal deformity. Cystic and loculated gaseous structures occupy right upper quadrant. Note that curvilinear densities are outlined in this area, suggesting pneumoperitoneum. **B,** delayed film shows hepatodiaphragmatic interposition of colon in which pneumatosis cystoides is present. Curvilinear densities represent summation of shadows of overlapping cyst walls, as described by Kenney.[14] (From Meyers et al., Gastrointest. Radiol. 2:91, 1977, with permission.)

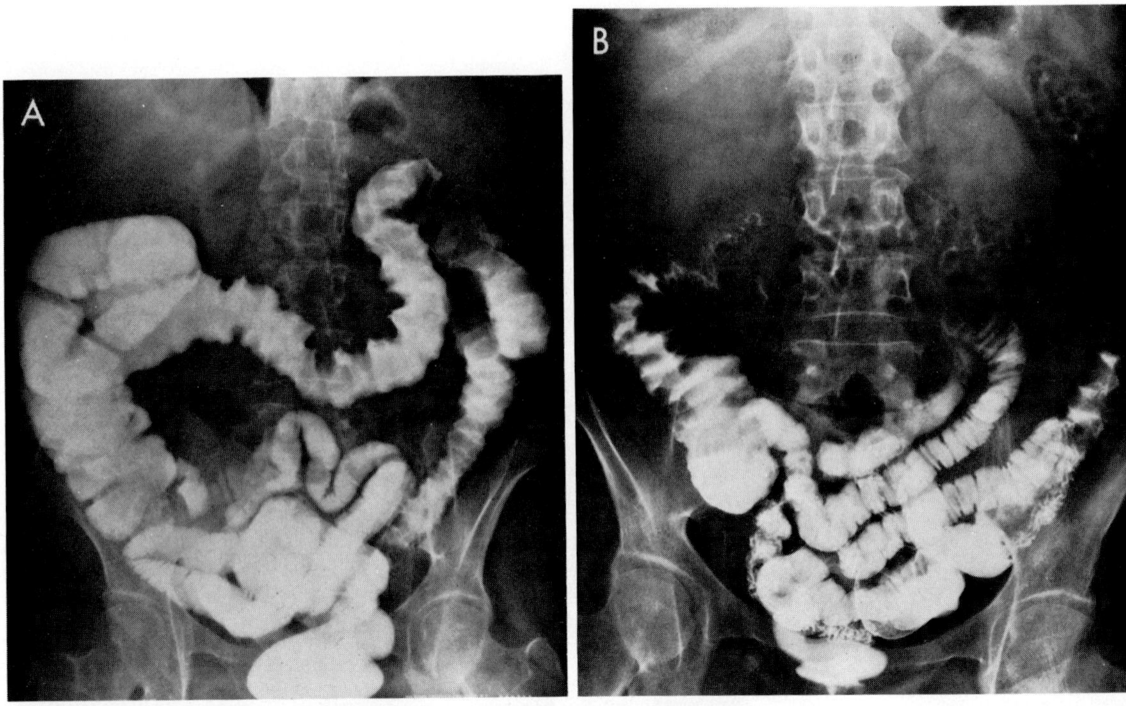

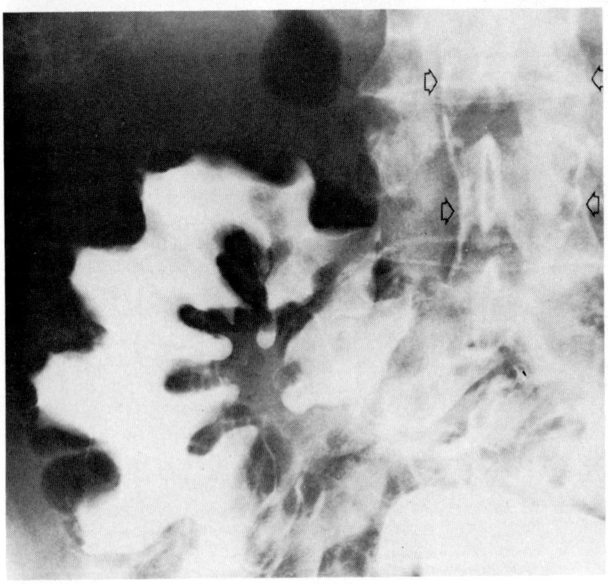

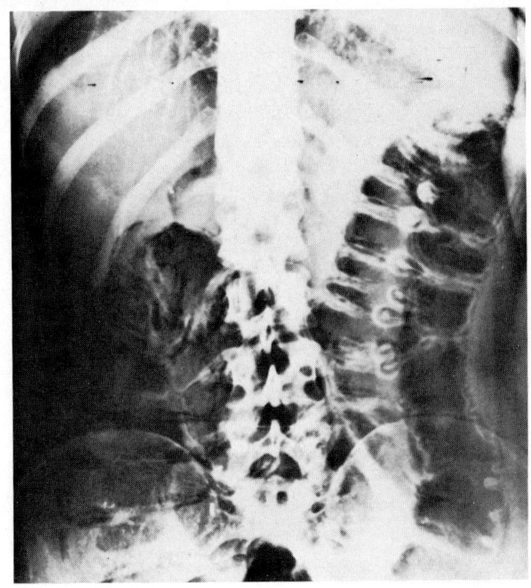

Fig 33–4 (top).—Pneumatosis cystoides coli accompanying ischemic colitis, following mitral valve replacement and postoperative coumadin. **A** and **B,** pneumatosis cystoides throughout transverse and descending colon, accompanying thumbprinting and transverse ridging of ischemic colitis. Ten days later, after conservative management and adequate anticoagulant therapy, there was virtually complete resolution of changes. (From Meyers et al., Gastrointest. Radiol. 2:91, 1977, with permission.)

Fig 33–5 (bottom left).—Pneumatosis coli accompanying ischemic colitis. Prominent cystic collections of intramural gas are associated with evidence of ischemic changes involving redundant sigmoid colon. Calcified aneurysmal dilatation of lower abdominal aorta is seen *(arrows).* Following anticoagulant therapy and oxygen administration by face mask, bloody stools and radiographic findings resolved. (From Meyers et al., Gastrointest. Radiol. 2:91, 1977, with permission.)

Fig 33–6 (bottom right).—Pneumatosis coli following proctoscopy. Linear intramural gas highlights haustra and septa of large intestine. Under medical observation, this episode resolved completely within 1 week. (From Meyers et al., Gastrointest. Radiol. 2:91, 1977, with permission.)

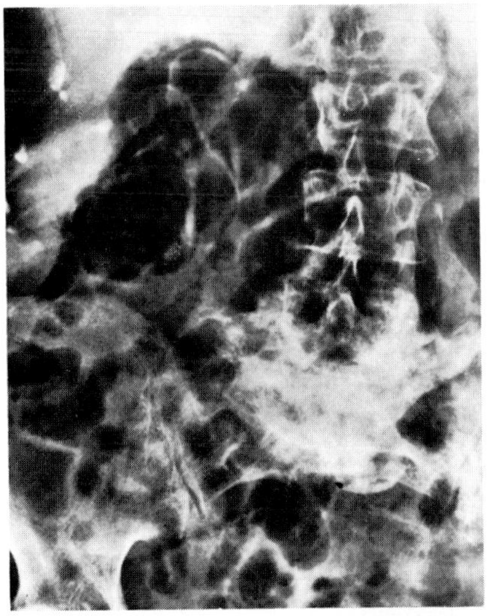

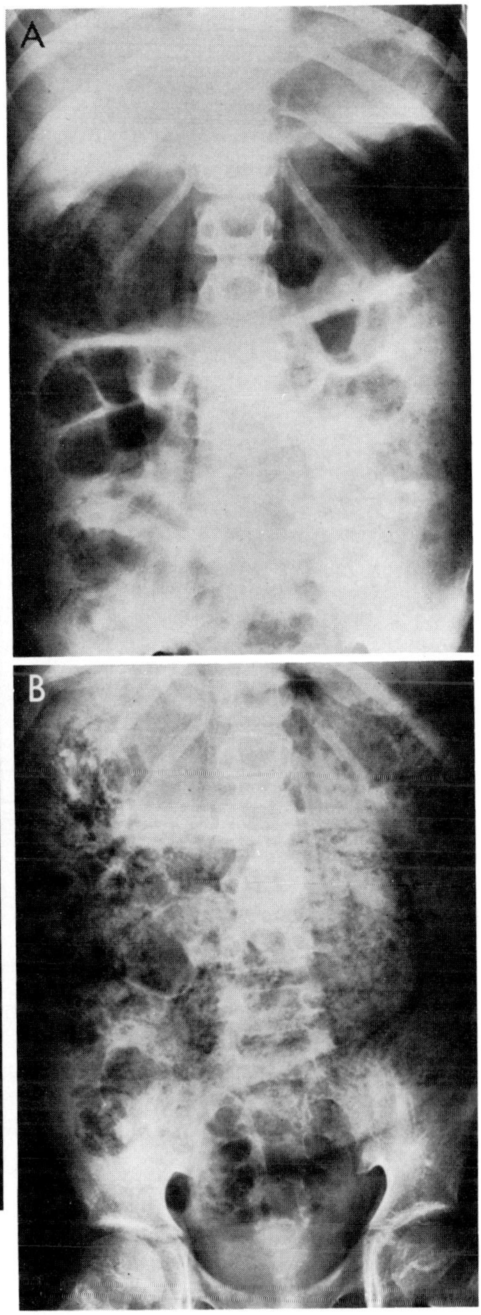

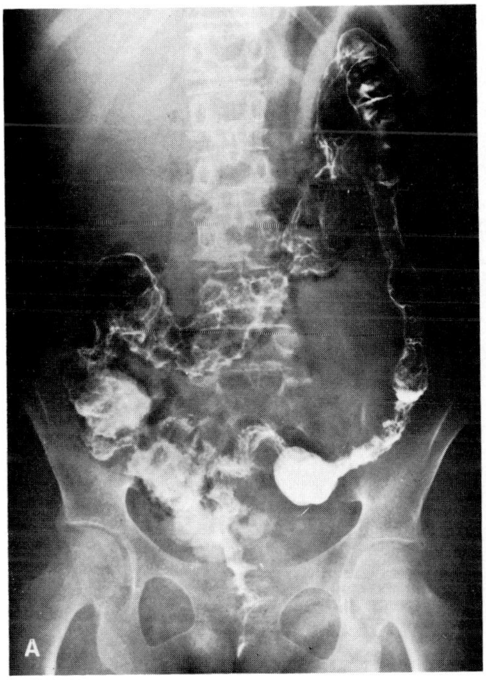

Fig 33–7 (top left). – Pneumatosis coli secondary to colonoscopy. Plain film following colonoscopy demonstrates pneumatosis of hepatic flexure of colon. (From Meyers et al., Gastrointest. Radiol. 2:91, 1977, with permission.)

Fig 33–8 (right). – Pneumatosis coli complicating toxic megacolon in girl, age 10. **A,** admission supine film demonstrates massive distention of transverse colon. Defects produced by pseudopolypoid changes of ulcerative colitis are evident. **B,** 24 hours later, extensive mottled gaseous collections are scattered throughout wall of grangrenous colon. (From Meyers et al., Gastrointest. Radiol. 2:91, 1977, with permission.)

Fig 33–9 (bottom left). – Pneumatosis coli associated with granulomatous ileocolitis in girl, age 17. Postevacuation barium enema film demonstrates mucosal ulcerations of sigmoid and colon proximal to splenic flexure. Latter segment is involved with pneumatosis coli. (From Ghahremani et al., Am. J. Dig. Dis. 19:315, 1974, with permission.)

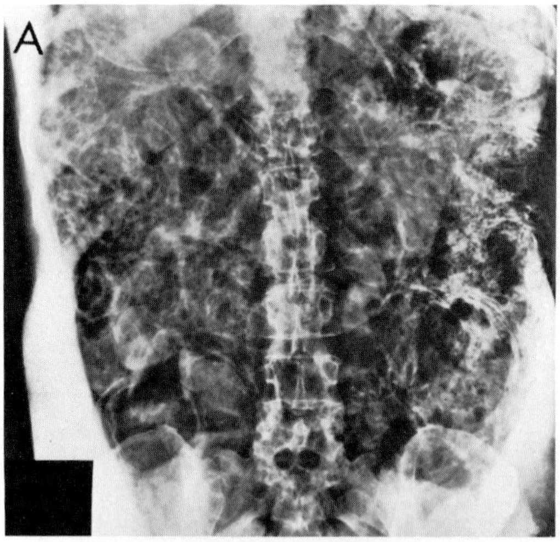

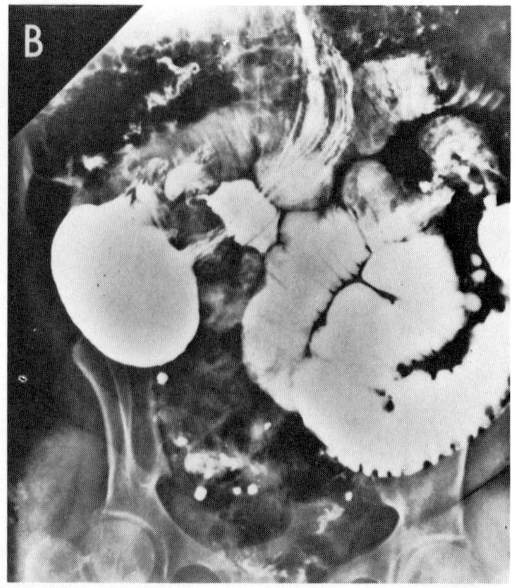

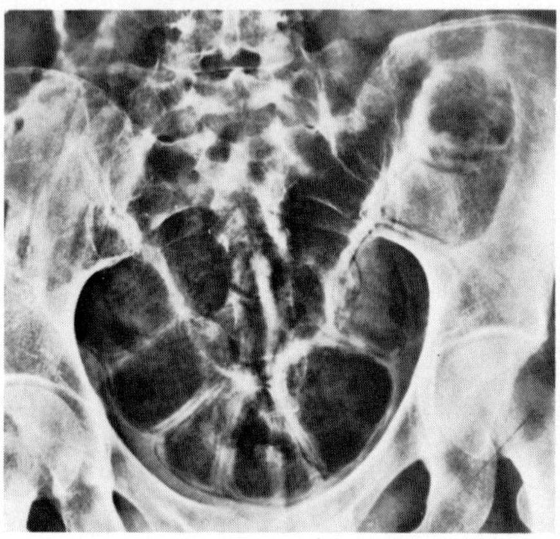

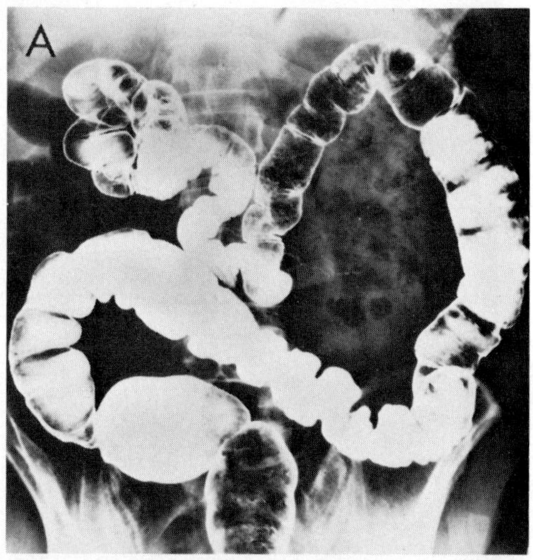

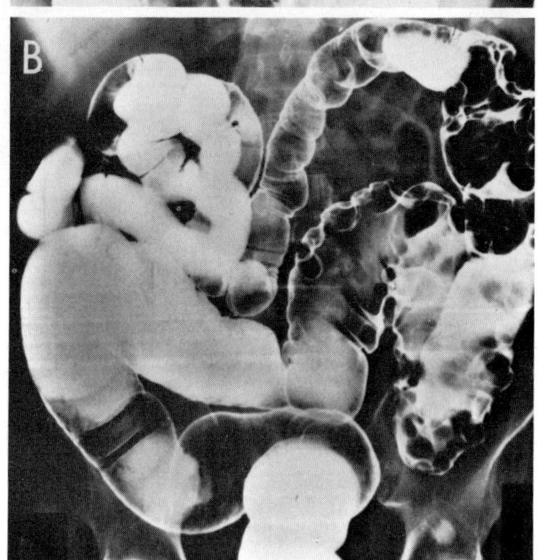

Fig 33–10 (top).—Pneumatosis coli secondary to scleroderma. **A,** plain film demonstrates extensive intestinal pneumatosis. **B,** small bowel series. Sclerodermatous involvement is shown by dilatation, stasis and pseudodiverticular formation. Pneumatosis involves both small and large intestine. (From Meyers et al., Gastrointest. Radiol. 2:91, 1977, with permission.)

Fig 33–11 (center left).—Pneumatosis coli in systemic lupus erythematosus. Plain film demonstrates extensive curvilinear collections of intramural gas within distal colon. This led to liquefaction necrosis secondary to vasculitis.

Fig 33–12 (center and **bottom right).**—Pneumatosis cystoides coli distal to surgical anastomosis. **A,** barium enema study following right hemicolectomy and ileotransverse colostomy demonstrates no other abnormalities. **B,** 20 months later, conspicuous gas cysts have developed over a considerable length in colon distal to anastomosis. (From Meyers et al., Gastrointest. Radiol. 2:91, 1977, with permission.)

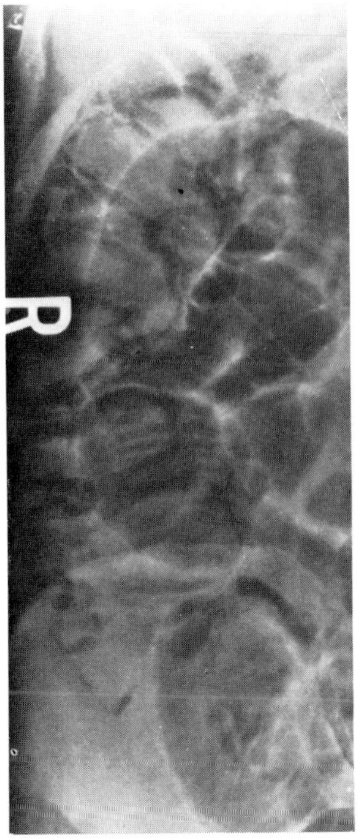

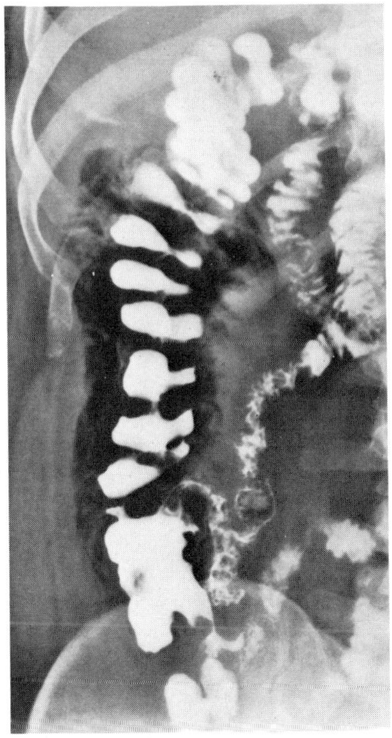

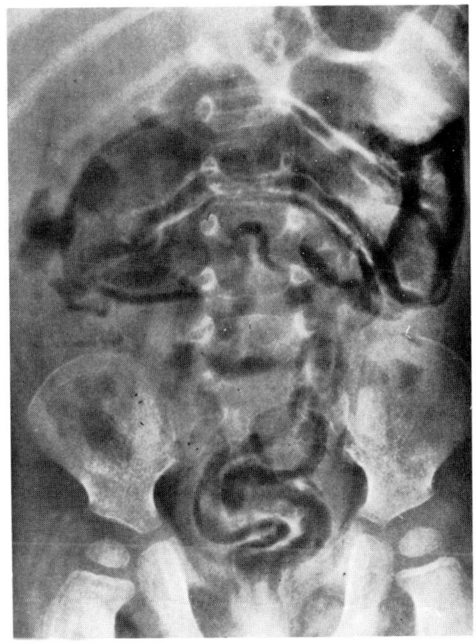

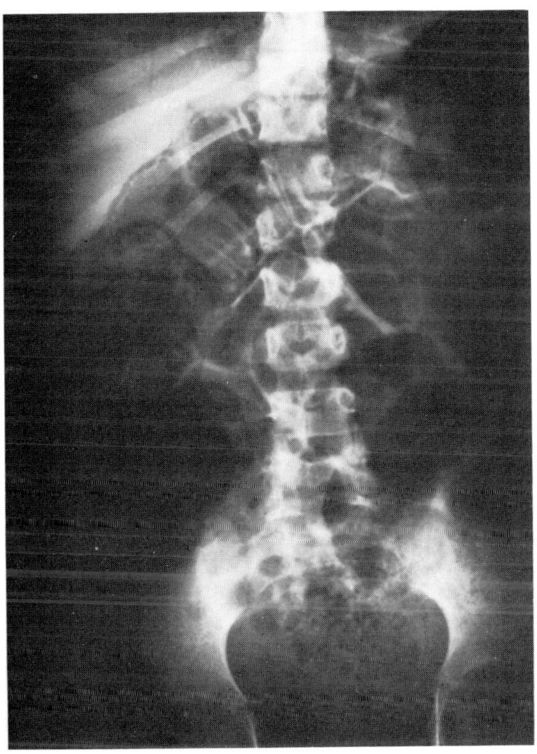

Fig 33–13 (top left).—Pneumatosis coli secondary to jejunoileal surgical bypass. Plain film shows intramural gas within ascending colon. (From Meyers et al., Gastrointest. Radiol. 2:91, 1977, with permission.)

Fig 33–14 (top center).—Pneumatosis coli secondary to jejunoileal surgical bypass. Delayed film of small bowel series demonstrates severe pneumatosis of ascending colon. (From Meyers et al., Gastrointest. Radiol. 2:91, 1977, with permission.)

Fig 33–15 (top right).—Pneumatosis coli in child with acute lymphatic leukemia on steroid therapy. Conspicuous intramural gas is present throughout left colon. Serial plain films showed complete resolution of pneumatosis by 6th day. (From Meyers et al., Gastrointest. Radiol. 2:91, 1977, with permission.)

Fig 33–16 (bottom).—Pneumatosis coli secondary to Hirschsprung's disease in a girl, age 6. Prominent intramural gas present within dilated transverse colon. There also is dilatation of intestinal loops due to fecal impaction in distal colon. Following pull-through operation, pneumatosis coli of unresected proximal colon showed gradual but complete regression. (From Meyers et al., Gastrointest. Radiol. 2:91, 1977, with permission.)

Chapter 34

Polypoid Lesions of the Colon

ROBERT N. BERK, M.D.

MUCH OF THE CONFUSION concerning the classification and malignant potential of colonic polyps is due to the indiscriminate use of terms. The word polyp has no specific histologic implications but indicates only that a circumscribed excrescence or mass protrudes from a mucosal surface. Such elevations may be either sessile (broad based) or have a pedicle (pedunculated). The term polypoid lesion is synonymous with polyp but is preferred because it emphasizes the heterogeneous nature of this group of tumors and pseudotumors. This is the term used in the present discussion, since the intention here is to review the radiologic features of all types of polypoid masses of the colon, whether they are actually neoplastic lesions or not.

TABLE 34-1. —CLASSIFICATION OF POLYPOID LESIONS OF THE COLON

Neoplastic polyps
Benign
Adenomatous
Villous
Lipoma
Leiomyoma
Neurofibroma
Hemangioma
Malignant
Adenocarcinoma
Lymphoma
Leukemic infiltration
Metastases
Nonneoplastic polyps
Hyperplastic
Hamartoma
Lymphoid hyperplasia
Pneumatosis coli
Pseudopolyposis

Histologically, polypoid lesions may be classified as neoplastic (benign and malignant) and nonneoplastic (Table 34-1). The two main varieties of benign neoplastic polyps (adenomatous polyps and villous adenomas) are of major importance because of their relationship to carcinoma.

Adenoma-Carcinoma Sequence

Although the subject of controversy for years, benign adenomas—both adenomatous polyps and villous adenomas—have been shown convincingly by accumulated data to be the precursors of most carcinomas of the colon[1-5] (Fig 34-1). Evidence for this adenoma-carcinoma sequence includes the fact that benign tumors occur in continuity with carcinoma.[5] Careful histologic study of malignant tumors reveals all gradations: from an adenomatous polyp, to an adenomatous polyp with a microscopic focus of invasive carcinoma, to an obvious cancer.[4] Varying proportions of adenomatous tissue were found in 14% of 1,961 colonic carcinomas studied by Muto et al.[5] Furthermore, Morson[6] reported that the incidence of the benign component of the carcinoma is inversely related to the degree of extension of the tumor through the bowel wall.[4-6] This suggests that, as the carcinoma grows, progressively more of the precursor adenoma is destroyed or is transformed into malignant tissue. Further evidence for the adenoma-carcinoma sequence is the fact that documented cases of de novo intramucosal carcinoma, unassociated with an adenoma in an otherwise normal colon, have not been observed.[1-3] In addition, carcinoma develops in nearly all patients with familial polyposis who do not have a colectomy.[6] Finally, the anticipated incidence of carcinoma is reduced in patients who undergo annual proctosigmoidoscopy and polypectomy.[7]

Since the incidence of polyps is much greater than that of carcinoma, the adenoma-carcinoma sequence must be relatively uncommon. However, not all polyps have an equal propensity to become carcinoma. Morson[3, 4] has shown that the malignant potential of adenomas is influenced by the size and histologic type of the polyp. Data from the St. Mark's Hospital in London show that the prevalence of carcinoma in adenomas less than 1 cm in size is only about 1%, whereas carcinoma occurs in 46% of adenomas over 2 cm in size.[3-5] Similarly, Morson[3, 4] and Muto et al.[5] showed that the incidence of carcinoma is much higher in patients with villous adenomas than in those with adenomatous polyps. However, these authors emphasize that, as adenomatous polyps grow, they have a tendency to assume a villous pattern and that, in addition, individual polyps have a spectrum of histologic appearances. Considering that benign hyperplastic polyps are 10 times more common than adenomatous polyps and that small adenomatous polyps (less than 1.5 cm in size) are 10 times more common than large adenomatous polyps, large adenomatous polyps represent only 1% of all colonic polyps.[2] Consequently, the adenoma-carcinoma sequence occurs with greater regularity in large adenomatous polyps than anticipated from the overall incidence of adenomatous polyps and carcinoma.

The stages of the sequence from adenoma to carcinoma include preinvasion, invasion, proliferation and penetration. The transformation probably requires 5 years or more in most cases, although the time involved is extremely variable[4] (Fig 34–2). This has obvious importance in the management of patients with polyps or in those with the propensity to develop them.

Radiologic Detection of Polypoid Lesions

The number of polyps discovered by barium enema examination varies considerably depending on the technique used. The frequency of polyps detected with the single contrast barium enema ranges from 1 to 8% but increases with the air contrast technique to 10–13%.[1] The latter figures compare with the average autopsy incidence of colonic polyps (12%) and indicate that the air contrast examination is more sensitive in detecting these lesions[1] (Fig 34–3). Up to 60% of polyps diagnosed by the air contrast examination are less than 5 mm in size, which confirms the ability of this procedure to reveal small lesions of the colon[8] (Figs 34–4 and 34–5). Although available figures favor the air contrast examination for detection of polyps, an adequately controlled study comparing the sensitivity of the two barium enema techniques has not been done.

A high index of suspicion of polyps must be maintained in patients with one or more additional risk factors for developing carcinoma of the colon (Table 34–2). An air contrast barium enema examination should be performed in this group of patients and in those with evidence of blood in the stool as shown by the hemoccult test. In others who are less likely to have polyps, and in the elderly or sick in whom the detection of polyps is less significant, a single contrast barium study is sufficient.

Accurate detection of colonic polyps depends on thorough cleansing of the colon.

TABLE 34-2.—RISK FACTORS IN COLORECTAL CARCINOMA

Age—over 40 years
Associated disease
Ulcerative colitis
Granulomatous colitis
Familial polyposis
Gardner's disease
Past history
Colonic polyps or cancer
Female genital or breast cancer
Family history
Colonic polyps or cancer
Familial polyposis
Gardner's disease

After Winawer, S. J., et al., Gastroenterology 70:783, 1976.

This prerequisite must not be ignored and requires vigorous preparation of the patient. This should include a low-residue diet, two sequential laxatives, hydration and properly administered cleansing enemas. The responsibility for preparation of the patient should be assumed by the radiologist, who must communicate its importance to the patient, the nursing staff and the referring physician. When necessary, cleansing enemas should be given by radiology personnel, either on the ward or in the radiology department.[9]

That adenocarcinoma of the colon nearly always arises in adenomatous polyps (adenoma-carcinoma sequence), in conjunction with the ability of the colonoscopist to resect polyps without resorting to laparotomy, places a new burden of responsibility on the radiologist to identify adenomatous polyps. Success depends on the skillful performance of the air contrast barium enema examination. Appropriate filling of the colon with air and barium in proper proportions under fluoroscopic guidance; careful spot filming; radiographs made in the proper positions with exacting radiographic technique; and scrupulous preparation of the colon are essential. Furthermore, since the malignant potential of a polypoid tumor varies with the size, presence and length of a stalk as well as the configuration (irregular, lobulated, smooth), these features must be fully evaluated on the barium enema study and carefully described in the written report.

Neoplastic Polyps

BENIGN POLYPOID TUMORS

Adenomatous Polyps

Although a precise histologic diagnosis is impossible on barium enema examinations, certain radiologic findings suggest a specific diagnosis (Figs 34-6 to 34-9). Of particular importance is detection of a stalk that, when longer than 1 cm, indicates that the polyp is adenomatous and nonmalignant.[10] The stalk consists of stroma, blood vessels and lymphatics pulled into the lumen by the force of peristalsis on the mucosa and submucosa. Adenomatous polyps tend to be nodular and to have a narrow base when they arise, so that the lesion and adjacent mucosa are readily pulled into a pedicle by peristalsis as the lesion enlarges. Pedicles are rare in villous adenomas, which are flat and have a wide base with less tendency to prolapse into the lumen. Invasion of the submucosa, which occurs early in carcinoma, fixes the lesion to the muscularis beneath the tumor, making pedicle development impossible.[10]

Adenomatous polyps and other types of tumors must be distinguished from fecal material, mucus, air bubbles and oil droplets (Figs 34-10 and 34-11). This usually is possible, based on identification of a constant relation between a polyp and the bowel wall on projections made in different positions. On the other hand, extraneous materials in the lumen move in relation to the bowel wall under the influence of gravity. Occasionally, fecal material may be tenacious and adhere to the mucosa, so that differentiation from tumor will be virtually impossible. In these cases a second barium enema examination, performed after better preparation of the colon, is required.

Diverticula can readily be distinguished from polyps, if they project beyond the lumen (Fig 34–12). A barium-coated, air-filled diverticulum superimposed on the bowel, however, may simulate a polyp. In these cases the ring of barium coating the diverticulum has a smooth, well-defined outer border and an irregular inner surface.[11] Conversely, the barium coating a polyp is smooth on its inner border and poorly defined on the outer. This difference occurs because the barium is inside the diverticulum but on the surface of the polyp.

Villous Adenomas

Villous adenomas often have a characteristic radiologic appearance[12,13] (Figs 34–13 and 34–14). These lesions have multiple frondlike outgrowths of epithelium over their surface that appear shaggy and irregular on barium studies. Barium in the interstices of the tumor surface produces unique striated, reticulated or lacelike radiographic features. This typical appearance is more frequent in villous adenomas on the left side of the colon than on the right.[13] In fact, most villous adenomas in the cecum and ascending colon are indistinguishable from adenomatous polyps and adenocarcinoma.

Stalks are unusual in villous adenomas and are almost never longer than 1 cm.[10] Hence, a polypoid lesion on a long stalk is far more likely to be an adenomatous polyp.

Lipomas

Although lipomas of the colon are second only to adenomatous polyps in frequency, they still are uncommon. Comfort and Stearns[14] report an incidence of 0.5% in a series of 3,934 autopsies. The lesion may occur in any part of the colon, but almost two-thirds occur on the right side, usually in the cecum and ascending colon.

The diagnosis of lipoma may be suspected when radiographic examination discloses a single, sharply defined, smooth intramural lesion of the colon[15,16] (Figs 34–15 to 34–17). When the tumor is on a pseudopedicle, the mass is intraluminal. The shape and sharpness of the tumor mass and the smooth surface, with normal pliability and distensibility of the bowel wall, are often sufficient to suggest the diagnosis of lipoma. The defect usually is spherical or oval, although occasionally it is irregular owing to lobulations in the mass. The pedicle is short and broad, and the lesion is mobile. Some lipomas reach large size without developing a pseudopedicle and becoming an intraluminal mass. This variety produces an intramural defect with sharp demarcation, broad base and smooth surface.

With proper spot radiograms, the soft consistency of the tumor may be detected by changes in tumor shape with compression. The relative radiolucency of the tumor rarely is appreciated on conventional barium enema examinations.

Simple surgical excision of uncomplicated colonic lipomas usually is recommended. Removal is necessary because, although the tumors are benign, they are not harmless. None of the tumors becomes malignant, but excision establishes a definite diagnosis and avoids the hazards of colonic obstruction, intussusception and bleeding.

Rare Benign Tumors

Leiomyomas are uncommon in the colon. They tend to maintain their intramural position more consistently than lipomas and therefore may remain asymptomatic until they become large. Mucosal folds overlying the lesion persist longer than with a lipoma and, as a result, the characteristic sharp demarcation of mural lesions may be absent. Specific differentiation from other extramucosal lesions usually is impossible. The broad-based, lobulated, smooth mass indicates only that the lesion arises in the bowel wall beneath the mucosa and that it is intramural.

Hemangiomas of the colon are rare submucosal tumors, which may be recognized radiographically by detection of calcified phleboliths within the tumor mass. Neurofibromas of the colon may occur alone or in association with generalized neurofibromatosis (Figs 34–18 to 34–20). In one series, 25% of patients with neurofibromatosis had a neurofibroma of the small bowel or colon, and 10% of these had intestinal neurofibrosarcoma.[17] The neurofibromas tend to be multiple and, in the small bowel at least, have a propensity to involve only one side of the bowel wall.[18]

MALIGNANT POLYPOID TUMORS

Polypoid Adenocarcinoma

Like other cancers of the gastrointestinal tract, adenocarcinoma of the colon may be polypoid, infiltrating or ulcerative. Each morphologic type has a characteristic radiologic appearance. In the polypoid variety, barium enema examination discloses a tumor mass with a rough, irregular, lobulated surface, which usually is distinct from the smooth configuration of benign submucosal lesions such as a lipoma (Fig 34–21). The stalk is not over 1 cm in length.[10] A contour defect in the barium column is characteristic[19] (Figs 34–22 to 34–24). This consists of an interruption in the margin of the colon produced by the desmoplastic reaction associated with the carcinoma. This retraction abnormality is an ominous sign and is of great importance in radiologic differential diagnosis between carcinoma and a benign polyp. Complications of adenocarcinoma include obstruction, perforation and intussusception (Fig 34–25).

Lymphoma

Lymphomas arise in lymphoid tissue in the submucosa of the colon and extend along the long axis of the bowel. Growth may be into the lumen or outside the bowel. Exophytic extension produces large tumor masses outside the bowel, extending into the mesentery. Tumors are often multiple. Because lymphosarcoma is a medullary tumor, the lesion may grow to a large size before obstruction develops, which then causes symptoms. Hemorrhage, perforation, intussusception, fistula and malabsorption may occur.

Marshak et al.[19] classify lymphosarcoma in five morphologic categories: nodular, infiltrating, polypoid, exo-endoenteric and mesenteric (Figs 34–26 to 34–28). Many cases have features of several forms of the disease.

In the nodular variety of lymphosarcoma, there are multiple intraluminal or intramural tumor masses of the same or varying size. The lesions are sharply defined and frequently extend across the ileocecal valve into the terminal ileum. The lumen of the bowel is normal or increased in diameter. Differentiation from multiple polyposis, metastatic disease and inflammatory conditions may be difficult. The cobblestone pattern of the mucosa in granulomatous colitis may simulate lymphosarcoma, although ulcerations, edema, narrowing of the lumen and exudate in the lumen are concomitant features of Crohn's disease that are absent in lymphosarcoma. The multiple nodules of familial polyposis may be indistinguishable from those of lymphosarcoma.

In the polypoid form of lymphosarcoma, the tumor grows into the lumen from its submucosal origin. The lesion is usually smooth and sharply demarcated and is typical of mural lesions of any cause. Peristalsis may create a pseudopedicle, or the mass may form the lead point for an intussusception (Fig 34–29). The tumor often reaches a large size without producing narrowing of the lumen. Multiple tumors are common.

Metastases and Leukemic Infiltration

Marshak et al.[20] divide metastatic disease of the bowel into three morphologic categories: (1) single or multiple lesions involving primarily the wall of the intestine, (2) lesions involving primarily the mesentery and (3) multiple lesions that involve both the bowel wall and mesentery. Ascites is common in the last group.

Discrete tumor masses that primarily involve the bowel wall produce well-defined mural lesions in the colon that are difficult to distinguish from other extramucosal lesions (Fig 34–30). The desmoplastic reaction associated with metastases often causes pleating of the mucosa, which is apparent on barium enema examination. Lesions are usually multiple, and ascites may be present.

The incidence of leukemic infiltration of the gastrointestinal tract varies between 10% and 60% in different series.[21] In lymphocytic leukemia, involvement usually is confined to the mucosa and submucosa. In the myelogenous variety, the infiltrate may be localized or diffuse, and the infiltrates may form plaques, nodules or masses. Rabin et al.[21] reported a case in which leukemic infiltrates produced diffuse nodular defects throughout the colon. On barium enema examination these resembled the defects of nodular lymphoid hyperplasia, familial polyposis and lymphosarcoma.

Nonneoplastic Polyps

Hyperplastic Polyps

Hyperplastic (metaplastic) polyps are nonneoplastic sessile, smoothly rounded elevations, almost always less than 5 mm in diameter. They are usually multiple and may be present in such large numbers that they mimic the radiologic appearance of familial polyposis. They are by far the most common variety of colonic polyp, and are 10 times more frequent than adenomatous polyps.[2, 4]

Hyperplastic polyps represent an alteration in maturation of normal mucosal epithelium and bear no relation to neoplastic polyps or carcinoma. They present with few or no clinical symptoms.

Hamartomatous Polyps

Hamartomas are composed essentially of normal tissue abnormally arranged. The most common variety in the colon is the juvenile polyp, the most frequent polyp in childhood (Fig 34–31). However, adult cases are not rare, so that the term juvenile polyp is not entirely accurate. Some authorities prefer inflammatory or retention polyp, based on the histologic appearance of the lesion.[4, 10] This consists of cystic dilatation of the glands, which contain inflammatory cells and tissue debris. The polyp is not a true neoplasm but rather is a hamartomatous malformation affecting the glands and lamina propria. Juvenile polyposis and the Canada-Cronkhite syndrome, two of the multiple polyposis syndromes in which the polyps are of the juvenile variety, will be discussed later in this chapter.

Hamartomatous polyps also occur in the Peutz-Jegher syndrome (to be discussed) and in multiple neurofibromatosis associated with von Recklinghausen's disease.

Lymphoid Hyperplasia

Lymphoid hyperplasia of the colon is characterized radiographically by small, uniform, umbilicated polypoid lesions involving all or part of the colon[22] (Fig 34–32). A fleck of barium in the center of the small polypoid mass represents the umbilication at the apex of the lymphoid nodule and is unique to lymphoid hyperplasia. Such umbilication has not been observed in juvenile polyps or multiple polyposis of the colon, and its presence permits a definitive diagnosis.

Double contrast study of the colon is necessary to demonstrate the umbilicated lesions. The nodules vary from 1 to 4 mm in diameter and are seen throughout the colon from the rectum to the cecum.

There is no agreement in the literature concerning the cause of lymphoid hyperplasia. There appears to be no single etiologic factor, lymphoid hyperplasia simply being a normal response to a variety of stimuli. Infection, allergy and dysgammaglobulinemia may play a role.

Lymphoid hyperplasia is a benign condition that does not undergo malignant transformation. The lesions must be distinguished

TABLE 34-3.—MULTIPLE POLYPOSIS SYNDROMES

DISEASE	TYPE	LOCATION	OTHER SIGNS	MALIGNANT POTENTIAL
Familial polyposis	Adenomatous	Colon	None	95%
Gardner's syndrome	Adenomatous	Colon	Osteoma, dental abnormalities, desmoids	95%
Peutz-Jegher syndrome	Hamartomas	Stomach, small bowel, colon	Pigmentation	Rare
Turcot's syndrome	Adenomatous	Colon	CNS tumor	Probable
Canada-Cronkhite syndrome	Juvenile	Stomach, small bowel, colon	Alopecia, nail dystrophy, hyperpigmentation	None

from those of familial polyposis, lymphosarcoma and inflammatory diseases of the colon in order to avoid unnecessary surgery.

Pneumatosis Cystoides Coli

Gas cysts in the wall of the colon may create polypoid masses that simulate multiple polyps radiographically (Fig 34-33). The causal factors of this condition are not clear. The disease is self-limited and usually requires no treatment. The radiologic diagnosis is based on recognition that the masses contain gas and are radiolucent in contrast to solid tumors.

Cystic Fibrosis of the Pancreas

Many older children and young adults with cystic fibrosis have a distinctive mucosal pattern throughout the colon on postevacuation barium enema examination[23] (Fig 34-34). This cobblestone pattern may simulate multiple small polypoid lesions. In these cases the mucosa is redundant and hyperplastic. Tenacious fecal material often clings to the mucosa, producing persistent marginal defects. Histologically the colonic mucosa shows dilatation and gaping of the crypts with goblet cell hyperplasia. The epithelium is replaced by goblet cells, which are distended with mucus.

Colonic mucosal abnormalities are fairly specific, and the diagnosis of cystic fibrosis can often be suggested on this basis alone. Lymphoid hyperplasia of the colon produces smaller, more discrete nodules that have a central umbilication. In lymphosarcoma and familial polyposis of the colon, the multiple nodules are usually larger and better defined. Occasionally, a coarse mucosal pattern is seen in normal patients, especially when the colon has been poorly cleansed and fecal material simulates adherent colonic mucus.

Pseudopolyposis

Inflammatory diseases of the colon may cause severe damage to the mucosal surface. The mucosa may be denuded over large areas, resulting in multiple ulcerations. Portions of the mucosa adjacent to these ulcers may become undermined and partially detached. After remission of the acute inflammatory condition, with healing of the ulcers, the abnormal mucosa consists of polypoid excrescences (pseudopolyposis or inflammatory polyps), similar to ashes remaining after a fire. Repeated exacerbations and remissions of the inflammatory process also cause irregular overgrowth of the mucosa. This occurs in chronic ulcerative colitis and, to a lesser extent, in Crohn's disease of the colon.

Inflammatory pseudopolyps vary in number, size and shape and may be round, bifid, filiform or massive.[24-27] Histologic examination shows irregularly arranged normal epithelium, an inflammatory infiltrate, chronic granulation tissue and varying amounts of fibrosis.

Barium enema examination discloses single or multiple, round or elongated, polypoid masses in the mucosa (Figs 34–35 to 35–41). In most cases the acute phase of the bowel disease has subsided, so that the radiologic manifestations of acute inflammation are no longer present. In these cases the length and caliber of the bowel, haustral architecture and mucosal pattern (except for the pseudopolyps) are normal.

The cobblestone pattern of Crohn's disease of the colon (Fig 34–42), the thumbprinting of ischemic colitis (Fig 34–43) and the flat mosaic of colonic urticaria[28] (Fig 34–44) occasionally simulate the radiologic appearance of polyposis and pseudopolyposis. However, the distinction is usually not difficult and is based on the presence of other radiologic features.

Intestinal Polyposis Syndromes

The intestinal polyposis syndromes (Table 34–3) may be hereditary or not.[29-32] All three major hereditary syndromes (familial polyposis, Gardner's syndrome and the Peutz-Jegher syndrome) are transmitted in an autosomal dominant pattern. Consequently, about half of the offspring of individuals with these syndromes will be affected, without sex predilection. Turcot's syndrome appears to be transmitted by an autosomal homozygous recessive inheritance, a feature that could partially account for its great rarity.[29] The Canada-Cronkhite syndrome is not familial, all reported cases being isolated and sporadic.[33] Most patients with juvenile polyposis have a negative family history, but some varieties of juvenile polyposis appear to have mendelian-dominant inheritance characteristics.

Dodds et al.[29, 30] emphasize the important role that radiologists play in the diagnosis and evaluation of intestinal polyposis syndromes. They point out that these syndromes should be considered when (1) an intestinal polyp is identified in a young patient, (2) two or more polyps are demonstrated in any patient, (3) a colon carcinoma is present in a patient under age 40 and (4) extraintestinal manifestations associated with one of the syndromes are present. A high index of suspicion is imperative because failure to recognize familial polyposis and Gardner's syndrome leads to premature death of the patient and unaware afflicted relatives.

Familial Polyposis Coli

Familial polyposis is a hereditary disease characterized by polyposis of the colon and eventual development of colonic carcinoma in untreated patients. About two thirds of affected individuals have a family history of colonic polyps or carcinoma.[32] The other one-third have no family history and represent spontaneous mutations. Only affected family members have affected children.

The polyps are not present at birth but usually appear at puberty, although there is considerable variation in age at onset.[29, 30] The average age at onset of symptoms is 32 years, but the first symptoms may appear at any time between age 5 and 55. Diarrhea is almost invariable for reasons that are unclear. On the average, 10 years elapse between the appearance of polyposis and recognition of the diagnosis on the basis of signs and symptoms.[29]

Colonic polyps are usually numerous, range from 1–2 mm in size to 1 cm or more and may be sessile or pedunculated[30] (Figs 34–45 to 34–48). The colon is often diffusely involved, but the disease may also be segmental. Frequently the colon is covered with hundreds of polyps or is carpeted with myriad polyps, too numerous to count. Other portions of the gastrointestinal tract are not involved. Histologically the lesions are adenomatous polyps, indistinguishable from the adenomatous polyps that occur in the general population.

Colon carcinoma usually complicates the disease about 15 years after onset of the polyps, at which time the patient is generally in the 3d or 4th decade. The incidence of carcinoma is not proportional to the number of polyps present, so that a patient with thousands of polyps may not yet have developed a cancer, whereas another patient with fewer than 100 polyps may have concomitant carcinoma. The number of patients who already have carcinoma increases with the age of the patient at the time of diagnosis of polyposis. If the disease is recognized before age 20, 15% of patients will already have a colon carcinoma[31]; when the diagnosis is made after age 30, carcinoma is already present in 66%. The tumor is often multifocal.[34]

Gardner's Syndrome

This syndrome is an autosomal dominant disease characterized in its most complete form by polyps of the colon; multiple osteomas; dental abnormalities; soft tissue tumors (fibromas, desmoids, epidermoid cysts, lipomas); and the propensity of untreated patients to develop carcinoma of the colon[30-32] (Fig 34–49). The potential for development of carcinoma appears to be as high as it is with familial polyposis of the colon.[32] The various concomitants of the disease may appear at different times without a constant sequence (variable expressivity). The Gardner syndrome gene is fully penetrant, but the probability of recognition of its manifestations depends in part on the age of the patient.

Patients with this syndrome often seek medical attention for cosmetic deformities associated with the soft tissue or bony abnormalities. The diagnosis may first be suggested when dental abnormalities are detected or when sinusitis occurs secondary to osteomas of the paranasal sinuses.

The fibrous tissue in patients with Gardner's syndrome often has a pronounced tendency toward excessive proliferation, resulting in desmoid tumors, keloids, mesenteric fibrosis and peritoneal adhesions (Fig 34–50). Recent studies of fibroblast cultures from skin biopsy specimens taken from affected patients have raised the possibility that abnormalities may be manifest in these cells before onset of the characteristic findings elsewhere.[35]

The intestinal polyps associated with the syndrome are usually limited to the colon and are similar to those of familial polyposis. In addition, however, polyps sometimes are found in other parts of the gastrointestinal tract, particularly the small intestine.[34] Like patients with familial polyposis, those with Gardner's syndrome invariably develop colonic carcinoma if they do not have surgical treatment. Recent reports indicate that Gardner's syndrome shows a predilection for duodenal, periampullary and pancreatic carcinoma[33-35] (Fig 34–51).

Peutz-Jegher Syndrome

Peutz and Jeghers independently described a syndrome consisting of multiple intestinal polyps (hamartomas) associated with mucocutaneous melanin pigmentation[29, 30] (Fig 34–52). The skin lesions are brown or black macules, 1–5 mm in size, occurring on the perioral and buccal mucosa. The soles and palms may be involved. About 50% of reported patients have a positive family history, and about 50% are cases that represent a new mutation.[31]

Clinical symptoms are usually related to the intestinal polyps, the most common of which is abdominal pain caused by intussusception. The small bowel is involved in more than 50% of cases, the colon and rectum in 30% and the stomach in about 25%.[29, 30] The lesions are hamartomas with no tendency to undergo malignant change. However, there is a 2–3% risk of development of carcinoma in the pancreaticoduodenal region, not necessarily associated with polyps.[34]

Turcot's Syndrome

An association between polyps of the colon and central nervous system tumors was first described by Turcot et al.[29] Seven patients with the syndrome have been documented.[30] Nearly all of the neural tumors have been supratentorial glioblastomas, and most patients have died as a result of the neurologic disease.

The colonic polyps are adenomatous polyps, which presumably have a propensity to become carcinomas if patients survive long enough.

Juvenile Polyposis and Canada-Cronkhite Syndrome

Babies with juvenile polyposis may have a clinical syndrome consisting of devastating protein-losing enteropathy, cachexia and electrolyte depletion,[36, 37] leading to death (Fig 34–53). There are no extraintestinal manifestations.

The Canada-Cronkhite syndrome includes generalized gastrointestinal polyposis in association with neuroectodermal changes consisting of alopecia, hyperpigmentation and atrophy of the nails.[29, 30, 38] Patients usually have polyps of the stomach and small intestine, as well as of the colon. The polyps are of the juvenile variety with no tendency to become malignant.

REFERENCES

1. Ott, D. J., and Gelfand, D. W.: Colorectal tumors: Pathology and detection, Am. J. Roentgenol. 131: 696, 1978.
2. Lane, N., and Fenoglio, C. M.: Observations on the adenoma as precursor to ordinary large bowel carcinoma, Gastrointest. Radiol. 1:111, 1976.
3. Morson, B. C.: Genesis of colorectal cancer, Clin. Gastroenterol. 5:505, 1976.
4. Morson, B. C.: Pathogenesis of Colorectal Cancer, in *Major Problems in Pathology, Vol. 10* (Philadelphia: W. B. Saunders Co., 1978).
5. Muto, T., Bussey, H. J. R., and Morson, B.: The evolution of cancer of the colon and rectum, Cancer 36:2251, 1975.
6. Bussey, H. J. R.: Gastrointestinal polyposis, Gut 11:970, 1970.
7. Gilbertson, V. A.: Proctosigmoidoscopy and polypectomy in reducing the incidence of rectal cancer, Cancer 14:936, 1974.
8. Andrea, L., Frieberg, S., and Welin, S.: Roentgen Diagnosis of Small Polyps in the Colon and Rectum, Acta Radiol. 43:201, 1955.
9. Miller, R. E.: The cleansing enema, Radiology 117: 483, 1975.
10. Welch, C. E.: Polypoid Lesions of the Gastrointestinal Tract, in *Major Problems in Clinical Surgery,* Vol. II (Philadelphia: W. B. Saunders Co., 1964).
11. Youker, J. E., and Welin, S.: Differentiation of true polypoid tumors of the colon from extraneous material: A new roentgen sign, Radiology 84:610, 1965.
12. Wolf, B. S.: Roentgen diagnosis of villous tumors of the colon, Am. J. Roentgenol. 84:1093, 1960.
13. Kaye, J. J., and Bragg, D. G.: Unusual roentgenologic and clinicopathologic features of villous adenomas of the colon, Radiology 91:799, 1968.
14. Comfort, M. W., and Stearns, M. W.: Submucous lipomata of the gastrointestinal tract, Surg. Gynecol. Obstet. 52:101, 1931.
15. Wolf, B. S., Melamed, M., and Khilnani, M. T.: Lipoma of the colon, MT. Sinai NY 21:8, 1954.
16. Berk, R. N., Scher, G. S., and Bode, D. F.: Unusual tumors of the gastrointestinal tract, Am. J. Roentgenol. 113:159, 1971.
17. Davis, G. B., and Berk, R. N.: Intestinal neurofibromas in von Recklinghausen's disease, Am. J. Gastroenterol. 60:410, 1973.
18. Ginsburg, L.: Eccentric polyposis of the small intestine, Radiology 116:561, 1975.
19. Marshak, R. H., Khilnani, M. T., and Eliasoph, J.: Roentgen findings in lymphosarcoma of the small intestine, Am. J. Roentgenol. 86:682, 1961.
20. Marshak, R. H., Khilnani, M. T., Eliasoph, J., and Wolf, B. S.: Metastatic carcinoma of small bowel, Am. J. Roentgenol 94:385, 1965.
21. Rabin, M. S., Bledin, A. G., and Lewis, D.: Polypoid leukemic infiltration of the large bowel, Am. J. Roentgenol. 131:723, 1978.
22. Capitanio, M. A., and Kirkpatrick, J. A.: Lymphoid hyperplasia of the colon in children, Radiology 94: 323, 1970.
23. Berk, R. N., and Lee, F. A.: The late gastrointestinal manifestations of cystic fibrosis of the pancreas, Radiology, 106:377, 1973.
24. Zegel, H. G., and Laufer, I.: Filiform polyposis, Radiology 127:615, 1978.
25. Hammerman, A. M., Shatz, B. A., and Susman, N.: Radiographic characteristics of colonic mucosal bridges, Radiology 127:611, 1978.
26. Fitterer, J. D., Cromwell, L. G., and Sims, J. E.: Colonic obstruction by giant pseudopolyposis, Gastroenterology 72:153, 1977.
27. Wills, J. S., and Han, S. S.: Localized giant pseudopolyposis complicating granulomatous ileocolitis, Radiology 122:320, 1977.
28. Berk, R. N., Scher, G. S., and Bode, D. F.: Unusual tumors of the gastrointestinal tract, Am. J. Roentgenol. 113:159, 1971.
29. Dodds, W. J.: Clinical and roentgen features of intestinal polyposis syndromes, Gastrointest. Radiol. 1:127, 1976.
30. Dodds, W. J., and Lydon, S. B.: Intestinal polyposis syndromes, CRC Crit. Rev. Clin. Radiol. Nucl. Med. 5:295, 1974.
31. Erbe, R. W.: Inherited gastrointestinal polyposis syndromes, N. Engl. J. Med. 294:1101, 1976.

32. McKusick, V. A.: Genetic factors in intestinal polyposis, J.A.M.A. 182:271, 1962.
33. Cronkhite, L. W., and Canada, J. W.: Generalized gastrointestinal polyposis: An unusual syndrome of polyposis, pigmentation, alopecia and onychotrophia, N. Engl. J. Med. 252:1011, 1955.
34. Erbe, R. W.: Clinicopathological exercises, N. Engl. J. Med. 299:1237, 1978.
35. Kopelovich, L., Conlon, S., and Pollack, R.: Defective organization of actin in cultured skin fibroblasts from patients with inherited adenocarcinoma, Proc. Natl. Acad. Sci. USA, 74:3019, 1977.
36. Ruyman, F. B.: Juvenile polyps with cachexia, Gastroenterology 57:431, 1969.
37. Berk, R. N., Rush, J. L., and Elson, E. C.: Multiple inflammatory polyps of the small intestine with cachexia and protein losing enteropathy, Radiology 95:611, 1970.
38. Johnson, G. K., Soergel, K. H., Hensley, G. T., Dodds, W. J., and Hogan, W. J.: Cronkhite Canada syndrome: Gastrointestinal pathophysiology and morphology, Gastroenterology 63:140, 1972.

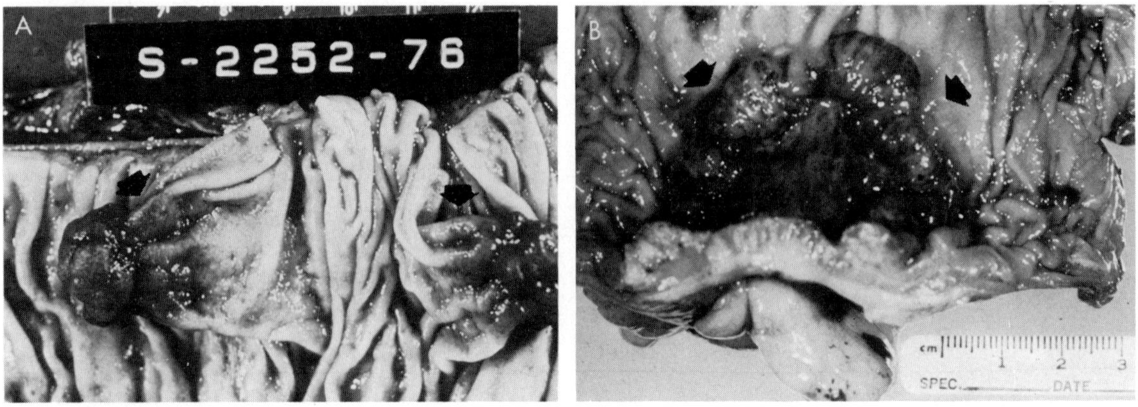

Fig 34-1.—**A,** photograph of colon viewed from mucosal surface showing two typical adenomatous polyps on short broad stalks *(arrows).* **B,** photograph of another colon viewed from the mucosal surface showing a characteristic infiltrating adenocarcinoma *(arrows).* Note the rolled edge of the tumor and the thickening of the colonic wall. Convincing evidence has now been accumulated to prove that adenomatous polyps are the precursor of carcinoma of the colon (the adenoma-carcinoma sequence). Malignant transformation of adenomatous polyps **(A)** accounts for most cases of adenocarcinoma of colon **(B).**

Fig 34-2.—Barium enema examinations in a 64-year-old man showing the sigmoid colon. **A,** initial exam discloses a 1.5-cm sessile polyp. Patient refused treatment and was lost to follow-up until melena occurred 6 years later. **B,** second study performed 6 years after initial examination shows typical apple core deformity of an infiltrating carcinoma encircling bowel. No metastases identified at surgery. The adenoma-carcinoma sequence requires 5 years or more in most cases, although the time interval is extremely variable. (Courtesy of Dr. James Bendon, San Diego, Calif.)

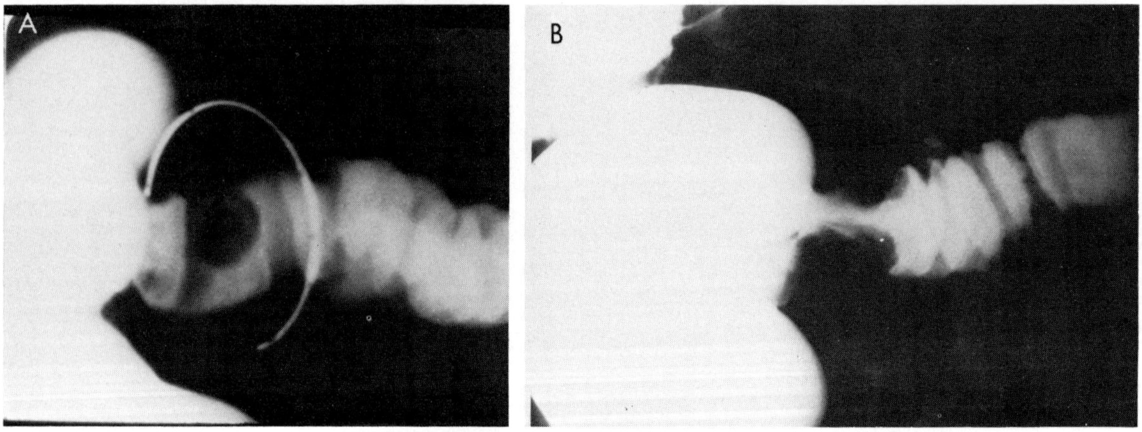

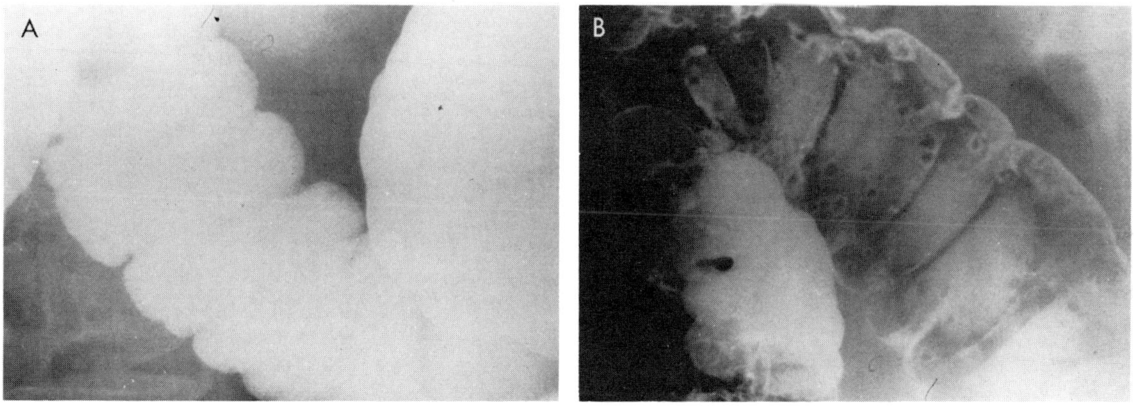

Fig 34–3.—Solid column **(A)** and air contrast **(B)** barium enema examination in man, age 27, with familial polyposis. Innumerable 5-mm polyps are visible in transverse colon only on air contrast study. Air contrast barium enema examinations are more accurate in detection of small polyps and are indicated in any patient in whom there is a high index of suspicion of polyps (see Table 34–2.)

Fig 34–4.—Air contrast barium enema examination in woman, age 69, showing 4-mm polyp in rectum. **A,** supine projection; **B,** lateral projection. Histologic examination following removal through sigmoidoscope indicated lesion was an adenomatous polyp. Lesions of this size are rarely detected on solid column barium enema studies, despite use of low-density barium and high kvp radiography.

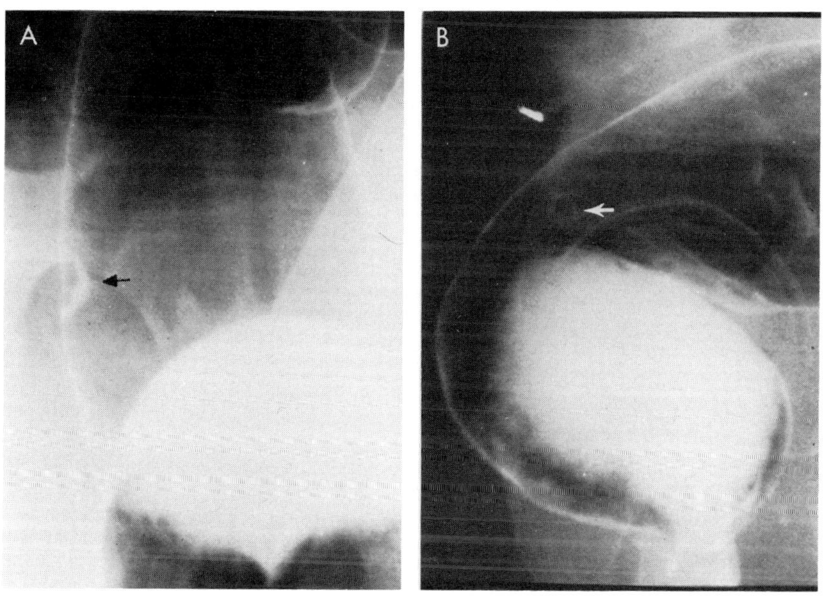

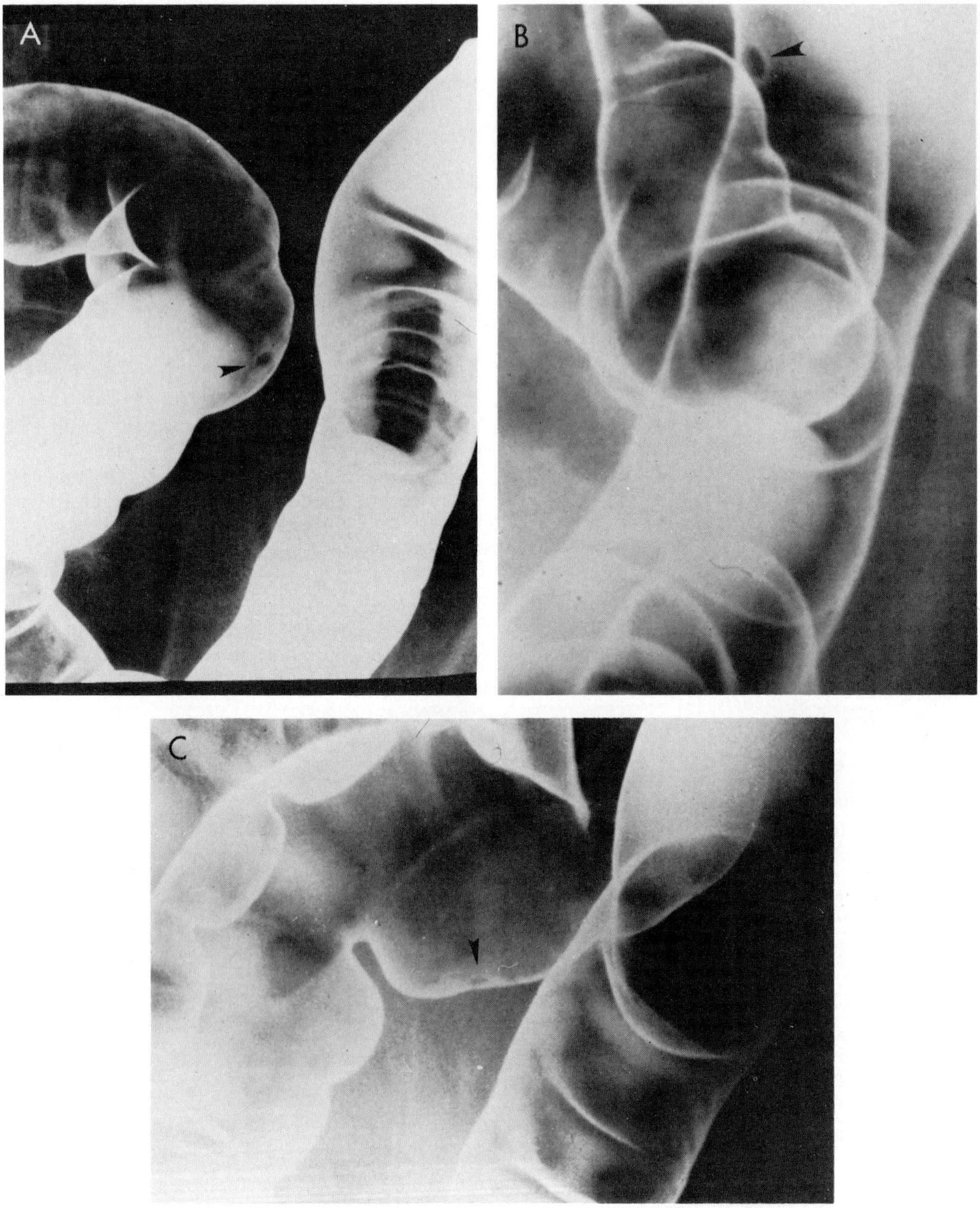

Fig 34–5.—**A, B** and **C,** air contrast barium enema examinations in 3 patients showing 5-mm adenomatous polyps in sigmoid colon *(arrow).* Diagnosis confirmed by histologic examination after removal of polyps through sigmoidoscope. Hyperplastic polyps are 10 times more common than adenomatous polyps, and small adenomatous polyps (less than 15 mm) are 10 times more common than large adenomatous polyps.

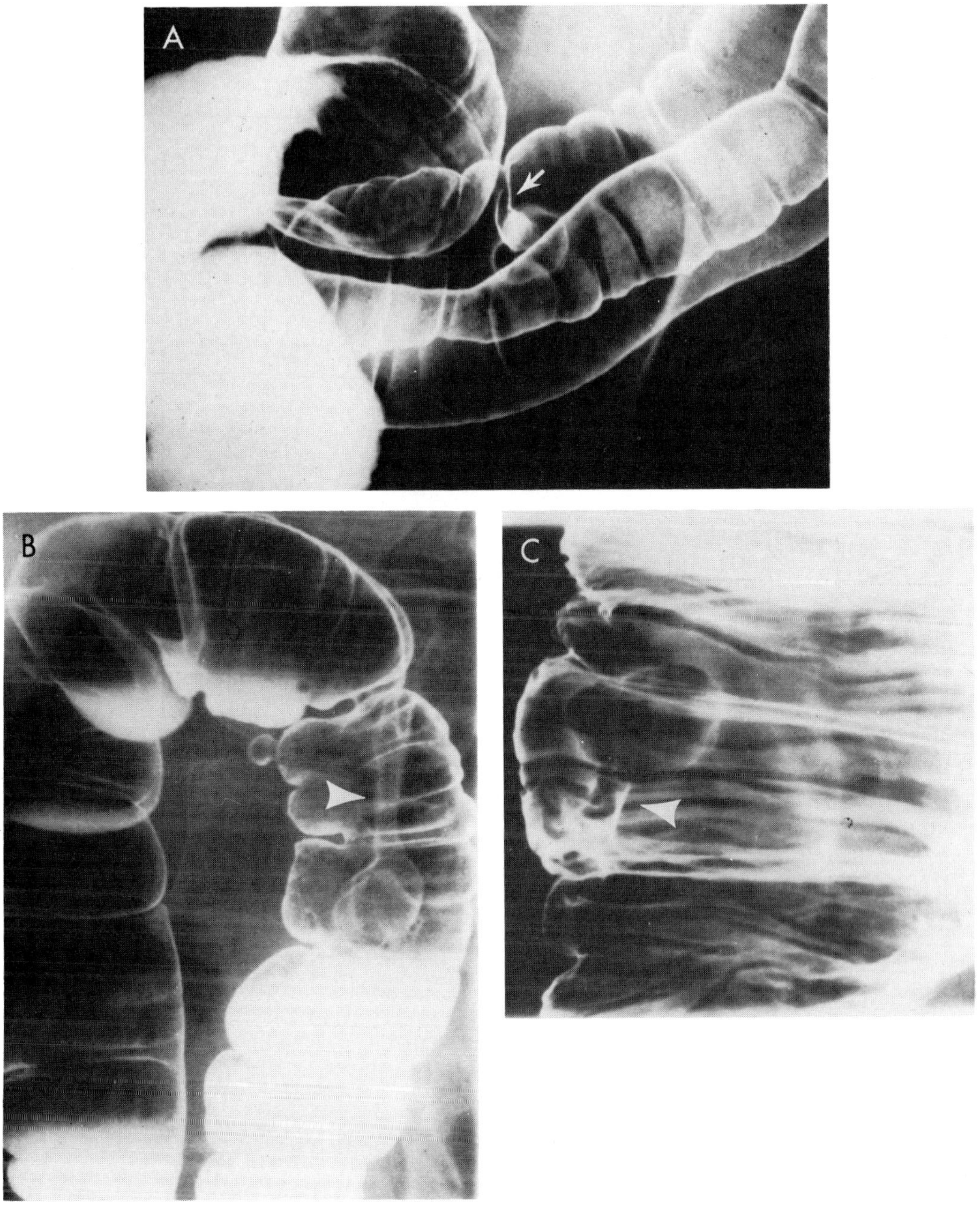

Fig 34–6.—Air contrast barium enema examinations in three patients showing adenomatous polyp on stalk *(arrows)*. **A**, sigmoid colon; **B**, splenic flexure; **C**, ascending colon. Identification of a stalk longer than 1 cm indicates that lesion is a benign adenomatous polyp.

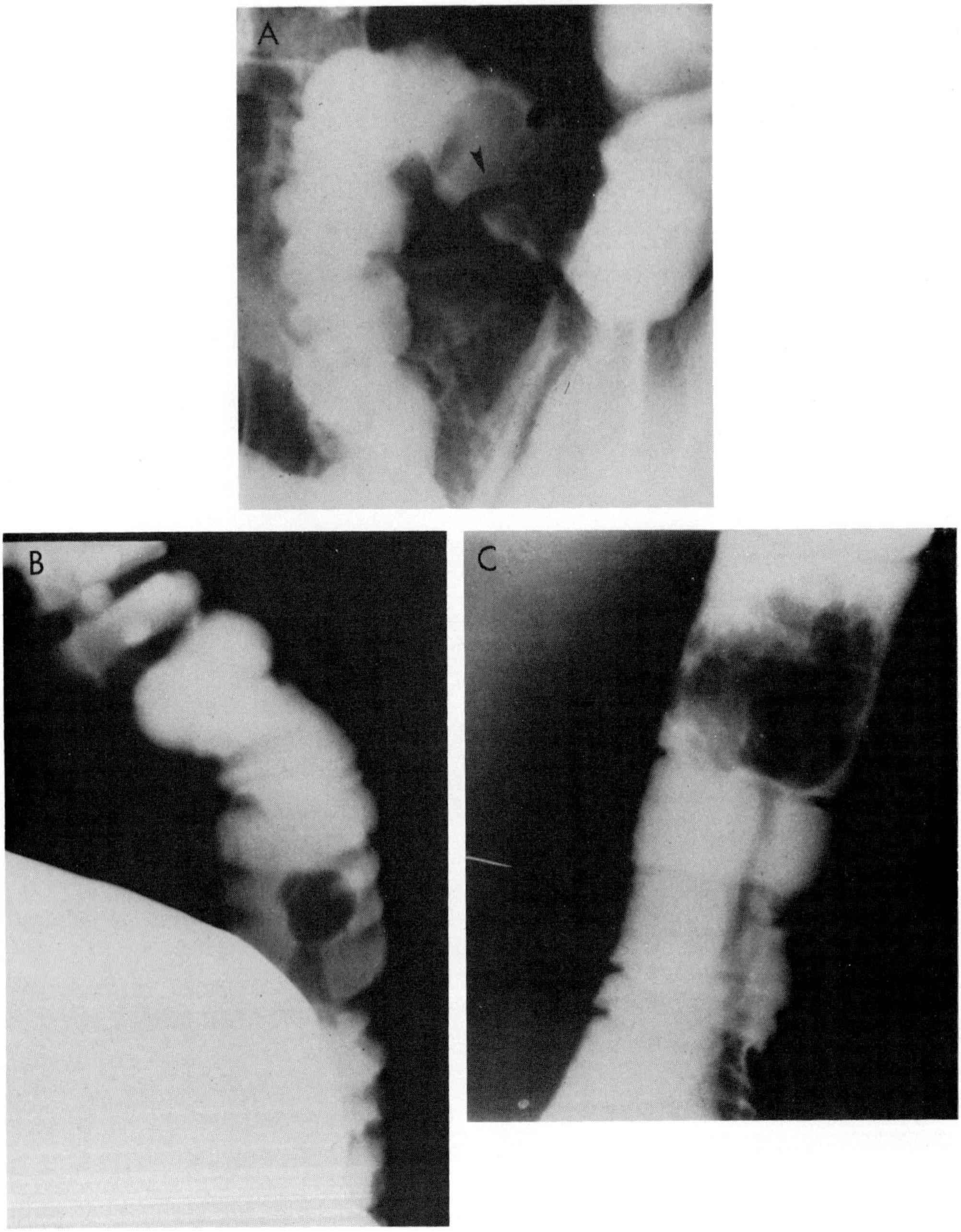

Fig 34–7.—Solid column barium enema examinations in three patients showing adenomatous polyp on a stalk. **A,** sigmoid colon; **B** and **C,** descending colon. Compression spot radiographs are usually necessary for optimal evaluation of polyps on solid column barium enema studies.

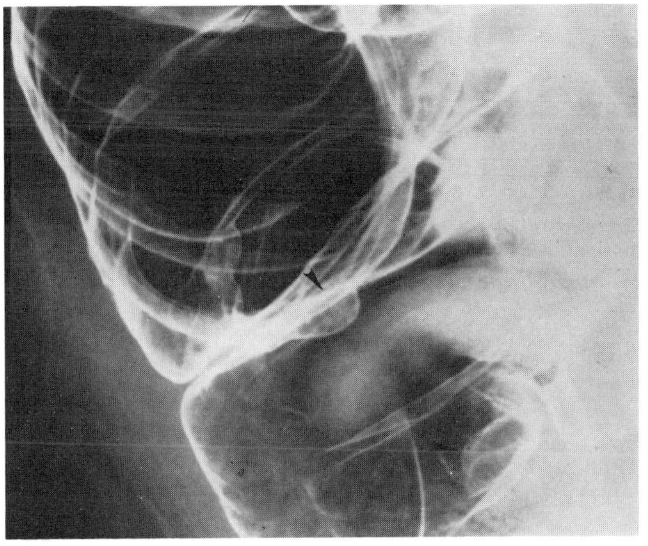

Fig 34–8.—Air contrast barium enema examination in man, age 49, showing 2 sessile adenomatous polyps *(arrow)*. One is attached to ileocecal valve; the other is in cecum adjacent to base of appendix. A third adenomatous polyp lies lateral and distal to polyp atttached to valve.

Fig 34–9.—**A,** air contrast barium enema examination showing lobulated, sessile, 2-cm polyp in sigmoid colon *(arrow)*. **B–C,** endoscopic views of lesion. Histologic examination after removal through sigmoidoscope indicated that tumor was an adenomatous polyp. Adenomatous polyps larger than 1.5 cm in size have greater incidence of malignant transformation than smaller adenomatous polyps and should be removed.

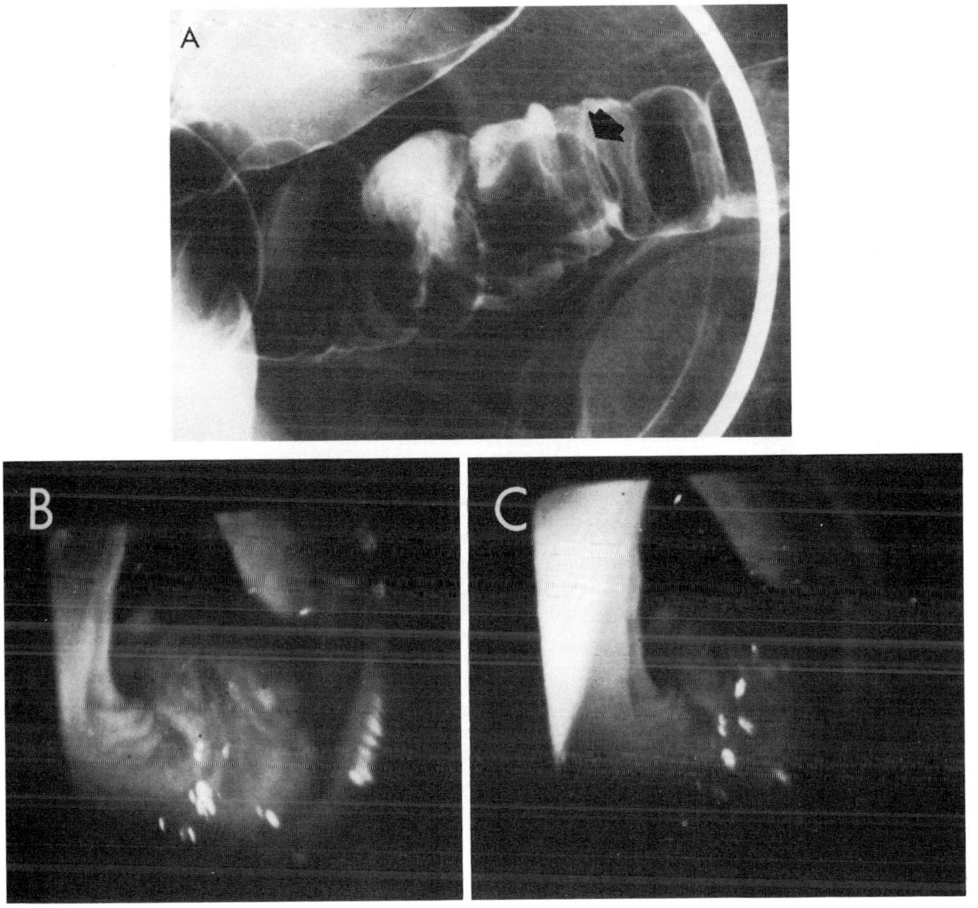

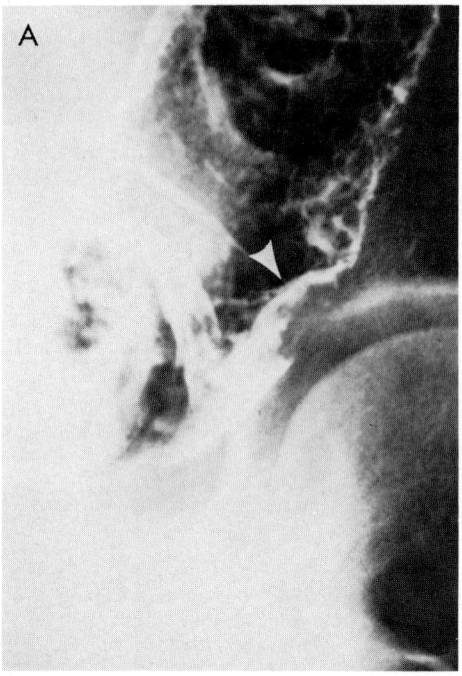

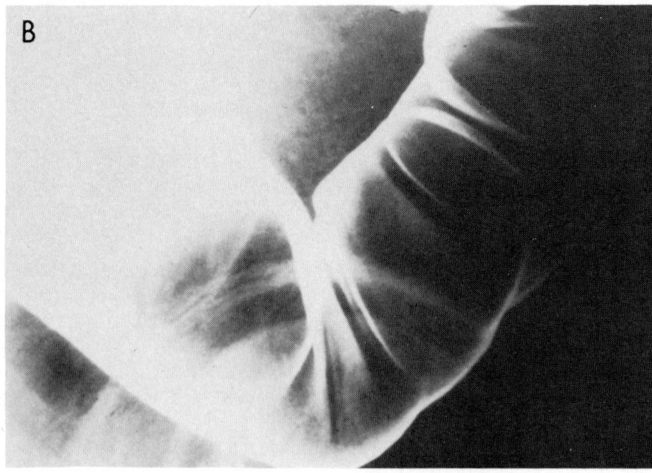

Fig 34–10.—Air contrast barium enema examinations on same patient done at different times, showing sigmoid colon. **A,** apparent mass in wall of bowel suggests presence of a tumor *(arrow).* Irregular coating of mucosa with barium indicates presence of fecal material. **B,** second examination performed after better cleansing of colon indicates that colon is normal. Thorough cleansing of colon is a prerequisite for an accurate diagnosis.

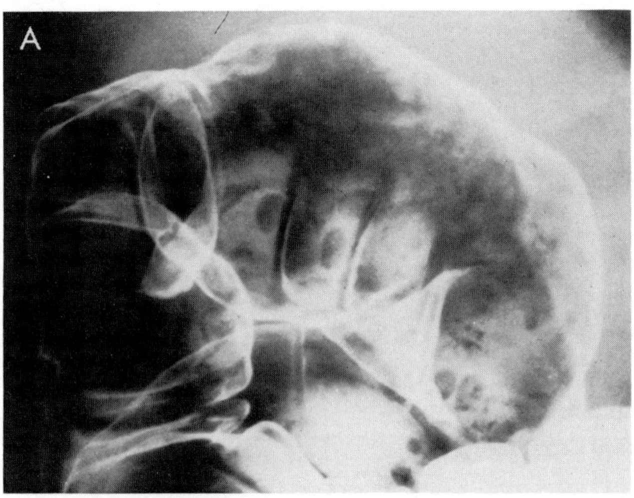

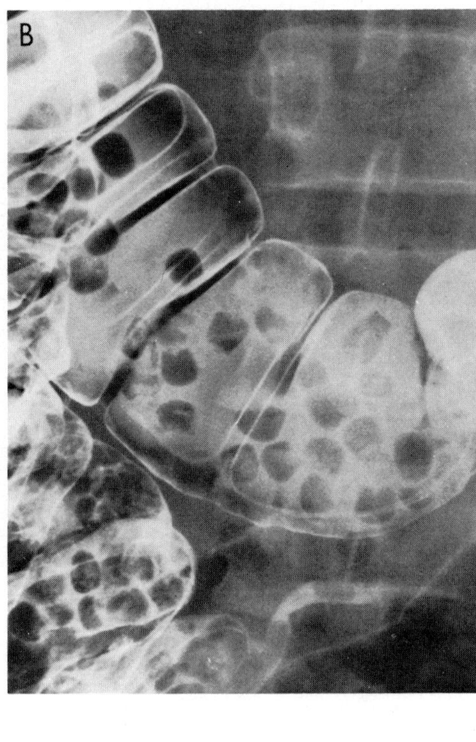

Fig 34–11.—**A,** air contrast barium enema showing hepatic flexure. Multiple small filling defects are all same size and shape due to numerous watermelon seeds in the lumen. Precise diagnosis is possible based on shape of seeds. Extraneous material in lumen bears no constant relation to colonic wall and moves in relation to gravity. **B,** undigested corn kernels in colon appearing as multiple radiolucencies simulating multiple polyposis. (From Dr. Harry C. Press, Jr., Ingested corn kernels simulating polyposis, Am. J. Roentgenol. 127: 1040, 1976, with permission.)

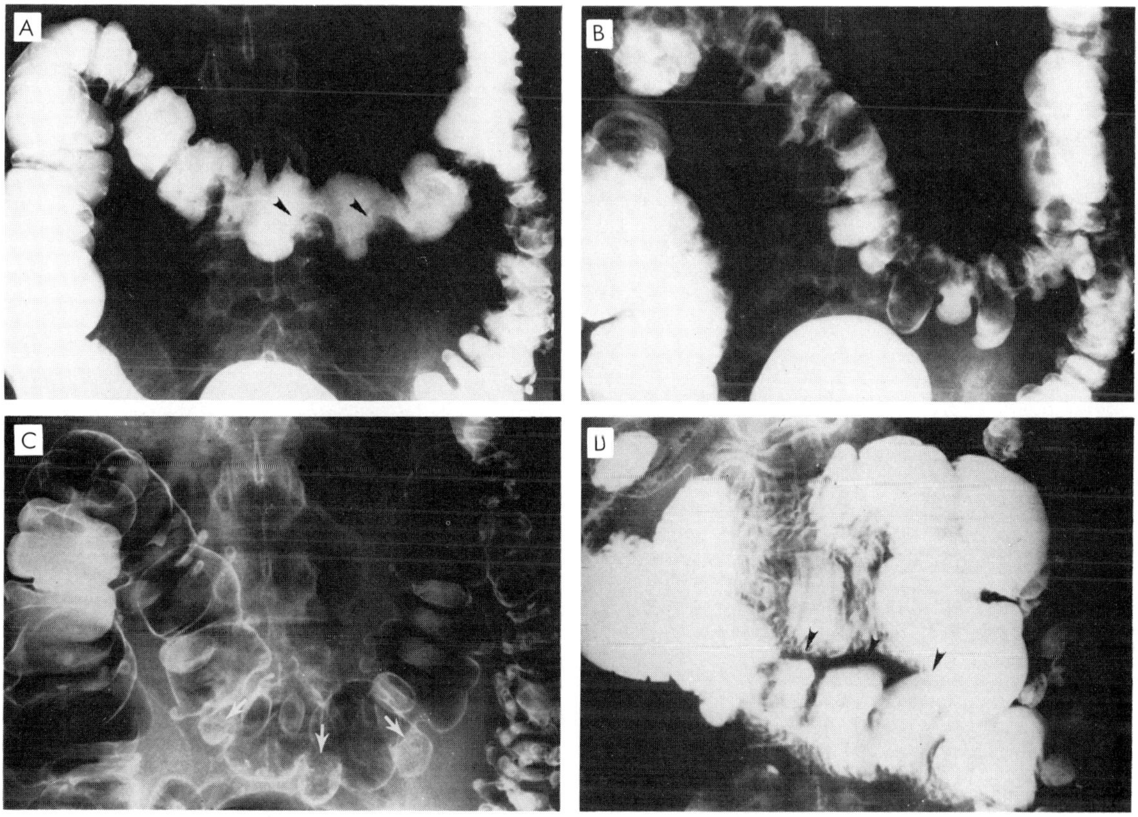

Fig 34–12.—Barium enema and small intestine examination in woman, age 38, with progressive systemic sclerosis. **A,** solid column barium enema examination shows several radiolucencies in transverse colon suggesting masses in bowel wall *(arrows)*. Diverticula are evident in descending colon. **B,** postevacuation radiograph shows that radiolucencies are caused by fecal material in wide-mouthed pseudodiverticula, which are characteristic of scleroderma. **C,** air contrast barium enema examination shows unusual diverticula (sacculations), which contain fecal material *(arrows)*. **D,** small bowel examination in same patient shows similar wide-mouthed pseudodiverticula in small intestine due to scleroderma *(arrows)*.

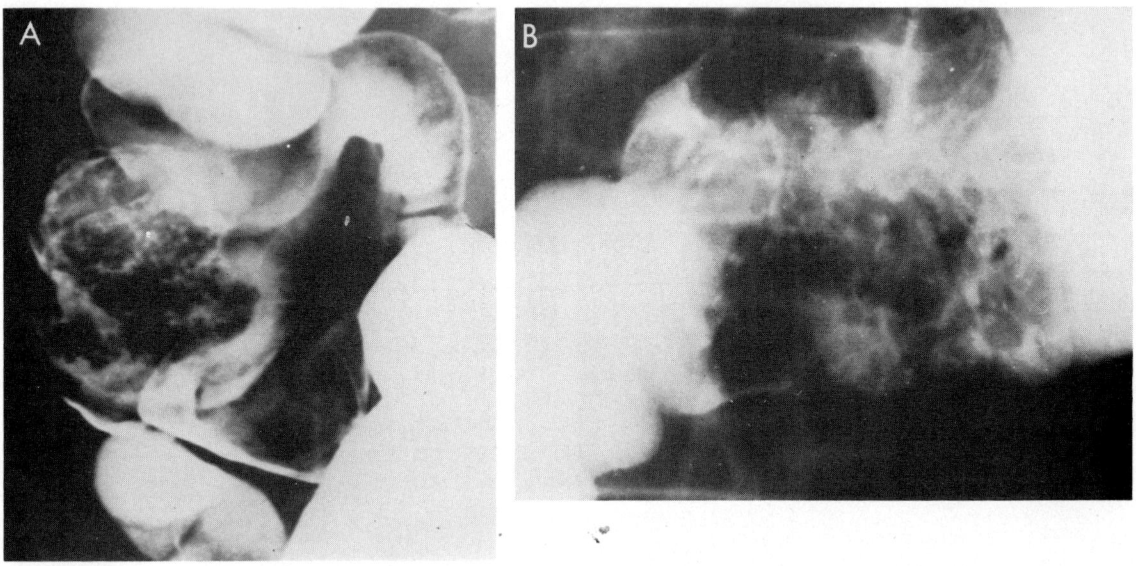

Fig 34-13.—Barium enema examination in 2 patients showing large villous adenomas of colon. **A,** cecum; **B,** transverse colon. Shaggy reticulated pattern of barium coating surface of tumor is characteristic of this lesion.

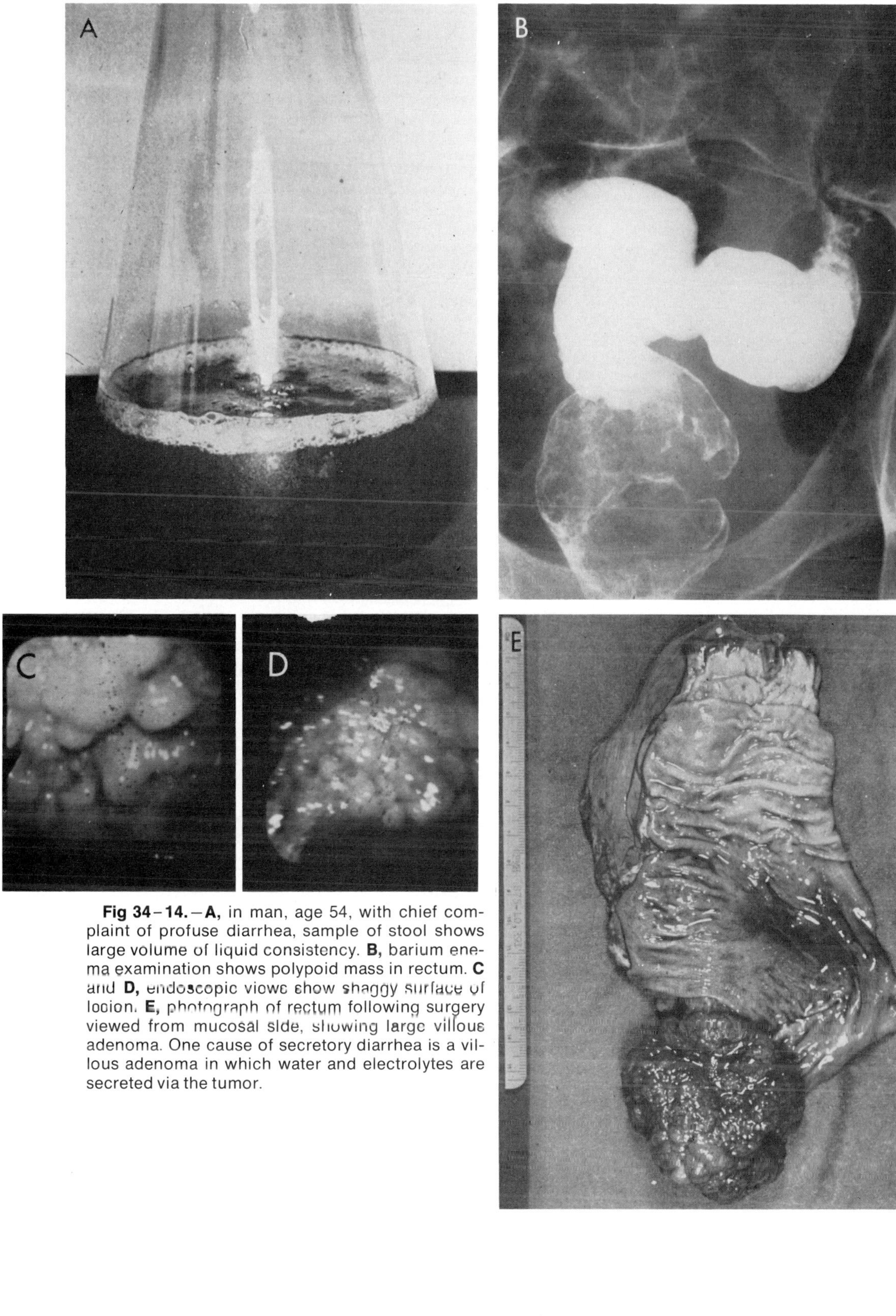

Fig 34–14.—**A,** in man, age 54, with chief complaint of profuse diarrhea, sample of stool shows large volume of liquid consistency. **B,** barium enema examination shows polypoid mass in rectum. **C** and **D,** endoscopic views show shaggy surface of lesion. **E,** photograph of rectum following surgery viewed from mucosal side, showing large villous adenoma. One cause of secretory diarrhea is a villous adenoma in which water and electrolytes are secreted via the tumor.

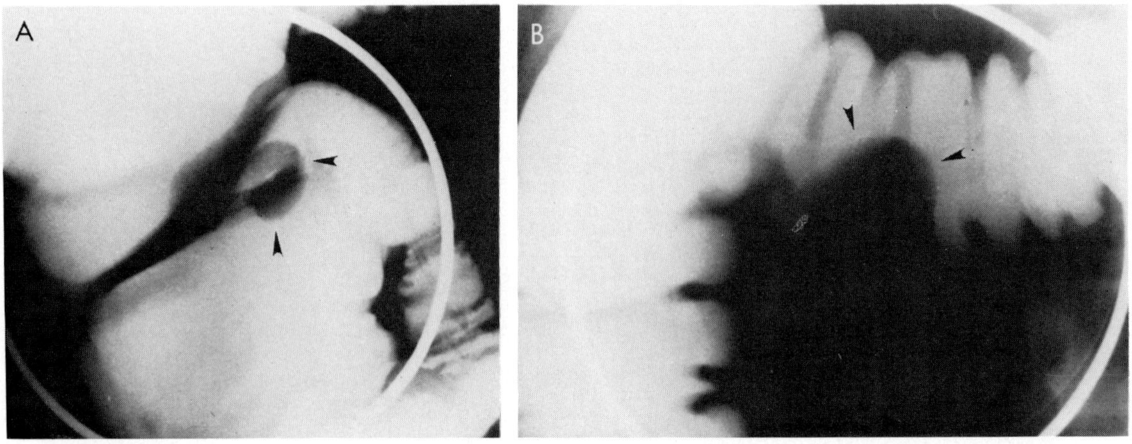

Fig 34–15.—Barium enema examinations in 2 patients showing typical lipomas of colon *(arrows)*. **A,** cecum; **B,** right side of transverse colon. Lipomas are mural lesions with a smooth surface and a tendency to grow into lumen of colon.

Fig 34–16. A–D, barium enema examination showing large lipoma of sigmoid colon adjacent to polypoid adenocarcinoma *(arrows)*. There is an air bubble between the two lesions in **B. C,** endoscopic view of lipoma, site of a biopsy is evident. **D,** endoscopic view of adjacent carcinoma. The lipoma has smooth surface both radiologically and endoscopically; the carcinoma has a rough, irregular surface with overhanging edges.

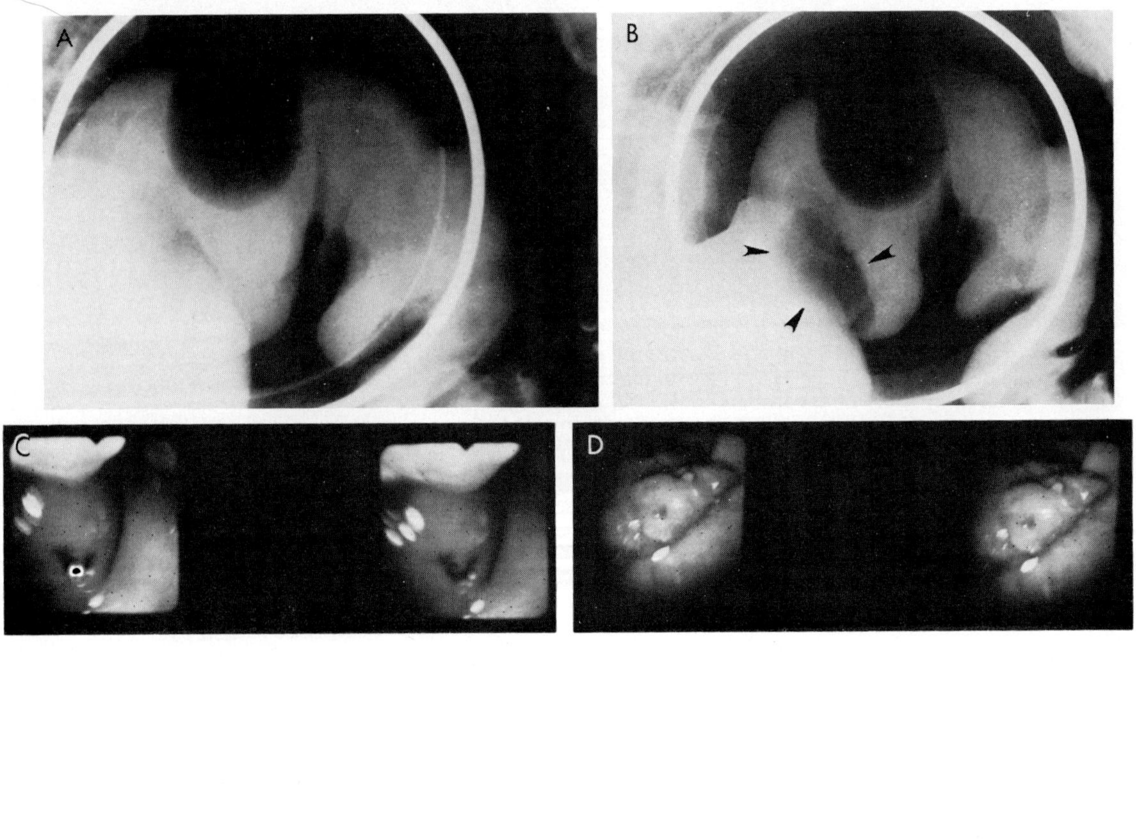

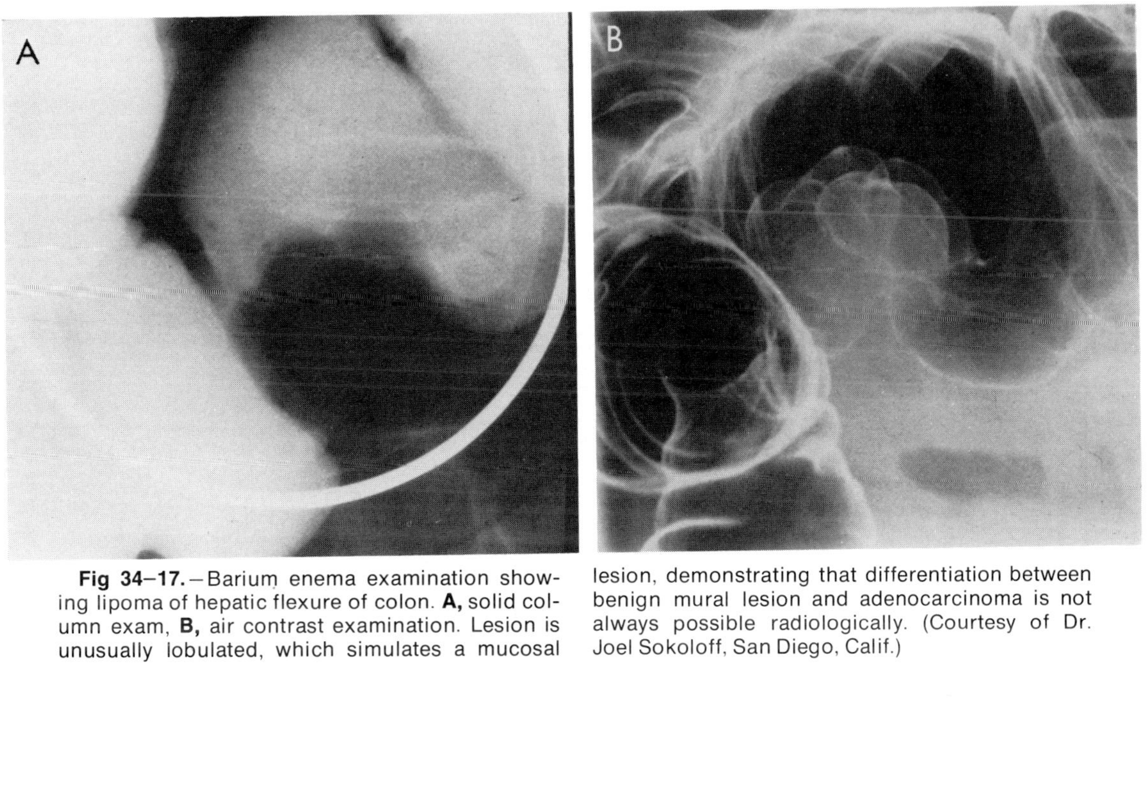

Fig 34–17.—Barium enema examination showing lipoma of hepatic flexure of colon. **A,** solid column exam, **B,** air contrast examination. Lesion is unusually lobulated, which simulates a mucosal lesion, demonstrating that differentiation between benign mural lesion and adenocarcinoma is not always possible radiologically. (Courtesy of Dr. Joel Sokoloff, San Diego, Calif.)

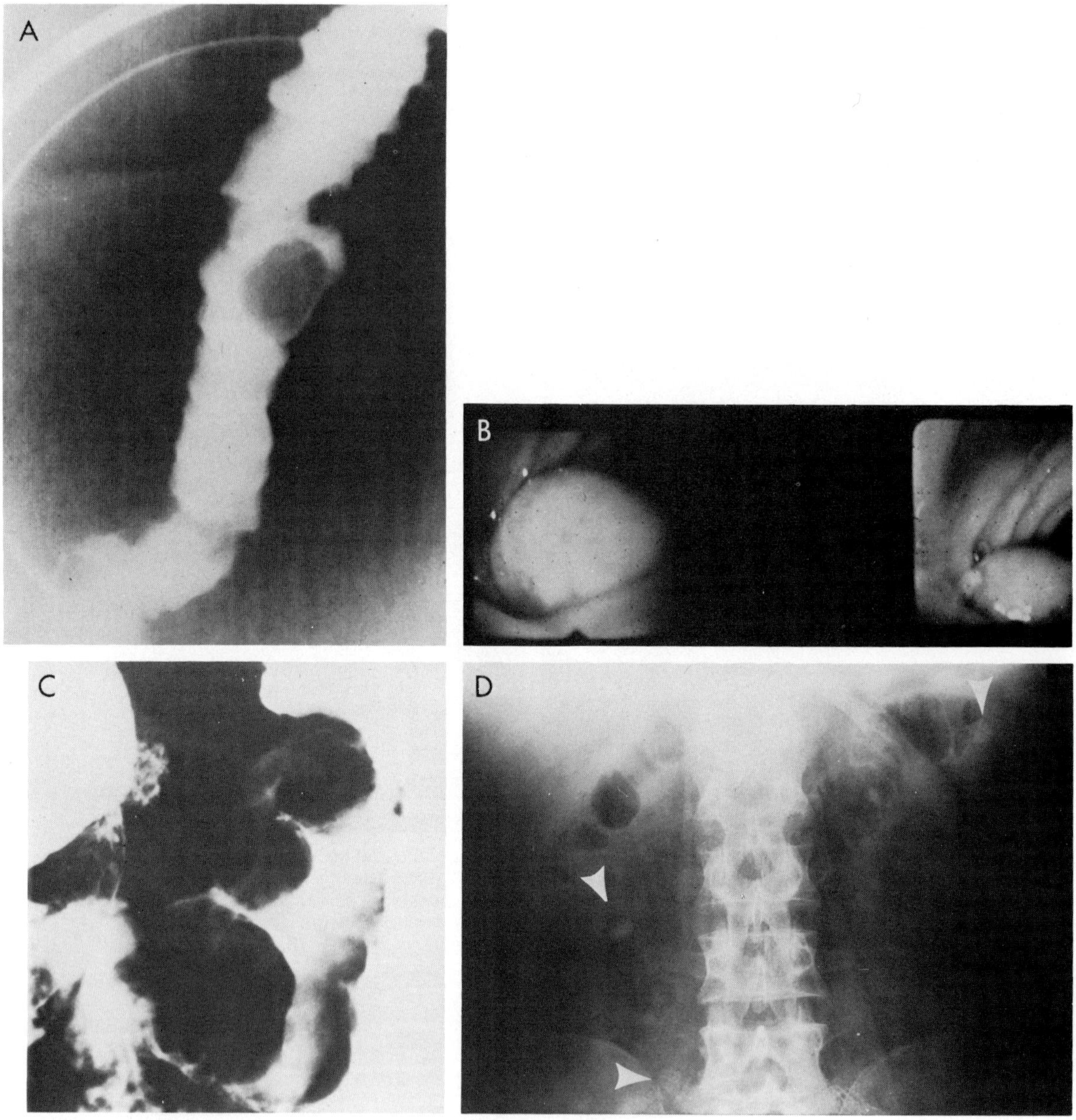

Fig 34–18.—Woman, age 24, with generalized neurofibromatosis with lesions in the colon, small intestine and skin. **A,** barium enema examination showing smooth mural mass in descending colon. **B,** endoscopic views of neurofibroma in descending colon. Smooth surface is characteristic of all submucosal mural lesions. **C,** small bowel study showing three neurofibromas of intestine. Tendency of lesions to be multiple and to involve one side of bowel wall is typical. **D,** plain abdominal radiograph showing multiple cutaneous neurofibromas *(arrows)*.

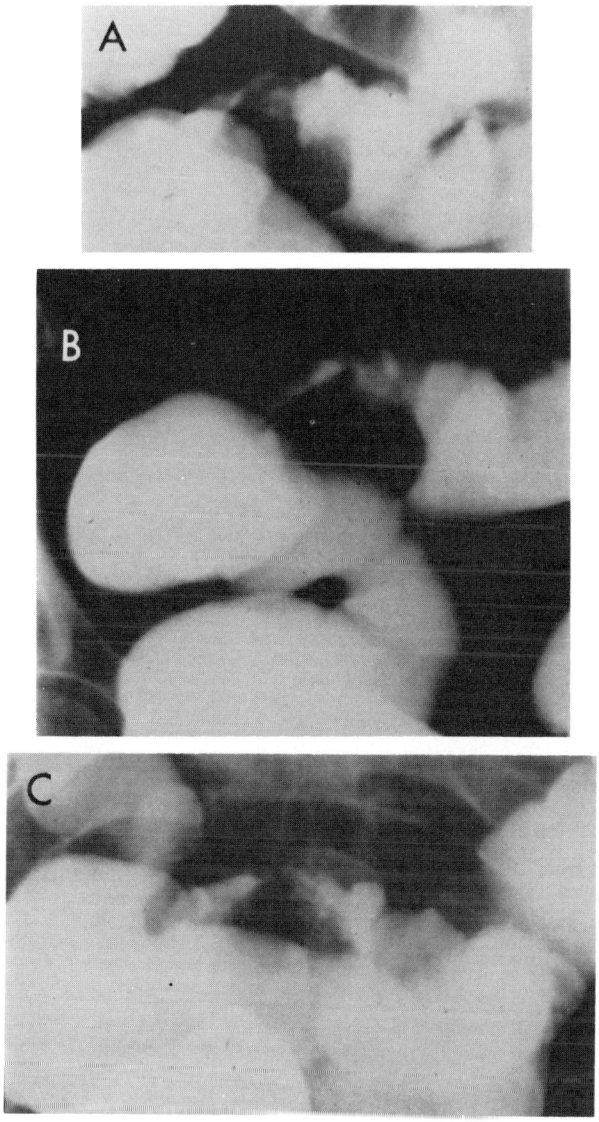

Fig 34–19.—**A–C,** barium enema examination showing endometriosis of sigmoid colon. Smooth mass is typical and is due to extensive desmoplastic reaction associated with endometrial implant on the bowel wall.

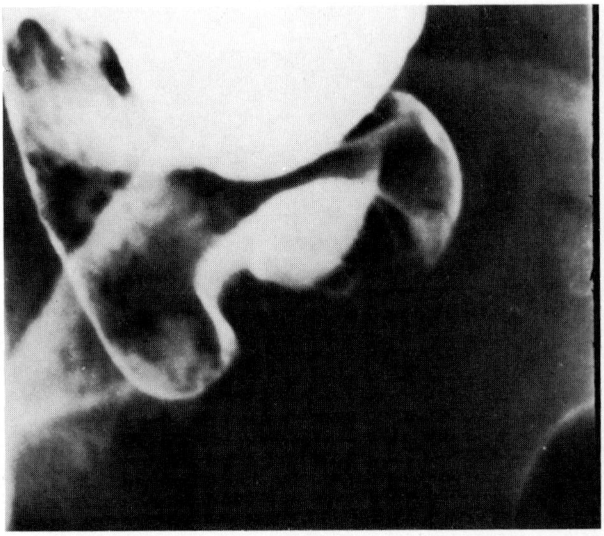

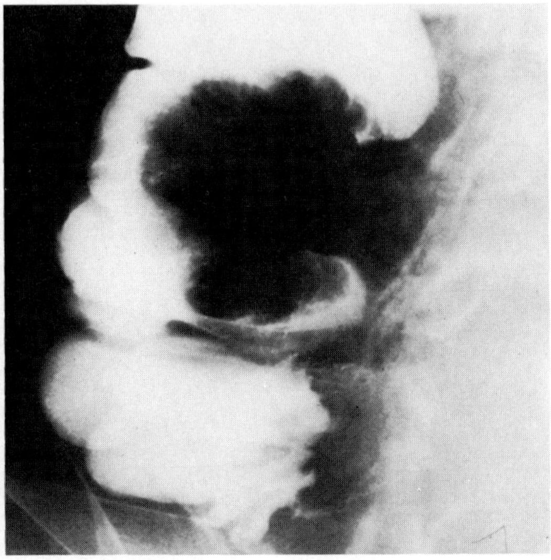

Fig 34–20 (left).—Double contrast barium enema examination in another patient with endometriosis. Similar smooth endometrioma is present in cecum.

Fig 34–21 (right).—Barium enema examination demonstrating typical polypoid adenocarcinoma of ascending colon. Rough irregular surface and overhanging margins are typical of malignant mucosal lesions.

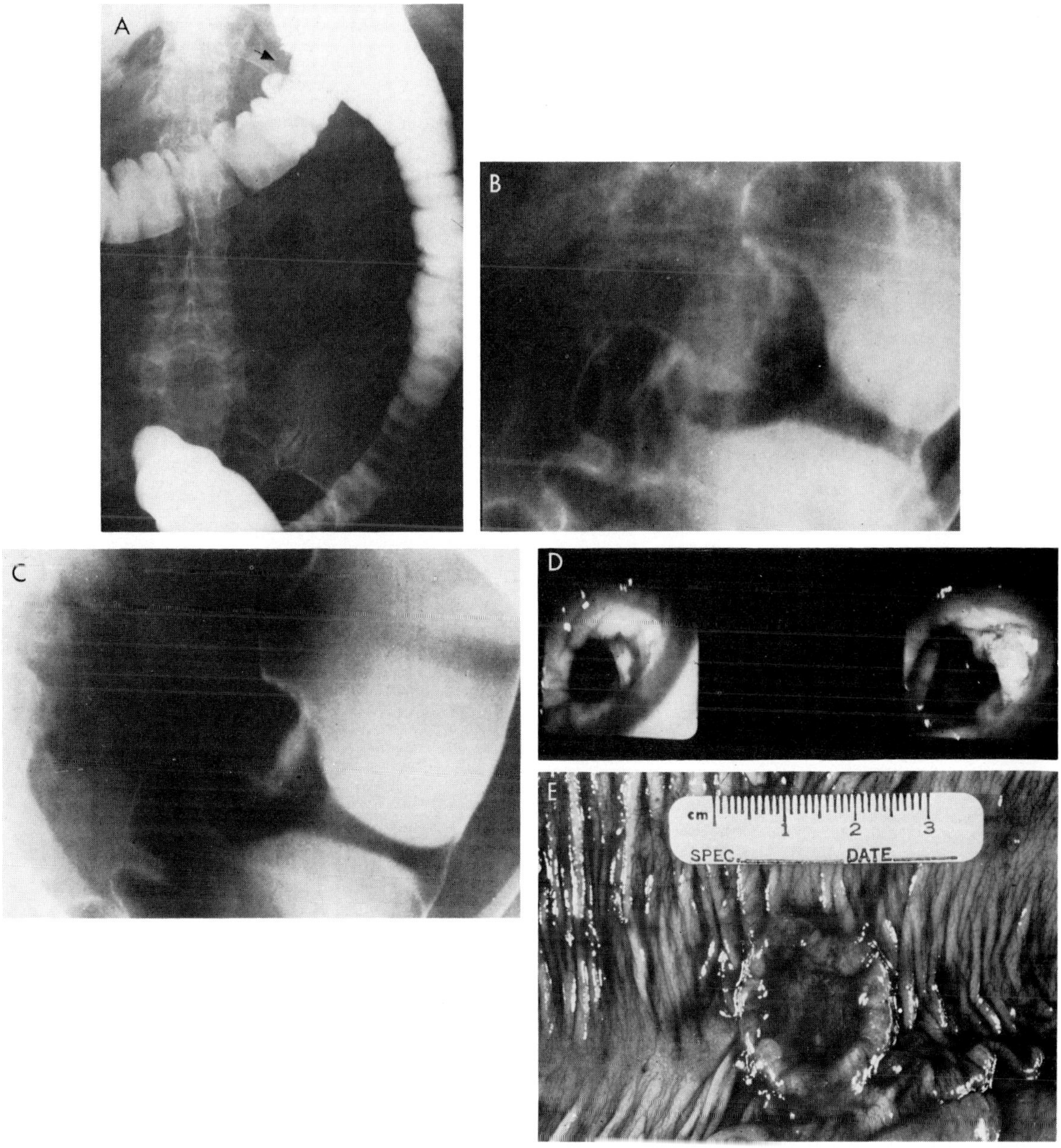

Fig 34–22.—**A,** barium enema examination showing typical contour defect in hepatic flexure due to adenocarcinoma *(arrow).* **B** and **C,** spot radiographs of lesion. **D,** endoscopic views of tumor in hepatic flexure demonstrating rolled edge of carcinoma. **E,** photograph of colon after resection viewed from mucosal side shows typical infiltrating carcinoma of colon. A contour defect is a characteristic radiograph feature of carcinoma and consists of interruption of margin of bowel wall due to scirrhous reaction associated with tumor. Note that abrupt rolled margin of carcinoma in **B** and **C** simulates smooth surface of a benign mural tumor.

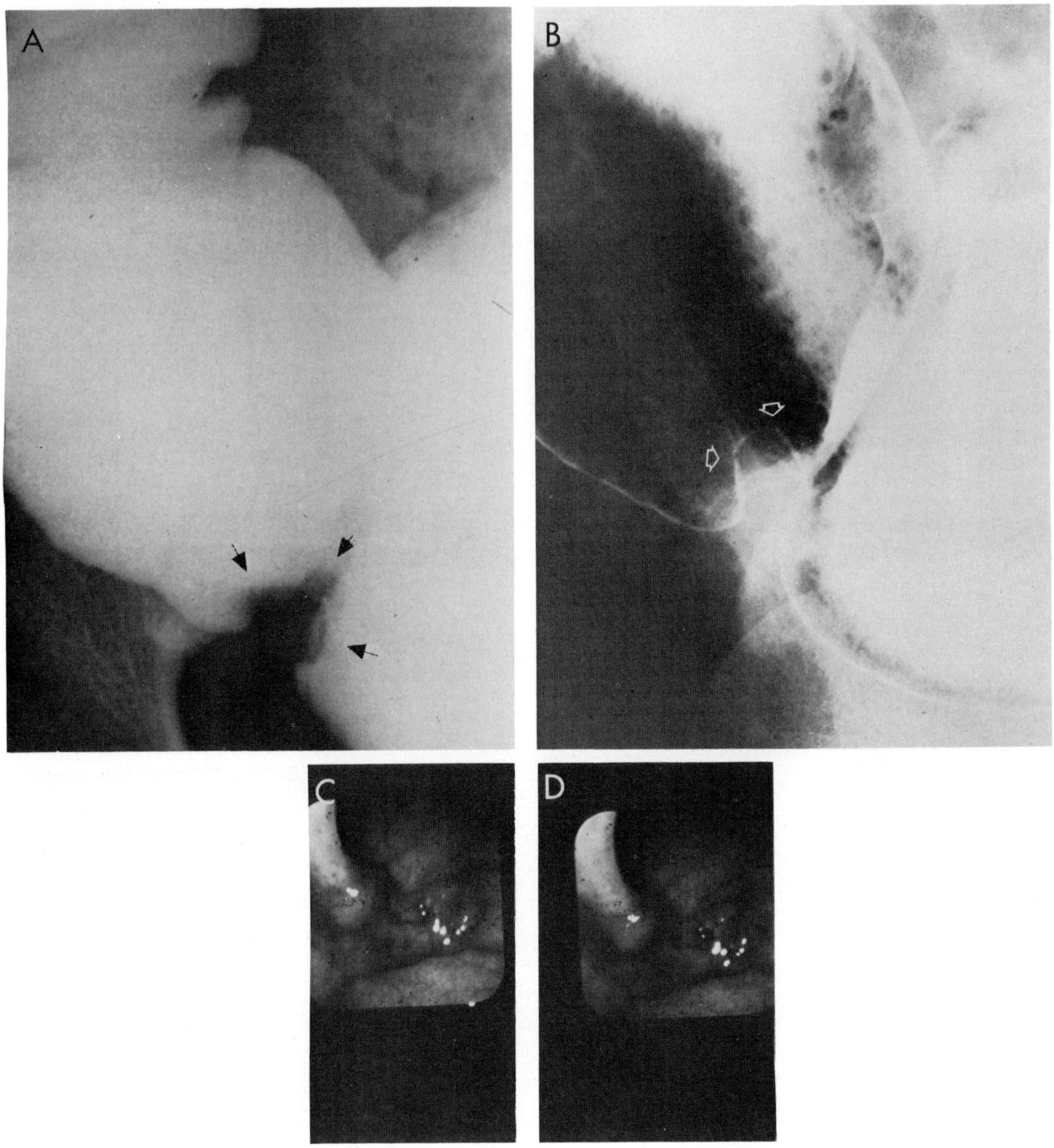

Fig 34–23.—Barium enema examination showing small adenocarcinoma of ascending colon opposite ileocecal valve *(arrows)*. **A,** solid column barium enema examination shows prominent contour defect, making diagnosis of carcinoma of colon likely. **B,** air contrast barium enema study does not show contour defect as well but discloses small, smooth, polypoid lesion, which is more characteristic of adenomatous polyp than adenocarcinoma. **C–D,** endoscopic view of carcinoma showing irregular surface of lesion. In this case the solid column barium enema demonstrated ominous nature of lesion better than double contrast examination.

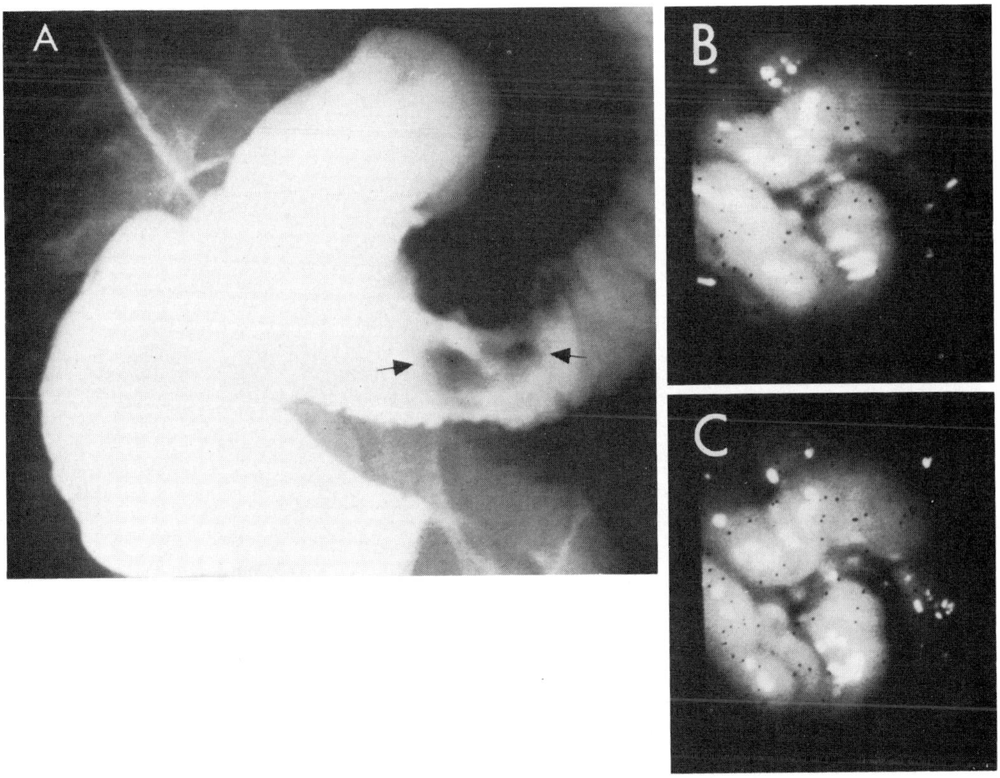

Fig 34–24.—Adenocarcinoma of colon in girl, age 12 years. **A,** barium enema examination showing polypoid carcinoma in sigmoid colon with contour defect in margin of bowel *(arrows)*. **B** and **C,** endoscopic view of tumor showing fungating nature of lesion. Diagnosis of carcinoma of colon should be considered in pediatric patients. Although the lesion is rare in this age group, it does occur.

Fig 34–25.—Barium enema examination demonstrating intussuscepting polypoid adenocarcinoma of cecum. Large mass in right portion of transverse colon is caused by intussusception. This complication of colonic carcinoma is not rare, particularly in association with polypoid cecal tumors.

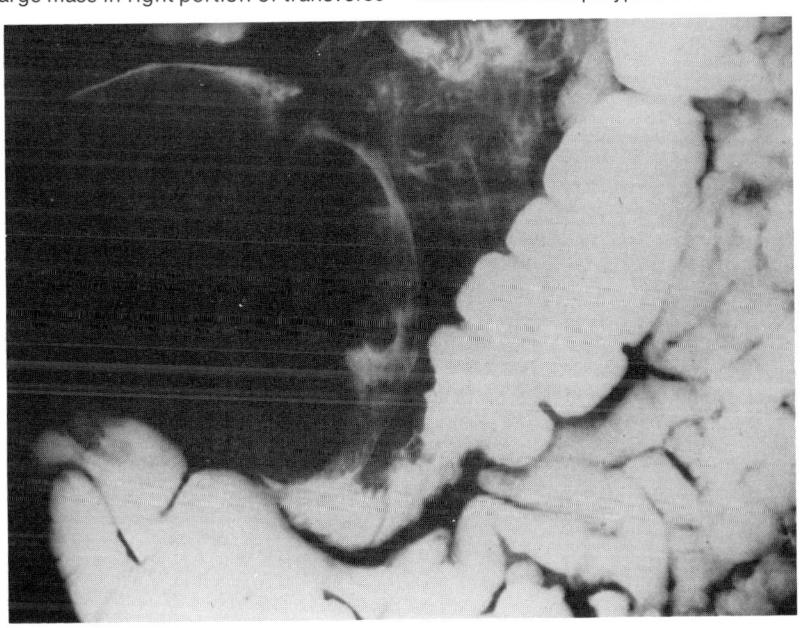

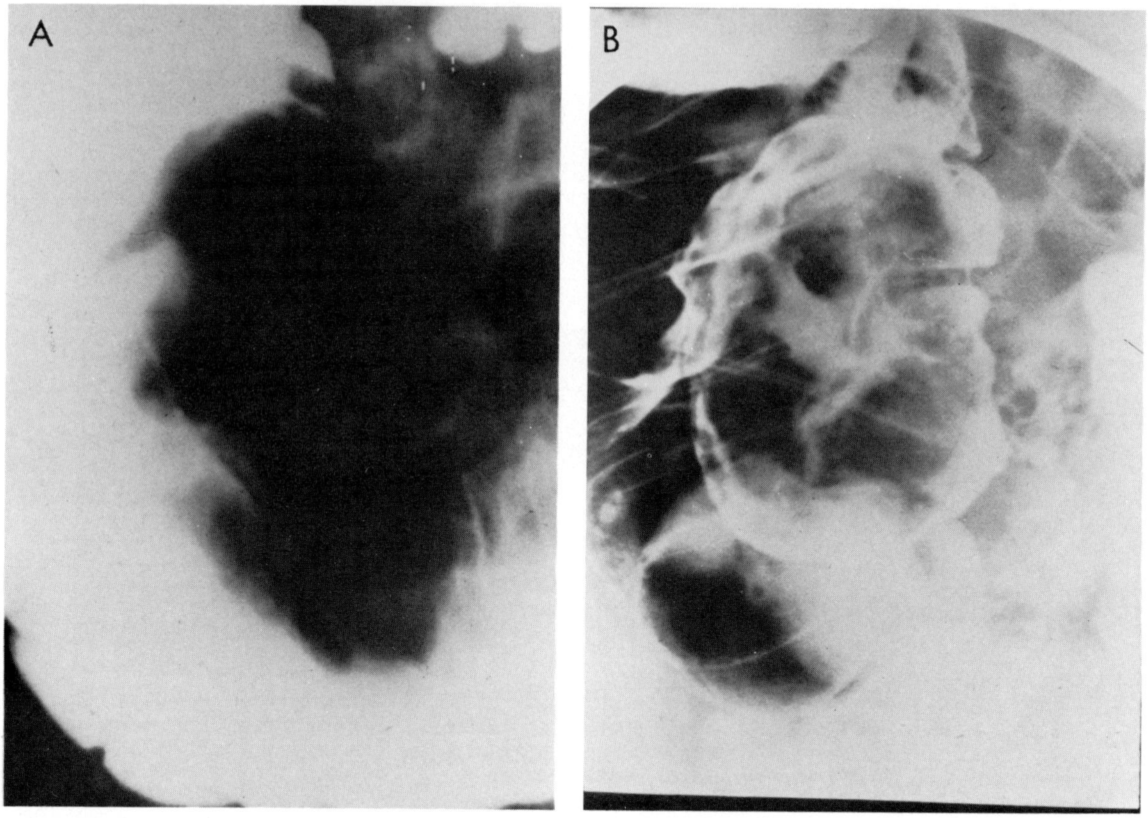

Fig 34–26.—Barium enema examination showing large polypoid lymphosarcoma of ileocecal valve in boy, age 12. **A,** solid column barium enema examination. **B,** double contrast barium enema study. Terminal ileum, ileocecal valve and cecum are commonly involved with lymphosarcoma. A polypoid mass in cecum is typical.

Fig 34–27.—Barium enema examination showing multiple nodular variety of lymphosarcoma. **A,** splenic flexure. **B,** transverse colon. Innumerable nodules up to 1 cm in size are visible. This variety of lymphoma is virtually indistinguishable radiologically from familial polyposis.

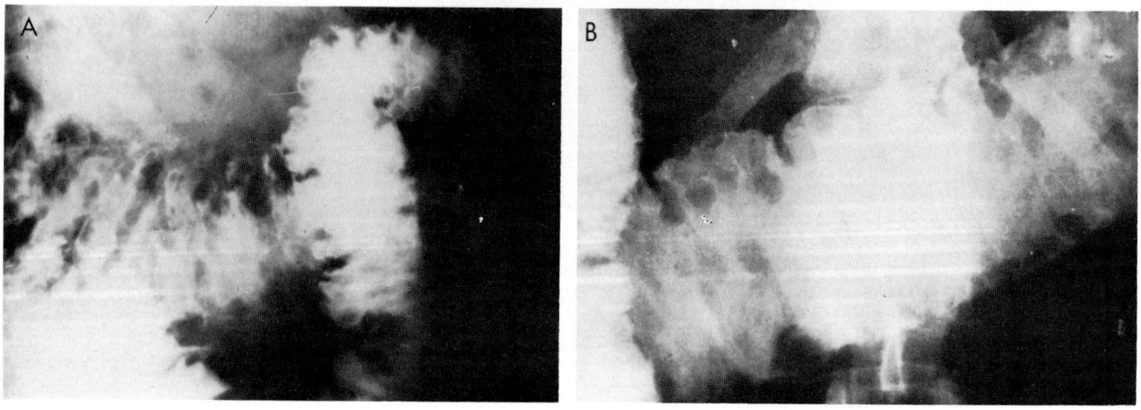

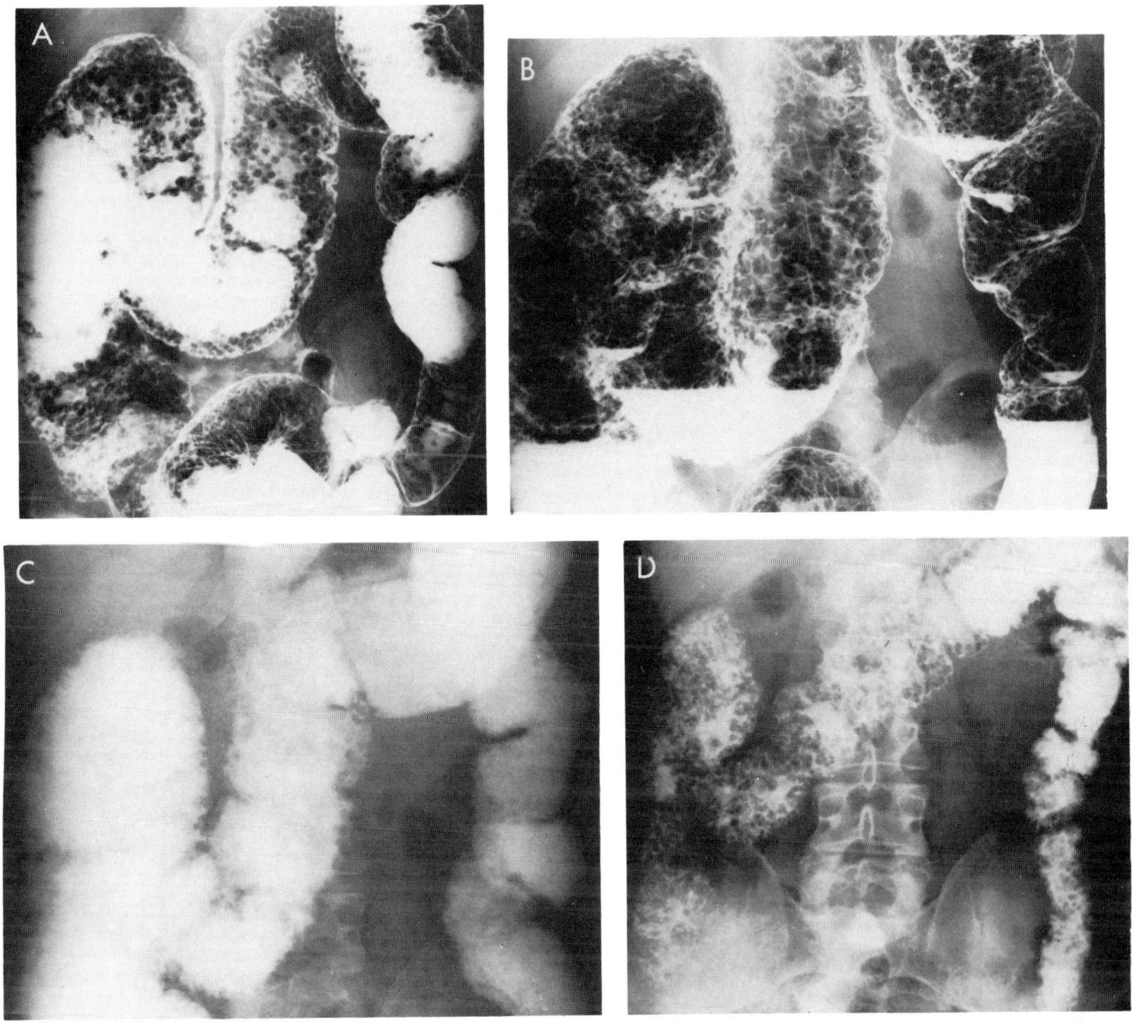

Fig 34–28. — Barium enema examination illustrating another example of nodular lymphosarcoma. **A** and **B**, air contrast barium enema examination showing innumerable nodules of same size uniformly distributed throughout bowel. **C** and **D**, solid column barium enema study in same patient demonstrating the lesions. **C**, preevacuation radiograph. **D**, postevacuation radiograph. Although diagnosis is possible using either technique, demonstration of lesions is better with air contrast procedure. (Courtesy of Dr. Steven Dorros, San Diego, Calif.)

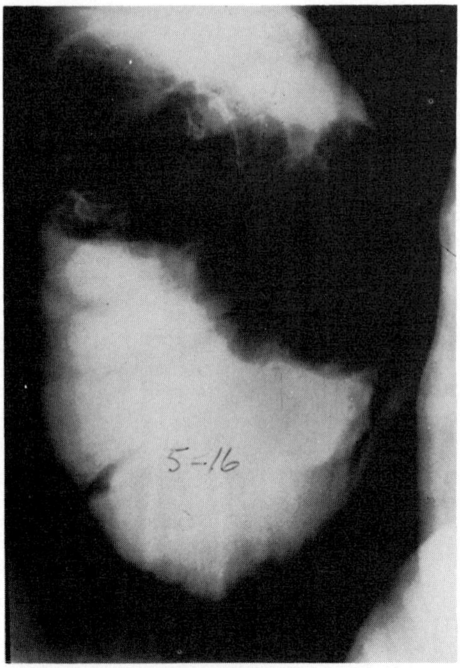

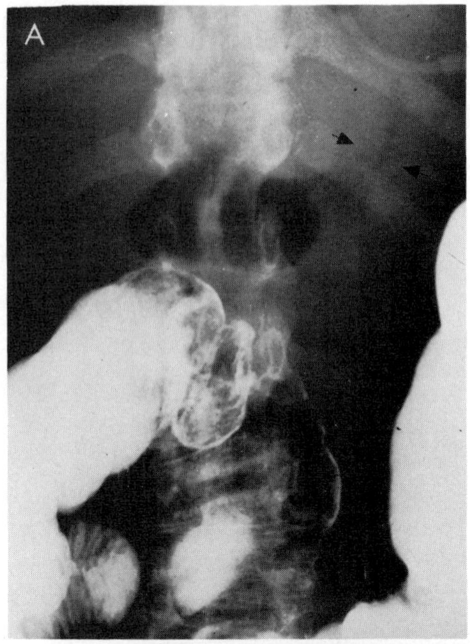

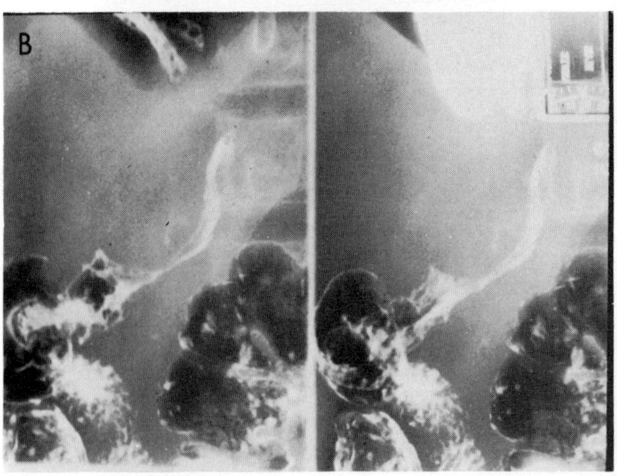

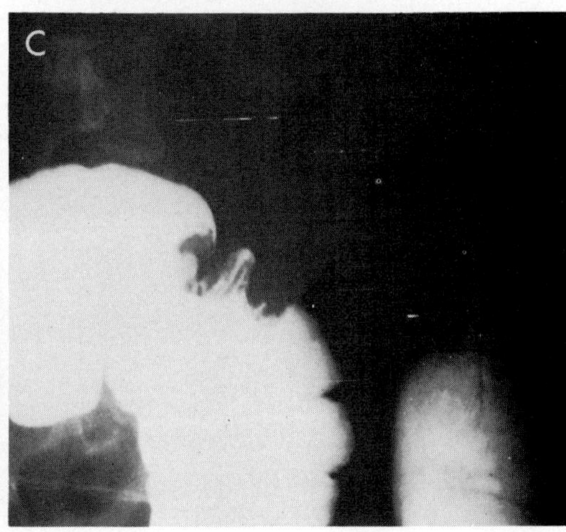

Fig 34–29 (top left). – Barium enema examination demonstrating ileocecal intussusception due to lymphosarcoma of terminal ileum in girl, age 9. Tubular configuration of cecal mass and its relation to ileocecal valve suggest diagnosis of intussusception.

Fig 34–30 (top right and **bottom).** – **A,** barium enema examination showing polypoid mass in hepatic flexure due to metastasis from adenocarcinoma of stomach. Primary tumor in stomach is apparent on radiograph because of abnormal configuration of air in stomach *(arrows).* Gastric antrum and duodenum appear normal. **B,** upper gastrointestinal examination in same patient showing linitis plastica of stomach with sparing of antrum. **C,** barium enema examination in another patient showing metastasis in hepatic flexure of colon. Pleating of bowel wall produced by scirrhous reaction associated with metastasis is evident on barium study and is characteristic of metastatic lesions.

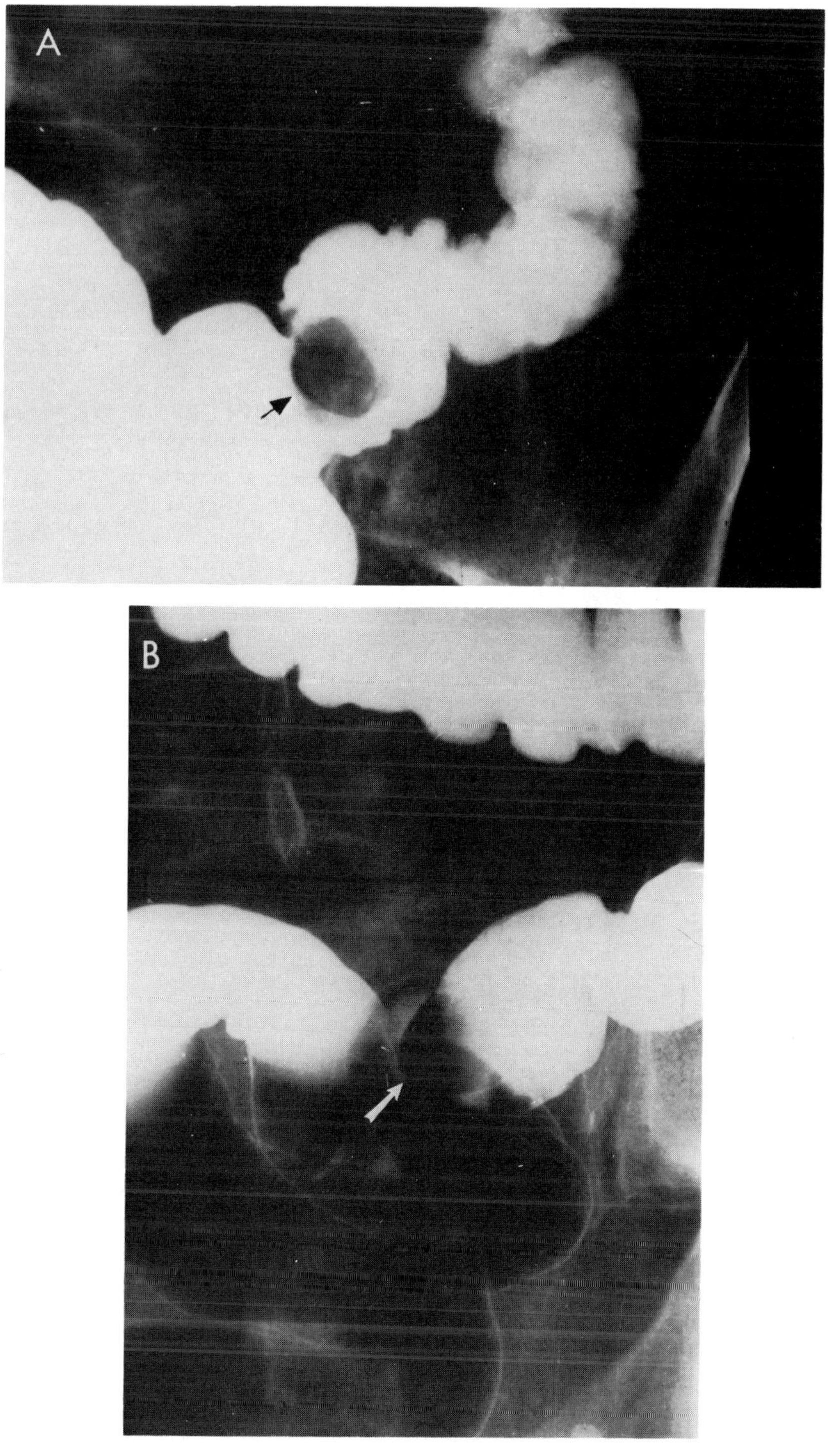

Fig 34–31.—Barium enema examination showing a 2-cm juvenile polyp in sigmoid colon *(arrows)* in boy, age 9. **A,** solid column barium enema. **B,** air contrast barium enema. Juvenile polyps are the most common variety in pediatric age group and have no malignant potential.

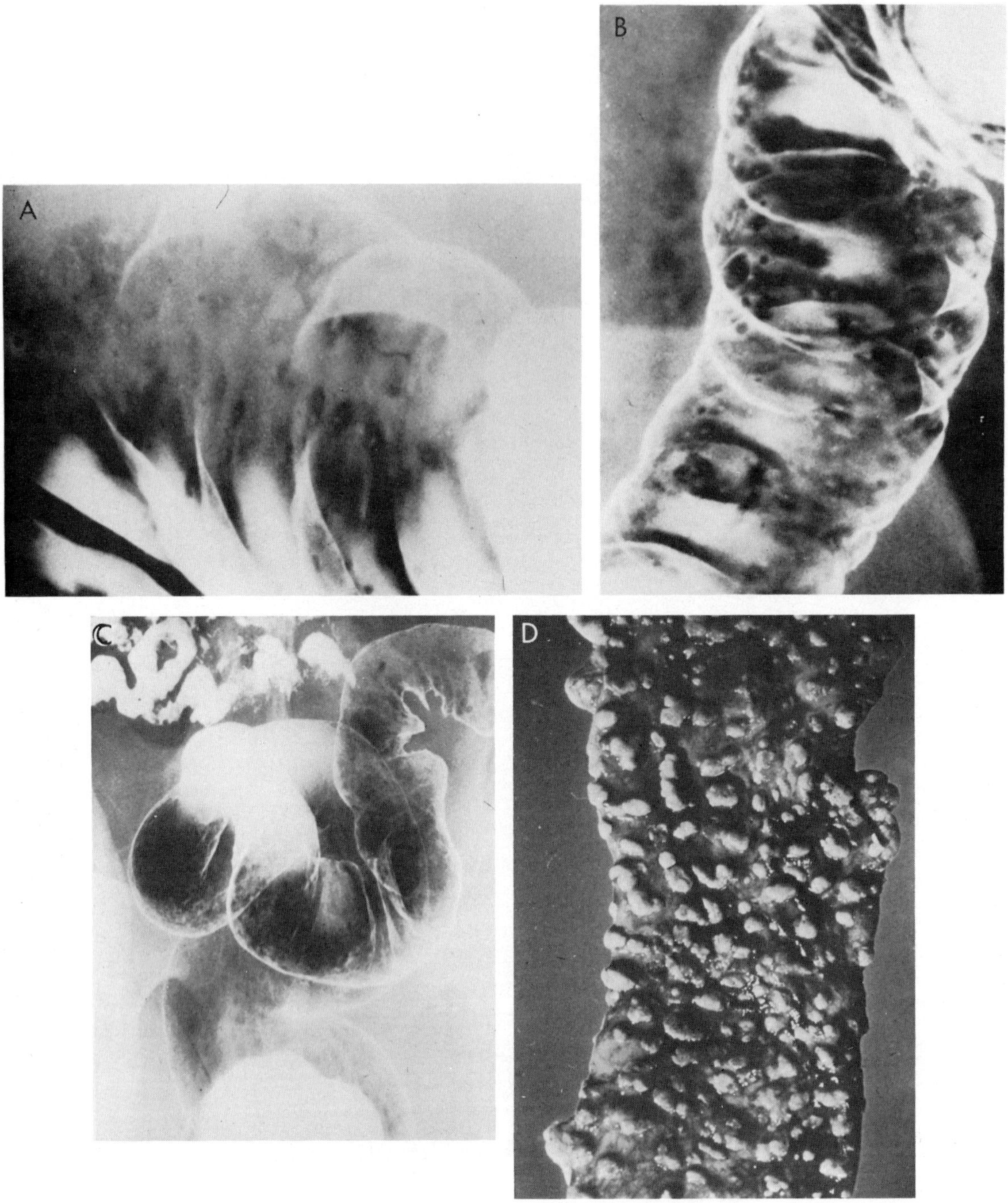

Fig 34–32.—Double contrast barium enema examination showing lymphoid hyperplasia. **A,** hepatic flexure. **B,** descending colon. Central umbilication filled with barium in small lymphoid nodules is readily apparent and typical of lymphoid hyperplasia. **C,** double contrast barium enema examination in another patient shows lymphoid hyperplasia of rectum and sigmoid colon. Lymphoid hyperplasia is rarely seen on solid column barium enema examinations. **D,** photograph of sigmoid colon in another case viewed from mucosal surface shows multiple nodules due to lymphoid hyperplasia. Colon was resected in Mexico because of an incorrect radiologic diagnosis of familial polyposis.

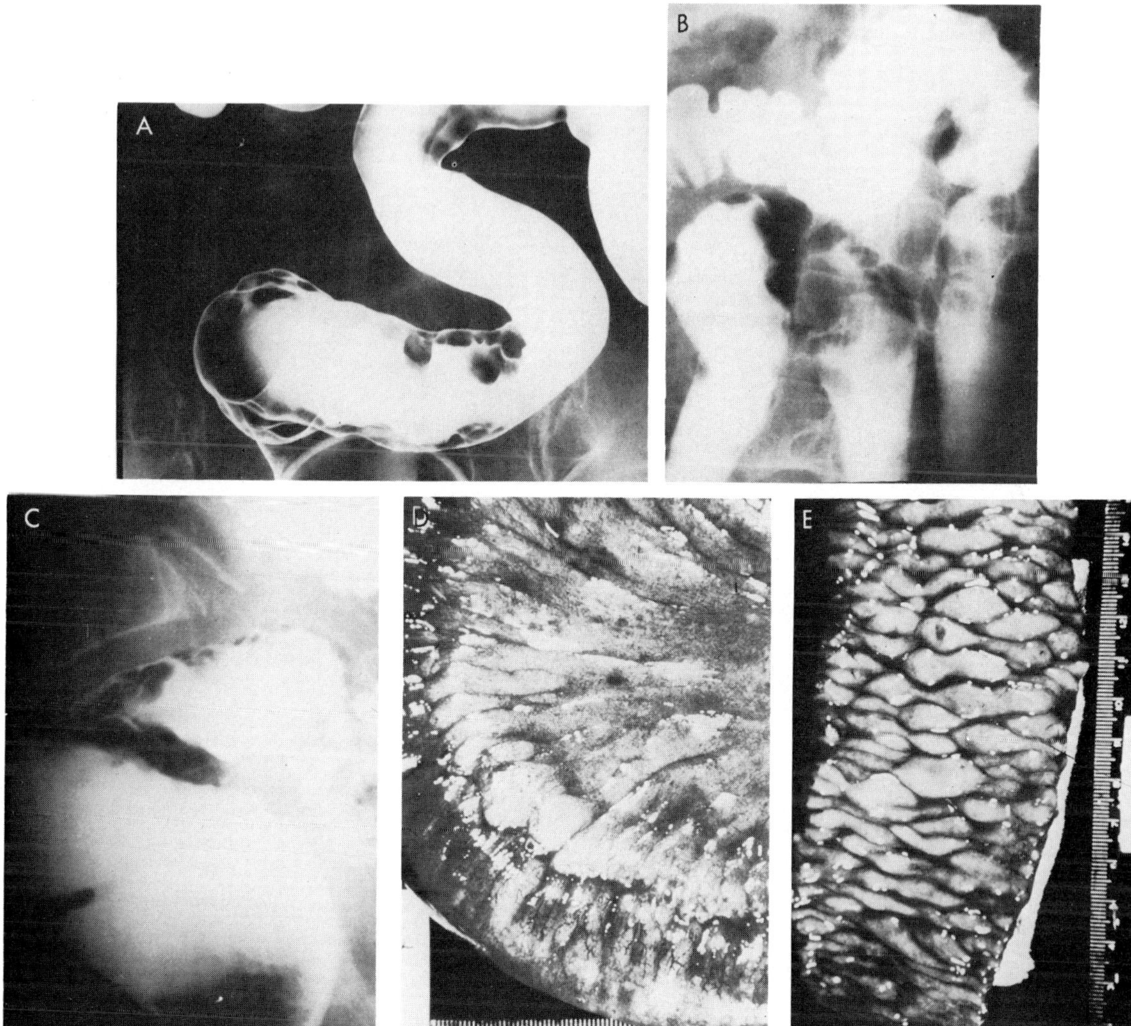

Fig 34-33.—**A**–**C**, barium enema examination in 3 patients with pneumatosis coli. **A**, sigmoid colon. **B**, splenic flexure. **C**, rectum. Relative radiolucency of the cysts compared to water-density tumor masses must be recognized to make the proper diagnosis and to differentiate pneumatosis from multiple polyps of colon. **D** and **E**, photographs of sigmoid colon from fourth patient showing pneumatosis of colon. **D**, specimen viewed from serosal side, showing multiple gas-filled cysts in mesentery. **E**, specimen viewed from mucosal side showing gas-filled cysts in submucosa.

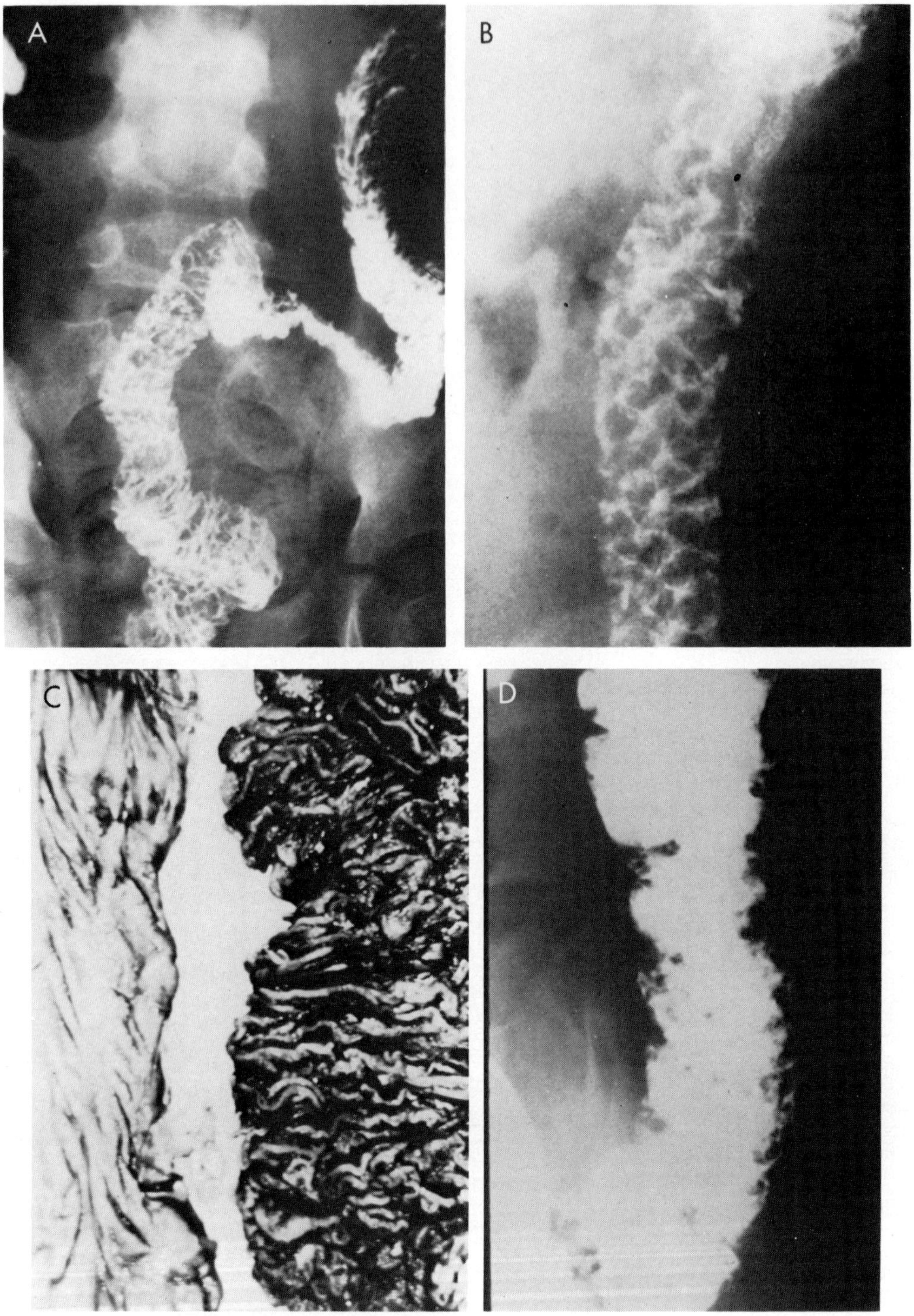

Fig 34–34.—**A** and **B,** postevacuation radiographs from barium enema in two patients with cystic fibrosis of pancreas. **A,** sigmoid colon. **B,** descending colon. Both cases show a coarse, nodular mucosal pattern typical of cystic fibrosis. **C,** photograph of sigmoid colon viewed from mucosal side in man, age 19, with cystic fibrosis, showing hyperplastic, redundant mucosa *(right)* compared to normal mucosa in another patient with normal colon *(left)*. **D,** barium enema examination in a third patient with cystic fibrosis showing adherent feces in descending colon. This finding is seen in many patients with poor preparation of the colon, but it is typical in patients with cystic fibrosis in whom the tenacious fecal material is not removed by routine methods used for cleansing the colon.

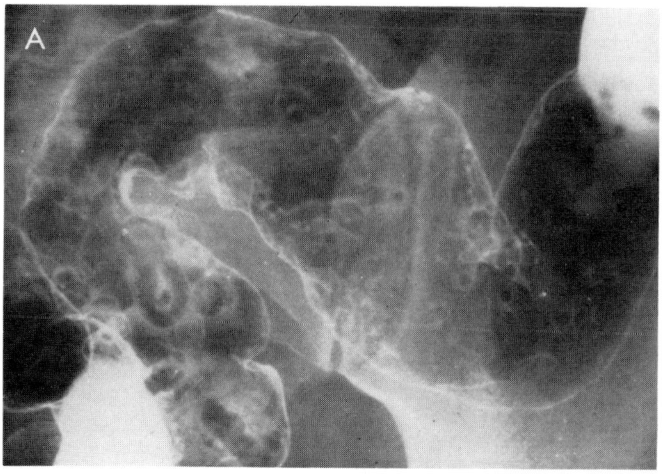

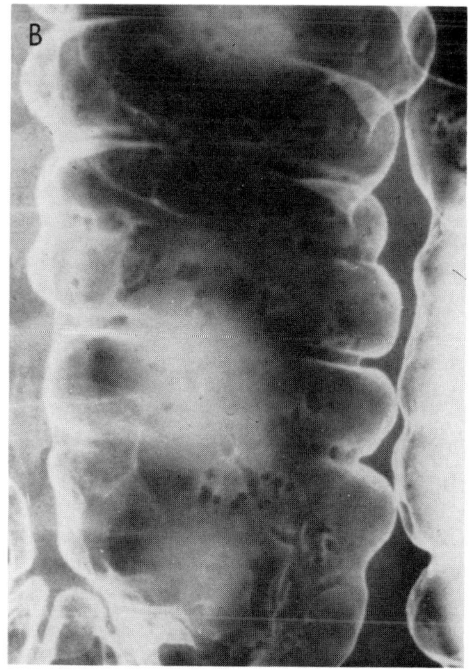

Fig 34–35.—Air contrast barium enema examination showing pseudopolyposis of colon due to ulcerative colitis of colon. **A,** sigmoid colon. **B,** left side of transverse colon. Numerous nodular and linear tags of mucosa are apparent. Length and diameter of bowel are normal, and haustral pattern is not disturbed, indicating that acute inflammatory process has subsided.

Fig 34–36.—Barium enema examination showing splenic flexure of colon in patient with pseudopolyposis of colon due to ulcerative colitis. **A,** preevacuation radiograph. **B,** postevacuation radiograph. Innumerable small nodules are present. Absence of associated inflammatory changes (ulcerations, exudate, spasm) indicate that acute ulcerative colitis has subsided, leaving abnormal mucosal pattern. (Courtesy of Dr. Ronald Saldino, San Diego, Calif.)

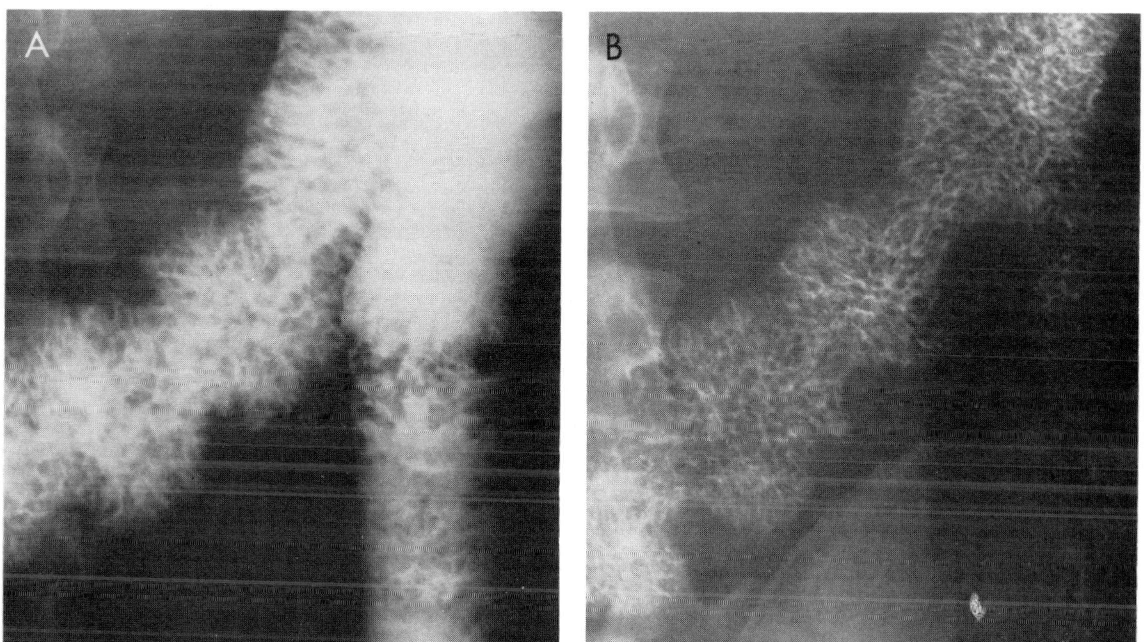

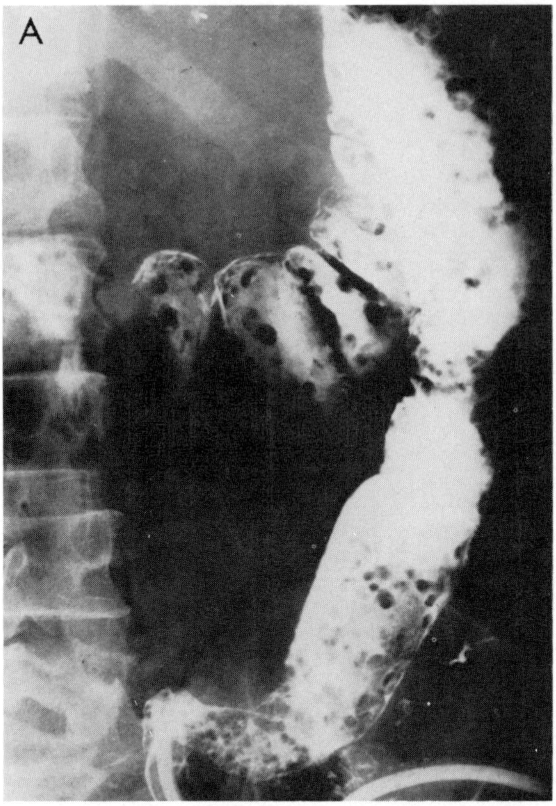

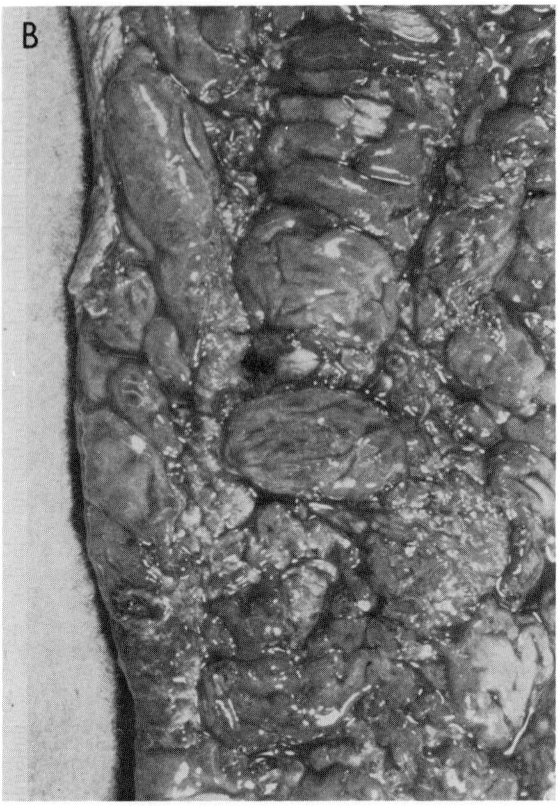

Fig 34–37.—**A,** barium enema examination showing left side of colon in patient with ulcerative colitis and pseudopolyposis. Numerous nodules due to pseudopolyposis are visible. **B,** photograph of colon after resection, showing descending colon viewed from mucosal surface. Islands of mucosa are evident surrounded by areas of ulceration. Histologically pseudopolyposis was due to mounds of normal mucosa, granulation tissue and inflammatory reactions. In this patient the acute inflammatory process had not subsided.

Fig 34–38.—Barium enema examination showing pseudopolyposis of sigmoid colon in patient with acute ulcerative colitis in remission. **A,** most of colon appears normal. **B,** several pseudopolyps are visible in sigmoid colon *(arrows)*. Note that sigmoid is narrowed and shortened. In this case the pseudopolyposis is present after acute inflammatory process had resolved.

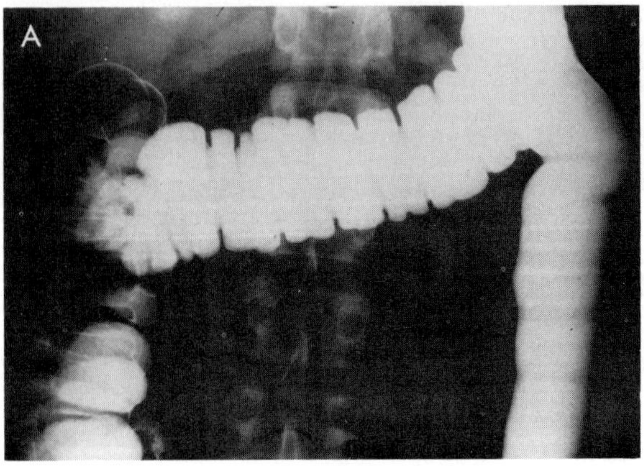

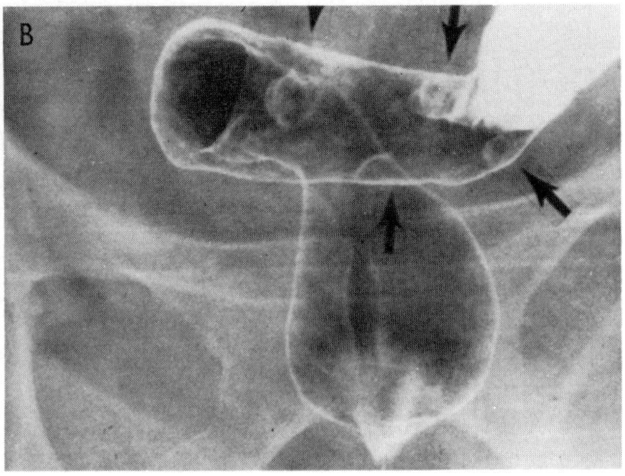

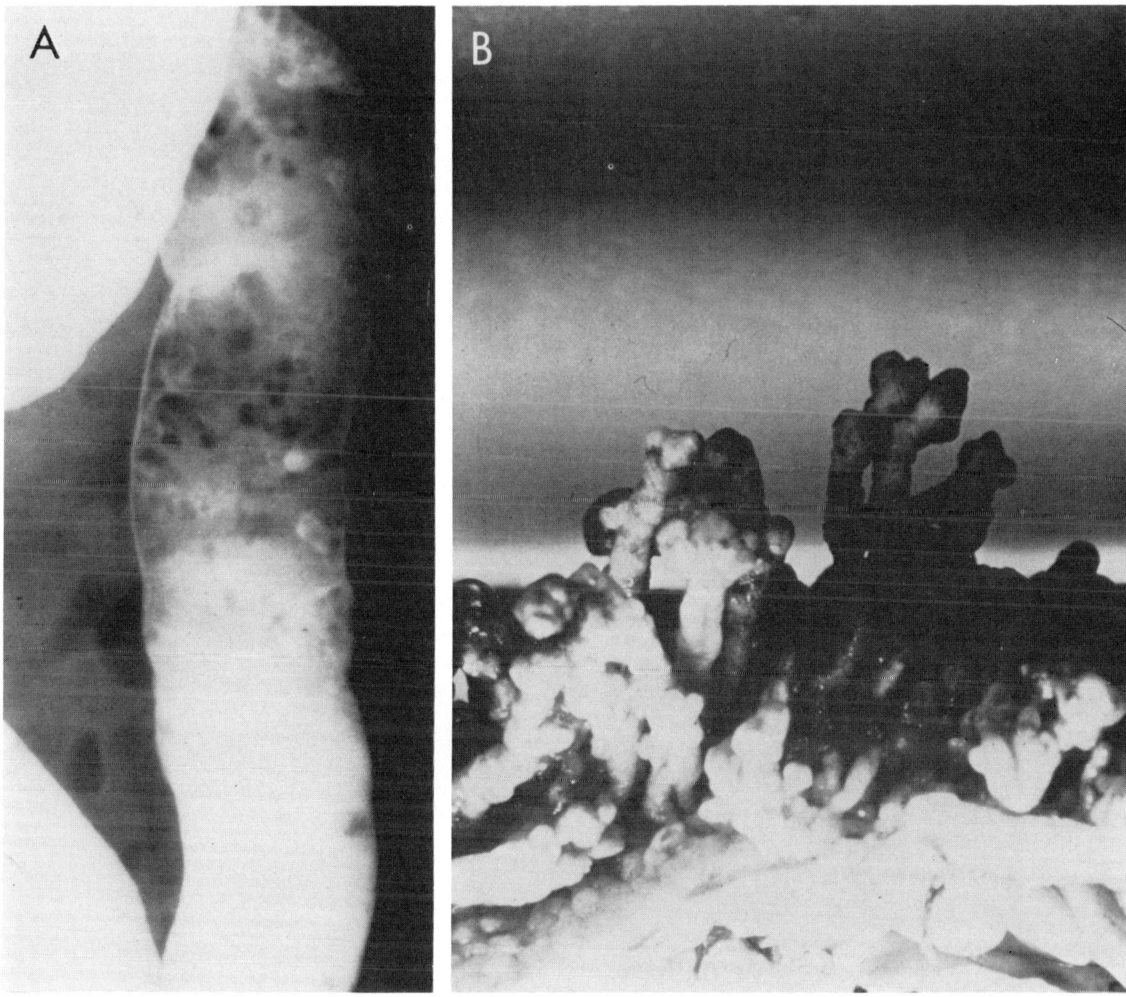

Fig 34–39.—**A,** barium enema examination showing filiform pseudopolyposis in descending colon in patient with ulcerative colitis. **B,** film of colon after surgery viewed from mucosal side showing filamentous pseudopolyps in colon. (Courtesy of Dr. John Fennessy, Chicago, Ill.)

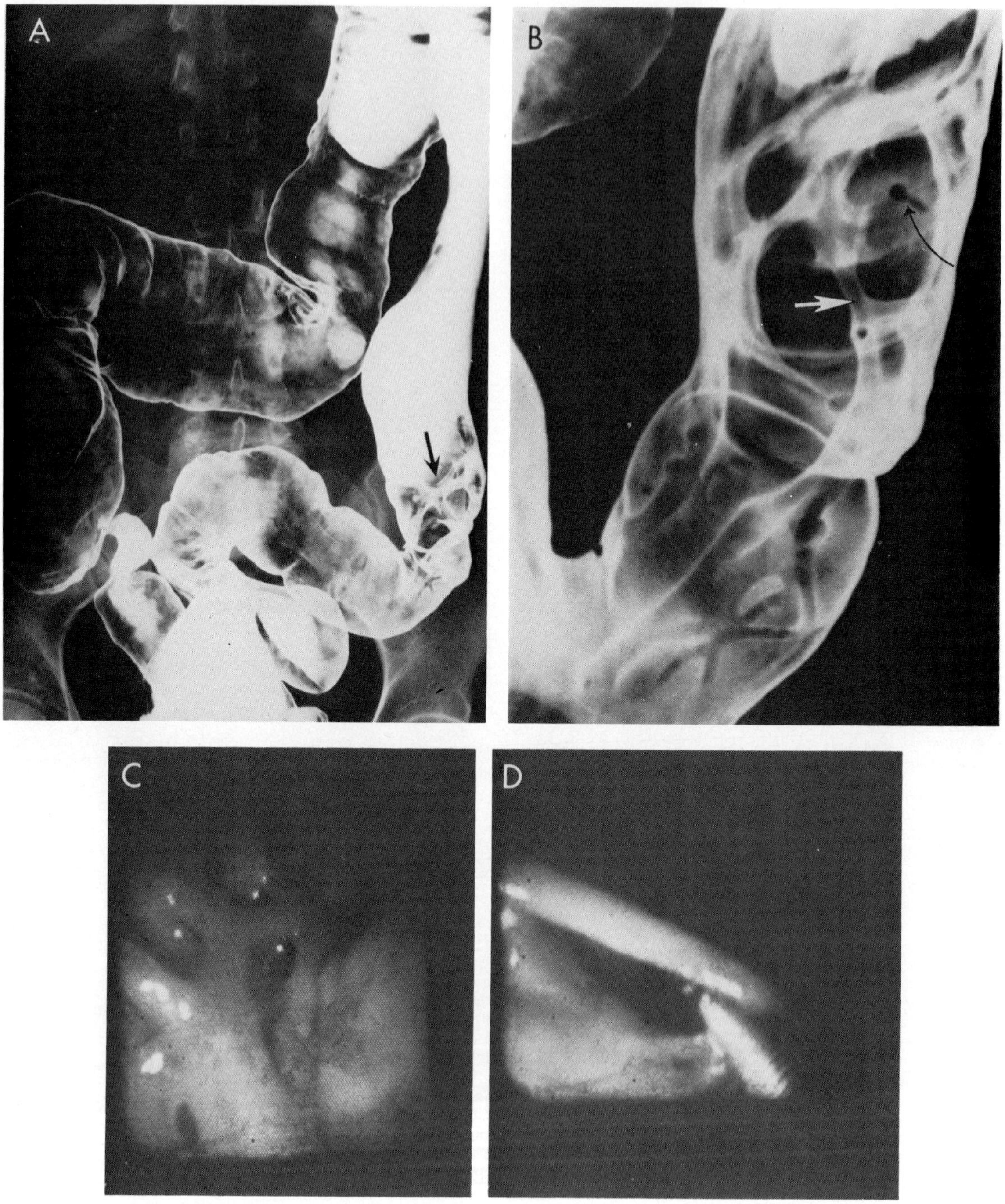

Fig 34–40. – **A** and **B,** air contrast barium enema examination showing filiform pseudopolyposis of descending colon in patient with ulcerative colitis *(arrows).* **C** and **D,** endoscopic view of pseudopolyps. In filiform variety of pseudopolyposis, linear strands of mucosa often bridge the bowel lumen. (Courtesy of Dr. Lawrence Goldberger, San Diego, Calif.)

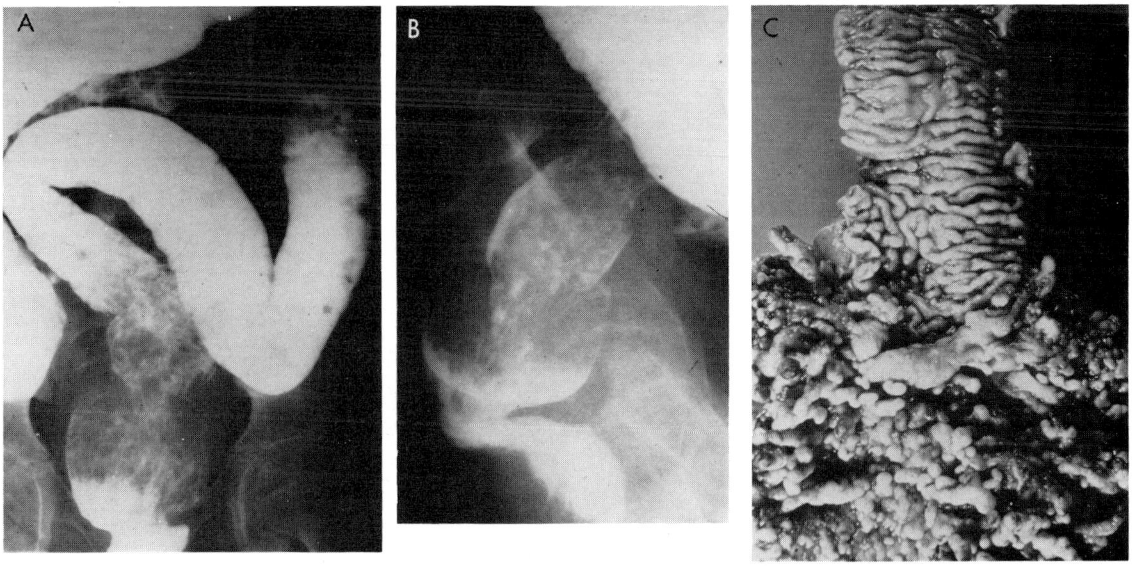

Fig 34–41. – **A** and **B,** barium enema examination in girl, age 9, showing polypoid mass in rectum due to giant pseudopolyposis. **(A,** anterior-posterior projection; **B,** lateral projection.) Lesion developed several years after symptoms of acute ulcerative colitis subsided. **C,** film of gross specimen after resection viewed from mucosal side. Histologically the mass consisted of exuberant granulation tissue, acute and chronic inflammation and normal mucosa.

Fig 34–42. – **A,** barium enema examination showing descending colon in patient with granulomatous colitis. There is a prominent cobblestone pattern of mucosa superficially resembling nodularity of polyposis or pseudopolyposis. **B,** film of colon after resection viewed from mucosal surface, showing nodular mucosa adjacent to linear ulcerations. Histologically, focal masses were due to submucosal edema and inflammation surrounded by deep ulcerations.

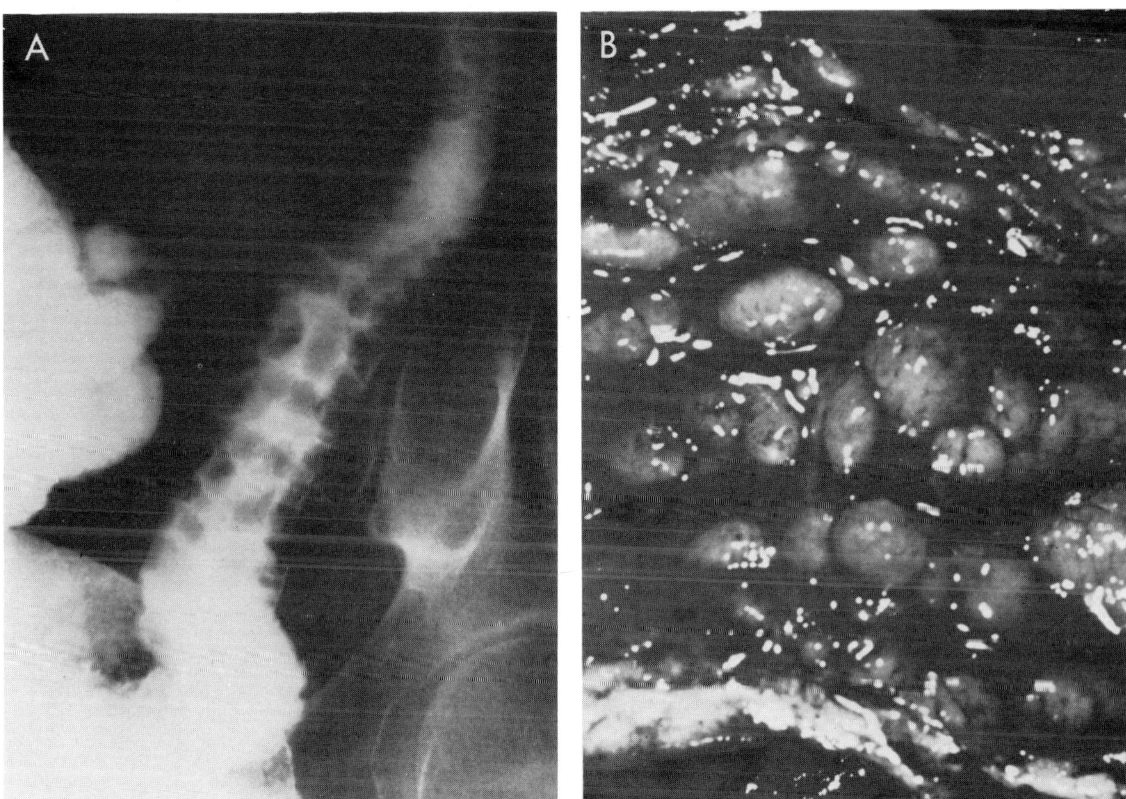

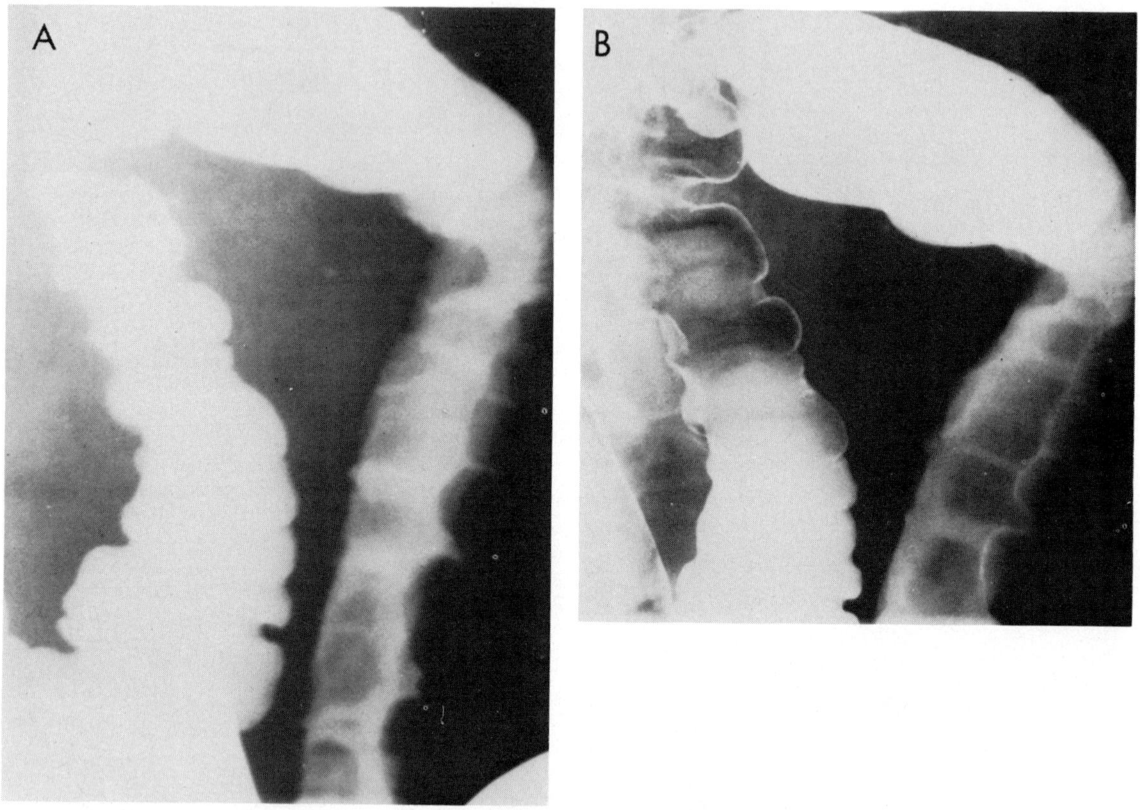

Fig 34–43. – **A** and **B,** barium enema examination showing splenic flexure in patient with ischemic colitis. Characteristic thumbprinting of barium column is visible in descending colon. Histologically these localized masses in bowel wall are due to hemorrhage and edema caused by ischemia. Ulcerations are visible in transverse colon **(A)** and are also typical of ischemic colitis.

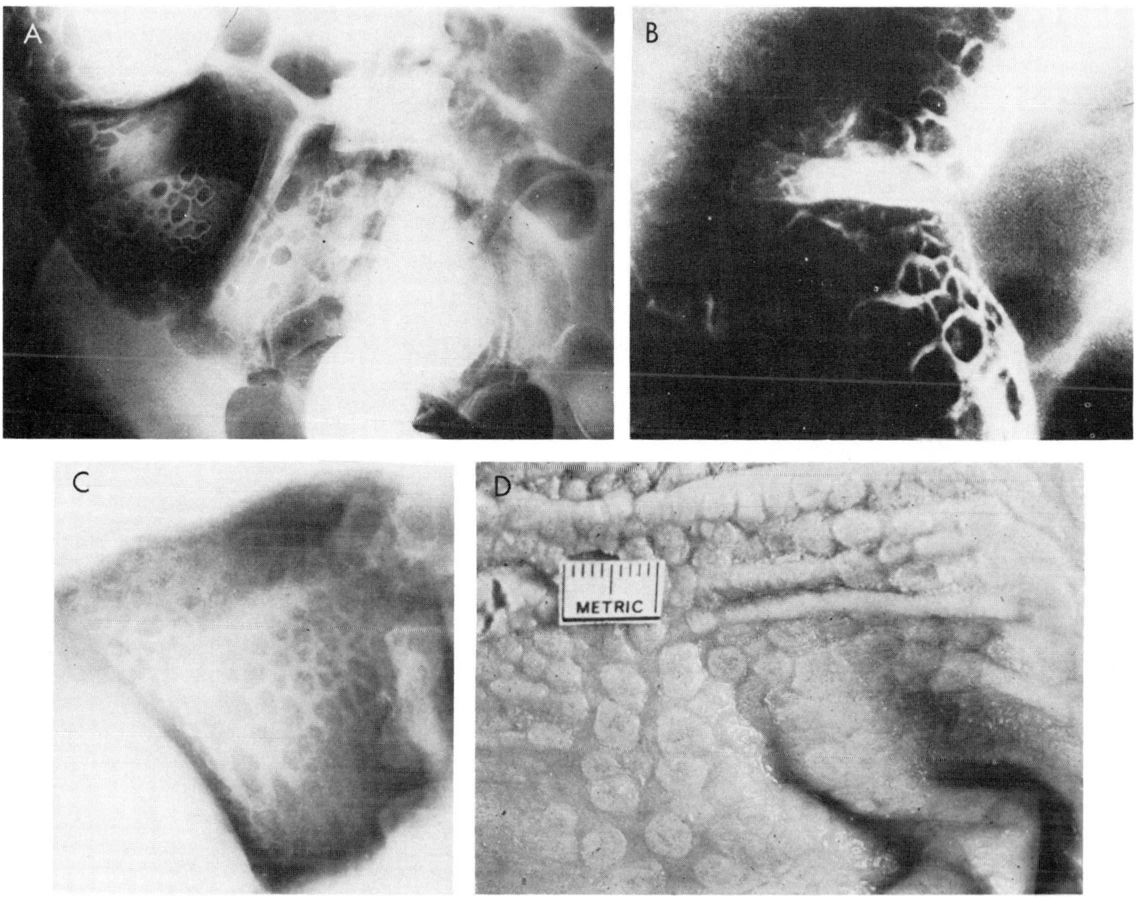

Fig 34-44.—**A-C,** barium enema examination in patient with urticaria of colon of unknown cause. Unusual mucosal pattern consisting of bizarre flat elevations is apparent. **A,** cecum and ascending colon. **B,** hepatic flexure. **C,** transverse colon. **D,** photograph of colon (same patient) at autopsy viewed from mucosal surface shows mosaic of flat elevations due to urticaria.

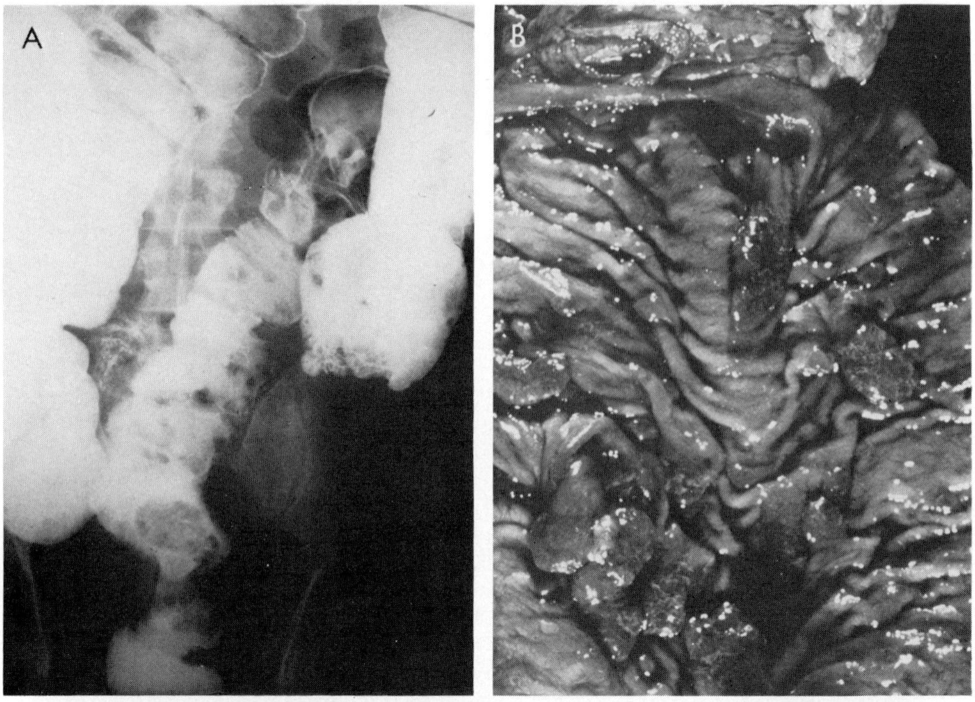

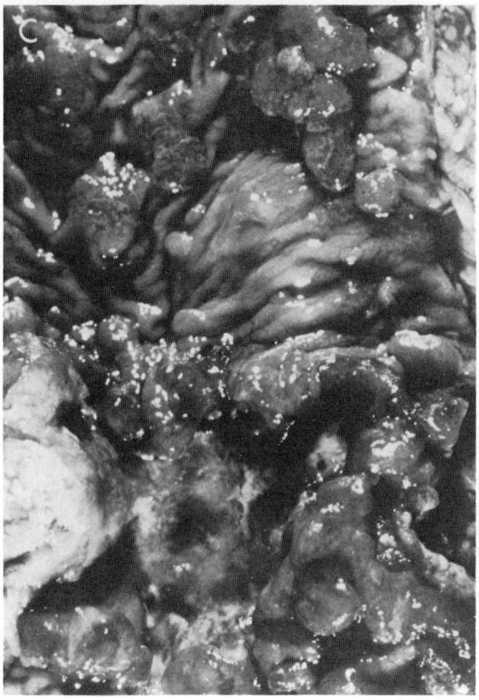

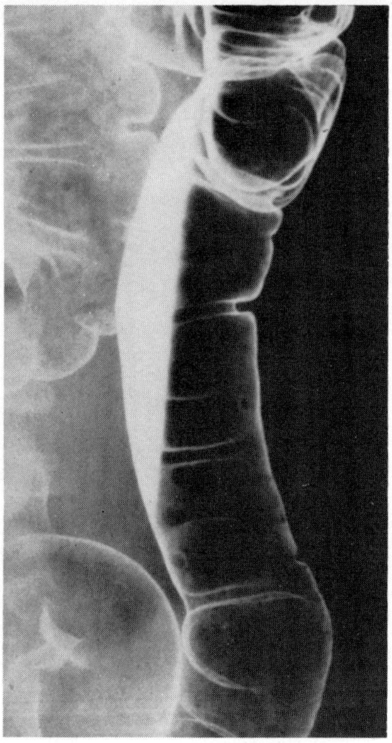

Fig 34–45 (top and bottom left).—**A,** barium enema examination in man, age 27, with known familial polyposis who had refused treatment. The radiograph shows numerous polyps in sigmoid colon and annular adenocarcinoma in rectum. **B** and **C,** photograph of specimen after surgery showing rectum viewed from mucosal side. Numerous adenomatous polyps are visible, many with short stalks. Infiltrating carcinoma is visible in lower one half of specimen in **C.**

Fig 34–46 (bottom right).—Decubitus projection from double contrast barium enema examination showing numerous small polyps in descending colon due to familial polyposis. Number and size of polyps in familial polyposis are variable and not proportional to incidence of carcinoma. Double contrast barium enema study is more accurate in detection of small polyps than solid column barium enema technique.

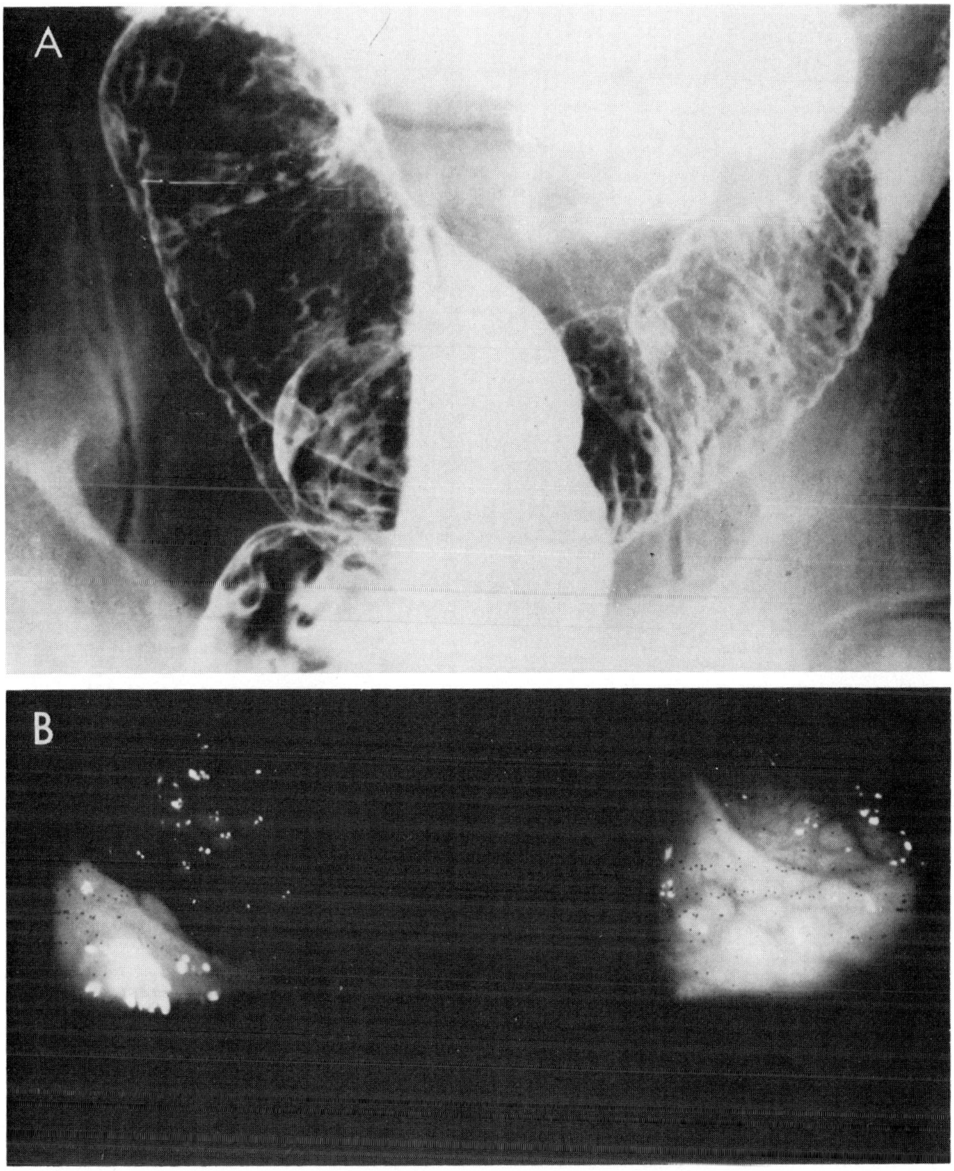

Fig 34-47. — **A,** decubitus projection from double contrast barium enema examination showing numerous adenomatous polyps in patient with familial polyposis. **B,** endoscopic views of colon showing carpet of small polyps, which covers mucosa.

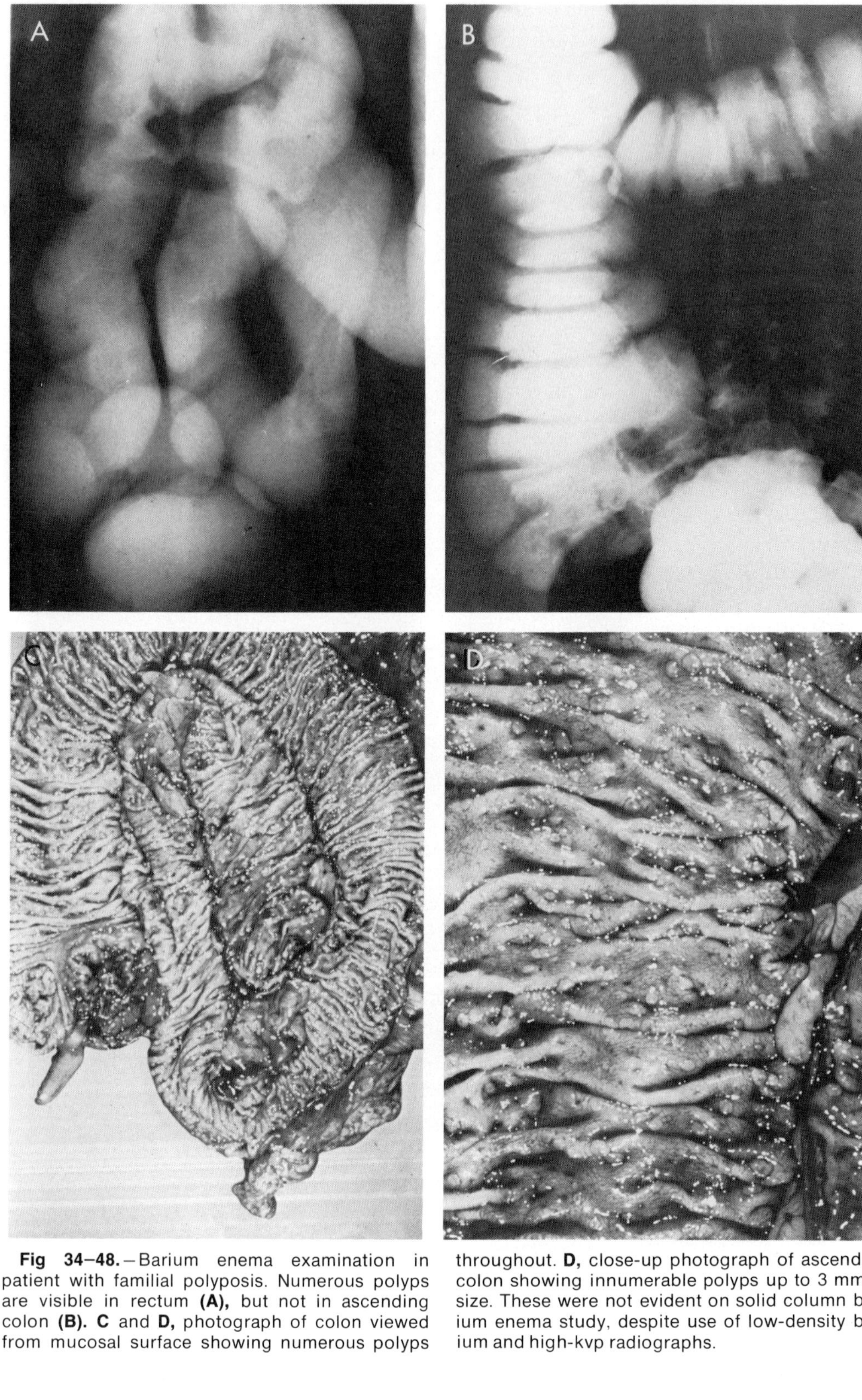

Fig 34–48. – Barium enema examination in patient with familial polyposis. Numerous polyps are visible in rectum **(A),** but not in ascending colon **(B). C** and **D,** photograph of colon viewed from mucosal surface showing numerous polyps throughout. **D,** close-up photograph of ascending colon showing innumerable polyps up to 3 mm in size. These were not evident on solid column barium enema study, despite use of low-density barium and high-kvp radiographs.

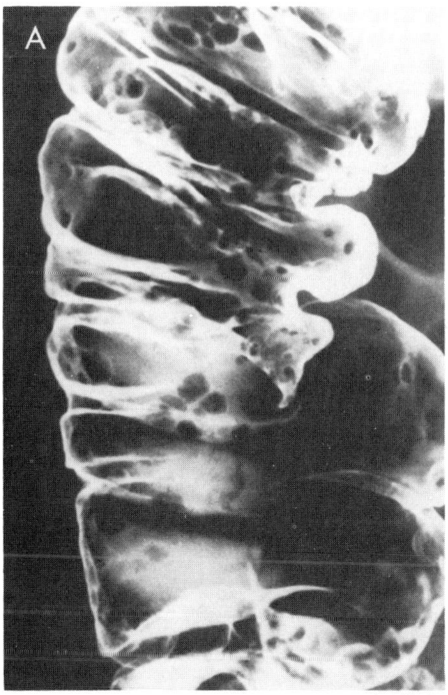

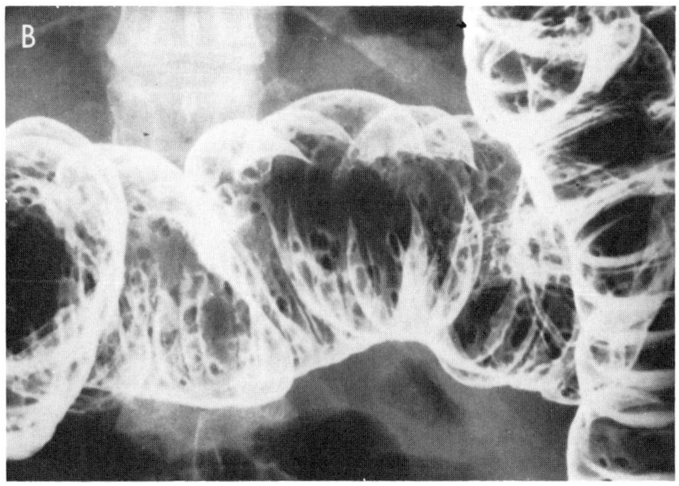

Fig 34–49.—Double contrast barium enema examination in patient with multiple adenomatous polyps of colon due to Gardner's syndrome. **A,** ascending colon; **B,** transverse colon. **C** and **D,** radiographs of paranasal sinuses showing osteomas in frontal **(C)** and maxillary sinuses **(D). C,** lateral projection. **D,** Waters' projection.

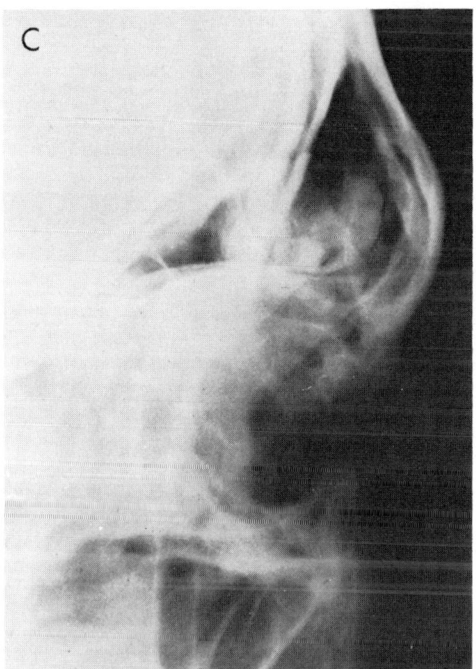

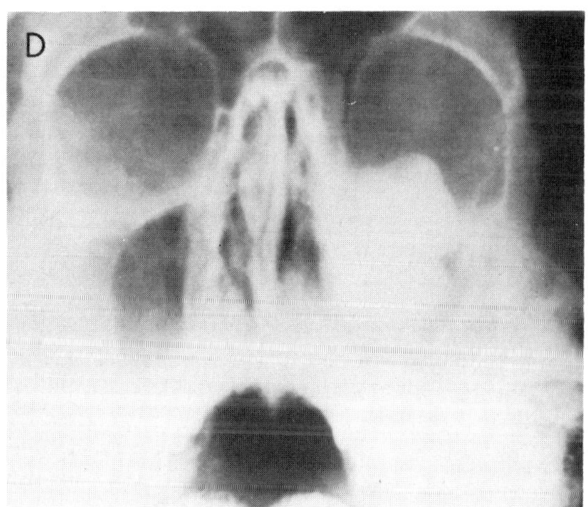

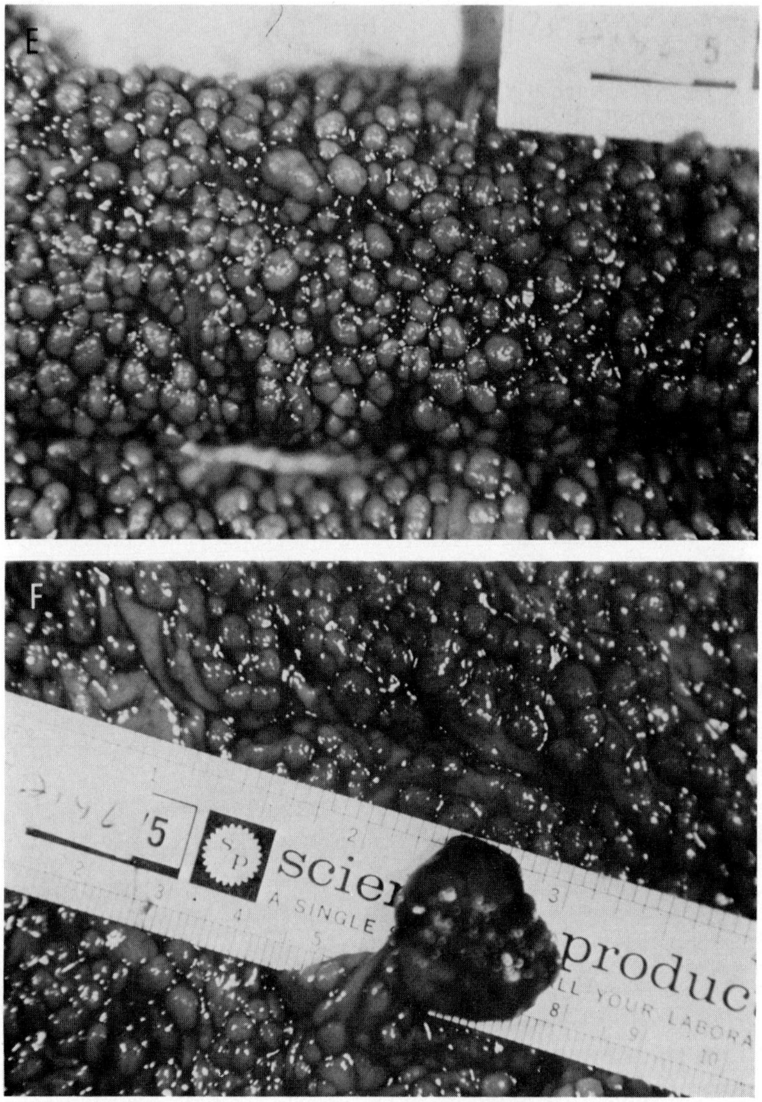

Fig 34–49 continued.—**E** and **F,** photograph of colon after resection viewed from mucosal surface. Myriad adenomatous polyps are visible. Large polyp on stalk is visible in **F.**

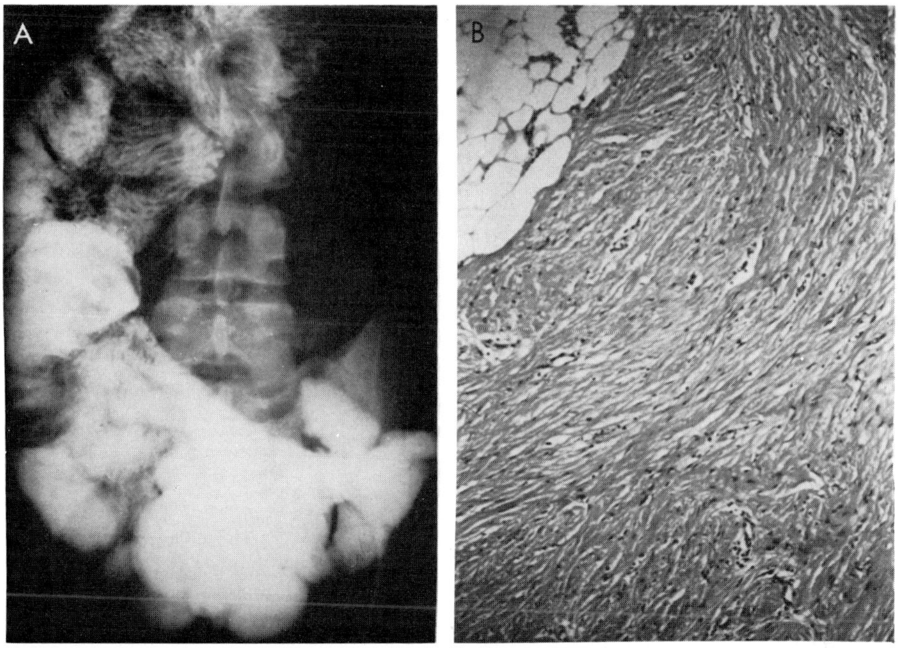

Fig 34–50.—**A,** small bowel examination in patient with Gardner's syndrome. Total colectomy had been performed earlier for multiple adenomatous polyps. Large mass fills left upper quadrant of abdomen, displacing small bowel downward and to the right. At surgery, this was found to be due to a huge retroperitoneal desmoid tumor. **B,** photomicrograph of tumor showing mature fibrous tissue. In Gardner's syndrome, fibrous tissue has a pronounced tendency to proliferate excessively.

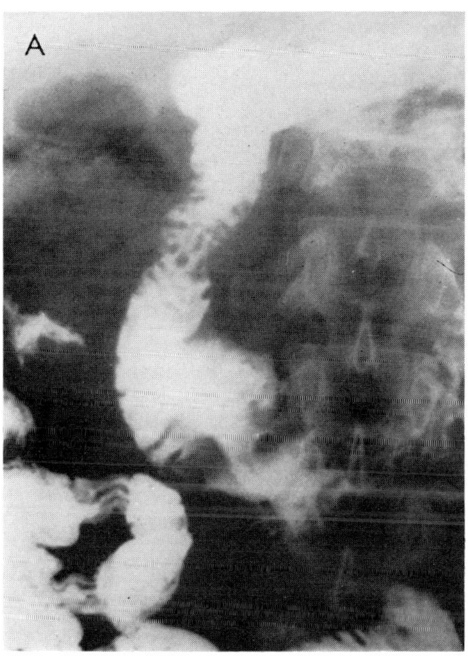

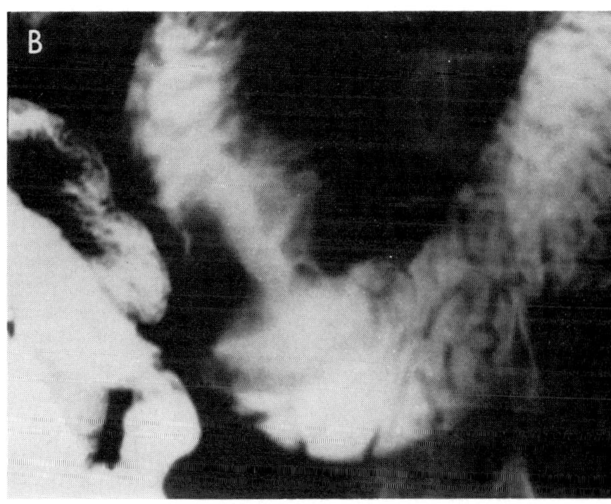

Fig 34–51.—**A** and **B,** upper gastrointestinal examination in another patient with Gardner's disease, showing annular carcinoma of second and third portions of duodenum. Patients with Gardner's syndrome have an increased incidence of carcinoma of duodenum, papilla of Vater and pancreas.

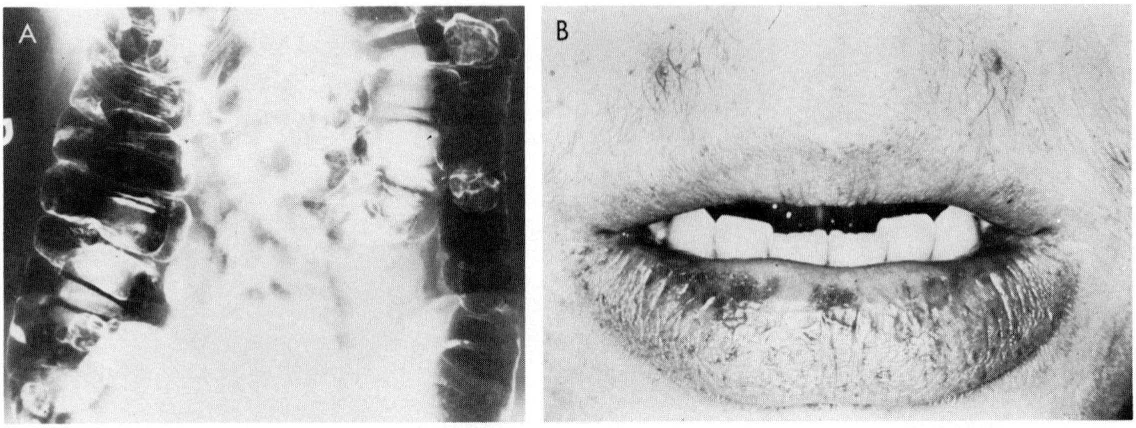

Fig 34–52.—**A,** air contrast barium enema examination showing multiple polyps of colon in boy, age 17, with Peutz-Jeghers syndrome. **B,** film of mouth showing melanin pigmentation of lips. Polyps in Peutz-Jeghers syndrome are hamartomas with no malignant potential. (Courtesy of Dr. William Bernstein, Minneapolis, Minn.)

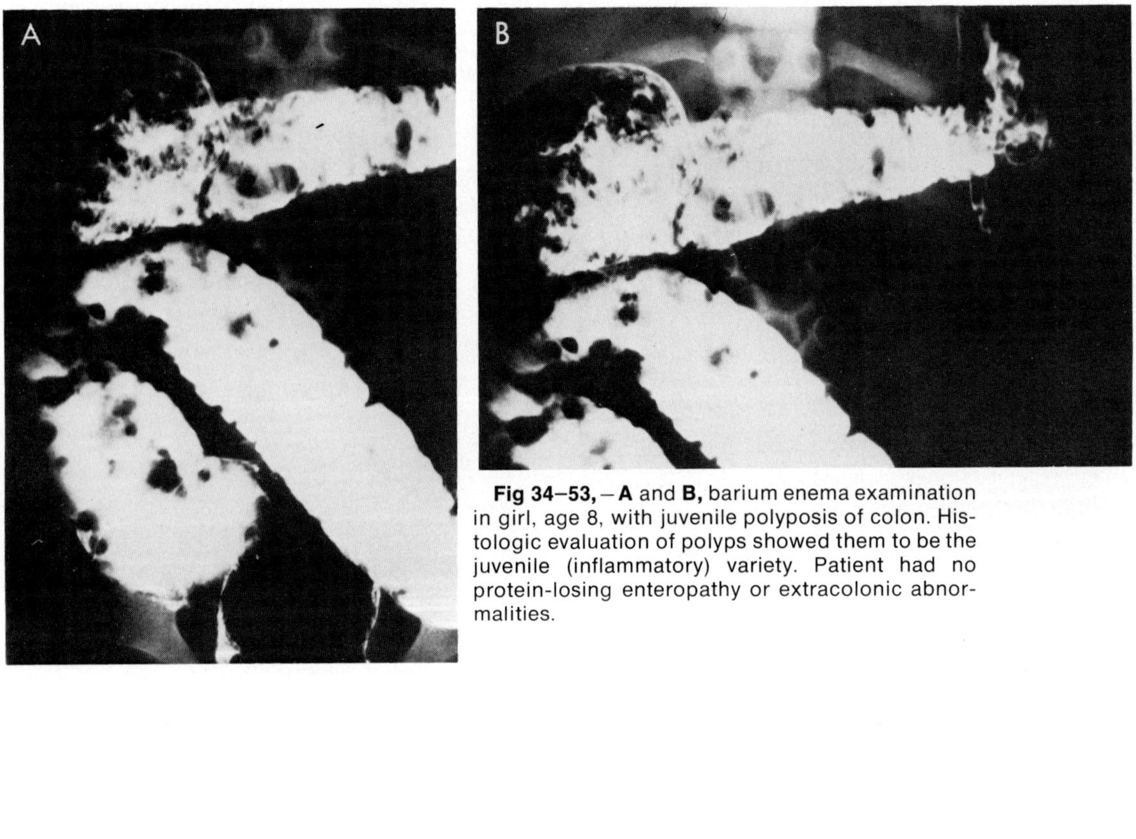

Fig 34–53,—**A** and **B,** barium enema examination in girl, age 8, with juvenile polyposis of colon. Histologic evaluation of polyps showed them to be the juvenile (inflammatory) variety. Patient had no protein-losing enteropathy or extracolonic abnormalities.

Chapter 35

Pseudomembranous Colitis

J. FRANK ARGUELLO, M.D.

ANTIBIOTIC-ASSOCIATED pseudomembranous colitis—a result of medical progress, a complication of modern therapy—has carried many names in the past: pseudomembranous enterocolitis, diphtheritic colitis, staphylococcal enterocolitis, antibiotic-associated pseudomembranous colitis, neonatal necrotizing enterocolitis and postoperative colitis. It has only been in the last decade that this entity has finally had some light shed upon it.

The first case of a pseudomembranous colitis-like syndrome was reported by Finney in 1893[1] in a patient who underwent an uncomplicated gastroenterostomy and 5 days later developed bloody diarrhea and hypotension and then died. For the next 40 years many cases of "diphtheritic colitis" and postoperative pseudomembranous colitis were reported.

Then in the 1950s *Staphylococcus aureus* enterocolitis was added to the list, further confusing the picture. However, for the first time a bacterial agent was implicated in the cause of the entity. This was reported as a consequence of the observation by some investigators that there was heavy growth of staphylococci in the stools of patients with antibiotic-associated pseudomembranous colitis. Therefore, it was postulated that antimicrobial agents altered the normal flora and favored growth of resistant pathogens, mainly *S. aureus*.

Etiology

When the term staphylococcal colitis was coined in the 1950s, staphylococci infections were rampant throughout hospital wards and so it was not unusual to culture it from any stool. Some observers later noted that 14–30% of all postoperative patients had staphylococci in their stools but seldom had pseudomembranes on sigmoidoscopy.[2] Several attempts to reproduce staphylococcal pseudomembranous colitis in animal models have failed, despite the fact that almost every other type of staphylococcal infection has been duplicated, including enterotoxin-producing staphylococcus.[3, 4] It is also now known that 30% of the normal population have staphylococci in their stool without being ill, whether or not treated with antimicrobials.[5, 6] The entity of staphylococcal pseudomembranous colitis is therefore now seriously questioned, though an infectious agent is still thought to be responsible for pseudomembranous colitis, i.e., a clostridium.

The first antibiotics associated with pseudomembranous colitis were tetracycline and chloramphenicol in the early 1950s. In the following decade, not much was reported in the way of antibiotic-associated colitis, but in the 1970s the subject once again became popular with the often quoted articles of Tedesco et al.[7, 8] The study of 200 patients treated with clindamycin (all routes: intravenous, oral, intramuscular) incriminated this drug as a major offender in the development of pseudomembranous colitis. The major findings were (1) an incidence of diarrhea of 21% (2) an incidence of pseudomembranous colitis of 10%, (3) absence of dose relationship in the syndrome, (4) increased risk from use of the oral route and (5) possibility of development of the syndrome even after discontinuance of the antibiotic.

Other studies found that the association between pseudomembranous colitis and clindamycin was not as great as originally thought. Lusk et al.,[9] in 104 patients, noted an incidence of 2%, with an incidence of diarrhea of 20%. Swartzberg et al.[10] in 1,000 patients receiving clindamycin found an incidence of diarrhea of 6.6% with no cases of pseudomembranous colitis. The incidence therefore of clindamycin-associated pseudomembranous colitis seems to be somewhere between 2% and 10%.

The other antibiotic commonly associated with pseudomembranous colitis is ampicillin. Most investigators, including Lusk et al.,[9] have found that it closely trails clindamycin in its association with pseudomembranous colitis. Many other antibiotics have also been reported to be implicated, including the cephalosporins, the penicillins (synthetic and nonsynthetic), chloramphenicol and the sulfas.[11-13]

Clinical Presentation

Antibiotic-associated pseudomembranous colitis presents at early onset with a watery, mucus-like diarrhea. Abdominal pain, most often crampy, accompanies the clinical picture. Leukocytosis and fever complete the features of the syndrome. By clinical signs and symptoms alone, pseudomembranous colitis can easily mimic ulcerative colitis, infectious enterocolitis (e.g., shigellosis, salmonellosis, amebiasis) or acute abdomen.

Endoscopy

In conjunction with a positive history of antibiotic usage, the most reliable method of diagnosis is sigmoidoscopy and/or colonoscopy. These examinations reveal a multitude of yellowish plaques, 3 – 4 mm in size, throughout the colon. The plaques often are confluent, forming a membrane-like structure. The underlying mucosa is very friable and edematous. In severe cases it may bleed from erosions underlying the membranes (Fig 35 – 1 and 35 – 2).

Pathology

An acute inflammatory infiltrate is the most common finding. Both polymorphonuclear leukocytes and some lymphocytes may be found. Fibrinoid necrosis of the epithelium and villous tips is commonly seen. Thrombosis of the mucosal or submucosal vessels is not seen. True ulcerations are rare.

Pseudomembranous Colitis, an Infectious Disease?

Because at one time it was thought that pseudomembranous colitis might be viral in origin, many studies have been carried out using tissue cultures. This has led indirectly to the finding of a cytopathic toxin that is inactivated by clostridial antitoxins. In late 1977 Larson and Price[14] described a toxin found in the feces of each of nine patients with pseudomembranous colitis and in two patients with antibiotic-associated nonspecific colitis. The toxin was neutralized by *Clostridium sordellii* antitoxin. Rifkin and others[15] also late in 1977, reported the same toxin and antitoxin relationships. Bartlett et al.[16] in early 1978 were able to produce an enterocolitis in hamsters by injecting intracecally the stool from patients who had pseudomembranous colitis and positive cultures for cytotoxicity. No intestinal disease was noted when hamsters were injected with stool from healthy subjects. In all cases cytotoxicity in tissue culture and enterocolitis in hamsters were neutralized by pretreatment with antitoxin.

In November 1978 Bartlett and others[17] provided even more convincing evidence that intestinal overgrowth of a cytotoxigenic strain of *Clostridium difficile* preceded the development of pseudomembranous colitis. They demonstrated that *C. difficile* was commonly isolated in stools from affected patients. It was also uniquely cytotoxigenic to human amnion cells. *C. sordellii* was rarely found. Stools from patients with neonatal necrotizing enterocolitis or ulcerative colitis and healthy controls all showed negative results of cytopathic assay. All these studies point to *C. difficile* as the major cause of antibiotic-associated pseudomembranous colitis.[18-20]

Roentgen Findings

The radiology of antibiotic-associated colitis was first reported in the early 1960s by Feinberg,[21] when he described plain film findings of this disease. In the mid and late 60s, barium enema findings were described in several case reports. Throughout the literature the general consensus was that the radiologic findings of antibiotic-associated colitis were fairly nonspecific and undistinguishable from the other colitides, such as ulcerative colitis, Crohn's colitis, ischemic colitis and the colitis of infectious etiology, e.g., shigellosis and amebiasis.

In the 70s several authors[22-24] attempted to associate the endoscopic and gross pathologic findings with what is seen radiologically. Roentgen examination in antibiotic-associated colitis may be divided into three stages: (1) plain films, (2) standard full-column barium enema, (3) air contrast barium enema.

PLAIN FILMS

Stanley et al.[25] in early 1976 described several criteria that were "highly suggestive" of antibiotic-associated colitis in patients deemed to be too ill to undergo a full barium enema. These patients all had antibiotic-associated colitis established either by endoscopy (sigmoidoscopy or colonoscopy) or pathologic criteria. This combination of findings has been supported by several other case reports.[26-29] The findings are as follows:

1. *Moderate bowel distention.*—Involvement mainly of the colon, not small bowel (contrary to Feinberg's original paper) (Fig 35–3, A).
2. *Markedly thickened colonic wall.*—Secondary to mural edema with severely decreased lumen diameter (see Fig 35–3, B).
3. *Thumbprinting.*—Secondary to colonic haustral edema, seen throughout the colon and usually associated with thickened transverse folds (see Fig 35–3, A and C).
4. *Marginal irregularities.*—Probably representing pseudomembranous plaques in profile (see Fig 35–3, D).
5. *Total colonic involvement.*—Nonsegmental; typical of severe pseudomembranous colitis.

FULL-COLUMN BARIUM ENEMA

Barium enema findings in antibiotic-associated pseudomembranous colitis vary considerably depending on the severity of the disease. The findings range from nonspecific patterns, e.g., small mucosal nodular irregularities on the surface (Fig 35–4, A) and better demonstrated by air contrast (Fig 35–5, A), to a full-blown picture of multiple rounded or oval filling defects (pseudomembranous plaques) seen throughout the entire mucosal surface (see Fig 35–4, B and C). Sometimes careful inspection is needed to appreciate the serrated appearance of the contour of the barium column produced by smaller plaques (see Fig 35–4, D).

As previously noted in the description of the plain films, the involvement with the pseudomembranous plaques is diffusely spread throughout the entire colon. The rectum and sigmoid are almost always involved, making sigmoidoscopic diagnosis very accessible. (see Fig 35–4, E and F).

AIR CONTRAST BARIUM ENEMA

Although more time consuming than the routine barium enema, the air contrast barium enema provides a definite advantage in diagnosis of antibiotic-associated pseudomembranous colitis. In this disease large amounts of mucus are found on the mucosal surface; good coating of the mucosa is therefore impaired, making it difficult to differentiate between ulcerations and plaques. Air contrast studies help to differentiate the pseudomembranous plaques in pseudomembranous colitis from the ulcerations of ulcerative colitis. Figure 35–5, A, demonstrates well the pseudomembranous plaques in the rectum and sigmoid, which would not have been visualized by routine barium enema alone.

Contrast studies are safe when carefully done and can demonstrate the pseudomembranous plaques in any part of the colon, both enface and in profile (see Fig 35–5, B). However, if characteristic plain film changes are present, a barium enema is best withheld and proctoscopy opted for to establish a diagnosis.

Therapy

The mainstay of therapy of antibiotic-associated pseudomembranous colitis is clearly discontinuation of all antibiotics plus general supportive therapy.

Tedesco and Markham[30] reported the use of oral vancomycin, 2 gm per day, in nine patients with pseudomembranous colitis. All had severe diarrhea and tissue culture evidence of a clostridial toxin. All patients showed a good clinical response.

Other investigators, such as Hofmann,[31] have suggested the use of cholestyramine, but further studies are needed to find the true place of this agent in the therapy of pseudomembranous colitis. Glucocorticosteroids have not been demonstrated to aid in treatment and may even be contraindicated if pseudomembranous colitis is truly an infectious process. As a last resort, surgical resection is indicated.[32]

REFERENCES

1. Finney, J. M.: Gastroenterostomy for cicatrizing ulcer of the pylorus, Johns Hopkins Med. J. 4:53, 1893.
2. Azar, H., and Drapanas, T.: Relationship of antibiotics to wound infection and enterocolitis in colon surgery, Am. J. Surg. 115:209, 1968.
3. Wood, J. S., et al.: Staphylococcal enterocolitis in chinchillas, Johns Hopkins Med. J. 98:454, 1956.
4. Shemano, I., and Hitchens, J.: Paradoxical intestinal inhibitory effects of staphylococcal enterotoxin, Gastroenterology 53:71, 1967.
5. Hummel, R. P.: Iatrogenic staphylococcal enterocolitis, Ann. Surg. 160:551, 1964.
6. Dearing, W. H., et al.: Studies on the relationship of Staphylococcus aureus to pseudomembranous enteritis, Gastroenterology, 38:441, 1960.
7. Tedesco, F. J.: Clindamycin and colitis: A review, J. Infect. Dis. 135:95, 1977.
8. Tedesco, F. J., et al.: Clindamycin-associated colitis, Ann. Intern. Med. 81:429, 1974.
9. Lusk, R. H., et al.: Gastrointestinal side effects of clindamycin and ampicillin therapy, J. Infect. Dis. 135 (suppl.):111, 1977.
10. Swartzberg, J. E., et al.: Clinical study of gastrointestinal complications associated with clindamycin therapy, J. Infect. Dis. 135:99, 1977.
11. Fee, H. J., et al.: Pseudomembranous colitis associated with Cephazolin therapy, Am. J. Surg. 133(2): 247, 1977.
12. Cameron, A., and Meiron, T.: Case report: Pseudomembranous colitis and co-trimoxazole, Br. Med. J. 1:1321, 1977.
13. Reiner, L., and Schlesinger, M. J.: Pseudomembranous colitis following Aureomycin and chloramphenicol, Arch. Pathol. 54:39, 1952.
14. Larson, H. E., and Price, A. B.: Pseudomembranous colitis. Presence of clostridial toxin, Lancet 2: 1312, 1977.
15. Rifkin, G., et al.: Intestinal and Systemic Toxicity of Fecal Extracts from Hamsters with Clindamycin-Induced Colitis (C.L.C.) (Abst.), University of Michigan, Ann Arbor.
16. Bartlett, J. G., et al.: Antibiotic-associated pseudo-

membranous colitis due to toxin-producing clostridia, N. Engl. J. Med. 1238:531, 1978.
17. Bartlett, J. G., et al.: Clindamycin-associated colitis due to a toxin-producing species of Clostridium in hamsters, J. Infect. Dis. 136:701, 1977.
18. Gorbach, S. L., and Bartlett, J. G.: Pseudomembranous enterocolitis: A review of its diverse forms, J. Infect. Dis. (suppl.) 135:89, 1977.
19. Dupont, H. L.: Etiology of antibiotic-associated colitis, Gastroenterology, 75:913, 1978.
20. George, W. L., Sutter, V. L., Finegold, S. M.: Antimicrobial agent-induced diarrhea—A bacterial disease, J. Infect. Dis. 136:822, 1977.
21. Feinberg, S. B.: The roentgen findings in severe pseudomembranous colitis, Am. J. of Roentgenol. 74:778, 1960.
22. Scott, A. J., and Nicholson, G. I.: The recognition of pseudomembranous colitis as a clinical entity, Aust. NZ J. Med. 4:502, 1974.
23. Stanley, R. J., et al.: The spectrum of radiographic findings in antibiotic-related pseudomembranous colitis, Radiology 111:519, 1974.
24. Shimkin, P. M., and Link, R. J.: Pseudomembranous colitis: A consideration in the barium enema differential diagnosis of acute generalized ulcerative colitis, Br. J. Radiol. 46:437, 1973.
25. Stanley, R. J., Melson, L., Tedesco, F., and Saylor, J.: Plain film findings in severe pseudomembranous colitis, Radiology 118:7, 1976.
26. Stanley, R. J., and Tedesco, F.: Antibiotic-associated pseudomembranous colitis, CRC Crit. Rev. Clin. Radiol. Nucl. Med. 8:255, 1976.
27. Ecker, J. A., Williams, R. G., and McKittrick, J. E.: Pseudomembranous enterocolitis—an unwelcome gastrointestinal complication of antibiotic therapy, Am. J. Gastroenterol. 54:214, 1970.
28. Sherbon, K. J.: Radiology in pseudomembranous colitis, Australas. Radiol. 16:66, 1972.
29. Tully, T. E., and Feinberg, S. B.: A reappearance of antibiotic-induced pseudomembranous colitis, Radiology 110:563, 1974.
30. Tedesco, F., and Markham, R.: Oral vancomycin for antibiotic-associated pseudomembranous colitis, Lancet 2:226, 1978.
31. Hofmann, A. F.: Bile Acids, diarrhea and antibiotics: Data, speculation and a unifying hypothesis, J. Infect. Dis. 135:s126, 1977.
32. Boyd, W. C., and DenBesten, L.: Subtotal colectomy for refractory pseudomembranous enterocolitis, J.A.M.A. 235:181, 1976.

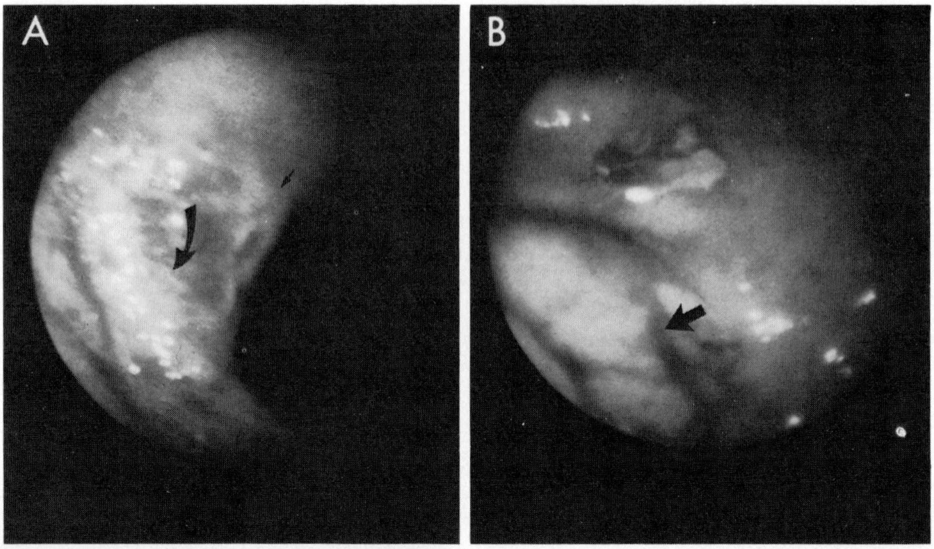

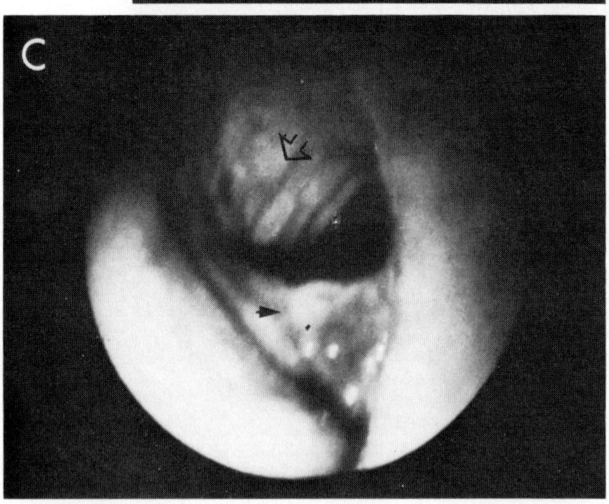

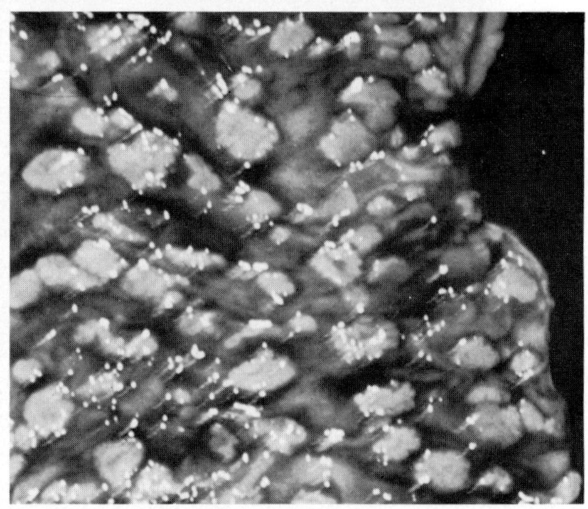

Fig 35–1 (top and **bottom left).**—**A,** colonoscopic view from descending colon demonstrating pseudomembranous plaques *(arrow).* Patient had received multiple antibiotics: aminoglycosides, penicillins and cephalosporins. **B** and **C,** same patient. Marked diffuse friability, as evidenced by bleeding *(arrows).* Patient subsequently died.

Fig 35–2 (bottom right).—Multiple pseudomembranous plaques ranging in size from 2 to 6 mm, taken from autopsy specimen. (Reprinted with permission from Stanley and Tedesco, CRC Crit. Rev. Clin. Radiol. Nucl. Med., September 1976. Copyright The Chemical Rubber Co., CRC Press, Inc.)

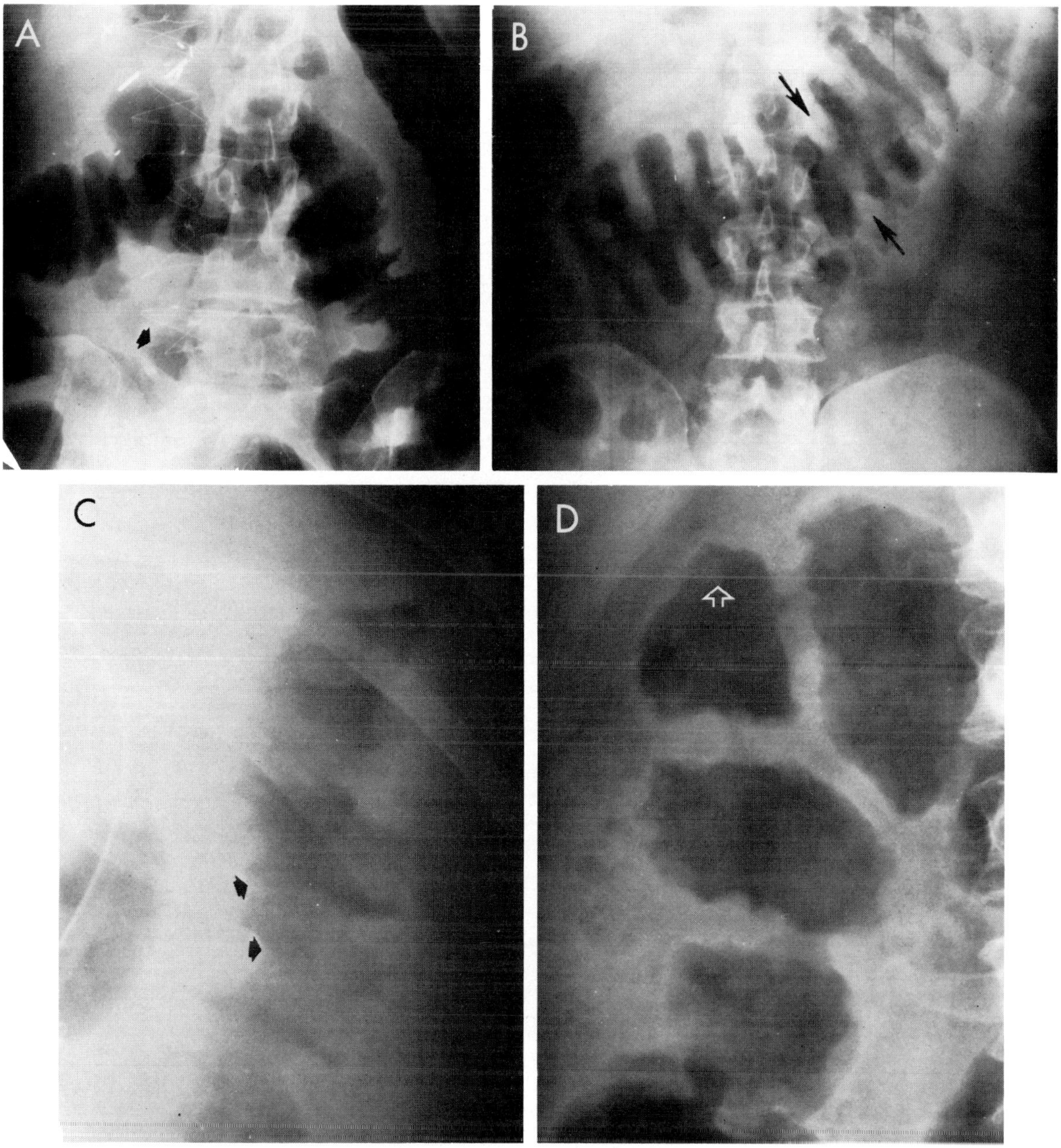

Fig 35–3.—A, anteroposterior plain film of patient with clindamycin pseudomembranous colitis. Colonic distention and relatively normal small bowel *(arrow)* are noted. Thumbprinting also seen. **B,** plain film of patient with pseudomembranous colitis. Thick colonic wall with wide bands severely narrowing lumen and almost obliterating it *(arrows)*. **C,** enlarged view of splenic flexure and descending colon of patient with ampicillin-associated pseudomembranous collits. Severe haustral edema and transverse bands densities are noted, producing thumbprinting *(arrows)*. **D,** enlarged view of hepatic flexure in plain film of patient with clindamycin-associated pseudomembranous colitis. Pseudomembranous plaques en face and in profile are seen *(arrow)*. (Reprinted with permission from Stanley and Tedesco, CRC Crit. Rev. Clin. Radiol. Nucl. Mod., September 1976. Copyright The Chemical Rubber Co., CRC Press, Inc.)

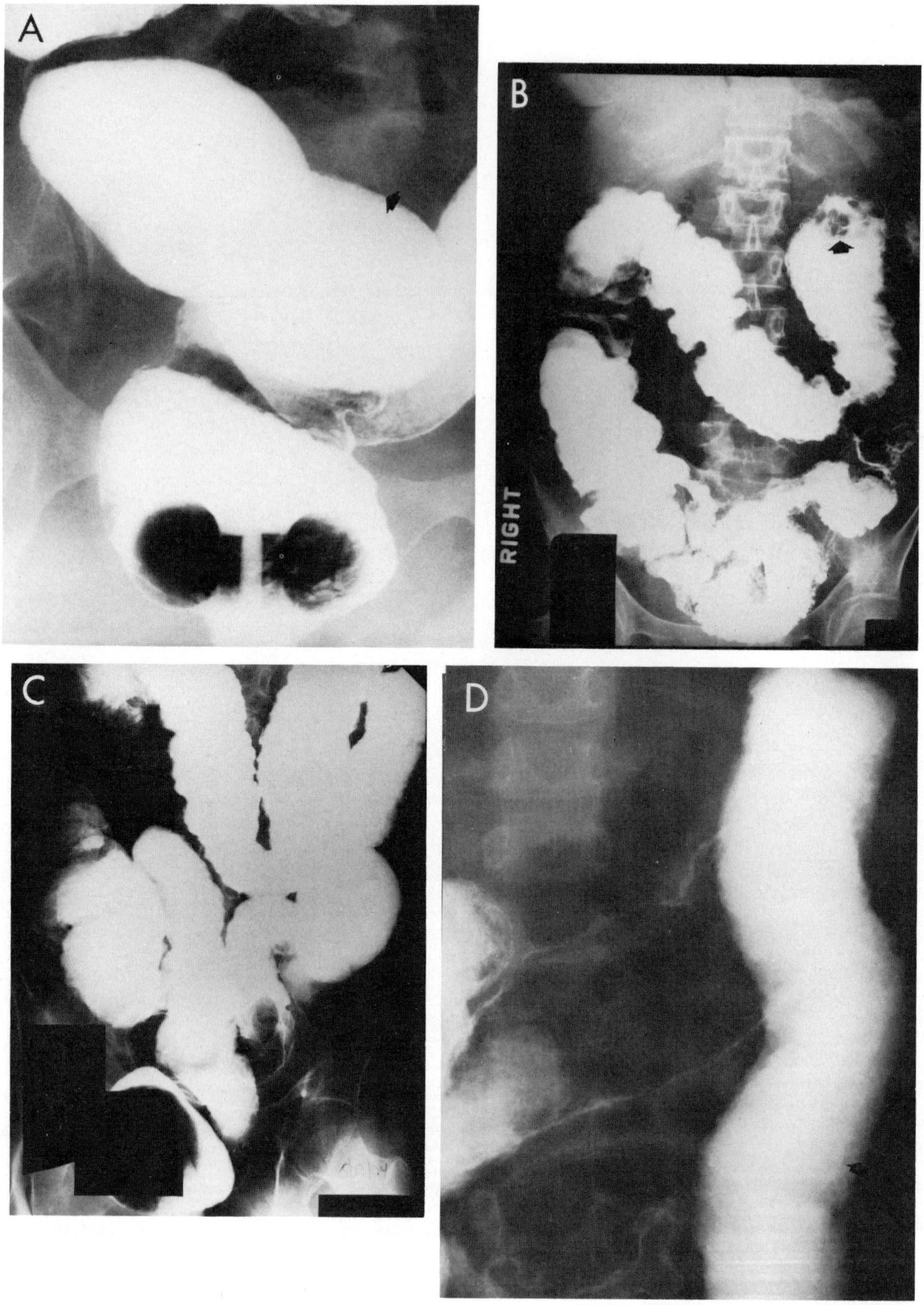

Fig 35–4.—**A,** barium enema of rectum and distal sigmoid colon, showing earliest changes of pseudomembranous colitis *(arrow).* Patterns are subtle and can be found in other colitides, e.g., ulcerative colitis. Plaques are better brought out by air contrast (see Fig 35–5, A). **B,** clindamycin-associated pseudomembranous colitis showing diffuse involvement of colon. Note round and oval filling defects created by pseudomembranous plaques *(arrow).* **C,** same patient as in **B,** different view. Small plaques cause marginal irregularity along colon contour. **D,** views of transverse and descending colon in patient, age 4 years, with ampicillin-associated pseudomembranous colitis. Note fine spiculations and serrated appearance *(arrow)* pro-

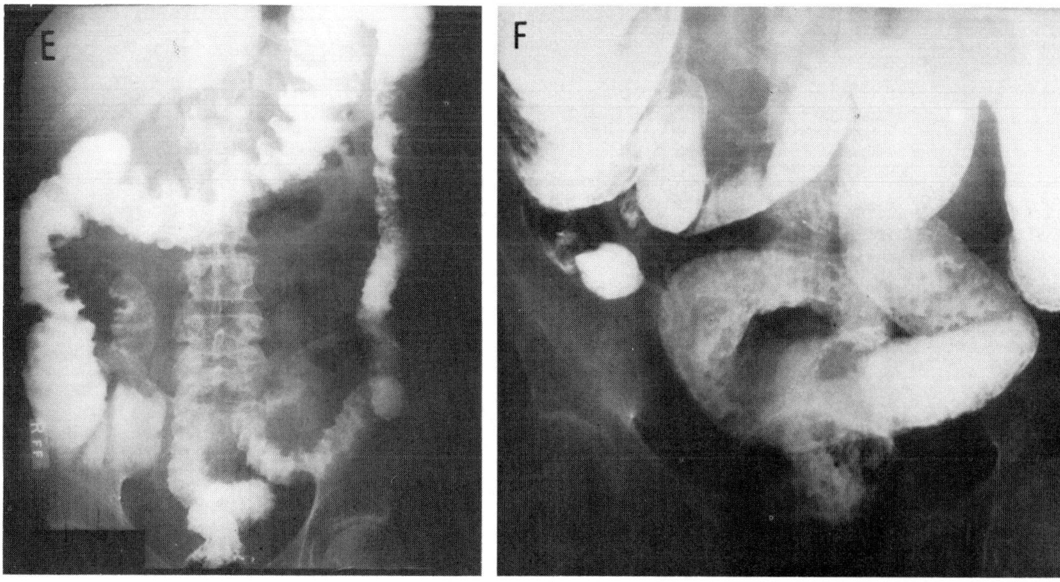

duced by small plaques. **E,** barium enema of patient treated with oxacillin and penicillin for hand cellulitis. Note diffuse involvement, with obvious rectal and sigmoid disease. Diffuse marginal irregularity caused by plaques. Edematous thickening of haustral folds also noted. **F,** barium enema using thin coating clearly demonstrates rectal and sigmoid pseudomembranous plaques. (**A, D** and **F** reprinted with permission from Stanley and Tedesco, CRC Crit. Rev. Clin. Radiol. Nucl. Med., September 1976. Copyright The Chemical Rubber Co., CRC Press, Inc.)

Fig 35–5. – **A,** air contrast barium enema of rectum and sigmoid, same patient as in Figure 35–4, A. Early changes of pseudomembranous colitis, not readily apparent with normal barium column, became obvious with air contrast. **B,** close-up view of descending colon using air contrast study. Innumerable pseudomembranous plaques are seen.

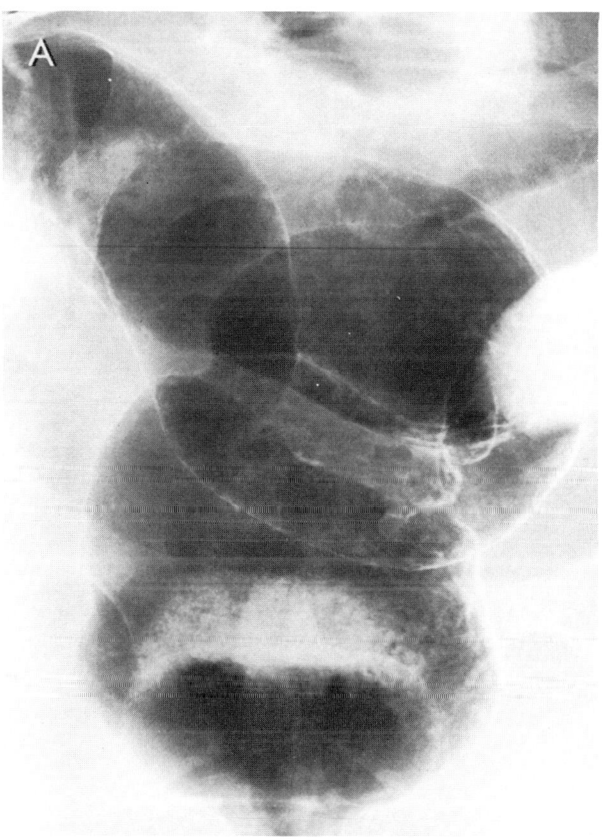

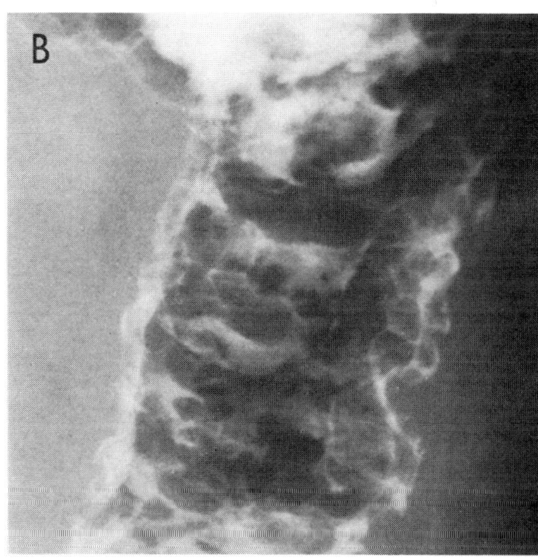

Acknowledgment. – The author wishes to express his gratitude to Robert J. Stanley, M.D. for his cooperation in the use of these photographs and for his review of the manuscript.

Chapter 36

Radiation Injury of the Colon and Rectum

BERNARD ROSWIT, M.D., F.A.C.R.

IN THIS DECADE striking advances in radiation therapy have significantly brightened the outlook for survival of patients with abdominopelvic cancer, when this therapy is used as an independent regimen or as an adjuvant to surgery and/or cancer chemotherapy. This is particularly true for patients with carcinoma of the cervix, uterus, bladder, testicle, prostate, colon or rectum.

Nevertheless, in all medical practice there are calculated risks—of reactions, changes and injuries, early and late—to normal structures in an uncompromising attack on a life-threatening disease. Radiation therapy is no exception. The radiosensitivity of the alimentary tract remains a principal barrier to further improvement of the cure rate by radiotherapy. There is as yet no way to significantly improve the limited radiation tolerance of the gastrointestinal viscera.

Clearly, in this decade and the next, diagnostic radiologists will need to recognize and evaluate radiation enteropathies with greater accuracy, and gastroenterologists and surgeons to manage them with greater skill. Unless recognized early and promptly treated, severe radiation damage to the bowel may give rise to acute and long-term suffering, disability and even death from malfunction, stricture, ulceration and perforation.

In the light of the current escalation of claims filed for alleged medical liability, it is timely and appropriate that we present the radiologic profile of colorectal radiation complications, a brief review of the pathogenesis, the iatrogenic factors of high risk, and recommendations for better clinical management. In previous communications we have offered guidelines for safer radiotherapeutic practice.[22-26]

The roentgenologist shoulders a grave responsibility for accurate diagnosis. An erroneous report of "severe radiation damage" places the therapeutic radiologist at high risk. In a recent poll, 24% of 348 therapeutic radiologists have had to face one or more claims, of which more than a third were prompted by a third party.[23] If, on the other hand, radiation pathology on x-ray is described as "recurrent cancer," the patient may be offered more radiation, compounding the damage or inviting surgical exploration, which may add its own burden of complications to a heavily irradiated abdomen or pelvis.[2-7, 14, 15, 17, 18, 29, 30]

Radiation pathology in the colon and rectum can readily be simulated by a number of entities, e.g., granulomatous colitis, post-ischemic colonic disease, primary sclerosing carcinoma, carcinoma metastatic to the bowel, chronic ulcerative colitis, parasitic disease, lymphopathia venereum. A perforation or fistula may be the outcome of an operative misadventure or secondary to recurrent ulcerating carcinoma. The roentgenologist confronted with a difficult differential diagnosis must give serious consideration to the radiologic and clinical factors of high risk in radiation therapy, e.g., treatment volume, dose fractionation scheme, cumulative dose, previous colonic pathology, operative history.

The most critical decision that therapeutic radiologists must face at the outset is selection of the optimal dose, time, treatment volume and fractionation regimen that offers the best chance for cure and the least probability of harm to vital normal structures, particularly the gastrointestinal viscera. The radiologists' prescription will reflect their training, experience and value judgment, as well as reliance on recognized standards of reference in the medical literature.[10, 19, 27, 28] Yet even after their best therapeutic effort, crowned with cure of the cancer, some patients' normal viscera may respond poorly.[1]

There is a variation in the complication rate that radiotherapists are able, or willing, to accept. Rubin and Casarett[27, 28] have suggested that the tolerance dose (TD) of exposed normal organs and tissues be expressed as the *minimum* and *maximum* injurious dose acceptable to the clinician in different clinical settings. In favorable settings, the radiation oncologist rarely is willing to risk a dose that would yield a 5% complication rate in 5 years (TD 5/5), in return for a better than 50% tumor control (Table 36 – 1). When confronted with a much more formidable setting, he may be willing to risk a dose closely approaching the maximum tolerance, with the possibility of a 50% chance of severe complications, in return for even a limited chance for a cure (TD 50/5). These values rest on a standard set of conditions such as supervoltage therapy, a fractionation regimen of 1,000 rads per week, five daily fractions and a weekend rest period.

In this decade we have come to accept still another standard for tolerance, expressed as the nominal standard dose (NSD), recorded in "rets" (roentgen equivalent therapy). The dimensions of this quantity are related to overall treatment time (in days), number of individual fractions and total dose. The NSD is generally accepted as the biologically equivalent dose, given individual variation in these treatment factors. It does not, however, include a factor for field size (Fig 36 – 1); therefore, the larger the field size, the lesser the tolerance and a somewhat lower value for the ret dose.

For the gastrointestinal viscera, the range for the NSD should be about 1,365 – 1,800 rets, as we move with increasing tolerance from the duodenum (the lowest) to the rectum (the highest) (see Table 36 – 1). Rarely are we likely to encounter significant radiation change below 1,365 rets, equivalent to about 4,000 rads in 26 days, with daily 200-rad fractions, unless massive portals are used.

The principal factors of high risk include dose fractions in excess of 300 rads, hyperintensive total dose, previous abdominal surgery, infection or radiotherapy, overlapping portals, poorly calibrated or uncalibrated dosimeters, inadequate vaginal packing during implants, single portal therapy or overlooking or masking signals of distress by overmedicating. These interacting factors, in our opinion, constitute the "formula fatale."[22-28]

Pathogenesis

In the large intestine, as in other organ systems, our principal interest is in the two major components: mucosal and vasculoconnective. We are concerned with the impact of radiation on the proliferative cells in the basal portion of the crypts; the maturing and matured functioning cells of the mucosa; the lamina propria projecting into the villi as a loose connective tissue mesh with a pleomorphic cell population, particularly the

TABLE 36-1.—RADIATION TOLERANCE DOSES (RADS) IN ABDOMINOPELVIC REGION

ORGAN	INJURY AT 5 YEARS	1-5% TD 5/5	25-50% TD 50/5	VOL. OR LENGTH
Skin	Ulcer, severe fibrosis	5,500	7,000	100 cm³
Esophagus	Ulcer, stricture	6,000	7,500	75 cm³
Stomach	Ulcer, perforation	4,500	5,000	100 cm³
Intestine	Ulcer, stricture	4,500	6,500	100 cm³
Colon	Ulcer, stricture	4,500	6,500	100 cm³
Rectum	Ulcer, stricture	5,500	8,000	100 cm³
Pancreas	Secretory functions		No data	
Liver	Liver failure, ascites	3,500	4,500	Whole
Biliary ducts	Stricture, obstructions		No data	
Kidney	Nephrosclerosis	2,300	2,800	Whole
Bladder	Ulcer, contracture	6,000	8,000	Whole
Ureters	Stricture, obstruction	7,500	10,000	5-10 cm
Testes	Permanent sterilization	500-1,500	2,000	Whole
Ovary	Permanent sterilization	200-300	625-1,200	Whole
Uterus	Necrosis, perforation	<10,000	<20,000	Whole
Vagina	Ulcer, fistula	9,000	<10,000	5cm
Bone				
Child	Arrested growth	2,000	3,000	10 cm³
Adult	Necrosis, fracture	6,000	15,000	10 cm³
Spinal cord	Necrosis, transection	5,000	<6,000	5 cm³
Adrenal	Hypoadrenalism	<6,000		Whole
Bone marrow	Hypoplasia	200	550	Whole
		2,000	4,000-5,000	Localized
Lymph nodes	Atrophy	3,500-4,500	7,000	
Lymphatics	Sclerosis	5,000	8,000	
Fetus	Death	200	450	

(From Rubin, P., and Casarett, G. W.: *Clinical Radiation Pathology, Vol. 1,* [Philadelphia: W. B. Saunders Co., 1968]) with permission.

lymphatic (Peyer's patches); the muscularis mucosa, a sentinel at the junction of the mucosa and submucosa; the submucosa, a dense connective tissue zone with abundant collagen and elastic fibers with a rich plexus of blood vessels, lymphatics and nerves; a smooth muscle layer, i.e., inner circular and outer longitudinal harboring medium-sized vessels from major mesenteric and serosal trunks; and finally the narrow zone of loose connective tissue designated as serosa[15, 16] (Figs 36-2 and 36-3).

Early enteropathy is principally due to epithelial and microvascular injury. As the principal functioning cells on the surface deteriorate from the impact of radiation, the proliferative cells respond within hours to signals of distress and begin to replenish the functional components. In time (1-3 weeks), there is progressive reduction in the crypt cells, with gross abnormalities in their mitotic pattern. Eventually the integrity of the epithelial barrier may be threatened with slough and ulceration, if the radiation regimen has been hyperintensive. During this period the capillaries and arterioles exhibit endothelial swelling and diminished luminal caliber, which may be a prelude to delayed effects (months to years).[32, 33] However, if the therapist fails to respect the tolerance of the normal bowel, the epithelium will not be reconstituted and the patient will be in more acute distress as ulcerations develop, associated with inflammation and narrowing of the intestinal lumen. With still more severe damage, the ulceration may penetrate through the muscle coats, terminating in perforation, with ileus or fistulization.

Months to years after overaggressive therapy, there will be profound changes in the supportive structures of the intestine. One sees vascular sclerosis with progressive ischemia, atrophy and scarring. Further, the surviving mucosa becomes flattened and shallow, without villous or glandular pattern, and the muscularis exhibits edema or fibrosis.[32, 33] The muscle layers are rarely normal, are generally atrophied and densely scarred, whereas the overlying delicate serosal membrane has become very thick and fibrotic. After intensive beam therapy, there is often so much lignification of the surrounding connective tissue structures within the pelvis that clinical differentiation from advancing carcinoma is difficult. This fibrotic process itself will greatly narrow the lumen and complicate surgical repair (Figs 36–4 and 36–5).

The Early Acute Clinical Syndrome

Rarely will the roentgenologist be called upon to perform an examination of a patient for radiation changes in normal bowel during a conventional course of radiation therapy for an abdominopelvic tumor. Radiation changes demanding his attention will not be encountered at dose levels below 4,000 rads, administered in a conventional fashion to fields of about 15×15 to 18×18 cm, with all fields treated daily.

Transient cramps and diarrhea of more or less severity are predictable in most cases, depending on anatomical volume exposed; size of the daily fraction, dose distribution, cumulative dose and, above all, a history of previous abdominopelvic surgery and/or infection.

After surgery, the small bowel, even a loop of sigmoid, may be pinioned by adhesions within the high-dose area. A barium study will reveal only increased irritability and motility of the small bowel, and little in the colon except a spastic area, representing a radiation hot spot a week or 10 days following an implant. This is particularly so in the anterior rectal or rectosigmoid wall during radioactive implant for carcinoma of the cervix or uterus.

Endoscopic examination will disclose an edematous, inflamed mucosa with multiple tiny bleeding points, but this angry landscape will quickly cool after completion of a moderate therapeutic regimen and leave no permanent clinical or radiologic stigmata. Most enteric pathology—at least 90%, early or late, mild or severe—is encountered in the management of gynecologic carcinoma. Even here, the usual incidence is well below 5%.[10, 19, 22, 24]

It has become our practice to perform a gastrointestinal study, a barium enema and sometimes a special small bowel study in patients presenting with formidable gynecologic or other pelvic tumors demanding a relatively high dose for control. The posterior cul-de-sac, particularly in a woman, is the place to look for a loop of ileum or sigmoid, with every effort made to avoid a hot spot at this site (Fig 36–6).

Treatment of the early syndrome is symptomatic and supportive, including use of antispasmodics, low-residue diet and especially corticosteroid enema, if there appears to be a risk of ulceration. If treatment is interrupted briefly (split course program), there is nearly always prompt recovery of the injured and reactive mucosa. Epithelial regeneration is rapid, and recovery may be complete, with normal villi in about 2–3 weeks. With hyperintensive dosage, epithelial integrity may be forever lost, and acute ulceration with luminal constriction may ensue within weeks of completion of therapy (Figs 36–7 to 36–9).

The Delayed, Severe Clinical Syndrome

Serious large bowel complications demand surgical correction or long-term, in-hospital management. They may be encountered 6 months to 2 years after treatment, or even several years later. We must emphasize here that the absence of early acute reactions in the course of therapy is no guarantee against severe late radiation pathology. Most commonly involved are the sigmoid colon and the rectum, with fixation, stenosis, ulceration and fistula (Figs 36–10 to 36–12). Associated damage to the terminal ileum and especially the urinary bladder, if included in the portal, is encountered in most cases and should always be looked for by the roentgenologist to help to confirm the diagnosis of radiation damage (Fig 36–13). Selective angiography may be helpful, revealing arterial and venous irregularity, beading and even focal obstructions of bowel wall vasculature, with crowded vessels because of the typical bowel foreshortening.[12]

Whereas mild early radiation enteropathy during treatment is the outcome of epithelial and microvascular injury with recovery, late severe changes are principally the response to progressive evolution of major vascular damage. A full spectrum of late changes may be expected in all of the structural divisions of the bowel wall (mucosa, submucosa, muscle, serosa).[32, 33] The patient complains of unrelenting lower abdominal cramps, obstipation and bouts of bleeding and diarrhea. Barium enema frequently reveals a rigid, smooth fibrotic segment resembling the aganglionic segment in Hirschsprung's disease. The involved area is straightened and elevated out of the pelvis (see Fig 36–4). Endoscopic examination becomes difficult. Early examination will reveal an angry, shallow mucosa, with many hemorrhagic points. In the more severe injuries, there are multiple ulcerations (see Figs 36–7 and 36–14). These patients, with ulceration and stenosis of the rectosigmoid, may be helped by an anterior resection and anastomosis. Stenosis low in the rectum must be handled by a permanent sigmoid colostomy. The radiation pathology in the rectosigmoid colon sometimes simulates carcinoma (pseudocarcinoma) because of filling defects created by heaped-up granulation tissue (Fig 36–15).

By far the most distressing complications are encountered low in the rectum following hyperintensive radiotherapy for gynecologic cancer (cervix, uterus, vagina) (Fig 36–16) involving teletherapy plus brachytherapy (radioactive implants).[11, 21] Anorectal pain, tenesmus and bleeding may become intolerable. A low rectovesical or rectovaginal fistula may develop, demanding surgical correction. Lateral and oblique views during initial barium filling will best demonstrate these communications (see Fig 36–13). Cystography will reveal a contracted and sometimes ulcerated bladder wall. There is a more than 50% probability of necrosis and/or perforation and fistula, if the combined dose to the bowel exceeds 8,000 rads. A sigmoid colostomy is mandatory, followed later by an effort at reparative surgery, if feasible. The radiologist should always investigate the small bowel as well as the large intestine prior to surgery because of the possibility of an associated ileorectovaginal fistula.

It is of the greatest importance to remind the surgeon contemplating reparative surgery that the small bowel, notably the ileum, is often involved in lower bowel enteropathy. The patient, by this time, is usually wasted, presenting most of the stigmata of the malabsorption syndrome. His small gut is kinked, twisted and matted, sometimes simulating massive involvement with recurrent carcinoma. Under these conditions the surgeon should stay out of the abdomen. However, if a surgical procedure must be seriously considered for relief, it should be extremely simple and conservative because these fragile, damaged loops will not survive manipulation. Adherent loops must not be freed; it is far better to provide a bypass or sidetracking anastomosis. The postoperative period may be stormy, and some patients may succumb in the 1st or 2d postoperative week.

Toxicity of Multimodal Therapy

Modern strategy in the treatment of cancer involves skillful integration from the outset of all methods—surgery, radiation, chemotherapy and even immunologic agents. This all-out effort invites the possibility of a significant escalation of risks, additive and/or potentiative. We have already discussed the dangers involved when abdominopelvic surgery is a prelude to radical radiation therapy or when the surgeon risks opening an abdomen after large volumes of bowel have received high radiation dosage (in excess of 5,000 rads). Today we are becoming increasingly more concerned, even fearful, of the effect of adjuvant chemotherapeutic agents on the lung, heart, liver, bone marrow and particularly the bowel, when used in combination with radiation therapy.[13]

Danjoux and Catton[4] were among the first to call attention to the delayed complications in colorectal carcinoma treated by a combination of radiotherapy and fluorouracil. Despite minimal early acute reactions, fully 29% of their patients experienced late serious and sometimes fatal complications about 8 months after treatment. Early studies by Falkson et al.[9] and Moertal et al.[16] indicated the very real possibility of chemotherapeutic potentiation of irradiation in rectal, pancreatic and gastric cancer.

Danjoux and Catton,[4] who were engaged in an Eastern Cooperative Oncology Group pilot study, emphasize that careful assessment of late bowel complications should be part of any pilot study of combination therapy before it is used in any large, controlled clinical trial, since the absence of early adverse reaction is no guarantee of safety.

Radiotherapy in Infancy and Childhood

The implications of late radiation damage in children are far more serious than in the mature adult because successful treatment today is followed by a life expectancy now measured in decades rather than years. Even small dosage can lead to grave functional and anatomical disturbances. The viscera of the very young are much more radiosensitive than those of adults. Vigilant surveillance and follow up of these patients for many years is mandatory. We must be alert for late disturbances in bowel function and nutrition, as well as in bone growth, gonadal deficiency, impairment of fertility and even oncogenesis. In children an intensive effort must always be made to exclude normal structures from the beam. Their future is in our hands.

Donaldson and her colleagues[8] were among the first to call attention to the syndrome of severe delayed radiation enteritis in children. These authors developed an effective dietary regimen that achieved marked clinical, histologic and functional improvement, which remained permanent. The diet consisted of fractionated low-residue, low-fat, gluten-free food, free of milk and milk products.

Donaldson et al.[8] made several other observations: notably, that infants and very young children appear to tolerate aggressive treatment less well than older children; that previous surgery and multiple surgical procedures often contribute to multiple adhesions and fibrosis; and that there is an association between the intensity of early intestinal symptoms and later bowel obstruction in children receiving concomitant chemotherapy, in particular, actinomycin D.

REFERENCES

1. Amory, H. I., and Brick, I. B.: Irradiation of the intestines following 1,000-kv. roentgen therapy. Evaluation of tolerance dose, Radiology 56:49, 1951.
2. Ashbaugh, P. G., and Owens, J. C.: Intestinal complications following irradiation for gynecologic cancer, Arch. Surg. 87:100, 1963.
3. Brick, I. B.: Effects of million volt irradiation on the gastrointestinal tract, Arch. Intern. Med. 96:26, 1955.
4. Danjoux, C. E., and Catton, G. E.: Delayed complications in colorectal carcinoma treated by combination radiotherapy and 5-Fluorouracil—Eastern Cooperative Oncology Group Pilot Study, Int. J. Radiat. Oncol. Biol. Phys. 5:311, 1979.
5. DeCosse, J. J., Rhodes, R. S., Wentz, W. B., et al.: The natural history and management of radiation-induced injury of the gastrointestinal tract, Ann. Surg. 170:369, 1969.
6. Dencker, H., Johnson, J. E., Liedberg, G., and Tibblin, S.: Surgical aspects of radiation injury to the small and large intestine, Acta Chir. Scand. 137: 692, 1971.
7. Deveney, C. W., Lewis, F. R., and Schrock, T. R.: Surgical management of radiation injury of the

small and large intestine, Dis. Colon Rectum 19:25, 1976.
8. Donaldson, S. S., Jundt, S., Ricour, C., Sarrazin, D., Lemerle, J., and Schweisguth, O.: Radiation enteritis in children, Cancer 35:1167, 1975.
9. Falkson, G., Sandison, A. G., Jacobs, E. L., and Fichart, T.: Combined telecobalt and 5-Fluorouracil therapy in cancer of the stomach, S. Afr. Med. J. 37:712, 1963.
10. Fletcher, G. H.: *Textbook of Radiotherapy* (Philadelphia: Lea & Febiger, 1973).
11. Friberg, L. G., and Johnsson, J. E.: Bladder and intestinal injuries following intracavitary irradiation of carcinoma of the uterine cervix, Acta Radiol. (Ther) 13(4):288, 1974.
12. Goldstein, H. M.: Diagnostic Roentgenology of Radiotherapy Change, in Lifshitz, H. I. (ed.): *Small Bowel and Colon* (Baltimore: Williams & Wilkins Co.), Chap. 7.
13. Henderson, I. W. D., Lipowska, B., and Lougheed, M. N.: Clinical evaluation of combined radiation and chemotherapy in gastrointestinal malignancies, Am. J. Roentgenol. 102:545, 1968.
14. Localio, A., Stone, A., and Friedman, M.: Surgical aspects of radiation enteritis, Surg. Gynecol. Obstet. 129:1163, 1969.
15. Marks, G.: Combined abdominal transsacral reconstruction of the radiation-injured rectum, Am. J. Surg. 131:54, 1976.
16. Moertel, C. G., Childs, D. S., Jr., Reitemeier, R. J., Colby, M. Y., Jr., and Holbrook, M. A.: Combined 5-Fluorouracil and supervoltage radiation therapy of locally unresectable gastrointestinal cancer, Lancet 2:865, 1969.
17. Mortenson, E., Nelsson, T., and Vesterhauge, S.: Treatment of intestinal injuries following irradiation, Dis. Colon Rectum 17:638, 1974.
18. Morgenstern, L., Thompson, R., and Friedman, N. B.: The modern enigma of radiation enteropathy: Sequelae and solutions, Am. J. Surg. 134:166, 1977.
19. Moss, W. T., Brand, W. N., and Battifora, H.: *Textbook of Radiation Oncology—Rationale, Technique, Results* (4th ed.; St. Louis: C. V. Mosby Co., 1973).
20. Palmer, J. A., and Rush, R. S.: Radiation injuries to the bowel associated with the treatment of carcinoma of the cervix, Surgery 80:458, 1976.
21. Powell-Smith, C.: Factors influencing the incidence of radiation injury in cancer of the cervix, J. Can. Assoc. Radiol. 16–17:132, 1965–66.
22. Roswit, B.: Complications of Radiation Therapy: The alimentary tract, Semin. Roentgenol. 9:51, 1974.
23. Roswit, B., and Bensel, F. P.: Medical liability in the practice of radiation oncology, Int. J. Radiat. Oncol. Biol. Phys. 2:553, 1977.
24. Roswit, B., Malsky, S. J., and Reid, C. B.: Radiation Tolerance of the Gastrointestinal Tract, in Vaeth, J. M. (ed.): *Frontiers of Radiation Therapy and Oncology, Vol. 6* (Baltimore: University Park Press, 1972), pp. 160–181.
25. Roswit, B., Malsky, S. J., and Reid, C. B.: Severe radiation injuries of the stomach, small intestine, colon and rectum, Am. J. Roentgenol. 114:460, 1972.
26. Roswit, B., Malsky, S. J., Reid, C. B., et al.: In vivo radiation dosimetry: Review of a 12-year experience, Radiology 97:413, 1970.
27. Rubin, P., and Casarett, G. W.: A Direction for Clinical Radiation Pathology—The Tolerance Dose, in Vaeth, J. M. (ed.): *Frontiers of Radiation Therapy and Oncology, Vol. 6,* (Baltimore: University Park Press, 1972, pp. 1–16.
28. Rubin, P., and Casarett, G. W.: *Clinical Radiation Pathology, Vol 1.* (Philadelphia: W. B. Saunders, 1968).
29. Sterns, E. E., Palmer, J. A., and Kergin, F. G.: The surgical significance of radiation injuries of bowel, Can. J. Surg. 7:407, 1964.
30. Sugg, W. L., Lawler, W. H., Ackerman, L. V., et al.. Operative therapy for severe irradiational injury to the enteral and urinary tracts, Ann. Surg. 157:62, 1963.
31. Wellwood, J. M., and Jackson, B. T.: The intestinal complications of radiotherapy, Br. J. Surg. 60:814, 1973.
32. White, D. C.: *An Atlas of Radiation Histopathology,* Division of Radiation Pathology, Armed Forces Institute of Pathology, Washington, D. C., 1975. Published by Technical Information Center, Office of Public Affairs, U.S. Energy and Development Administration.
33. White, D. C., and Persing, R. L.: The rectal mucosa as a biologic indicator of radiation injury. 1. Preliminary cytopathologic observations, Med. Ann. DC 34:68, 1965.

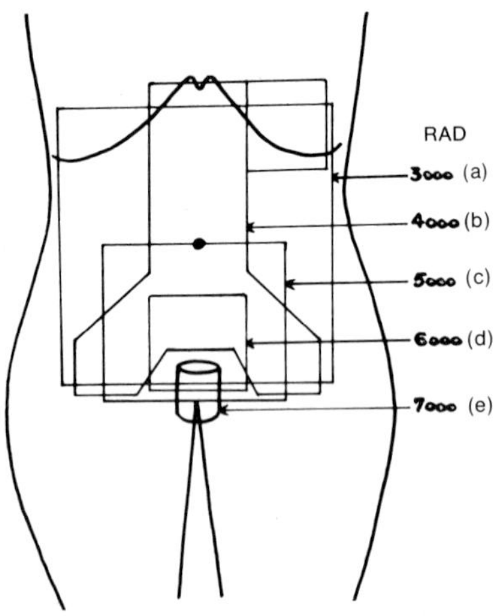

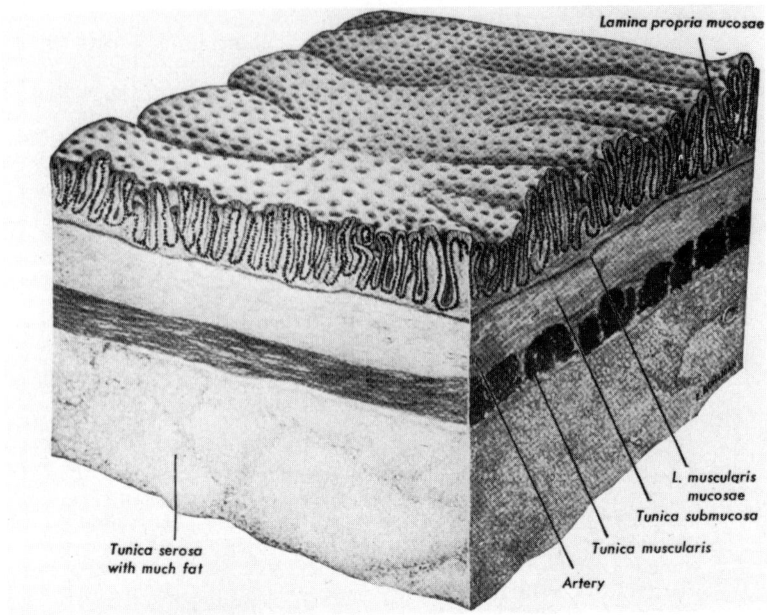

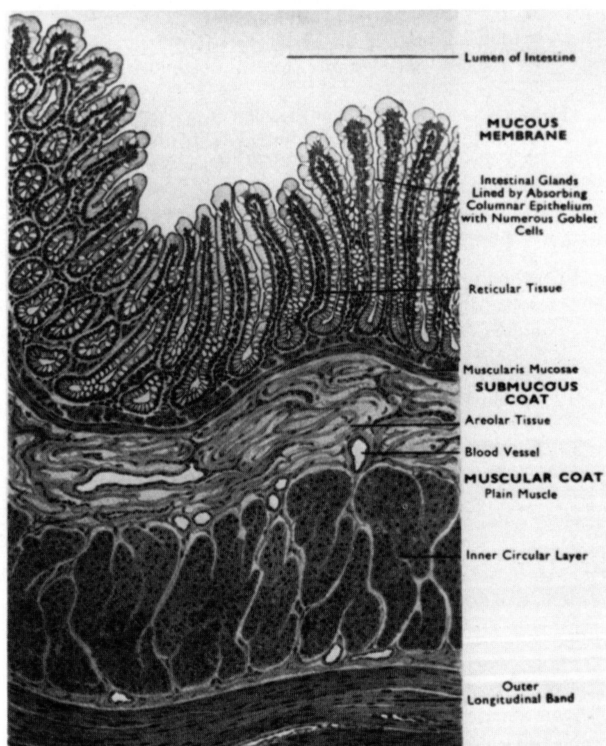

Fig 36–1 (top left).—Anatomical drawing to illustrate correlation between typical irradiated volumes for several major neoplasms and acceptable tumor dose values for these compartments. *a,* disseminated ovarian carcinoma; *b,* inverted "Y" for pelvic lymphoma; *c,* pelvic portal for carcinoma of cervix; *d,* reduced pelvic portal for advanced local pelvic carcinoma; *e,* rotational portal for early prostatic carcinoma. (From Roswit, B.: Complications of radiation therapy—The alimentary tract, Semin. Roentgenol. 9:51, 1974, with permission.)

Fig 36–2 (top right).—Drawing of block from human colon. Note single muscle layer. Openings of glands of Lieberkühn clearly shown, ×24. (From Bloom, W., and Fawcett, D. W. (eds.): *Textbook of Histology* [Philadelphia: W. B. Saunders Co., 1962], with permission.)

Fig 36–3 (bottom).—Longitudinal section of large intestine, ×75. (From Gillison, M. (ed.): *Histology of the Body Tissues* [Baltimore: Williams & Wilkins Co., 1962], with permission.)

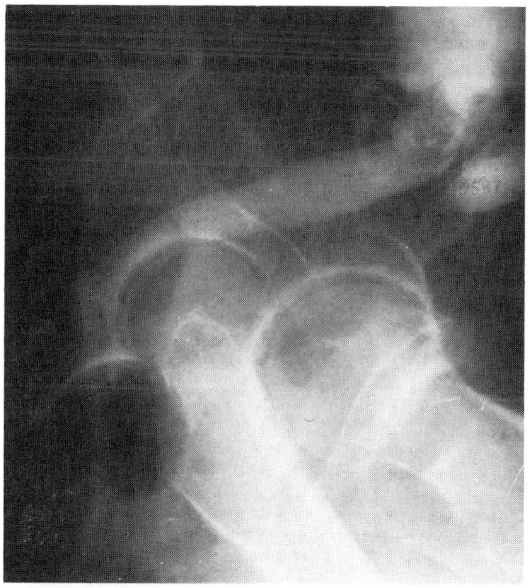

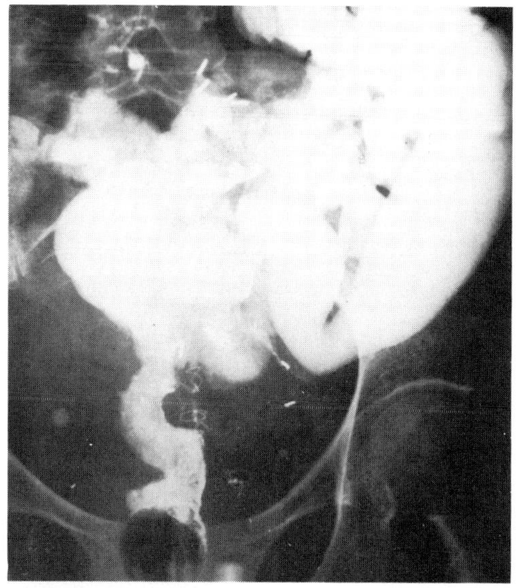

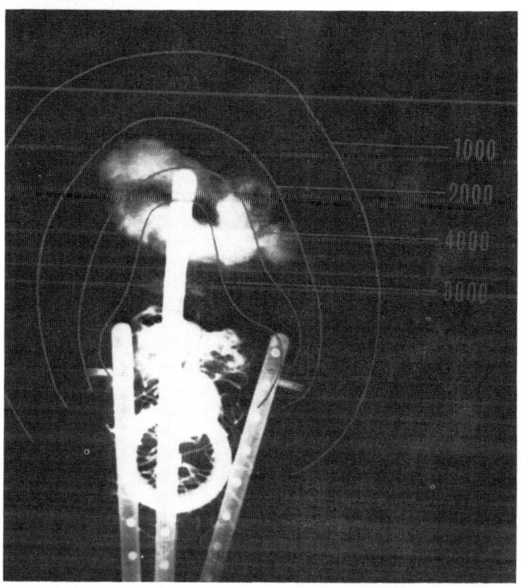

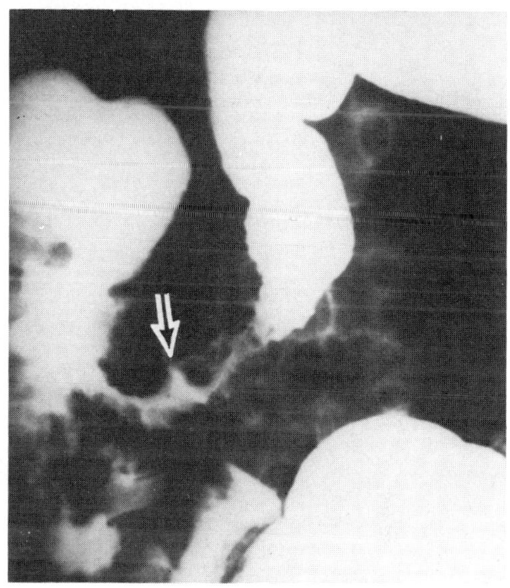

Fig 36–4 (top left).—Rigid rectosigmoid loop nearly 1 year following 33 Mev betatron x-ray therapy (7,000 rad) for locally advanced prostatic cancer involving bladder neck. (From Roswit, Complications of radiation therapy—The alimentary tract, Semin. Roentgenol. 9:51, 1974, with permission.) (Courtesy of Dr. Thomas Beneventano, Montefiore Hospital, New York.)

Fig 36–5 (top right). Severe radiation proctitis with ulceration of mucosa, contraction and rigidity after hyperintensive radiotherapy for far-advanced carcinoma of cervix. Transverse colostomy became imperative to relieve intractable tenesmus and bleeding. (From Roswit, B.: Complications of radiation therapy—The alimentary tract, Semin. Roentgenol. 9:51, 1974, with permission.) (Courtesy of Dr. Thomas Beneventano, Montefiore Hospital, New York.)

Fig 36–6 (bottom left).—Radiograph of radium implant for cervical cancer using afterloading Henschke applicator. It was patient's good fortune that residual barium remained in a sigmoid loop deep in posterior cul-de-sac several days after barium study for intestinal problem. Note hazardous position of sigmoid loop in high intensity treatment zone (8,000 rads) revealed by computer. Treatment plan was promptly modified when this verification film was reviewed and patient spared a disastrous complication. (From Roswit, B.: Complications of radiation therapy—The alimentary tract, Semin. Roentgenol. 9:51, 1974, with permission.)

Fig 36–7 (bottom right).—Severe radiation colitis, transverse colon, with ulceration, stenosis and shortening, fully 3 years after 5,760 rad in 6 weeks (300-rad fractions), single portal, 1 mv resonance generator. Patient treated at military hospital for retroperitoneal nodes from embryonal testicular carcinoma, after orchiectomy. Differential diagnosis from segmental granulomatous colitis would be extremely difficult without appropriate radiation history of treatment regimen well beyond tolerance. This segment was excised, with successful end-to-end anastomosis, but patient also required partial gastrectomy for radiation gastric ulcer. (From Roswit, B.: Am. J. Roentgenol. 114:460, 1972, with permission.)

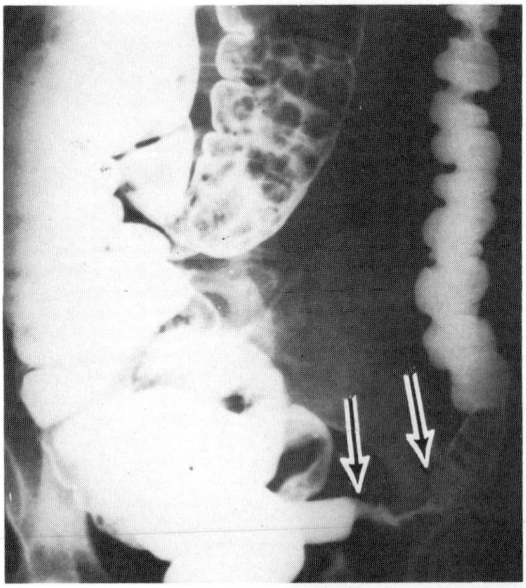

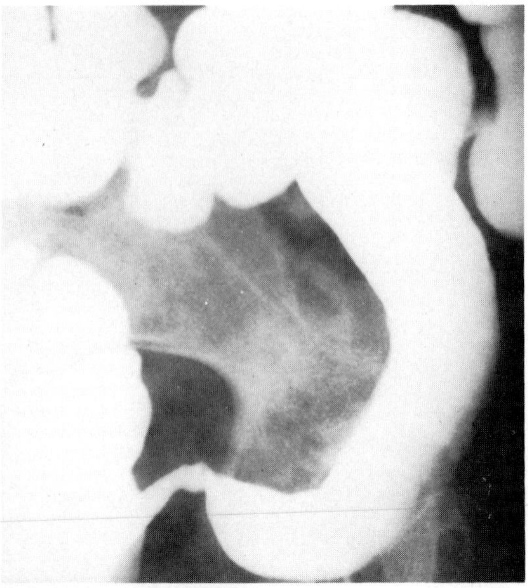

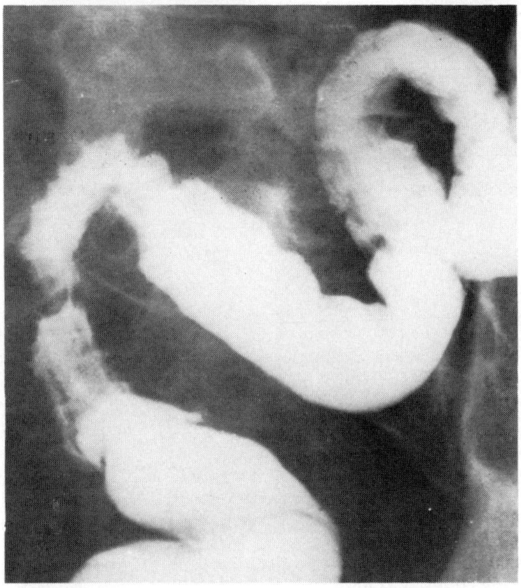

Fig 36–8 (top left). – Barium study of a woman, age 47, showing severe stricture of sigmoid colon. Patient was treated in hospital in 1960 for in situ carcinoma of cervix, with intensive cobalt beam therapy plus intravaginal and intrauterine radium implant. By 1961, she had a radiation neuropathy of right femoral nerve that ended in paralysis of right lower extremity. Severe gastrointestinal symptoms led to narcotic addition necessitating colostomy. (Courtesy of Dr. Martin Edelman, Memorial-Sloan Kettering Medical Center, New York.)

Fig 36–9 (top right). – Classic pipestem loop of rectosigmoid following cobalt and radium therapy for far-advanced cervical carcinoma. Patient survives and appears reasonably well 4 years after treatment. (From Roswit, B.: Complications of radiation therapy – The alimentary tract, Semin. Roentgenol. 9:51, 1974, with permission.) (Courtesy of Dr. Thomas Benevantano, Montefiore Hospital, New York.)

Fig 36–10 (bottom). – Chronic radiation injury of rectosigmoid colon 7 months after treatment for advanced endometrial carcinoma, involving 4,500 rad in 33 days with 33 Mev betatron x-rays plus high-dose intrauterine Heyman Capsules. (Reproduced with permission from Roswit, B.: Complications of Radiation Therapy – The Alimentary Tract, in Felson, B. [ed.]: *Seminars of Roentgenology, Vol. 9,* [New York: Grune & Stratton; Copyright 1974].) (Courtesy of Dr. Thomas Beneventano, Montefiore Hospital, New York.)

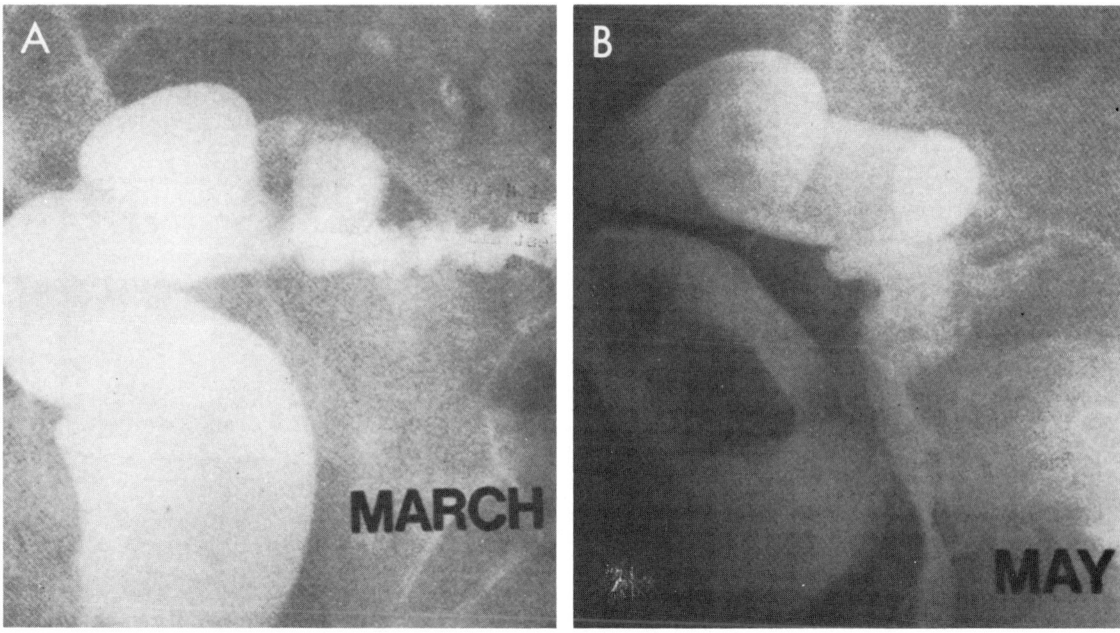

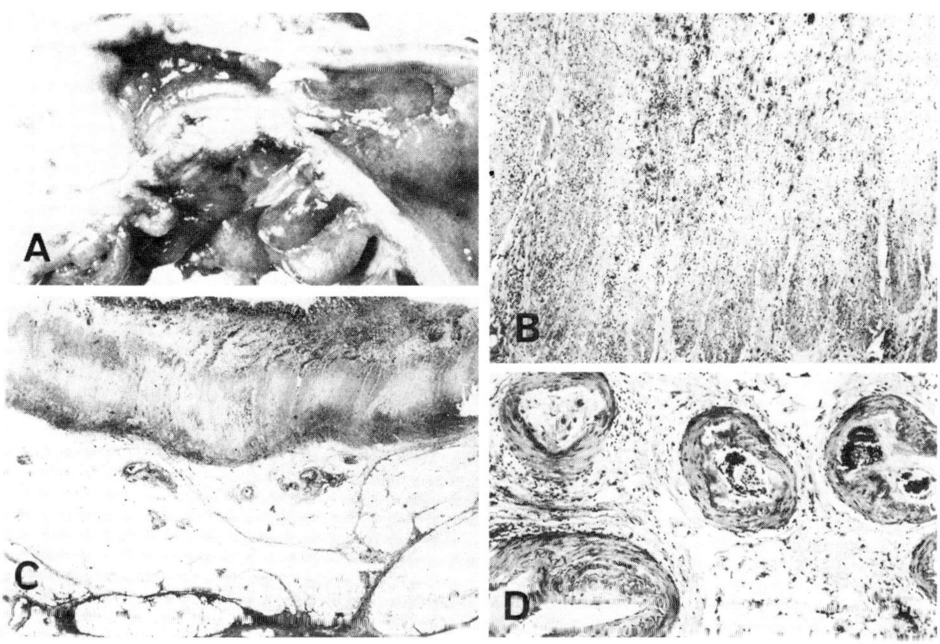

Fig 36–11 (top). – **A,** striking ulcerative and stenotic pathology in distal rectosigmoid colon following high x-ray dose to pelvis – 5,250 rad with betatron x-ray, plus 4,000 rad with intracavitary cesium 137 implant – total 9,250 rad. **B,** same patient 2 months later with perforation and rectosigmoid-vaginal fistula. (From Palmer, J. A., and Bush, R. S.: Surgery 80:461, 1976, with permission.)

Fig 36–12 (bottom). – **A,** stenosis of rectosigmoid colon. **B,** prominent submucosal thickening and fibrosis of serosa. **C,** destruction of intestinal smooth muscle. **D,** profound alterations in small arteries. Note subintimal fibrosis, medial calcification and huge fat-filled endothelial cells characteristic of radiation injury. (From Sugg, W. L., et al., Ann. Surg. 157:62, 1963, with permission.)

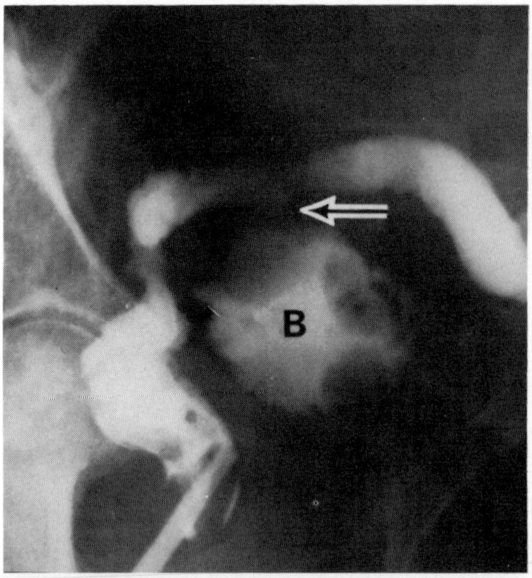

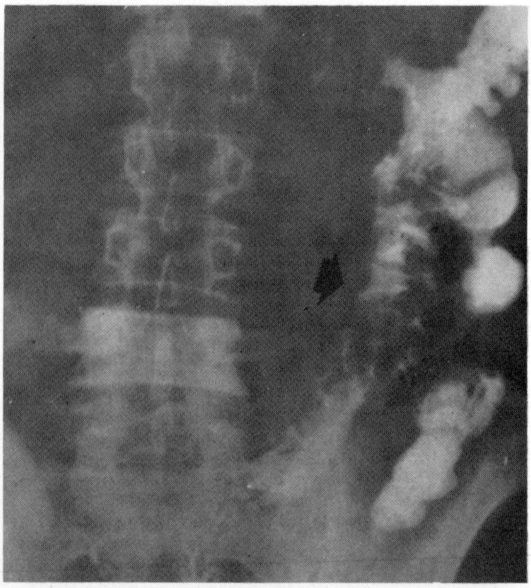

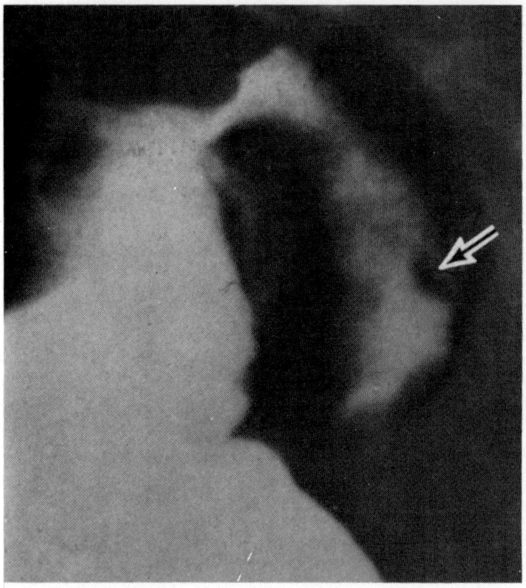

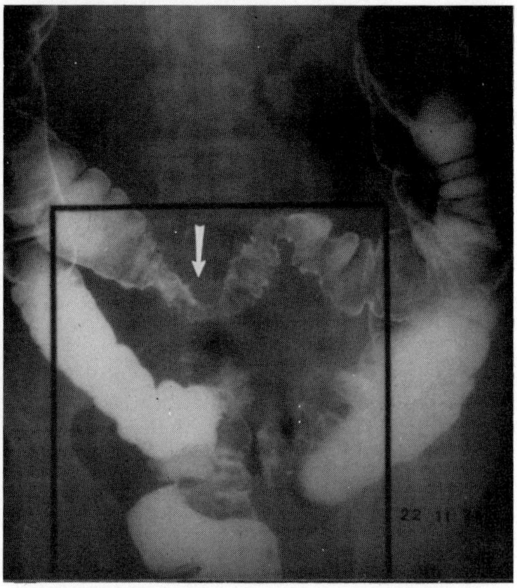

Fig 36–13 (top left). – Colovesical fistula and late, severe ulcerative and constrictive pathology in sigmoid colon and rectum. Note profound changes in bladder *(B)* with thumbprints simulating carcinoma of bladder. Patient was a woman, age 52, treated at age 18 for inoperable adenocarcinoma of cervix, with extension to base of bladder. She was treated with orthovoltage x-ray through 6 portals plus intravaginal "radium bomb." She survives without tumor but has bilateral nephrostomy and transverse colostomy. (Courtesy of Martin Edelman, Memorial Sloan-Kettering Medical Center, New York.)

Fig 36–14 (top right). – Severe radiation colitis in transverse colon and descending colon 1 year following postoperative irradiation to left upper abdomen following nephrectomy for hypernephroma of left kidney. Patient complained of rectal bleeding and abdominal cramps controlled by conservative management. (From Rubin, P., and Casarett, G. W.: In-Radiation Pathology [Philadelphia: W. B. Saunders Co., 1968], with permission.)

Figure 36–15 (bottom left). – Late severe radiation reaction at rectosigmoid junction masquerading as recurrent, advancing carcinoma of cervix. Note irregular, heaped-up granulation tissue simulating filling defects of carcinoma, referred to as "pseudocarcinoma." Patient had hyperintensive dose of 9,500 rads to rectal wall from external radiation and implant for stage I carcinoma of cervix. (From Rubin, P., and Casarett, G. W.: *In-Radiation Pathology* [Philadelphia: W. B. Saunders Co., 1968], with permission.)

Fig 36–16 (bottom right). – Woman, age 79, had a hysterectomy for carcinoma of uterus in 1965. In 1966 she returned with advanced carcinoma of rectum, Dukes C, treated with radiation therapy (6,000 rads in three split courses) combined with 5 Fluorouracil (500 mg M^2 delivered intravenously). Six months later, without early signals of distress, stenosis of transverse colon *(arrow)* developed. She survives but has distressing chronic diarrhea. (From Danjoux, and Cotton, Int. J. Radiat. Oncol. Biol. and Phys. 4:1979, with permission.)

Chapter 37

Retroperitoneal Fibrosis and Rectosigmoid Stricture

GERALD J. GELFORD, M.D.
DAVID K. CROMWELL, M.D.

A RELATIONSHIP between long-term methysergide therapy and retroperitoneal fibrosis appears to be well established,[2-4, 8, 9, 13] although the incidence is certainly low. Only about 50–60 cases have been reported in the literature, although more than 500,000 patients with migraine have taken the drug.[5] Ureteral obstruction with medial deviation usually is present bilaterally (Fig 37–1). Fibrotic stricture of the aorta, inferior vena cava and other major vessels of the abdomen and pelvis occurs in some cases (Fig 37–2). In others there are vasospastic narrowings of major arteries, not associated with fibrosis.[7, 11] Other roentgenographically detectable complications associated with methysergide therapy include severe and extensive inflammatory fibrotic lesions of the lung, pleura, aorta and heart, the latter resulting in both stenosis and regurgitation of the mitral and aortic valves.

Other side effects and complications of methysergide include nausea, vomiting, diarrhea, abdominal pain, minor neurologic manifestations, vertigo, muscle spasm and thrombophlebitis. Both the minor and the major complications usually are promptly alleviated by stopping the drug. In patients with severe fibrotic lesions, the improvement may be gradual over a period of many weeks (Figs 37–2 and 37–3). In some patients with retroperitoneal fibrosis, permanent irreversible renal damage remains, even though the fibrotic process has subsided and the ureteral obstruction has been relieved following cessation of the drug. Surgical decompression of the obstructed ureters generally is ineffectual if the patient continues taking the drug,[7] although there is a single published exception to this rule.[3]

The patient presented was experiencing increasing constipation over a 3-month period, as well as increasing swelling of her left lower leg, the latter due to occlusion of the left common iliac vein. She also had bilateral ureteral obstruction without oliguria. Barium enema revealed an abrupt short severe stricture at the rectosigmoid, which could readily be mistaken for either a primary rectosigmoid adenocarcinoma or a rectal shelf from peritoneal carcinomatosis. The associated findings of rectosigmoid stricture and major pelvic vascular occlusion suggest

---

This chapter, as "Methysergide, Retroperitoneal Fibrosis and Rectosigmoid Stricture," was published in the American Journal of Roentgenology 104:566–570, 1968, copyright 1968 American Roentgen Ray Society. It also appeared in the *Yearbook of Radiology* 1970.

widespread malignant disease; but retroperitoneal fibrosis should always be considered, as demonstrated in this case.

No therapy was provided other than withdrawal of the offending medication. The progressive constipation subsided completely, and a subsequent barium enema provided clear objective evidence of regression of the inflammatory mass. The laparotomy could have been avoided had the causal relationship of methysergide therapy been recognized. No decompression of the rectosigmoid was attempted at laparotomy.

Methysergide probably is the most effective available agent for prevention of migraine.[4, 7] Severe complications are not common and can be minimized by observing the contraindications,[8] by periodic cessation and by specialized periodic physical examination, as described by Graham.[7]

The retroperitoneal fibrosis associated with methysergide is indistinguishable from the idiopathic variety. Both types on pathologic study disclose a fibrotic process with associated vasculitis.

Idiopathic retroperitoneal fibrosis has produced severe fibrotic strictures of the duodenum,[1, 12] rectosigmoid,[10] common bile duct and pancreas or pancreatic duct system.[12]

REFERENCES

1. Chew, C. K., Jarzylo, S. V., and Valberg, L. S.: Idiopathic retroperitoneal fibrosis with protein-losing enteropathy and duodenal obstruction successfully treated with corticosteroids, Can. Med. Assoc. J. 95:1183, 1966.
2. Conley, J. E., Boulanger, W. J., and Mendeloff, G. L.: Aortic obstruction associated with methysergide maleate therapy for headaches, J.A.M.A. 198: 136, 1966.
3. Gelford, G. J., Wilets, A. J., Nelson, D., and Kroll, L. L.: Retroperitoneal fibrosis and methysergide: Report of three cases, Radiology 88:976, 1967.
4. Graham, J. R.: Methysergide for prevention of headache: Experience in five hundred patients over three years, N. Engl. J. Med. 270:67, 1964.
5. Graham, J. R.: Cardiac and pulmonary fibrosis during methysergide therapy for headache, Am. J. Med. Sci. 254:23, 1967.
6. Graham, J. R.: Personal communication, 1968.
7. Graham, J. R.: CCXXX-methysergide, Curr. Ther. 198:302, 1967.
8. Graham, J. R., Suby, H. I., LeCompte, P. R., and Sadowsky, N. L.: Fibrotic disorders associated with methysergide therapy for headache, N. Engl. J. Med. 274:359, 1966.
9. Johnson, D. A., and Ballinger, W. M.: Headache: Methysergide therapy complicated by retroperitoneal fibrosis: Report of case, Med. Ann. DC 35:75, 1966.
10. Leffall, L. D., Jr., White, J. E., and Mann, M.: Retroperitoneal fibrosis: Two unusual cases, Arch. Surg. 89:1070, 1964.
11. Rackley, C. E., Mengel, C. E., Pomerantz, M., and McIntosh, H. D.: Vascular complications with use of methysergide, Arch. Intern. Med. 117:265, 1966.
12. Schneider, C. F.: Idiopathic retroperitoneal fibrosis producing vena caval, biliary, ureteral and duodenal obstructions, Ann. Surg. 159:316, 1964.
13. Suby, H. I., Kerr, W. S., Graham, J. R., and Fraley, E.: Retroperitoneal fibrosis: Missing link in chain, J. Urol. 93:144, 1965.

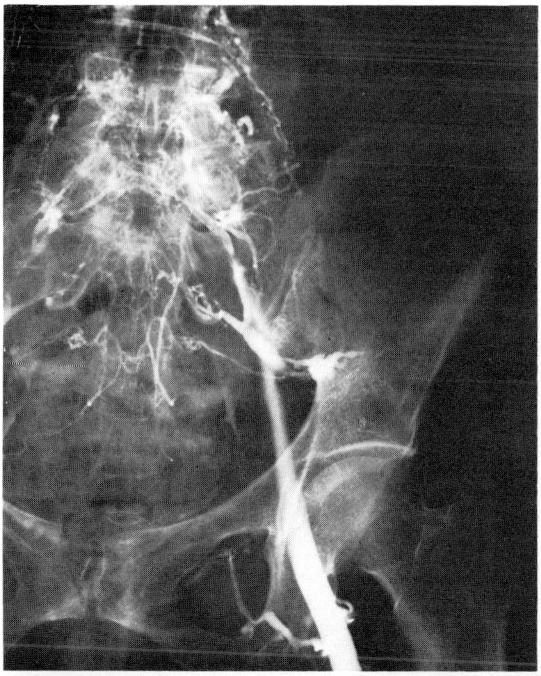

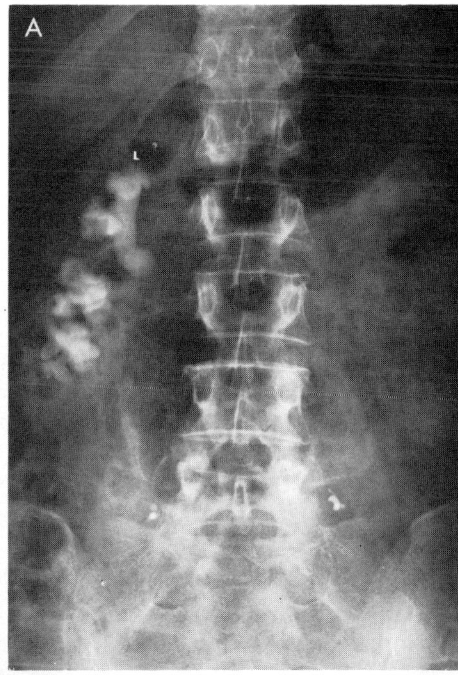

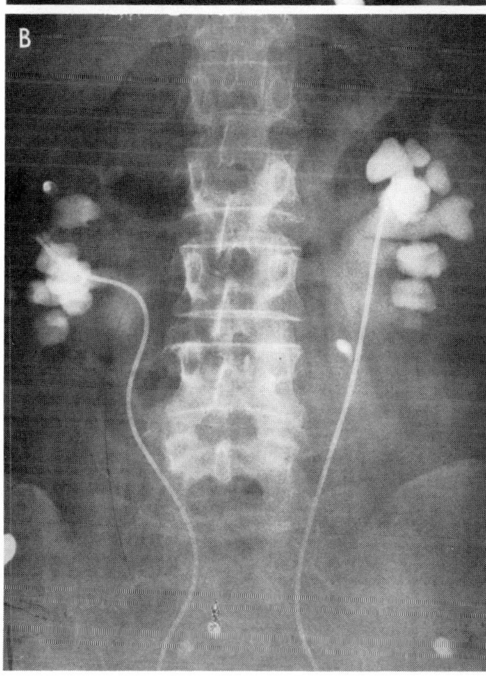

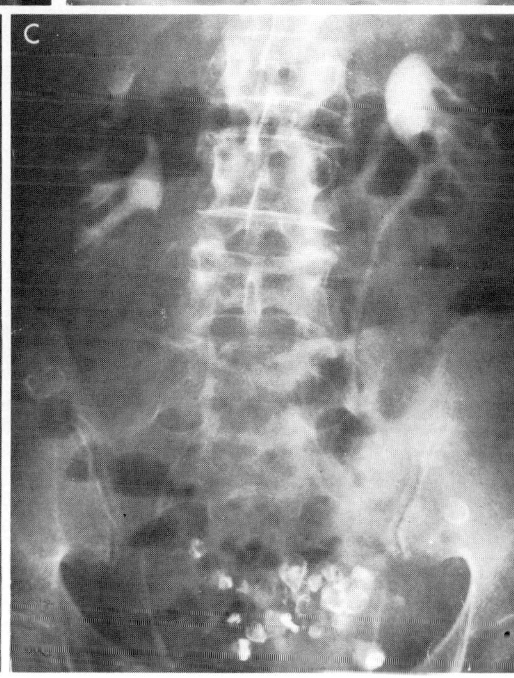

Fig 37–1 (top right and bottom).—**A,** excretory urogram shows severe bilateral obstruction *(arrow),* most marked on left, where only nephrogram is present. Film was exposed 10 minutes following injection. **B,** 5 days later, retrograde urogram demonstrates bilateral medial deviation of lower portions of ureters and dilated renal collecting systems. This combination of findings strongly suggests presence of retroperitoneal fibrosis. **C,** about 3 months later intravenous pyelogram following cessation of methysergide shows return to normal appearance, the usual result of merely stopping the drug. (From Am. J. Roentgenol. 104:566, 1968, with permission. Copyright 1968, American Roentgen Ray Society.)

Fig 37–2 (top left).—Venogram reveals tapering constriction of left common iliac vein and rather extensive venous collateral vessels. (From Am. J. Roentgenol. 104:566, 1968, with permission. Copyright 1968, American Roentgen Ray Society.)

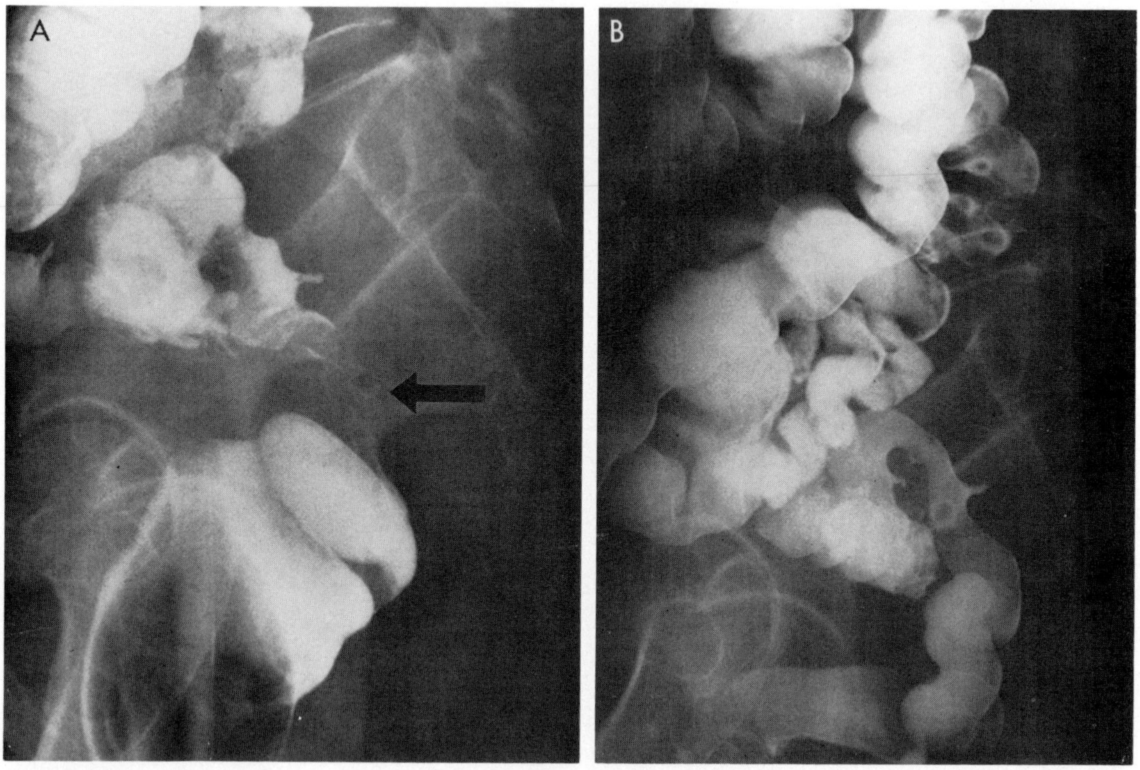

Fig 37–3. – **A,** lateral roentgenogram of rectosigmoid area on barium enema examination shows sharply defined narrowing apparently of extrinsic origin. Since there was no clinical or roentgenographic evidence of other causes (e.g., ulcerative colitis), widened presacral space is presumably secondary to known obstruction of major pelvic venous channel. **B,** lateral roentgenogram of rectosigmoid area 10 weeks following discontinuation of methysergide shows relief of narrowing and return to near-normal appearance. (From Am. J. Roentgenol. 104:566, 1968, with permission. Copyright 1968, American Roentgen Ray Society.)

Chapter 38

Retrorectal Space

STEVEN K. TEPLICK, M.D.

THE RETRORECTAL SPACE is the site of a variety of pathologic entities that may involve the rectum, sacrum and any of the intervening soft tissue structures. Lesions occur at any age and in either sex. The following discussion deals mainly with presacral lesions in adults.

Opinions differ concerning the value of routinely obtaining a lateral view of the barium-filled rectum during barium enema examinations.[1, 2] Teplick et al.[3] believe that it is an important part of the examination because it can provide useful information about the sacrum and presacral space. In addition, it helps to discern minimal and early inflammatory changes of the rectosigmoid, as well as to follow the course of ulcerative colitis and other inflammatory bowel diseases.[4, 5] The lateral is also the best projection to show the anterior rectosigmoid surface where the peritoneal reflection forms the pouch of Douglas, a frequent site of seeding from intraperitoneal carcinomatosis.

Gross Anatomy

The retrorectal area is a potential space bounded in front by the posterior wall of the rectum and behind by the ventral surface of the sacrum (Fig 38–1). The inferior extent is formed by the pelvic floor composed mainly of the levator ani and coccygeus muscles. The rectum is fixed as it passes through the floor. Cranially the space is limited by the peritoneal reflection at the rectosigmoid junction, adjacent to about the third sacral segment. The rectum measures 12–14 cm in length.

The presacral space has two fascial layers: (1) the fascia pelvis parietalis interna, or Waldeyer's fascia, covers the anterior sacral surface, and (2) the fascia propria covers the posterior rectum. These enclose retrorectal fat, areolar tissue, lymph nodes and hemorrhoidal vessels. Between the two fascial layers is the presacral space. In it are branches of the sacral and hypogastric nerve plexuses and the median sacral and iliolumbar arteries.[6, 7]

Normal Radiographic Anatomy

Normally the barium-filled rectum closely parallels the hollow of the sacrum, separated by only a few millimeters of soft tissue (Fig 38–2). Variations from this appearance should be questioned. Several methods have been described to measure the presacral space.[2, 1, 6] For this it is generally agreed to use the shortest distance between the barium-filled rectum and the anterior surface of the sacrum at the third to fifth sacral segments. Measurements at S5 are considered more

Part of the material in this chapter is republished with permission from Clin. Radiol. 29:177, 1978.

accurate, since at this level there is less chance that the rectum will be off midline than at S3. Any displacement from midline can falsely enlarge the presacral space. Probably an underfilled normal rectum will falsely widen the space. However, Gardiner[2] stated that the degree of rectal distention did not make a significant difference in his measurements.

Edling and Eklof[4] observed that the normal presacral space measured 0.5 cm or less in 95 of 100 examinations. They considered greater than 1 cm abnormal, 1–2 cm a moderate enlargement and greater than 2 cm a marked enlargement. Chrispin and Fry[6] stated that an area of 1.5 cm is suspicious, but greater than 2 cm is definitely abnormal. Gardiner[2] in a series of 2,000 consecutive barium enemas found only 75 cases (3%) in which the presacral area was 2 cm or larger. Only four of these were due to pathologic conditions. In five of these 75 cases, the space measured 4 cm, and all five variations were normal. The retrorectal space measured 1 cm or greater in 11% of his cases. Teplick et al.[3] in a series of 99 cases in which the presacral space measured 1.5 cm or greater found that nearly 40% were normal variations (no pathology). Some normal spaces measured considerably greater than 2 cm. Most (74%) normal variations occurred in large or obese patients, but a significant number (26%) were in average-sized individuals (Fig 38–3).

It should be emphasized that a wide presacral space per se is not necessarily pathologic. Other associated roentgenographic findings can help to determine if a true abnormality exists. These include a localized mass as well as sacral or rectal abnormalities.

Statements concerning the incidence of the type of pathology in the retrorectal area vary depending on the institution and type of patients evaluated. Castro[8] reported an incidence of tumor in the presacral space of 1 per 1,000, but this was at a clinic specializing in gastrointestinal tract surgery. Most of these tumors were in adults, and over 50% of them were dermoids or developmental cysts. Teplick et al.[3] found an almost equal percentage of inflammatory lesions and tumors (Table 38–1).

TABLE 38–1.—REPORTED CAUSES OF ENLARGED RETRORECTAL SPACE

Normal variations (no pathologic features)
Inflammatory conditions
Ulcerative colitis
Granulomatous colitis (Crohn's disease)
Infectious proctitis (tuberculosis)
Radiation proctitis
Ischemic colitis
Idiopathic proctosigmoiditis
Diverticulitis
Perforated appendix
Idiopathic presacral abscess
Tumors
Developmental cysts (dermoids, duplications, postanal gut)
Primary rectal tumors (adenocarcinoma, lymphomas, sarcomas, cloacogenic carcinoma)
Secondary rectal tumors (prostate, ovary, bladder)
Neurogenic (schwannomas, neurofibromas, chordomas)
Multiple myeloma and solitary plasmacytomas
Lipomas and hemangioendotheliomas
Teratomas*
Anterior sacral meningoceles*
Primary sacral tumors (osteogenetic sarcomas, chondrosarcomas, giant cell)
Metastases to sacrum
Miscellaneous lesions
Associated with inguinal hernias
Amyloidosis
Pelvic lipomatosis
Pneumatosis cystoides intestinalis
Following partial sigmoid resection
Inferior vena cava obstruction
Cushing's disease

*Usually occur in pediatric age group.
From Teplick et al., Clin Radiol. 29:177, 1978.

Inflammatory Conditions

ULCERATIVE COLITIS

Ulcerative colitis[2, 4-6] commonly causes a widened retrorectal space. Usually there is a generalized increase without evidence of a focal mass. The sacrum is not affected, and acute or chronic inflammatory changes of the rectum are usually present (Fig 38–4). Proctitis from other causes such as ischemia, radiation, tuberculosis or amebiasis may have a similar appearance.

The enlarged presacral space in ulcerative colitis is due to several factors. These include thickening of the bowel wall, edema of the presacral soft tissues, diminished distensibility of the rectal lumen and shortening of the bowel, which may pull the rectum away from the sacrum.

An enlarged space may develop at any time during the course of the disease. It seems more prevalent in the older age groups and in patients with more severe, chronic and extensive colitis. The size of the retrorectal area at any given time is not of prognostic significance, but an increasing width indicates progression of the disease. The retrorectal area either remains unchanged or enlarges during the course of the disease. It does not become smaller even during remissions.

GRANULOMATOUS COLITIS (CROHN'S DISEASE)

Involvement of the rectum by granulomatous colitis[9] may result in the formation of retrorectal fistulas or sinus tracts. These may be demonstrated on barium enema examination. Abscesses develop, which can be seen as focal presacral masses that may or may not fill with barium. Sacral osteomyelitis is an occasional complication (Fig 38–5). Diffuse widening also occurs. This is due to fibrosis as well as to edema and lymph node enlargement. In contrast to ulcerative colitis, the widening may decrease during the course of the disease.

Other causes of retrorectal abscesses include infected dermoids, extension from infected crypt glands at the dentate margin, diverticulitis and perforated carcinomas (Fig 38–6).

Tumors

Retrorectal tumors[8, 10, 11] (Fig 38–7) frequently are asymptomatic, discovered during routine rectal, proctoscopic or barium enema examinations. As the tumor enlarges, symptoms owing to pressure develop. A feeling of fullness in the pelvis, constipation and difficulty in urinating are common complaints. Low back pain is frequent; it is important to do a rectal examination in all patients with this complaint. Pressure on nerves can cause pain and numbness in the perineum and legs, as well as fecal and urinary incontinence.

The most common tumors in the retrorectal space are developmental cysts. Most of these are dermoid cysts, less commonly enteric (duplication) cysts or postanal gut cysts. Most occur in adults, and more often in females. Some cysts are discovered during routine physical examinations or during childbirth. They rarely become large enough to produce pressure symptoms. Many become infected and present as recurrent retrorectal abscesses with draining sinuses and fistulas to adjacent organs. The diagnosis can be suggested preoperatively if contrast material injected into a sinus tract enters a cavity. Malignancy or calcification is rare in these cysts.

Histologically dermoids are lined by stratified squamous epithelium. The wall may contain dermal appendages, e.g., hair follicles, sweat and sebaceous glands. These differ from teratomas, which contain all three germ layers. Teratomas usually are found in infants and frequently contain calcium.[12]

Uncomplicated large cysts produce a smooth extrinsic pressure indentation on the posterior wall of the barium-filled rectum. Usually the sacrum is normal, but smooth bony erosions from pressure may occur[7] (Fig 38–8). When cysts become infected, complete surgical removal is difficult and recurrent infection is common.

Tumor from adjacent tissues may enter

and enlarge the retrorectal space. Adenocarcinomas of the rectum and prostate are among the most common invaders. Sacral destruction from a primary carcinoma of the rectum is uncommon. However, sacral destruction may occur from recurrent carcinoma of the rectum. Recurrent tumor should be considered a cause of low back pain that develops after surgical removal of a primary rectal cancer.[13]

Prostatic carcinoma may extend posteriorly to involve the rectum and the presacral space.[14] Most commonly it envelops the rectum, causing narrowing and occasionally obstruction. Less often it involves only the anterior surface of the rectum. Rarely it simulates primary rectal carcinoma, with mucosal destruction and shelf formation.[15] Differentiation from primary rectal carcinoma is important for treatment purposes. Commonly, bone metastasis and urinary tract involvement are present at the time of rectal involvement. The barium enema usually shows eccentric circumferential narrowing of the rectum or rectosigmoid with normal or edematous mucosa, no overhanging edges and a widened presacral space (Fig 38–9).

One half of all chordomas[7, 11, 16] occur in the sacrococcygeal region (Fig 38–10). They originate from remnants of the notochord and usually grow slowly. The average age at onset is 50, and they are more frequent in males. Trauma may be a predisposing factor. In most cases a soft tissue mass can be demonstrated radiographically. The mass usually extends in front of the sacrum and may displace the rectum anteriorly. The rectal mucosa usually is normal. Amorphous calcifications are present in about 50% of sacrococcygeal chordomas. The common bone findings are sacral expansion and destruction, which usually begins near the midline and extends laterally. The tumor may engulf bone fragments and carry them along as sequestra.

Neurogenic tumors (Fig 38–11) comprised 15% of retrorectal lesions in the series of Jackman et al.,[7] but only 2% in those of Teplick et al.[3] These tumors may become quite large before discovery. They often displace the rectum anteriorly but do not invade the bowel wall. Bone changes owing to pressure may occur and are smooth erosions with well-defined sharp margins. Neurofibromas arising in a sacral foramen can widen and distort the foramen.

Miscellaneous Lesions

Most of the lesions in the miscellaneous category do not often cause enlargement of the retrorectal space (Fig 38–12). Left-sided inguinal hernias that contain sigmoid colon may widen the presacral area, possibly by exerting a constant pull on the rectum. Involvement of the colon by amyloid frequently resembles colitis.[17] It is not known if the widened space is caused only by amyloid infiltrating the rectal wall and narrowing the lumen, or if amyloid actually is present in the presacral soft tissues.

REFERENCES

1. Craig, J. O. M. C., Highan, J. H., and Palmer, F. J.: The lateral view in the radiology of the rectum and rectosigmoid, Br. J. Surg. 58:908, 1971.
2. Gardiner, G. A.: Routine lateral view of the barium filled rectum: Is it worthwhile? A review of 2500 consecutive examinations, Am. J. Roentgenol. 104: 571, 1968.
3. Teplick, S. K., Stark, P., Clark, R. E., et al.: The retrorectal space, Clin. Radiol. 29:177, 1978.
4. Edling, N. P. G., and Eklof, O.: The retrorectal soft tissue space in ulcerative colitis. A roentgen diagnostic study, Radiology 80:949, 1963.
5. Fennessy, J. J., Sparberg, M., and Kirshner, J. B.: Early roentgen manifestations of mild ulcerative colitis and proctitis, Radiology 87:848, 1966.
6. Chrispin, A. R., and Fry, I. K.: The presacral space shown by barium enema, Br. J. Radiol. 36:319, 1963.
7. Jackman, R. J., Clark, P. L., and Smith, N. D.: Retrorectal tumors, J.A.M.A. 145:956, 1951.
8. Castro, A. F.: Presacral tumors, South. Med. J. 54: 319, 1961.
9. Eklof, O., and Gierup, J.: The retrorectal soft tissue space in children: Normal variations and appearance in granulomatous colitis, Am. J. Roentgenol. 108:624, 1970.
10. Mather, B. S.: Presacral dermoid cyst, Br. J. Surg. 52:198, 1965.

11. Campbell, W. L., and Wolff, M.: Retrorectal cysts of developmental origin, Am. J. Roentgenol. 117: 307, 1973.
12. Eklof, O.: Roentgenologic findings in sacrococcygeal teratoma, Acta Radiol. (Diag) 3:41, 1965.
13. Jarvis, L. J.: Involvement of the sacrum by recurrent carcinoma of the rectum, Am. J. Roentgenol. 84:339, 1960.
14. Gengher, L., Baer, J., and Finby, N.: Rectal and sigmoid involvement secondary to carcinoma of the prostate, Am. J. Roentgenol. 125:910, 1975.
15. Shin, M. S., and Witten, D. M.: Unusual involvement of the rectum by carcinoma of the prostate, Dig. Dis. 20:42, 1975.
16. Utne, J. R., and Pugh, D. G.: The roentgenologic aspects of chordoma, Am. J. Roentgenol. 74:593, 1955.
17. Seliger, G., Krassner, R. L., Beranbaum, E. R., et al.: The spectrum of roentgen appearance in amyloidosis of the small and large bowel: Radiologic pathologic correlation, Radiology 100:63, 1971.
18. Williams, I.: Innominate grooves in the surface of mucosa, Radiology 84:877, 1965.

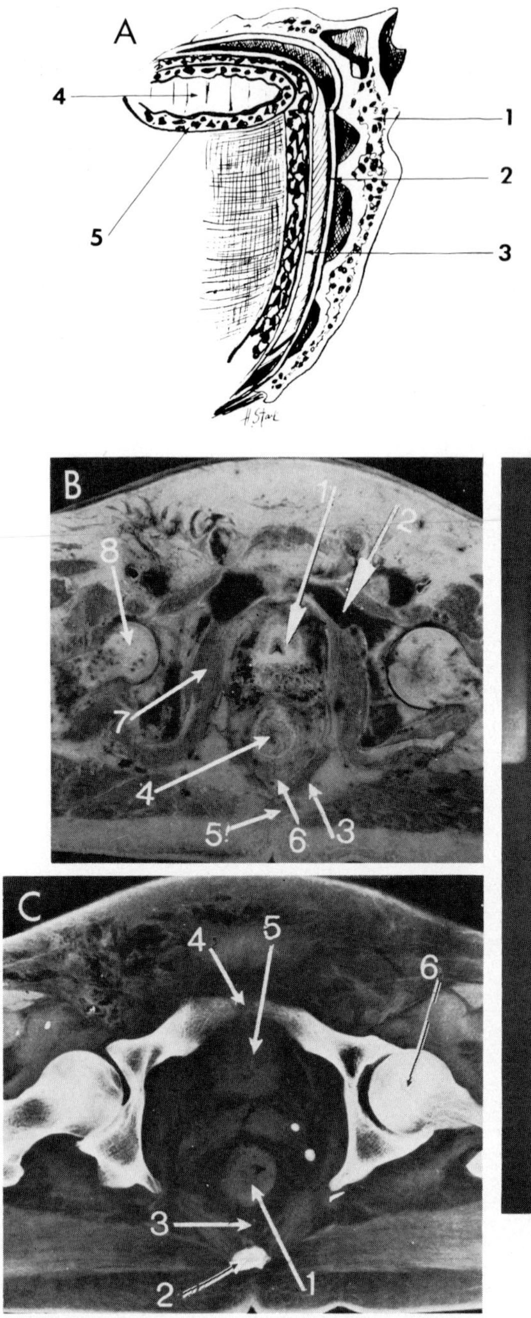

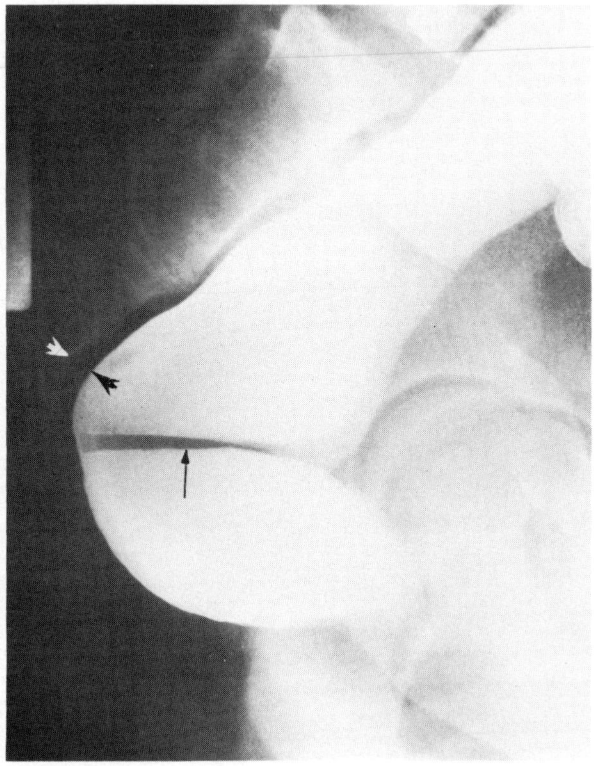

Fig 38–1 (left). — **A,** normal gross anatomy (lateral view). *1,* sacrum; *2,* Waldeyer's fascia; *3,* posterior limiting membrane; *4,* rectal lumen; *5,* rectal wall. Retrorectal space lies between *2* and *3*. **B,** cross-sectional gross anatomy. Section at level of lower rectum: *1,* prostate; *2,* pubis; *3,* levator ani muscle; *4,* rectum; *5,* coccyx; *6,* retrorectal space; *7,* internal obturator muscle; *8,* femoral head. **C,** cross-sectional radiographic anatomy. Radiogram of **B:** *1,* rectum; *2,* coccyx; *3,* retrorectal space; *4,* pubic symphysis; *5,* prostate; *6,* femoral head. (**B** and **C** Courtesy of Dr. Lawrence R. Goodman. Reprinted from *Transverse Anatomy of the Human Thorax, Abdomen and Pelvis,* copyright 1978, Little, Brown and Company.)

Fig 38–2 (right). — Normal radiographic anatomy (lateral view). Barium-filled rectum has smooth posterior border and closely follows sacral contour. Presacral space is only several millimeters wide *(arrowheads).* Note normal Houston fold *(arrow).*

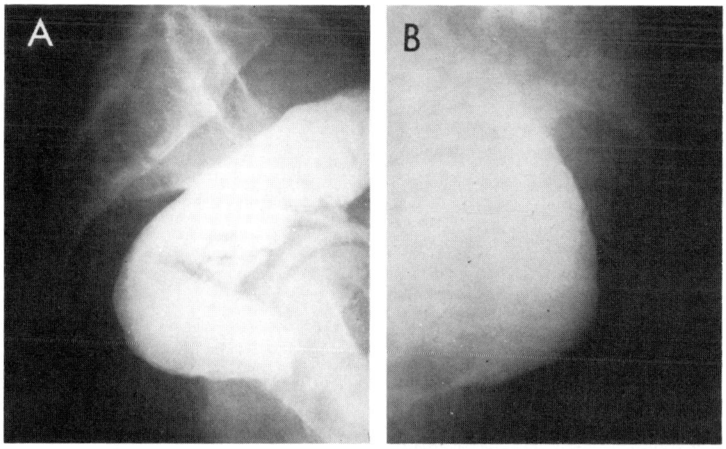

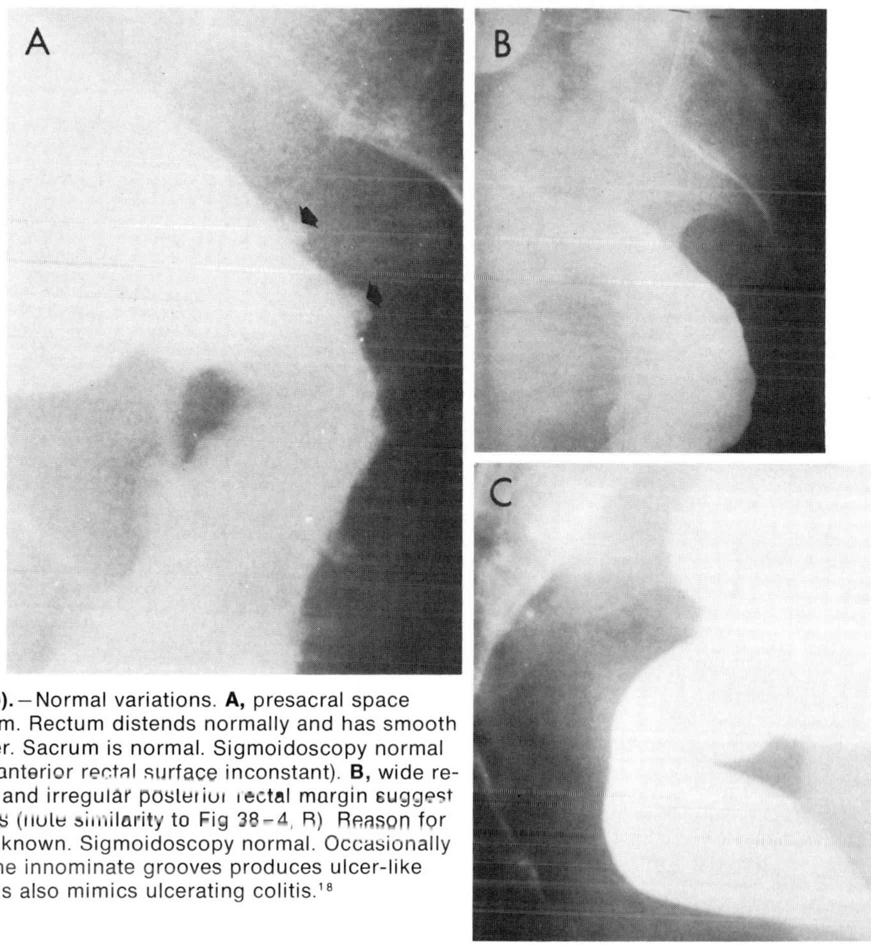

Fig 38–3 (top).—Normal variations. **A,** presacral space measures 2.5 cm. Rectum distends normally and has smooth posterior border. Sacrum is normal. Sigmoidoscopy normal (irregularity of anterior rectal surface inconstant). **B,** wide retrorectal space and irregular posterior rectal margin suggest ulcerative colitis (note similarity to Fig 38–4, B). Reason for irregularity not known. Sigmoidoscopy normal. Occasionally barium filling the innominate grooves produces ulcer-like projections. This also mimics ulcerating colitis.[18]

Fig 38–4 (bottom).—Ulcerative colitis. **A,** acute proctosigmoiditis with large ulcerations *(arrows)*. **B,** acute proctosigmoiditis. Appearance is identical to that of Fig 38–3, B. History and sigmoidoscopy are needed to distinguish normal from abnormal. **C,** chronic ulcerative colitis. Presacral space is uniformly widened, and rectum lacks distensibility. (**A** and **B** courtesy of Dr. Ervin Philippe, Boston University Medical School.)

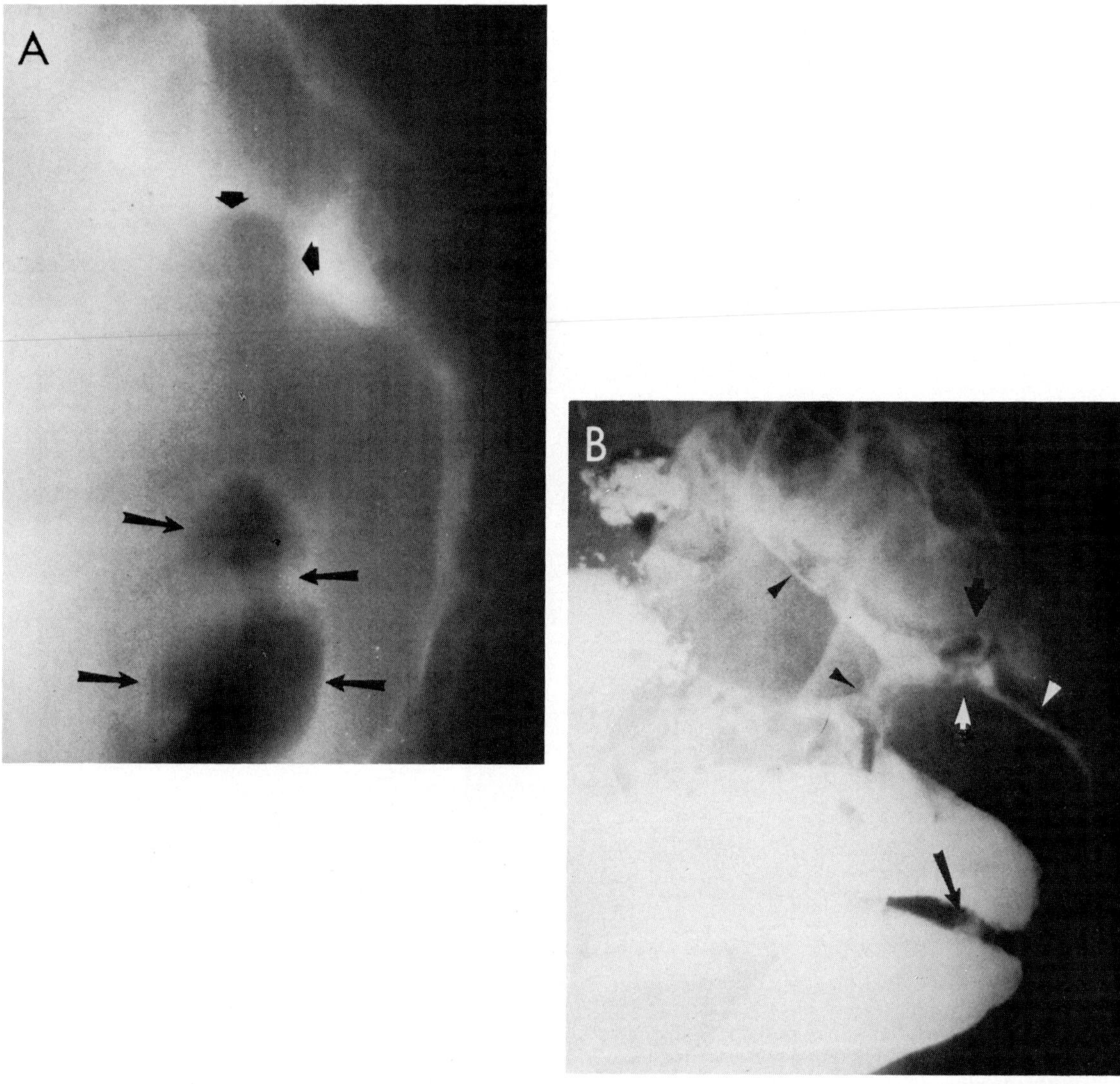

Fig 38–5.—Granulomatous colitis with sacral osteomyelitis. **A,** tomogram of sacrum showing erosion on anterior border of S2–3 *(short arrows).* Rectal gas pattern is abnormal *(long arrows).* **B,** barium outlines retrorectal sinus tracts *(arrowheads)* and collects in abscess at sacral defect *(short arrows).* Presacral space is enlarged. There is stricture of rectum *(long arrow).*

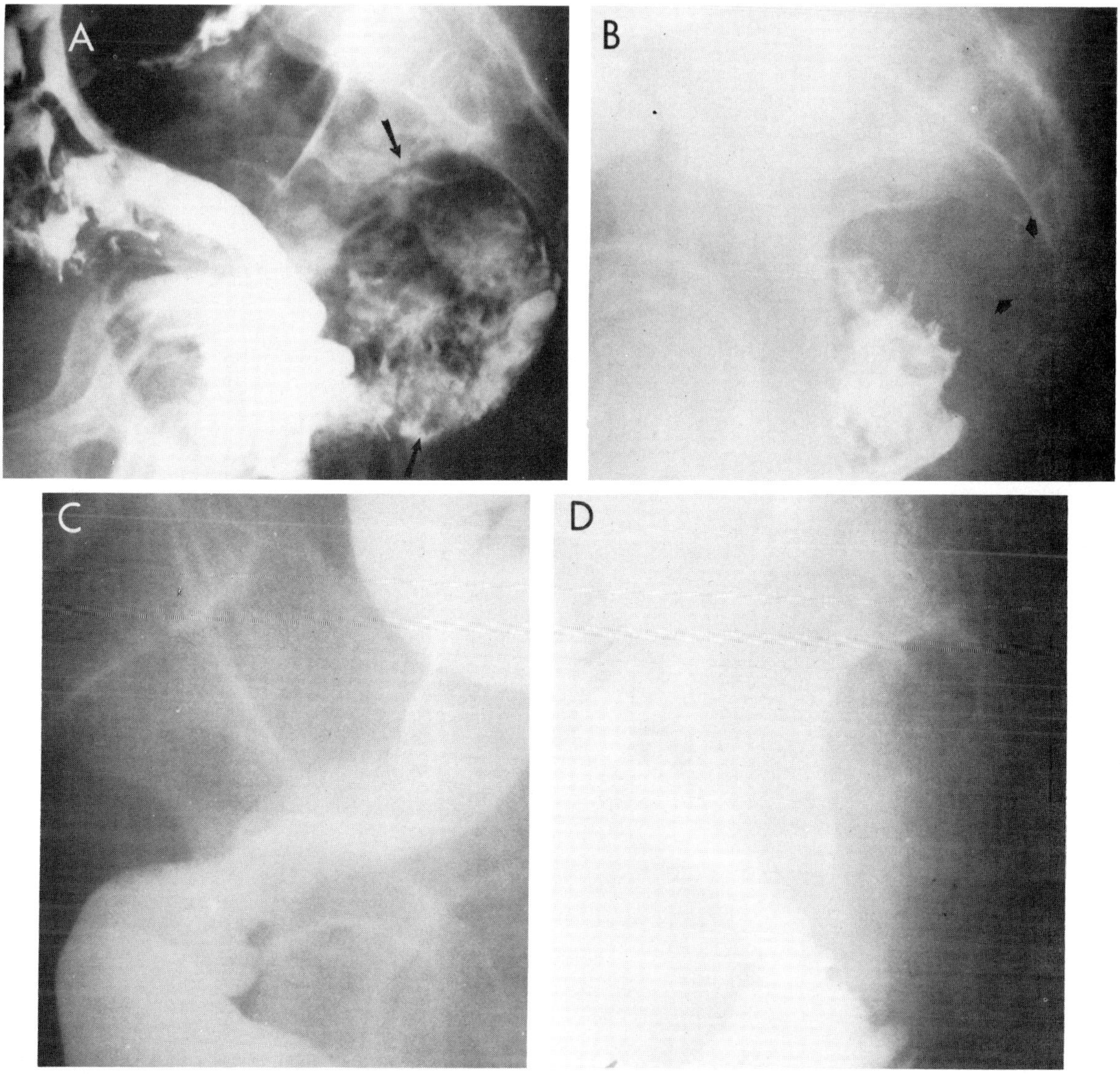

Fig 38–6.—**A,** diverticulitis with presacral abscess. Marked widening of retrorectal space with large collection of barium in abscess *(arrows).* Site of perforation clearly demonstrated on other projections. **B,** perforating adenocarcinoma. Unusually long primary adenocarcinoma of rectosigmoid. Presacral space enlarged. Small amounts of barium anterior to sacrum are from perforation *(arrows).* Other views (not shown) were more diagnostic of primary carcinoma. **C,** diverticulitis and presacral abscess. Diverticulitis of proximal sigmoid resulted in presacral abscess displacing bowel anteriorly. Secondary inflammatory changes of distal rectosigmoid resulting from adjacent abscess. No barium entered retrorectal abscess. **D,** idiopathic abscess. Large presacral mass causing inflammatory changes of rectosigmoid. No site of extravasation or other colon pathology. Abscess probably originated from infected crypt gland. (**A** courtesy of Dr. Harvey Borden, Weymouth, Massachusetts.)

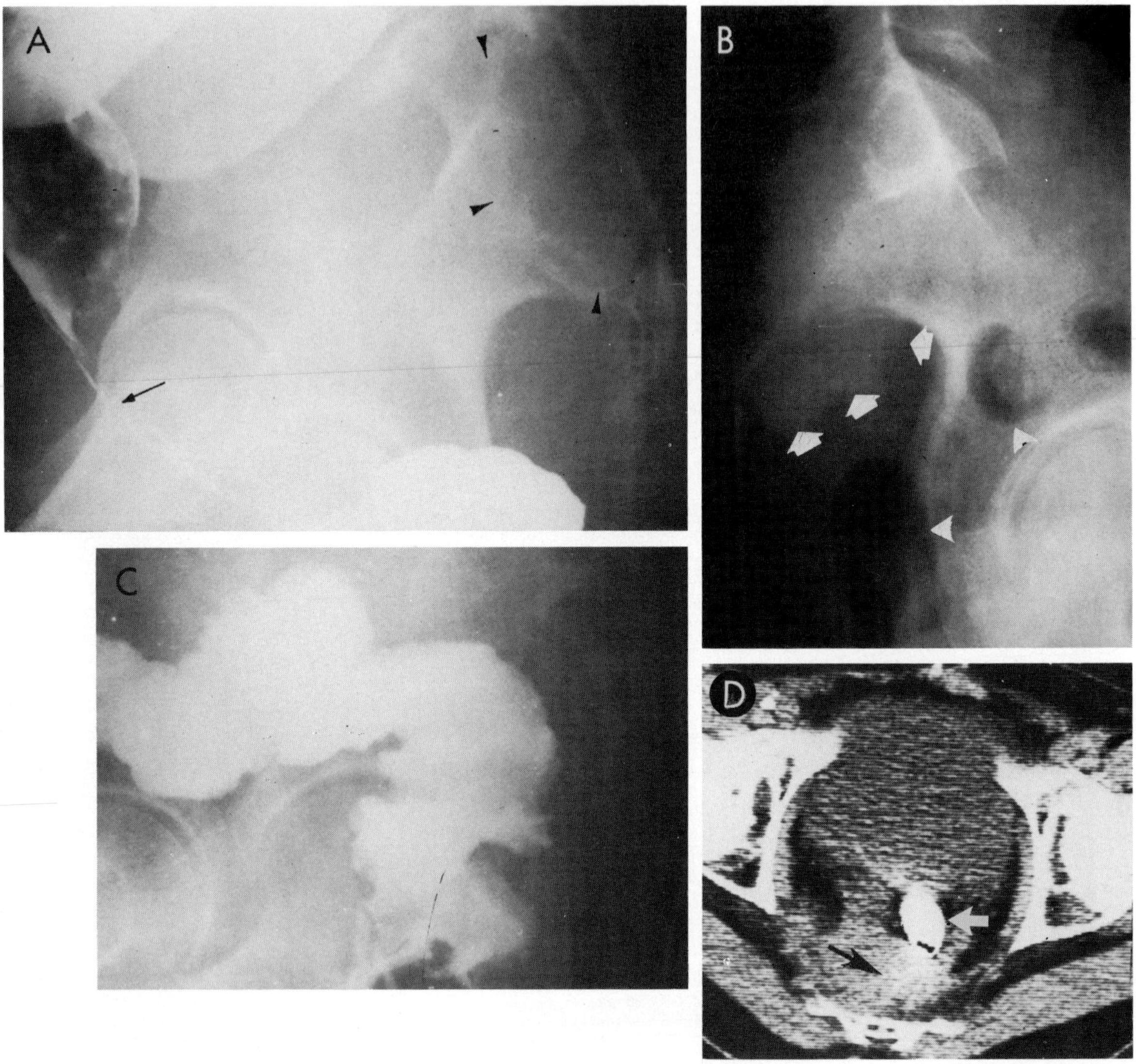

Fig 38–7.—**A,** fibrosarcoma. Huge retrorectal mass displacing rectosigmoid *(arrow)* anteriorly. Well-defined areas of sacral destruction *(arrowheads)* indicate slow growth. **B,** solitary plasmacytoma. Extensive destruction of sacrum, and soft tissue mass invading retrorectal space *(arrows)*. Rectum is displaced anteriorly *(arrowheads)*. **C,** primary lymphoma. Tumor is producing irregularity of rectosigmoid and widening of presacral area. **D,** recurrent colon carcinoma. CT scan of pelvis in patient who had prior resection of sigmoid for carcinoma. Recurrent carcinoma in presacral space *(black arrow)* is displacing opacified rectum *(white arrow)*. (**D** Courtesy of Dr. Herbert Y. Kressel, Reprinted with permission from Radiology 129:451, 1978).

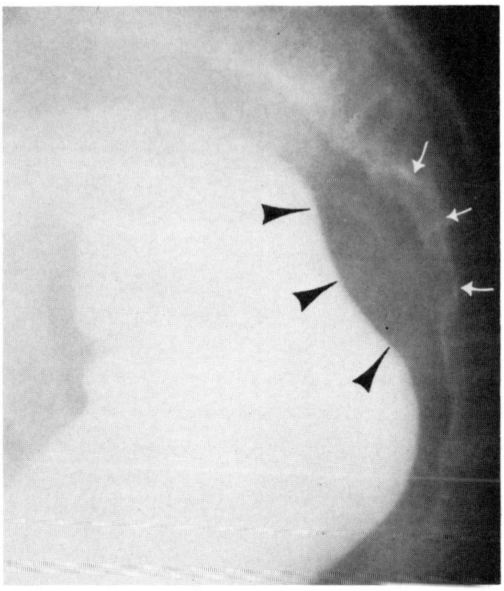

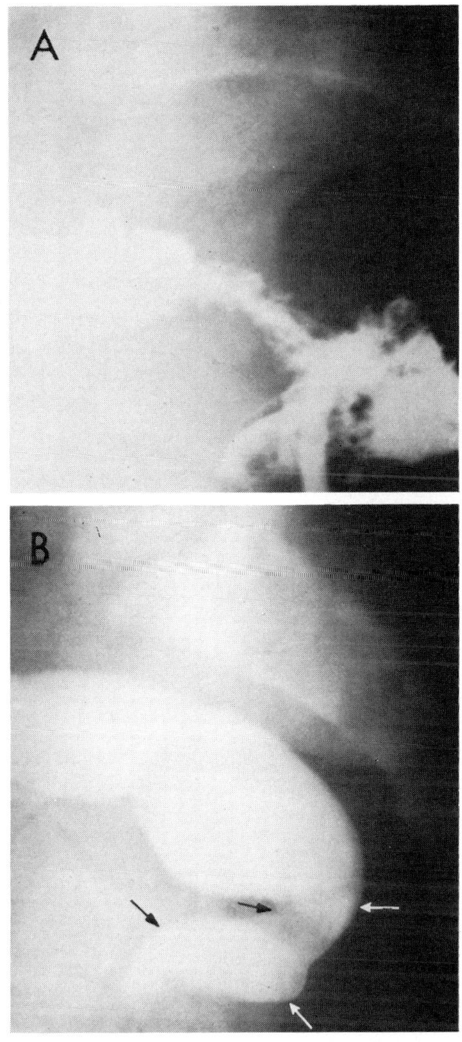

Fig 38–8 (left). Probable developmental cyst with sacral erosion. Asymptomatic focal mass causing smooth extrinsic indentation on posterior rectal surface *(arrowheads)* and pressure erosion of sacrum *(arrows).*

Fig 38–9 (right).—**A,** carcinoma of prostate. Tumor encircles rectosigmoid and extends into presacral area. Rectal mucosa is not destroyed. Bones are dense from skeletal metastasis. **B,** carcinoma of prostate. Tumor envelops distal rectum *(arrows)* and extends into presacral space. Osteoblastic metastases present.

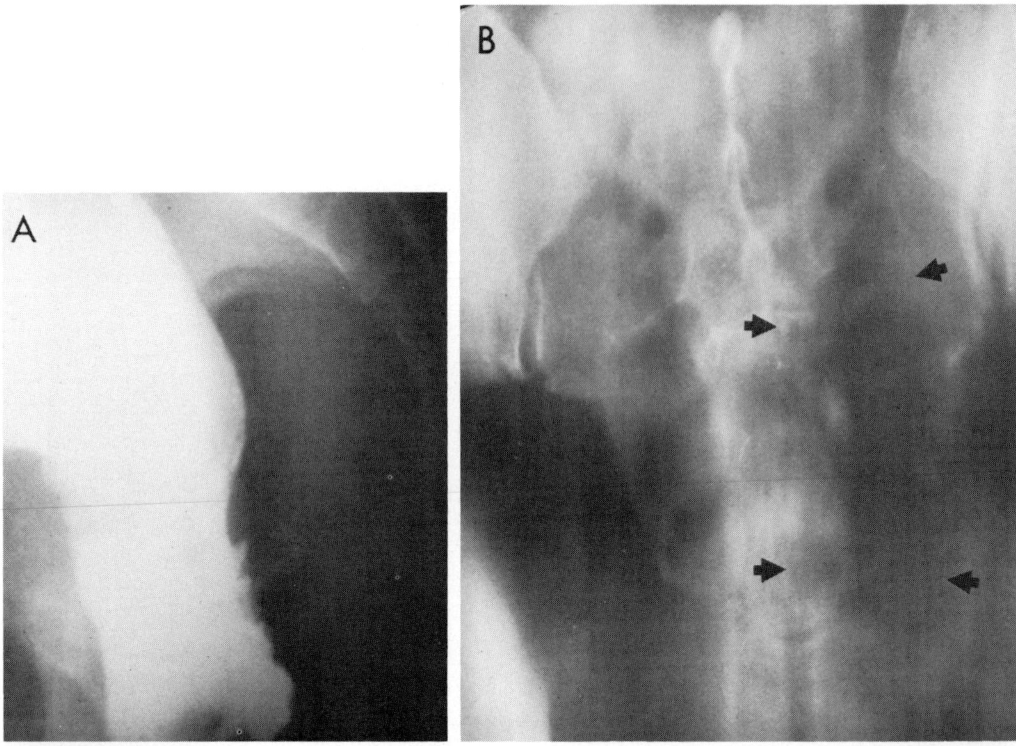

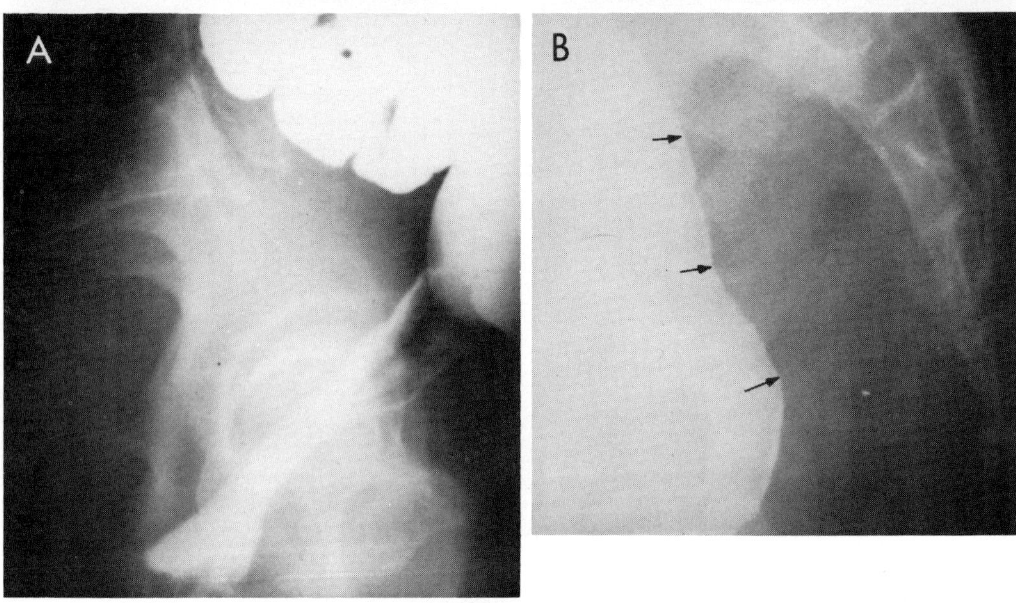

Fig 38–10 (top).—Chordoma. **A,** large noncalcified soft tissue mass pushing rectum anteriorly. Mucosa edematous but not invaded. Tumor was easily separated from bowel. **B,** AP tomogram showing destruction of sacrum mainly on left *(arrows).*

Fig 38–11 (bottom).—Schwannomas. **A,** huge presacral soft tissue mass displacing but not invading rectosigmoid. No calcifications or bone destruction. Pelvic angiogram (not shown) demonstrated hypervascularity from left internal iliac artery. **B,** large noncalcified mass *(arrows)* pushing rectum anteriorly. No bone destruction.

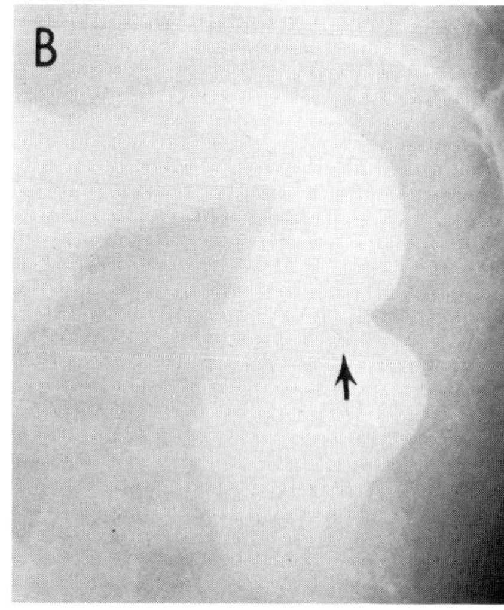

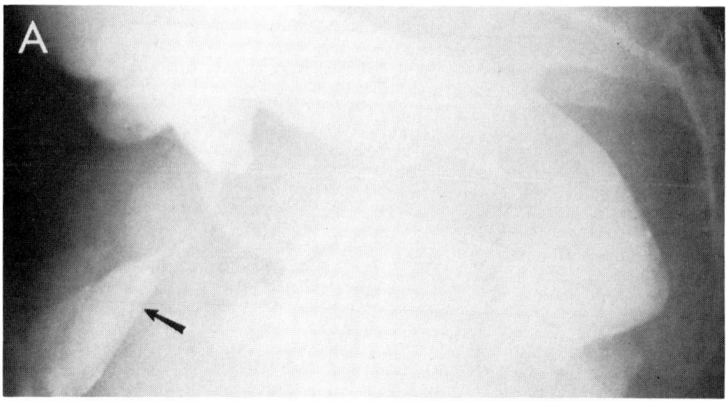

Fig 38–12.—Inguinal hernia. **A,** normal variation? Enlarged retrorectal space. Normal sigmoidoscopy. Left inguinal hernia containing sigmoid colon *(arrow)* **B–D,** miscellaneous lesions. **B,** amyloidosis. Widened presacral space, finely spiculated posterior rectosigmoid surface, diminished distensibility and thickened Houston fold *(arrow)* resemble ulcerative colitis. Amyloid of colon frequently resembles colitis. **C,** pneumatosis cystoides intestinalis. Gas-containing cysts *(arrows)* cause apparent enlargement of presacral space. **D,** pelvic lipomatosis. Fatty tissue surrounds rectosigmoid, causing diminished distensibility and widened retrorectal space.

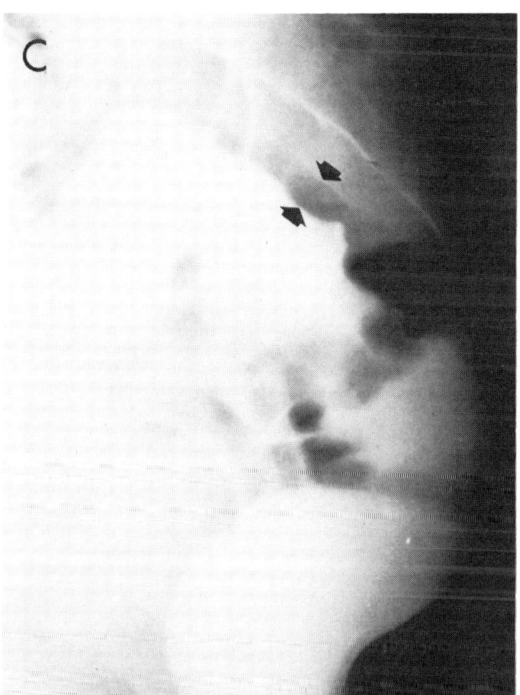

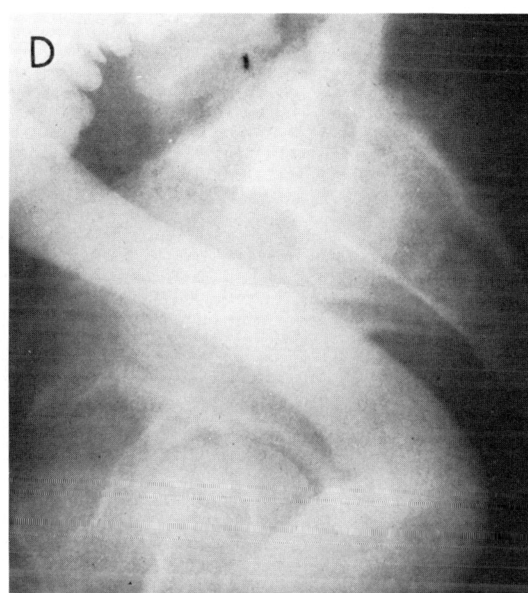

Chapter 39

Right Lower Quadrant Disease

ROBERT E. KOEHLER, M.D.

THE ILEOCECAL VALVE, appendix, cecum and ascending colon are portions of the large intestine that normally lie in the right lower abdominal quadrant. Sufficient air is often present in the right colon to permit determination of its position and caliber on plain films of the abdomen. The proximal colon is sometimes difficult to examine adequately on barium enema because of its large volume and because the barium column tends to push residual fecal material back to the cecum. Whenever possible, spot films should be obtained with sufficient abdominal compression to partially flatten the cecum. High kvp technique should be used to allow penetration of the barium column in this area.

The air contrast barium enema technique is particularly useful in this region of the colon, as it alleviates the necessity of penetrating the large volume of barium in the cecum. Retention of feces in the right colon is sometimes less of a problem with this technique as well, since on decubitus views particles of stool tend to flow with the barium away from the area being examined by double contrast.

Using either enema technique, adequate distention of the right colon should be achieved. Glucagon, 0.5 mg, may be administered intravenously when spasm prevents complete filling of the cecum. With well-distended views of the cecum, either type of barium enema becomes a sensitive indicator of large and small intraluminal mass lesions and of impressions by extrinsic right lower abdominal masses.

The air contrast examination in particular can provide exquisitely detailed views of the surface of the colonic mucosa in this region. The pattern of normal innominate grooves is often seen as a network of fine lines covering the surface of the colon[1, 2] and should not be confused with inflammatory bowel disease and other pathology. With this technique the colonic lymphoid follicules are frequently visible as numerous, uniform 1–3-mm nodules studding the colonic surface (Fig 39–1). These often are seen in both children and adults and, if confined to colon and terminal ileum, represent a normal appearance.

Portions of the colon that usually lie in the right lower quadrant may be involved by the variety of diseases that affect the colon, but they are also the site of conditions that rarely, if ever, affect the remainder of the colon. It is important to remember that, in patients with congenital malrotation of the bowel or those in whom a portion of the ascending colon is suspended on a mesentery, signs and symptoms of ileocecal or appendiceal disease may be centered in other quadrants of the abdomen. Also of importance in patients with a mobile cecum is that volvulus of the cecum can occur and may lead to ascending colon obstruction. In this situation there are signs of small bowel obstruction, and the markedly dilated, gas-filled cecum fills the midabdomen, its tip pointing toward the left upper quadrant.

Cecum and Ascending Colon

The cecum and ascending colon may be involved by ulcerative or granulomatous colitis and, in general, the radiographic features of cecal involvement by these diseases are similar to those seen when more distal portions of the colon are affected.[3] Ulcerative colitis rarely involves the cecum or ascending colon in the absence of contiguous involvement of the left colon and rectum. By comparison, Crohn's disease frequently affects the right colon, usually in contiguity with disease of the adjacent terminal ileum. When the left colon also is implicated, the disease may be continuous or show intervening "skip areas" of uninvolved colon. In the early stages, the cecum and other areas may show only small discrete aphthoid ulcers.[4]

When the right colon is involved, a helpful clue in distinguishing ulcerative colitis from granulomatous colitis is the appearance of the ileocecal valve and terminal ileum. In patients with ulcerative colitis the ileum often is normal. Alternatively, backwash ileitis may be present, causing a flaccid, dilated terminal ileum. If ileal fold thickening is present, it usually is mild and confined to a short segment immediately adjacent to the ileocolic junction (Fig 39–2). Narrowing and ulceration over a longer segment of ileum may occur in patients with ulcerative colitis but are rare. Typically the ileocecal valve is patulous and may be fixed in the open position (Fig 39–3). Its lips are thin or nonexistent and fistulas do not occur.

By way of contrast, the ileum and ileocecal valve take on a very different appearance in patients in whom the cecum shows granulomatous colitis (Figs 39–4 to 39–7). In these patients the terminal ileum usually but not always is involved as well. The ileocecal valve tends to be thickened, and its lumen usually is narrowed. The ileum shows thickening and distortion of mucosal folds and ulceration and thickening of the bowel wall and adjacent mesentery. Strictures and fistula formation are common and are typical of Crohn's disease. Fistula formation virtually never occurs in patients with ulcerative colitis.

Inflammatory disease of the bowel also may arise on an infectious basis. Tuberculosis, amebiasis, typhoid fever and infection with *Yersinia enterocolitica* all have a predilection for the ileocecal area.

The cecum and terminal ileum are the most common sites of gastrointestinal infection by tuberculosis. In the United States the usual route in patients with active pulmonary tuberculosis is thought to be swallowing of infected sputum.[5] In most instances both cecum and ileum are affected, but cecal involvement alone occurs in about 20% of cases.[6] Ileal involvement with sparing of the cecum is rare. Radiographically edema, spasm and irritability of the cecum and adjacent ileum may be seen. Ulceration may be evident, and fibrosis may lead to shortening and stricture formation (Fig 39–8). The ileocecal valve may be fixed in the open position or may take on a narrowed appearance more typical of that usually seen in patients with Crohn's disease. In the hyperplastic form of cecal tuberculosis, a mass of inflammatory and granulomatous tissue (tuberculoma) may mimic a carcinoma. The distinction between carcinoma and tuberculoma is often suggested on the basis of the ileal involvement in tuberculosis, which is rare in cecal carcinoma.

Amebiasis, usually caused by *Entamoeba histolytica,* may infect the entire colon and may mimic the clinical features of ulcerative colitis or Crohn's disease[7]. In 3–5% of patients, however, the disease is confined to the ileocecal area. Characteristic radiographic findings include spasm and irritability of the cecum and the presence of ulcers, which may be small and superficial or may coalesce to form deep flask-shaped ulcers. As the disease progresses and fibrosis sets in, the cecum may take on the classic cone-shaped appearance. The ileocecal valve is often patulous. Unlike tuberculosis or Crohn's disease, amebiasis rarely involves the ileum, and this feature may permit its distinction from these other conditions. As in patients with intestinal tuberculosis, a mass of proliferative granulomatous tissue (ameboma) may develop, usually in the cecum.

Y. enterocolitica infection has been recognized with increasing frequency in recent years, usually in children. Clinically this disease mimics acute appendicitis, and many patients are diagnosed at surgery. When radiograms are obtained, ulceration and thickening and distortion of mucosal folds may be seen in the terminal ileum. Similar changes occasionally occur in the colon but are usually confined to the cecum and ascending colon.[8, 9] In typhoid fever, which has become rare in the United States, radiographically visible signs of inflammation are usually confined to the distal ileum.

The cecum and terminal ileum also may be the site of involvement of other inflammatory conditions. Necrotizing colitis of the cecum known as leukemic typhlitis may occur in children with acute leukemia, usually those in severe or terminal stages. The pathogenesis is not fully understood and more than one mechanism may be involved. Leukemic infiltration, localized inflammation and hemorrhage all may be features of the disorder. Because of the patients' moribund condition, barium enema is rarely performed. Plain abdominal films may show a paucity of gas in the right lower quadrant, indicative of small bowel obstruction, or a right lower quadrant, soft tissue density owing to distention of an atonic, fluid-filled cecum.[10]

The cecum may be the site of an isolated ulcer. The cause of nonspecific cecal ulcers is not well understood.[11] In some cases they may be stercoraceous; in others, local ischemic changes may play a role. If the ulcer is small or superficial, there may be no radiographic abnormalities on barium enema. Often a cecal mass will correspond to edema and other inflammatory response around the ulcer, although the actual crater may not be identifiable. The diagnosis is usually confirmed colonoscopically.

Diverticula occur in the cecum and ascending colon, often at a younger age than is typical of sigmoid diverticulosis. This observation, coupled with the fact that cecal diverticula often contain all three layers of the colonic wall, lead most authors[6] to conclude that most diverticula seen in this region are congenital. Diverticulitis with localized perforation may occur and usually presents radiographically as an isolated mural or pericolic inflammatory mass with or without extravasation of barium. Filling the appendix with barium helps to distinguish this entity from appendicitis, which has a similar presentation. Differentiation of the radiographic features from those of carcinoma may be difficult if not impossible, especially when spasm and irritability are not prominent and other diverticula are not noted.

The other major complication of right colonic diverticulosis is bleeding; some authors[12] have concluded that diverticula are the most common cause of severe rectal bleeding in the elderly. The bleeding may be repeated occult bleeding or massive exsanguinating hemorrhage. Since it usually occurs in the absence of diverticulitis, there usually are no radiographic findings except diverticulosis on barium enema. Arteriography is sometimes helpful in locating the bleeding site. If the patient is studied when active bleeding is occurring at a rate in excess of about 1 ml per minute, visible extravasation may be seen.

Arteriography also may be the only radiographic means of localizing the site of another cause of colonic bleeding. Angiodysplasias (vascular ectasias) represent abnormalities of small vessels of the mucosa of the right colon. They are usually found after age

60 and are probably acquired on a degenerative basis.[13] Characteristic arteriographic findings include a small tuft of ectatic submucosal capillaries and veins and dense, early opacification of the vein draining the angiodysplasia (Fig 39–9).

As in the area of the rectum, congenital colonic duplications occasionally occur in relation to the cecum. If the duplication communicates with the bowel lumen, it usually resembles a diverticular outpouching. If there is no communication, it takes the form of a cystic mass in the bowel wall (Fig 39–10).

Benign and malignant tumors that involve the right lower quadrant portions of the colon are similar to those in the remainder of the large intestine. Benign polypoid lesions of mucosal origin usually represent adenomas of tubular, villous or mixed histologic type. Radiographic detection is important because of the presence of foci of malignancy in some of these tumors, particularly those exceeding 1 cm in size. As in other areas of the colon, villous adenomas often have an irregular frondlike surface, although this is less frequently seen than with villous adenomas of the left colon[14] (Figs 39–11 and 39–12). Radiographic detection of small polypoid or plaque-like lesions of the cecum is facilitated by use of the air contrast technique (Fig 39–13). Irrespective of which enema technique is used, the ileocecal valve must be identified with certainty and polypoid lesions distinguished from the normal valve.

Adenocarcinoma of the cecum and ascending colon is a problem of increasing magnitude. There is epidemiologic evidence that the proportion of colonic carcinomas in the proximal colon has been rising in recent years.[15] For this reason digital rectal and proctoscopic examinations now detect a lower percentage of colonic malignancies than in the past, and radiographic and colonoscopic techniques have taken on greater importance. Because tumors in this location rarely obstruct the bowel lumen before they are quite large, clinical signs and symptoms often appear rather late (Fig 39–14).

The radiographic appearance of adenocarcinoma of the cecum is similar to that of carcinoma elsewhere in the colon. When early, the tumor usually appears as a small polypoid or plaque-like lesion (Fig 39–15). As the disease progresses, it may become annular and constricting or may take on the appearance of a polypoid intraluminal mass (Figs 39–16 and 39–17). Uncommonly, carcinoma of the cecum may be predominantly extrinsic, with only a small area of cecal abnormality evident radiographically. Extension across the ileocecal valve to the ileum is unusual. Occasionally differentiation from a periappendiceal abscess is difficult (Fig 39–18).

The most common intramural tumor of the right colon is lipoma. These tumors most often are single and vary considerably in size. Although they usually are submucosal in origin, they may grow to develop a pseudopedicle owing to stretching of the overlying and adjacent mucosa. Radiographically they appear as smoothly outlined, sharply demarcated, intramural or intraluminal lesions usually spherical or ovoid in shape (Fig 39–19). By applying manual compression to the abdomen, the radiologist sometimes can demonstrate the softness and pliability of these tumors. Leiomyomas of the colon are less common. They have a similar radiographic appearance but are less pliable.

Lymphoma occasionally may involve the colon, usually as a site of secondary involvement but sometimes as an isolated primary tumor. Secondary colonic involvement by lymphoma tends to be somewhat more frequent on the left side.[16] Primary colonic lymphoma, on the other hand, occurs most commonly in the cecum. The usual radiographic appearance of cecal lymphoma is that of an intraluminal mass, often large, without an obstructive component (Fig 39–20). The mass usually involves the ileocecal valve and may be associated with colocolic intussusception. Other forms of colonic lymphoma, e.g., diffuse small nodules, large excavated masses or annular lesions, may occur in the cecal region but are less common. Extension of lymphoma across the ileocecal valve to involve the ileum is not uncommon and helps to distinguish this tumor from the more common adenocarcinoma.

Metastatic tumor also may localize to the right lower quadrant and cause abnormalities visible on barium enema examination. Extension of carcinoma of the pancreas[17] or other gastrointestinal organs[18] to the right lower quadrant may occur via the mesenteric reflections or by flow of tumor cells in intraperitoneal fluid along the mesenteric root to the ileocecal region and right paracolic gutter. Tumors of ovarian origin are also prone to intraperitoneal spread. Embolic spread of tumor, usually from a primary tumor of lung, breast or melanoma, also may involve the right colon. Characteristically, mesenteric or intraperitoneal spread results in extrinsic masses impressing the medial cecal tip and adjacent ileum (Fig 39–21); spread up the paracolic gutter tends to affect the posterolateral aspect of the right colon. Hematogenously disseminated deposits appear as submucosal nodules, which may show a central depression or umbilication.

Some patients with endometriosis exhibit cecal involvement, usually in the form of a mural nodule.[19] Kinking of the bowel owing to fibrosis and annular constricting or intramural lesions also occur.

Ileocecal Valve

The normal ileocecal valve appears as a round or oval mound of tissue in the cecum. On barium enema examination, it usually is possible to see the ileum entering the colon at the center of the valve. When viewed en face, the folds on the surface of the valve converge on the central lumen in the form of a rosette. The size of the normal ileocecal valve varies considerably. The upper limit of normal for the vertical dimension of the ileocecal valve has been stated as 3 cm by some authors and as high as 5 cm by others.[20] The smaller of these two values is probably more reasonable. It should be remembered that the valve is larger when the cecum is empty than when the cecum and ileum are fully distended.

The most common cause of enlargement of the ileocecal valve is lipomatosis or fatty infiltration. This is most common in women and usually occurs after age 40.[21] There is debate as to whether lipomatosis of the ileocecal valve can lead to symptoms through intermittent production of ileocecal intussusception or obstruction, but the condition is probably asymptomatic in most persons.

Radiographic distinction between lipomatosis and a neoplasm involving the ileocecal valve is often difficult. Although fatty infiltration may give the valve a somewhat lobulated contour (Fig 39–22), the mucosal surface remains smooth. Change in the size and shape of an enlarged ileocecal valve with abdominal compression and with varying degrees of cecal distention provides further evidence that enlargement of the valve is due simply to fatty infiltration. Fatty infiltration usually involves both labia of the valve, generally in a symmetric fashion (Fig 39–23). Thus, localized enlargement of the valve should raise suspicion of a tumor. Infiltration of the ileocecal valve by hyperplastic lymphoid tissue has also proved a cause of smooth symmetric enlargement of the ileocecal valve in children.[22]

Prolapse of ileal mucosa into the cecum can also cause prominence of the ileocecal valve. This may occur with or without associated lipomatosis, and the radiographic appearance of these two entities can easily be confused. Prolapse extensive enough to simulate a tumor is rare but may occur. Attempts should be made on barium enema examination to demonstrate the relationship of the ileal lumen to the polypoid mass in the cecum. If the folds of the rosette pattern can be shown to converge at the center of the valve and its surface is smooth, the presence of a carcinoma or other tumor is unlikely.

The spectrum of tumors involving the ileocecal valve is similar to that affecting the adjacent colon. Lipoma constitutes the most common benign tumor of the ileocecal valve and differs from lipomatous infiltration in that a pathologically definable capsule surrounds the tumor. Radiographically lipomas have a smooth surface and appear round or slightly lobulated (Fig 39–24). The mucosa covering them is usually intact. They may reach large size without causing obstruction or symptoms. As with lipomatous infiltration, films or fluoroscopic examination with abdominal compression may demonstrate the soft and pliable nature of the lipoma.

Adenomas of tubular or villous histologic type may arise from the ileocecal valve. Their appearance and significance do not differ from those of similar tumors of the adjacent colon. Adenomas, particularly villous, may have a rougher surface appearance than do lipomas.

Carcinoid tumors also may arise in the ileocecal region and may involve the ileocecal valve. They are often incidental findings in asymptomatic patients but, in patients with hepatic metastases, the carcinoid syndrome may be evident. Carcinoid tumors of the ileocecal valve have a tendency to develop in areas covered by ileal mucosa. As a result, they often arise at the center of the valve rather than on one of its lips. The carcinoid may develop in the lumen of the ileocecal valve and cause smooth, symmetric enlargement of the valve, indistinguishable from fatty infiltration.

Of adenocarcinomas of the colon, 1.5–2% arise from the ileocecal valve. These tumors commonly cause obstruction of the lumen (Fig 39–25), but this occasionally appears late because of the fluid nature of the bowel contents at this level. As with benign tumors of the ileocecal valve, intussusception may occur (Fig 39–26). In contrast to lipomatosis or benign tumors, surface irregularity owing to mucosal destruction and ulceration is common (Fig 39–27). As with carcinoma arising elsewhere in the cecum, the tumor may have abrupt, overhanging margins or an annular configuration. Spread to involve the adjacent cecum is common. Involvement of the terminal ileum with adenocarcinoma of the ileocecal valve is unusual, and this finding should suggest the possibility of lymphoma, which most often involves the terminal ileum in contiguity with valvular and colonic involvement.

As is true for the cecum, metastatic tumor can reach the ileocecal valve via hematogenous, intraperitoneal or mesenteric spread (Fig 39–28).

Appendix

There are multiple variations in the length, diameter and position of the normal human appendix. The appendix often lies intraperitoneally and may project medially or inferiorly from its site of origin at the cecal tip. In as high as 26–65% of cases,[23, 24] however, the appendix is retrocecal, either intra- or extraperitoneal. When the appendix does not fill with barium, its position may be inferred from the position of the ileocecal valve.[25] In patients with an intraperitoneal appendix that points inferiorly, the ileocecal valve lies in its customary position on the medial aspect of the cecum. When the ileocecal valve lies posteriorly, the appendix usually ascends in a retrocecal orientation.

Occasionally intussusception of the appendix leads to partial, or rarely, complete invagination of the appendix into the cecum. On barium enema an invaginated appendix may be discovered incidentally as a finger-like filling defect in the cecum at the anticipated site of origin of the appendix (Fig 39–29). In some patients the intussusception will reduce spontaneously during barium enema. Alternatively, appendiceal intussusception may present as an acute abdominal emergency, and surgery may be performed without preliminary barium studies.

A somewhat similar radiographic aspect may be presented by the defect caused by an inverted appendiceal stump following appendectomy. The inverted stump usually appears as a smooth, rounded filling defect, up to 1 cm in size, arising from the medial wall of the cecum. Occasionally an inverted appendiceal stump may be as large as 3 cm in diameter, particularly in the several weeks following appendectomy (Figs 39–30 and 39–31). Although the surface of the stump defect is usually smooth, it may be somewhat irregular or lobulated, and differentiation from a polypoid neoplasm may not be possible on radiographic grounds alone.

Acute inflammation of the appendix is usually associated with obstruction of the appendiceal lumen by a fecalith, which may or may not be calcified. In unusual cases the appendiceal obstruction may be due to Crohn's disease, tumor of the cecum or appendix (Fig 39–32), a foreign body (Fig 39–33) or other cause. In most cases, the diagnosis is strongly suspected on clinical grounds, and a preoperative barium enema is not performed.

Many patients undergo plain film examination of the abdomen, and recognition of the plain film findings of appendicitis is important. Plain abdominal radiograms are normal in about half of patients with appendicitis,[24] so that a normal plain film examination must not be taken as evidence against the presence of appendiceal inflammation. Accumulation of fluid in the cecum with a visible air-fluid level is observed frequently in patients with appendicitis but is not highly specific, since it is commonly seen in normal individuals. Air-fluid levels in the ileum are also often seen in patients with appendicitis and, particularly if dilatation also is noted, indicate a right lower quadrant abnormality with greater reliability. Generalized small bowel dilatation is occasionally observed in patients with appendicitis. This can be due to an adynamic ileus or to mechanical obstruction resulting from adhesions surrounding the inflammatory process. Asymmetry of the fat bordering the margin of the psoas muscles is difficult to evaluate radiographically, since overlying bowel contents and minor degrees of obliquity may make a psoas margin indistinct. However, if the margin of the upper portion of the right psoas is sharply delineated but the margin of its lower portion indistinct, right lower quadrant inflammatory disease should be suspected.[26] Obliteration of the margin of the right obturator internus muscle carries similar significance. If a periappendiceal abscess is present, there may be radiographic evidence of a soft tissue mass in the right abdomen with or without the presence of stippled lucencies indicating gas within the abscess (Figs 39–34 to 39–36). Perforation of the appendix, resulting in free intraperitoneal air, is occasionally seen. In some patients, gas may be seen in the lumen of the obstructed appendix. This sign lacks specificity, however, since gas in the appendix is sometimes seen in normal individuals, particularly when the appendix is in an ascending orientation.

An important radiographic sign of appendicitis is a calcified fecalith in the right lower abdomen. Appendicoliths usually present radiographically as round or oval laminated densities, which average 1 cm in size (Figs 39–37 and 39–38). When multiple, appendicoliths may lie in a linear or curvilinear orientation.

Data from a variety of series[27-29] indicate that fecaliths are visible radiographically in about 10% of patients with appendicitis. The finding of a calcified fecalith in the right lower quadrant in a patient with signs and symptoms of appendicitis should be considered strongly confirmatory. There is less certainty about the significance of a calcified appendiceal fecalith in an asymptomatic patient. Because of the significant risk of subsequent development of appendicitis and because of the greater likelihood of perforation and other serious complications in patients with appendicitis in whom a fecalith is present, many authors have recommended prophylactic appendectomy in this situation.[30, 31]

In patients suspected of having appendicitis but in whom the clinical evaluation and plain radiographic findings are not conclusive, the barium enema sometimes is helpful. Adequate visualization of a normal cecum with filling of the appendix to its smooth, rounded tip excludes the diagnosis of appendicitis. Nonfilling of the appendix usually is observed in patients with appendicitis, but this finding alone is not conclusive since the appendix may not fill on barium enema in as high as 20% of normal patients. Much more conclusive evidence of appendicitis is provided by nonfilling of the appendix associated with an extrinsic or intramural mass impressing the medial aspect of the cecum (Figs 39–39 to 39–42). The mass is caused by abscess or inflammatory reaction surrounding the inflamed appendix and may be associated with some spasm or irritability of the adjacent cecum. The terminal ileum may be displaced or narrowed by the adjacent inflammatory mass and there may be thickening of the mucosal folds of the terminal ileum. Occasionally barium will extravasate into a periappendiceal abscess (Fig 39–43).

Care must be taken in interpreting the appearance of barium in the appendix, as partial filling may occur in the presence of appendicitis. Irregularity of the contour of the appendiceal lumen, draping of the barium-filled appendix around a mass and abrupt termination of the barium column in the appendix should raise the possibility of appendicitis (Figs 39–44 and 39–45). Unless the appendix fills out completely to a smoothly rounded tip, the diagnosis cannot be excluded with certainty.

Obstruction of the appendix without acute inflammation or perforation results in development of a mucocele, in which mucoid material accumulates in the distended appendiceal lumen to form a cystic mass. The condition is often asymptomatic and sometimes is detectable on plain films of the abdomen by presence of calcification in the wall of the mucocele. On barium enema a smooth, rounded impression on the cecum is typical (Fig 39–46). Edema, spasm and irritability of the adjacent cecum and appendix are usually absent. Myxoglobulosis of the appendix is a form of mucocele in which calcified globules form within the mucocele. The radiographic findings are characteristic and consist of numerous round or oval, rimlike calcifications in the right lower quadrant, ranging up to 1 cm in size. Myxoglobulosis may be an incidental finding in an asymptomatic patient.

Tumors of the appendix are rare. Most common are benign tumors, predominantly leiomyomas, neuromas or lipomas.[24] These usually are small and discovered incidentally at surgery or autopsy. Carcinoid tumors arise in the appendix in 0.5% of persons. They also tend to be small. Metastases causing the carcinoid syndrome are rare.

Adenocarcinoma of the appendix usually results in obstruction and presents clinically as appendicitis. As these tumors are often of the mucinous type, calcification is often visible radiographically (Fig 39–47).

REFERENCES

1. Matsuura, K., Nakata, H., Takeda, N., Nakata, S., and Shimoda, Y.: Innominate lines of the colon, Radiology 123:581, 1977.
2. Cole, F. M.: Innominate grooves of the colon: Morphological characteristics and etiologic mechanisms, Radiology 128:41, 1978.
3. Kelvin, F. M., Oddson, T. A., Rice, R. P., Garbutt, J. T., and Bradenham, B. P.: Double contrast barium enema in Crohn's disease and ulcerative colitis, Am. J. Roentgenol. 131:207, 1978.
4. Laufer, I., and Costopoulos, L.: Early lesions of Crohn's disease, Am. J. Roentgenol. 130:307, 1978.
5. Mitchell, R. S., and Bristol, L. J.: Intestinal tuberculosis: An analysis of 346 cases diagnosed by routine intestinal radiography on 5,529 admissions for pulmonary tuberculosis, 1924–49, Am. J. Med. Sci. 227:241, 1954.

6. Berk, R. N., and Lasser, E. C.: *Radiology of the Ileocecal Area* (Philadelphia: W. B. Saunders Co., 1975).
7. Cardoso, J. M., Kimura, K., Stoopen, M., Cervantes, L. F., Elizondo, L., Churchill, R., and Moncada, R.: Radiology of invasive amebiasis of the colon, Am. J Roentgenol. 128:935, 1977.
8. Shrago, G.: *Yersinia enterocolitica* ileocolitis findings observed on barium examination, Br. J. Radiol. 49:181, 1976.
9. Lachman, R., Soong, J., Wishon, G., Maenza, R., Hanelin, L., and St. Geme, J.: Yersinia colitis, Gastrointest. Radiol. 2:133, 1977.
10. Sherman, N. J., and Wooley, M. M.: The ileocecal syndrome in acute childhood leukemia, Arch. Surg. 107:39, 1973.
11. Brody, P. A., Hill, R. P., and Baron, S.: Benign ulceration of the cecum, Radiology 122:323, 1977.
12. Meyers, M. A., Volberg, F., Katzen, B., Alonso, D., and Abbott, G.: The angioarchitecture of colonic diverticula, Radiology 108:249, 1973.
13. Boley, S. J., Sammartano, R., Adams, A., DiBiase, A., Kleinhaus, S., and Sprayregen, S.: On the nature and etiology of vascular ectasias of the colon, Gastroenterology 72:650, 1977.
14. Kaye, J. J., and Bragg, D. G.: Unusual roentgenologic and clinicopathologic features of villous adenomas of the colon, Radiology 91:799, 1968.
15. Rhodes, J. B., Holmes, F. F., and Clark, G. M.: Changing distribution of primary cancers in the large bowel, J.A.M.A. 238:1641, 1977.
16. O'Connell, D. J., and Thompson, A. J.: Lymphoma of the colon: The spectrum of radiologic changes, Gastrointest. Radiol. 2:377, 1978.
17. Joffe, N.: Medial cecal defect associated with metastatic pancreatic carcinoma, Radiology 111:297, 1974.
18. Meyers, M. A., and McSweeney, J.: Secondary neoplasms of the bowel, Radiology 105:1, 1972.
19. Thierstein, S. T., and Allen, E.: A comparative analysis of the diagnosis and treatment of endometriosis, including a report of 53 cases of intestinal endometriosis, Am. J. Obstet. Gynecol. 51:635, 1946.
20. Short, W. F., Smith, B. D., and Hoy, R. J.: Roentgenologic evaluation of the prominent or the unusual ileocecal valve, Med. Radiogr. Photogr. 52:2, 1976.
21. Boquist, L., Bergdahl, L., and Andersson, A.: Lipomatosis of the ileocecal valve, Cancer 29:136, 1972.
22. Selke, A. C., Jona, J. Z., and Belin, R. P.: Massive enlargement of the ileocecal valve due to lymphoid hyperplasia, Am. J. Roentgenol. 127:518, 1976.
23. Wakeley, C. P. G.: The position of the vermiform appendix as ascertained by the analysis of 10,000 cases, J. Anat. 67:277, 1933.
24. Collins, D. C.: 71,000 human appendix specimens. A final report, summarizing forty years' study, Am. J. Proctol. 14:365, 1963.
25. Meyers, M. A., and Oliphant, M.: Ascending retrocecal appendicitis, Radiology 110:295, 1974.
26. Frimann-Dahl, J.: *Roentgen Examinations in Acute Abdominal Diseases* (Springfield, Ill.: Charles C Thomas, 1960).
27. Felson, B.: Appendiceal calculi: Incidence and clinical significance, Surgery 25:734, 1949.
28. Steinert, R., Hareide, I., and Christiansen, T.: Roentgenologic examination of acute appendicitis, Acta Radiol. 24:13, 1943.
29. Faegenburg, D.: Fecaliths of the appendix: Incidence and significance, Am. J. Roentgenol. 89:752, 1963.
30. Brody, B. M., and Carroll, D. S.: Significance of calcified appendiceal enterolith, Radiology 68:648, 1957.
31. Copeland, E. M., and Long, J. M.: Elective appendectomy for appendiceal calculus, Surg. Gynecol. Obstet. 130:439, 1970.

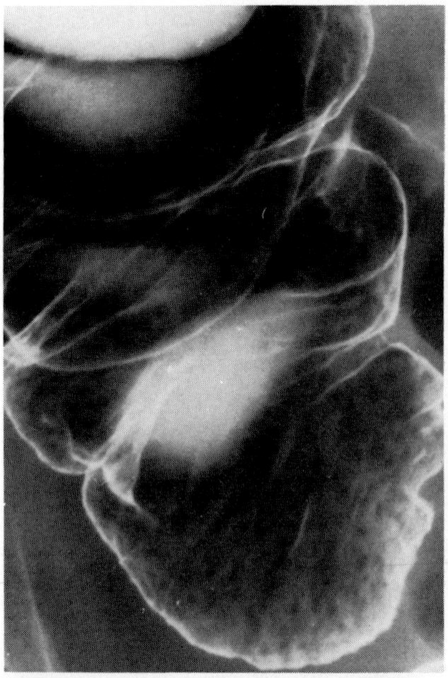

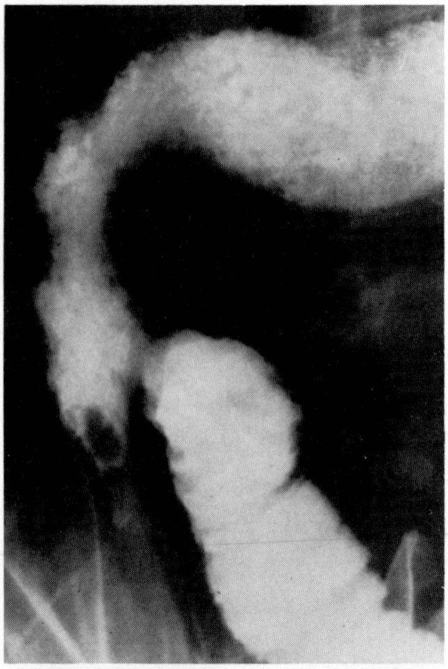

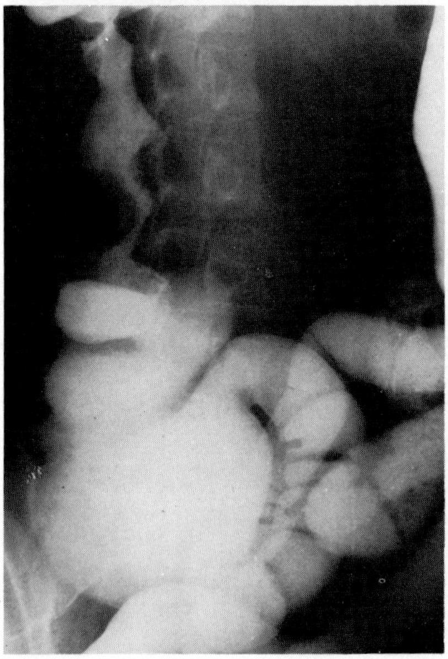

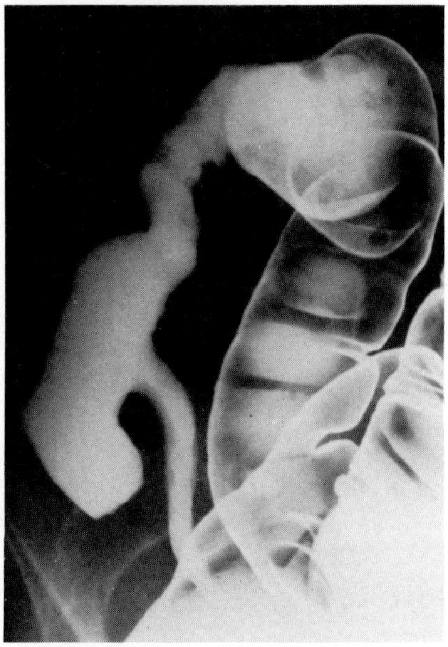

Fig 39–1 (top left).—Prominent but normal lymphoid follicles in cecum in man, age 55, without evidence of colon disease or immunoglobulin deficiency. Individual nodules are uniform and 2 mm in diameter. Lymphoid follicules were visible but less obvious in remainder of colon.

Fig 39–2 (top right).—Young man with ulcerative colitis of 10 years' duration. Entire colon is narrowed, shortened and ulcerated. Ileum and ileocecal valve are dilated, and there is slight thickening and irregularity of mucosal folds in distal few centimeters of ileum. Polyp at cecal tip was a benign adenoma, but there were foci of macroinvasive carcinoma in ascending colon.

Fig 39–3 (bottom left).—Woman, age 39, with long-standing ulcerative colitis had been advised repeatedly to undergo colectomy. She was found to have large constricting carcinoma of right colon. Patulous ileocecal valve and dilated terminal ileum are typical of backwash ileitis.

Fig 39–4 (bottom right).—Crohn's disease of ileum and cecum. Patulous appearance of ileocecal valve is unusual for this disease and more common with ulcerative colitis, but radiologic distinction from ulcerative colitis is possible, based on ileal narrowing and lack of involvement of remainder of colon.

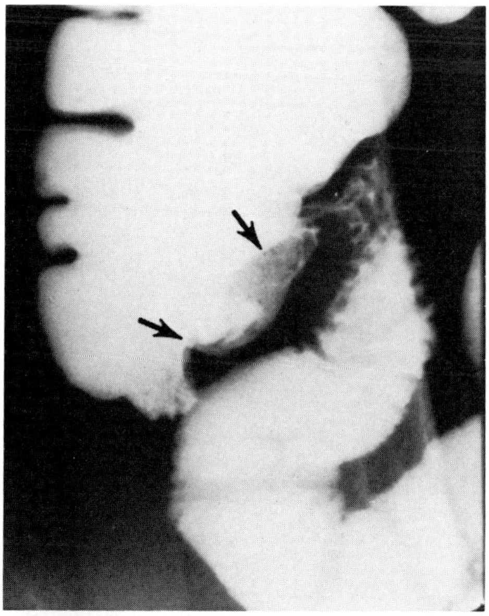

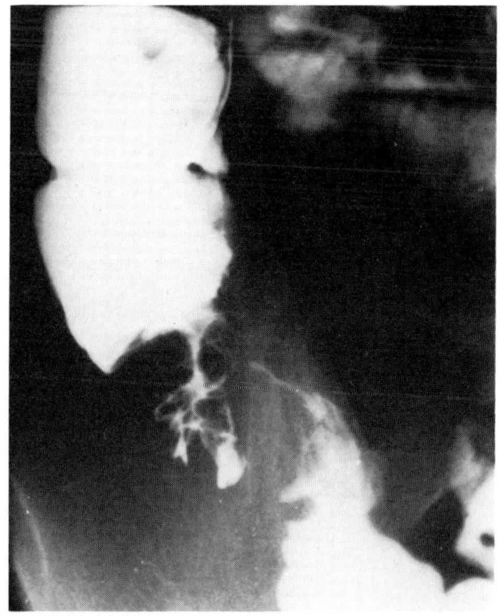

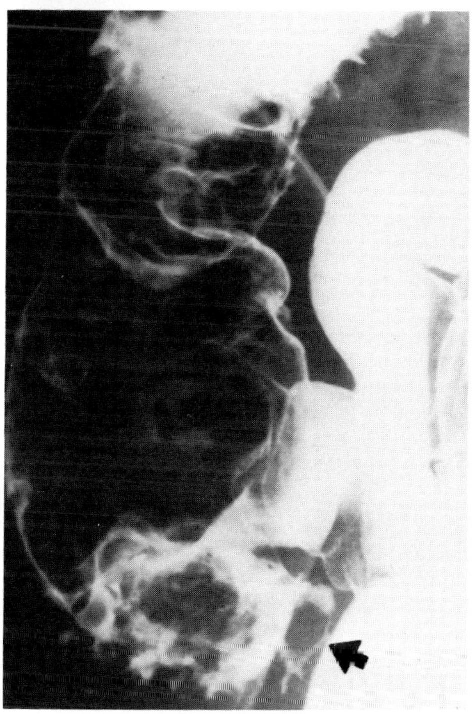

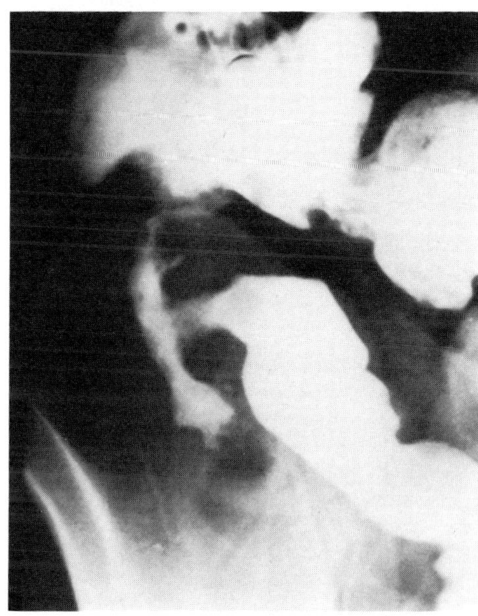

Fig 39–5 (top left).—Unusual appearance of granulomatous colitis involving only the cecum, originally interpreted as appendicitis. At surgery, 3-cm defect in medial cecal wall *(arrows)* was found to represent Crohn's disease.

Fig 39–6 (top right).—Narrowing and irregularity of cecum and terminal ileum in patient with Crohn's disease limited to this region.

Fig 39–7 (bottom left).—Woman, age 25, with granulomatous colitis of 5 years' duration. Ascending and transverse portions of colon were shortened and irregular. Colon is ulcerated, and widespread inflammatory polyps and fistulas arise from cecal tip *(arrow)*.

Fig 39–8 (bottom right).—Ileocecal tuberculosis resulting in marked narrowing of cecum and terminal ileum, associated with palpable right lower abdominal mass, in patient with tuberculous cervical adenitis.

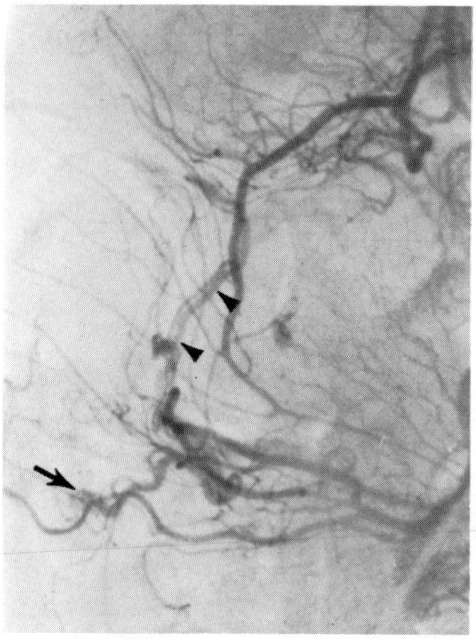

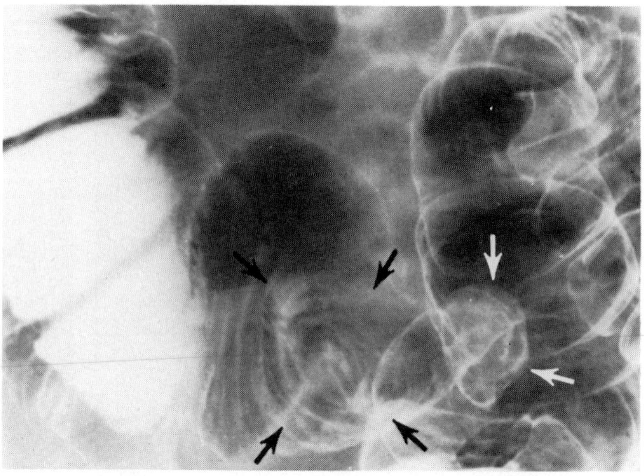

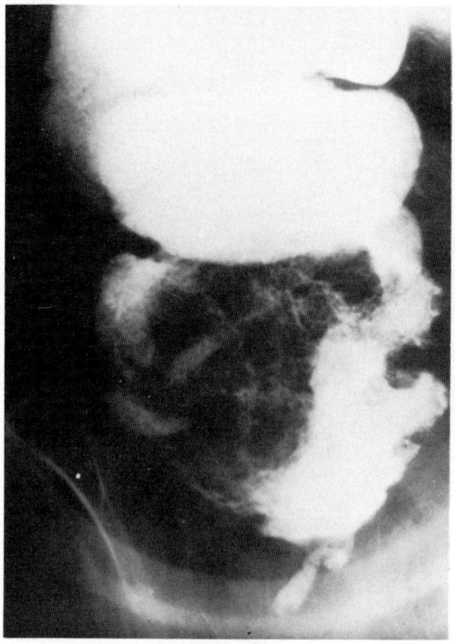

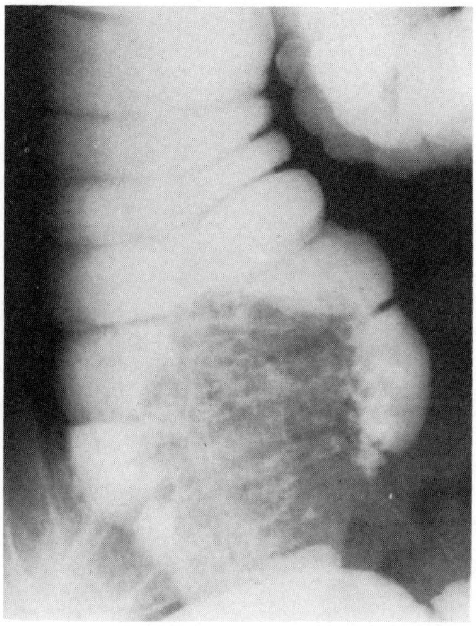

Fig 39–9 (top left).—Superior mesenteric arteriogram in elderly woman with recurrent, unexplained gastrointestinal bleeding. Tuft of small vessels *(arrow)* indicates site of angiodysplasia. Note early opacification of vein *(arrowheads)* draining lesion.

Fig 39–10 (top right).—Air contrast view showing concentric pattern of mucosal folds surrounding duplication cyst *(black arrows)* arising from cecum and adherent to adjacent sigmoid colon. Cyst was lined with colonic mucosa. Inflammatory polyp present in sigmoid *(white arrows)* at site of attachment of duplication cyst.

Fig 39–11 (bottom left).—Large mass filling cecum represents mixed villoglandular polyp with several foci of adenocarcinoma. Irregular, frondlike surface of lesion attests to partially villous nature.

Fig 39–12 (bottom right).—Large villous adenoma with very shaggy irregular surface virtually fills cecum. Surface irregularity is typical, but that pathologist could find no foci of malignancy in villous adenoma of this size is unusual.

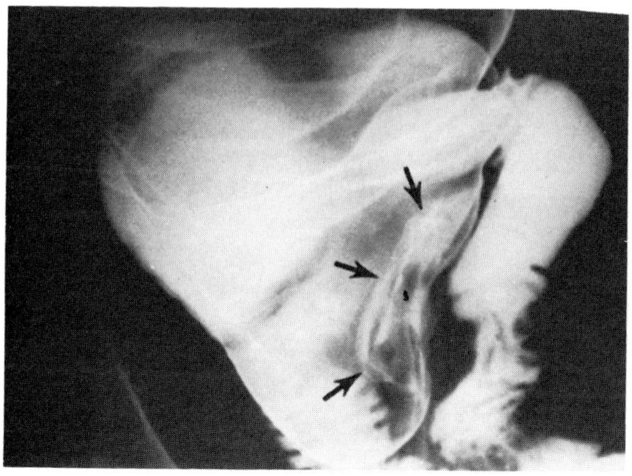

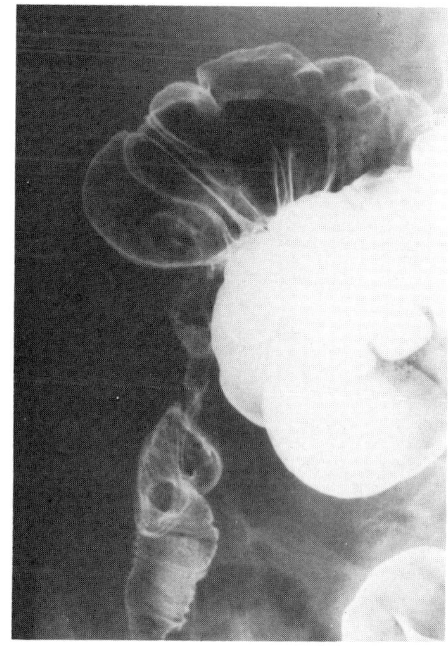

Fig 39–13 (left).—Small plaque-like adenocarcinoma of cecum *(arrows)* seen on air contrast barium enema. Lesion not visible on barium-filled views of cecum from same examination.

Fig 39–14 (right).—Large, constricting carcinoma virtually obliterates lower ascending colon, cecum and ileocecal valve in elderly man with abdominal pain of few weeks' duration.

Fig 39–15 (left).—A 2-cm polypoid carcinoma *(arrow)* arises from lateral wall of ascending colon. Tumor mimics ileocecal valve seen on adjacent medial cecal wall. At surgery, tumor had not yet penetrated muscular layer of colon.

Fig 39–16 (right).—Large polypoid carcinoma *(arrows)*. Surface of tumor is unusually smooth.

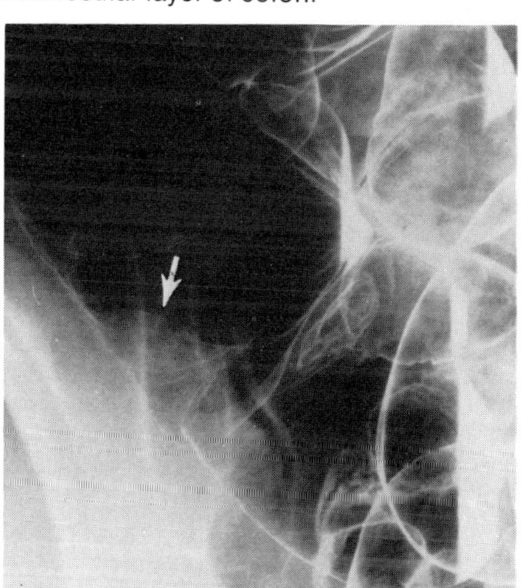

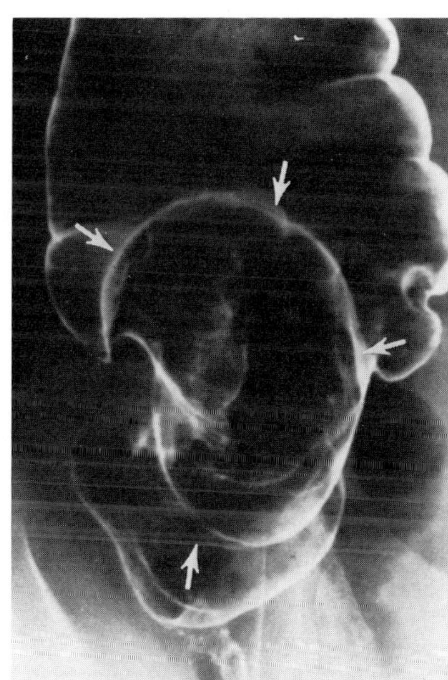

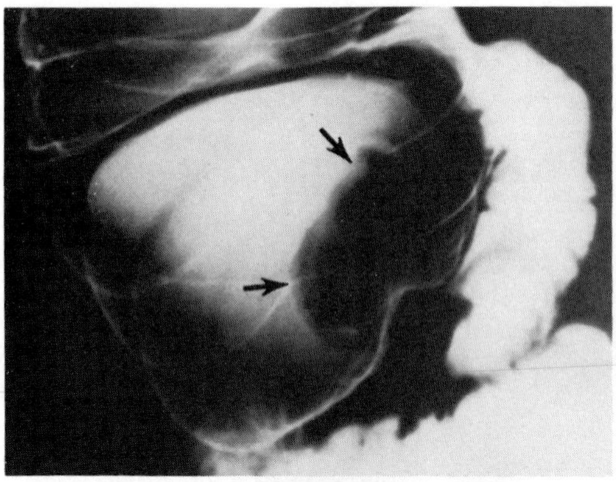

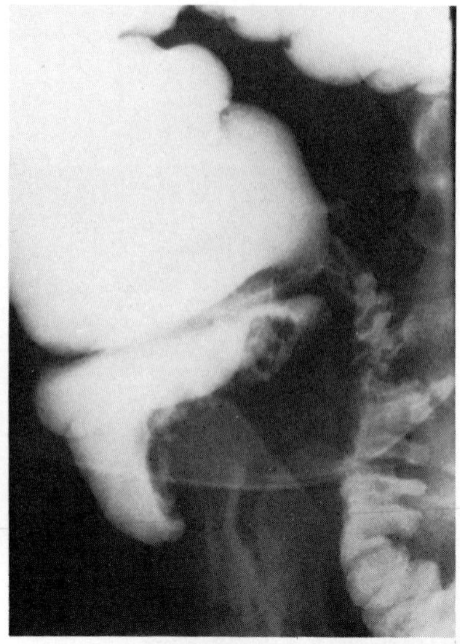

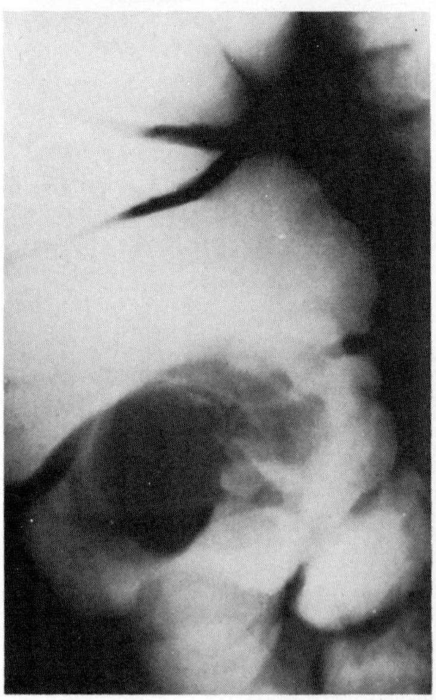

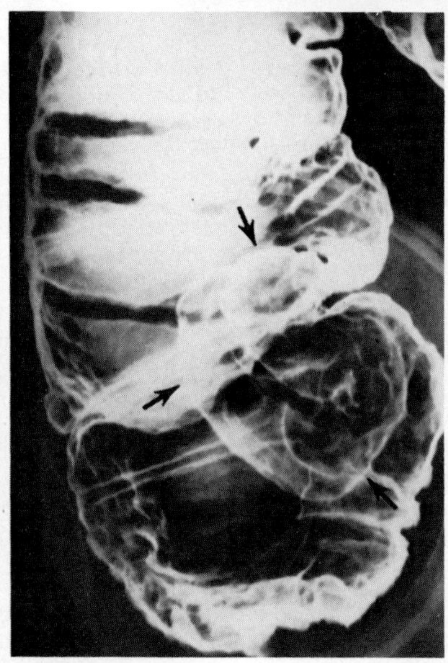

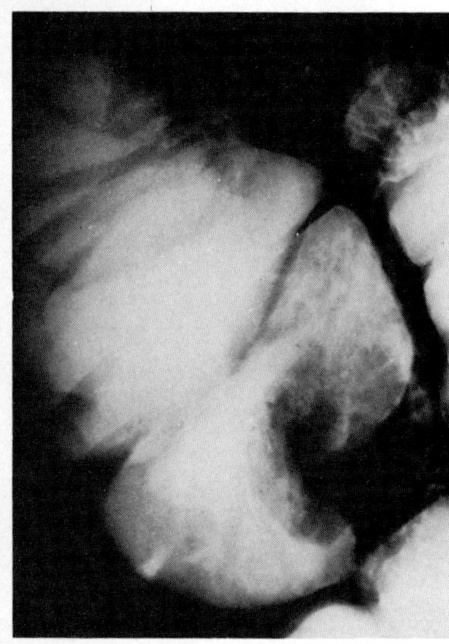

Fig 39–17 (top left).—Small polypoid adenocarcinoma of cecum *(arrows)* detected in man, age 70, with occult gastrointestinal blood loss.

Fig 39–18 (top right).—Mass impresses tip of cecum, and there is minimal effacement of mucosal folds on lateral aspect of terminal ileum. Single diverticulum is seen and appendix does not fill with barium. Clues to correct diagnosis of cecal carcinoma were history of occult bleeding and abrupt shelflike margins of mass. Radiographic appearance is also consistent with periappendiceal abscess, however.

Fig 39–19 (bottom left).—Large smooth mass in cecum in elderly women with rectal bleeding. Lesion represents 6-cm lipoma arising from ileocecal valve.

Fig 39–20 (bottom center).—Colonic lymphoma discovered incidentally in man, age 60, with previous rectal polyps. Lymphoma represented both by large mass *(arrows)* and innumerable small nodules that studded mucosa of entire colon.

Fig 39–21 (bottom right).—Extrinsic mass impressing medial aspect of cecal tip represents metastatic ovarian carcinoma in patient with widespread intra-abdominal involvement.

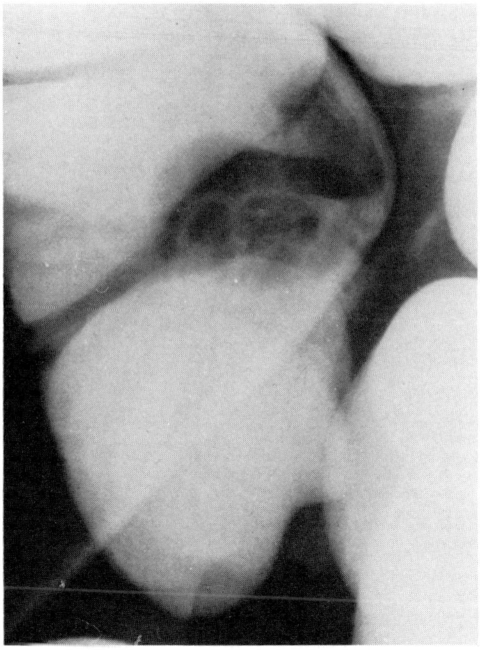

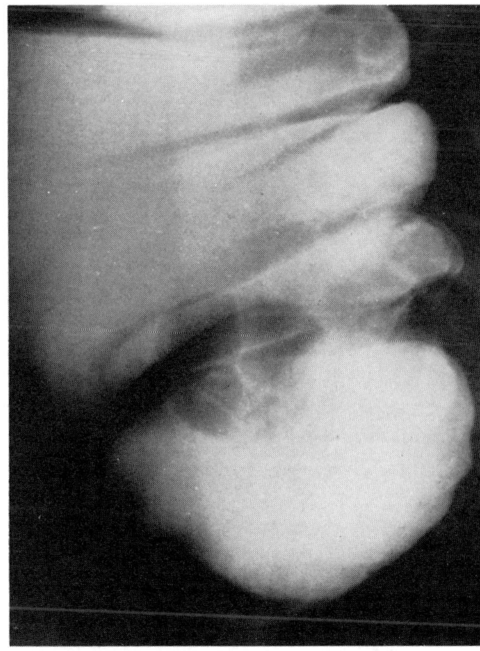

Fig 39–22 (left).—In elderly patient with abdominal pain eventually ascribed to cholecystitis, inferior lip of ileocecal valve looked thickened and nodular on some views, relatively normal on others. Lipomatosis of ileocecal valve found at surgery.

Fig 39–23 (right).—Fatty infiltration of ileocecal valve in elderly woman. Upper and lower lips of valve each measured 1.5 cm in thickness, and valve was unchanged in size and appearance over 2-year period.

Fig 39–24 (left).—Lipoma of ileocecal valve presenting as smooth, well-marginated 2-cm mass *(arrow)* on inferior lip of valve. (Courtesy of Dr. Edward I. Greenbaum, Los Angeles, Calif.)

Fig 39–25 (right).—Postevacuation view in patient with carcinoma of ileocecal valve *(arrowheads)*. Note obstruction of small bowel, which often occurs early in this disease.

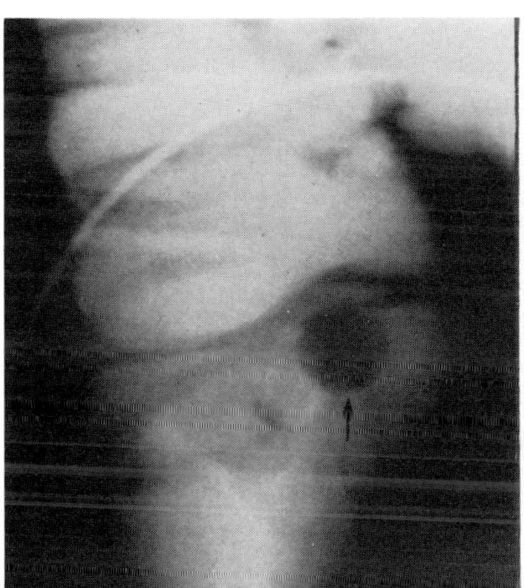

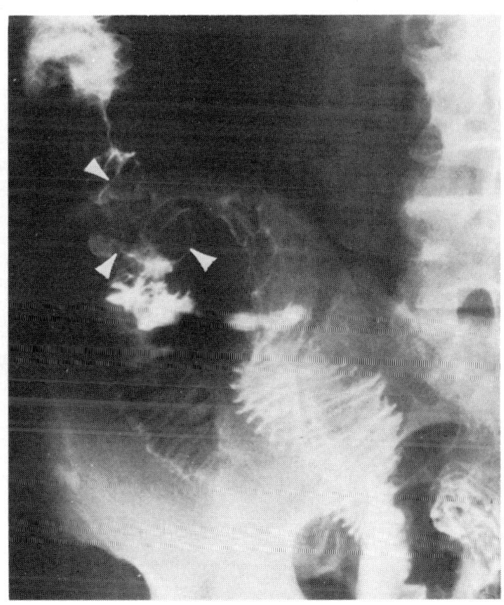

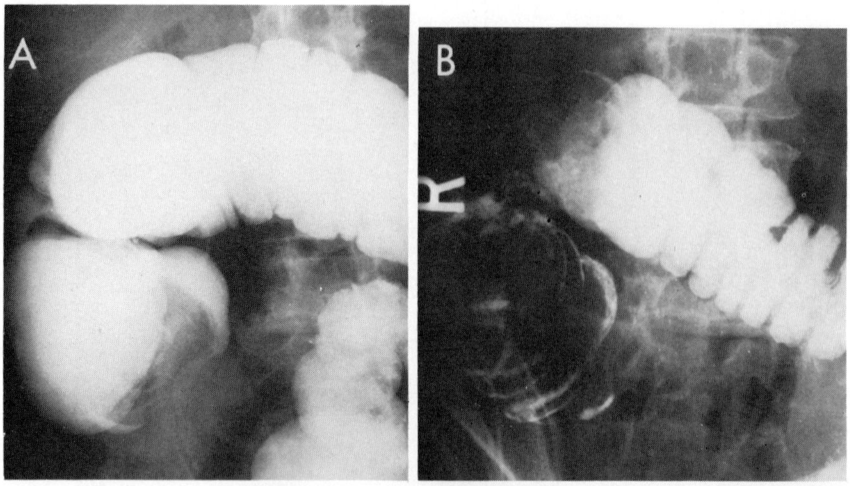

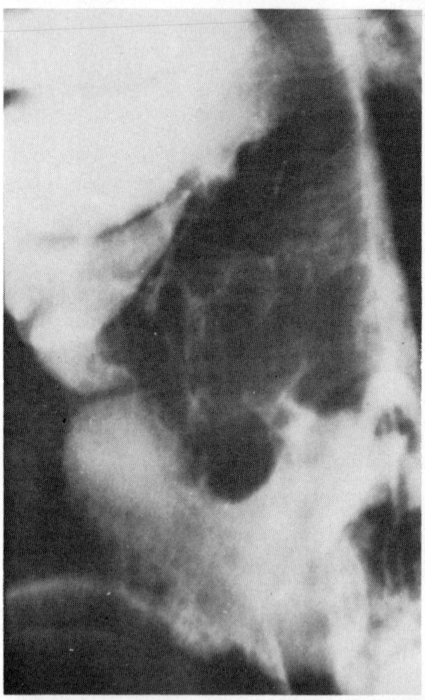

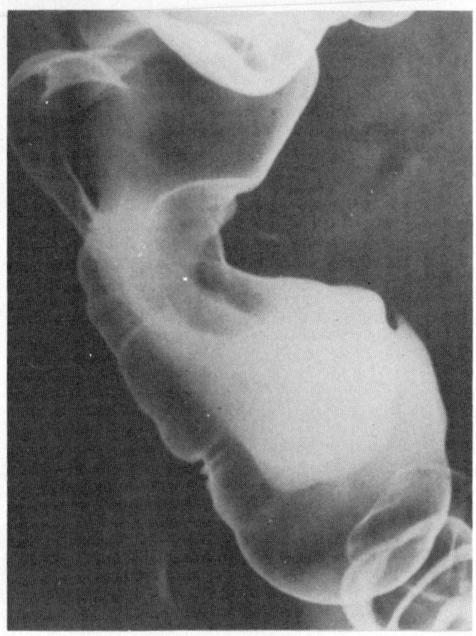

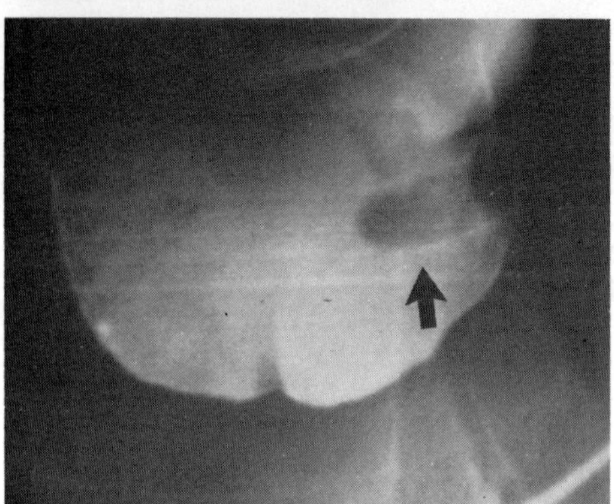

Fig 39-26 (top).—**A,** carcinoma of ileocecal valve causing intussusception. **B,** postevacuation view in same patient shows coiled-spring appearance typical of intussusception. (From Berk and Lasser, *Radiology of the Ileocecal Area* [Philadelphia: W. B. Saunders Co., 1975], with permission.)

Fig 39-27 (center left).—Ileocecal valve has been replaced by irregular polypoid adenocarcinoma. There was no evidence of small bowel obstruction, unusual for ileocecal valvular carcinoma of this size.

Fig 39-28 (center right).—Smooth enlargement of ileocecal valve with some narrowing of adjacent colon due to involvement with metastatic ovarian carcinoma. Several areas of colon similarly affected.

Fig 39-29 (bottom).—Intussusception of appendix presenting as oblong filling defect within lumen of cecum *(arrow)*. (Courtesy of Dr. Edward I. Greenbaum, Los Angeles, Calif.)

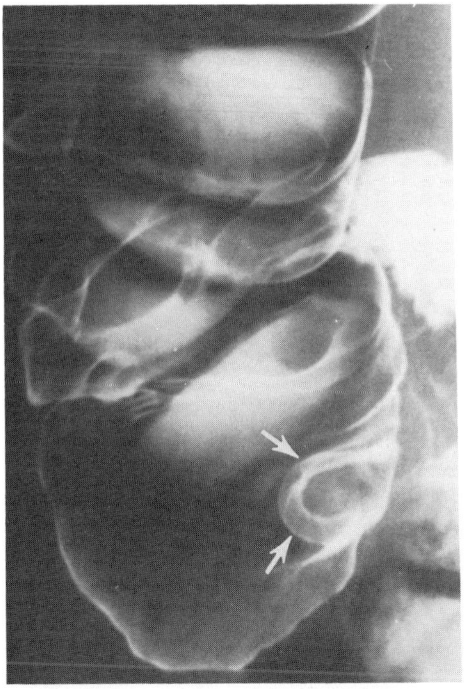

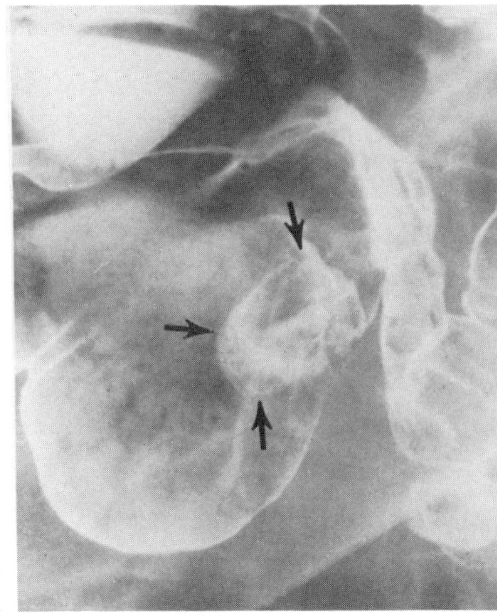

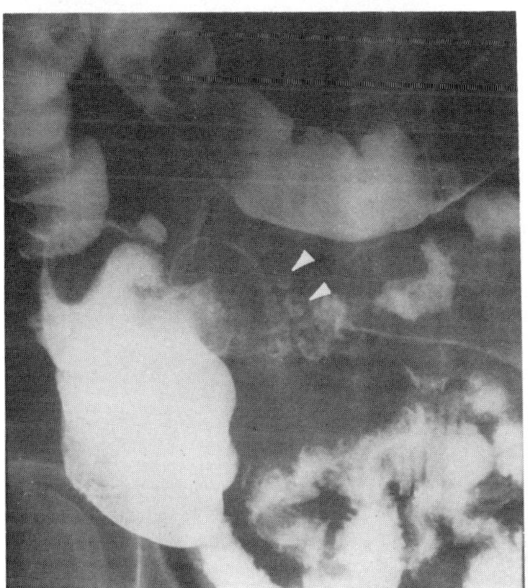

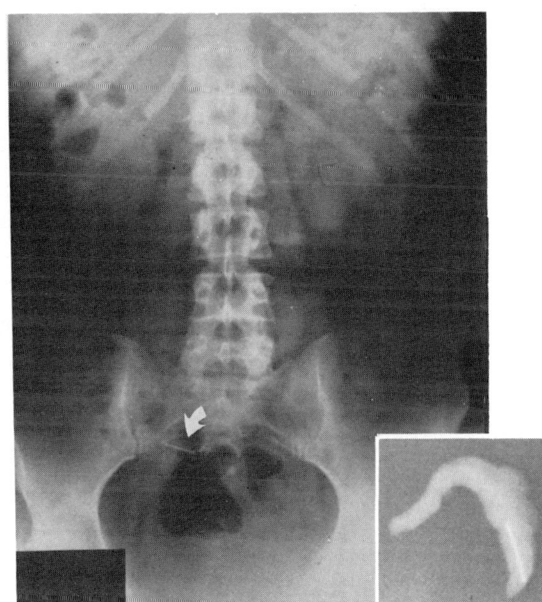

Fig 39–30 (top left). Typical appendiceal stump defect *(arrows)* 5 weeks after uncomplicated appendectomy.

Fig 39–31 (top right). – Smoothly outlined inverted appendiceal stump *(arrows)* measuring 2.5 cm in greatest diameter. Lesion was removed at time of cholecystectomy because of concern that it might represent a neoplasm.

Fig 39–32 (bottom left). – Postevacuation film in woman, age 64, with abdominal pain and diarrhea for 5 days. Appendiceal diverticula *(arrowheads)* present, and tip of appendix is not filled with barium. Configuration of small bowel in lower abdomen suggests presence of right lower abdominal mass. At surgery, tip of appendix was perforated and there was a surrounding inflammatory mass. A 2-cm mucinous adenocarcinoma of appendix was found at site of perforation.

Fig 39–33 (bottom right). – Straight pin *(arrow)* in appendix is seen overlying sacrum on right. At surgery, perforated appendix was noted. **Inset,** pathologic specimen showing pin within appendiceal lumen. Specimen showed evidence of appendicitis with exudate extending to serosal surface. (Courtesy of Dr. Edward I. Greenbaum, Los Angeles, Calif.)

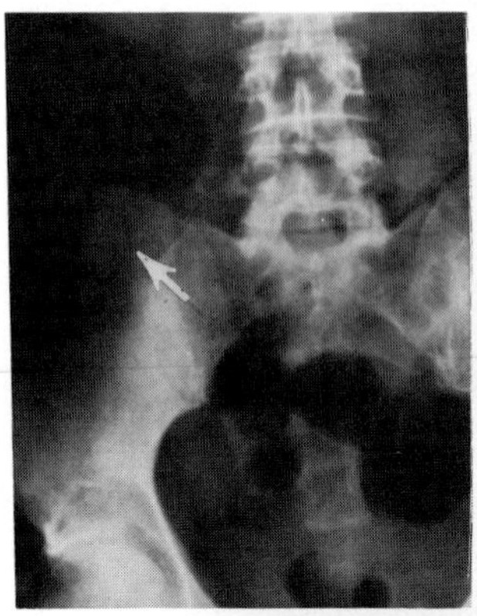

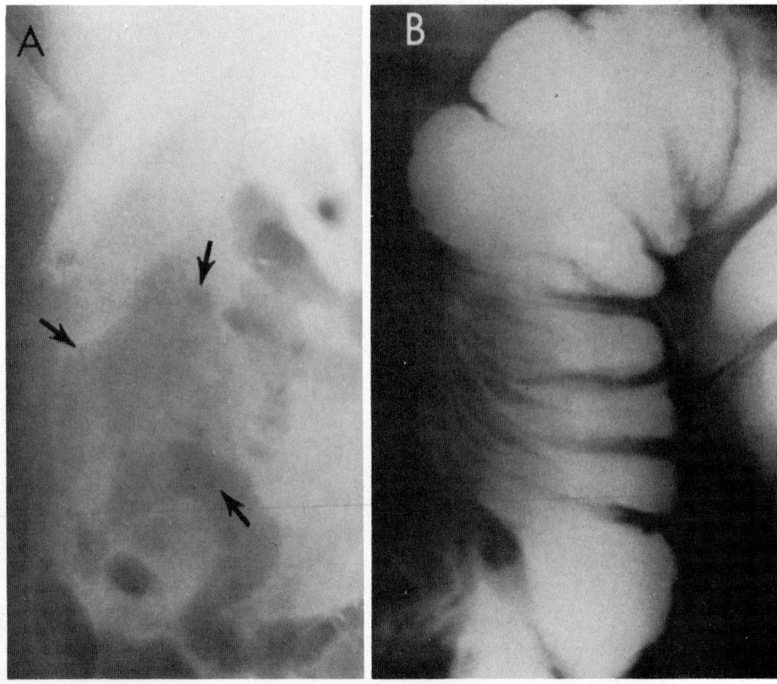

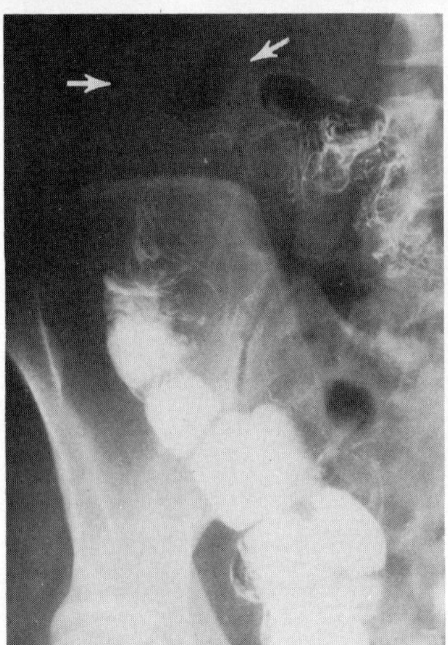

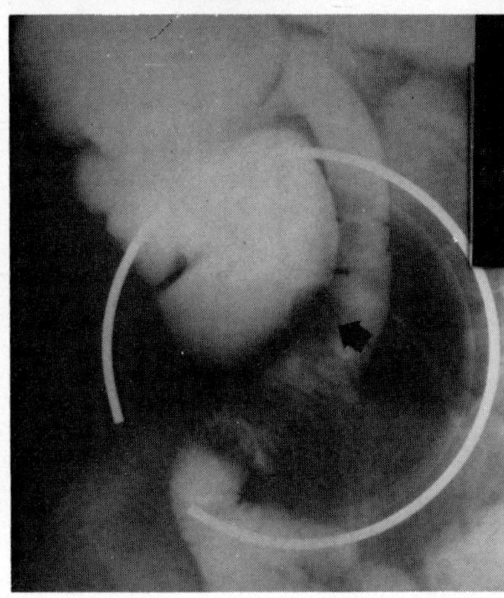

Fig 39–34 (top left).—Perforated appendicitis with surrounding mass *(arrow)* impressing medial aspect of cecum. Cecal dilatation also noted. (Courtesy of Dr. Edward I. Greenbaum, Los Angeles, Calif.)

Fig 39–35 (top right).—Man, age 38, with right abdominal pain. **A,** plain film shows unusual gas pattern in right midabdomen. Some gas *(arrows)* lies outside gastrointestinal tract. **B,** barium enema shows extrinsic mass posterolateral to ascending colon, with prominence and spiculation of adjacent mucosal folds. Retrocecal appendiceal abscess found at surgery.

Fig 39–36 (bottom left).—In woman, age 50, with right upper quadrant pain, postevacuation film shows gas *(arrows)* between hepatic flexure and liver. Abscess was suspected and at surgery was found due to perforation of tip of long retrocecal appendix.

Fig 39–37 (bottom right).—Laminated appendicolith *(arrow)* adjacent to cecal tip. Note lack of appendiceal filling. (Courtesy of Dr. Edward I. Greenbaum, Los Angeles, Calif.)

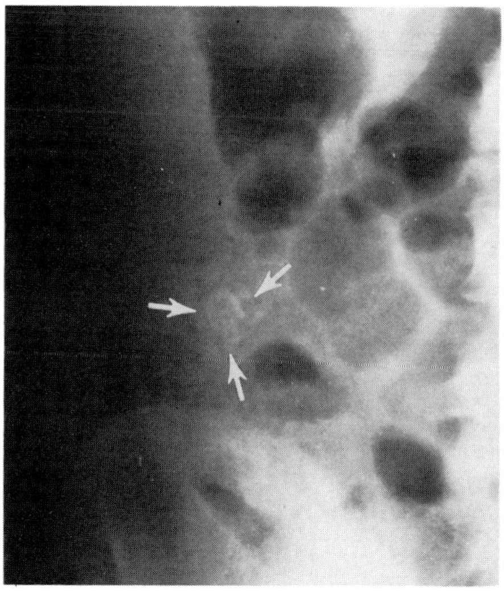

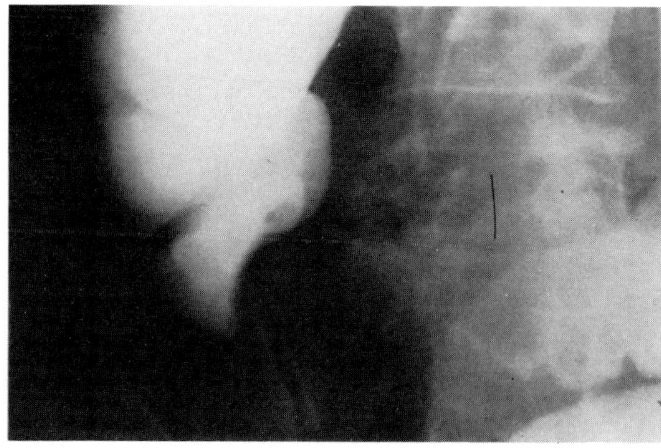

Fig 39-38 (left).—In boy, age 9, with right lower abdominal pain, calcific density and small, ill-defined densities surrounding it *(arrows)* represent calcified fecalith. Small collections of gas surrounding calcifications lie within periappendiceal abscess.

Fig 39-39 (right).—Appendicitis with periappendiceal abscess, which causes smooth impression on inferomedial aspect of cecum. (Courtesy of Dr. Edward I. Greenbaum, Los Angeles, Calif.)

Fig 39-40 (left).—Elderly man with epigastric pain for 24 hours. Smooth defect impressing tip of cecum initially thought to represent mucocele or carcinoid tumor. At surgery, periappendiceal abscess due to impacted fecalith in appendix was found.

Fig 39-41 (right).—Periappendiceal abscess. Appendix is not filled and a mass impresses tip of cecum. Note similarity to findings in cecal carcinoma (see Fig 39-18). Margins of mass are less distinct, and inflammatory changes of terminal ileum are more marked than with adenocarcinoma.

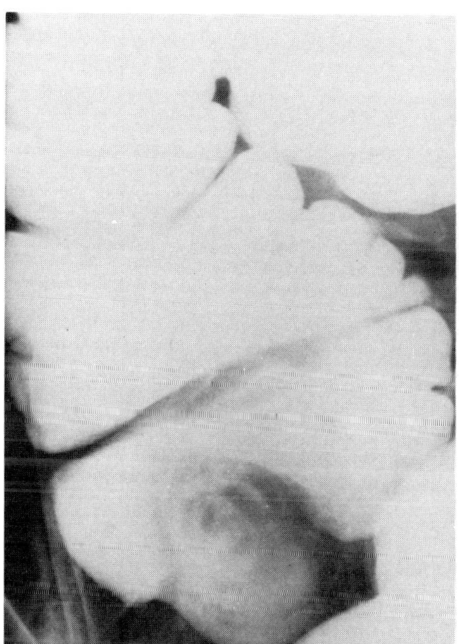

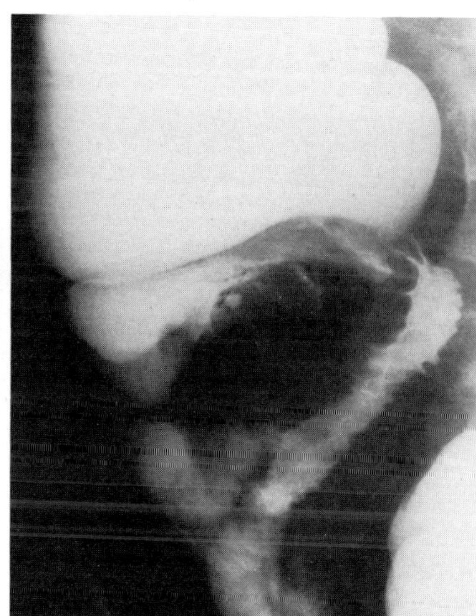

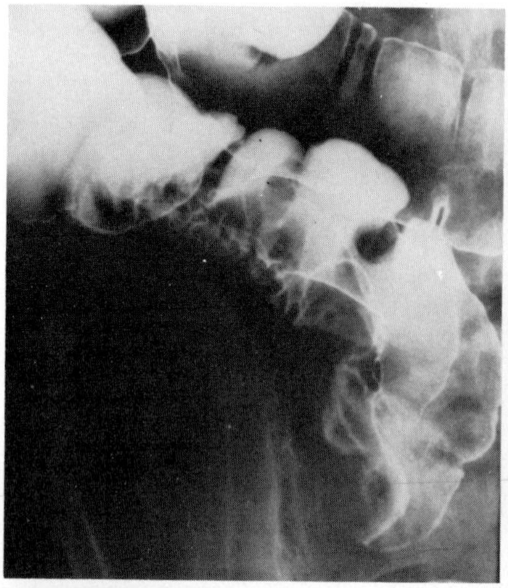

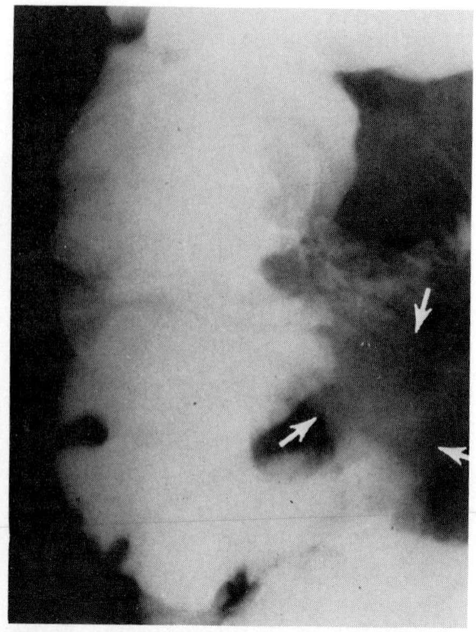

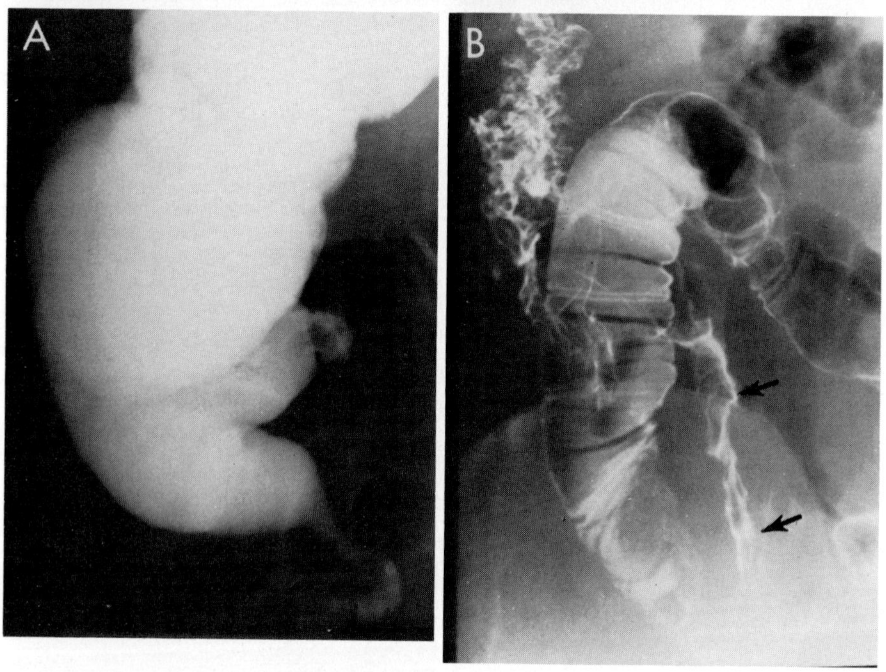

Fig 39–42 (top left).—Chronic, indolent periappendiceal abscess presenting as palpable right lower quadrant mass. Although somewhat abrupt margins and central excavation suggested that findings might be due to carcinoma, mass was found to consist of fibrous and chronic inflammatory tissue in which appendix was imbedded.

Fig 39–43 (top right).—Irregularity of cecum and distal ileum and a collection of extravasated barium *(arrows)* lying outside gastrointestinal tract. At surgery, subacute appendicitis with perforation was found.

Fig 39–44 (bottom).—Patient with right lower quadrant pain of 2 weeks' duration. **A,** filled film from barium enema shows filling of appendix, tip of which is irregular. Also a diverticulum of cecum. **B,** on postevacuation view, appendix has emptied and barium now outlines narrowed, edematous distal ileum *(arrows)* with partial small bowel obstruction. Initially, inflammatory disease of ileum was thought most likely but, at surgery, appendix was obstructed by fecalith near its tip and periappendiceal abscess accounted for radiographic findings.

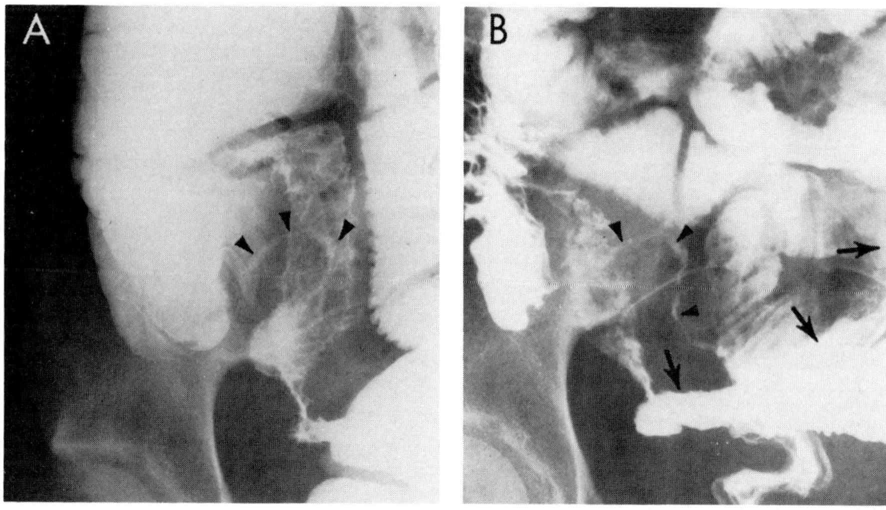

Fig 39-45.—Man, age 19, with diarrhea and mild abdominal pain. **A,** mass impressing cecum and thickened folds and narrowing of terminal ileum. Appendix *(arrowheads)* is partially filled. **B,** after evacuation, appearance of ileum indicates large abdominal mass *(arrows)*; 9-cm length of appendix *(arrowheads)* is filled but appears very irregular. Findings were due to perforation of tip of appendix. Remainder of appendix and distal ileum were draped over surrounding inflammatory mass.

Fig 39-46 (left).—Asymptomatic appendiceal mucocele discovered in patient with carcinoma of sigmoid colon. Smooth but lobulated mass indenting cecum was initially thought to represent second carcinoma, but its true nature was discovered at surgery.

Fig 39-47 (right).—Mucin-producing adenocarcinoma of appendix, which presented as large pelvic mass with calcifications *(arrowheads)*. There is an impression on medial cecum and on right lateral aspect of rectosigmoid colon.

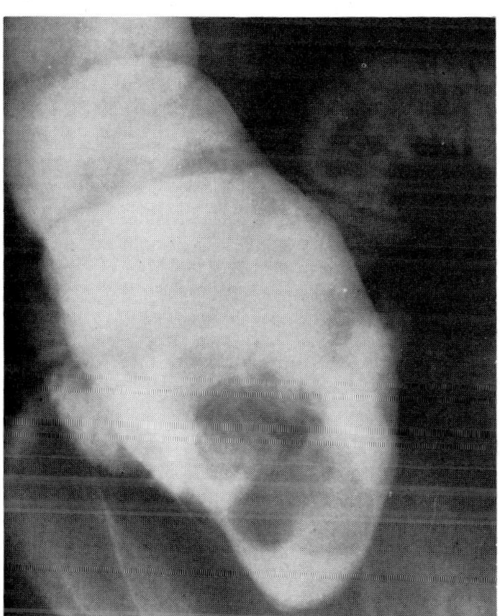

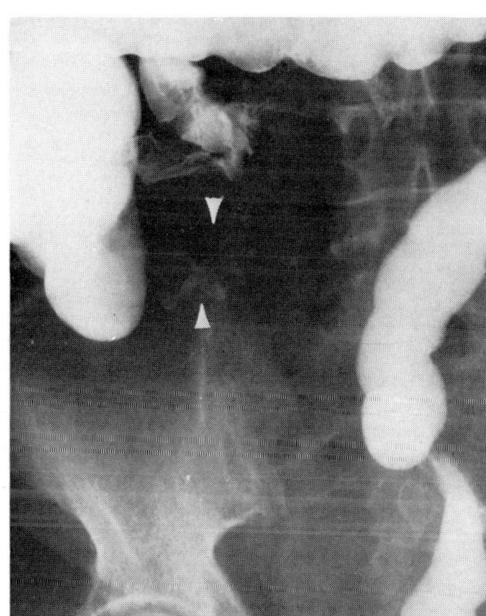

Chapter 40

Technique of Colon Examination

ROSCOE E. MILLER, M.D.

EXAMINATION OF THE COLON in its entirety is accomplished best and most economically by roentgenology. Ancillary methods are sigmoidoscopy, colonoscopy, arteriography and scintigraphy. Radiologic methods include (1) plain films of the abdomen; (2) contrast studies using various contrast materials such as barium sulfate suspensions, water-soluble contrast materials, water alone, air and combinations of the above; (3) selective arteriography; and (4) scintigraphy with ^{99m}Tc-sulfur colloid.

The two most common but separate methods are (1) introduction of a full column of low density barium sulfate suspension (about 2,000 ml) to fill the colon, and (2) introduction of a small quantity (about 400 ml) of a high density barium sulfate suspension to coat the mucosa, followed by filling and distention of the colon by insufflation with air—the double contrast enema. Both types of barium enema are highly accurate when properly performed and individualized to answer specific questions raised by the referring physician.

Selective arteriography to locate the site of bleeding in the colon, a roentgenographic method used less frequently than the barium enema, is valuable in certain patients.[3] A less invasive technique for colonic bleeding, and even more sensitive, is the use of ^{99m}Tc-sulfur colloid.[1, 4, 50]

The single most important aspect of the colon examination is assumption by the examiner of complete responsibility—moral, legal and technical—for preparation of the patient, technique of examination and interpretation. Part of this responsibility is to obtain precise clinical information from both patient and referring physician to determine (1) the purpose of the examination, (2) any limitations or restrictions imposed by the patient's condition and (3) all questions posed by the referring physician.

Contraindications to the examination must be carefully considered. These include suspected perforation of the colon, toxic megacolon and biopsy of the colon after sigmoidoscopy or colonoscopy. An exception is after a superficial mucosal biopsy of a large exophytic lesion. Barium examinations also are contraindicated if there is definite evidence of *acute* diverticulitis or other *acute* inflammatory bowel disease. Barium enemas should be delayed for a period of several days (10–14) to allow medical management to quiet the inflammation.

I routinely perform air contrast examinations after sigmoidoscopy or colonoscopy, since I add much more air than has been introduced by these procedures. I do not like to do "routine" full column barium enemas after such procedures because of the confusion caused by air bubbles. If there is no evidence of perforation, emergency unprepared examinations for complete obstruction of the colon are carried out at any time. These examinations are done, however, only after careful consideration of the desirability of performing colonoscopy, arteriography or scintigraphy prior to any enema. Barium enemas to localize the site of bleeding from diverticula not only are useless but seriously interfere with the more diagnostic methods of colonoscopy, arteriography and scintigraphy. The full column method is excellent, however, to localize the site of complete or partial obstruction or fistulas.

The radiologist must assume the major responsibility for finding early lesions. He has the proved tools at hand if he will but assume the responsibility for proper preparation and technique. He can no longer delegate this to some well-meaning, but perhaps ill-informed, referring physician. He does not do this in angiography or endoscopy, and he must not do it for gastrointestinal examinations. Most missed lesions in the colon are due to poor preparation, faulty technique and inadequate attention to detail rather than to an inherent invisibility.

Preparation for Examination

The colon must be well prepared. Except in emergencies, this is a primary requirement for all colon examinations. Fecal matter simulating polyps will be seen in any type of examination if the colon is not clean. A combination of diet, laxatives and enemas must be used for successful cleansing.

A low-residue or clear-liquid diet is adhered to on the day before the examination and for 2 or 3 days, if possible, preceding the study.

Two laxatives should be taken the day before the examination. Two ounces (60 ml) of castor oil at noon or shortly thereafter plus 2½ oz (75 ml) of X-Prep liquid at 4 P.M. is my preference and usually reliable. I sometimes substitute 10 oz of magnesium citrate or 20 gm of magnesium sulfate for one or the other of these cathartics (e.g., in diabetic patients). A large volume of oral liquids also must be given to assist an effective purge. I urge a full 8-oz glass of clear liquids, one each hour for 8 hours on the day preceding the examination. This totals about 2 L.

In addition to laxatives, a single 2,000-ml tap-water enema is given in the x-ray department on the morning of the study.[29] This combination has proved as effective as any method I have tried for obtaining a clean colon. The statement "enemas until clear" is worthless. One carefully done 2,000-ml enema is far better and less traumatic than 15 to 20 "enemas until clear." The patient, too, must be given precise, written instructions, not only about the cathartic, the necessity for a clear liquid diet and fluid intake the day before examination, but also about the reasons for following them closely. We do this by giving each patient a printed pamphlet written and furnished by the radiology department (pp. 524–525). The patient must also be given instructions and encouragement just before and during administration of the cleansing enema.[29]

Good evacuation usually follows the 2,000-ml tap-water enemas, whereas a 500–1,000 ml enema may be retained in the rectum and sigmoid. I allow a full 30 minutes for evacuation before giving glucagon.[25, 35] Rarely some water is retained in the colon, but this can be tolerated because of the high radiographic density of the barium suspension, especially in air contrast studies.

The nature of the two specific laxatives is not nearly as important as relentless application of the inflexible rule that the colon must be clean before the examination is started. As an adjunct to enforcement, I routinely schedule the upper gastrointestinal tract first when both examinations are requested. Barium from the upper gastrointestinal tract is used as a "marker" to see if the colon is clean before starting the colon study. Infrequently this means that I must bring the patient back the next day for the study after having wasted 5 minutes on a preliminary film or 5 seconds on preliminary fluoroscopy. Almost invariably this residual barium is a clue that the patient did *not* follow instructions. We then give him another of our printed instruction pamphlets and reinforce the necessity for compliance. I agree with Eyler[6] that the colon report must read either positive or negative—or the study must be repeated.

The reports of Welin,[45, 46] Carlile,[5] Rogers[39] and Eyler,[6] in addition to my own,[26] have shown that the colon can be cleansed in the department of radiology. In fact, the cleansing enema can be done in any department of radiology. I originally gave the cleansing enema on the x-ray table, but it is much easier and more convenient for the patient and for the attendant if it is administered in a special room equipped with bedpans, wash bowl and toilet. In almost any department, two adjacent dressing cubicles with the separating panel removed may be used. A plywood board with a 2–4 inch foam rubber mattress covered with a plastic sheet will serve as an adequate table on which to give the enema. A cleansing enema done in the radiology department results in far fewer repeat examinations and is literally a lifesaving measure.

It is the radiologist who should be responsible for this aspect of the examination. A tumor should not be missed because the radiologist does not take full responsibility for a clean colon, including a cleansing enema, in his department.

Using this colon cleansing technique, our radiology department reports under 5% of people with all types of conditions who do not have satisfactorily clean colons on the first attempt. In these few failures, the technique is repeated the next day, generally with a change in the type of cathartic used; a repeat 2,000-ml cleansing enema also is given.

The radiologist needs, deserves and must demand as clean a colon as does the colonoscopist. The latter may give cathartics for 3 nights, a liquid diet for 48 hours plus a high colonic enema 1–3 hours prior to examination. All colonoscopists use a combination of all three methods to insure a liquid diarrhea and a clean colon.[14, 41] If the attending physician resists using our standard preparation (1 day), we will agree to using the colonoscopist preparation, but nothing less. We refuse to do poor radiology and poor medicine.

DRUGS

During barium enema examinations, when the colon does not fill properly because of muscle spasm or for other reasons, anticholinergic drugs often have been administered. In 1958 and 1967 Welin[45, 46] recommended that, with few exceptions, these drugs be given routinely to patients prior to air contrast studies of the colon. The anticholinergic purportedly reduced smooth muscle spasm and prevented vasovagal reflex, allowing the radiologist to accomplish a more detailed and complete examination with less discomfort to the patient.[23] However, adverse effects[7-9, 10, 21, 24] of propantheline bromide or atropine sulfate in colon examinations may persist long after the examination has been completed. We now use 0.5–0.75 mg glucagon intravenously immediately prior to the examination.

The short action of glucagon, with excellent relaxation and few side effects, leads us to agree with Ferrucci and Benedict[7] that hypotonic examination of the colon is useful in some situations. Their indications for a hypotonic barium enema examination are as follows:

1. Lesions with diffuse painful spasm: ulcerative or granulomatous colitis or functional disorders.
2. Areas of localized narrowing: spasms vs. constricting lesions, colonic valves or sphincters or evaluation of strictures in colitis.
3. Diverticular disease, with sigmoid spasm.
4. Need for decrease in smooth muscle

tone for adequate distention during air contrast study.

5. Functional inability to retain the enema, seen especially in aged patients.

Because glucagon relaxes the colon and makes the patient more comfortable during barium enema examination, it is useful for hypotonic barium enema examination in the situations listed above. It is better than atropine sulfate as a hypotonic agent because it produces better relaxation with fewer side effects. We believe that glucagon should be used in patients who have any of the above indications. These indications occur more commonly in older patients.

Occasionally in older, debilitated, arthritic patients or those having chronic pain or extreme anxiety, we have used diazepam and rarely also in addition meperidine HCl to make the examination more comfortable. This is done in consultation with the referring physician.

EQUIPMENT

The image-intensified fluoroscope with automatic collimation and photo-timed spot filming devices are mandatory. It is important that these instruments have high ratio 12:1 or 6:1 crisscross grids in the spot film device for either conventional or 105 mm spot films.[10] I also use and recommend a 12:1 linear grid for table-top Bucky films and a 6:1 crisscross aluminum (A1) interspaced grid for the lateral decubitus apparatus, which can be attached to any fluoroscopic table for lateral decubitus films.[17] This device permits decubitus films to be made easily in a few seconds. Short exposures are desirable, and therefore the generator should be capable of delivering exposure in the 120 kvp or higher range with high milliamperage output to reduce the time of exposures. Compression devices are extremely helpful. At times I use an old wooden butter paddle as well as several gauze pads—some round, some flat, some square—for compression. In addition, an inflatable rubber balloon paddle is kept in each fluoroscopic room. These are in addition to the usual plastic compression device found on the fluoroscope.

I also prefer a disposable plastic bag, tubing and tip, with large-bore 1/2 inch internal diameter tubing and a flexible enema tip.*

In difficult patients, retention balloons may be needed, but these always should be attached to the enema tip and not allowed to be inserted far into the rectum. I never use the flexible Bardex type of inflatable balloon because they may rise above the peritoneal reflection, and fatalities with its use have been reported.[36]

Plain Films of the Abdomen

Preliminary films of the abdomen are most useful in examination of the colon. Certainly this is a part of the usual examination of the acute abdomen prior to any emergency colon examination. Calcifications and unusual air or fat collections, as well as fluid-filled loops, fecal collections in the colon and contrast material remaining in the stomach or bowel from previous examinations, may be noted. This easily solves many problems that may arise either during fluoroscopy or after the roentgenograms are developed. Residual contrast material at times may cause great confusion in determining whether fistulas or other lesions exist, if preliminary films are not available for comparison. Frequently this film may be one of those taken shortly before examination in an acute abdominal series or with excretory pyelograms. In any event, careful fluoroscopic scanning of the abdomen before the contrast material starts to flow is mandatory in any examination of the colon. With proper equipment, preliminary spot films may be substituted for the usual overhead radiograms. I agree with Margulis[13] that the advantages of a permanent record over

---

*E–Z–EM Company, Inc., 7 Portland Avenue, Westbury, New York 11590.

the memorized impressions of even an expert fluoroscopist are so obvious that they need no further discussion.

Full Column Techniques

I prefer full column technique for unprepared and emergency examinations for bowel obstruction, reduction of intussusception or volvulus and in young patients investigated for diarrhea or constipation. I use 15% w/v barium sulfate with 110 kvp single-phase units or 100 kvp three-phase equipment. This is optimal for the average patient (27.5 mm A1 1/20 value layer). In suspected abscess or fistula from perforated diverticula below the peritoneal reflection, a water-soluble contrast material such as diatrizoate (Hypaque) diluted 3:1 may be used. This special type of examination should be evaluated and approached most carefully. If there is suspected perforation above the peritoneal reflection, and certainly if any pneumoperitoneum is present, enemas should not be done at all.[19, 22]

Water enemas may be used for diagnosis of lipomas, but I prefer air contrast techniques with compression to show change in shape of the lesion.

Using full column techniques, Miller has shown with the use of phantoms and human volunteers that 1 cm tumors in a 10 cm diameter colon or rectum could not be seen in any patient of 29 cm thickness with any equipment at any energy level. These tumors also would be missed in noncompressible colon segments in patients over 21 cm in thickness.[30]

Evaluation and Choice of Radiographic Method

The diagnostic yield in radiographic colon examinations depends primarily on a reliable technique. Although human factors play an important role in all x-ray examinations, the efforts of a competent examiner may be wasted if he does not know and use the best available techniques. Because a high percentage of malignant lesions found in the colon are operable and resection of early lesions usually means cure, technique in finding a tumor becomes extremely important. Selected studies reports an 81% 5-year survival rate after surgery for localized disease.[44]

Roentgenologic technique to detect colon cancer is limited to recognition of macroscopic disease, but it can even detect lesions that measure only a few millimeters in diameter.[5, 26, 27, 32, 39, 45] Currently a 4–5 mm tumor in any part of the colon from the anus to the appendix is detectable. This is the present limitation of diagnostic roentgenology for colon carcinoma, and it also is the goal of proficiency toward which the radiologist should continually aspire.[26, 40] Because the end result of missing a cancer of the colon is so serious, any physician performing a barium enema should be held to the standard demanded of the expert.

Air Contrast Techniques

To achieve adequate air contrast studies, five requirements must be fulfilled, all attainable:

1. A clean colon (adequate preparation).
2. A suitable barium suspension that will coat well and not bubble or "flake out."
3. Adequate insufflation of the bowel.
4. Drainage of excess barium from the rectum.
5. An adequate number of films with good radiologic technique.

BARIUM SUSPENSION

I use a liquid ready-to-use barium suspension for air contrast colon examinations (HD-85* or Liquid Polybar†). This assures quality control.

---

*Lafayette Pharmacal Company, Inc., 522 Earl Street, Lafayette, Indiana 47902.

†E-Z-EM Company, Inc., 7 Portland Avenue, Westbury, New York 11590.

AIR INSUFFLATION

Adequate insufflation adds greatly to the visibility of lesions and adds little to patient discomfort after bowel relaxation with intravenous injection of 0.5–0.75 mg of glucagon. A total of 2,500 cc or more of air usually is necessary in adults. This equals 70 or more full compressions of a sphygmomanometer bulb.

It is important to note that, just as the gravid uterus rises out of the pelvis when it becomes enlarged, so do distended loops of the rectosigmoid colon. These loops then become clearly visible. Furthermore, additional air may be instilled at any point in the examination. This is especially true during spot filming of questionable lesions.

DRAINAGE

Excellent demonstration of the rectum and distal sigmoid lesions is one of the superior aspects of good air contrast studies. This simply requires drainage of excess barium through the enema tip before air instillation and a short final check just before film exposure. It is a simple and rewarding maneuver. If it is not done, excess barium in the rectum will hide obvious lesions. Drainage is achieved by placing the enema bag below the table top and releasing the tubing clamp. This sometimes is helped by elevating the head of the fluoroscopic table.[33] Evacuation of the rectum is observed and controlled by fluoroscopy. Some air also may escape, but this is easily reinstilled, especially when using the "Miller" air tip*.[16] This tip allows complete control of barium, air and rectal drainage at any point during the examination. Since the tube for instilling the air extends to the end of the enema tip, instillation of air does not force residual barium in the enema tubing into the patient.

The importance of rectosigmoid films cannot be overemphasized. Though it has been customary to consider the rectum and lower sigmoid the responsibility of the proctosigmoidoscopist, this is no longer true. Andren and Freiberg,[2] Welin,[45, 46] Carlile[5] and Miller[15, 20] have demonstrated convincingly that the radiologist should take responsibility for the total colon examination, including the sigmoid and rectum. Because these areas cannot be compressed, lesions here are notoriously missed by full column techniques. However, multiple studies have shown that bleeding benign polyps, cancer, villous adenomas and other lesions of the rectum—all within reach of the sigmoidoscope and finger—have been missed by competent physicians but diagnosed on adequate air contrast colon examinations with drainage of the rectum.[34] The reverse sometimes is true and each method is a check on the other, much to the benefit of the patient. Although I agree completely that radiologic examination of this area is not a substitute for the digital or sigmoidoscopic examination, it is certainly complementary. The radiologists must take responsibility for the entire colon from anus to appendix.

Adequate radiograms in sufficient number are necessary to obtain reliable information on all segments of the colon. As opposed to conventional barium enema techniques, the barium should be instilled with the patient in the prone position. This prevents barium from entering the ileum for the first five critical radiograms of the rectum and rectosigmoid area. After the colon is inflated, the patient may be rotated with little risk of barium reflux into the small bowel, if care is used to keep him prone during the first stage of the examination when barium is in the cecum.

Steps in Colon Examination

The 85% w/v barium water mixture is squeezed into the colon immediately after intravenous injection of glucagon, the patient remaining prone until barium reaches the

---

*E-Z-EM Company, Inc., 7 Portland Avenue, Westbury, New York 11590.

splenic flexure. At that point, the enema bag is quickly dopped to the floor and the barium drained from the rectum. As the air is insufflated, the table may be tilted, first with the head down, then with the feet down, while rotating or turning the patient so that the barium can flow to the dependent uncoated part of the colon. This is best done by watching the head of the barium column and following the course of the colon. The barium can easily be manipulated so that it runs its course by gravity to the cecum. At this point, care must be used not to fill the terminal ileum with barium. Air in front of the barium should cause no concern because this lifts the ileocecal valve and prevents barium from entering the terminal ileum. When the colon is distended with air, accordion-like folds also are straightened and the barium flows easily and quickly. The patient is not sent to the toilet for evacuation either before instillation of air or at completion of the study. Standing upright and then sitting and straining during defacation might force barium into the terminal ileum and ruin an otherwise competent study. The proper procedure is to instill more air.

Drainage or instillation of more barium may be carried out from time to time in order to obtain the optimal distribution and amount of barium in the colon. The patient may be rotated, turned and placed head down or head up, as necessary (just as one would tip and turn a Chinese puzzle in order to place a small lead shot at the end of a maze).[51] Rarely it is necessary to have the patient sit up, or to use manual palpation. In every case without complete obstruction, the cecum must be coated with barium. If too much barium has accidentally been allowed to enter the colon, it can be drained back into the enema bag. All of this usually is not necessary after a little experience.

One aspect of double contrast colon studies that is seldom stressed is the sequence of filming.[37] The technologist cannot be left to decide this because vast differences in film quality will result. The initial or first stage of the examination concludes with the patient prone. Filming should begin with the PA view made with a perpendicular central ray. This film demonstrates the rectum to good advantage and often provides additional visualization of the sigmoid. To include the rectum, the lowest point of the cassette should be placed about one inch (2.54 cm) below the gluteal fold.

The patient should then be turned in a 15-degree RAO position and the tube angled 35 degrees toward the feet. To compensate, the tube must be lowered from 40 (101 cm) to 33 inches (84 cm) above the plane of the Bucky. With oblique positioning, the natural tendency is to bend the right leg. This must not be done, as the added soft tissue density of the thigh degrades imaging of the sigmoid. In addition to decreasing distance, compensation for increased part thickness because of the angulation may be accomplished by doubling the milliamperage per second (mAs) or increasing kvp by 10.

Next the patient is rolled into a right lateral position and a 10×12 inch (25×30 cm) film of the rectum is exposed.

Next, the 20 degree RPO film is obtained, with the top of the film at the xiphoid. Even in large patients, the films should not be turned transversely. This view is made primarily to visualize the distal transverse and descending colon, and these areas must be fully covered. In some patients the ascending and proximal transverse colon will not be included on the film, but the overlapping of these segments makes their visualization of little benefit.

The patient should now be rolled supine and into a left lateral position for 10 seconds to allow drainage of barium and air distribution into the right colon. When the patient is placed in this position, air will rise into the transverse colon and cecum. To prevent the sigmoid from collapsing, between five and 10 additional pumps of air should be administered at this time. This additional air also tends to elevate the sigmoid out of the pelvis.

The patient is then rolled back into a 45-degree LPO position, and a film exposed to include the hepatic flexure. In almost every patient the rectum and sigmoid also can be included on this film.

At this point, the patient is placed in a 15-degree LPO position and an exposure made with the central ray angled 35 degrees toward the head. The centering point for most patients is the right anterior superior iliac spine, but in large patients this should be moved to the left slightly.

The final overhead films are made in the decubitus position. Once again the sequence is important. As the first spot film will be of the cecum, the left lateral decubitus film is exposed last. This assures optimal air/barium distribution, draining and inflating the right colon. The absolute necessity of first quality decubitus films must be emphasized. With the technical modifications first described by Miller,[17] this is an easily accomplished task.

Following the right and left lateral decubitus views, the patient is placed in a supine Trendelenburg position and a compression spot film of the cecum obtained. Slight degrees of obliquity are often useful to demonstrate the cecum to best advantage. At times it may be necessary to use a compression balloon or wooden paddle to move sigmoid loops away from the cecum. The value of compression in decreasing body thickness to give better quality spot films is extremely important.

Finally, the table is elevated and, with the patient upright, compression spot films are made of the flexures and transverse colon. At this stage the patient is placed prone and the table returned to a horizontal position. If a rectal balloon has been used, it may be deflated at this point. After redraining the rectum and insufflating air, a spot film will now demonstrate any pathologic features covered by the retention device. The tubing clamp is released and air will now flow into the bag, thus relieving some of the patient's fullness. At this time the radiologist should examine the films to determine whether additional spot or overhead films are necessary. This is possible, even an hour later, if proper barium is used.

We have also adapted these techniques to the high kilovoltage full column barium enema. Gas is often present in the colon in large quantities, especially if an examination is performed following sigmoidoscopy. Even small gas bubbles can be annoying. The combination of prone and supine radiograms described can be of great help in solving this problem. The decubitus films will be of little benefit and may be eliminated. The spot films, naturally, should be obtained in the recumbent position with compression.

The single major exception to our routine procedure is in the examination of the sigmoid colon. In patients with a long initial sigmoid loop crossing far to the right, the PA and AP angled views are superior to the 15-degree oblique films. The RAO and LPO angled views cause an increase rather than a decrease in overlapping with this anatomical variation. This type of sigmoid pattern is easily recognized at fluoroscopy and the angled views modified to obtain the superior views.

There is a minimum number of films that must be obtained as well as a proper order in which to take them:

1. PA view to include rectum-perpendicular central ray.
2. 15-degree RAO view with 35-degree caudad central ray.
3. Right lateral view – 25×30 cm film.
4. 20-degree RPO to include descending and splenic flexure.
5. 45-degree LPO view with perpendicular central ray (after left lateral position for 10 seconds during which time 10 pumps of additional air are given).
6. 15-degree LPO view with 35-degree cephalad central ray.
7. Right lateral decubitus view to include rectum (after #7 turn patient through the prone position to obtain #8.

8. Left lateral decubitus view to include rectum.

9. Supine compression spot of cecum (often in some degree of obliquity and Trendelenburg).

10. Upright compression spots of flexures and transverse colon. (Occasionally these cannot be made in completely upright position but should be made as erect as possible.)

The order of filming is most important. However, it should be obvious that any of the above overhead films may be taken on spot films or remote controlled apparatus, if appropriate equipment for beam angulation and direction is available. The above system can be followed on the simplest radiographic fluoroscopic units.

Some colon anatomy may be adequately demonstrated on two or three views, but the large majority of patients can be well evaluated only by a minimum of eight overhead and four spot radiograms. Occasionally, redundancy and anatomical variations will be encountered and even this number of films will not totally evaluate a given segment of the colon. The views described not only represent a reduction in the number of films originally advocated by Miller,[28, 30] but they result in an even more precise examination. The number of films to be scrutinized is lower and they are easier to interpret because of reduced superimposition. Any further reduction will result in a compromised examination.

CRITICAL INITIAL REVIEW OF RADIOGRAMS

These radiograms must be evaluated carefully by the radiologist before the patient leaves the department in case additional overhead or spot films are required to evaluate suspicious or frankly abnormal areas. The pliability of this barium preparation allows a thorough radiographic examination without haste. The barium will not clump for at least an hour, and the colon can easily be reinflated. In most cases the review is made before any air escapes from the patient, and little or no additional air is needed.

FLUOROSCOPY

Fluoroscopy with spot films and compression is still an important part of examining the colon. We simply reverse the usual order, reserving intensive fluoroscopy and additional spot films for suspicious areas seen on the initial 12 radiograms. Fluoroscopy with compression is as valuable in the air contrast technique as in the conventional filled colon study. It has enabled us to confirm or reject many suspicious lesions.

Comment

Obviously, it takes the desire, a little effort and some know-how on the part of the examiner to develop a reliable and consistent air contrast technique. I have outlined one such technique above. Are the results of high quality air contrast studies worth these efforts? The facts, not opinions, are as follows:

In a series of 182 patients having both barium enemas and colonoscopy, Williams et al.[49] reported that the regular barium enemas missed 43% more tumors than the air contrast technique. He also showed that the air contrast technique revealed 98% of all tumors over 1 cm. Theoni and Menuck,[43] two gastrointestinal radiologists, find a 45.2% error rate with the single contrast dilute barium high kv technique – a 33.5% higher error rate than with the air contrast technique. I believe that these are significant percentages. To date, no other examination has been proved to give such precise information of the entire colon as does a good air contrast technique. In addition, inflammatory lesions in the mucosa will show up earliest and in great detail with air contrast studies.[11, 12, 47]

At the very least, there is a high-risk group of patients who I believe should have an air contrast colon examination as the primary examination. This group comprises patients with any of the following findings:

1. Rectal bleeding for any reason or a history of bleeding.
2. Polyps on proctoscopic examination.
3. Previous history of polyps or carcinoma.
4. Strong family history of polyps or carcinoma.
5. Age over 40.
6. Change in bowel habits, weight loss, unexplained anemia, previous ureterosigmoid anastomosis,[38, 48] long-standing (10 years) inflammatory bowel disease, hemoccult-positive stools or other signs, on the basis of which the clinician or radiologist should have a high index of suspicion for carcinoma.

The question sometimes arises as to whether both a conventional barium enema and air contrast enema can be done on the same day. To do both enemas well and combine them is certainly a rare exception, because these are two entirely different types of examination.[30] In rare instances the air contrast enema may follow the conventional barium enema, i.e., when no barium enters the terminal ileum and there is good evacuation. The conventional barium enema is then used as a cleansing enema. Only in these unusual circumstances, rare in my experience, can a satisfactory air contrast enema with dense barium and a bowel relaxant follow a conventional barium enema. The use of just one or two films after thin low density barium and a little air will not suffice and is an abuse of an excellent method.

Summary

The radiologist must assume complete responsibility for the preparation and examination of the entire colon, including the rectum. Some diagnostic radiologists argue that they do not have the time to do air contrast studies. There was also a time in Semmelweis' life when doctors said that they did not have the time to wash their hands in an antiseptic solution between autopsies and the examinations that preceded the delivery of babies.[42] If one can do a barium enema in an x-ray department, one can give a cleansing enema and do an air contrast examination in that same department on the same table. One may do fewer studies, admittedly, but these will be better diagnostic studies, requiring fewer repeat examinations. *All* scientific evidence to date reveals that good air contrast studies are superior to full column or so-called combined techniques for detecting small tumors in the high-risk carcinoma group. Look at the scientific evidence: imperfect as it may be, it is subtantial.[30, 31, 43, 49] There is *no* controlled evidence to the contrary.

REFERENCES

1. Alavi, A., Dann, R. W., Baum, S., and Biery, D. N.: Scintigraphic detection of acute gastrointestinal bleeding, Radiology 124:753, 1977.
2. Andren, I., and Freiberg, A.: Roentgen diagnosis of the rectum, Gastroenterology 31:566, 1956.
3. Athanasoulis, C. A., Baum, S., Waltman, A. C., et al.: Control of acute gastric mucosal hemorrhage, N. Engl. J. Med. 290:597, 1974.
4. Barry, J. W., and Engle, C. V.: Detection of hemorrhage in a patient with cecal varices using ^{99m}Tc-sulfur colloid, Radiology 129:489, 1978.
5. Carlile, T.: The Roentgenologic Diagnosis of Carcinoma of the Colon, in *Cancer of the Gastrointestinal Tract* (Chicago: Year Book Medical Publishers, Inc., 1967), pp. 187–211.
6. Eyler, W.: In *Detection of Colon Lesions, First Standardization Conference, 1969* (Chicago: American College of Radiology, 1973), p. 108.
7. Ferrucci, J. T., Jr., and Benedict, K. T., Jr.: Anticholinergic-aided study of the gastrointestinal tract, Radiol. Clin. North Am. 9:23, 1971.
8. Friedland, G.: Colon Preparation, in *Detection of Colon Lesions, First Standardization Conference, 1969* (Chicago: American College of Radiology, 1973), p. 107.
9. Gelfand, D. W., and Moskowitz, M.: Massive gastric dilatation complicating hypotonic duodenography. A report of three cases, Radiology 97:673, 1970.
10. Hayt, D. B., Simon, D. F., and Collica, C. J.: Grid choice in high-kilovoltage 70 mm. radiographic spotfilming, Radiology 93:135, 1969.
11. Laufer, I., Mullens, J. E., and Hamilton, J.: Correlation of endoscopy and double-contrast radiography in the early stages of ulcerative and granulomatous colitis, Radiology 118:1, 1976.
12. Laufer, I.: The radiologic demonstration of early

changes in ulcerative colitis by double contrast technique, Can. Assoc. Radiol. 26:116, 1975.
13. Margulis, A.: Examination of the Colon, in *Alimentary Tract Roentgenology, Vol. 2* (2d ed.; St. Louis: C. V. Mosby Co. 1973), pp. 923–924.
14. Marks, G.: Flexible fiberoptic colonoscopy, J.A.M.A. 228:1411, 1974.
15. Miller, R. E.: Barium enema examination with large bore tubing and drainage, Radiology 82:905, 1964.
16. Miller, R. E.: A new enema tip, Radiology 92:1492, 1969.
17. Miller, R. E.: Simple apparatus for decubitus films with horizontal beam, Radiology 97:682, 1970.
18. Miller, R. E., and Lehman, G.: Localization of small bowel hemorrhage: Complete reflux small bowel examination, Am. J. Dig. Dis. 17:1019, 1972.
19. Miller, R. E.: The technical approach to the acute abdomen, Semin. Roentgenol. 8:267, 1973.
20. Miller, R. E.: Examination of the Rectum, in *Detection of Colon Lesions, First Standardization Conference, 1969* (Chicago: American College of Radiology, 1973), pp. 162–171.
21. Miller, R. E., Chernish, S. M., Rosenak, B. D., and Rodda, B.: Hypotonic duodenography with glucagon, Radiology 108:35, 1973.
22. Miller, R. E.: The radiological evaluation of intraperitoneal gas (pneumoperitoneum), CRC Crit. Rev. Clin. Radiol. Nucl. Med. 4:61, 1973.
23. Miller, R. E.: Shock following saline barium enema in elderly patient, J.A.M.A. 228:1169, 1974.
24. Miller, R. E., Chernish, S. M., Skucas, J., Rosenak, B., and Rodda, B.: Hypotonic roentgenography with glucagon, Am. J. Roentgenol. 121:264, 1974.
25. Miller, R. E., Chernish, S. M., Skucas, J., Rosenak, B., and Rodda, B.: Hypotonic colon examination with glucagon, Radiology 113:555, 1974.
26. Miller, R. E.: Detection of colon carcinoma and the barium enema, J.A.M.A. 230:1195, 1974.
27. Miller, R. E., and Lehman, G.: The barium enema: Is it obsolete?, J.A.M.A. 235:2842, 1976.
28. Miller, R. E.: Die vollstandige Colonuntersuchung, Radiologie 15:410, 1975.
29. Miller, R. E.: The cleansing enema, Radiology 117: 482, 1975.
30. Miller, R. E.: Examination of the colon, Curr. Probl. Radiol. 5:3, 1975.
31. Miller, R. E.: The barium enema in the high-risk carcinoma patient (Letter to the Editor), Radiology 123:813, 1977.
32. Miller, R. E.: The barium enema in the high-risk carcinoma patient – Epilogue (Letter to the Editor), Radiology 127:271, 1978.
33. Miller, R. E., and Peterson, G. H.: Drainage of the rectum: A simple maneuver to improve the accuracy of colon examinations, Radiology 128:506, 1978.
34. Miller, R. E., and Lehman, G.: Polypoid colonic lesions undetected by endoscopy, Radiology 128: 295, 1978.
35. Miller, R. E., Chernish, S. M., Brunelle, R. L., and Rosenak, B. D.: Double blind roentgenographic study of dose response to I. V. glucagon for hypotonic duodenography, Radiology 127:55, 1978.
36. Noveroske, R.: Perforation of the rectosigmoid by a Bardex balloon catheter, Am. J. Roentgenol. 96: 326, 1966.
37. Peterson, G. H., and Miller, R. E.: The barium enema. A reassessment looking towards perfection, Radiology 128:315, 1978.
38 Preissig, R. S., Barry, W. F., Jr., and Lester, R. G.: The increased incidence of carcinoma of the colon following ureterosigmoidostomy, Am. J. Roentgenol. 121:806, 1974.
39. Rogers, C. W.: Early discovery of cancer of the colon. A radiographic method, South. Med. J. 65: 957, 1972.
40. Sherman, R. S.: The roentgenologist as a consultant, Radiology 75:293, 1960.
41. Shinya, H.: Fiberoptic Colonoscopy for Diagnosis and Treatment of Colonic Disease, in *Surgery of the Gastrointestinal Tract* (New York: Intercontinental Medical Book Corporation, 1974), pp. 455–462.
42. Slaughter, F. G.: *Immortal Magyar. Semmelweis, Conqueror of Childbed Fever* (New York: Henry Schuman, 1950), p. 79.
43. Theoni, R. F., and Menuck, L.: Comparison of barium enema and colonoscopy in the detection of small colonic polyps, Radiology 124:631, 1977.
44. Turnbull, R. B., Jr.: The no-touch isolation technique of resection, J.A.M.A. 231:1181, 1975.
45. Welin, S.: Modern trends in diagnostic roentgenology of the colon, Br. J. Radiol. 31:453, 1958.
46. Welin, S.: Results of the Malmo technique of colon examination, J.A.M.A. 199:369, 1967.
47. Welin, S., and Brahme, F.: The double contrast method in ulcerative colitis, Acta Radiol. 55:257, 1961.
48. Whitaker, R. H., Pugh, R. C. B., and Dow, D.: Colonic tumours following ureterosigmoidostomy, Br. J. Urol. 43:562, 1971.
49. Williams, C. B., Hunt, R. H., Loose, H., Riddell, R. H., Sakai, Y., and Swarbrick, E. T.: Colonoscopy in the management of colon polyps, Br. J. Surg. 61:673, 1974.
50. Malmud, L. S.: Scintigraphic detection of intestinal bleeding, Gastrointest. Radiol. In press.
51. Miller, R. E.: Solution for the "air block" problem during fluoroscopy, Am. J. Roentgenol. 132:1020, 1979.

RECOMMENDED FOODS

DAYS 1 and 2 — MINIMAL RESIDUE

Foods Permitted

1) Strained fruit juices — orange, apple, grapefruit, pineapple, grape.
2) Cereal — cream of wheat, farina, or Rice Krispies.
3) Eggs — any style.
4) Cottage cheese — dry, not creamed.
5) Meat — canned baby meats, baked skinless fish, finely chopped canned tuna.
6) Macaroni, spaghetti, noodles or rice — in clear broth or buttered if desired.
7) Oil, butter or margarine — 1 to 2 tablespoons daily if desired.
8) Sweets and sugar — plain gelatin (jello) desserts without added fruit or vegetables, moderate amount of sugar or strained honey, marshmallows, arrowroot or vanilla wafers or sugar wafers.
9) Seasonings — moderate amounts.
10) Beverages — clear broth or bouillon, tea, weak coffee or Sanka, carbonated beverages (cola drinks, 7-Up), Gatorade, Kool-Aid or other synthetic drink mixes. Several tablespoonfuls of cream may be used if desired with cereals.

NO bread, fruit, vegetables or milk.

DAY 3 — CLEAR LIQUIDS

Foods Permitted — Use **only** these foods.

1) Synthetic juices, Kool-Aid, Gatorade, carbonated beverages, weak coffee or Sanka, or tea with sugar.
2) Clear broth, bouillon or consomme .
3) Gelatin dessert (jello without added fruits or vegetables).
4) Moderate amount of sugar.
5) Hard candies — lemon drop type.

NOTE: Use Day #3 (Clear Liquids) the day before the X-ray examination of the colon. Drink at least one (1) eight (8) ounce glass of water each hour starting at 11:00 a.m. until 8:00 to 10:00 p.m. the day before the X-ray examination.

FOLLOW THESE INSTRUCTIONS CAREFULLY

THEY CAN PREVENT A REPEAT EXAMINATION

BEFORE THE COLON EXAMINATION:

1) A minimal residue diet for three (3) days is preferable. (If not possible, start as soon as your colon study is scheduled). See the suggested foods enclosed with this pamphlet.

THE DAY BEFORE:

1) Hydration and Lavation — Drink fluids - a large eight (8) ounce glass of clear liquid each hour from 11:00 a.m. to 8:00 or 10:00 p.m. Check each space as you drink your fluid:

☐ 11:00 a.m. ☐ 12:00 noon ☐ 1:00 p.m. ☐ 2:00 p.m.
☐ 3:00 p.m. ☐ 4:00 p.m. ☐ 5:00 p.m. ☐ 6:00 p.m.
☐ 7:00 p.m. ☐ 8:00 p.m. ☐ 9:00 p.m. ☐ 10:00 p.m.

2) For **all** meals, a clear liquid diet starting with breakfast.

3) Take two (2) ounces of castor oil or four (4) ounces of NEOLOID soon after the noon meal.

☐ check when taken

4) Take two and one-half (2½) ounces of X-Prep Liquid, one (1) bottle at 4:00 p.m. the evening before the examination.

☐ check when taken

(If the two (2) ounces of castor oil cannot be given at noon, then two (2) ounces of castor oil between 3:00 and 5:00 p.m. should be taken. Take X-Prep Liquid four (4) hours later.)

THE NIGHT BEFORE:

1) Take only sweetened, strained fruit juice, coffee or tea with sugar but no cream. **Do not drink milk.**

2) Nothing by mouth after midnight until the end of the examination.

IN THE MORNING:

1) No breakfast on the day of the examination.

Report to X-ray at ____________ a.m.

on ____________ .

Your Doctor Has Ordered An X-Ray Barium Enema

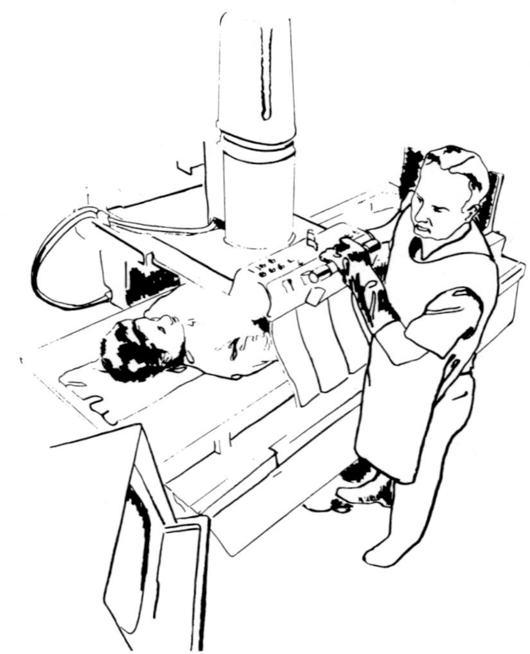

INDIANA UNIVERSITY MEDICAL CENTER
INDIANAPOLIS, INDIANA

THE REASON FOR YOUR STUDY:

Your physician has made an appointment with the X-ray Department to examine your colon. The colon can also be referred to as large bowel or large intestine. This examination may be called by various names: Barium Enema, Lower G.I. (Lower Gastro-Intestinal) or Large Bowel X-rays.

This pamphlet is designed to make you familiar with this test and what the physician will require of you in the X-ray Department, and to acquaint you with the equipment.

HOW TO PREPARE YOUR COLON

The accuracy of the X-ray study of the colon by the barium enema method depends to an extreme degree on the care that is taken in preparing the colon for the examination. The purpose of the preparation is to have the colon completely free from all waste matter or fecal content. Feces or waste matter will displace the barium and appear on an X-ray film similar to a tumor. The colon can be made free from fecal content by a **combination** of four procedures: (1) By selected diet for several days. (2) By hydration/and lavation from drinking large amounts of fluid. (3) By cathartics. (4) By cleansing enemas.

(1) Diet

Those foods that leave a residue (indigestible) in the colon are the fibers of meat, vegetables, fruits, and nuts. Milk and all milk products such as cheese also have an indigestible residue. The following diet is largely non-residue:

1) Jello without the addition of fruit.
2) Eggs (hard boiled and scrambled well done).
3) Butter, but **no bread**.
4) Polished rice.
5) Farina, macaroni, noodles (plain boiled).
6) Dry cottage cheese.
7) Strained lean meat and liver (baby food).
8) Fruit or vegetable juices, strained to remove all solids or fibers.
9) Soups; canned, dried, or homemade (made or diluted with water and each strained to remove all solids or fibers).
10) Jelly (but no jam).
11) Soft drinks such as Coca-Cola, grape juice, 7-Up, ginger ale, and Gatorade.
12) Tea or coffee with sugar and a small amount of cream (not milk).

See other suggested foods at the end of this pamphlet.

(2) Hydration and Lavation

Drink plenty of water or other fluids such as soft drinks. It takes water to flush the colon, just as it takes water to flush the toilet.

(3) Cathartics

Castor oil is the cathartic or laxative of choice to cleanse the upper bowel. The average dose is two (2) ounces. Castor oil is best taken in ½ glass of strained orange juice with a pinch of baking soda stirred into the mixture, and drunk while fizzing or effervescing. To remove the taste of castor oil, drink a bottle of coca-cola, 7-UP, or some drink containing citric acid. Two and one-half (2½) ounces of X-Prep Liquid (extract of senna) is also used to clean the lower colon. Four (4) ounces of NEOLOID may be taken for the castor oil.

(4) Cleansing Enema or Bowel Irrigation

This procedure is done in the X-ray Department before the X-ray examination. This is the final step to insure a clean colon. A single two thousand (2,000) ml. tap water cleansing enema will be given in the X-ray Department by trained personnel one-half to one hour before the X-ray procedure. If you are in the hospital when the X-ray Department is ready to do your examination, the nurse will notify you. You will be taken to the department and asked to change into a gown provided by X-ray. Any type of metal on your body will show on the X-ray and so it should be removed (for example, belts, medals or brassiere).

THE EXAMINATION:

In the examination room, you will be asked to lie down on a large X-ray table. The X-ray tube, which will record the actual activity, contour and size of the colon, is located directly above your abdomen. The dye that will outline the colon is Barium, a white liquid, and it will be given to you gently by a tube into the rectum in the same manner as an enema would be given. Sometimes only fluid is given (regular Barium enema), sometimes both fluid and air is instilled through the rectal tube (double contrast enema). This depends upon what you have told your doctor and what condition needs investigation. You may be given a medication to relax your colon.

If you have difficulty in holding the Barium, you should take deep breaths in and out like a dog panting This will relieve the urge to spill the liquid. The Barium will pass through the colon, allowing the Radiologist (X-ray doctor) to note the actual passage of the liquid and record it on film. In order to obtain a complete view of the colon, the camera and X-ray table will move. The Radiologist will also ask you to move from one side to another on the X-ray table during the examination.

After the Radiologist has completed his study, you will be allowed to go to the bathroom and eliminate the Barium. A post-elimination film will be taken.

The examination will last approximately one hour. The X-ray films will be quickly reviewed by the Radiologist. If satisfactory, your examination is completed and you will be dismissed or taken to your room and allowed to eat and drink.

AFTER THE EXAMINATION:

The Barium should pass out of your body in one or two days, resulting in "white" stool. Your physician may order a laxative to ease the passage of the Barium. If you do not have a bowel movement within three days, please inform your physician.

The Radiologist will interpret the examination later in. the day and a report will be sent to your physician.

Ideally, abdominal radiological examination of a woman of childbearing age should be performed during the first few (approximately 10) days following the onset of menses to minimize the possibility of irradation of an embryo. In practice, medical needs should be the primary factors in deciding the timing of the examination. If there is **any possibility** you may be pregnant, please inform your physician.

Please Follow the Checklist on the Last Page of this Pamphlet

Chapter 41

Technique and Interpretation of the Barium Enema Examination

EDWARD I. GREENBAUM, M.D.

IN RADIOLOGY NO TECHNIQUE is more important than that used in examination of the colon. Indeed, examination of the colon is a complex function. Each step from preparation of the patient to completion of the examination must be done with exquisite care. If there is a breach of technique in any of these steps, lesions slip by unnoticed. Saunders and MacEwen,[1] in reviewing 500 cases of colonic carcinoma, indicate that over 9% (47 cases) of carcinomas of the colon are completely missed on the initial barium enema examination. Lauer et al.,[2] in an analysis of 707 colonic cancers, reported a false negative error rate of 4%. Carcinomas were missed because of poor preparation of the patient (Fig 41–1) and because of observer and technical errors (Figs 41–2 and 41–3).

Although there is considerable variation in preparation techniques in different institutions, the patient should have verbal and written instructions in a language he understands. At our institution we have modified Miller's[3] protocol slightly to include a *routine* 3-day, low-residue diet with a clear-liquid dinner the evening before the examination. Fluids are encouraged on the day before the examination, and at noon 60 cc of castor oil is administered, following which, at 4 P.M., 75 cc of X-Prep liquid (see Chapter 40) is administered. Specific instructions are sent to the patient with regard to proper enema techniques, and he is instructed to use cleansing enemas consisting of 2,000 cc (i.e., 2 quarts) of tap water on the morning of the examination.

Counseling of the nurses, with repeated mini-courses in enema techniques, is of great value, since many of the nursing assistants who are actually performing the enemas are not aware of proper enema technique. In training the nurses, it is important to emphasize that the patient is first turned on his left side, following which the second half of the enema is done with the patient right side down so as to facilitate filling of the right colon.

Absolute contraindications to barium examination of the colon include (1) toxic megacolon and (2) biopsy immediately after sigmoidoscopy or colonoscopy. In the latter case, it should be ascertained what kind of biopsy was performed; if, for example, there is an exophytic mass, with biopsy only of a superficial portion of the mass, careful examination may be performed. If the patient had sigmoidoscopy or colonoscopy on the same day and inordinate amounts of air are present, the examination is cancelled and the patient is rescheduled for another day. If there is a suspicion of perforation of the colon, Gastrografin is preferred as the contrast medium.

The barium enema examination should begin only after a preliminary discussion of the history and physical examination and review of the KUB. The examination is done very carefully without undue hydrostatic pressure applied and with inflation of the rectal balloon under fluoroscopic control and only when absolutely necessary. The time-honored indications such as Guiac-positive stools is no longer honored, and the clinician is requested when possible to use hemoccult slide testing, since the latter is far more specific. The KUB is reviewed for retained fecal material, but its major function is to serve as a guide for technique and should bé reviewed with the technologist before overhead films are performed. The film should be dark with preferably a gray-black background density in the region of the soft tissues. This KUB should be obtained in the same room using the same technique (110–120 kv) as will be used with the subsequent barium enema.

We use a 15–20% barium suspension, the barium being thin enough so that the high kilovoltage technique can penetrate the barium column (Fig 41–4). Care must be taken so that the mixture is not too thin (Fig 41–5). The bag must be adequately shaken so that the barium will remain in suspension. We train our technicians to make sure that the osseous structures are clearly seen through the filled column of barium. Although dense barium and contrasty x-rays may please certain clinical nonradiologic colleagues, this dense barium will mask cancer (Figs 41–6 and 41–7). We train our residents to judge the quality of the barium during fluoroscopy and, if the mixture is too watery, the examination is stopped and more barium is added to the bag; conversely, if the mixture is too thick, more water is added to the bag so that the overhead films may be done with optimal technique.

Although Bardex balloons are in common use, it should be remembered that the balloon may obscure lesions in the rectum (Figs 41–8 and 41–9). Every attempt should be made to do the examination without inflation of the Bardex balloon; it should be inflated only if the clinician has excluded carcinoma of the rectum via digital examination. Inflation of the balloon in the face of a rectal carcinoma may cause perforation (Fig 41–10).

When the fluoroscopic techniques are set up, the density settings should be regulated so the spot films register gray-black shades in the soft tissues. I prefer a 9½ × 9½ spot film rather than 70 mm or 105 mm spot film, since small polyps are much easier to appreciate on the larger films. Several films of the sigmoid colon are taken at the beginning and at the end of the examination with and without compression in the prone and supine positions. This allows shift of any extraneous material so that a persistent defect is more easily recognizable. The sigmoid, right colon and any redundant loops should be compressed; otherwise, small polyps will be overlooked and even annular lesions may be lost in a redundant, coiled sigmoid (Figs 41–11 and 41–12).

Polyp detection in a filled colon is much like x-raying a marble in a glass of barium. Visualization of the marble as a negative defect will not be possible if the marble is too small or the diameter of the glass too large, the barium too thick or thin or the kilovoltage too low. Although we can control the kilovoltage and barium consistency and the size of the container for example, the ascending colon or the cecum can only be affected by compression.

Careful distinction between a point of physiologic narrowing, e.g., Canon's point, and a neoplastic lesion must be made (Fig 41–13). The colon examination is not complete until there is filling of the appendix, the terminal ileum or definite identification of the ileocecal valve (Fig 41–14).

Overhead films utilizing high kilovoltage technique must include an AP, PA, lateral rectum, RPO, LPO angled sigmoid and postevacuation views.

The controversy as to the superiority of a single versus a double contrast technique will be covered elsewhere; however, at the First Standardization Conference, 1969, in the *Detection of Colon Lesions*,[4] it was stated that "there is more than one technique that is satisfactory for the examination of the colon."

In performing the double contrast examination, we use a high viscosity barium sulfate suspension (Polibar)* especially formulated for double contrast examination, which provides excellent mucosal coating and therefore is recommended. In employing the double contrast technique, several pitfalls must be kept in mind. Subtle contour defects may be overlooked. We have shared Figiel's[5] experience when, in the process of performing an air contrast study to confirm the presence of a lesion, we have been unable to identify the lesion and have had to revert to a repeat single contrast examination for confirmation (Fig 41–15). Air contrast examination is particularly difficult in the presence of numerous diverticula, and frank early carcinomas may be missed, especially when the observer is not experienced in the use of this technique.[6,7] On the other hand, I have seen single contrast work done with optimal technique where "no pathology is found" and, 1 year later, a large exophytic mass is seen (Fig 41–16). Since it is known that, by doubling times of tumors, the lesion had to have been present on the first examination, it goes without saying that the air contrast technique might have been effective in detection of this lesion.

In the literature and among many experienced radiologists, there is an ongoing dispute as to which of these techniques is superior. Miller[8,9] and Marshak[10] appear to disagree on the validity and application of the results described in the article by Williams et al.[11] in which they reported a 43% error rate with single contrast barium examination. Marshak states, "citing Williams'[11] article in detailing a 43% error rate in barium enema examination is insulting to any competent radiologist. The statistics at his hospital are regrettable."

Miller also quotes Cooley et al.[12] who, in a retrospective study, showed that 25% of 179 carcinomas were missed on the first barium enema and that over 85% were of the single contrast type. In reviewing Table 1 of Miller's article,[8] it would appear that 34 of the 45 missed carcinomas cited by Cooley were within the rectum and well within the reach of the proctosigmoidoscopist. If these patients had had complementary proctosigmoidoscopy and these rectal lesions had been detected, only 11 cancers would have been missed, for an error rate of about 6%.

It should be remembered that some lesions of the rectum may be overlooked and, although we agree that the radiologist should not abrogate his responsibility in this area, sigmoidoscopy and colonoscopy are complementary and should not be omitted in the quest for expediency.

Theoni and Menuck[13] found 219 polyps in 112 patients. They found a miss rate of 45% with single contrast examinations compared to 11.7% with double contrast examinations. Although this certainly would appear to be an indictment of single contrast techniques, several factors should be kept in mind. First, the polyps in question averaged 0.5 cm in size and the single contrast examinations were done without any cleansing enemas on the day of the examination. There appears to be no question as to the superiority of air contrast techniques in lesions 1 cm or less (Fig 41–17), but what is to be said about those over 1 cm, particularly if single contrast techniques are combined with proctosigmoidoscopy?

Although strong answers to this question are controversial and interesting, I agree

*E-Z-Em Co. Inc., 7 Portland Avenue, Westbury, N.Y. 11590.

with Dodds et al.,[14] who state that "it seems clear that the pneumocolon and single contrast barium examinations need to be individually compared with colonoscopy as well as with each other in a prospective, well-designed investigation."

In the last analysis, however, the report issued from the radiologic department will be the "final word" so far as the average clinician is concerned, and the present ongoing discussion as to the superiority of one technique over another is not likely to interest the average busy practitioner.

In reporting the examination, the radiologist is responsible for the examination being technically adequate and, if this is not the case, he should state that no conclusion is possible and suggest a repeat examination. When we hedge a report, the clinician is lulled into a false sense of security and an unwarranted amount of time is lost before the examination is repeated, if indeed it ever is. Since in localized malignancy of the colon there is an opportunity for an 81% 5-year survival,[15] the radiologist should never relax his vigil.

REFERENCES

1. Saunders, C. G., and MacEwen, D. W.: Delay in diagnosis of colonic cancer—a continuing challenge, Radiology 101:207, 1971.
2. Lauer, J. D., Carlson, H. C., and Wollaeger, E. E.: Accuracy of the roentgenologic examination in detecting carcinoma of the colon, Dis. Colon Rectum 8:190, 1965.
3. Miller, R. E.: Examination of the colon, Curr. Probl. Radiol. 5:5, 1975.
4. Youker, J. E.: In *Detection of Colon Lesions, First Standardization Conference, 1969* (Chicago: American College of Radiology, 1973), p. 209.
5. Figiel, S.: In *Detection of Colon Lesions, First Standardization Conference, 1969* (Chicago: American College of Radiology, 1973), p. 187.
6. Youker, J. E.: In *Detection of Colon Lesions, First Standardization Conference, 1969* (Chicago: American College of Radiology, 1973), p. 188.
7. Ho, Chia-sing, and Rubin, E.: Linear shadows in the air-contrast barium enema, Radiology 127:621, 1978.
8. Miller, R. E.: The barium enema in the high-risk carcinoma patient (Letter to the Editor), Radiology 123:813, 1977.
9. Miller, R. E.: The barium enema in the high-risk carcinoma patient (Epilogue), Radiology 127:271, 1978.
10. Marshak, R. H.: The barium enema in the high risk carcinoma patient (Letter to the Editor), Radiology 125:549, 1977.
11. Williams, C. V., Hunt, R. H., Loose, H., et al.: Colonoscopy in the management of colon polyps, Br. J. Surg. 61:673, 1974.
12. Cooley, R. N., Agnew, C. H., and Rios, G.: Diagnostic accuracy of the barium enema in carcinoma of the colon and rectum, Am. J. Roentgenol. 84: 316, 1960.
13. Theoni, R. R., Menuck, L.: Comparison of barium enema and colonoscopy in the detection of small colonic polyps, Radiology 124:631, 1977.
14. Amberg, J. R., Berk, R. N., Burhenne, H. J., Clemett, A. R., Dodds, W. J., Friedland, G. W., Goldberg, H. I., Goldstein, H. M., Laufer, I., Lawson, T. L., Margulis, A. R., Marshak, R. H., Miller, R. E., Short, W. F., Stewart, E. T., Youker, J. E., Zboralske, F. F.: Colon polyp detection: Role of roentgenography and colonoscopy, Radiology 125: 255, 1977.
15. Turnbull, R. B., Jr.: The no-touch isolation technique of resection, J.A.M.A. 231:1181, 1975.

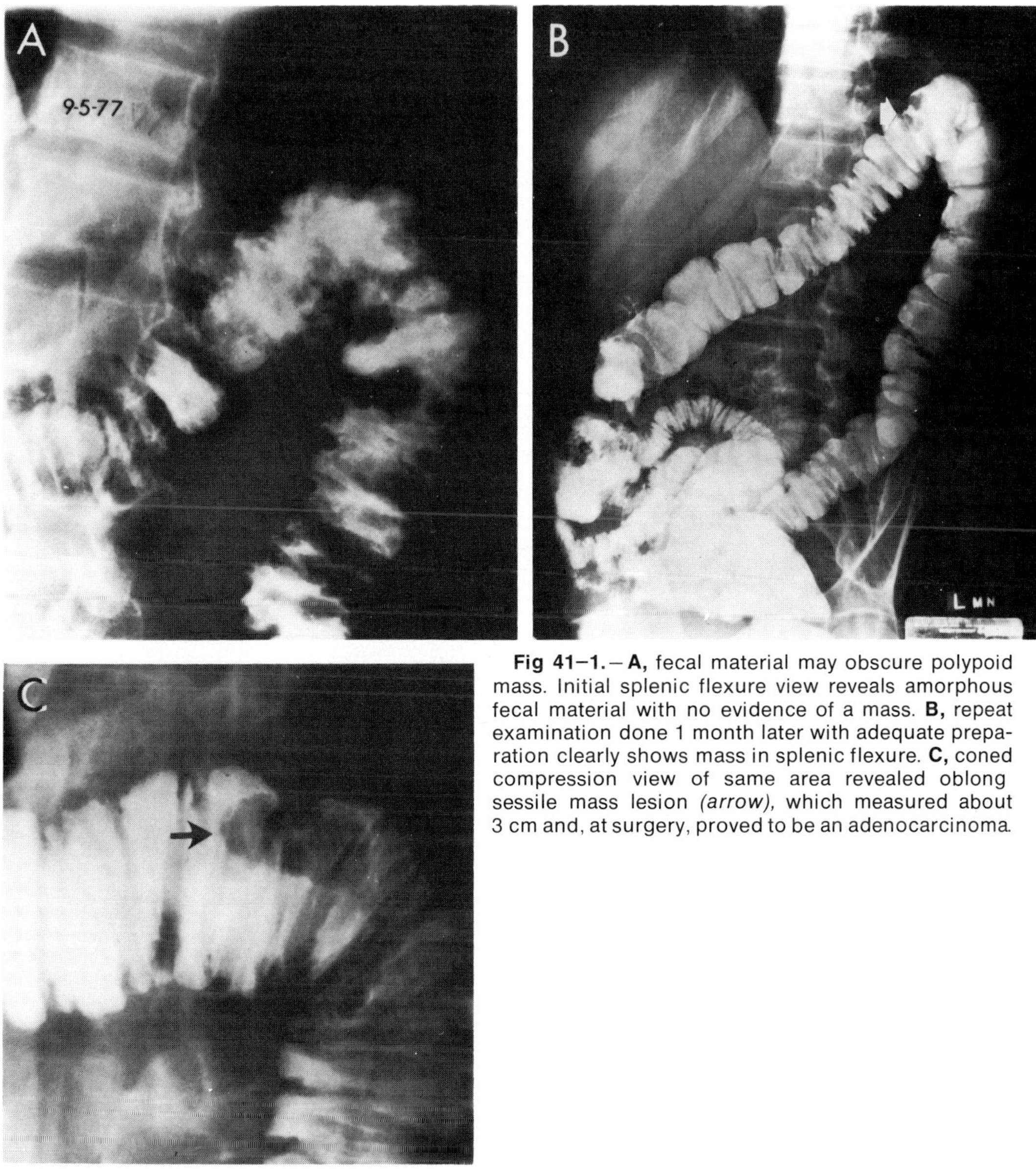

Fig 41–1.—**A,** fecal material may obscure polypoid mass. Initial splenic flexure view reveals amorphous fecal material with no evidence of a mass. **B,** repeat examination done 1 month later with adequate preparation clearly shows mass in splenic flexure. **C,** coned compression view of same area revealed oblong sessile mass lesion *(arrow),* which measured about 3 cm and, at surgery, proved to be an adenocarcinoma.

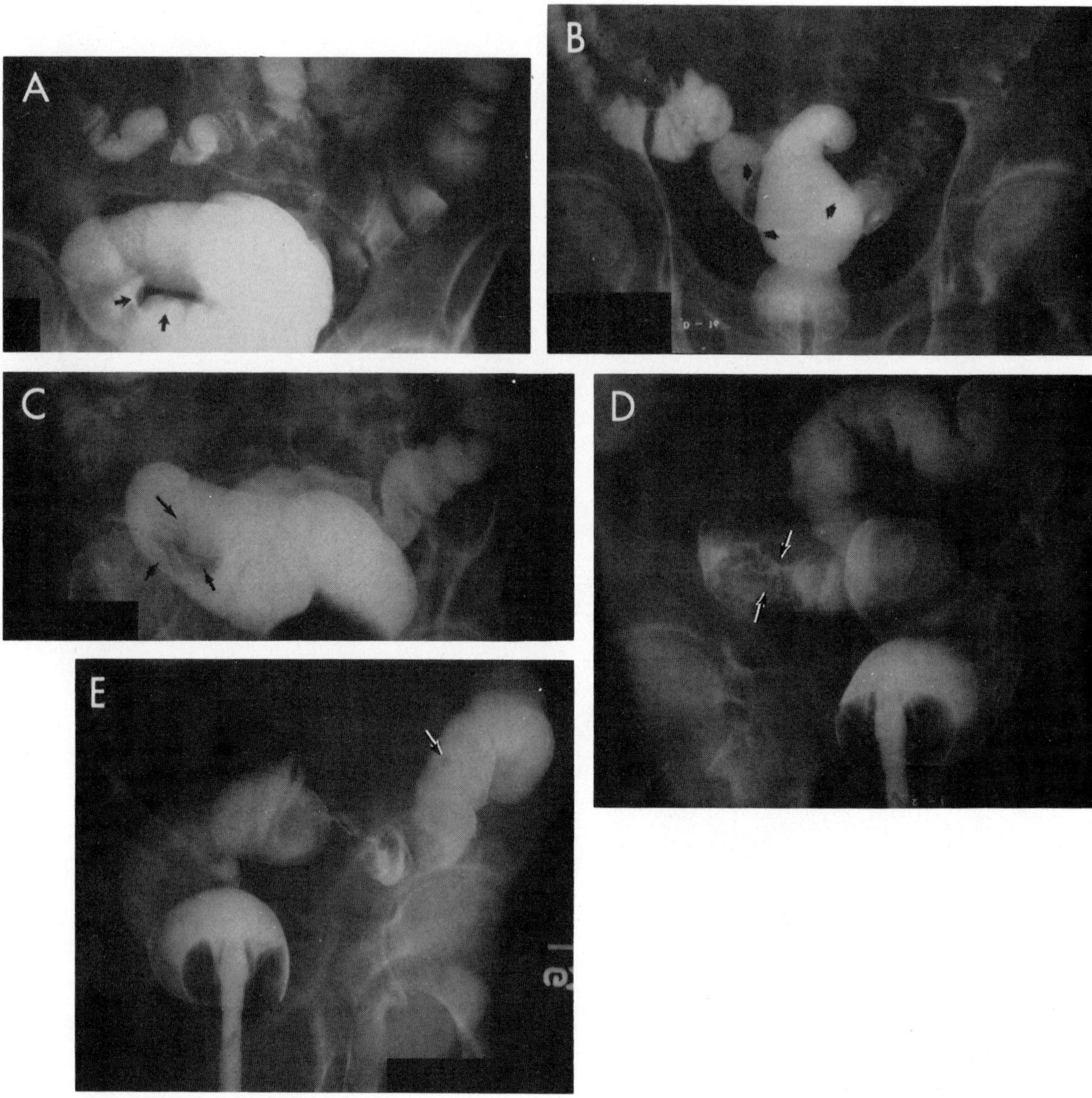

Fig 41–2.—**A,** observer error is major cause in delay in diagnosis of carcinoma of colon. A $1\frac{1}{2}$-cm broad-based mass lesion is seen in sigmoid colon *(arrows)* that was not detected at time of initial barium enema examination. **B** and **C,** AP and RPO views done 15 months later showed that mass *(arrows)* had grown to 4 cm, but it was again overlooked by resident physician doing barium enema. **D** and **E,** RPO and LPO views done 21 months after original barium enema reveal annular adenocarcinoma (*arrows* in **D**), confirmed at surgery; *arrow* in **E** points to additional small polyp.

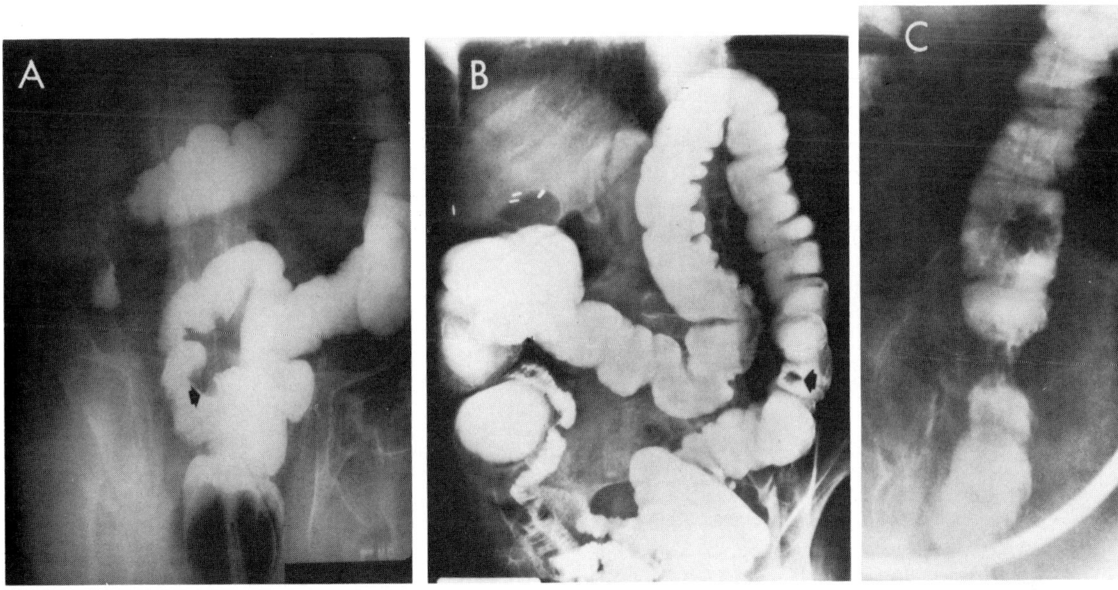

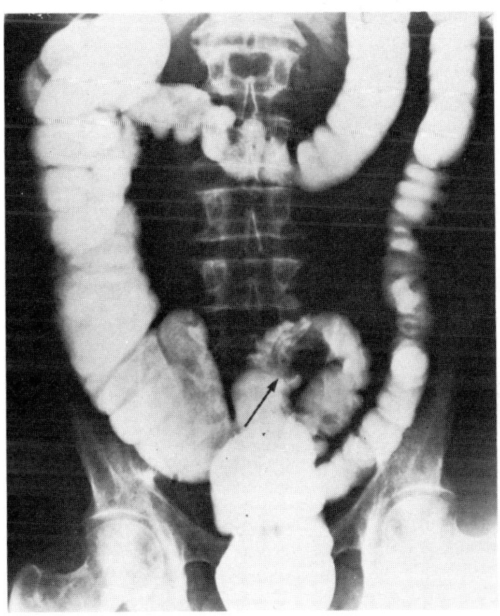

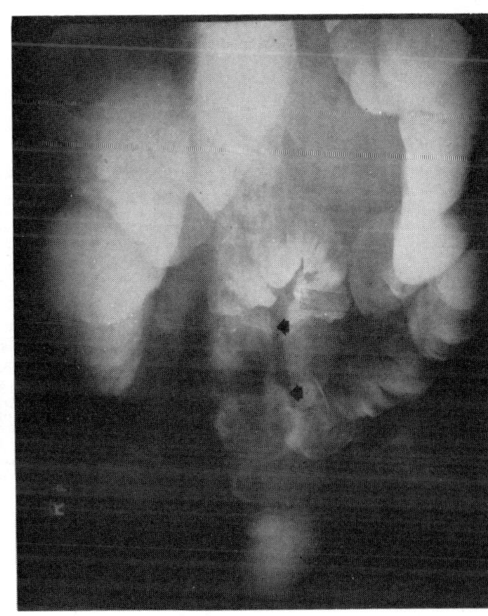

Fig 41-3 (top).—Observer error resulting in delay of diagnosis. **A,** obvious contour defect *(arrow)* seen on angled sigmoid view was overlooked, this examination being called normal. Nine months later, patient reappeared with rectal bleeding, and adenocarcinoma of rectosigmoid was removed. **B,** $1\frac{1}{2}$-cm villous adenoma, noted in descending colon, was originally interpreted at another hospital as being extraneous fecal material. **C,** 1 year later a repeat barium enema with coned compression views of descending colon once again reveals villous adenoma, which had shown no growth since previous examination. At this time, surgical resection showed lesion to be benign.

Fig 41-4 (bottom left).—With high kilovoltage techniques, background densities should be dark gray-black so that osseous structures may be clearly seen through filled barium column. Note that lumbar spine can be visualized through barium-filled transverse colon. Large sessile cauliflower mass seen in midsigmoid *(arrow)*.

Fig 41-5 (bottom right).—Watery, thin barium mixture was used in this examination, causing observer to almost miss obvious annular lesion of rectosigmoid *(arrows)*. Other views did not show this lesion, and it was only because observer knew sigmoidoscopic findings that lesion was detected.

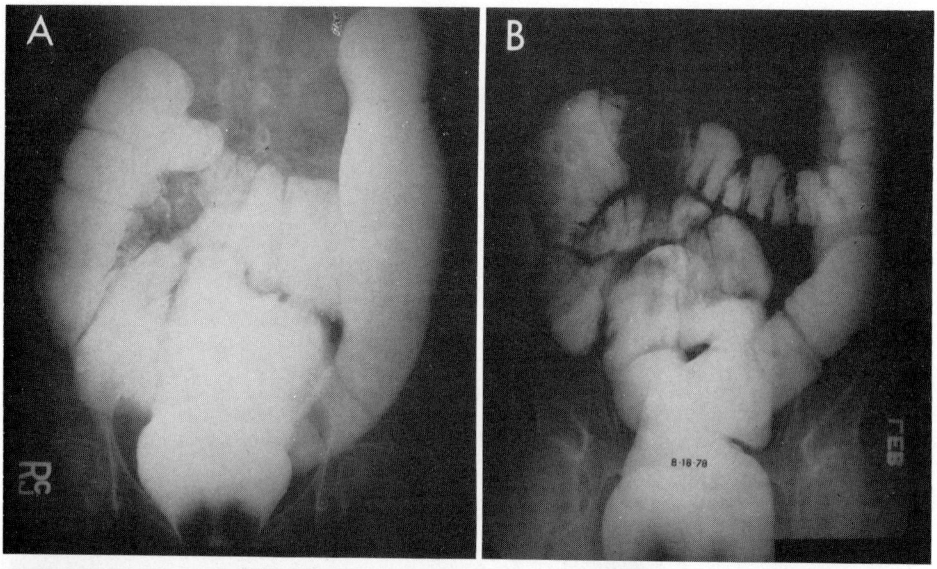

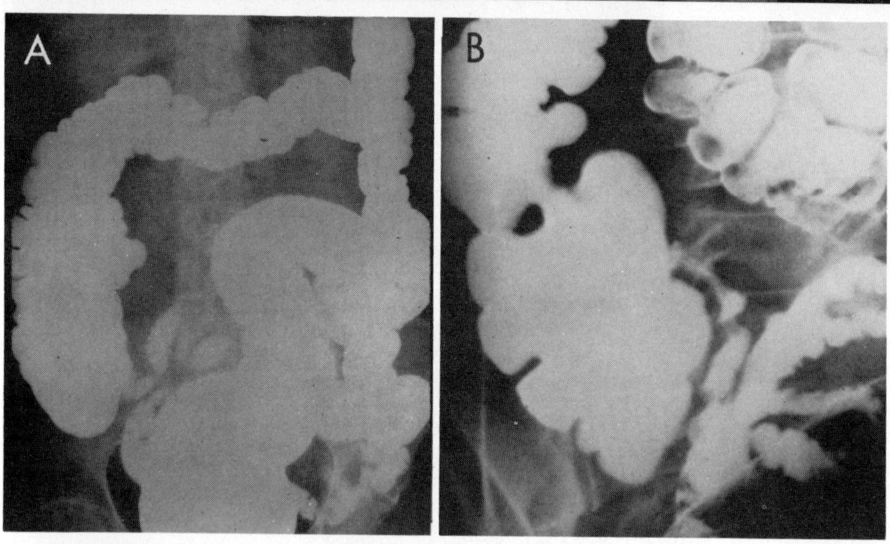

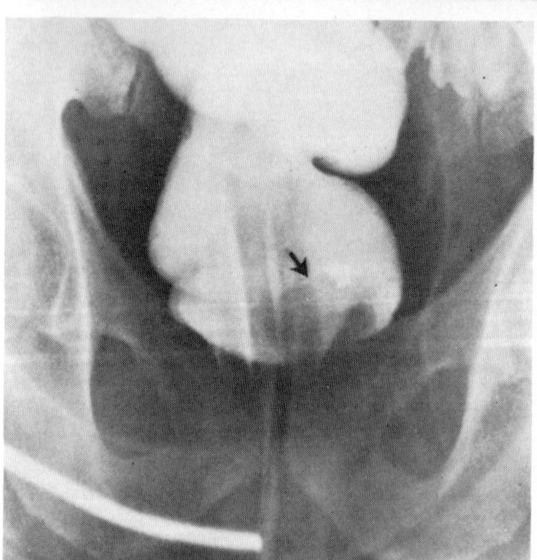

Fig 41–6 (top).—**A,** barium used in this examination is too dense, as it obscured adenocarcinoma, present at colonoscopy in proximal aspect of transverse colon. **B,** repeat barium enema examination 3 months later, using more optimal barium mixtures and high kilovoltage technique, revealed obvious carcinoma in proximal transverse colon, later confirmed at surgery.

Fig 41–7 (center).—**A,** barium enema examination done with dense undiluted barium obscured adenocarcinoma in right ascending colon. Examination was called normal. **B,** 6 months later an obvious annular carcinoma was seen in ascending colon and adenocarcinoma was confirmed at surgery.

Fig 41–8 (bottom).—Cloacogenic tumor *(arrow)* noted in rectum, which might easily have been obscured by an inflated Bardex balloon.

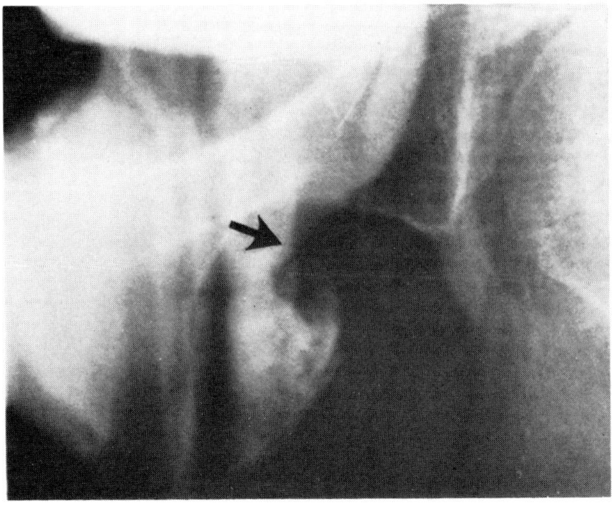

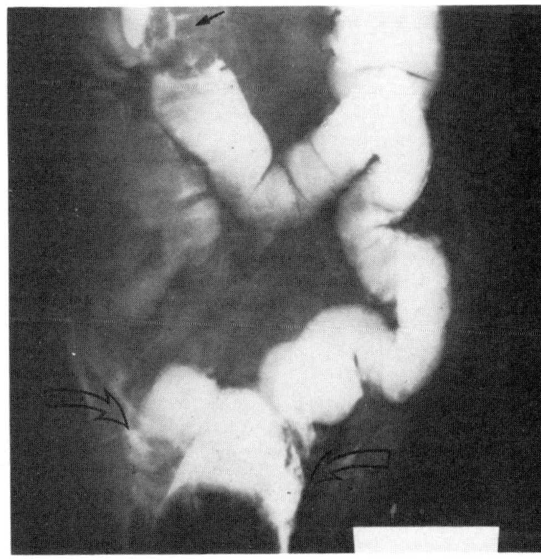

Fig 41-9 (left).—Contour defect *(arrow)* in left lateral wall of rectum could be seen tangentially only under fluoroscopic control. Lesion proved to be an adenocarcinoma and might have been obscured had Bardex balloon been inflated.

Fig 41-10 (right).—Adenocarcinoma of hepatic flexure *(black arrow)* with second synchronous carcinoma in rectum. This later carcinoma had perforated secondary to inflation of Bardex balloon; barium is extravasated into perirectal tissues *(open arrows)*.

Fig 41-11.—**A,** redundant loops of sigmoid colon and overlapping distal small bowel obscure sessile adenocarcinoma in sigmoid colon. **B,** above lesion was clearly demonstrated with use of compression paddle *(arrow)*.

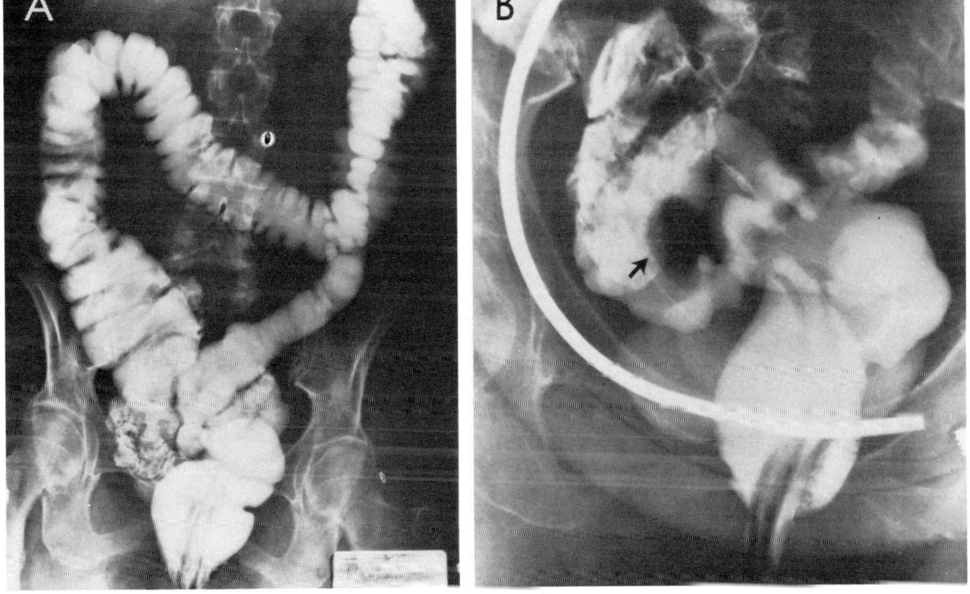

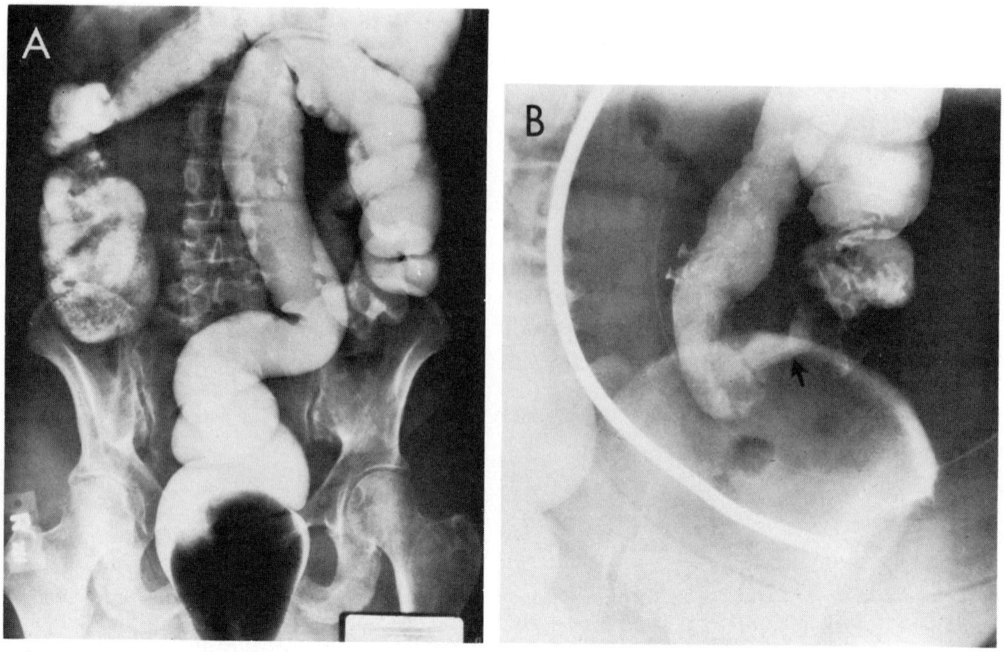

Fig 41–12. – **A,** redundant loops of large bowel at junction of sigmoid and descending colon obscure lesion in this area. **B,** with use of compression paddle, annular adenocarcinoma *(arrow)* was clearly demonstrated.

Fig 41–13. – **A,** Canon's point, physiologic narrowing in region of hepatic flexure *(arrow)*. **B,** overhead view with barium enema taken in LPO position shows that previously narrowed area has now returned to normal caliber. Case was misdiagnosed as adenocarcinoma of hepatic flexure; at surgery, no pathology was found.

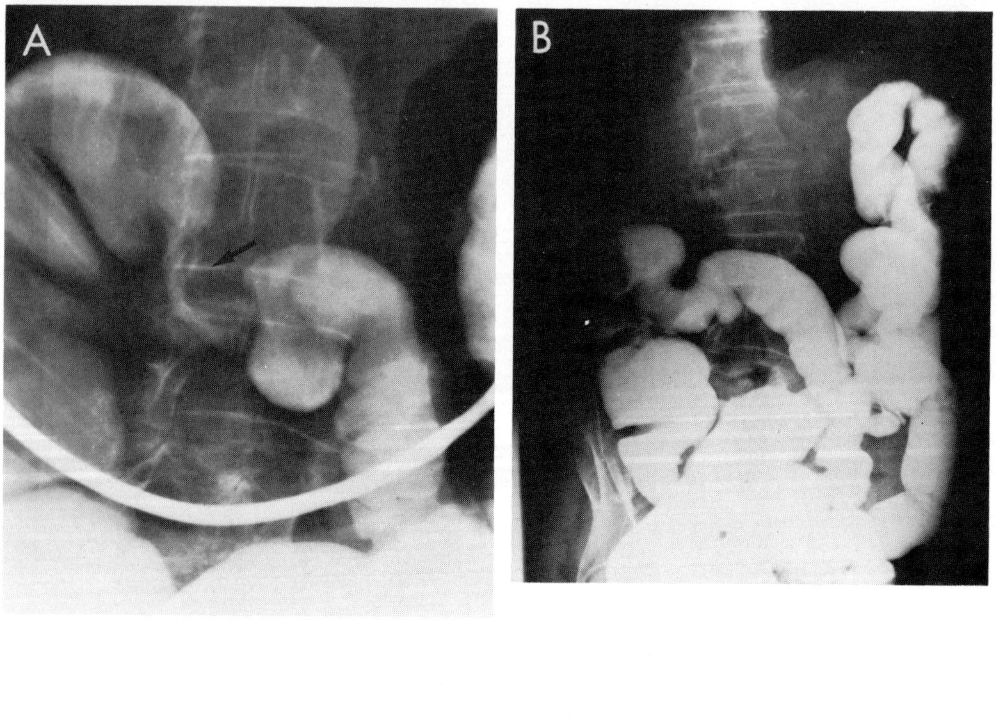

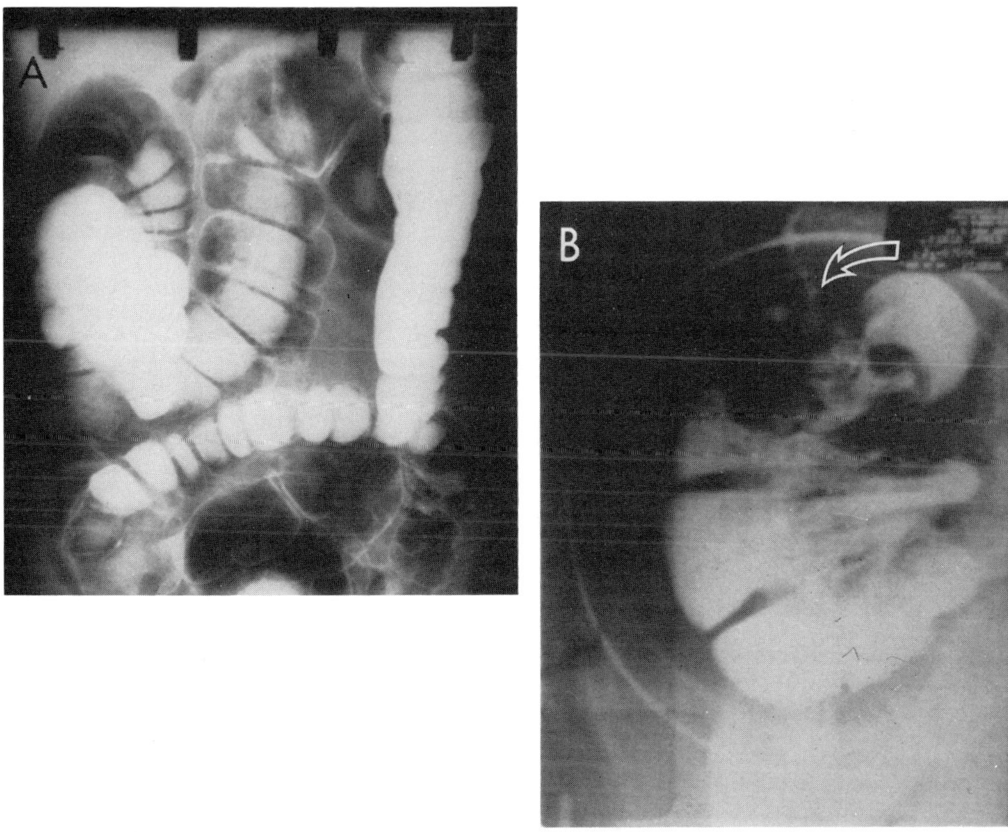

Fig 41-14.—**A,** patient had been examined at several institutions where on two examinations a diagnosis of a normal colon had been made. This examination revealed no filling of appendix and terminal ileum and no demonstration of ileocecal valve. Therefore cecum was considered incompletely examined and oral barium meal was suggested. **B,** small bowel examination with spot filming of ileocecal area shows filling of cecum with constricting adenocarcinoma of ascending colon *(arrow)* immediately superior to region of ileocecal valve.

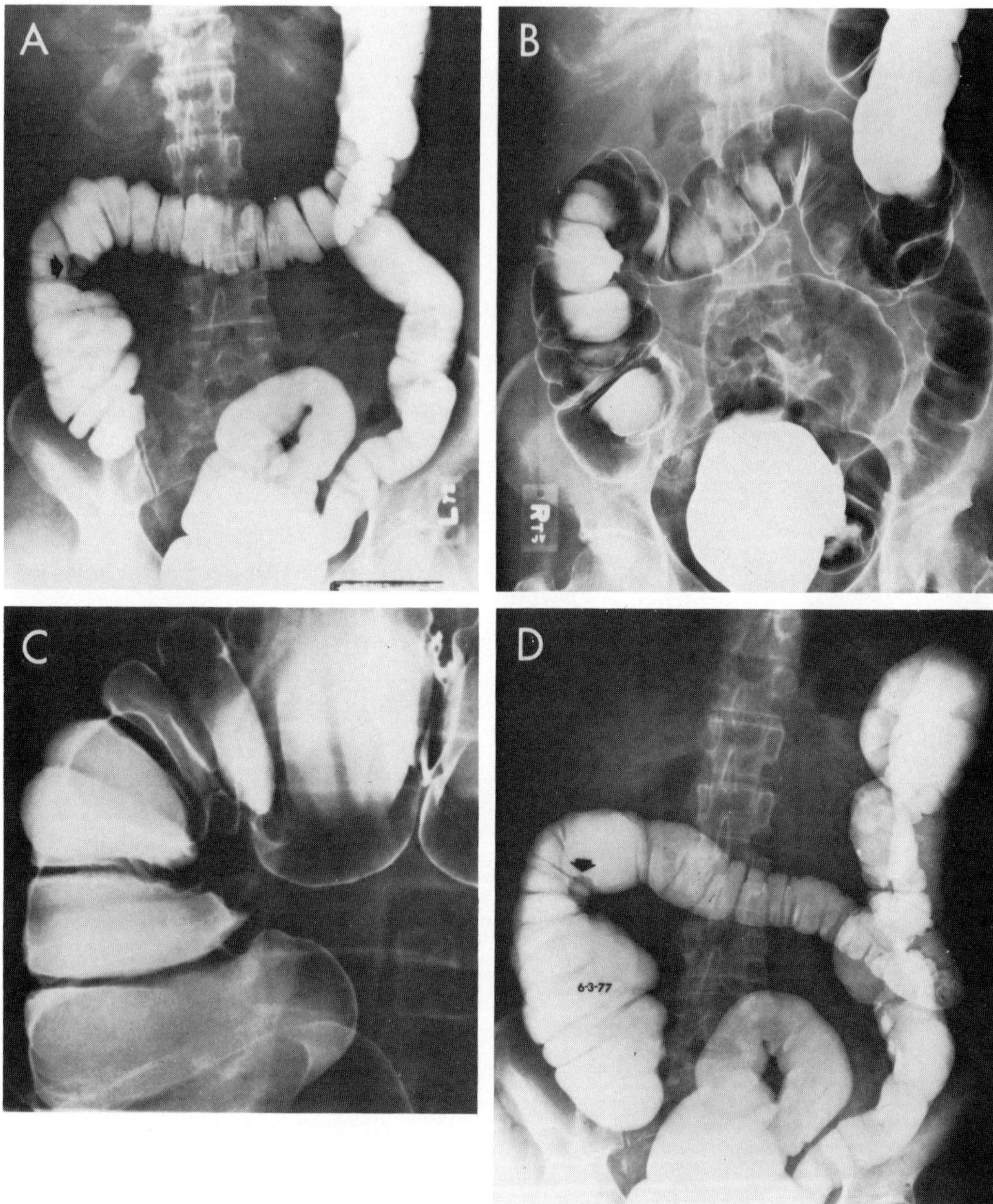

Fig 41-15.—**A,** barium enema reveals small (1.5 cm) mass lesion *(arrow)* at medial aspect of hepatic flexure. **B** and **C,** air contrast barium enema appears to obscure lesion. Although lesion was thought to be present, a diagnosis could not be established with certainty. **D,** repeat barium examination confirmed presence of small mass *(arrow)* in hepatic flexure, which at surgery was found to be ovarian carcinoma growing inward from serosal surface.

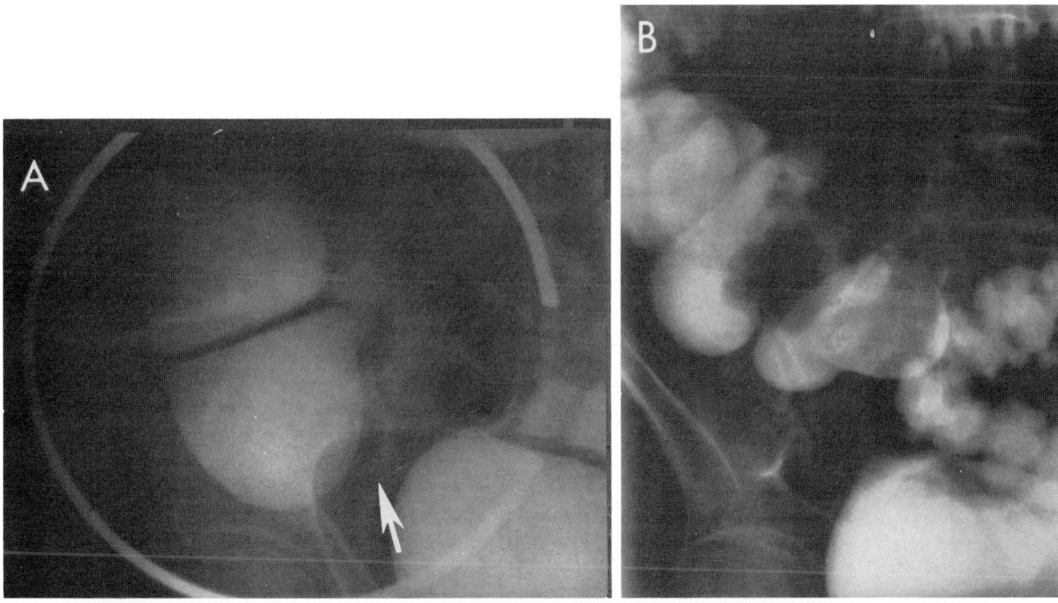

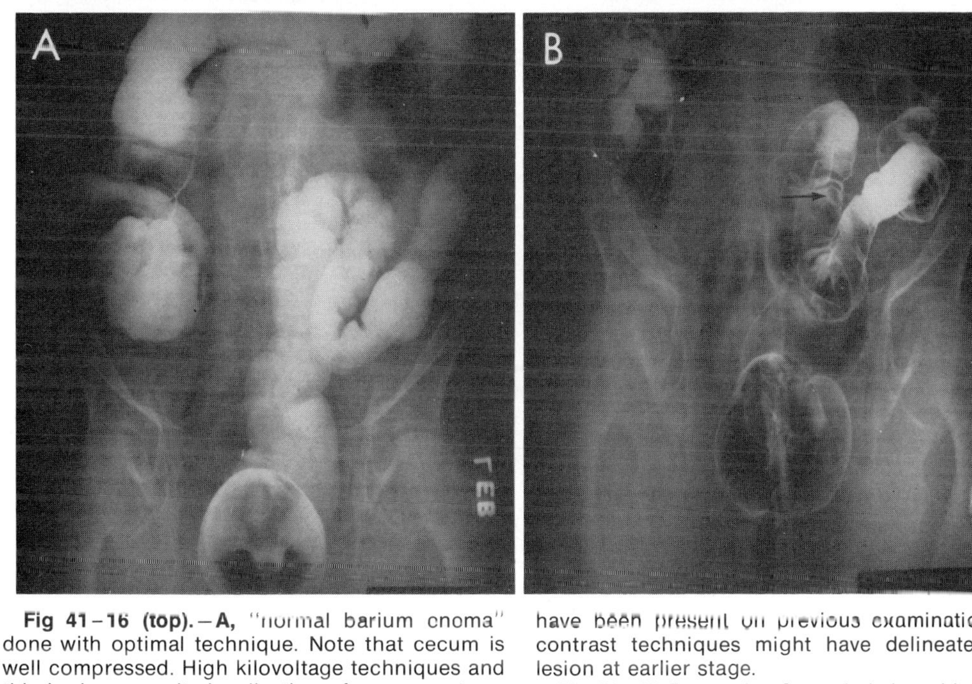

Fig 41–16 (top).—**A,** "normal barium enema" done with optimal technique. Note that cecum is well compressed. High kilovoltage techniques and thin barium permit visualization of osseous structures through filled cecum. Note filled appendix *(arrow)*. **B,** 5-cm lobular mass in cecum was noted 1 year later. According to studies on growth characteristics of colon carcinoma, this lesion must have been present on previous examination. Air contrast techniques might have delineated this lesion at earlier stage.

Fig 41–17 (bottom).—**A,** angled sigmoid view of rectosigmoid with single contrast technique failed to reveal pathology. **B,** repeat examination done within 1 week using air contrast technique shows 1 cm polyp in midsigmoid *(arrow)*.

Chapter 42

Trauma to the Colon and Rectum

ALLEN J. COHEN, PH.D., M.D.
JEFFERSON O. JANES, M.D.

IN THE UNITED STATES trauma is the fourth ranking cause of death and the leading cause below age 40. Although trauma to the colon is relatively uncommon, constituting 3 – 5% of all abdominal injuries,[1] the injury is often severe and may be life threatening. Violent trauma to the colon occurs most frequently in motor vehicle accidents, shootings or stabbings. Nonviolent accidental trauma often is caused by foreign bodies forced into the colon from below. Iatrogenic colonic trauma fortunately has occurred infrequently but has been reported in both the radiologic and nonradiologic literature.

Classification

Colonic injuries may be classified in several ways. Westcott and Smith[2] suggest the following based on anatomical location: (1) bowel lacerations (complete, seromuscular or mucosal), (2) intramural hematomas and (3) mesenteric lacerations associated with hematoma or major vessel injury. A classification based on the cause of the trauma is offered below to clarify the radiologic picture associated with certain types of trauma.

1. *Accidental trauma: violent.*—Blunt or penetrating.
2. *Accidental trauma: nonviolent.*
3. *Iatrogenic trauma: radiologic.*—Normal or abnormal bowel.
4. *Iatrogenic trauma: nonradiologic.*

ACCIDENTAL TRAUMA: VIOLENT

Blunt Trauma

In a series of patients sustaining 25 separate surgically treated blunt colon injuries, motor vehicle accidents and assaults constituted the most frequent clinical settings[3] (Fig 42 – 1). Three patients in this series sustained colon trauma after a fall, and the most frequent type of injury was "hemorrhagic contusion." In the latter injury there are subserosal hemorrhage and edema of the bowel wall without apparent disruption of the serosa or peritoneum.

In a series of animal experiments, Williams and Sargent[4] showed that the primary mechanism of bowel injury in blunt trauma resulted from compression and laceration of the bowel and mesentery between abdominal wall and spine, i.e., that portion of the bowel and mesentery midline at the instant of trauma. The high percentage of transverse colon injuries noted by Howell et al.[3] can be explained by this mechanism. The site of injury could not be directly related to a rise in intraluminal pressure or fixed bowel attachments. It has been suggested that the frequent injuries to the sigmoid result from compression and laceration between the abdominal wall and iliac crest.[3]

The introduction of automobile lap seat belts decreased the accident mortality by 35%,[5] but introduced the lap belt injury[3, 5, 6]

(Fig 42–2). Lap belt injury to the colon is produced by direct trauma to or compression of the bowel against the lumbar spine, with consequent contusion, hematoma and frequently a serosal tear.[7] Laceration of the mesenteric vessels is the most common colonic injury in seat belt trauma.[5] Whereas small vessel laceration usually produces only hematoma (Fig 42–3), major vessel laceration causes acute blood loss or ischemia[2] (Fig 42–4). Acute colonic intramural hematomas usually present with severe pain rather than obstruction.[8] Conversely, chronic hematomas will cause obstructive symptoms several weeks to several years posttrauma,[2, 9] with delayed stenosis owing to ischemia of the involved bowel segment[2] or organization of the hematoma (Fig 42–5). Delayed rupture of the colon with cutaneous fistula formation secondary to blunt trauma has also been reported.[10]

Pelvic trauma has been associated with trauma to the rectum.[11] An unrecognized rectal tear associated with a traumatic diastasis of the symphysis pubis, resulting in death of the patient, has been reported[12] (Fig 42–6). In this case the pubococcygeus muscle attachment to the nonfractured separated pubic symphysis tore the rectum at the anorectal junction. The clinical setting of pelvic trauma, therefore, mandates a search for retroperitoneal air on the plain radiograph.

Penetrating Trauma

Violent trauma to the colon is caused most often by penetrating objects. In a series of 415 patients with colon and rectal trauma, 96% suffered stab or gunshot wounds and only 4%, blunt trauma.[13] Gunshot wounds are explored surgically, whereas stab victims are usually evaluated clinically for peritoneal involvement. The use of contrast studies rarely is necessary because plain films of the abdomen in penetrating trauma frequently show a pneumoperitoneum. Water-soluble contrast enemas are performed, if necessary, to prevent peritoneal spill of barium.

Colonic trauma must also be suspected in cases of lower chest wall trauma. An unusual case of a fecothorax occurring 2½ days after a stab in the left lower chest wall, which punctured the hemidiaphragm and splenic flexure, has been reported[14] (Fig 42–7).

ACCIDENTAL TRAUMA: NONVIOLENT

In a review of more than 300 cases of gastrointestinal tract perforation by ingested foreign bodies,[15, 16] ingested items included pins, nails, bones, toothpicks, pencils and dental appliances.[17] Use of complete dentures decreases the sensitivity of the palate, increasing the risk of foreign body ingestion.[18] Alcohol intoxication also adds to this risk.[19] Perforation of the colon may result in abscess, fistula formation, hemorrhage or free perforation causing peritonitis. In most instances of chicken bone perforation, the diagnosis was not established preoperatively.[20] Berk and Reit[19] presented two cases in which the bone was seen on the initial radiograph prior to surgery (Fig 42–8).

Compressed air injury of the colon has been reported.[21, 22] Most of these accidents occur as practical jokes by workers using compressed air. The induced perforation occurs most often in the sigmoid or rectum above or below the peritoneal reflection. Rosenberg and Smiddy[21] showed experimentally that the pressure within the bowel from a compressed air nozzle falls off rapidly with distance from the nozzle and that cloth positioned more than 1 cm from the nozzle reduced the pressure to below bursting levels. It was concluded, therefore, that purposeful action was necessary to produce injury.

Insertion of foreign bodies into the rectum has been reported mainly in children or psychiatric patients.[23] Recently anal sexual stimulation has been reported,[24] especially in male homosexuals.[25] Extravasation of water-soluble contrast secondary to a rectal perforation caused by a plunger handle is shown in Figure 42–9. This patient died of septic complications. Figure 42–10 shows a metallic dildo, which perforated the sigmoid colon (the falciform ligament is seen, indicating massive pneumoperitoneum; see Fig 42–10, A).

IATROGENIC TRAUMA: RADIOLOGIC

Although the barium enema is a safe radiologic procedure, complications occurring only rarely, the radiologist must be aware of potential problems in order to further reduce the risk.

Normal Bowel

Seaman and Wells[26] have reviewed complications of the barium enema. Most complications were caused by improper enema tip placement, excessive intraluminal pressure within the enema tip and inflation of a balloon within a colostomy or were secondary to recent sigmoidoscopy with biopsy. Introduction of the enema tip traumatizes the rectum. Nelson et al.[27] reviewed nine cases of rectal complication, all related to rectal balloon use. The balloons were shown experimentally to deform easily on inflation. Shearing forces of the enema tip, as it is forced against the colon wall, is the mechanism of injury. Rectal submucosal barium in a sigmoidoscopically "normal" patient in whom a balloon catheter was not used has been seen[28] (Fig 42–11). A transverse striated pattern, probably produced by barium dissecting among inner circular layer of muscle fibers, is seen (see Fig 42–11, A and C). Although minor intramural dissection of barium causes pain and local tenderness,[28] there usually is little or no toxic reaction to the barium sulfate.[29]

Other regions of normal colon are not immune to intramural barium dissection (Fig 42–12). One incomplete cecal rupture was probably caused by an abnormal increase in intraluminal tension secondary to the enema.[28] Retention of water-soluble contrast in the colon has been shown to cause cecal perforation[30] (Fig 42–13). The hypertonicity of the retained contrast medium caused a large amount of fluid to collect in the obstructed colon, which eventually lead to perforation. It seems advisable in the acutely ill patient to drain such water-soluble media in the radiology department.

Complete perforation of the normal colon during air contrast barium enema has been reported rarely, but the mortality is high.[31, 32] A patient with a 10-cm longitudinal perforation of the right transverse colon and a massive barium/fecal spill after an air contrast study (Fig 42–14) died of septic complications, whereas a patient with a 5-cm longitudinal cecal perforation, but minimal barium and fecal spill, recovered completely.[31] Since examinations in both patients failed to demonstrate reflux into the terminal ileum, it may be speculated that a closed loop obstruction occurred, increasing intraluminal pressures beyond the point of rupture. Kiser et al.[33] have reported one colonic perforation in a series of 2,150 barium enemas. Two deaths from myocardial infarction and cerebral vascular accidents directly related to the enema procedure also were noted.

Abnormal Bowel

Abnormal bowel increases the risk of colonic trauma by barium enema. Most cases of induced colonic perforation have occurred in carcinoma, ulcerative colitis, diverticulitis, tuberculous enterocolitis or amebiasis.[34] A location especially prone to perforation is that of a distal rectal carcinoma. Enema tip trauma is the usual cause. These perforations may be either above or below the peritoneal reflection (Figs 42–15 and 42–16).

The attendant risk of carcinoma in longstanding cases of ulcerative colitis[35] mandates periodic barium enemas.[36] However, the abnormally friable mucosa predisposes to intramural dissection of barium, with formation of barium granuloma[37] (Fig 42–17). Toxic megacolon following a barium enema in a patient with quiescent chronic ulcerative colitis has been reported.[36] Therefore, a barium enema in chronic ulcerative colitis should be performed slowly to prevent rapid rises in pressure that could precipitate acute toxic dilatation. Instances of toxic megacolon occurring after barium enema in patients with acute ulcerative colitis are well known.[38] Any contrast study of the colon in the acute colitides should be seriously questioned and performed only if absolutely necessary.

Development of fatal septicemia in a patient with acute leukemia has been reported,[39] confirming a well-founded maxim that immunologically compromised patients should undergo as few procedures as possible. Intravenous extravasation of barium carries a high mortality.[40] Barium extravasation into the portal venous system is usually due to sigmoid diverticulitis. Following radiation therapy to the abdomen for malignancy of the cervix, ovary or bladder, the patient may have symptoms of anorexia, diarrhea, abdominal cramping and rectal bleeding. Contrast examination may show radiation-induced colonic and rectal abnormalities, which must be distinguished from recurrent malignancy.[41]

IATROGENIC TRAUMA: NONRADIOLOGIC

Whenever the colon is invaded with a medical instrument, there is a small but significant risk of trauma. The 1974 American Society for Gastrointestinal Endoscopy Survey showed that the most common complication of diagnostic colonoscopy (0.22%) was perforation.[42] Factors causing perforation during colonoscopy are thought to be (1) volume of insufflated air, (2) rate of insufflation, (3) location of the area involved and (4) stretching of the bowel wall during insertion of the colonoscope.[43] Definite contraindications to colonoscopy are recent biopsy and toxic megacolon.

Surgical procedures in the region of the colon and rectum may inadvertently lead to bowel trauma. In a series of over 3,000 gynecologic surgical patients in whom the abdomen was entered, the colon was injured 0.25% of the time.[44] These injuries occurred during dissection of the uterus or adnexae and all were above the peritoneal reflection. In the same series, 0.35% of more than 1,900 vaginal operations resulted in rectal injuries during dissection of the posterior vaginal wall from perirectal fascia.

Cardiopulmonary resuscitation has the well-known attendant risks of sternal and rib fracture and the associated risk of liver or splenic trauma. Unrecognized ruptured transverse colon with subsequent abscess formation has been reported in a patient resuscitated after a myocardial infarction.[45]

Ileocolonic perforation has been reported to occur in 4.4% of renal transplant patients.[46] High-dose steroids have been implicated as an important etiologic agent in these perforations by decreasing bowel wall resistance to bacterial invasion. When a perforation has occurred, the steroid-induced immunosuppression masks signs and symptoms, causing a greatly increased morbidity.[47]

Iatrogenic perforation of the colon and rectum has been reported in a series of 10 newborn infants.[48] The causes of perforation included enemas to relieve constipation, examination of the anus and rectum for patency with a firm catheter or use of a rectal thermometer. In nine of these infants, diffuse peritonitis developed, resulting in four deaths. Greenbaum et al.[49] presented two cases of thermometer-induced rectal perforation; both infants survived (Fig 42–18). In newborn infants, the distance between anus and peritoneal reflection is less than 3 cm. Failure to direct the rectal thermometer posteriorly after advancing it 3 cm will cause penetration of the anterior rectal wall.

Iatrogenic perforation of the rectum is not limited to newborn infants. Radiographs in a nursing home patient who suffered a rectal perforation from a cleansing enema tip are shown in Fig 42–19. The fixed extraperitoneal air adjacent to the descending colon reveals the site of perforation to be below the rectal peritoneal reflection.

Summary

Various classes of trauma to the colon and rectum have been presented. Sharp penetrating trauma is by far the most common clinical setting. Less common types of trauma must also be recognized promptly. Lap belt injury, pelvic trauma, foreign body ingestion and rectal foreign body insertion are conditions in which early diagnosis may significantly reduce morbidity and mortality. The radiologist has a further responsibility to help prevent traumatic injury to the colon induced by necessary diagnostic procedures. Prompt recognition in such situations allows timely and appropriate therapy.

REFERENCES

1. Burrell, M., Toffler, R., and Lowman, R.: Blunt trauma to the abdomen and gastrointestinal tract, Radiol. Clin. North Am. 11:561, 1973.
2. Westcott, J. L., and Smith, J. R. V.: Mesentery and colon injuries secondary to blunt trauma, Radiology 114:597, 1975.
3. Howell, H. S., Bartizal, J. F., and Freeark, R. J.: Blunt trauma involving the colon and rectum, J. Trauma 16:624, 1976.
4. Williams, R. D., and Sargent, F. T.: The mechanism of intestinal injury in trauma, J. Trauma 3:288, 1963.
5. Williams, J. S., and Kirkpatrick, J. R.: The nature of seat belt injuries, J. Trauma 11:207, 1971.
6. Towne, J. B., and Coe, J. D.: Seat belt trauma of the colon, Am. J. Surg. 122:683, 1971.
7. Williams, J. S., Lies, B. A., Jr., and Hale, H. W., Jr.: The automotive safety belt: In saving a life may produce intra-abdominal injuries, J. Trauma 6:303, 1966.
8. Nance, F. C., and Crowder, V. H.: Intramural hematoma of the colon following blunt trauma to the abdomen, Am. Surg. 34:85, 1968.
9. Mays, E. T., and Noer, R. J.: Colonic stenosis after trauma, J. Trauma 6:316, 1966.
10. Wightman, J. A. K.: Delayed traumatic rupture of colon with colocutaneous fistula, Br. Med. J. 2:93, 1967.
11. Wanebo, H. J., Hunt, T. K., and Mathewson, C., Jr.: Rectal injuries, J. Trauma 9:712, 1969.
12. Berman, A. T., and Tom, L.: Traumatic separation of the pubic symphysis with associated fatal rectal tear: A case report and analysis of mechanism of injury, J. Trauma 14:1060, 1974.
13. Bartizal, J. F., Boyd, D. R., Folk, F. A., Smith, D., Lescher, T. C., and Freeark, R. J.: A critical review of management of 392 colonic and rectal injuries, Dis. Colon Rectum 17:313, 1974.
14. Das, P. B.: Penetrating injury of the diaphragm with herniated colon leaking into the left pleural space, Int. Surg. 62:463, 1977.
15. Maleki, M., and Evans, W. E.: Foreign-body perforation of the intestinal tract, Arch. Surg. 101:475, 1970.
16. MacManus, J. E.: Perforations of the intestine by ingested foreign bodies, Am. J. Surg. 53:393, 1941.
17. Cleator, I. G. M., and Christie, J.: An unusual case of swallowed dental plate and perforation of the sigmoid colon, Br. J. Surg. 60:163, 1973.
18. Bunker, P. G.: The role of dentistry in problems of foreign body in the air and food passage, J. Am. Dent. Assoc. 64:782, 1962.
19. Berk, R. N., and Reit, R. J.: Intra-abdominal chicken-bone abscess, Radiology 101:311, 1971.
20. Kimbrell, F. T., Jr., Tepas, J. J., and Mullen, J. T.: Chicken bone perforation of the sigmoid colon: A report of three cases, Am. Surg. 41:814, 1975.
21. Rosenberg, I. L., and Smiddy, F. G.: Insufflation injury of the bowel, Arch. Surg. 105:113, 1972.
22. Thiele, B. L.: Compressed air injury of the colon: A report of two cases, Aust. NZ J. Surg. 43:49, 1973.
23. Wolf, L., and Geraci, K.: Colonoscopic removal of balloons from the bowel, Gastrointest. Endosc. 24: 41, 1977.
24. Turell, R.: Sexual problems as seen by proctologist, NY State J. Med., 74:697, 1974.
25. Saghir, M. T., and Robins, E.: *Male and Female Homosexuality* (Baltimore: Williams & Wilkins Co., 1973), p. 52.
26. Seaman, W. B., and Wells, J.: Complications of the barium enema, Gastroenterology 48:728, 1965.
27. Nelson, J. A., Daniels, A. U., and Dodds, W. J.: Rectal balloons: Complications, causes and recommendations, presented at the Society of Gastrointestinal Radiologists, 1978 Annual Meeting, Osage Beach, Missouri.
28. Seaman, W. B., and Bragg, D. G.: Colonic intramural barium: A complication of the barium-enema examination, Radiology 89:250, 1967.
29. Lull, G. F., Jr., Bryne, J. P., and Sanowski, R. A.: Barium sulfate granuloma of the rectum, J.A.M.A. 217:1102, 1971.
30. Seltzer, S. E., and Jones, B.: Cecal perforation associated with Gastrografin enema, Am. J. Roentgenol. 130:997, 1978.
31. Kahn, S. P., Lindenauer, S. M., and Wojtalik, R. S.: Perforation of the normal colon during barium contrast examination, Am. Surg. 42:789, 1976.
32. Yudis, M., Cohen, A., and Pearce, A. E.: Perforation of the transverse colon during barium enema and air-contrast studies, Am. Surg. 34:334, 1968.
33. Kiser, J. L., Spratt, J. S., Jr., and Johnson, C. A.: Colon perforations occurring during sigmoidoscopic examinations and barium enemas, Mo. Med. 65: 969, 1968.
34. Hamit, H. F.: Perforation of the colon after barium

enema and air contrast studies, Am. Surg. 21:1226, 1955.

35. Marshak, R. H., and Lindner, A. E.: Ulcerative and Granulomatous Colitis, in Margulis, A. R., and Burhenne, H. J. (eds.): *Alimentary Tract Roentgenology, Vol. 2* (St. Louis: C. V. Mosby Co., 1967).
36. Wruble, L. D., and Bronstein, M. W.: Toxic dilatation of the colon following barium enema examination during the quiescent stage of chronic ulcerative colitis, Am. J. Dig. Dis. 13:918, 1968.
37. Carney, J. A., and Stephens, D. H.: Intramural barium (barium granuloma) of colon and rectum, Gastroenterology 65:316, 1973.
38. Silverberg, D., and Rogers, A. G.: Toxic megacolon in ulcerative colitis, Can. Med. Assoc. J. 90: 357, 1964.
39. Richman, L. S., Short, W. F., and Cooper, W. M.: Barium enema septicemia, J.A.M.A. 226:62, 1973.
40. Juler, G. L., Dietrick, W. R., and Eisenman, J. I.: Intramesenteric perforation of sigmoid diverticulitis with non-fatal venous intravasation, Am. J. Surg. 132:653, 1976.
41. Mason, G. R., Dietrich, P., Friedland, G. W., and Hanks, G. E.: The radiological findings in radiation-induced enteritis and colitis. A review of 30 cases, Clin. Radiol. 21:232, 1970.
42. Meyers, M. A., and Ghahremani, G. G.: Complications of gastrointestinal fiberoptic endoscopy, Gastrointest. Radiol. 2:273, 1977.
43. Livstone, E. M., and Kerstein, M. D.: Serosal tears following colonoscopy, Arch. Surg. 111:88, 1976.
44. Given, F. T., Jr., Old, L., Jr., and Lehew, W. L.: Colon and rectal injuries in gynecological surgery, Va. Med. 93:320, 1966.
45. Tobias, S.: Perforation of the transverse colon following external cardiac massage, Arch. Surg. 94: 335, 1967.
46. Thompson, W. M., Seigler, H. F., and Rice, R. P.: Ileocolonic perforation: A complication following renal transplantation, Am. J. Roentgenol. 125:723, 1975.
47. Thompson, W. M., Meyers, W., Seigler, H. F., and Rice, R. P.: Gastrointestinal complication of renal transplantation, Semin. Roentgenol. 13:319, 1978.
48. Fonkalsrud, E. W., and Clatworthy, H. W., Jr.: Accidental perforation of the colon and rectum in newborn infants, N. Engl. J. Med. 272:1097, 1965.
49. Greenbaum, E. I., Carson, M., Kincannon, W. N., and O'Loughlin, B. J.: Rectal thermometer-induced pneumoperitoneum in the newborn, Pediatrics 44: 539, 1969.

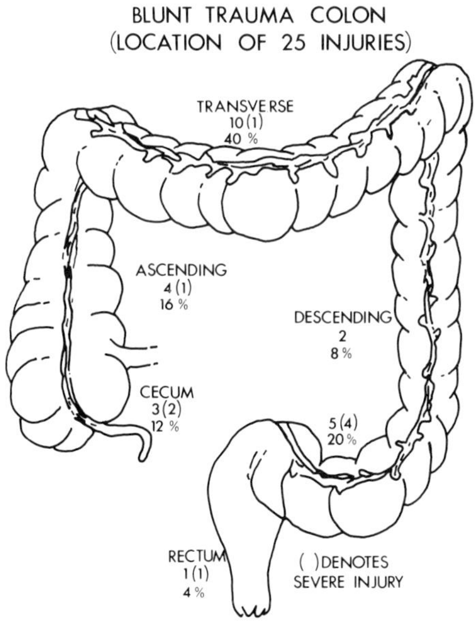

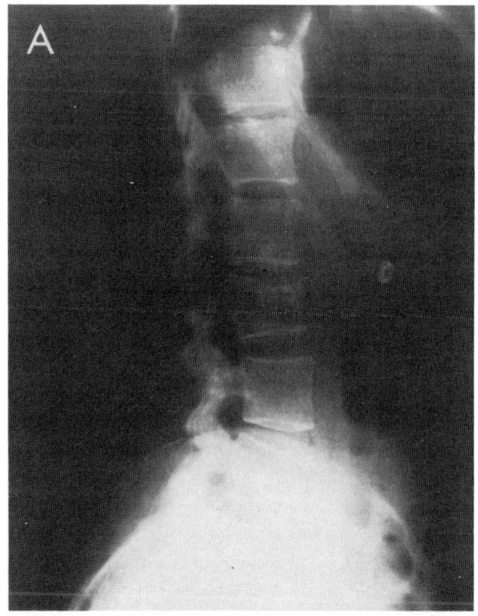

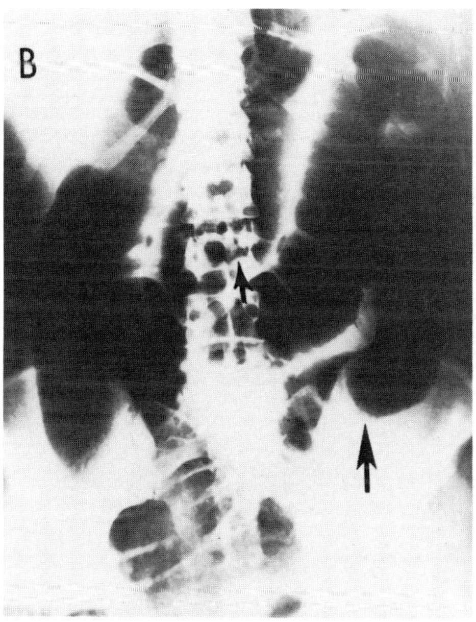

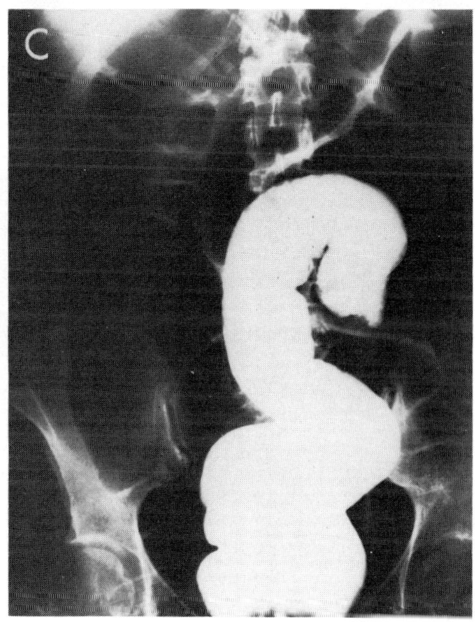

Fig 42–1 (top left).—Location, incidence and severity of 25 colon injuries in 19 patients who sustained blunt trauma. (From Howell, Bartizal and Freeark, J. Trauma 16:624, 1976. Copyright 1976, The Williams & Wilkins Co. Reprinted with permission.)

Fig 42–2 (top right and bottom).—Lap belt trauma. **A,** lateral lumbar spine: compression fracture of L3. **B,** plain film: large bowel obstruction down to level of sigmoid (*large arrow*). Also note horizontal splitting fracture through posterior elements L3 (*small arrow*). **C,** barium enema: transected sigmoid, which sealed spontaneously proximally and was plugged with omentum distally. No peritoneal spill of barium. (From Howell, Bartizal and Freeark, J. Trauma 16:624, 1976. Copyright 1976, The Williams & Wilkins Co. Reprinted with permission.)

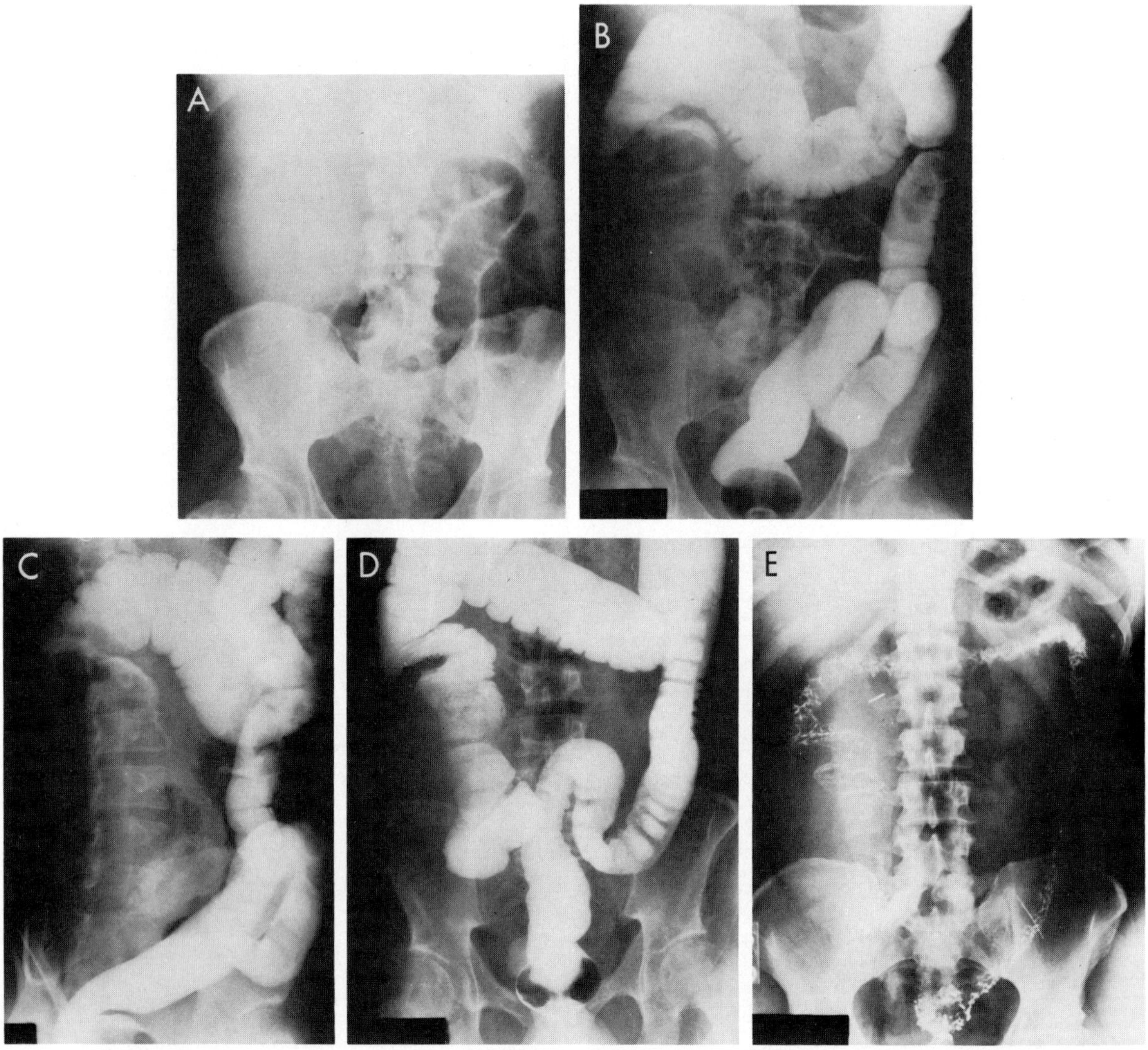

Fig 42-3.—Pericolonic hematoma with both pain and obstruction in man who ran into fire hydrant while intoxicated. **A,** plain film: right-sided abdominal mass and small bowel obstruction. **B,** Gastrografin enema: almost complete obstruction below hepatic flexure. **C,** Gastrografin enema: LPO view showing mass effect and obstruction. **D,** barium enema 1 month later: obstructive symptoms resolved. Mass effect of pericolonic hematoma seen displacing ascending colon and cecum toward midline. **E,** postevacuation film: barium enema. Mass effect again seen.

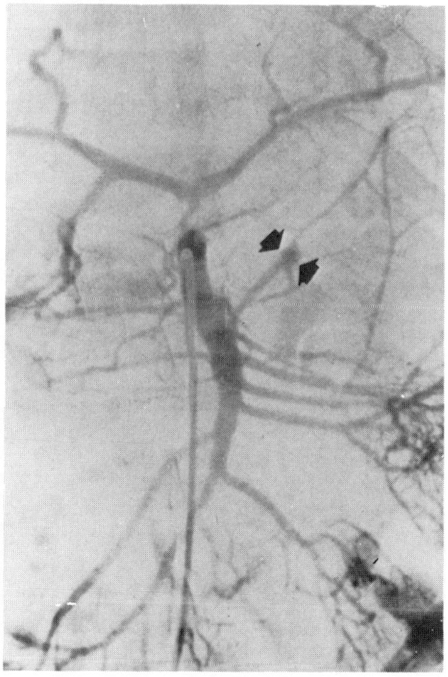

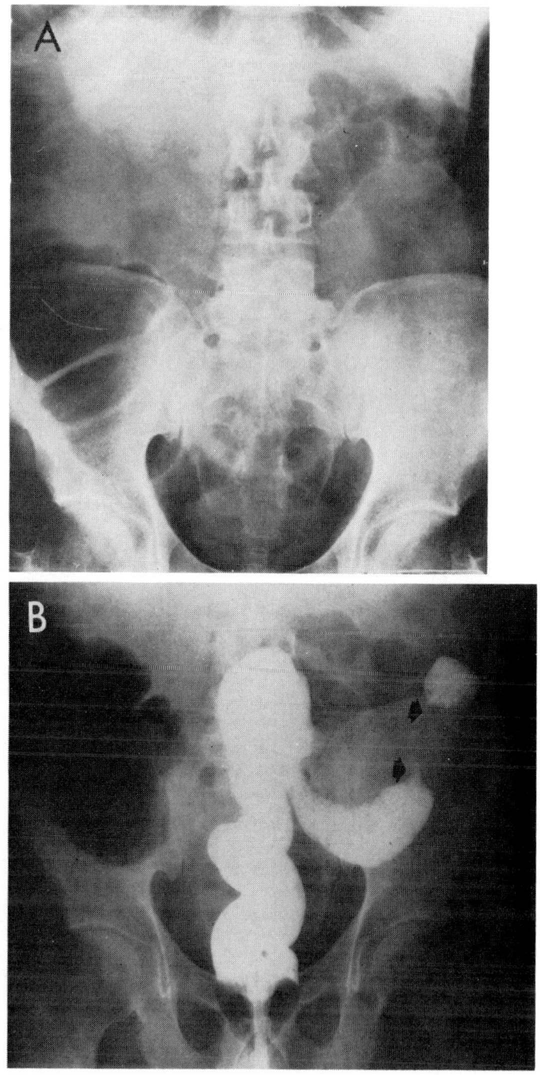

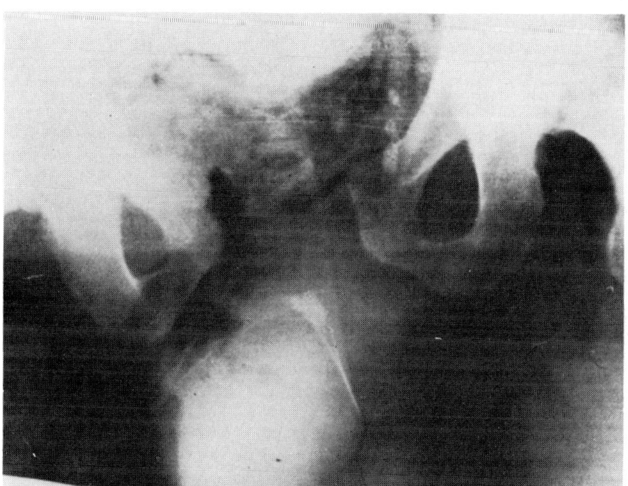

Fig 42–4 (top left).—Superior mesenteric artery angiogram. False aneurysm *(arrows)* of middle colic artery in automobile accident victim with signs of blood loss and abdominal pain. At surgery, large hematoma of left mesocolon and old blood in abdominal cavity were found. (From Westcott and Smith, Radiology 114:597, 1975, with permission.)

Fig 42–5 (right).—Chronic intramural hematoma caused by steering wheel trauma. **A,** plain film: dilatation of colon from cecum to lower descending colon. Obstructive symptoms developed 2 weeks post trauma. **B,** barium enema: almost complete obstruction by intramural hematoma *(arrows)* 4 weeks post trauma. (From Westcott and Smith, Radiology 114:597, 1975, with permission.)

Fig 42–6 (bottom left).—Anorectal-cutaneous fistula with soft tissue emphysema from rectal tear accompanying traumatic diastasis of symphysis pubis. (From Berman and Tom, J. Trauma 14:1060, 1974. Copyright 1976, The Williams & Wilkins Co. Reprinted with permission.)

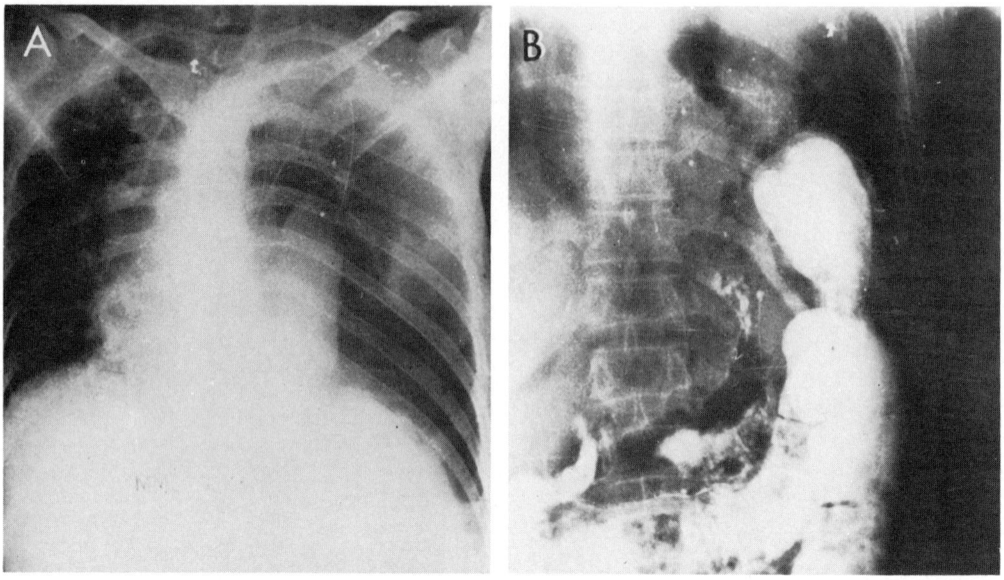

Fig 42-7—Herniation of colon into thorax following stab wound to left lower chest wall. **A,** tension pneumothorax 2 days posttrauma. **B,** herniation of colon into thorax 12 hours after insertion of left chest tube. High intrathoracic pressures prior to chest tube insertion probably prevented bowel from herniating earlier. (From Das, Int. Surg. 62: 463, 1977, with permission.)

Fig 42-8.—Chicken bone perforation of sigmoid in edentulous patient. **A,** plain film: chicken bone *(arrows)* seen in pelvis. **B,** postevacuation film (barium enema examination): displacement of sigmoid by mass *(arrowheads)* containing the bone *(arrow)*. The bone perforated a diverticulum and produced perisigmoid abscess. (From Berk and Reit, Radiology 101:311, 1971, with permission.)

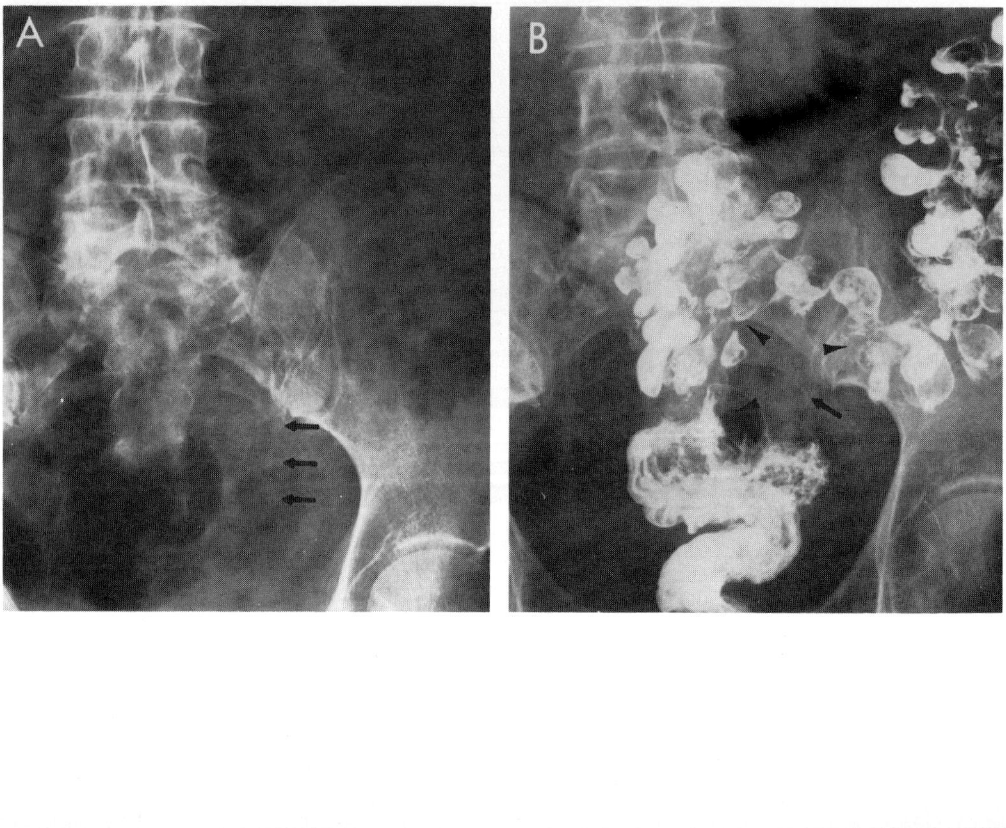

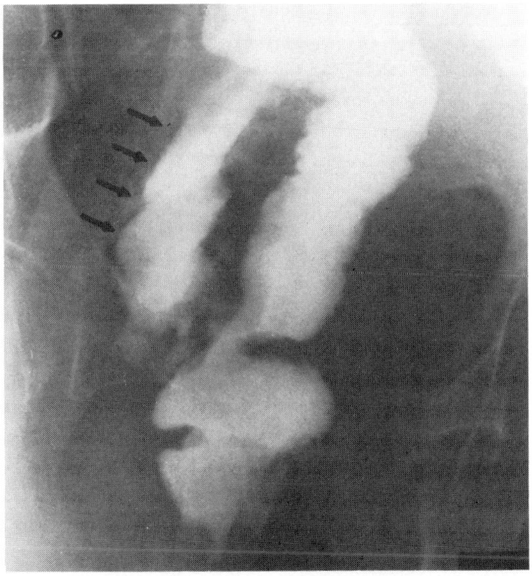

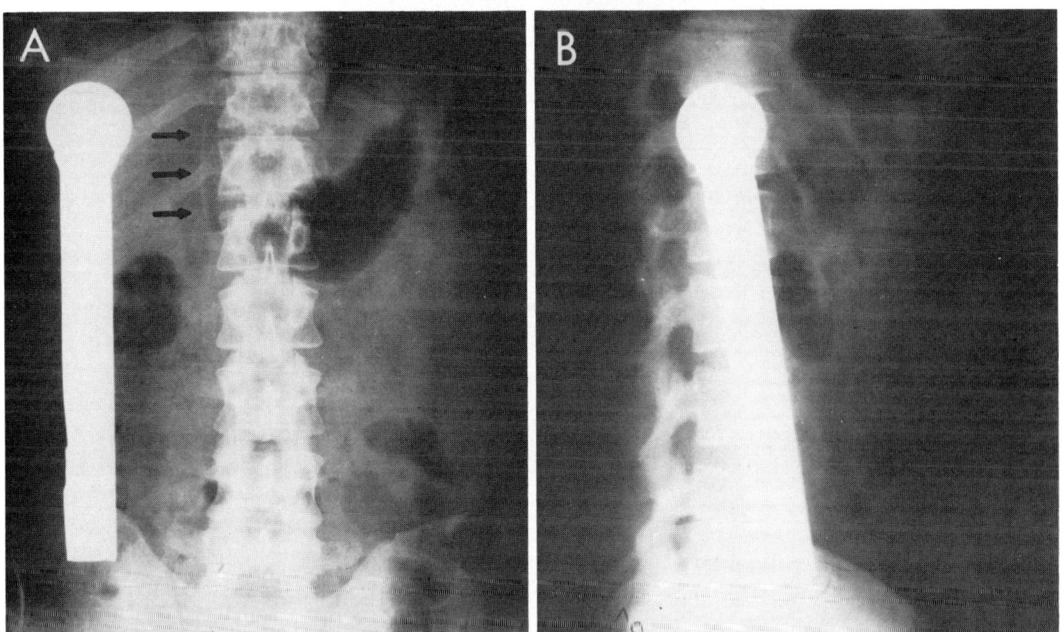

Fig 42–9 (top).—Water-soluble contrast enema. Extravasation of contrast *(arrows)* into peritoneal cavity after plunger handle induced rectal trauma.

Fig 42–10 (bottom).—**A,** plain film: metallic dildo free in abdominal cavity. Falciform ligament *(arrows),* indicating massive pneumoperitoneum, is seen. **B,** lateral projection: showing intra-abdominal position of metallic dildo. (Courtesy of Dr. E. R. Dana, Orange, Calif.)

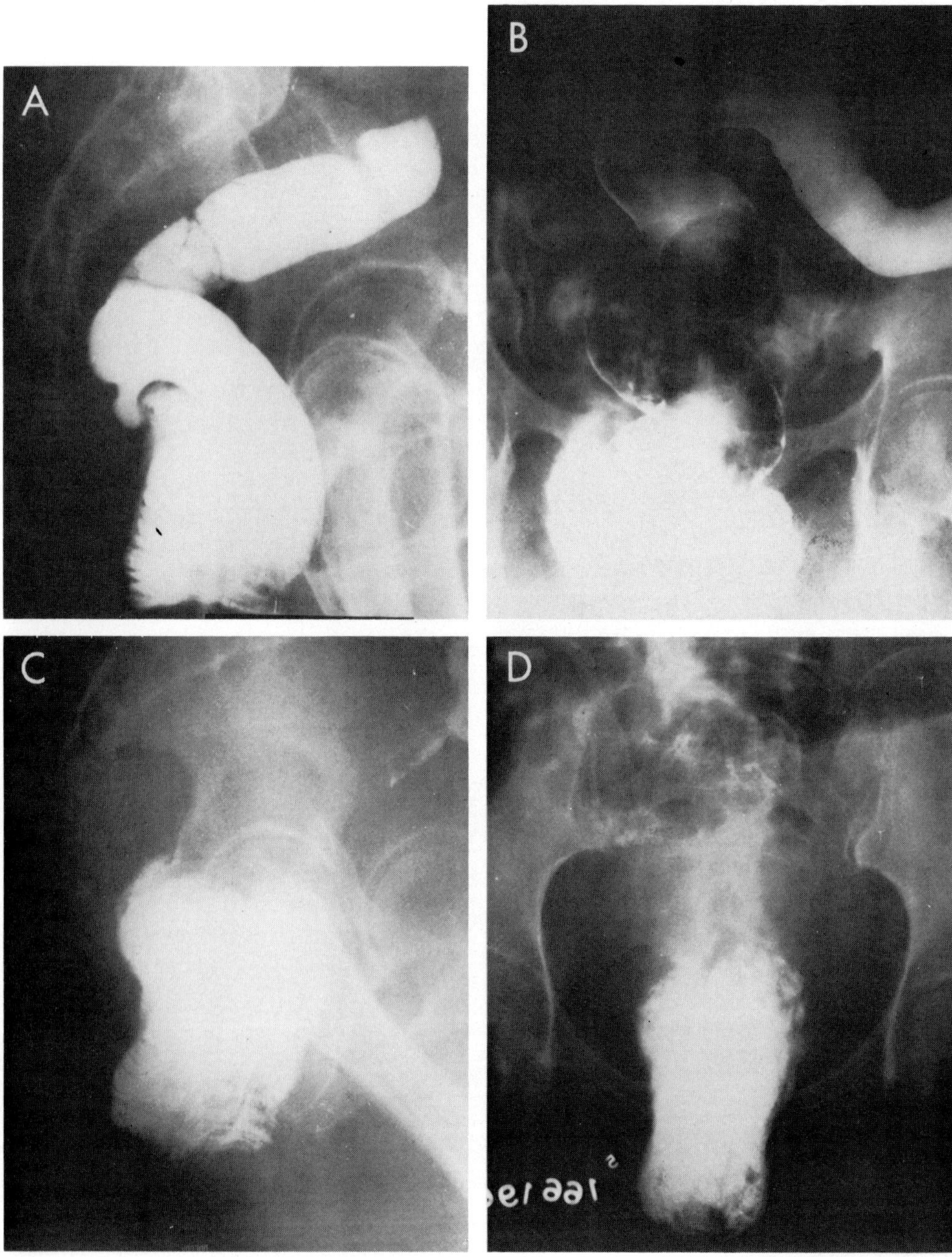

Fig 42–11.—Intramural barium following barium enema. **A,** lateral view of rectum: intramural dissection of barium seen in inner circular muscle fiber layer. **B,** frontal view of rectum: intramural barium. **C,** lateral view of rectum: post evacuation retention of intramural barium. **D,** frontal view of rectum: persistence of perirectal barium 4 days post procedure. (From Seaman and Bragg, Radiology 89:250, 1967, with permission.)

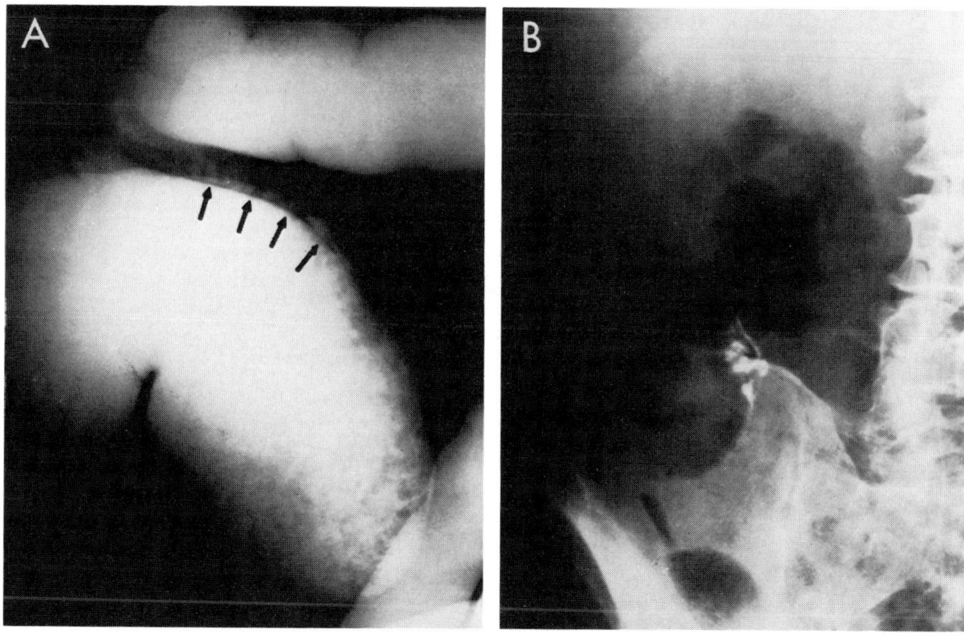

Fig 42-12.—Intramural barium following barium enema. **A,** intramural barium in medial wall of radiologically normal cecum *(arrows)*. **B,** residual intramural barium 5½ months post procedure. (From Seaman and Bragg, Radiology 89:250, 1967, with permission.)

Fig 42-13.—Cecal perforation associated with Gastrografin enema. Hypertonic solution in closed loop caused progressive distension and rupture. **A,** Gastrografin enema showing partial colonic obstruction by fecaloma *(arrowhead)* at rectosigmoid junction. **B,** abdominal film 24 hours later showing progressive cecal enlargement. Large amount of Gastrografin is retained. Later the same day cecum perforated and at laparotomy fecal soiling of peritoneum was noted. (From Seltzer and Jones, Am. J. Roentgenol. 130:997, 1978, with permission.)

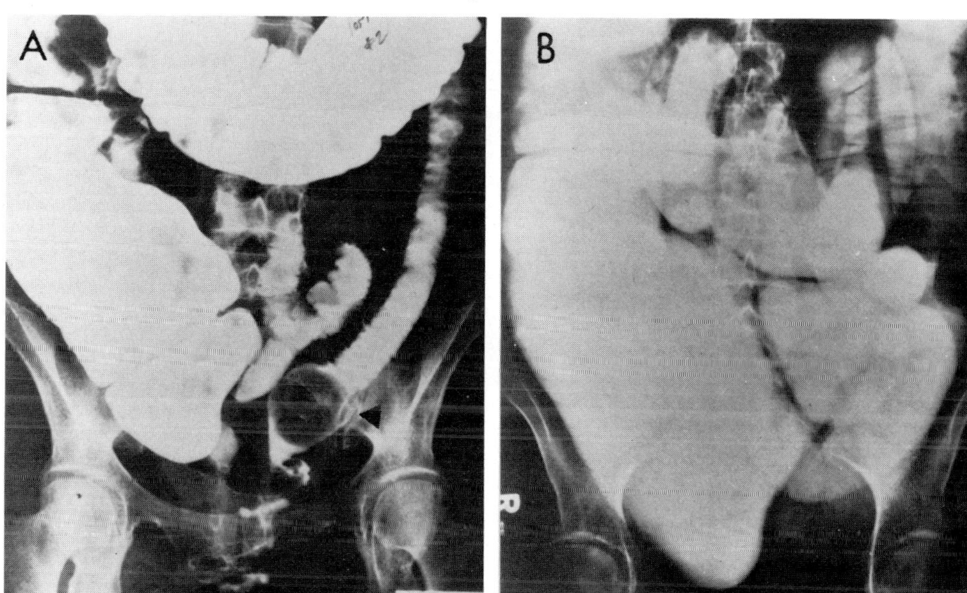

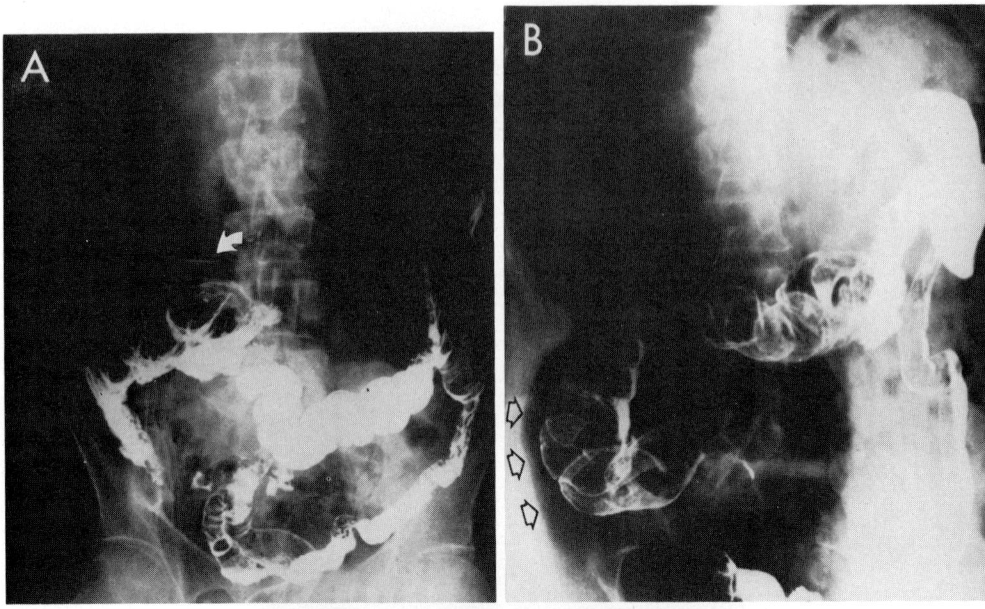

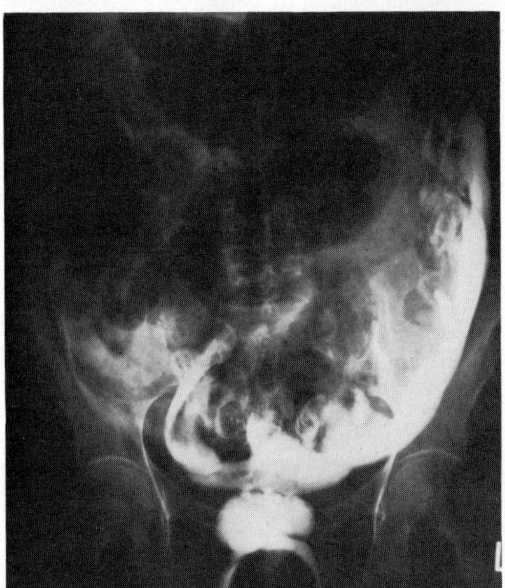

Fig 42–14 (top).—Air contrast barium enema-induced colonic perforation. **A,** air contrast barium enema: thin streak of intraperitoneal barium *(arrow)* seen above hepatic flexure. Massive amount of air in upper quadrants. **B,** left decubitus view, same patient. Large amount of air seen outlining cecum *(arrows)*. (From Kahn, Lindenauer and Wojtalik, Am. Surg. 42:789, 1976. Copyright 1976, J. B. Lippincott Co. Reprinted with permission.)

Fig 42–15 (bottom).—Contrast enema. Intraperitoneal extravasation of water-soluble contrast from rectal carcinoma perforation above peritoneal reflection.

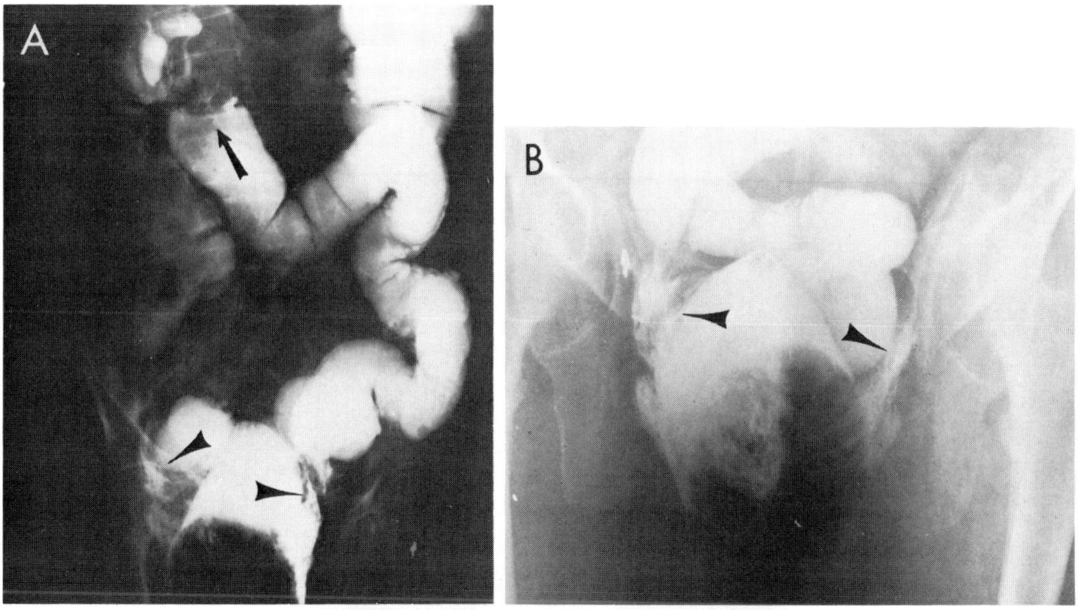

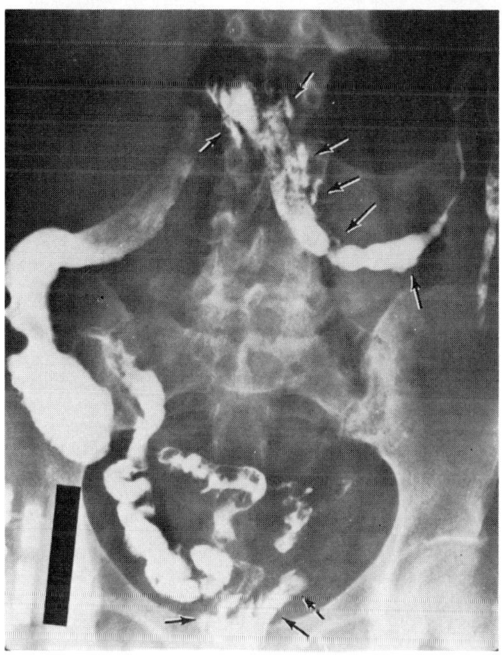

Fig 42–16 (top).—**A,** barium enema: retroperitoneal extravasation of barium *(arrowheads)* from rectal carcinoma perforation below peritoneal reflection. Note another carcinoma at hepatic flexure *(arrow).* **B,** Ferguson view: retroperitoneal barium extravasation *(arrowheads)* seen in different projection. (Courtesy of E. I. Greenbaum, Los Angeles, Calif.)

Fig 42–17 (bottom).—Barium enema in patient with transverse colon colostomy secondary to surgical procedure for ulcerative colitis. Intramural barium is seen in both transverse colon and rectum *(arrows).* Narrowing of colon caused by ulcerative colitis is evident. (From Carney and Stephens, Gastroenterology 65:316, 1973. Copyright 1973, The Williams & Wilkins Co. Reprinted with permission.)

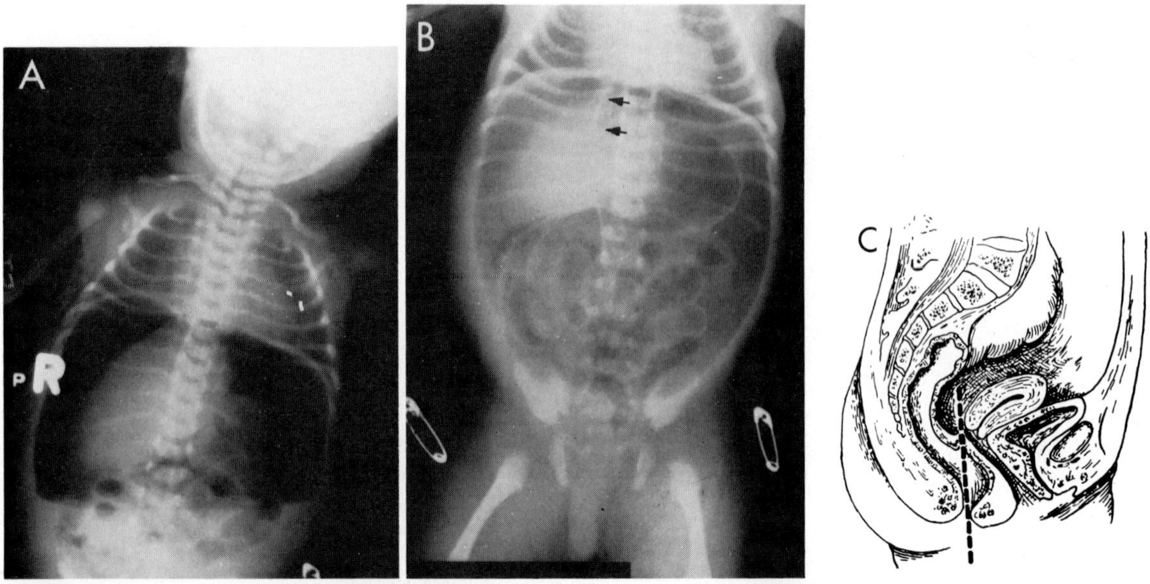

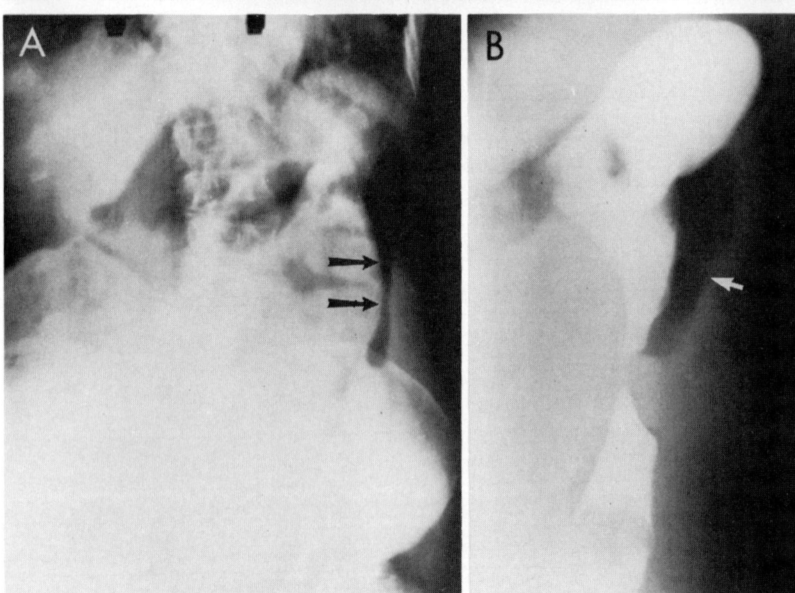

Fig 42–18 (top).—Rectal thermometer-induced colonic perforation. **A,** upright abdomen: massive amount of free air. **B,** supine abdomen: air outlines liver; falciform ligament *(arrows)* seen. Inner and outer walls of hollow viscera are outlined with air. **C,** line drawing of abdomen at midsagittal plane. In newborn infants, distance between anus and peritoneal reflection is less than 3 cm. If rectal thermometer is advanced past 3 cm and not directed posteriorly, it will penetrate anterior wall of rectum above peritoneal reflection. (From Greenbaum et al., Pediatrics 44:539, 1969, by permission. Copyright 1969, American Academy of Pediatrics. Reprinted with permission.)

Fig 42–19 (bottom).—Cleansing enema tip-induced rectal perforation. **A,** supine abdomen: extraperitoneal air *(arrows)* adjacent to descending colon. **B,** water-soluble contrast study: splenic flexure and extraperitoneal air seen in detail *(arrow)*. Perforation of rectum distal to peritoneal reflection seen on other views. (Courtesy of Dr. Edward I. Greenbaum, Los Angeles, Calif.)

Chapter 43

Tuberculosis of the Colon

S. CHAWLA, M.D.

HIPPOCRATES considered tuberculous enteritis a very serious complication of pulmonary tuberculosis and noted that "Phthisical persons, the hairs of whose head fall off, die if diarrhoea sets in . . . . diarrhoea attacking a person with phthisis is a mortal symptom."[30]

One of the earliest references to tuberculosis of the gastrointestinal tract is that of Virordt,[45] who in 1643 reported the finding in Louis XIII of an ulcerative, inflammatory process of the intestine in association with a large pulmonary cavity.

The use of radiologic methods for diagnosis of intestinal tuberculosis was first reported by Stierlin[42] in 1911.

Tuberculosis of the Intestinal Tract

PATHOGENESIS

Tuberculosis of the intestinal tract may occur either by ingestion of infected sputum or by swallowing infected food containing tubercle bacilli.[31, 32] These organisms make entry from the intestinal mucosa and colonize in the lymphoid follicles. Macroscopically the tuberculous lesion presents as either the hypertrophic, ulcerative or ulcerohypertrophic type.[1, 36]

The serous surface of the bowel may be studded with tubercles or covered with plastic exudate. Mesenteric lymph nodes may be enlarged, caseated or calcified. The hypertrophic type commonly affects the ileocecal region, but solitary or multiple lesions in the ileum and large bowel are also found. The cecum, adjacent ascending colon and terminal ileum are contracted and thickened and form a tumor-like mass. The ileum proximal to the lesion is dilated and rigid. In the ulcerative type, the ulcers are small and shallow and circumferentially placed. Perforation is not common. Healing occurs by fibrosis, producing strictures. In the ulcerohypertrophic type, the ulcers heal by fibrosis and there is thickening of the intestinal wall.

Histologically the tubercular granuloma is characterized by central caseation surrounded by epithelioid cells and Langhans' giant cells, with peripheral collection of lymphocytes, plasma cells and fibroblasts. The neighboring blood vessels show endarteritic changes. The typical tubercular lesion may be seen only in the draining mesenteric lymph nodes, whereas nonspecific changes may be present in the intestinal wall (Fig 43–1).

CLINICAL FEATURES

The incidence of the disease is highest from the 2d to the 4th decades of life, and it occurs more often in females and in people of low socioeconomic status.[26, 36, 47] General systemic disorders lower body resistance and render the person more susceptible to tuberculous infection.

Clinical manifestations are variable. Abdominal pain, weight loss, pyrexia, diarrhea, nausea and abdominal distention are the usual presenting features. Passage of blood per rectum is uncommon except in tubercular lesions of the distal colon.

Rarely the patient may present with acute intestinal obstruction, perforation or intussusception.

The patient may be malnourished and chronically ill if tuberculosis of the intestinal tract is associated with an extensive pulmonary lesion. Peripheral lymph nodes may be enlarged. Abdominal examination may reveal a doughy abdomen; abdominal tenderness; or a tender, fixed mass in the right iliac fossa since the ileocecal region is the most common site of involvement. Signs of subacute or chronic intestinal obstruction are often present.

The Mantoux test and erythrocyte sedimentation rate may only occasionally be of diagnostic value.[9] Sputum examination may fail to demonstrate tubercle bacilli,[16] or it may be positive, owing to endobronchial tuberculosis, although the chest x-ray may be normal.[7]

Diagnosis of intestinal tuberculosis is confirmed by culture and animal inoculation of suspected tissue, demonstration of acid-fast bacilli in the lesion or the presence of tubercles with caseation necrosis in the bowel wall or in mesenteric lymph nodes.

RADIOLOGIC DIAGNOSIS

Stierlin[42] in 1911 reported nonfilling of the cecum and ascending colon in cases of ileocecal tuberculosis 6 or 7 hours after ingestion of barium meal while the terminal ileum and transverse colon were filled. The importance of barium enema examination in radiologic diagnosis of abdominal tuberculosis and the necessity of doing barium meal study and barium enema examination under fluoroscopy was emphasized in 1946.[2]

The routine radiologic investigations required in suspected cases of tuberculosis of the colon are radiogram of the chest, plain x-ray of the abdomen, barium enema with or without double contrast and a barium meal follow-up study.

X-ray of the chest may be normal in a patient with abdominal tuberculosis. In about 20% of patients, associated active pulmonary tuberculosis has been observed.[19, 46]

Plain X-ray of the Abdomen

In patients presenting with subacute or acute obstruction at the ileocecal region or in the distal colon, erect and supine films show distention and air-fluid levels in the proximal bowel. Absence of gas shadows in the right iliac fossa or distortion of gas shadow of the cecum and ascending colon is commonly found in the presence of an ileocecal mass.

Associated small bowel strictures and ascites may be seen as dilated small bowel loops, with increased distance between the adjacent loops and general haziness and blurring of bowel outline on plain x-ray.

Free perforation is uncommon in tuberculosis of the colon but, when present, is seen as air under the domes of the diaphragm.

Enteroliths may be seen in small bowel or in colon proximal to an obstruction (Fig 43–2).

All the above radiologic signs are nonspecific. Associated pulmonary lesions or calcified abdominal lymph nodes favor the diagnosis of tuberculosis (see Fig 43–28, A).

Contrast Study of the Colon

Large bowel lesions are best delineated by conventional barium enema or double contrast study. However, filling of the cecum can be confirmed only if there is spill into the terminal ileum, which does not always occur.

The importance of ingested barium in study of ileocecal lesions has been emphasized.[10, 24, 25, 27] In colonic tuberculosis, antegrade barium study is an especially useful adjunct to barium enema, as it helps to outline not only the cecum and the terminal ileum but also the associated lesions in the proximal small bowel.

Ileocecal Tuberculosis

The incidence of ileocecal tuberculosis has been reported in 80–90% of all cases of intestinal tuberculosis.[3, 4, 26, 37]

As early as 1849 Rokitansky[41] emphasized that the first tubercles investing the intestinal tract are found in the lymphoid tissue and that this tissue, being abundant in the region of the cecum and the terminal ileum, explains the predilection of tuberculosis for the ileocecal region.

RADIOLOGIC SIGNS

In a predominantly hypertrophic lesion, barium enema may reveal a complete obstruction, and differentiation from malignancy may be impossible (Fig 43–3). If obstruction is incomplete, a streak of barium may outline all that is left of the lumen of the ascending colon. Associated fibrosis and contraction help to make a correct preoperative diagnosis (Fig 43–4).

More often there is no obstruction to the flow of barium but, rather, nonfilling of the cecum, stenosis and contraction of the ascending colon, with pulling up of the dilated terminal ileum, giving the radiologic appearance of the terminal ileum's being continuous with the hepatic flexure (Fig 43–5). The terminal ileum may be normal, dilated or ulcerated (Figs 43–6 to 43–10).

Hypertrophic lesions may result in a conical cecum with filling defects and a stenosed ascending colon (Fig 43–11).

The hypertrophied masses may project into the lumen of the cecum and ascending colon; the coexisting contraction helps to make a correct diagnosis (Fig 43–12).

In ileocecal tuberculosis, the ileocecal valve may show a tendency to gape because of ulceration or granulation that progresses to fibrosis and results in retraction of the valve lips. Radiologically this may be seen as a patulous opening of the terminal ileum into the cecum (Fig 43–13) or as a broad-based, triangular appearance of the terminal ileum, with the base toward the cecum—Fleischner's sign[22]. The ileocecal angle may become altered owing to fibrosis, and the ileum may appear to enter the cecum at a right angle (Fig 43–14) or to make an angle of 180 degrees with the ascending colon (see Figs 43–6, A, and 43–7).

In 19% of cases, ileocecal tuberculosis is associated with small bowel strictures.[4, 19] Any part of the small bowel may be involved, but the lesion is more common in the distal ileum. Barium enema may outline these lesions, but antegrade barium studies are essential for better delineation (Fig 43–15). Rarely, instead of a localized stricture, a long segment of the ileum may be involved, with loss of mucosa. The segment may resemble a narrow, rigid tube (Fig 43–16).

There may be marked stasis and dilution of the ingested barium in the small intestine (Fig 43–17).

Enterolithiasis

Enteroliths may form proximal to mechanical obstruction in the small or large bowel. The stenosis may be the result of Crohn's disease, malignancy, tuberculosis or previous surgery.[8, 12, 21, 28, 33, 40]

Enterolith formation proximal to tubercular strictures have been reported.[11, 38, 44] The incidence has been placed at 3.25% in intestinal tuberculosis.[17] The chemical composition of an enterolith is related to the site of formation. All enteroliths high in the intestine contain nonopaque choleic acid; those found at lower levels contain mostly calcium salts and hence are radiopaque. The enteroliths may be differentiated from other abdominal and pelvic opacities by their wide mobility and scattered distribution.[17]

Although plain x-ray of the abdomen reveals the presence of radiopaque enteroliths, contrast study of the gastrointestinal tract is essential to outline the stenosis (Figs 43-18 and 43-19). Rarely ileocecal tuberculosis with associated enlarged mesenteric glands and adhesions may cause extrinsic pressure on the duodenum and present as duodenal obstruction (Fig 43-20).

In tuberculosis of the cecum, the adjacent ascending colon is commonly involved. However, the lesion in the ascending colon may be remote from the involved ileocecal region, a normal segment intervening (Fig 43-21). The hypertrophied lesion may involve the ascending colon, whereas the cecum may be normal (Fig 43-22).

Tuberculosis of the Distal Colon

The tubercular process may involve colon distal to the cecum and ascending colon. In the absence of ileocecal tuberculosis, diagnosis of colonic tuberculosis is exceedingly difficult. It is probable that segmental involvement of the distal colon by tuberculosis is not as uncommon as the paucity of reported cases suggests. A total of 77 cases of segmental tuberculosis of the distal colon were reported in the English literature up to 1971. Ten additional cases were reported in the same year.[18] The lesion may occur anywhere in the colon. Of the 63 cases collected from the world literature, the sigmoid colon was involved in 37, followed in order of frequency by the transverse colon and descending colon. Multiple lesions were seen in three cases.[26] In India, where tubercular enterocolitis is not an uncommon disease, in a series of 24 patients with involvement of the distal colon, the transverse colon was the most common site of involvement, followed by the descending colon and rectosigmoid.[19]

The lesion may be solitary or multiple (Figs 43-23 and 43-24). Chronic obstruction may lead to enterolith formation in the proximal segment of the intestine (Fig 43-25). Although the tubercular strictures usually are smooth and concentric, they may be eccentric and irregular with an adjacent colon that appears normal (Fig 43-26).

Diffuse enterocolitis due to tuberculosis has been reported infrequently. Three cases have been reported in young patients with normal chest x-rays. Radiologic appearances suggested ulcerative colitis, but the rectum was normal.[13, 23] Diffuse colitis of tubercular cause usually is associated with an ileocecal lesion. The extent of colonic involvement is variable: it may be limited (Fig 43-27) or extensive, up to the splenic flexure (Fig 43-28) or up to middescending colon (Fig 43-29).

The radiologic appearances of contraction, loss of haustrations and pseudopolyps may simulate extensive ulcerative colitis (Figs 43-30 and 43-31), except that the lesion is right-sided, involving the ileocecal region and sparing the rectum.

In localized involvement of the distal colon, the sigmoid is the most common site (Fig 43-32);[26, 39] the rectum rarely is involved.[20] Recently five cases of tuberculosis of the sigmoid have been reported from Nigeria and South Africa.[34, 46] The radiologic appearance may simulate Crohn's disease[39] or ulcerative colitis. However, internal fistulas are a rare complication of intestinal tuberculosis.[35, 39]

Differential Diagnosis

Radiologic appearances in tuberculosis of the large bowel may closely resemble Crohn's disease, malignancy, amebiasis, ulcerative colitis, ischemic colitis, actinomycosis and nonspecific granulomas.[5, 6, 14, 15, 43] Coexistence of tuberculosis and carcinoma in the colon has been reported.[29]

Diagnosis in some cases may be difficult or impossible. Since chest x-ray may be normal, the final diagnosis can be made only by demonstration of *Mycobacterium tuberculosis*, on biopsy or culture of biopsy.

Although tuberculosis of the intestine is more prevalent in the developing countries, radiologists encounter it occasionally in all parts of the world.

REFERENCES

1. Abrams, J. S., and Holden, W. D.: Tuberculosis of the gastrointestinal tract, Arch. Surg. 89:282, 1964.
2. Adams, R., and Miller, W. H.: Surgical treatment of intestinal tuberculosis, Surg. Clin. North Am. 26: 656, 1946.
3. Aird, I.: *A Companion in Surgical Studies* (2d ed.; Edinburgh and London: E. & S. Livingstone, Ltd., 1957).
4. Anand, S. S., and Pathak, I. C.: Surgical treatment of abdominal tuberculosis with special reference to ileo-caecal tuberculosis. A record of 100 cases treated surgically, J. Indian Med. Assoc. 37:423, 1961.
5. Anscombe, A. R., Keddie, N. C., and Schofield, P. F.: Caecal tuberculosis, Gut 8:337, 1967.
6. Aronson, A. R., and Slattery, L. R.: Tuberculosis of the transverse colon: Report of case simulating carcinoma, Gastroenterology 36:698, 1959.
7. Ashken, M. H., and Baron, J. H.: Ulcerative tuberculous ileo-colitis with normal chest radiograph, Br. J. Surg. 49:454, 1962.
8. Atwell, J. D., and Pollock, A. V.: Intestinal calculi, Br. J. Surg. 47:367, 1960.
9. Bentley, G., and Webster, J. H. H.: Gastrointestinal tuberculosis, Br. J. Surg. 54:90, 1967.
10. Beranbaum, S. L., and Subbarao, K.: Normal ileocaecal valve, Am. J. Dig. Dis. 22:254, 1955.
11. Bery, K., Virmani, P., and Chawla, S.: Enterolithiasis with tubercular intestinal strictures, Br. J. Radiol. 37:73, 1964.
12. Blix, G.: 1935. Cited by Fowweather, 1955.
13. Bockus, H. L., Tumen, H., and Kornbloom, K.: Diffuse primary tuberculous enterocolitis: Report of 2 cases, Ann. Intern. Med. 13:1461, 1940.
14. Brombart, M., Massion, J., Bodart, P., Dive, C., and Van Trappen, G.: Radiologic differences between ileo-caecal tuberculosis and Crohn's disease, Am. J. Dig. Dis. 6:622, 1961.
15. Cavin, E.: Primary intestinal tuberculosis, United States Armed Forces Med. J. 3:903, 1952.
16. Chandra, A., and Basu, A. K.: Cicatrizing lesions of the ileo-caecal region, Indian J. Surg. 29:645, 1967.
17. Chawla, S., Bery, K., and Indra, K. J.: Enterolithiasis complicating intestinal tuberculosis, Clin. Radiol. 17:274, 1966.
18. Chawla, S., Mukerjee, P., and Bery, K.: Segmental tuberculosis of the colon (a report of ten cases), Clin. Radiol. 22:104, 1971.
19. Chawla, S.: Radiology of abdominal tuberculosis, Indian J. Radiol. 31:260, 1977.
20. Davis, J. W.: Hyperplastic tuberculosis of the rectum, Am. J. Surg. 93:490, 1957.
21. Fowweather, F. S.: True enteroliths of the small intestine, Br. Med. J. 2:1010, 1955.
22. Fleischner, F. G.: 1923. Quoted by Paustian, 1964.
23. Glenn, P. M., and Read, H. S.: Tuberculous ulcerative colitis or ulcerative colitis with superimposed tuberculous infection, Gastroenterology 6:9, 1946.
24. Golden, R.: *Diagnostic Roentgenology, Vol. II* (Baltimore: Williams & Wilkins Co., 1959).
25. Gottlieb, C., Beranbaum, S. L., and Dorfman, M.: Roentgen features of non-malignant periappendiceal and ileo-caecal lesions, Am. J. Dig. Dis. 18:79, 1951.
26. Hancock, D. M.: Hyperplastic tuberculosis of the distal colon, Br. J. Surg. 46:63, 1958.
27. Heitzman, E. R., and Berne, A. S.: Roentgen examination of the caecum and proximal ascending colon with ingested barium, Radiology 76:415, 1961.
28. Hellström, J.: 1929. Cited by Atwell and Pollock, 1960.
29. Hickinbotham, P.: A case of tuberculosis of the colon with carcinoma of the rectum, Br. J. Surg. 37: 360, 1950.
30. Hippocrates quoted by Walsh, J.: Diagnosis of intestinal tuberculosis, Trans. Nat. Assoc. Prev. Tuberc. London 5:217, 1909.
31. Hoon, J. R., Dockerty, M. B., and Pemberton, J., deJ.: Ileo-caecal tuberculosis including a comparison of this disease with non-specific regional enterocolitis and noncaseous tuberculated enterocolitis, Int. Abst. Surg. 91:417, 1950.
32. Horn, R. C., Jr.: Alimentary Tract, in Anderson (ed.): *Pathology, Vol. II* (6th ed.; St. Louis: C. V. Mosby Co., 1971).
33. Kelly, R. E.: Three enteroliths in a single coil of jejunum, Br. J. Surg. 20:168, 1932.
34. Kolawole, T. M., and Lewis, E. A.: A radiologic study of tuberculosis of the abdomen (gastrointestinal tract), Am. J. Roentgenol. 123:348, 1975.
35. Lewis, E. A., and Kolawole, T. M.: Tuberculous ileo-colitis in Ibadan: A clinico-radiological review, Gut 13:646, 1972.
36. Paustian, F. F., and Bockus, H. L.: So-called primary ulcerohypertrophic ileo-caecal tuberculosis, Am. J. Med. 27:509, 1959.
37. Paustian, F. F.: Tuberculosis of the Intestines, in Bockus, H. L. (ed.): *Gastroenterology Vol. II* (2d ed.; Philadelphia and London: W. B. Saunders Co., 1964).
38. Prakash, A., Bapna, B. C., Rao, B. S., and Chawla, R. C.: Enterolithiasis with multiple tubercular strictures, Can. J. Surg. 6:359, 1963.
39. Patel, M. P., and De, I.: Segmental tuberculosis of the colon with entero-colic fistula, Br. J. Radiol. 45:150, 1972.
40. Richards, H. J.: Enteroliths of small intestine, Br. Med. J. 2:1384, 1951.
41. Rokitansky, C.: 1849. Quoted by Paustian, 1964.
42. Stierlin, E.: 1911. Quoted by Paustian, 1964.
43. Stock, F. E., and Li, F. W. P.: Granulomas of the large bowel simulating malignant disease, Br. J. Surg. 51:898, 1964.

44. Taneja, O. P.: Enterolithiasis of the ileum associated with multiple tuberculous strictures, Indian J. Surg. 22:173, 1960.
45. Virordt: 1643. Quoted by Harris, W. C.: Intestinal tuberculosis with stenosis and obstruction, Tubercle 33:50, 1952.
46. Werbeloff, L., Novis, B. H., Bank, S., and Marks, I. N.: The radiology of tuberculosis of the gastrointestinal tract, Br. J. Radiol. 46:329, 1973.
47. Wig, K. L., Chitkara, N. L., Gupta, S. P., Kishore, K., and Manchanda, R. L.: Ileo-caecal tuberculosis with particular reference to isolation of *Mycobacterium tuberculosis,* Am. Rev. Respir. Dis. 84:169, 1961.

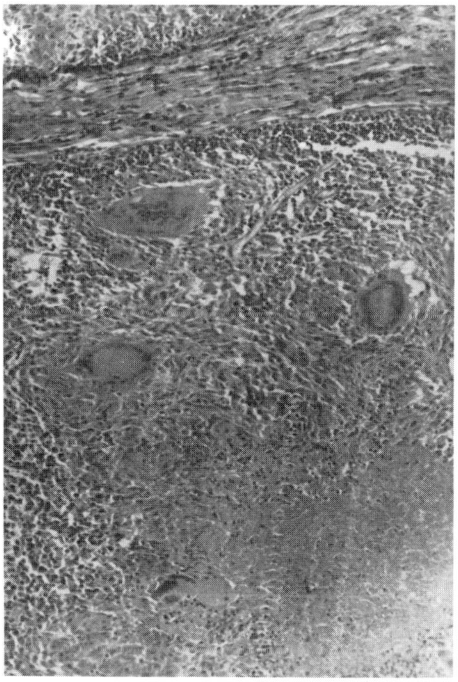

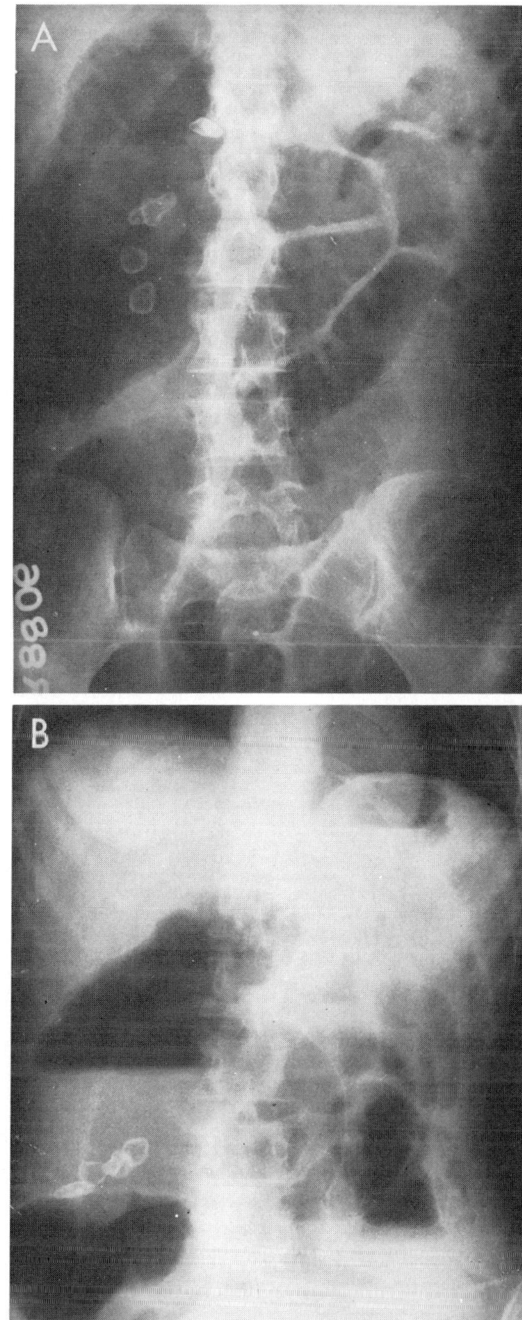

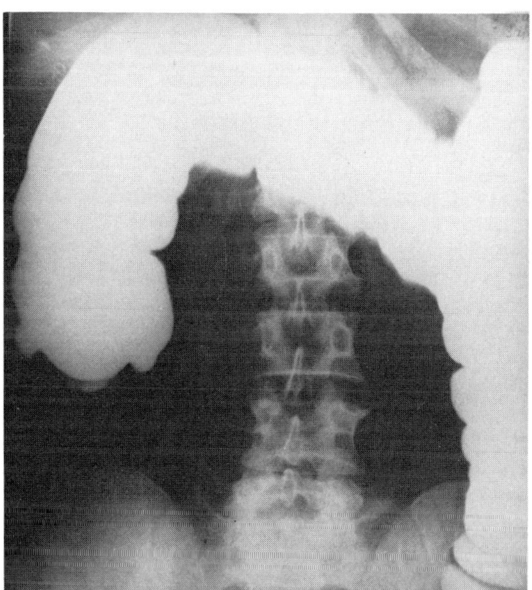

Fig 43–1 (top left).—H & E ×100, microphotograph of section from colonic wall showing confluent tubercles comprised of caseation, epithelioid cells, Langhans' giant cells and rim of lymphocytes.

Fig 43–2 (right).—**A** and **B,** plain x ray abdomen, erect and supine films showing intestinal obstruction and multiple opacities scattered over right abdomen. In woman, age 20, chest x-ray showed tubercular focus. At surgery, ileocecal tuberculosis and enteroliths were confirmed.

Fig 43–3 (bottom left).—Barium enema. Complete obstruction at midascending colon due to hypertrophied ileocecal tubercular mass, confirmed at surgery.

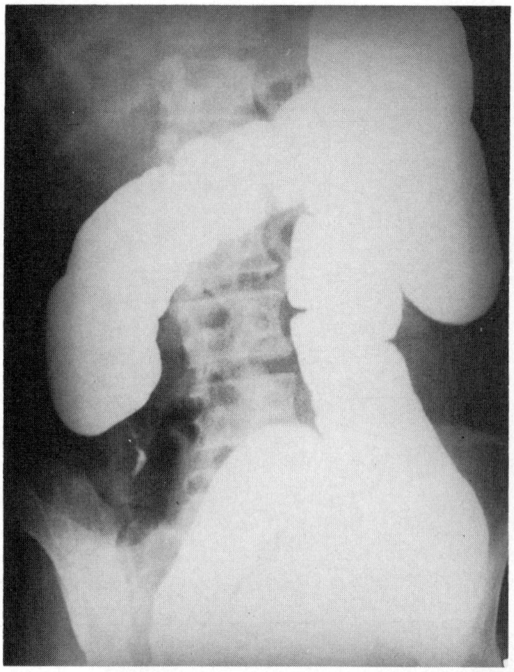

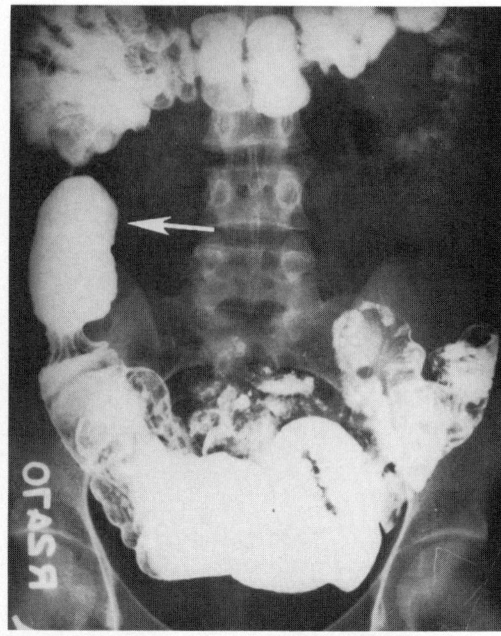

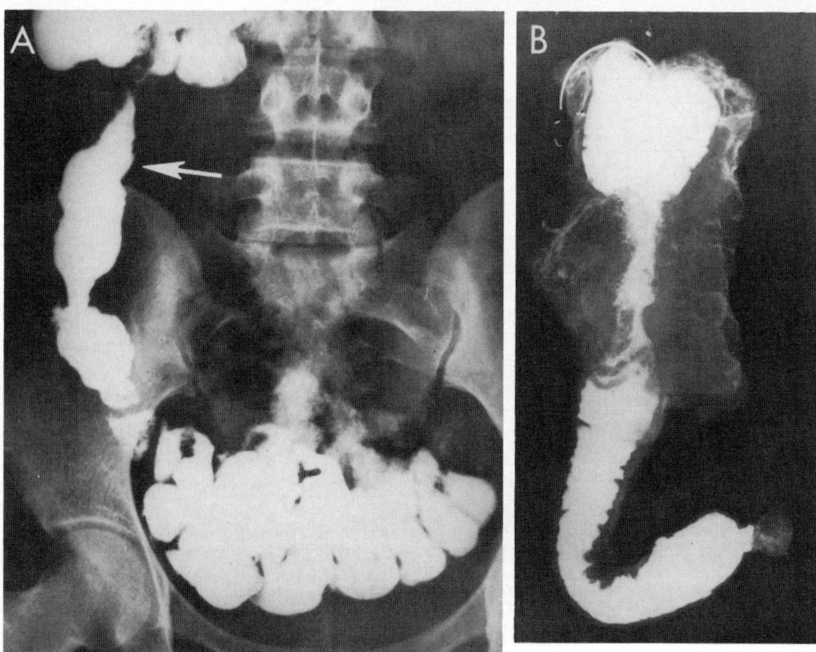

Fig 43–4 (top left).—Ileocecal tuberculosis. Barium enema examination shows streak of barium outlining ascending colon. Note pulled-down hepatic flexure.

Fig 43–5 (top right).—Barium meal, late film showing dilated pulled up terminal ileum *(arrow)* continuous with hepatic flexure; complete skipping of cecum.

Fig 43–6 (bottom). Woman, age 24, with history of subacute intestinal obstruction. **A,** barium meal: 8-hour film showing normal lumen of terminal ileum continuous with narrow, contracted ascending colon *(arrow)*. Complete skipping of cecum. **B,** barium-filled surgical specimen showing loss of ileocecal angle. Terminal ileum forms an angle of 180 degrees with ascending colon. Gross hypertrophy of walls.

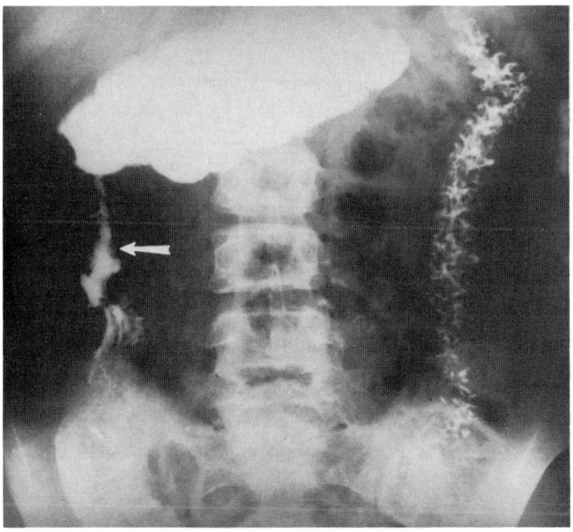

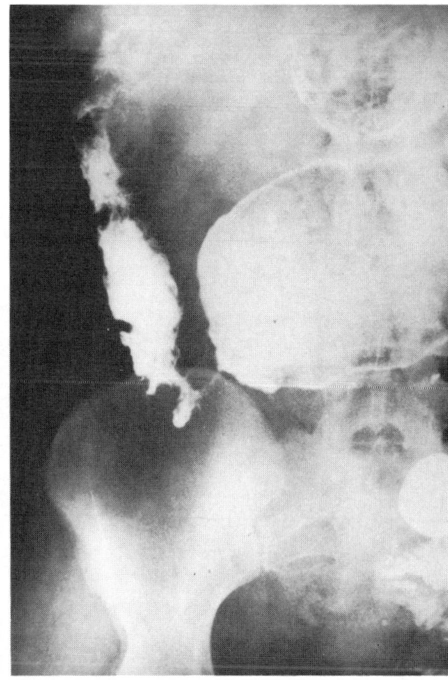

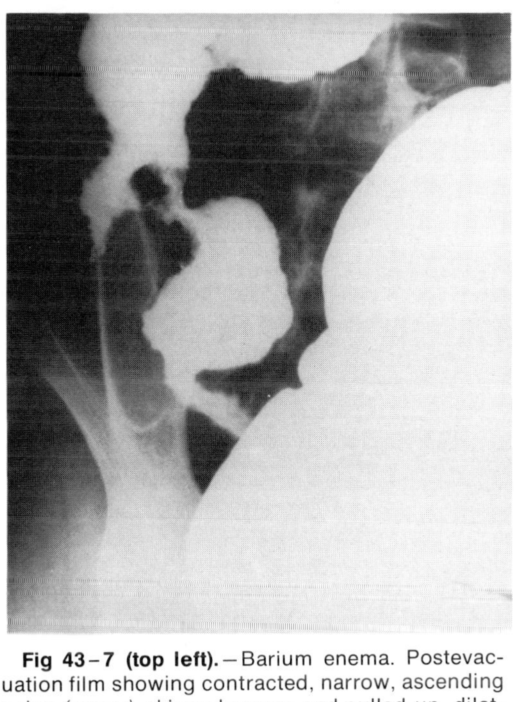

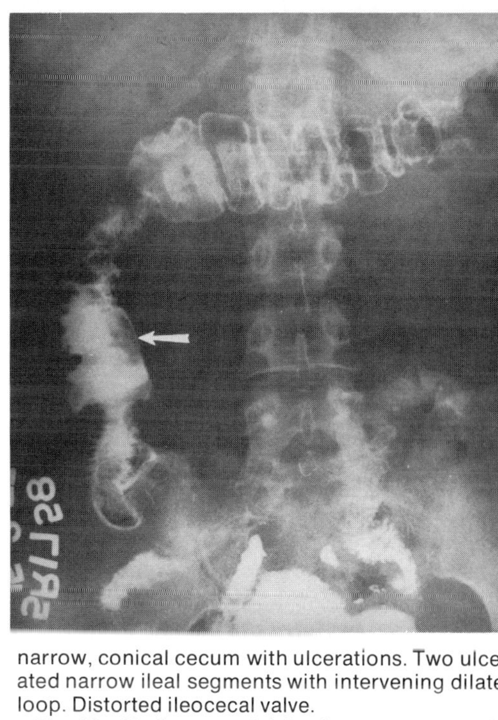

Fig 43-7 (top left).—Barium enema. Postevacuation film showing contracted, narrow, ascending colon *(arrow)*, skipped cecum and pulled-up, dilated terminal ileum. Right hemicolectomy done.

Fig 43-8 (top right). Barium meal, late film. Grossly dilated terminal ileum with stenosis at ileocecal junction and entering narrow, contracted cecum at abnormal angle.

Fig 43-9 (bottom left).—Ulcerohypertrophic ileocecal tuberculosis. Barium enema film showing narrow, conical cecum with ulcerations. Two ulcerated narrow ileal segments with intervening dilated loop. Distorted ileocecal valve.

Fig 43-10 (bottom right).—In woman, age 23, ileotransverse anastomosis done 2 years before for ileocecal tuberculosis. Patient received intermittent antituberculous chemotherapy; symptoms have recurred. Barium meal showing ulcerohypertrophic lesion involving terminal ileum *(arrow)*.

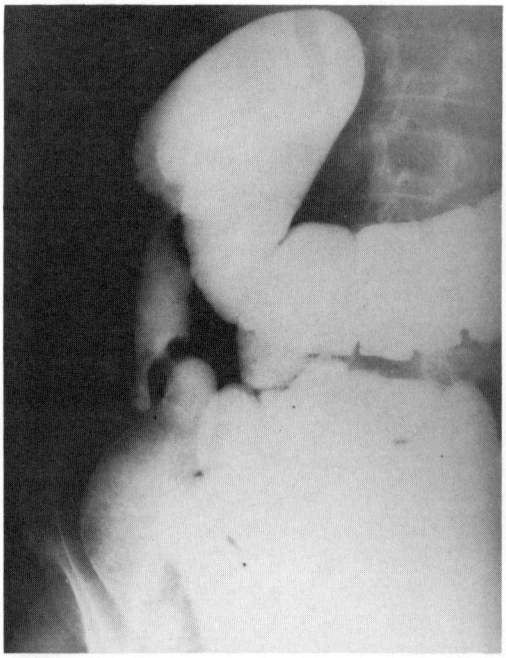

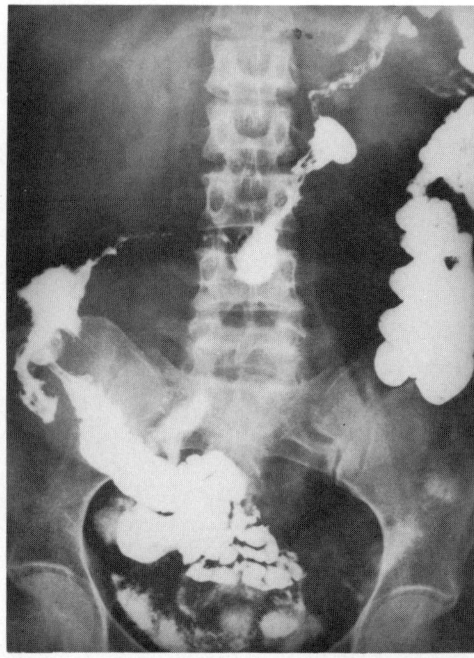

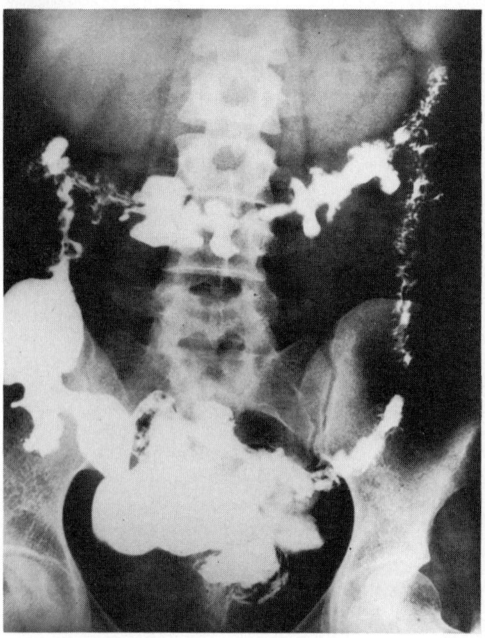

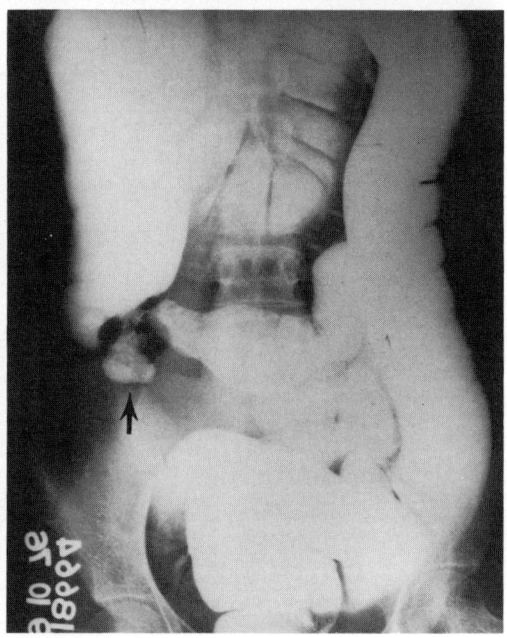

Fig 43–11 (top left).—Barium enema showing dilated terminal ileum, filling defects around ileocecal valve, conical cecum and narrow, contracted ascending colon. Hypertrophic ileocecal tuberculosis confirmed at surgery.

Fig 43–12 (top right).—Barium meal follow-through film showing ulcerations in terminal ileum, deformed cecum and polypoid filling defects in contracted ascending colon.

Fig 43–13 (bottom left).—Ileocecal tuberculosis with patulous ileocecal valve. Barium enema showing hypertrophied masses projecting into cecum.

Fig 43–14 (bottom right).—Barium enema. Dilated terminal ileum entering cecum at right angle. Cecum *(arrow)* pulled up, contracted and conical in appearance.

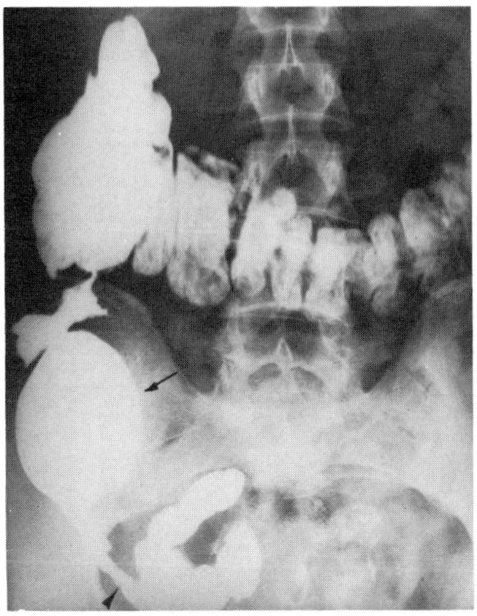

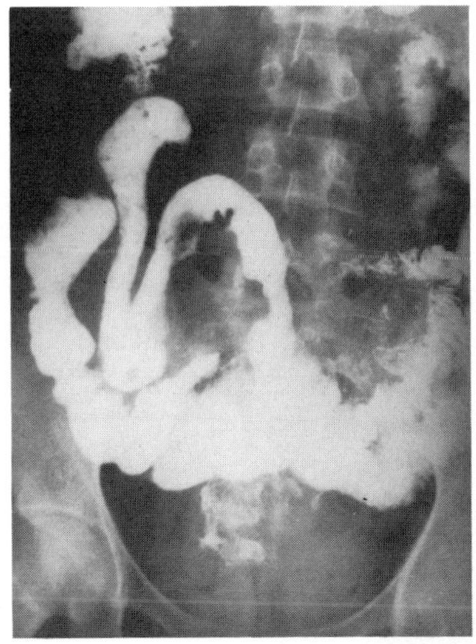

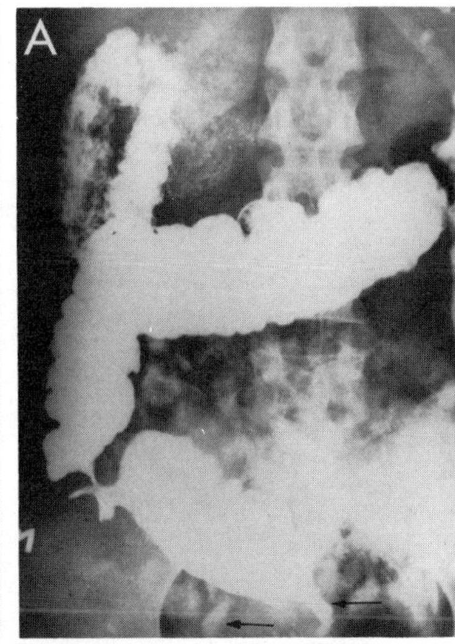

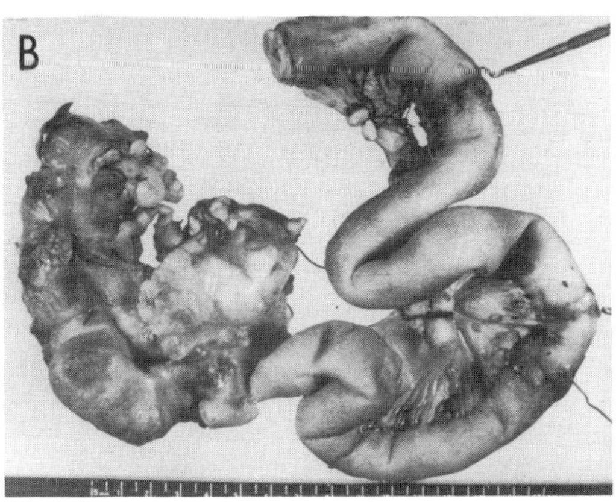

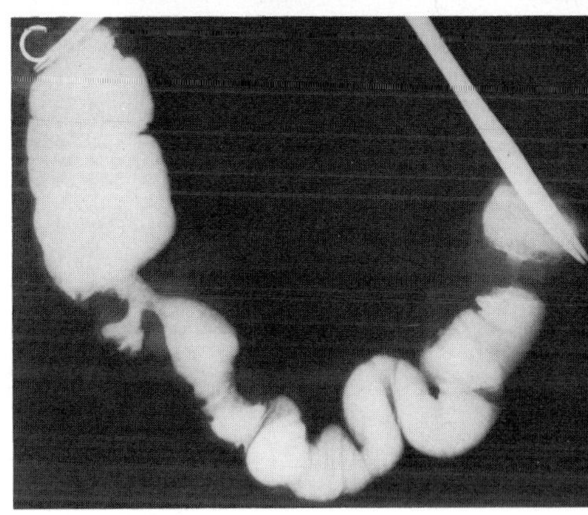

Fig 43–15 (top left).—Barium meal follow-through film showing dilated terminal ileum *(arrow)* patulous opening into abnormally contracted, narrow cecum and ascending colon. Long, narrow ileal segment *(arrowhead)* proximal to dilated terminal ileum.

Fig 43–16 (top center). Woman, age 28, with history of low grade fever and diarrhea. Barium meal, late film showing long, narrow, rigid segment of ileum with smooth margins and associated ileocecal lesion. At surgery, long segment of distal ileum along with ileocecal mass was resected.

Fig 43–17 (top right and bottom).—Young patient with subacute intestinal obstruction. **A,** barium meal, follow-through, 7-hour film shows stasis and dilution of barium in ileal loops. Ileal stricture *(arrows)* proximal to dilated terminal ileum, patulous ileocecal opening and deformed cecum. **B,** macroscopic appearance of resected segment showing hypertrophied ileocecal mass, multiple strictures in ileum and enlarged lymph glands. **C,** radiogram of barium-filled specimen showing ileal strictures and hypertrophied ileocecal lesion. Histopathology confirmed diagnosis of tuberculosis.

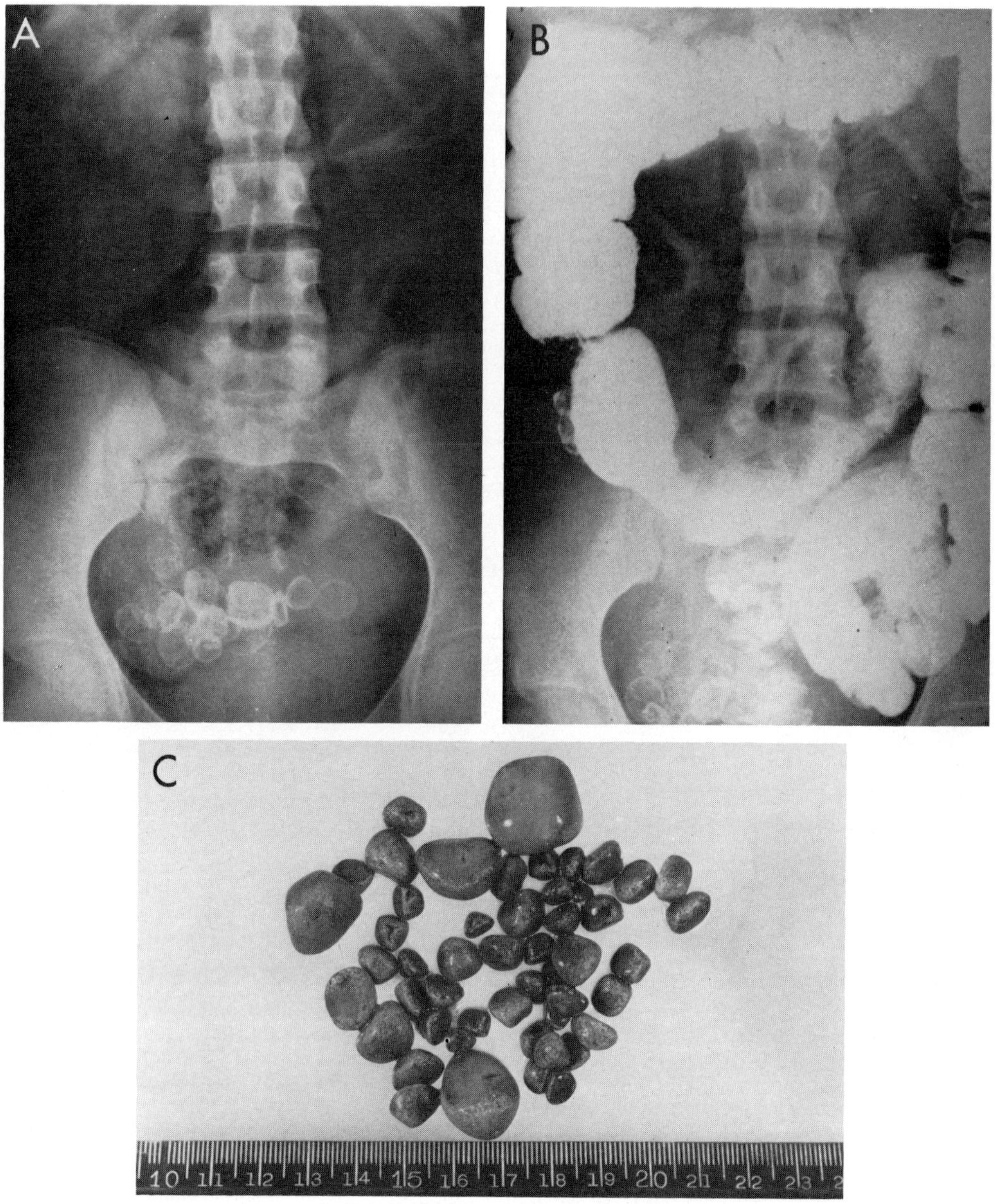

Fig 43–18.—Woman, age 25, with abdominal pain, vomiting and loss of weight for 2 years. Mass in right iliac fossa. **A,** plain x-ray abdomen showing multiple opacities with translucent centers, lying in pelvis. **B,** barium enema showing contracted ascending colon, skipped cecum and dilated terminal ileum. Opacities outside colon. Note change in position of enteroliths. **C,** enteroliths of varying sizes and shapes, removed from dilated ileal loop. Ileocecal tuberculosis confirmed. (From Chawla, Bery and Indra, Clin. Radiol. 17:274, 1966, with permission.)

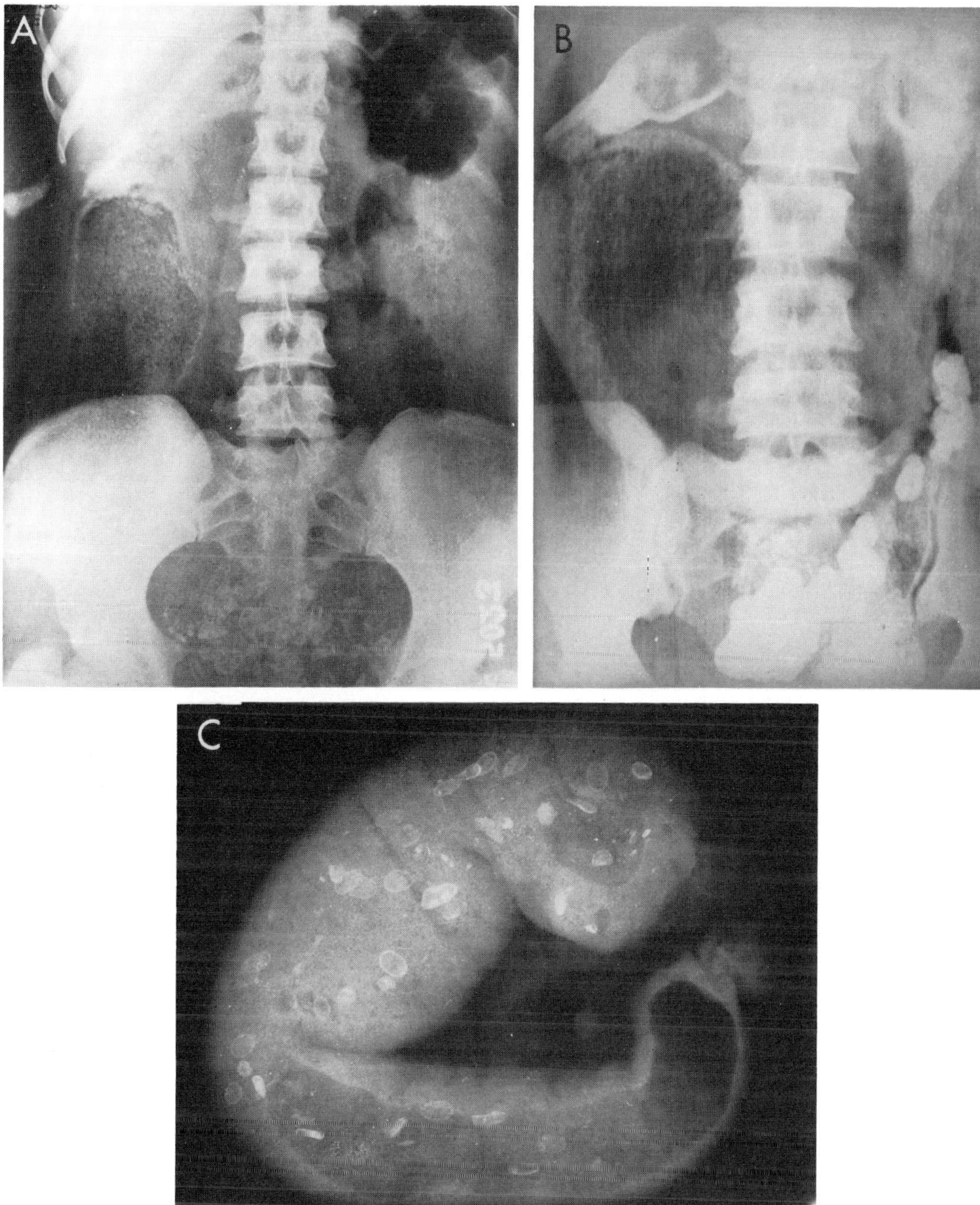

Fig 43–19.—**A,** plain x-ray abdomen showing multiple enteroliths in pelvic with grossly dilated loop of small bowel full of fecal matter lying in right abdomen. **B,** barium meal showing loop continuous with pulled-down hepatic flexure; cecum and ascending colon not visualized. Opacities are obscured by ingested barium. Ileocecal tuberculosis confirmed at surgery. **C,** radiogram of surgical specimen showing multiple enteroliths in dilated ileal loop with marked thickening of walls. Note enlarged lymph node. (From Chawla, Bery and Indra, Clin. Radiol. 17:274, 1966, with permission.)

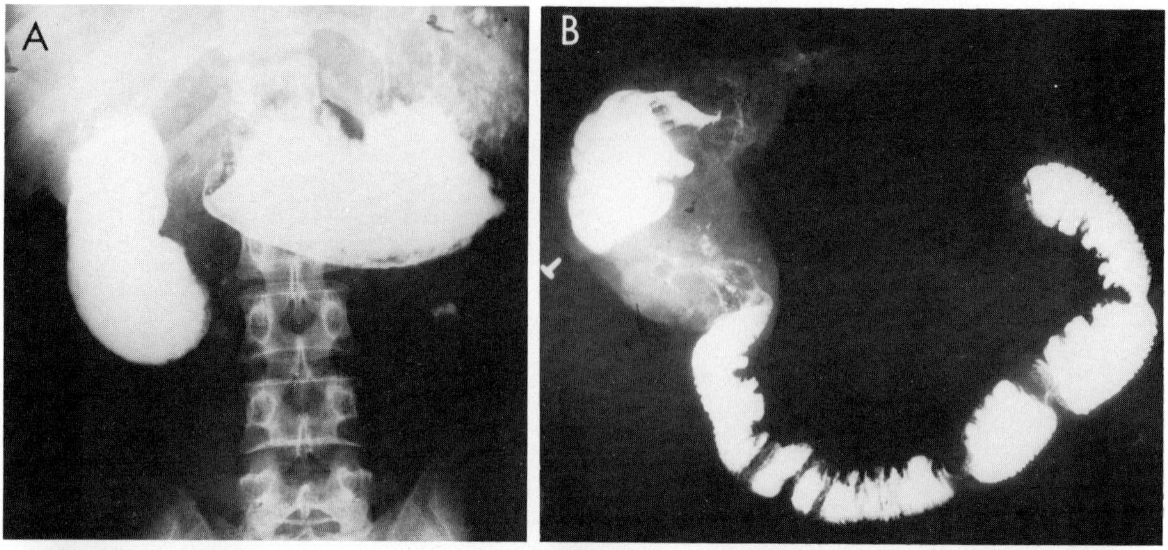

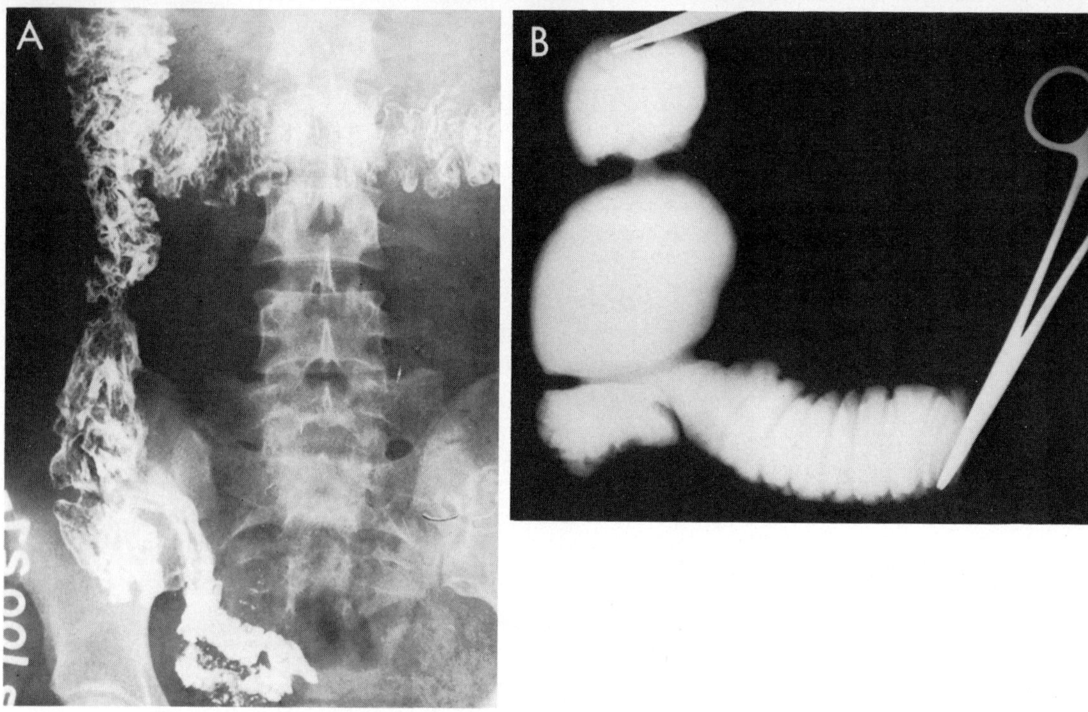

Fig 43–20 (top).—Woman, age 30, was investigated for colicky abdominal pain, diarrhea, occasional vomiting and a moving lump in upper abdomen for 3 months. **A,** stomach full of food residue, dilated second part of duodenum with nonfilling of first and obstruction at third part. At laparotomy, large hypertrophic ileocecal mass with adhesions, multiple small bowel strictures and matted mesenteric lymph nodes were causing extrinsic pressure on duodenum. **B,** barium-filled surgical specimen showing multiple strictures in lower ileum with hypertrophied ileocecal mass and narrowing of lumen. (From Chawla and Bery, Clin. Radiol. 20:99, 1969, with permission.)

Fig 43–21 (bottom).—**A,** barium meal follow-through film showing filling defect in cecum and annular stricture at middle of ascending colon. **B,** barium-filled resected specimen showing filling defect in cecum and centrally placed annular stricture in ascending colon owing to hyperplastic tubercular lesion.

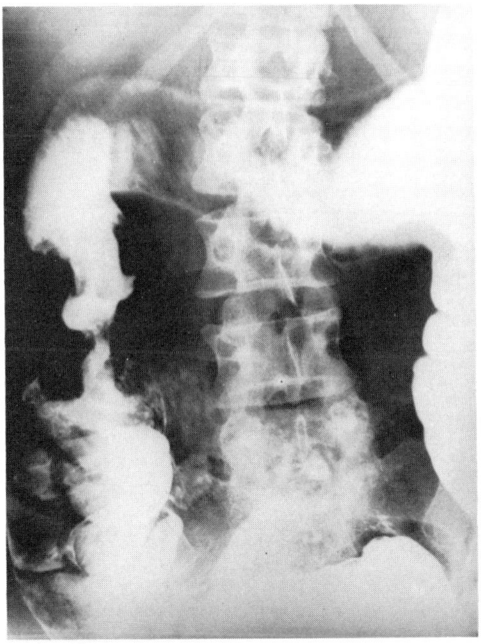

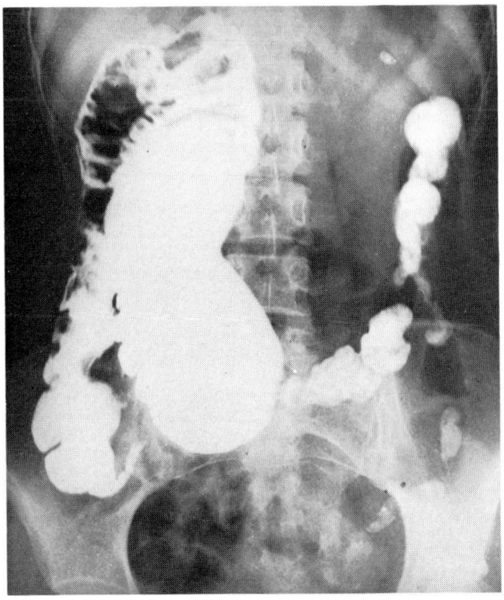

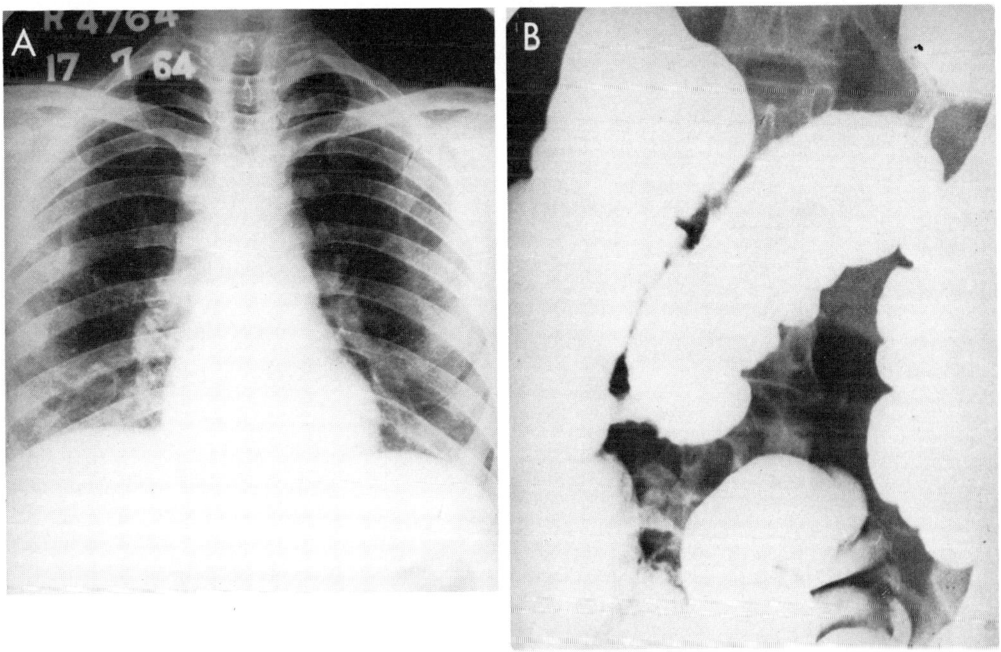

Fig 43-22 (top left). – Barium enema. Normal cecum, large hypertrophic polypoid masses projecting into lumen of ascending colon from both walls, hepatic flexure pulled down. Young female with normal chest radiogram.

Fig 43-23 (top right). – Woman, age 22, clinically diagnosed as having ileocecal tuberculosis, chest clear. Routine barium meal follow-through series did not reveal any abnormality; 24-hour film showed tight annular stricture in midtransverse colon, indistinguishable from other causes of stenosis. Stricture was resected and proved to be histopathologically tubercular.

Fig 43-24 (bottom). – **A,** chest film (PA): mediastinal and hilar lymphadenopathy. Soft infiltration at right midzone in patient, age 23. **B,** barium enema: two narrow segments, one at each end of transverse colon. At surgery, two strictures were seen in transverse colon, 15 cm apart. Mesenteric lymph nodes were enlarged. Colon was resected. (From Chawla, Mukerjee and Bery, Clin. Radiol. 22: 104, 1971, with permission.)

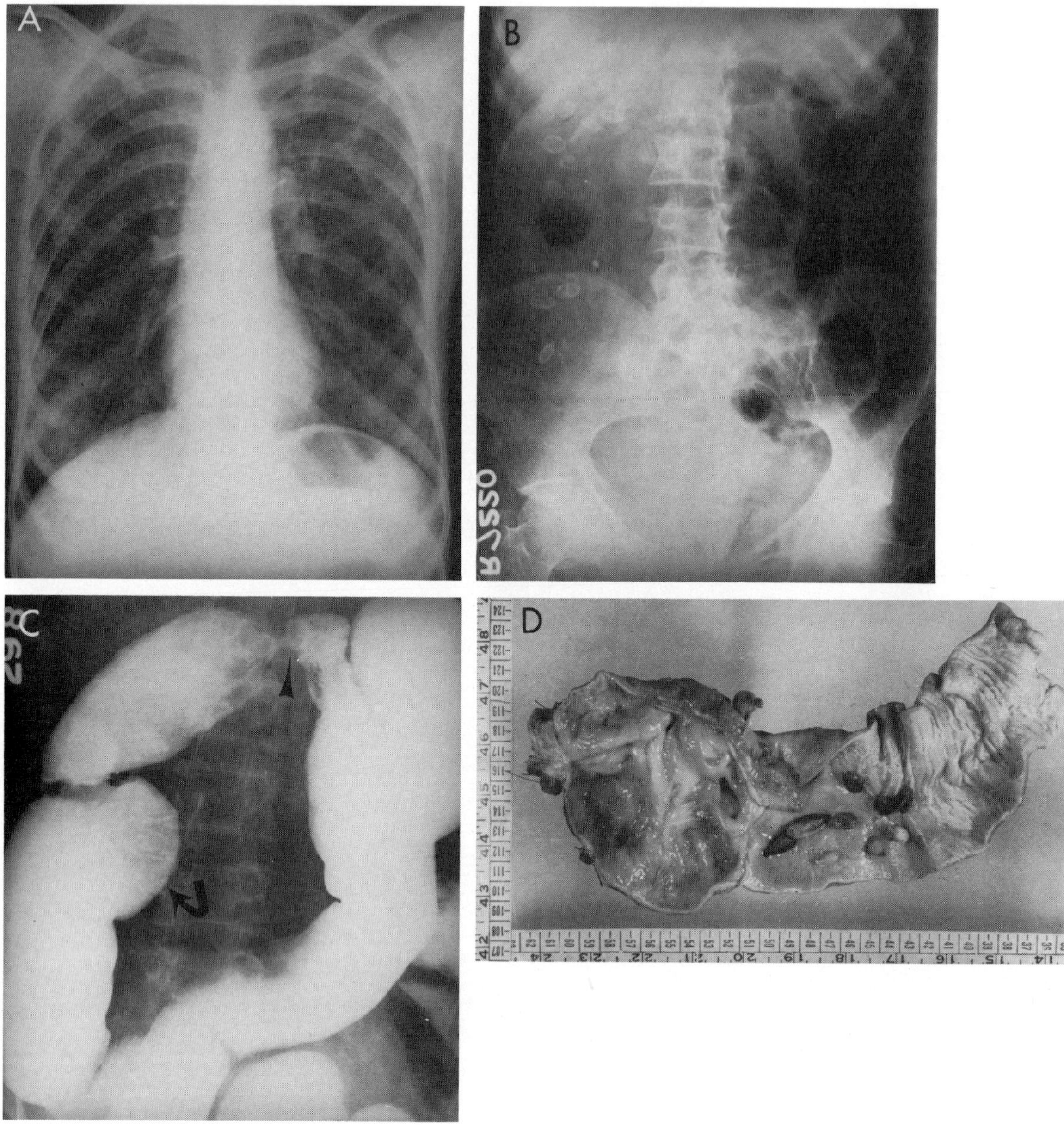

Fig 43–25.—Enterolithiasis proximal to midtransverse colon stricture. **A,** PA view of chest: soft opacities in left upper zone. **B,** plain x-ray of abdomen: multiple enteroliths in right abdomen. **C,** barium enema: smooth central stricture at midtransverse colon *(arrowhead).* Enteroliths seen as translucent filling defects in proximal transverse colon. Hepatic flexure pulled down and continuous with dilated pulled-up terminal ileum *(arrow).* **D,** macroscopic appearance of resected specimen showing enteroliths and lesions.

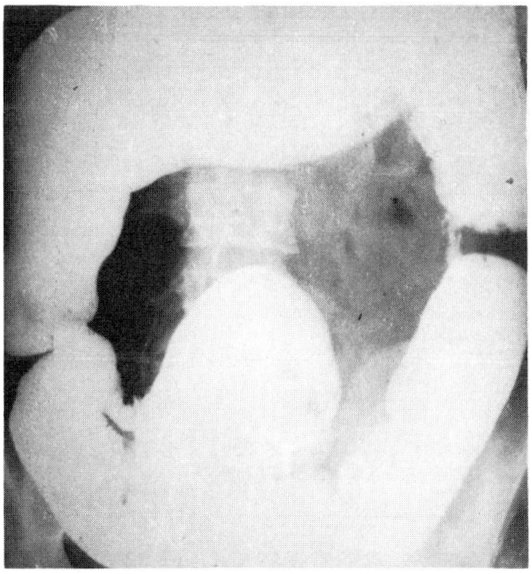

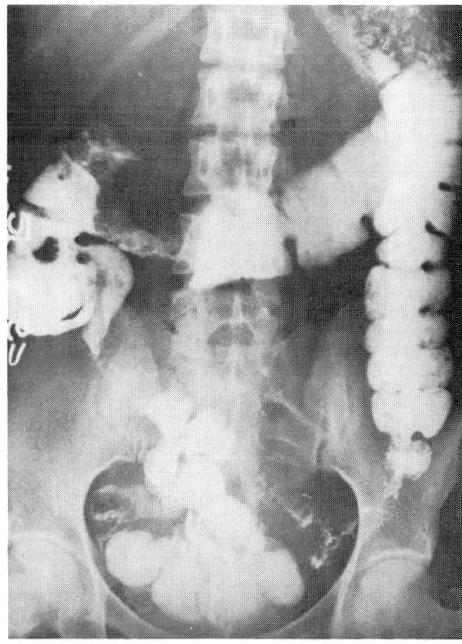

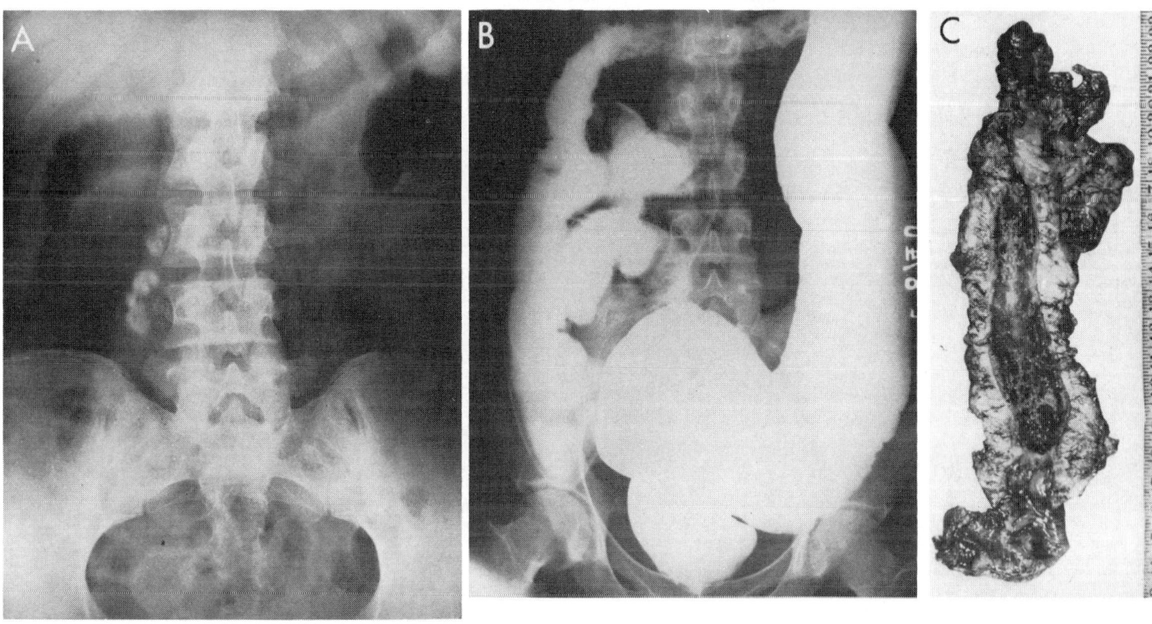

Fig 43-26 (top left).—Woman, age 20, was investigated for fever, swelling of feet, pain and mobile abdominal mass. Chest radiogram showed right pleural effusion and extensive soft infiltration, left upper zone. Barium enema showing eccentric stricture 2.5 cm long in middle of descending colon. Adjacent colon appears normal. At surgery, transverse colon was thickened and dilated. Stricture was found 6 cm distal to splenic flexure. Para-aortic and mesenteric groups of lymph glands were enlarged. Left hemicolectomy done. (From Chawla, Mukerjee and Bery, Clin. Radiol. 22:104, 1971, with permission.)

Fig 43-27 (top right).—Barium enema postevacuation film showing pulled-up terminal ileum and contracted ascending colon. Hepatic flexure and proximal transverse colon show narrow lumen with multiple pseudopolypoid filling defects. Note sharp transition between normal and abnormal segments. Chest was normal. At surgery, tubercular lesion was found involving small bowel, mesentery, omentum and large bowel up to midtransverse colon.

Fig 43-28 (bottom).—Patient, age 19, with history of loss of weight and diarrhea. Chest x-ray was normal. **A,** plain x-ray of abdomen. Calcified mesenteric lymph nodes. Narrow transverse colon outlined by gas; hepatic flexure pulled down. **B,** barium enema. Extensive involvement of colon up to splenic flexure. Colon is narrow, with loss of haustra and pseudopolypoid filling defects. **C,** macroscopic appearance of resected colon, showing hypertrophic masses projecting into lumen. Thickened walls. Diagnosis of tuberculosis confirmed histologically.

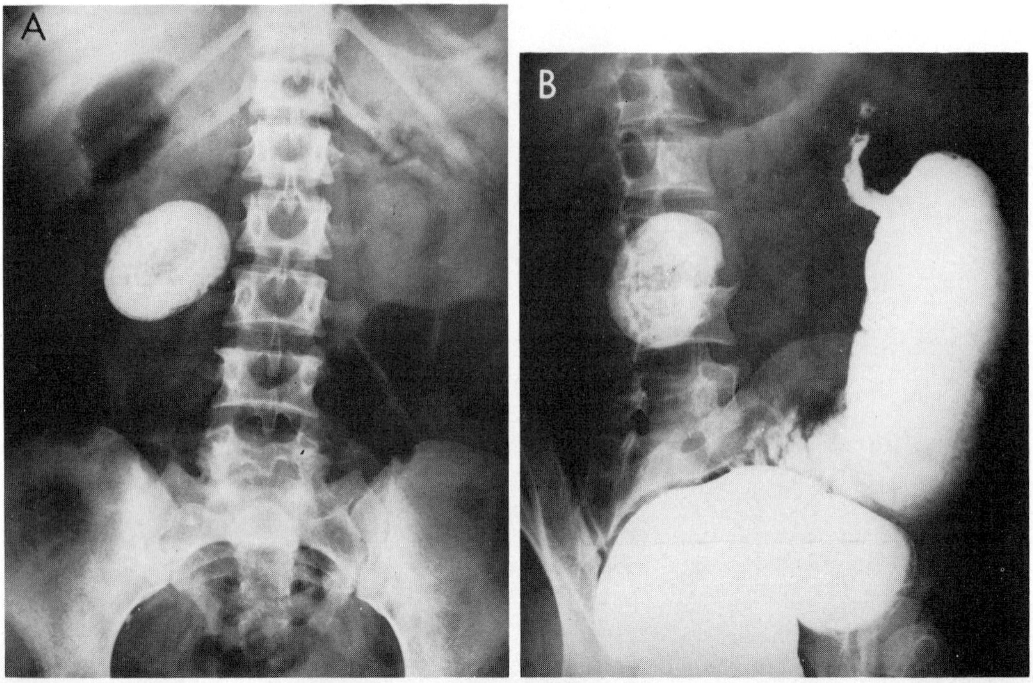

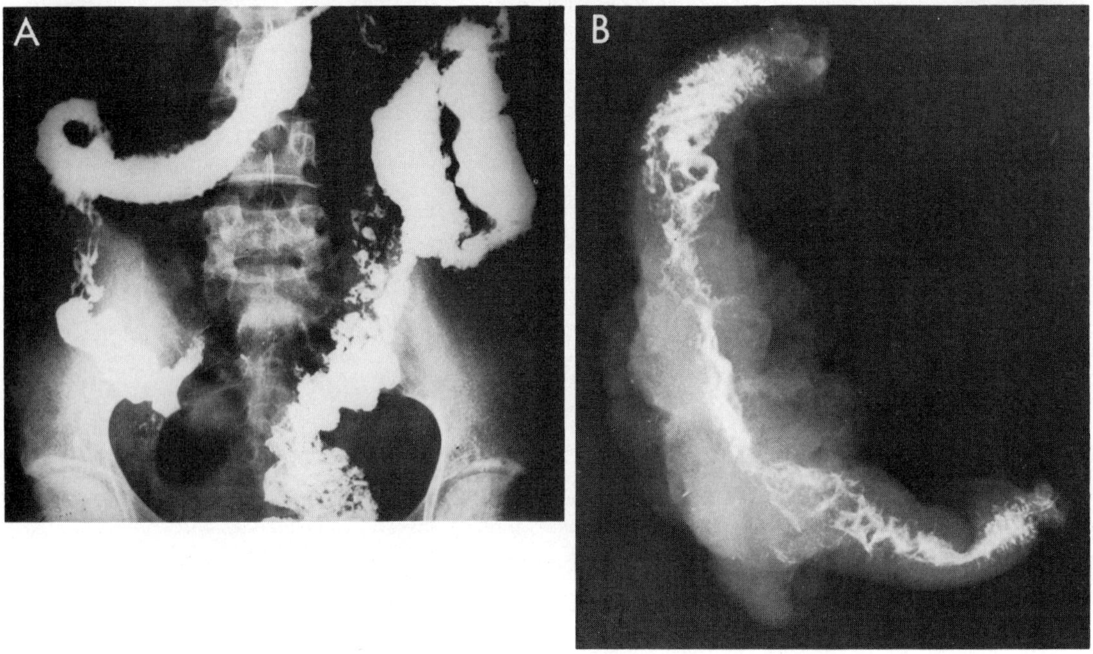

Fig 43–29 (top).—**A,** plain x-ray of abdomen showing large oval lamellated opacity in right abdomen, outside right renal shadow. **B,** barium enema. Long, narrow, irregular segment in descending colon near splenic flexure. No barium passed beyond it. At surgery, large enterolith was found in dilated ileum. Ileocecal region and entire colon up to middescending colon was involved and resected.

Fig 43–30 (bottom).—**A,** barium enema showing contracted, narrow colon with pseudopolypoid filling defects. **B,** barium-filled surgical specimen confirming extent of involvement. Note gross thickening of walls and filling defects. Tuberculosis confirmed histopathologically.

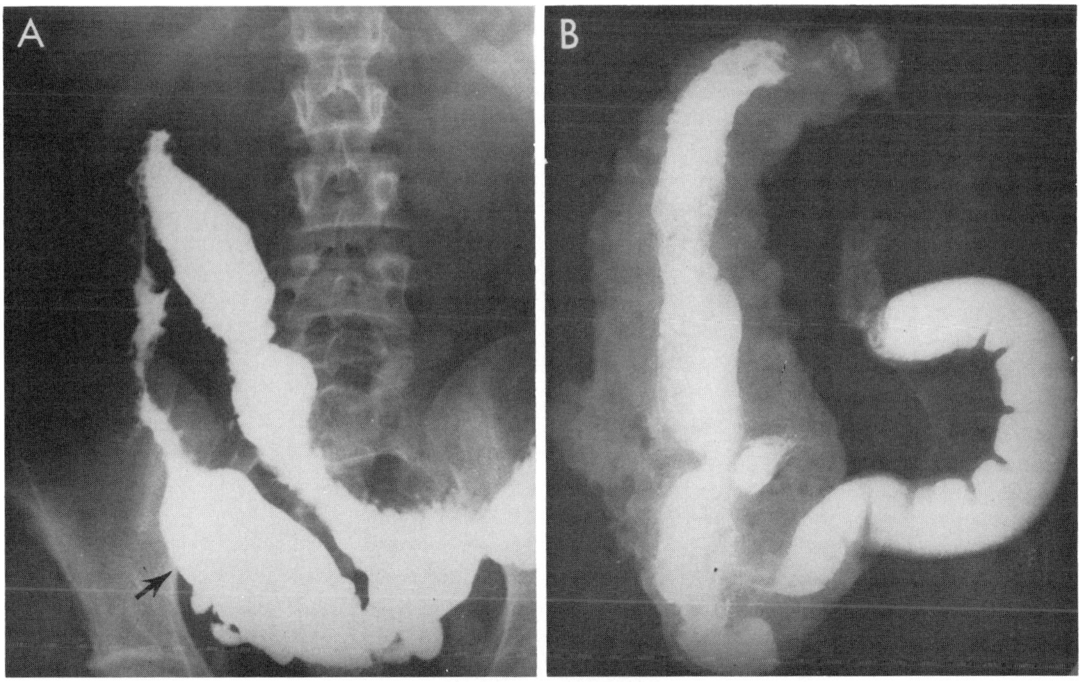

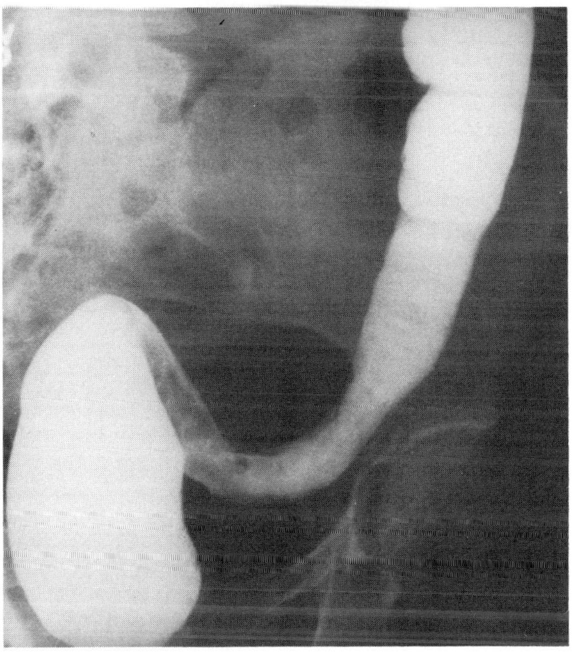

Fig 43–31 (top).—**A,** barium meal showing dilated terminal ileum *(arrow)* with narrow, ulcerated cecum and extensive involvement of colon. **B,** barium-filled surgical specimen confirming lesion.

Fig 43–32 (bottom).—Barium enema. Rectum not fully distensible. Narrowing of sigmoid colon with filling defects. Rest of large bowel normal. Chest x-ray showed healed tubercular focus. Rectal biopsy showed tubercular granuloma.

Chapter 44

Ulceration of the Cecum

PHILIP A. BRODEY, M.D.

BENIGN ULCERATION of the cecum is an uncommon entity of uncertain cause, first described by Cruveilhier in 1832.[9] Nonspecific ulceration may occur throughout the colon, but in 50% of cases it affects the cecum and ascending colon in the region of the ileocecal valve.[15, 16] The ulceration usually is solitary, but more than one ulcer may be present. The ulcer is of variable size and usually is located on the antimesenteric bowel wall in contrast to diverticula, which occur along the mesenteric border.[4, 14, 16]

In the extensive review by Hardie and Nicoll,[14] the histologic diagnosis of nonspecific ulceration of the cecum was accepted only after excluding such specific entities as ulcerative colitis, Crohn's disease, ulceration due to pathogenic bacteria or parasites, diverticulitis, cecitis or ulceration secondary to inflammation of adjacent viscera or neoplastic disease. Anatomically, the ulcer had to occur within the cecum or proximal ascending colon within 2 cm of the ileocecal valve to be included in the review.

Although there are numerous proposed causes, including cecal ulceration secondary to inflammation of a diverticulum[1] and thrombosis in the microcirculation of the cecal wall,[14] there is no commonly accepted etiologic explanation.

There are no specific clinical characteristics of this entity. Symptoms may be acute, similar to those of appendicitis,[1, 3, 6, 7, 14, 18] or chronic, with blood loss the presenting manifestation.[14, 16, 19] Occurrence is almost equal in the sexes, with perhaps a slight male predominance. Age at onset ranges from 18 to 70, the highest incidence in those between 25 and 50 years of age. There is a clinically palpable mass in only 30% of patients. Complications include hemorrhage,[6, 8, 10, 11, 17] perforation with peritonitis or subsequent abscess formation and stricture.[4, 12, 16]

In most reported cases in which a barium enema examination was obtained, the primary finding was a mass affecting the cecum.[4, 16, 19] The preoperative radiographic diagnosis on the basis of the barium enema usually was carcinoma.

The variability in the radiographic appearance of the cecum, shown on barium enema examination, is demonstrated in the illustrations. These findings include a cecum that is fully distensible (Fig 44–1, B), incompletely distensible (Fig 44–2, A) or fixed and nondistensible even after the use of glucagon (Fig 44–3, A). The terminal ileum is normal (Figs 44–1, B, 44–2, B, and 44–3, B). There is no extrinsic mass effect on the barium-filled colon or terminal ileum. The appendix fills

---

This chapter, including illustrations, previously published in Radiology 122:323–327, 1977. Reprinted with permission of the author and the Radiological Society of North America, Inc.

inconsistently. Single or multiple ulcers may be demonstrated; however, this may be difficult to appreciate if there are surrounding inflammatory changes.

Pathologically, either single or multiple areas of superficial ulceration or erosion can be demonstrated. This often is not identified radiographically, even with double contrast technique.

The difficulty in differentiation of a benign ulceration of the colon from a malignant process has been noted previously in the radiologic literature[4, 5] (Fig 44–4). The rarity of barium enema examinations performed in this condition probably is accounted for in part by the usual acute onset of the disease process and the clinical symptoms, which are compatible with the diagnosis of acute appendicitis.

Previous reports of hemorrhage from documented cecal ulcer have been described by both Corey et al[8] and Sutherland et al.[17]

Baer and Ryan[2] recently evaluated the vascular anatomy of the cecum in regard to vascular malformations. They found that most vascular malformations occur on the antimesenteric border, the same location in which cecal ulcerations typically occur.[16] Although several articles on vascular dysplasia of the right colon have described ulceration associated with vascular dysplasia,[2, 8, 10, 13] the possible relationship of benign cecal ulceration to vascular dysplasia of the right colon remains uncertain.

In the appropriate clinical setting, acute ulceration of the cecum should be included in the radiologic differential diagnosis when an abnormal cecum is shown on barium enema examination or bleeding is demonstrated angiographically in the cecal region.

REFERENCES

1. Anscombe, A. R., Keddie, N. C., and Shofield, P. F.: Solitary ulcers and diverticulitis of the cecum, Br. J. Surg. 54:553, 1967.
2. Baer, J. W., and Ryan, S.: Analysis of cecal vasculature in the search for vascular malformations, Am. J. Roentgenol. 126:394, 1976.
3. Benninger, G. W., Honig, Z. J., and Fein, H. D.: Nonspecific ulceration of the cecum, Am. J. Gastroenterol. 55:594, 1971.
4. Berk, R. N., and Lasser, E. C.: *Radiology of the Ileocecal Area* (Philadelphia: W. B. Saunders Co., 1975), pp. 242–244.
5. Bravo, A. J., Lowman, R. M.: Benign ulcer of the sigmoid colon, Radiology 90:113, 1968.
6. Brodey, P. A., Hill, R. P., and Barron, S.: Benign ulceration of the cecum, Radiology 122:323, 1977.
7. Butsch, J. L., Dockerty, M. B., McGill, D. B., et al.: Solitary nonspecific ulcers of the colon, Arch. Surg. 98:171, 1969.
8. Corry, R. J., Bartlett, M. K., and Cohen, R. B.: Erosions of the cecum, Am. J. Surg. 119:106, 1970.
9. Cruveilhier, J.: Un beau cas de cicatrisation d'un ulcère de l'intestin gaele datant d'une douzaine d'années, Bull. Soc. Anat. 7:1, 1832.
10. Eisenberg, H., Laufer, I., and Skillman, J. J.: Arteriographic diagnosis and management of suspected colonic diverticular hemorrhage, Gastroenterology 64:1091, 1973.
11. Eusebio, E. B., and Kaplan, A. P.: Idiopathic colonic ulcer, Dis. Colon Rectum, 17:763, 1974.
12. Fung, W. P., Tan, A. Y. O., and Kho, K. M.: Idiopathic ulceration and strictures of colon with unusual vascular changes, Am. J. Dig. Dis. 18:613, 1973.
13. Genant, H. K., and Ranninger, K.: Vascular dysplasias of the ascending colon, Am. J. Roentgenol. 115:349, 1972.
14. Hardie, I. R., and Nicoll, P.: Localized ulceration of the cecum due to microcirculatory thrombosis, Aust. NZ J. Surg. 43:149, 1973.
15. Margulis, A. R., and Burhenne, H. J.: *Alimentary Tract Roentgenology* (St. Louis: C. V. Mosby Co., 1967), p. 125.
16. Slesenger, M. H., and Fordtran, J. S.: *Gastrointestinal Disease* (Philadelphia: W. B. Saunders Co., 1973), pp. 1510–1514.
17. Sutherland, D., French, R. S., Weil, R., et al.: The bleeding cecal ulcer: Pathogenesis, angiographic diagnosis and nonoperative control, Surgery 71: 290, 1972.
18. Williams, A. M.: Inflammatory masses of the cecum, Ann. Surg. 165:697, 1967.
19. Zer, M., Wolloch, Y., Chaimoff, C. H., et al.: Benign lesions of the cecum simulating carcinoma, Am. J. Proctol. 25:52, 1974.

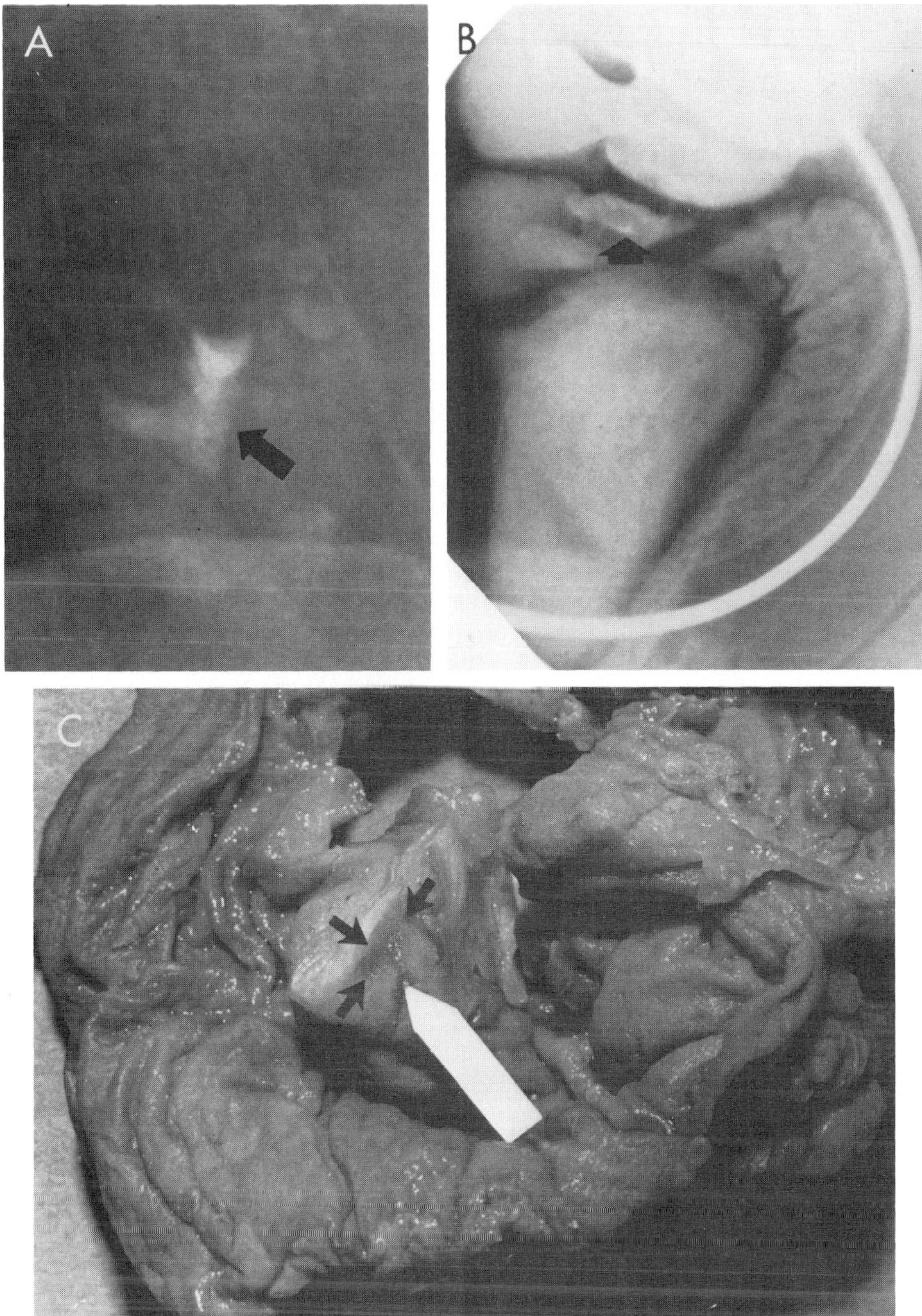

Fig 44-1. **A,** selective superior mesenteric angiogram in early arterial phase with extravasation *(arrow)* of contrast medium in region of cecum. **B,** barium enema with persistent collection of barium adjacent to ileocecal valve, representing acute ulcer *(arrow)*. Cecum is well distended. Terminal ileum is normal. Appendix removed previously. **C,** pathologic specimen showing ulceration *(arrow)* at ileocecal valve. No diverticula. Appendix removed previously. (Reprinted from Radiology 122:323, 1971, with permission.)

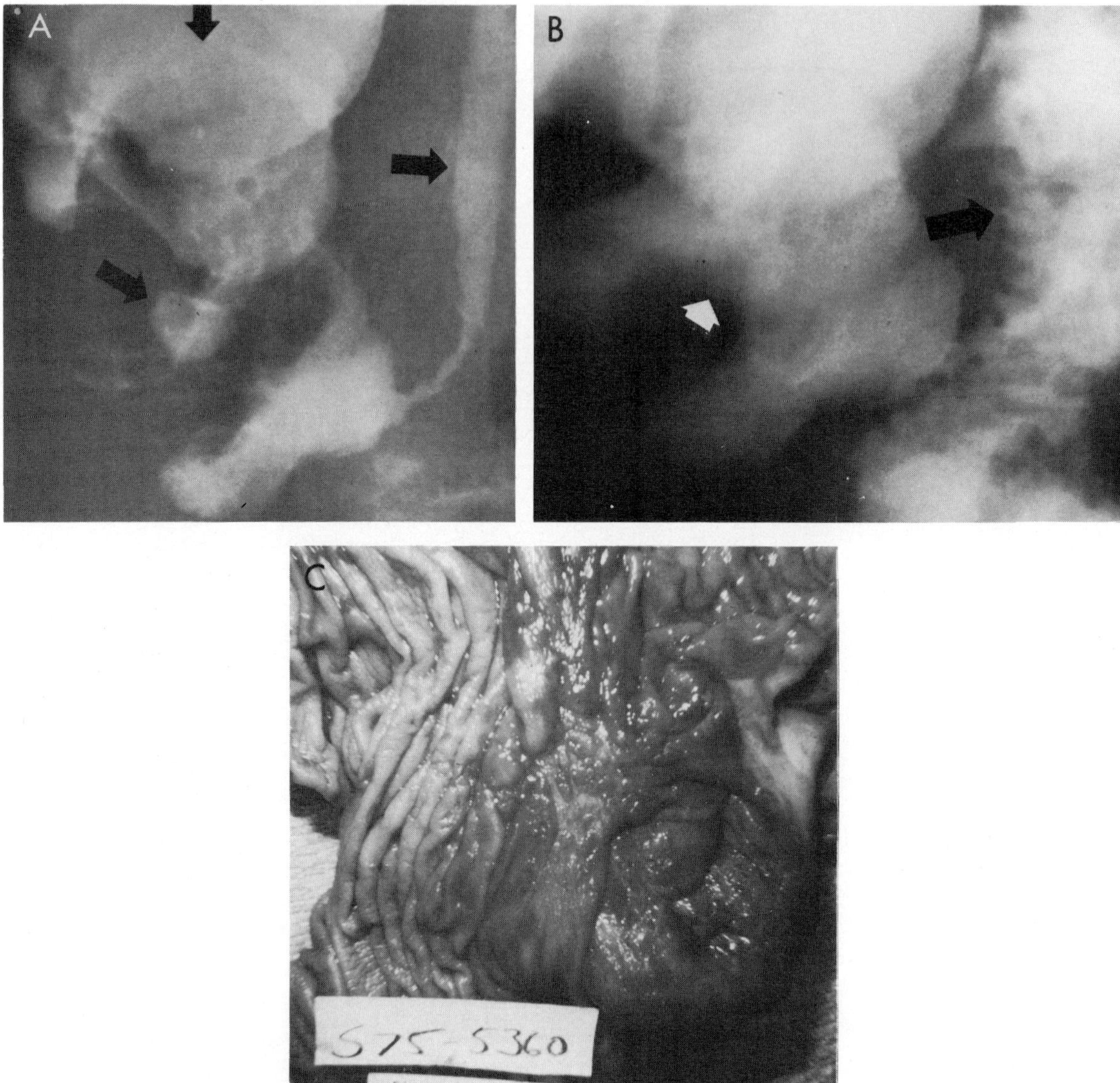

Fig 44-2. – **A,** distorted, incompletely distended cecum, which is not fixed in appearance, despite apparent masslike effect (see **B**). *Upper arrow* points to superior surface of inflammatory mass. *Slanted arrow* points to persistent collection of barium representing an ulcer. *Horizontal arrow* points to partially filled appendix. Base of appendix is narrowed and irregular. **B,** cecum is more distended than in **A,** indicating that distortion is not fixed. *Small arrow* points to same collection of barium as in **A.** *Large arrow* points to normal terminal ileum with no adjacent mass effect. **C,** pathologic specimen. Close-up view of cecum with numerous areas of superficial erosion. No single large ulcer identified; appendix normal; no diverticula.

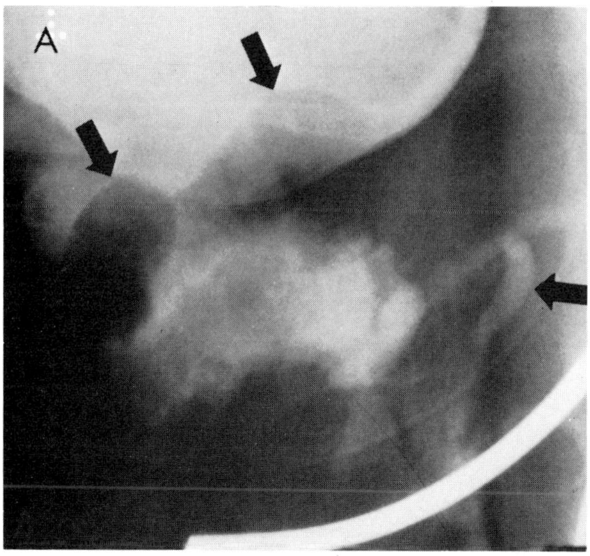

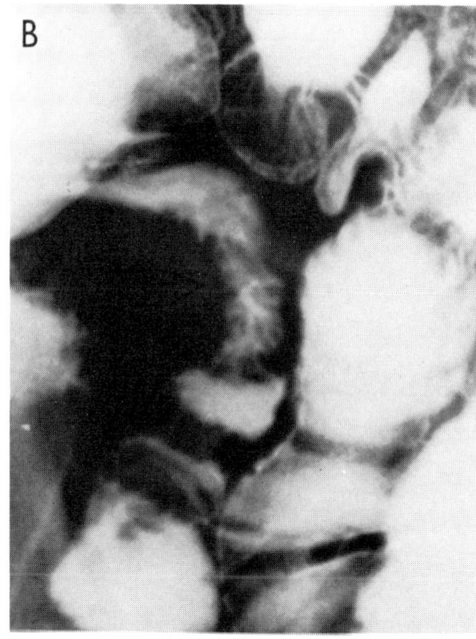

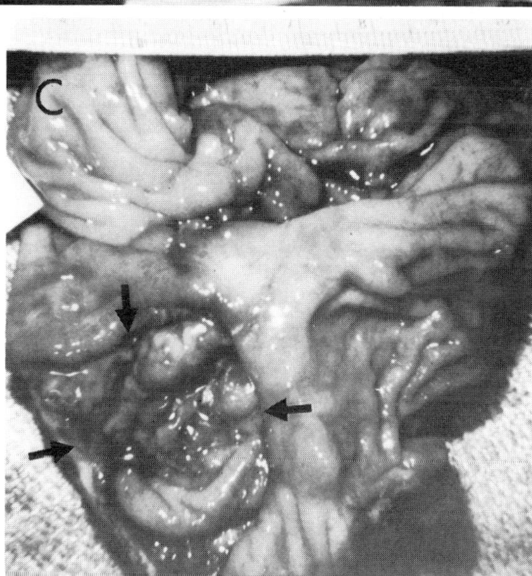

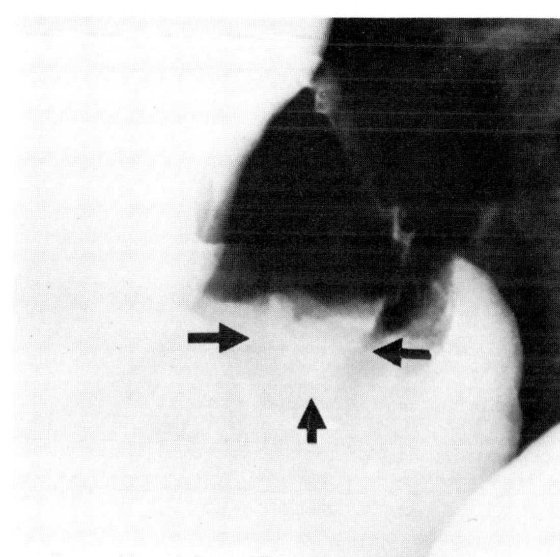

Fig 44–3 (top and bottom left).—**A,** contracted, nondistensible cecum with irregular nodular contour. Intravenous administration of glucagon failed to change appearance. *Upper arrows* point to superior surface of inflammatory mass. *Horizontal arrow* points to completely filled appendix. Terminal ileum did not fill. **B,** small bowel examination shows terminal ileum to be normal without any mass effect. **C,** pathologic specimen of cecum with solitary, large ulcer *(arrows)*. Appendix normal. No diverticula.

Fig 44–4 (bottom right).—Large ulceration *(arrows)*. Ulcer is within a mass, which did not change in appearance. Appendix is filled. Small bowel examination not performed. Surgery revealed carcinoma of cecum.

Chapter 45

Ulcerative Colitis

MARVIN WEINER, M.D.
BARBARA M. KADELL, M.D.

FOLLOWING THE ORIGINAL description of ulcerative colitis in 1875,[1] many of the noninfectious inflammatory diseases of the large intestine were included in this pathologic entity. With the recognition in 1960[2] of Crohn's disease involving the colon and the characterization of ischemic colitis in 1963,[3] criteria for the radiographic diagnosis of ulcerative colitis came into clearer focus. More recently, it has become apparent that considerable overlap in diagnostic signs exists among the various colitides.[4] Nevertheless, many radiographic criteria of ulcerative colitis are typical, if not pathognomonic.

Clinical Features

The etiologic factors in ulcerative colitis remain unknown. Immunologic, genetic and infectious causes have been suggested but have not been clearly established. The onset of symptoms usually is in the 3d or 4th decade and the disease occurs with near equal frequency in both sexes.[5] The primary clinical symptoms are diarrhea, rectal bleeding and abdominal pain. The most common associated extracolonic manifestations are arthritis, uveitis, erythema nodosum and pyoderma gangrenosum.[5] Onset may be insidious or abrupt and the clinical course may be chronic or of the relapsing-remitting type. Major complications include toxic megacolon (1 – 3%), massive colonic hemorrhage (1 – 3%), colonic perforation (2 – 3%) and development of colonic carcinoma.[6-8] The risk of carcinoma is related mainly to duration of the disease, and also to the age at onset and the extent of involvement. The overall incidence of carcinoma in patients with ulcerative colitis is about 3.5%

Pathology

The disease is characterized by an inflammatory process that primarily involves the mucosa and submucosa of the colon. Initially the mucosa is diffusely edematous, friable and frequently hemorrhagic. Small ulcerations are caused by coalescence of multiple microabscesses.[5] Linear extension and further coalescence of these shallow ulcers may isolate intact islands of mucosa, resulting in mucosal tags called pseudopolyps. Larger ulcers may occur, and abundant granulation tissue commonly appears in the denuded areas. During remissions the ulcerated areas may completely re-epithelialize. Hypertrophy of the muscularis mucosa is often seen in patients with long standing disease. Fibrosis occurs somewhat less frequently and is limited to the submucosa. When the entire colon is involved, the disease process may extend into the terminal ileum and produce similar pathologic changes (backwash ileitis).

Radiology

Plain films of the abdomen frequently yield useful information in patients with ulcerative colitis. The intraluminal colonic gas pattern may reveal pseudopolyps, shortening of the colon or haustral loss (Fig 45–1). In toxic megacolon, abdominal radiograms will demonstrate massive colonic distention associated with an abnormal mucosal contour (Fig 45–2). This dilatation most frequently is seen in the transverse colon. Colonic perforation may occur with or without toxic megacolon and can be diagnosed by detection of intraperitoneal air (Fig 45–3). The pneumoperitoneum associated with colonic perforation is usually massive.

The findings on barium enema examination vary with the stage and severity of the disease. The earliest mucosal changes are best seen with double contrast studies.[9] Even before ulcers appear, mucosal edema produces a fine granular appearance when viewed en face (Figs 45–4 and 45–5). In the normal distended colon, the mucosa is perfectly smooth. When ulcerations first appear, a fine stippled appearance of the mucosa is seen en face, a hazy spiculated contour in profile. When the ulcerations become confluent and the mucosa is replaced by granulation tissue, double contrast techniques reveal a characteristic coarsely granular appearance (Figs 45–6 and 45–7). On full column barium studies, the earliest changes are a fuzzy or finely spiculated contour secondary to the minute ulcerations and haustral widening and distortion due to edema. With further progression and increased severity of the disease, deeper ulcers may be seen that penetrate the muscularis mucosa (Figs 45–8 and 45–9). These may be shaggy or flask shaped but are rarely long and linear, such as those seen in Crohn's disease.

Pseudopolyps are the consequence of severe mucosal disease and present as multiple filling defects of varying size (Figs 45–12 to 45–15).[10] They may develop rapidly and tend to persist even when the disease is quiescent. Pseudopolyps are radiographically indistinguishable from true adenomas, and larger ones may mimic colonic carcinoma.[11] Occasionally, mucosal bridges are formed, which may be demonstrated on barium studies.[12] These are believed to be part of the spectrum of pseudopolyps, probably formed by complete undermining of mucosal segments with attached edges.

The radiographic changes described above may involve the entire colon (Figs 45–16 and 45–18), but when the disease is segmental it usually affects only the left side (Fig 45–10). Rectal sparing is rare, occurring in only 5% of cases. With incomplete colonic involvement, the transition between the normal and abnormal segment tends to be gradual. Skip lesions (multifocal involvement) are unusual. The diseased segment is usually circumferentially rather than asymmetrically affected. With increased severity and duration, the involved colon may narrow, shorten and lose its normal redundancy and haustral architecture (Fig 45–20). Rectal narrowing is easily demonstrated in the lateral projection by an increase in retrorectal space (Fig 45–11). These changes are more often due to spasm and hypertrophy of the muscularis but in long-standing disease may be caused by fibrosis. With remission, it is not uncommon to see a return to normal caliber and length and at times normal haustration (Figs 45–22 and 45–23).

When the entire colon is involved, changes in the terminal ileum may be seen (backwash ileitis) (Figs 45–16, 45–17, 45–19). In these cases, the ileocecal valve is patulous, and the affected segment of ileum is dilated rather than narrowed. The mucosa may be smooth, or fine ulcerations may be seen. Pseudopolyps involving the terminal ileum may at times be demonstrated.[13]

The reported incidence of benign strictures varies from 1 to 11%. These strictures usually occur in patients with long-standing disease and are found predominantly in the left side of the colon. Localized strictures are more often due to muscular hypertrophy than to fibrosis. They are typically smooth in contour, are concentric and have fusiform, tapered margins (Fig 45–24).[14]

Carcinoma complicating ulcerative colitis is usually annular and may at times be difficult to differentiate from a benign stricture. Often, however, they cause eccentric, nodular narrowing with shouldered edges (Fig 45–26). Multiple carcinomas are not unusual. Nearly one half of these neoplasms are not detected clinically or radiographically but are diagnosed at the time of colectomy or autopsy.

REFERENCES

1. Wilks, S., and Moxon, W.: *Lectures on Pathological Anatomy* (2d ed.; London: J. & A. Churchill, Ltd., 1875).
2. Lockhart-Mummery, H. E., and Morson, B. C.: Crohn's disease (regional enteritis) of the large intestine and its distinction from ulcerative colitis, Gut 1:87, 1960.
3. Schwartz, S., et al.: Roentgenographic aspects of reversible vascular occlusion of the colon and its relationship to ulcerative colitis, Radiology 80:625, 1963.
4. Margulis, A. R., et al.: The overlapping spectrum of ulcerative and granulomatous colitis: A roentgenographic-pathological study, Am. J. Roentgenol. 113(2):325, 1971.
5. Cello, J. P., and Meyer, J. H.: Ulcerative Colitis, in Sleisenger, M. H., and Fordtran, J. S. (eds.): *Gastrointestinal Diseases, Vol. II* (Philadelphia: W. B. Saunders Co., 1978).
6. Marshak, R. H., et al.: Toxic dilatation of the colon in the course of ulcerative colitis, Gastroenterology 38(2):165, 1960.
7. Lennard-Jones, J. E., et al.: Cancer in colitis: Assessment of the individual risk by clinical and histological criteria, Gastroenterology 73(6):1280, 1977.
8. Roth, J. L. A.: Ulcerative Colitis, in Bockus, H. G. (ed.): *Gastroenterology, Vol. II* (Philadelphia: W. B. Saunders Co., 1964).
9. Laufer, I.: Air contrast studies of the colon in inflammatory bowel disease, CRC Crit. Rev. Radiol. 9(4):421, 1977.
10. Marshak, R. H., and Lindner, A. E.: Ulcerative and Granulomatous Colitis, in Margulis, A. R., and Burhenne, H. J. (eds.): *Alimentary Tract Roentgenology, Vol. II* (St. Louis: C. V. Mosby Co., 1973).
11. Keating, J. W., Jr., and Mindell, H. J.: Localized giant pseudopolyposis in ulcerative colitis, Am. J. Roentgenol. 126:1178, 1976.
12. Goldberger, L. E., et al.: Large mucosal bridges. An unusual roentgenographic manifestation of ulcerative colitis, Gastrointest. Radiol. 3(1):81, 1978.
13. Gardiner, G. A.: "Backwash ileitis" with pseudopolyposis, Am. J. Roentgenol. 129:506, 1977.
14. Goulston, S. J. J., and McGovern, V. J.: The nature of benign strictures in ulcerative colitis, N. Engl. J. Med. 281(6):290, 1969.

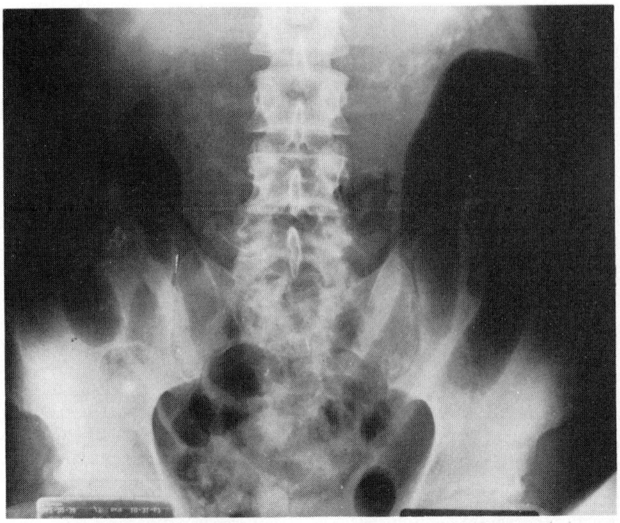

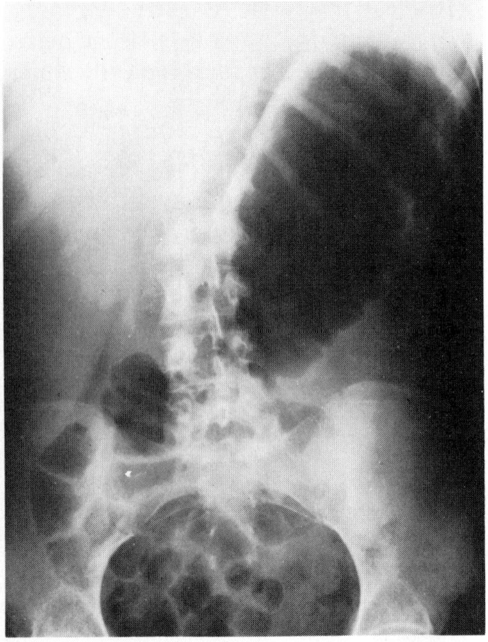

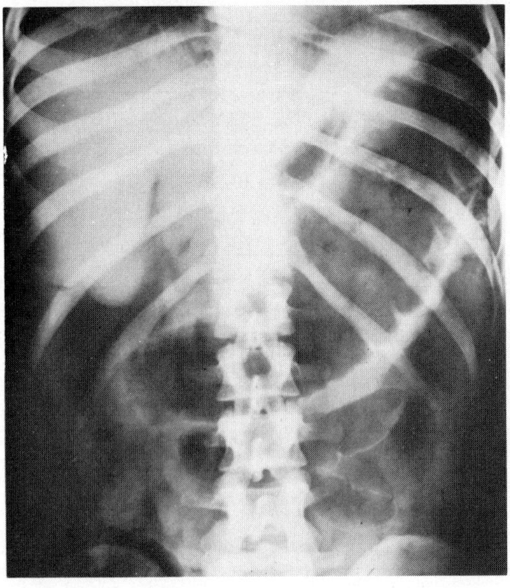

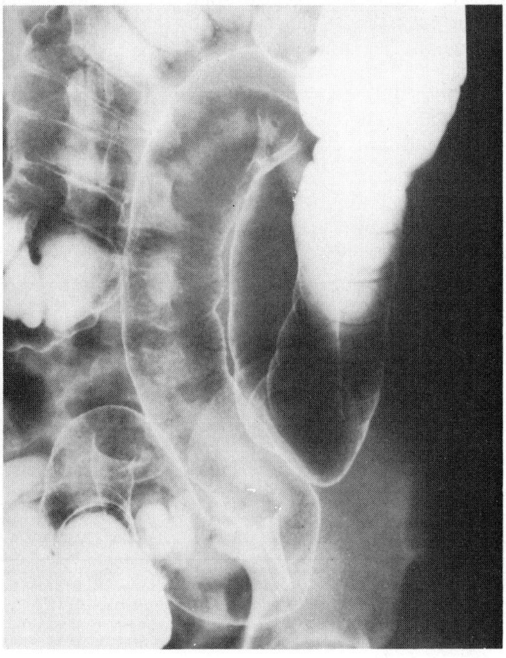

Fig 45–1 (top left).—Plain film of abdomen in ulcerative colitis. Intraluminal colonic gas demonstrates smooth, ahaustral, tubular-appearing colon.

Fig 45–2 (top right).—Plain film of abdomen in toxic megacolon. Transverse colon is massively distended and contains multiple rounded filling defects representing pseudopolyps.

Fig 45–3 (bottom left).—Plain film of abdomen in toxic megacolon with colonic perforation. Dilated gas-filled colon has nodular contour. Free intraperitoneal air outlines inferior margin of liver and gallbladder. Perforation of splenic flexure found at surgery.

Fig 45–4 (bottom right).—Early ulcerative colitis. Double contrast study demonstrates fine stippling and granularity of distal sigmoid colon. Transition zone to normal colon is gradual rather than abrupt.

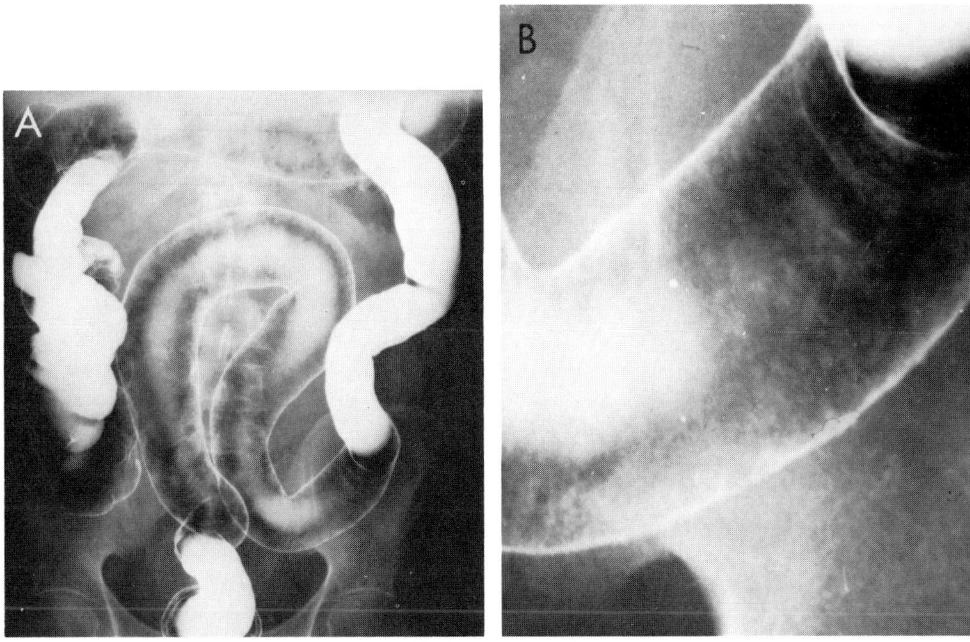

Fig 45-5.—Early ulcerative colitis. **A,** double contrast study reveals total colonic involvement. **B,** magnification view shows fine granular, stippled mucosal pattern with spiculated contour, representing superficial ulcerations.

Fig 45-6.—Chronic ulcerative colitis. **A,** double contrast study shows loss of haustral architecture. **B,** magnification reveals coarse granular mucosal pattern typical of ulcerative colitis.

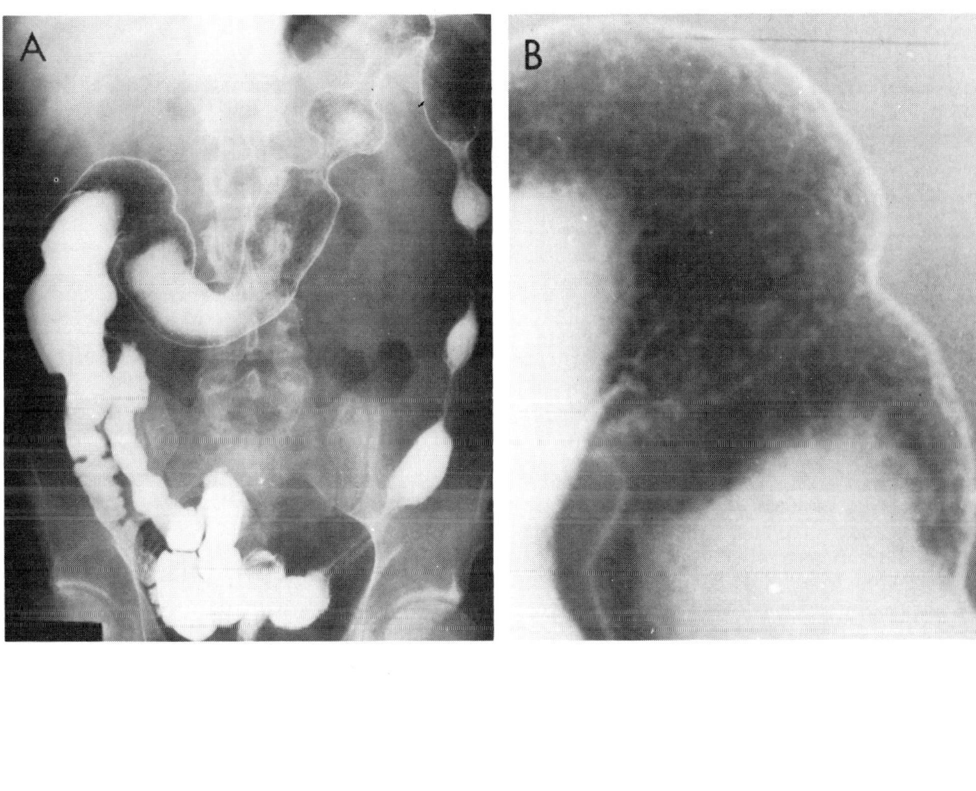

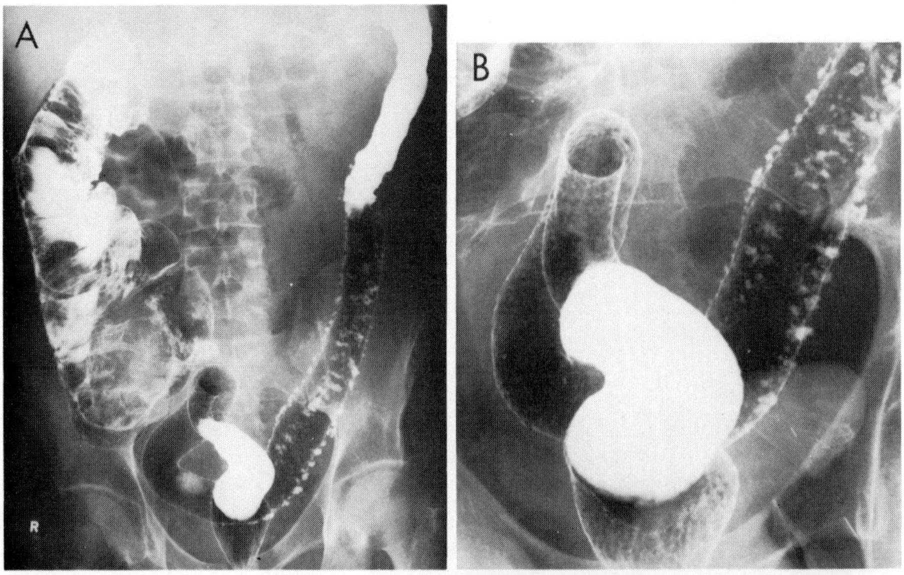

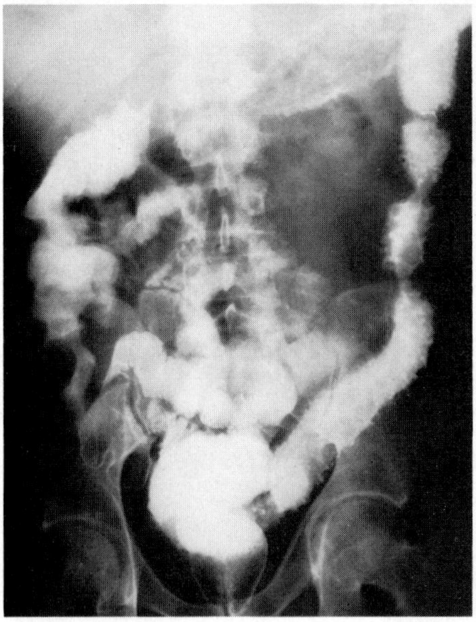

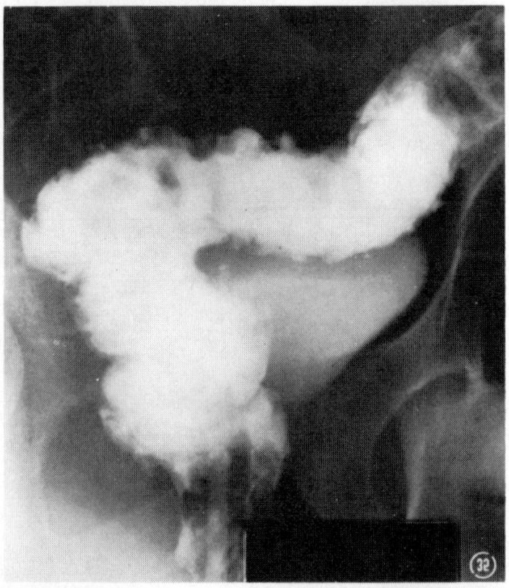

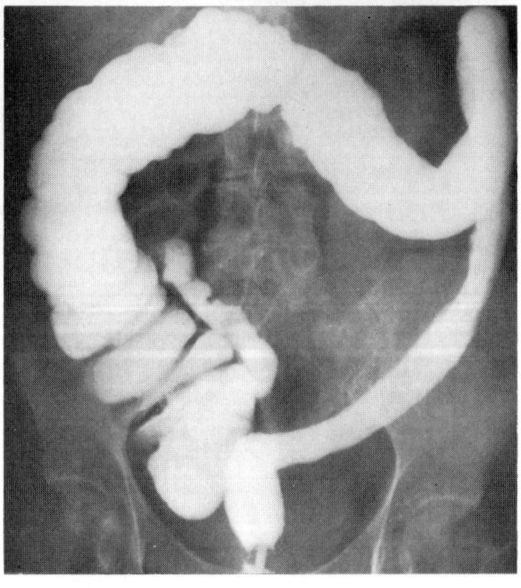

Fig 45-7 (top).—Acute ulcerative colitis. **A,** double contrast study reveals severe disease of left colon. **B,** spot film demonstrates deep undermining ulcers in descending colon and coarse granular mucosal pattern in rectosigmoid.

Fig 45-8 (center left).—Acute ulcerative colitis. Entire colon is involved. Deep ulcerations present in transverse and descending colon. Areas of spasm present in descending colon. No significant shortening.

Fig 45-9 (center right).—Acute ulcerative colitis. Rectosigmoid area shows extensive ulceration and pseudopolyposis. Ulcerations are deep and undermine mucosa.

Fig 45-10 (bottom).—Left-sided ulcerative colitis. Disease extends from midtransverse colon to rectum, with mucosal ulceration, loss of haustration, decreased distensibility and marked shortening of sigmoid colon. Transition zone between normal and involved colon is indistinct.

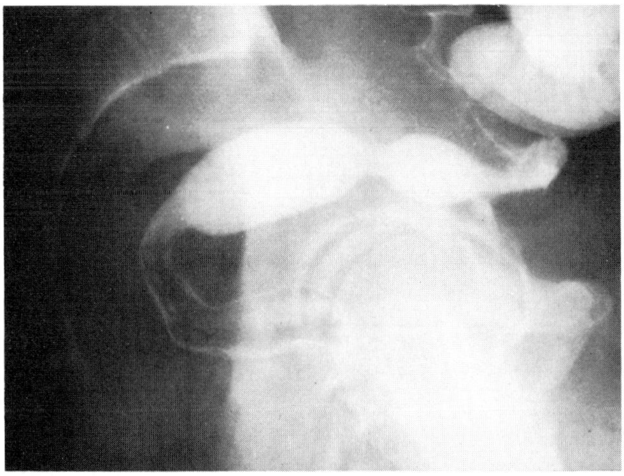

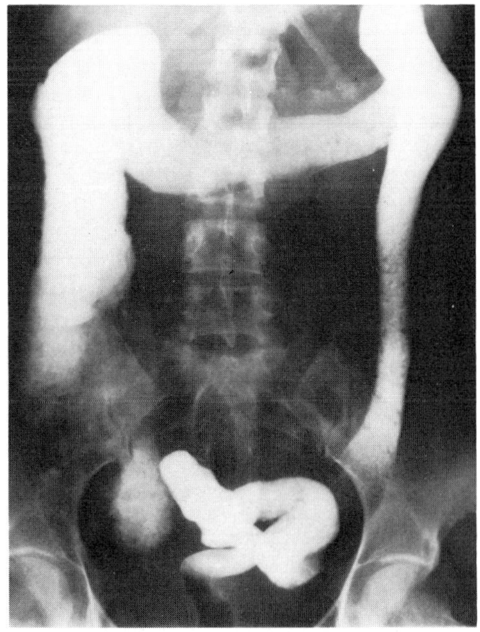

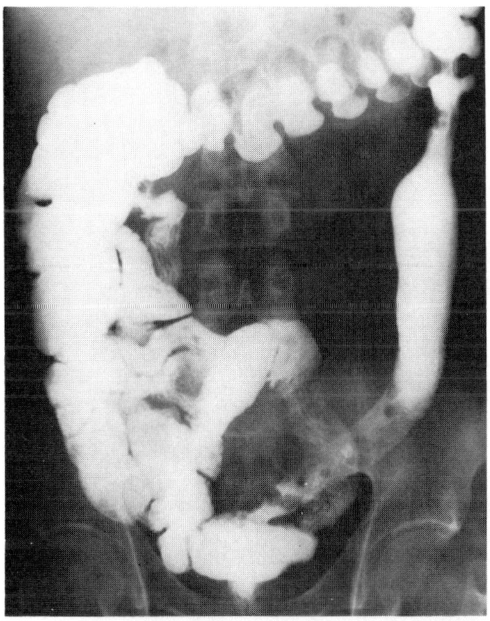

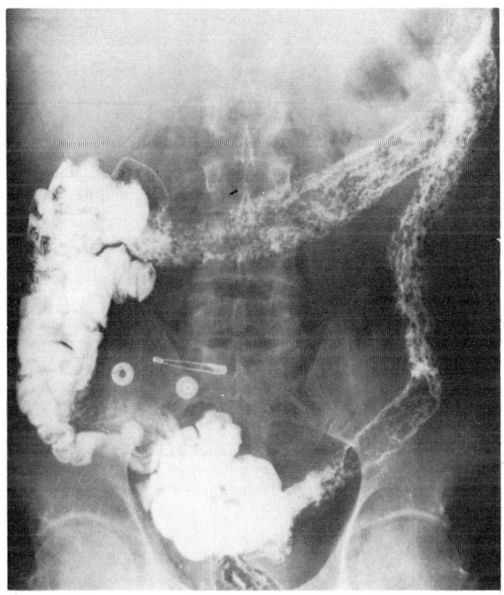

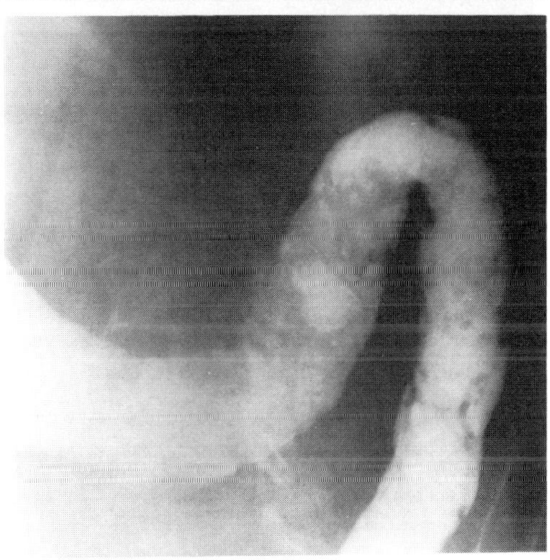

Fig 45–11 (top left). —Chronic ulcerative colitis. Lateral film of rectum demonstrates tubular narrowing of rectum with marked increase in retrorectal space.

Fig 45–12 (top right). —Chronic ulcerative colitis with pseudopolyposis. Colon is ahaustral, and multiple small rounded filling defects, representing pseudopolyps, are seen throughout large intestine, most prominent in descending colon.

Fig 45–13 (center left). —Chronic left-sided ulcerative colitis with pseudopolyposis. Examination performed during clinical remission. No ulcerations, but left colon is shortened and contains multiple large pseudopolyps.

Fig 45–14 (bottom right). —Ulcerative colitis with extensive pseudopolyposis. Postevacuation film shows carpeting of colon with multiple polypoid filling defects.

Fig 45–15 (bottom left). —Chronic ulcerative colitis with multiple mucosal bridges. Bandlike lucencies represent mucosal bridges present in splenic flexure.

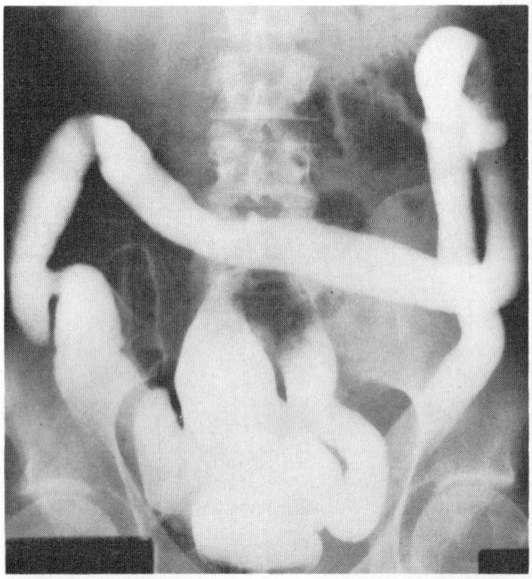

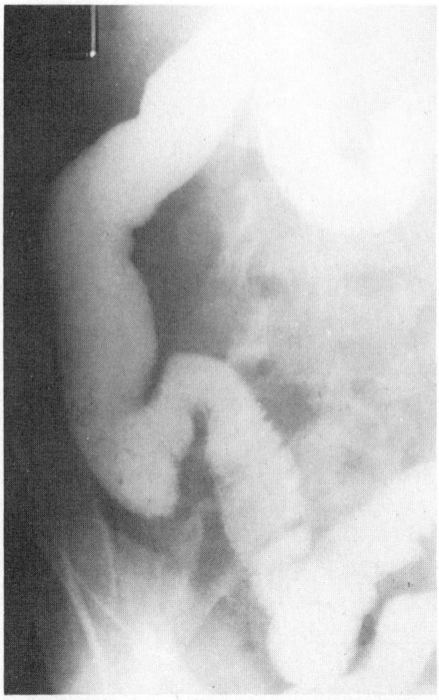

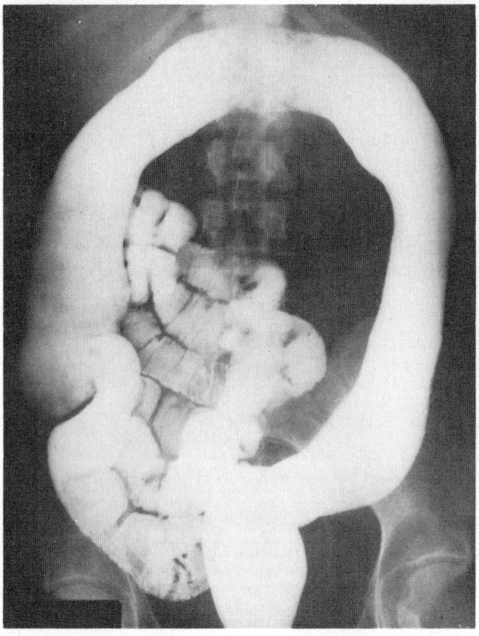

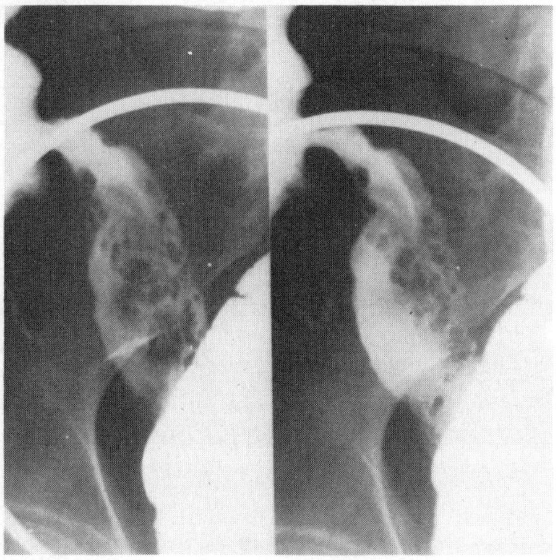

Fig 45–16 (top left).—Chronic ulcerative colitis with backwash ileitis. Colon is ahaustral and lacks distensibility. Ileocecal valve patulous and terminal ileum dilated and smooth.

Fig 45–17 (top right).—Chronic ulcerative colitis with backwash ileitis. Ileocecal valve is patulous, and distal few centimeters of terminal ileum is devoid of mucosal folds, in contrast to normal, more proximal ileum.

Fig 45–18 (bottom left).—Chronic ulcerative colitis. Colon completely devoid of haustral markings and, although significant shortening has occurred, distensibility appears normal.

Fig 45–19 (botton right).—Chronic ulcerative colitis. Backwash ileitis with pseudopolyposis. Multiple nodules of various size in patulous terminal ileum.

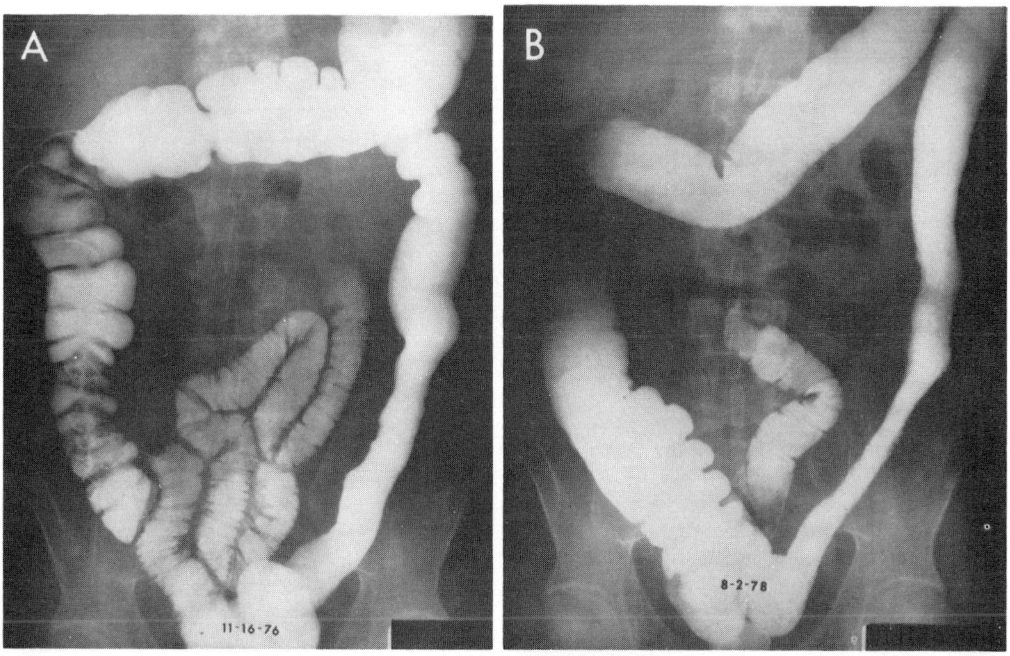

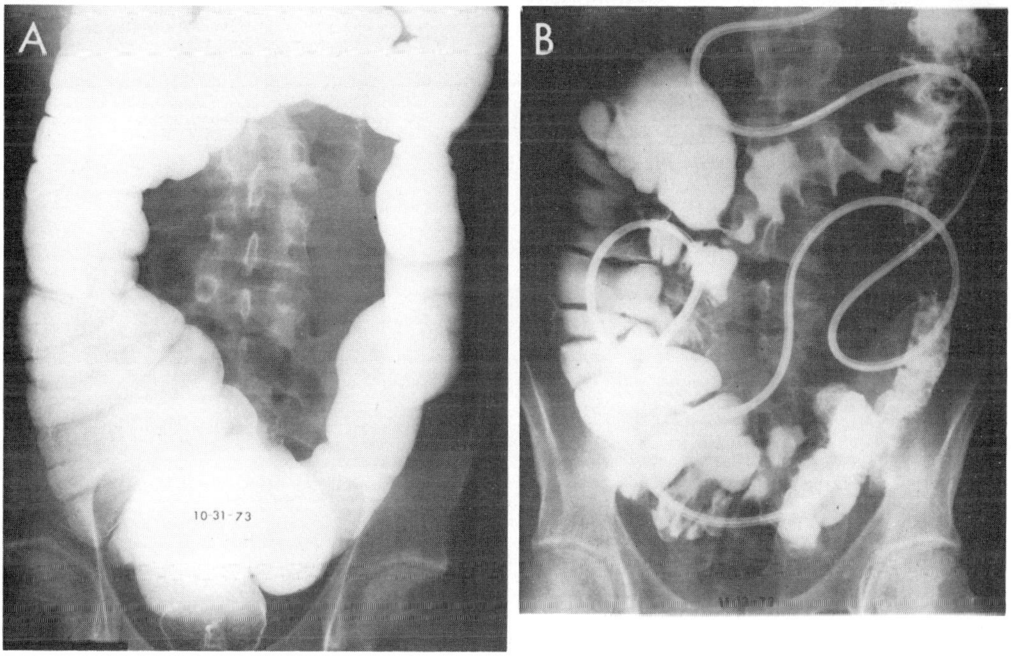

Fig 45–20 (top).—Ulcerative colitis with progression. **A,** initial study shows minimal lack of distensibilty and diminished haustrations in descending colon. **B,** examination 21 months later reveals progression in severity and extent of involvement.

Fig 45–21 (bottom).—Fulminant ulcerative colitis. **A,** initial examination shows only fine shallow ulcerations involving rectum. **B,** 2 weeks later, entire left colon severely involved, with edema and pseudopolyps. Patient refractory to medical therapy, necessitating colectomy

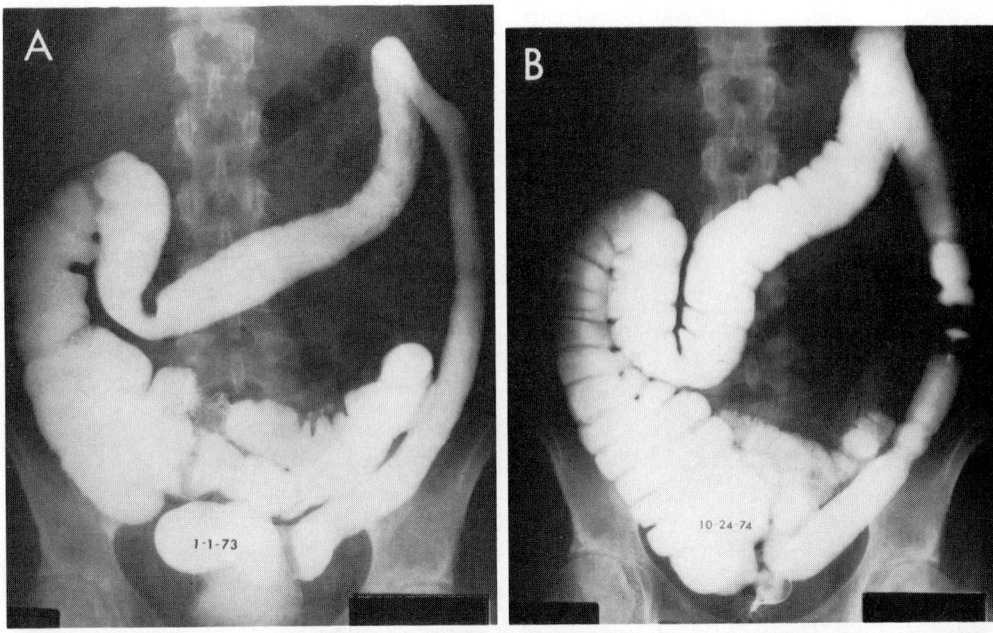

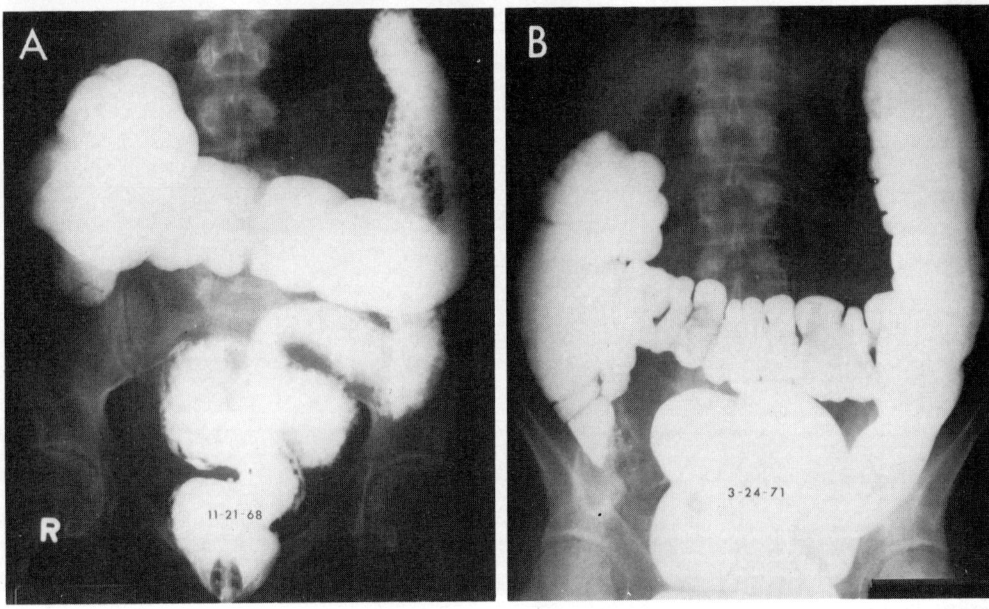

Fig 45–22 (top).—Ulcerative colitis with significant radiographic remission. **A,** initial study shows loss of haustration, decreased distensibility and scattered pseudopolyps from hepatic flexure distally. **B,** return to normal haustration and distensibility in transverse colon on follow-up examination.

Fig 45–23 (bottom).—Ulcerative colitis with complete remission. **A,** initial examination shows extensive deep longitudinal ulcerations undermining mucosa, with severe polyposis confined to left side of colon. **B,** following medical therapy, radiographic remission is complete.

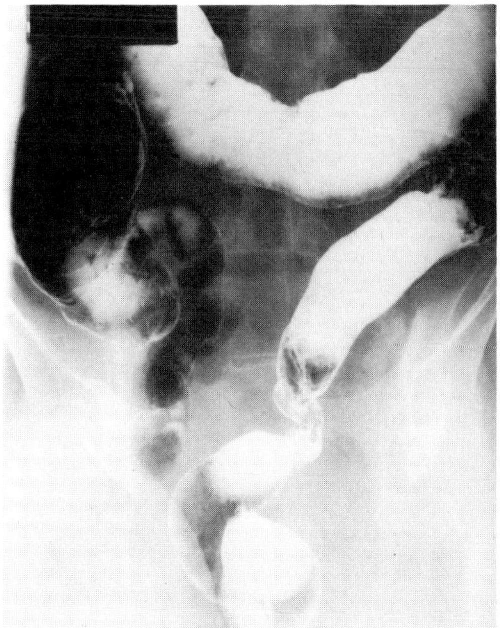

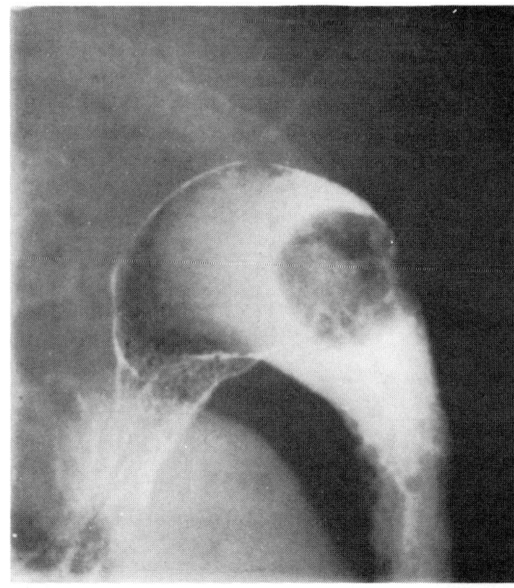

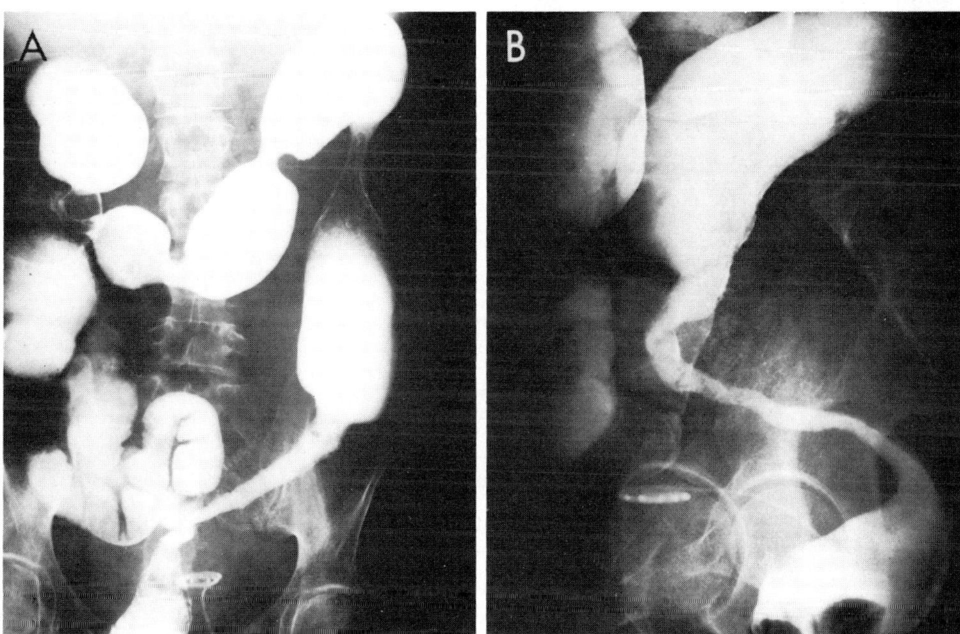

Fig 45–24 (top left).—Chronic ulcerative colitis with benign stricture. Zone of narrowing demonstrated in rectosigmoid area in patient with long-standing disease. Colectomy was performed and stricture proved benign on pathologic examination.

Fig 45–25 (top right).—Chronic ulcerative colitis with benign adenomatous polyp. A 2.5 cm finely lobulated filling defect is demonstrated in splenic flexure in patient with long-standing disease. Pathologic examination revealed benign adenoma with no evidence of malignancy.

Fig 45–26 (bottom).—Calcifying mucinous adenocarcinoma in chronic ulcerative colitis. **A,** long segment of irregular narrowing surrounded by punctate calcification in sigmoid colon. **B,** at surgery, mucinous adenocarcinoma was found that had widely metastasized.

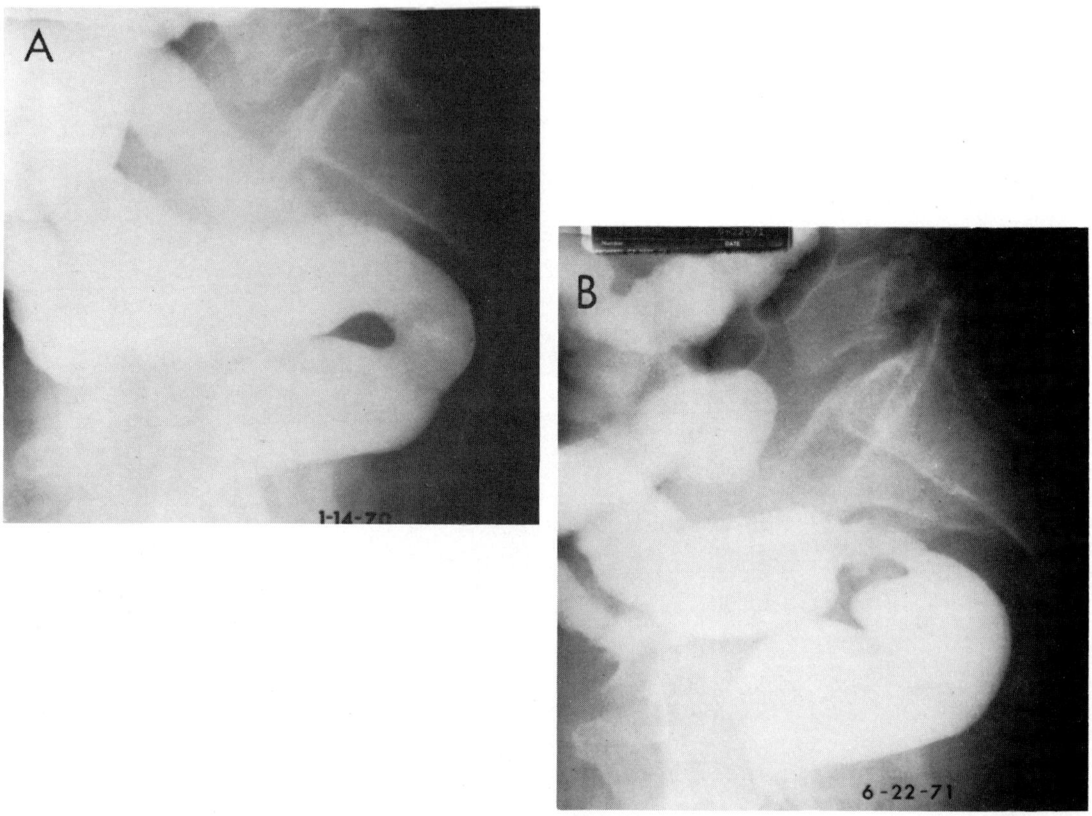

Fig 45–27.—Adenocarcinoma in chronic ulcerative colitis. Patient had chronic ulcerative colitis, which had been stable for 13 years. **A,** initial study shows minimal involvement of rectum. **B,** within 17 months, annular constricting lesion appeared in rectosigmoid area, which on biopsy proved to be adenocarcinoma.

Chapter 46

Ultrasonography of the Colon

STEPHEN J. HANDLER, M.D.

SINCE ITS FIRST CLINICAL application in the late 1950s, ultrasound has become an important tool in diagnosing diseases of the abdomen and pelvis and has also undergone extraordinary technical advances. New technology has given rise to increased instrument sensitivity, which has dramatically improved the imaging and interpretation of many disease processes. Ultrasound has become well established in its ability to detect abdominal and retroperitoneal structures[1-4] and now faces a new challenge in the gastrointestinal tract, specifically the colon.

It has only been within the past few years that the awareness and association of ultrasound with gastrointestinal lesions has been made. Recent papers by several authors elucidate their common experiences with respect to gastrointestinal tumors primarily confined to the gastric antrum.[5-8] For many years the gastrointestinal tract has been considered a "no man's land" for ultrasonographers because of bowel gas, which is impermeable to high frequency sound. It is my intent to present a variety of clinical cases in which ultrasound has definite applicability in diagnosing or aiding in the revelation of colonic pathology. Owing to its widespread community availability and its innocuous nature, ultrasound should be used more often in the search for gastrointestinal diseases.

Techniques of Examination

Discussion of basic ultrasonic techniques and instrumentation may be found both in standard ultrasound textbooks and in the recent radiologic literature.[9] Evaluation of the colon should include a systematic examination of the entire abdomen, with a complete set of transverse and longitudinal scans performed at 2-cm intervals, or a survey of the abdomen conducted with a real-time scanner. Of course, particular attention should be paid to any palpable masses or clinically suspicious regions. The ultrasound examination is routinely performed in the supine position; however, both left and right lateral decubitus positions should be used. Coronal scans of the abdomen are performed in the decubitus position and may provide additional information that would otherwise have been impossible to obtain, e.g., identification of the common bile duct.[10] The real-time scanner has particular importance in assisting in identification of normal or abnormal loops of bowel. Demonstration of peristalsis by real-time confirms the presence of bowel that could be confused with an abscess or cyst.

In addition to examination of the colon by ultrasound, the new field of computerized tomography (CT) of the abdomen also has application, as discussed in a recent article by Kressel et al.[11] The advantages of CT include an unobscured view of the air-filled colon and the use of dilute sodium diatrizoate enemas to define the colonic lumen; the disadvantages are its limited availability, increased cost and use of ionizing radiation.

Ultrasound may be used as the first diagnostic tool in the investigation of colon pathology, but should not replace conventional barium studies, proctoscopy or colonoscopy. It is well documented that the presence of barium in the gastrointestinal tract is detrimental to abdominal ultrasonography.[12, 13] For this reason and because of its expediency, it is advantageous to perform the ultrasound examination prior to the barium study.

A recent new technique of pelvic and colonic ultrasound examination has been described by Ruben et al.[14] Their paper described a technique of pelvic ultrasound that uses a distended bladder in combination with a water enema. The water-filled rectosigmoid colon can serve as an anatomical marker to help distinguish feces-filled colon from a significant pelvic mass. The feces-filled bowel has a characteristic stippled appearance, and this subsequently aids in alleviating confusion over pelvic masses versus normal sigmoid colon. This technique is potentially useful in outlining the caudal extent of the intraperitoneal space, e.g., the pouch of Douglas, not normally seen in the absence of ascites.[15] This water enema method is comparable to that used in CT, which utilizes intravenous contrast to fill the bladder and dilute enemas of sodium diatrizoate solution.[11] It must be added that in a busy ultrasound practice, it is sometimes difficult to use the water enema technique, and proper facilities must be close by.

Appearance of Normal Bowel

In order to recognize and comprehend the ultrasonic appearances of normal or pathologic bowel, one must be familiar with the overall presentation of the gastrointestinal tract. Figure 46–1 demonstrates a variety of these appearances in which the bowel is collapsed, air filled or fluid filled. The convention of display of the ultrasound images will be the following:

> The transverse scans are viewed with the patient's right side on the reader's left and the patient's left side on the reader's right; the longitudinal or parasagittal scans appear with the patient's head located to the reader's left and the patient's feet to the reader's right.

Normal collapsed bowel is exemplified by the gastric antrum (see Fig 46–1, A). The antral wall is primarily sonolucent and consists of a thin rim, which surrounds the collapsed echogenic lumen. The central echogenicity is caused by the intraluminal mucus. If the bowel is gas filled, it presents as an echogenic region with characteristic posterior acoustic shadowing (see Fig 46–1, B). Fluid-filled loops of bowel usually appear as multiple circular or cylindric structures with a finely irregular wall and with evenly distributed, weakly echoing material within them (see Fig 46–1, C and D). Sometimes in a distended, fluid-filled colon, one can also observe the colonic haustral pattern. The collapsed colon has an ultrasonic appearance similar to that of the gastric antrum (see Fig 46–1, E), and usually can be differentiated from the stomach by its location.[16] Fluid-filled loops of bowel must be distinguished from abnormal abdominal fluid collections; this usually is done on the basis of the following observations: the fluid-filled loops show a multiplicity of fluid collections, they are fairly uniform in size and they display a distinct change in size when undergoing peristalsis. This latter feature can be readily recognized with real-time ultrasound and, even though it is more difficult, it can still be appreciated during conventional B-scanning. The solitary fluid-filled loop of bowel may present a problem, and its distinction from an abnormal fluid collection, e.g., a pancreatic pseudocyst or an abscess, may be exceedingly difficult.

In examination of the colon, one must be aware of the so-called pseudotumor, which represents a feces-filled colon. This pseudotumor, usually well recognized on conventional radiograms, is demonstrated by ultrasound in Figure 46–2. In this particular example, the patient returned to the ultrasound laboratory 24 hours following purgative enemas and the mass disappeared.

Inflammatory and Neoplastic Diseases

INFLAMMATION

Inflammatory diseases such as Crohn's colitis or diverticulitis primarily affect the colon; however, pericolic extension is common. Pericolic extension may manifest itself as an inflammatory mass or, in a more acute state, as an abscess. In the examples of Crohn's disease shown in Figures 46–3 and 46–4, abnormally thickened loops of bowel were identified and appeared atonic on the real-time examination. The atonicity was due to the reflex ileus. The bowel wall, represented by the thickened sonolucent rim, is infiltrated by the inflammatory process. Although the configuration of affected bowel loops can be identified, an inflammatory mass may also be imaged as a solid inhomogeneous structure (see Fig 46–4, B). In Crohn's disease perforations and fistulous tracts are notoriously common to the disease process, and ultrasound can be beneficial in localizing these abscesses or inflammatory masses. Therapeutic surgical drainage or puncture and aspiration under ultrasound guidance can then be performed.[17-19]

In acute diverticulitis (Figs 46–5 to 46–7) with perforation, clinicians may choose not to perform colonoscopy because the introduction of air may further disseminate the infection. A water-soluble enema may be performed, but it too has limitations. In this clinical setting, ultrasonography can help to define the limits of the pericolic abscess and give clinicians some idea of the extent of bowel involvement. This is extremely important to the surgeon, who would consider localized resection of the involved colon if there were no demonstrable spread across the midline.

Although infrequent, a clinical situation may arise in which the patient presents with signs and symptoms of acute diverticulitis, and yet the barium enema is normal. This poses a difficult diagnostic dilemma, and it is during this early stage of evolving diverticulitis that a pericolic abscess may be present but undetected by conventional barium enema. In this situation, ultrasound can provide the definitive diagnosis by demonstrating a pericolic abscess; however, a negative examination does not exclude its presence. In the more advanced diseased state, there may be peritonitis resultant from colonic perforation despite the lack of x-ray findings of free air on examination. Ultrasound may be useful in detecting subphrenic abscesses that have occurred due to perforation and dissemination along the pericolic gutters. It is in these clinical situations that ultrasound plays an important and vital diagnostic role.

Figure 46–8, which illustrates a case of acute appendicitis and periappendiceal abscess, denotes the limit of the abscess cavity and also shows involvement of the cecum and terminal ilium. Figure 46–9 shows the ultrasonic appearance of a perirectal abscess, along with CT correlation. The abscess appears as a sonolucent mass, with thick irregular margins and good through-transmission. The perirectal abscess is represented by a complex mass rather than by the usual cystic appearance, which is a classic feature in about 70% of abscesses.[20] Since air filled structures reflect 99% of the ultrasound beam, they are impervious and cannot be imaged. In a recent article by Kressel and Filly,[21] gas-containing abscesses were diagnosed and imaged by ultrasound in spite of this "reflecting" phenomenon (see Fig

46–10, C). Other authors[22, 23] refer to the "micro-bubble" theory to explain ultrasonically imaged abscesses that appear as strongly echogenic masses but without characteristic posterior acoustic shadowing. The micro-bubble theory may further be used to explain the dense echoes commonly seen within the gastrointestinal lumina on ultrasound. These sonodense echoes represent mucus and small bubbles of air that have not coalesced; under these conditions, there is no posterior acoustic shadowing.

NEOPLASIA

Figures 46–10 through 46–16 provide ultrasonic, radiographic and CT examples of colonic neoplasms. The typical sonographic appearance of bowel malignancies consists of a mass lesion with an almost entirely sonolucent or echo-free periphery and sonodense central echoes. This ultrasonic pattern for carcinoma appears to hold true for any portion of the alimentary tract in which the lesion directly involves the bowel wall (Fig 46–17). Concentric thickening of the infiltrated bowel wall gives this sonolucent appearance. The strong central echoes arising from the lumen are usually a combination of mucus and intraluminal air. This pattern of carcinoma was first described by Freimanis and Ascher[24] in 1970. Others have since reported similar findings.[5-8]

The ultrasonic appearance of bowel wall infiltration with a sonolucent mantle seems typical of tumors of the gastrointestinal tract, and yet other benign and inflammatory diseases may produce similar findings, as previously demonstrated. It has been my experience and that of others that gastrointestinal neoplasms must be large in order to produce the typical sonographic pattern and involve about one-half the circumference of the bowel wall.[5-8] The size of these lesions strongly suggests an exophytic component, and this degree of mantle thickening is not usually seen in inflammatory or benign conditions.[6] In addition to demonstrating various lesions, ultrasound may disclose other helpful abnormalities, such as metastases to the liver (see Fig 46–17, E). If considerable obstruction exists, a large fluid collection can be demonstrated proximal to the lesion. Although this principally occurs in the stomach, lesions of the colon can also show proximal fluid-filled bowel loops.

With the advent of CT of the abdomen, in the mid 1970s, its application to the alimentary tract has only recently been demonstrated. Although abdominal CT has had its principal application and success in evaluation of the liver, spleen, pancreas and retroperitoneum, the studies of Kressel and Callen[11] and others[25-27] demonstrated that CT can provide valuable information about the extraluminal extent of gastrointestinal lesions. Although there are advantages and disadvantages to both ultrasound and CT, they are complementary procedures and must be tailored to the individual patient. Ultrasound and CT are valuable in assessing resectability of gastrointestinal tumors, monitoring tumor response to radiation or chemotherapy and evaluating postoperative patients for suspected recurrent disease.

Diagnosis of colon carcinoma will still depend on the barium enema study, colonoscopy and proctoscopy, and biopsy. The size of the smallest but still ultrasonically detectable colon carcinoma has yet to be determined, and a negative ultrasound examination does not exclude a colonic carcinoma. Knowledge of the ultrasonic appearance of the colon in both inflammatory and neoplastic diseases is especially important when a neoplastic or infectious process is unsuspected.

Miscellaneous Conditions Affecting the Colon

Segmental narrowing of the colon is a common pathologic entity seen during a barium enema. The causes of narrowing are numerous and may be primary or secondary malignancy, inflammatory or ischemic processes or pressure by external masses.[28-30] The rectosigmoid and sigmoid colons are the most frequent areas of the colon to be affected by these processes and are especially prone to compression within the relatively narrow bony pelvis.

Pelvic lipomatosis is a relatively rare benign disorder of unknown cause and was first described by Engels[31] in 1959. About 58 cases have been reported in the English literature, none diagnosed by ultrasound. A case of pelvic lipomatosis diagnosed by ultrasound examination is presented in Figure 46–18. This case involves the bladder in an asymmetric rather than symmetric fashion, the latter being the typical presentation. Gerson et al.[32] reported two cases of pelvic lipomatosis that were confirmed by CT. A more detailed discussion of pelvic lipomatosis is contained in Chapter 31.

Other cases presenting with narrowing of the rectosigmoid colon due to carcinoma of the prostate and with recurrent leiomyosarcoma of the small bowel are demonstrated in Figures 46–19 and 46–20, respectively. An unusual cause of narrowing of the rectosigmoid colon is external compression by an enlarged urinary bladder.[33, 34] In the article by Kleinhaus and Kaftori,[33] the rectosigmoid colon shows a gradual biconcave narrowing on lateral projection of the barium enema (Fig 46–21, A). This narrowing is largest at the level of the sacral promontory. The compression of the colon exists because the distended bladder is located between the sacrum and the colon. This anatomical relationship is demonstrated nicely by CT (see Fig 46–21, B). In the frontal projection (see Fig 46–21, C) in the barium enema, there may be irregular lateral margins of the rectosigmoid colon. This finding may lead the radiologist to suggest an organic stricture but, according to Kleinhaus and Kaftori,[33] it is due to incomplete filling of the bowel because of extrinsic compression. Since the urinary symptoms may be absent or few, pseudostenosis should be part of the differential diagnosis. Allowing the patient to void or undergo bladder catheterization will confirm the diagnosis. Another simple method of confirmation is to perform a real-time ultrasound examination of the lower pelvis, with or without a concomitant saline enema.

Narrowing of other portions of the colon occur; involvement of the proximal descending colon is seen in Figure 46–22. The patient was a young black man, who presented with a stab wound to the upper abdomen and underwent an immediate exploratory laparotomy. The intraoperative and immediate postoperative periods were uneventful, but 3–4 days later, the patient complained of left upper quadrant pain, and a mass was palpated in that region. The patient underwent an ultrasound examination, which demonstrated the findings seen in Figures 46–22, B and C. Figure 46–22, C, represents a longitudinal scan with the patient in the right lateral decubitus position, permitting a coronal section of the left upper quadrant of the abdomen. In this case, a coronal view was of particular importance because the descending colon was well visualized and located medial to the predominantly sonolucent collection seen on the transverse scans. A barium enema correlated the ultrasound findings. The patient returned to the ultrasound laboratory and, under ultrasound guidance, 300 cc of hemorrhagic fluid was aspirated. This was thought to represent a postoperative hematoma and it was almost entirely drained. The patient experienced relief of symptoms and the remainder of his postoperative course was unremarkable.

Ultrasound has application in suspected cases of intussusception.[35-38] Adult intussusception is rare but is relatively common in young children. During infancy it is the most common cause of acquired intestinal obstruction, the intussusception being either ileocolic or ileo-ileocolic.[39] Five cases of ultrasonically diagnosed adult ileocolic intussusception have been reported in the medical literature.[35-38] Although the ultrasonic findings are very similar to the previously discussed changes in bowel loops seen in inflammatory and neoplastic diseases, Holt and Samuel[38] have suggested a characteristic multiple concentric ring shadow appearance in intussusception: longitudinal sonograms of the intussusception demonstrated multiple concentric shadows not previously appreciated. This ultrasonic finding may strongly suggest the presence of an intussusception rather than a colon carcinoma or inflammatory process.

It is in pediatrics that ultrasound can be especially helpful in diagnosing intussuception. In the realization that pediatric intussusceptions are dynamic phenomena and may undergo spontaneous reduction, ultrasound can be an important adjunct prior to the conventional barium enema. Since ultrasound experience is limited in diagnosing adult or pediatric intussusceptions, we must await further clinical correlation before a definitive statement of efficacy can be made.

Conclusion

Ultrasound of the colon, and of the gastrointestinal tract in general, is one of the newer applications of this diagnostic method. The ultrasonic appearance of normal bowel within the abdomen is commonplace in any abdominal or pelvic examination. Inflammatory or neoplastic diseases of the colon have certain characteristics that should be recognized, especially in unsuspected cases. Although the primary diagnosis of colonic lesions will depend on clinical examination, proctoscopy and colonoscopy, conventional radiographic procedures and biopsy, ultrasound is an important adjunct in defining the presence and extent of colonic pathology. Since ultrasound is still in the incipient stages of application to the colon, more widespread awareness and usage are needed before its present and future reliability can be accurately determined.

REFERENCES

1. Cooperberg, P. L., and Cohen, M. M.: Gray-scale ultrasound in the diagnosis of abdominal mass lesions, Can. J. Surg. 20:361, 1977.
2. Green, B., Bree, R. L., and Goldstein, H. M.: Gray-scale ultrasound evaluation of hepatic neoplasms: Patterns and correlations, Radiology 124:203, 1977.
3. Bhimiji, S. D., Cooperberg, P. L., Naimen, S., Morrison, R., and Shergill, P.: Ultrasound diagnosis of splenic cysts, Radiology 122:787, 1977.
4. Leopold, G., and Ascher, M. M.: *Fundamentals of Abdominal and Pelvic Ultrasound,* (Philadelphia: W. B. Saunders Co., 1975).
5. Peterson, L. R., and Cooperberg, P. L.: Ultrasound demonstration of lesions of the gastrointestinal tract, Gastrointest. Radiol. 3:303, 1978.
6. Lutz, H., and Petzoldt, R.: Ultrasonic patterns of space occupying lesions of the stomach and the intestines, Ultrasound Med. Biol. 2:129, 1976.
7. Walls, W. J.: The evaluation of malignant gastric neoplasms by ultrasound B-scanning, Radiology 118:159, 1976.
8. Kremer, H., Lohnoeller, G., and Zollner, N.: Primary ultrasonic detection of a double carcinoma of the colon, Radiology 124:481, 1977.
9. Bartrum, R. J., and Crow, H. C.: *Gray-Scale Ultrasound: A Manual for Physicians and Technical Personnel* (Philadelphia: W. B. Saunders Co., 1977).
10. Kazam, E., and Behan, M.: Sonography of the common bile duct: Value of the right anterior oblique view, Am. J. Roentgenol. 130:701, 1978.
11. Kressel, H. Y., Callen, P. W., Montagne, J. P., Korobkin, M., Goldberg, H. I., Moss, A. A., Arger, P. H., and Margulis, A. R.: Computerized tomographic evaluation of disorders affecting the alimentary tract, Radiology 129:451, 1978.
12. Leopold, G. R., and Ascher, W. M.: Deleterious affects of G.I. contrast material on abnormal echography, Radiology 113:714, 1971.
13. Sarti, D. A., and Lazere, A.: Re-examination of deleterious effect of G.I. contrast material on abdominal echography, Radiology 126:231, 1978.
14. Ruben, C., Kurtz, A. B., and Goldberg, B. B.: Water enema: A new ultrasound technique in defining pelvic anatomy, J. Clin. Ultrasound 6(1):28, 1978.
15. Yeh, H., and Wolf, B. S.: Ultrasonography in ascites, Radiology 124:783, 1977.
16. Walen, J. P., Evans, J. A., and Shanser, J.: Vector principal in the differential diagnosis of abdominal masses: The left upper quadrant, Am. J. Roentgenol. 113:104, 1971.
17. Holm, H. H., Pedersen, J. F., Kristensen, J. K., Rasmussen, S. N., Hancke, S., and Jensen, F.: Ultrasound guided percutaneous puncture, Radiol. Clin. North Am. 13:493, 1975.
18. Holm, H. H., Rasmussen, S. N., and Kristensen,

J. K.: Ultrasound guided percutaneous technique, J. Clin. Ultrasound 1:27, 1973.
19. Smith, E. H., and Bartrum, R. J.: Ultrasonically guided percutaneous aspiration of abscesses, Am. J. Roentgenol. 122:308, 1974.
20. Doust, B. D., and Doust, D. L.: Ultrasound diagnosis of abdominal abscess, Am. J. Dig. Dis. 21:569, 1976.
21. Kressel, H. Y., and Filly, R. A.: Ultrasonographic appearance of gas-containing abscesses in the abdomen, Am. J. Roentgenol. 130:71, 1978.
22. Yeh, H. C., and Wolf, B. S.: Ultrasonic contrast study to identify stomach tap water "micro-bubbles," J. Clin. Ultrasound 5:170, 1977.
23. Gramiak, R., Shaw, P. H., and Kramer, D. H.: Ultrasound cardiography: Contrast studies in anatomy and function, Radiology 92:939, 1969.
24. Freimanis, A. K., and Ascher, W. M.: Development of diagnostic criteria in echographic studies in abdominal lesions, Am. J. Roentgenol. 108:747, 1970.
25. Alfidi, R. J., Haaga, J. R., Meaney, T. F., MacIntyre, W. J., Leopold, G., Tarar, R., Zelch, M. G., Boller, M., Cook, S. A., and Jelden, G.: Computerized tomography of thorax and abdomen: A preliminary report, Radiology 117:257, 1975.
26. Sagel, S., Stanley, R. J., and Evens, R. G.: Early clinical experiences with motionless whole body computed tomography, Radiology 119:321, 1976.
27. Stanley, R. J., Sagel, S. S., and Levitt, R. G.: Computerized tomography of the body: Early trends in application and accuracy of the method, Am. J. Roentgenol. 127:53, 1976.
28. Marshak, R. H.: Extrinsic lesions affecting the rectosigmoid, Am. J. Roentgenol. 58:439, 1947.
29. Simpkins, K. C., and Young, A. C.: The differential diagnosis of large bowel strictures, Clin. Radiol. 22: 449, 1971.
30. Love, L.: Large bowel obstruction, Semin. Roentgenol. 8:299, 1973.
31. Engels, E. P.: Sigmoid colon and urinary bladder in high fixation: Roentgen changes simulating pelvic tumor, Radiology 72:419, 1959.
32. Gerson, E. S., Gerzof, S. G., and Robbins, A. H.: Computerized tomographic confirmation of pelvic lipomatosis: 2 cases, Am. J. Roentgenol. 129:338, 1977.
33. Kleinhaus, U., and Kaftori, J.: Rectosigmoid pseudostenosis due to urinary retention, Radiology 127: 645, 1978.
34. Bryk, D.: Barium enema examination in the evaluation of large pelvic masses, Am. J. Roentgenol. 101: 970, 1967.
35. Weissberg, D. L., Scheible, W., and Leopold, G. R.: Ultrasonographic appearance of adult intussusception, Radiology 124:971, 1977.
36. Uhland, H., and Parshley, P. F.: Obscure intussusception diagnosed by ultrasonography, J.A.M.A. 239:224, 1978.
37. Burke, L. F., and Clark, B.: Ileocolic intussusception—a case report, J. Clin. Ultrasound 5(5):346, 1977.
38. Holt, S., and Samuel, A. E.: Multiple concentric ring sign in the ultrasonographic diagnosis of intussusception, Gastrointest. Radiol. 3:307, 1978.
39. Caffey, J.: *Pediatric X-ray Diagnosis* (6th ed.; Chicago: Year Book Medical Publishers, Inc., 1973).

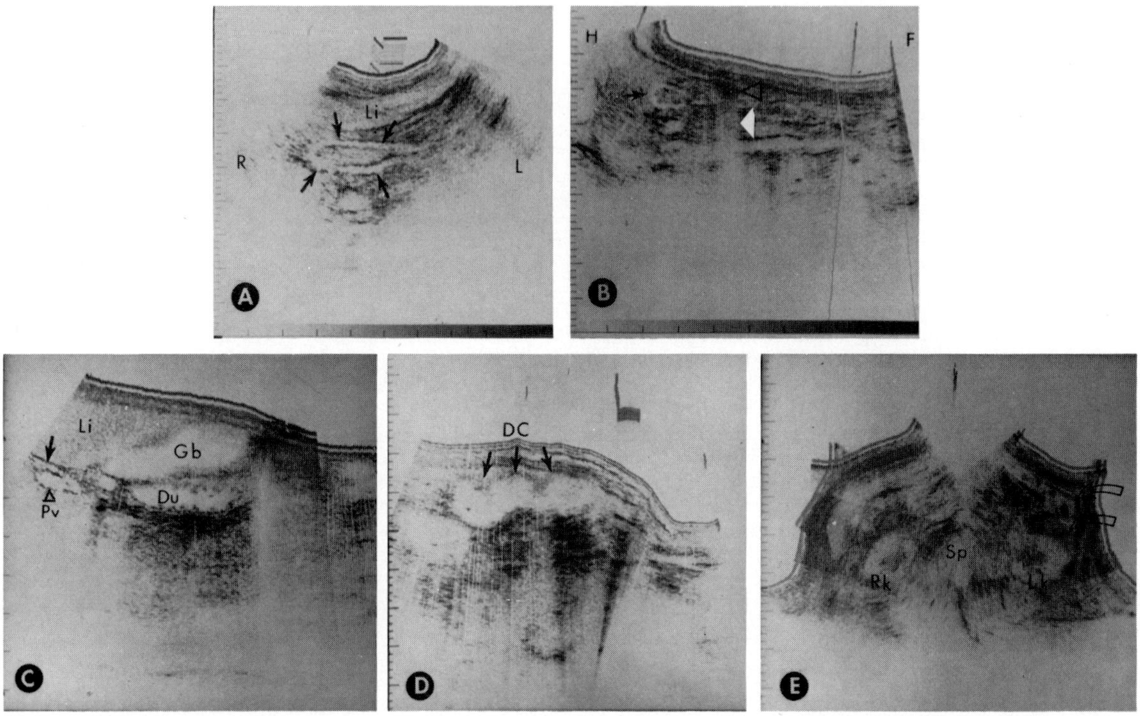

Fig 46–1.—Normal anatomy. **A,** limited transverse scan of midabdomen: gastric antrum. Note thin sonolucent rim of echoes representing antral wall *(arrows)* and gastric contents with mucus (light gray echoes). *Li* = liver, *R* = patient's right, *L* = patient's left. **B,** longitudinal scan in same region as **A.** *Black arrow* = antrum; *open arrowhead* = transverse colon containing air; *white arrowhead* = posterior acoustic shadowing caused by colonic air. **C,** longitudinal scan. Example of fluid-filled duodenum. Mucosal projections can be seen protruding into fluid-filled lumen. *Li* = liver; *Gb* = gallbladder; *Du* = duodenum; *Pv* = portal vein; *arrow* = common bile duct. **D,** longitudinal scan 8 cm to left of midline. Fluid-filled descending colon *(DC)* can be identified, along with haustral demarcations *(arrows).* **E,** transverse scan at level of kidneys. Descending colon, with central mucus *(black arrow),* is seen. *Open arrows* = descending colon; *RK* = right kidney; *LK* = left kidney; *SP* = spine.

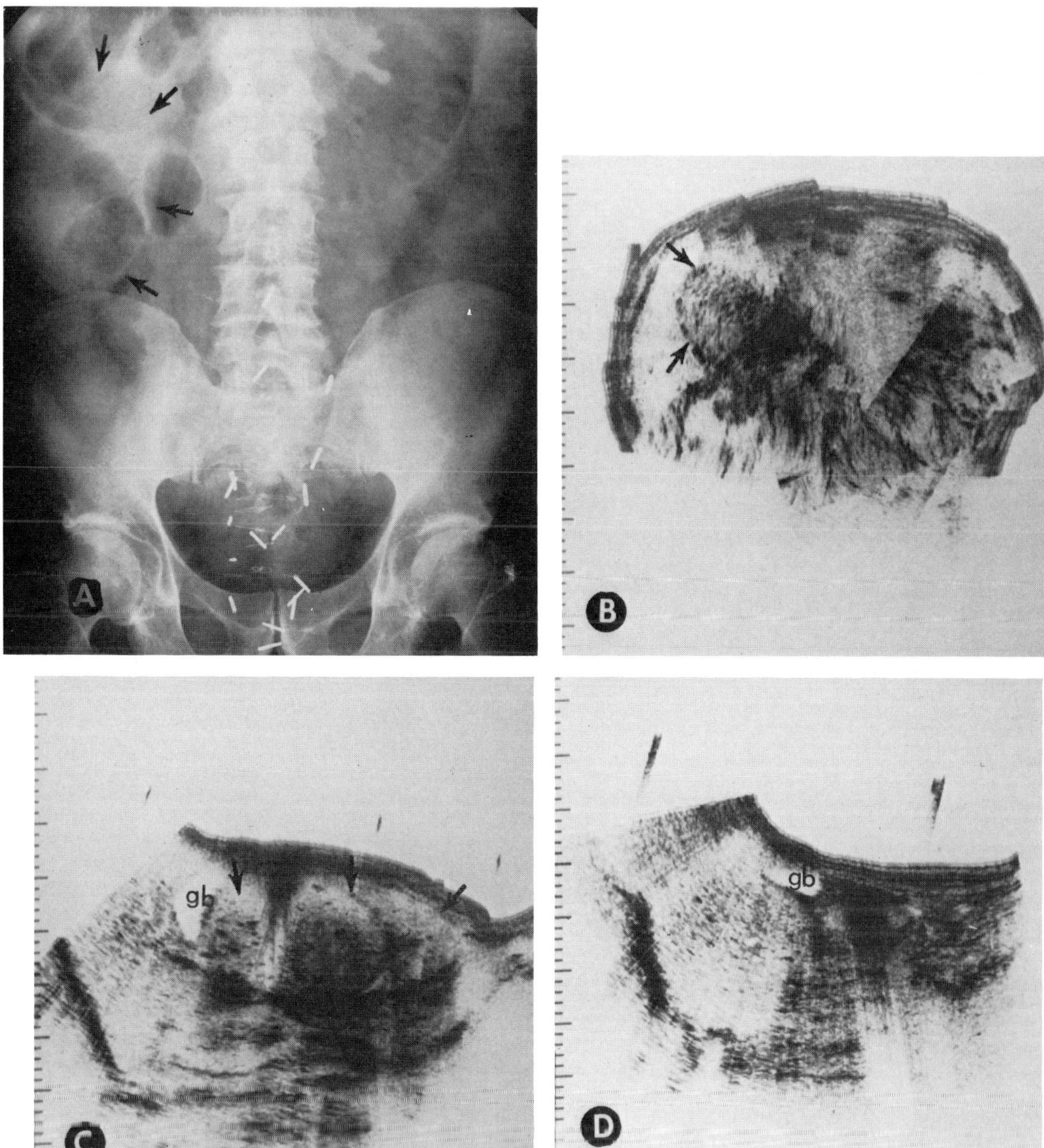

Fig 46–2.—Pseudotumor. Mass in right upper quadrant of abdomen. **A,** a KUB in postoperative patient. *Arrows* = soft tissue mass. **B,** transverse scan at level of palpated mass. Solid inhomogeneous mass *(arrows)* medial to liver. **C,** longitudinal scan to right of midline. Very large mass is confirmed *(arrows).* Note right kidney posterior to mass. *Gb* = gallbladder. **D,** longitudinal scan made 24 hours later; previously documented mass no longer present. Mass = focal pseudotumor. *Gb* = gallbladder.

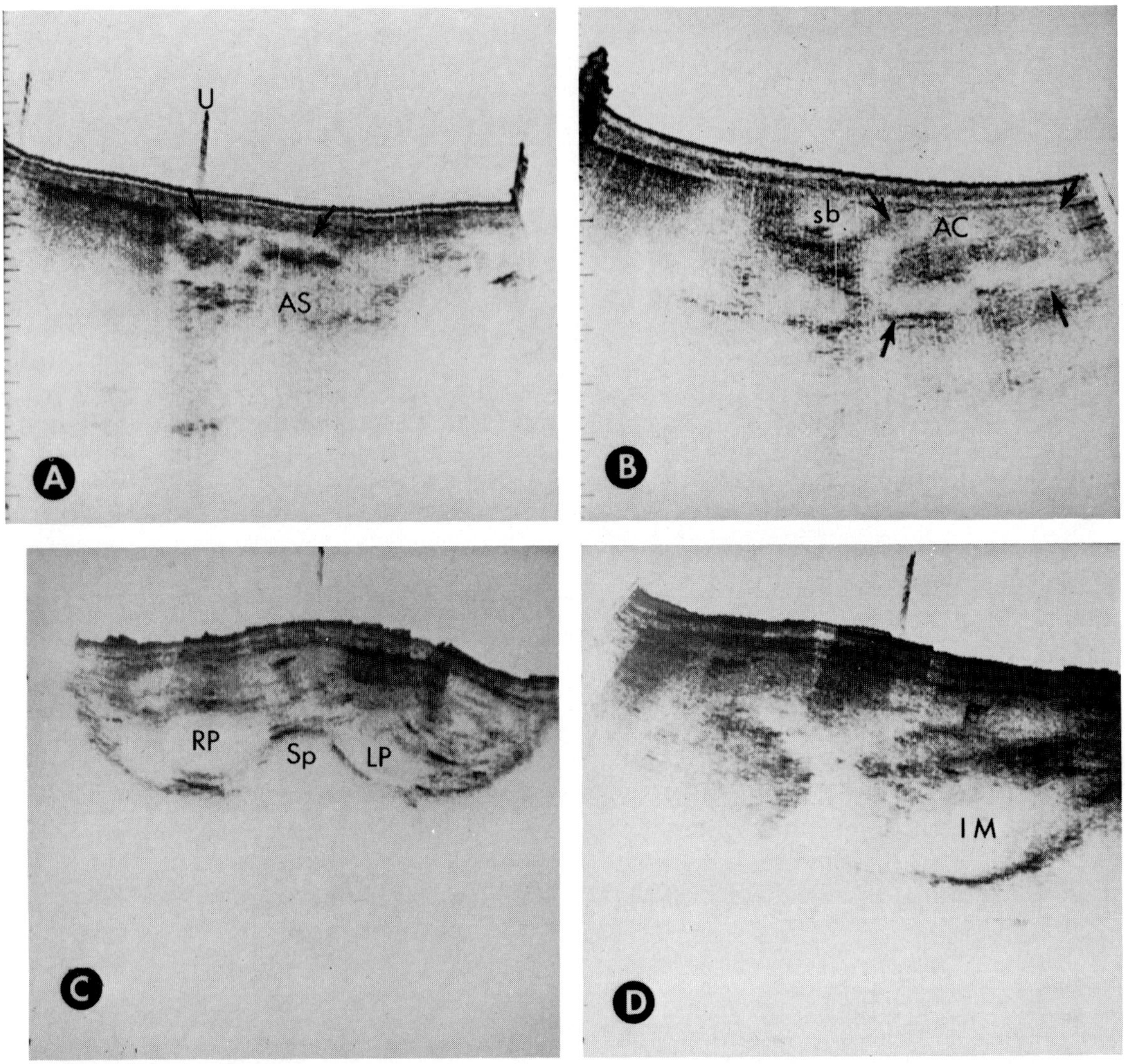

Fig 46–3.—Perforated Crohn's ileocolitis. Man, age 51, with known Crohn's disease and acute right lower quadrant pain. **A,** longitudinal scan of right flank with 8-cm-long segment of irregularly inflamed thick-walled bowel. *Arrows* = abnormal bowel (colon); *U* = umbilicus; *AS* = acoustic shadows. **B,** magnified longitudinal view of bowel *(arrows)* in **A.** Note fluid-filled loop of bowel (probably small bowel) superior to colon. *AC* = ascending colon; *Sb* = small bowel. **C,** transverse scan of lower abdomen. Right psoas muscle is markedly larger and more sonolucent than left. *RP* = right psoas muscle; *LP* = left psoas muscle; *Sp* = spine. **D,** angled longitudinal scan of right psoas muscle. Findings are consistent with right retroperitoneal inflammatory mass (surgically proved) affecting right psoas muscle. *IM* = inflammatory mass.

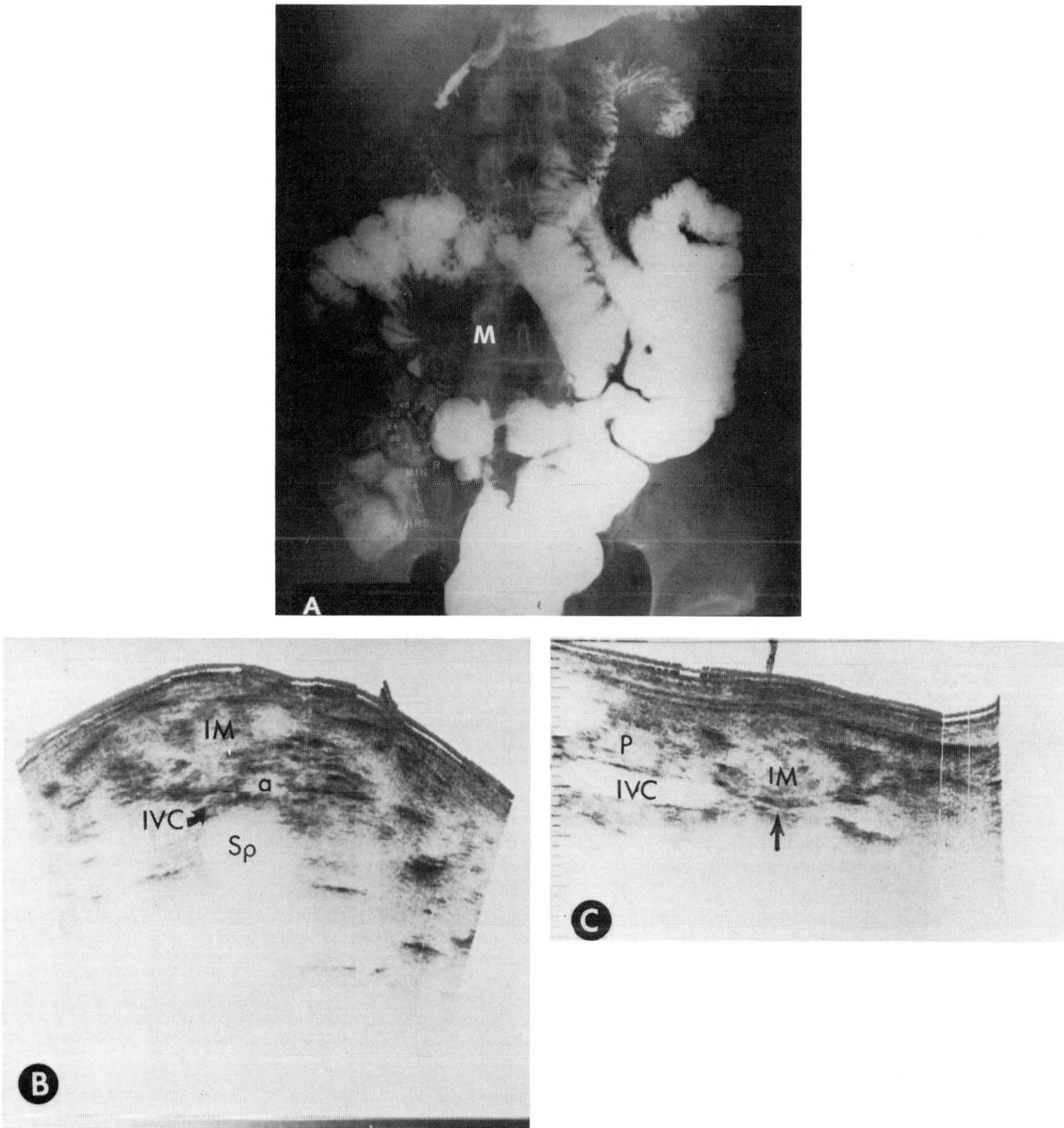

Fig 46–4.—Crohn's disease. White man, age 30, with 11-year history of Crohn's disease presented with right lower quadrant pain for 2 months. **A,** 40-minute film from small bowel follow-through demonstrating lower midabdominal mass and abnormal small bowel loops. *M* – mass. **B,** transverse scan of mid-lower abdomen. A 7×4×6 cm predominantly solid mass is identified to right of midline. Mass is compressing inferior vena cava *(IVC)*. *IM* – inflammatory mass; *a* = aorta; *Sp* = spine. **C,** longitudinal scan 1 cm to right of midline. Compression of inferior vena cava *(IVC)* by mass can be better appreciated. Pancreas is sonolucent, consistent with pancreatitis. Surgically proved case of Crohn's inflammatory mass *(IM)*. *P* = pancreas, *arrow* = narrowed *IVC*.

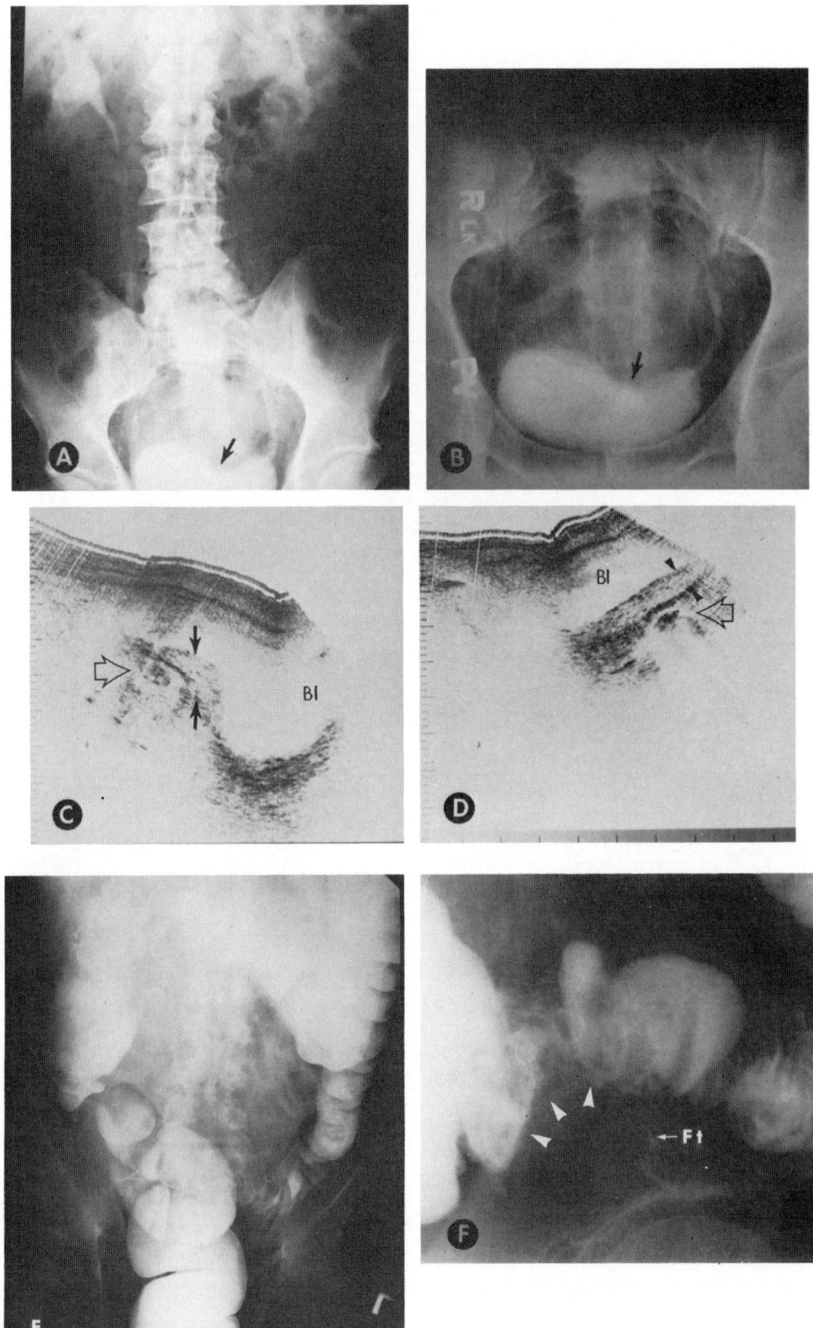

Fig 46–5.—Diverticulitis. Patient presented with 6-month history of chronic cystitis of unknown cause. **A,** intravenous urogram showing soft tissue mass *(arrow)* compressing left superior aspect of bladder. **B,** cone-down bladder view from **A.** Some irregularity of bladder contour *(arrow)* also seen superiorly. **C,** longitudinal ultrasound scan 1 cm left of midline. Note thickening of both posterior aspect of bladder (cystitis) and adjacent sigmoid colon. *Bl* = bladder; *arrows* = thickened bladder wall; *large open arrow* = inflamed sigmoid colon. **D,** transverse scan at level of dome of bladder *(Bl).* Persistent loop of bowel *(open arrow)* adjacent to thickened bladder wall *(arrowheads).* Posterior acoustic shadowing from luminal colonic air is seen. Ultrasound suggested diverticulitis. **E,** barium enema. Abnormal appearance of transverse sigmoid colon. **F,** cone-down view of sigmoid colon. Note irregular, though intact, sigmoid mucosa with regions of spasm. Pericolic mass *(arrowheads)* with extravasation and small fistulous tract *(Ft).* Surgery confirmed diagnosis of diverticulitis with small "colovesical fistula."

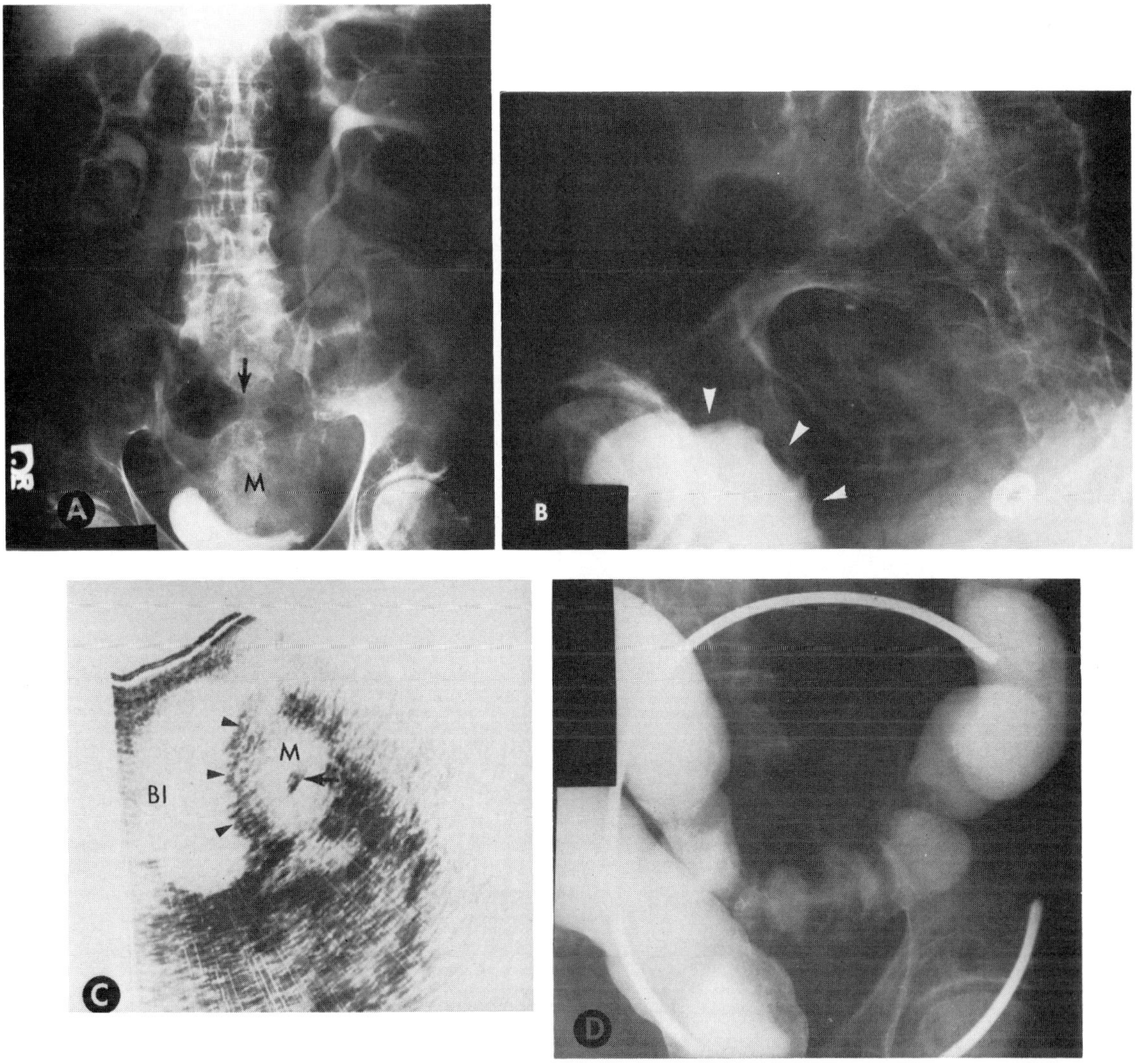

Fig 46–6.—Diverticulitis. Man, age 58, with left lower quadrant pain. **A,** intravenous urogram. Soft tissue mass indenting left lateral and superior aspect of bladder dome. *M* = mass; *arrow* = narrowed segment of air-filled sigmoid colon. **B,** cone-down bladder view of **A,** RPO position. Note irregular posterior and superior contours of bladder, suggesting infiltrative process. *Arrowheads* = bladder contour. **C,** transverse ultrasound scan of pelvis. Bladder *(Bl)* is asymmetric, with mass effect on left caused by abnormally thickened loop of bowel. Left lateral wall of bladder is thickened. *M* = mass (thickened bowel wall); *arrow* = mucus in bowel tumor; *arrowheads* = thickened bladder wall. **D,** barium enema. Spot film of sigmoid colon. long segmental zone of narrowing with intact, irregular mucosa. Surgery revealed diverticulitis with pericolic inflammatory mass involving transverse sigmoid colon and bladder.

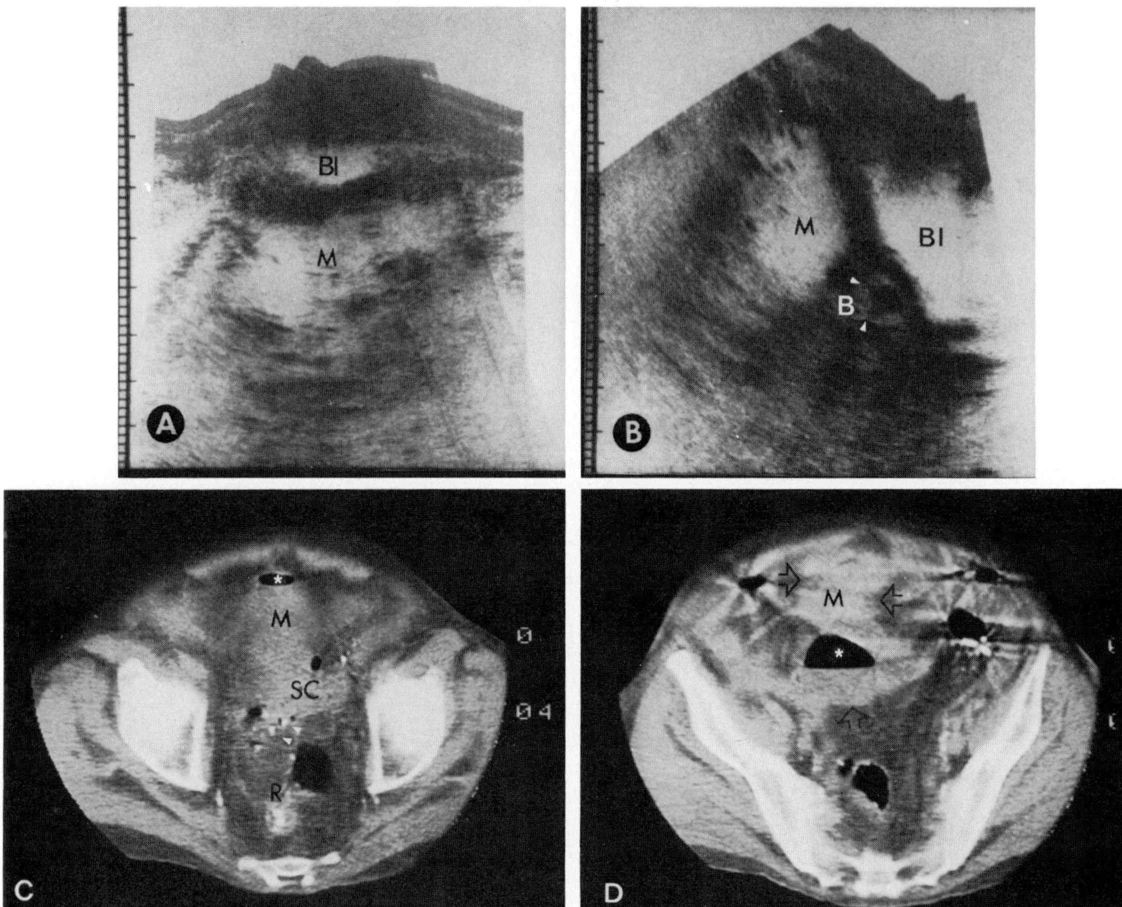

Fig 46–7.—Diverticulitis in man, age 58. Status: postcoronary artery bypass with left lower quadrant pain and fever of unknown origin. **A,** transverse ultrasound scan in lower pelvis. Large elongated complex mass *(M)* with internal echoes, moderate through-transmission and irregular walls, located posterior to bladder *(Bl)*. **B,** longitudinal scan 2 cm right of midline. Mass *(M)* extends superior to dome of bladder *(Bl)*. *B* = bowel (rectosigmoid colon). **C,** CT of lower pelvis just superior to bladder. A soft tissue density mass *(M)* with air fluid level (*) is located anterior to transverse sigmoid colon *(SC)*. *R* = rectum; *white arrowheads* = barium and air-filled rectosigmoid diverticula. **D,** CT scan of midpelvis. Mass *(M)* extends superiorly into abdomen. *Open arrows* = outline of abscess cavity, (*) = large air-fluid level in abscess. At surgery, diverticulitis with large pericolic abscess extending superiorly into abdomen was found. (Courtesy of Dr. Robert T. Reinke, Long Beach, Calif.)

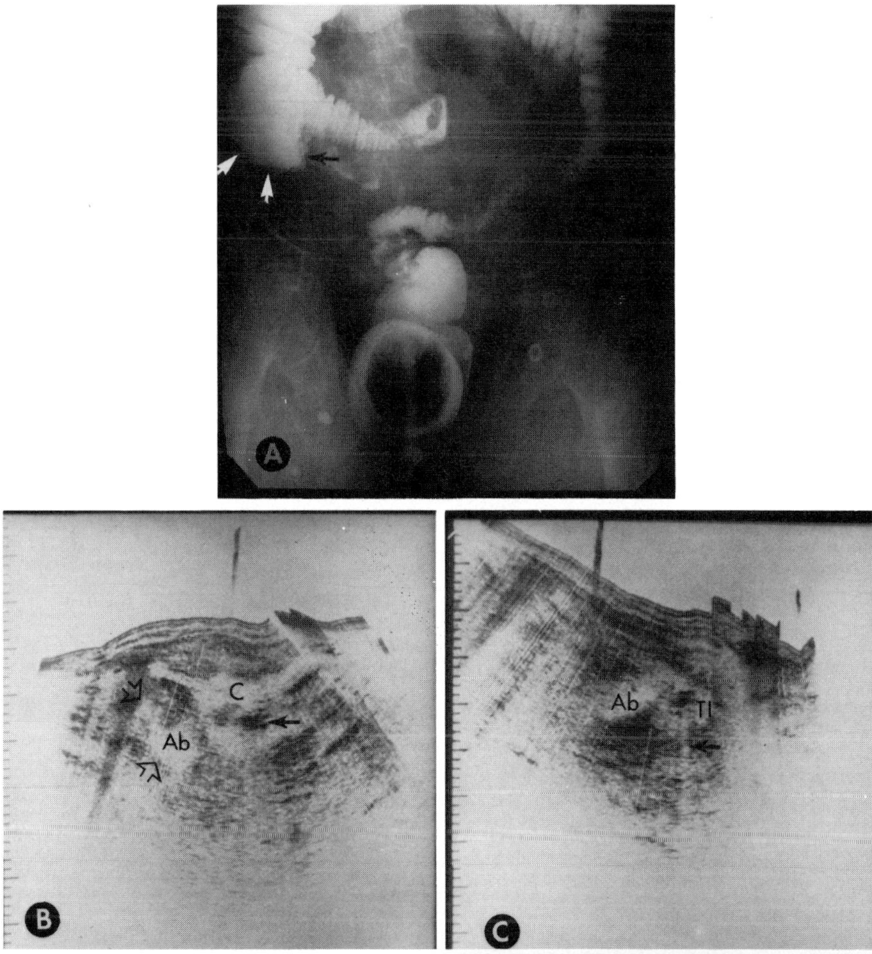

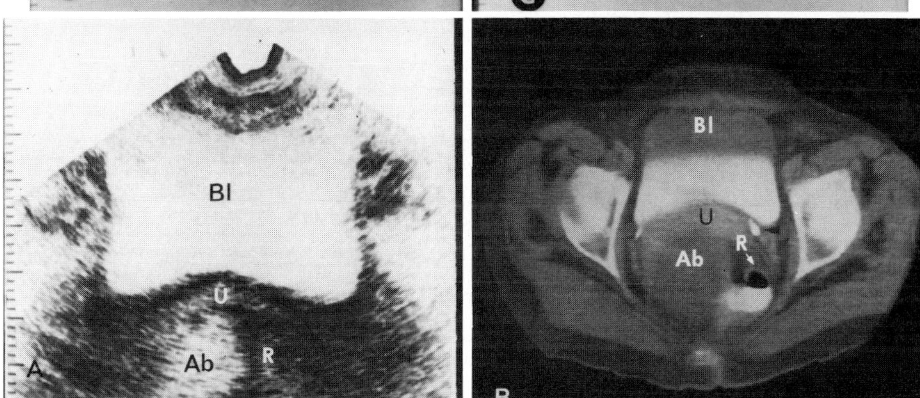

Fig 46–8 (top and center) – Perforated appendicitis. Fever, acute right lower quadrant pain. **A,** water-soluble contrast enema. Extrinsic compression of cecum along inferior, medial and lateral surfaces *(arrows)*. **B,** transverse ultrasound scan of right lower quadrant. Thickened persistent loop of bowel was identified (cecum), along with sonolucent region laterally (other scans showed better through-transmission). *C* = cecum; *Ab* = abscess collection; *Open arrow* delineates margin of periappendiceal abscess. *Black arrow* indicates mucus and air in lumen of cecum. **C,** sagittal scan medial to cecum. Region of terminal ileum *(TI)* is seen, and abscess collection *(Ab)* is located superiorly. *Arrow* = acoustic shadow caused by air.

Fig 46–9 (bottom). – Perirectal abscess. Woman, age 67, with vague lower abdominal pain and mass on pelvic examination. **A,** transverse ultrasound scan of lower pelvis. Abnormal 4×3 cm complex mass (primarily sonolucent with good through-transmission), posterior and separate from uterus *(U)*. *Ab* = abscess, R = rectum; *Bl* = bladder. **B,** CT scan at level comparable to **A.** Mass with decreased attenuation posterior to uterus (cul-de-sac) displacing rectum *(R)* to left. Note excreted intravenous contrast material layering dependently in bladder *(Bl)*. Rectum contains introduced dilute water-soluble contrast material. *Ab* = perirectal abscess; *U* = uterus; *arrowhead* = left ureter. (Courtesy of Dr. Robert T. Reinke, Long Beach, Calif.)

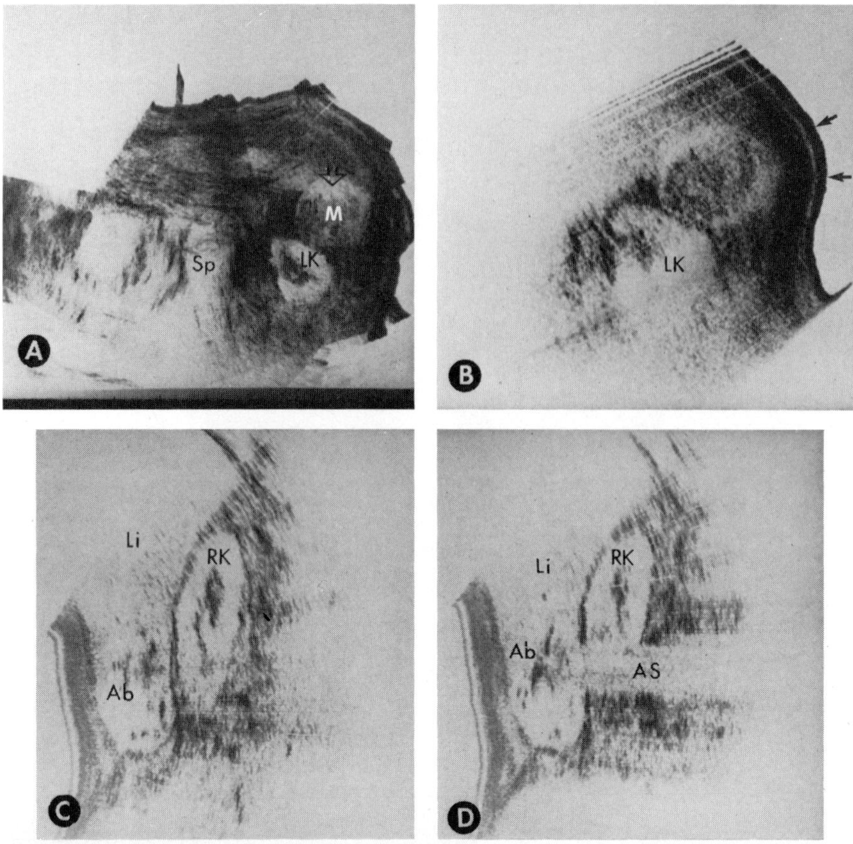

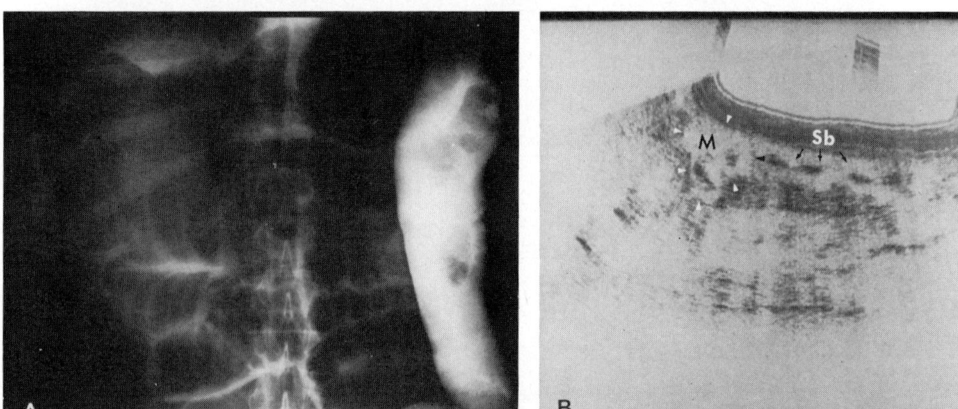

Fig 46–10 (top and middle).—Splenic flexure carcinoma. Man, age 60, presented with fever and right lower quadrant pain. Exploratory laparotomy demonstrated ruptured cecum secondary to obstructing splenic flexure adenocarcinoma. Cecostomy and diverting colostomy performed. **A,** transverse scan at level of kidneys with **(B)** cone-down sector-scan of left upper quadrant. Demonstration of 7-cm diameter, palpable mass *(M),* which is echogenic and has sonolucent rim, being thickest superiorly *(open arrow).* (Not typical appearance of colon carcinoma.) Note mass effect on skin surface *(arrows). LK* = left kidney; *Sp* = spine. **C,** coronal scan (patient in left lateral decubitus position) of right upper quadrant. Spiking fever 3 days postoperatively. Note complex mass with internal echoes, lateral to right kidney *(RK)* and subhepatic. Difficult to separate from liver edge. *Ab* = abscess; *Li* = liver. **D,** coronal scan slightly posterior to **B.** Note acoustic shadowing *(AS)* from gas in abscess *(Ab).* At surgery, subhepatic abscess drained. AS = acoustic shadow; *RK* = right kidney; *Li* = liver.

Fig 46–11 (bottom).—Adenocarcinoma of the splenic flexure. Man, age 58, presenting with diffuse abdominal pain. **A,** barium enema. Complete obstruction by annular splenic flexure carcinoma (not well seen on this view). Massively dilated loops of proximal bowel. **B,** oblique parasagittal scan. Mass *(M)* with posterior exophytic extension *(arrowheads).* Note edematous loops *(arrows)* of small bowel *(Sb).*

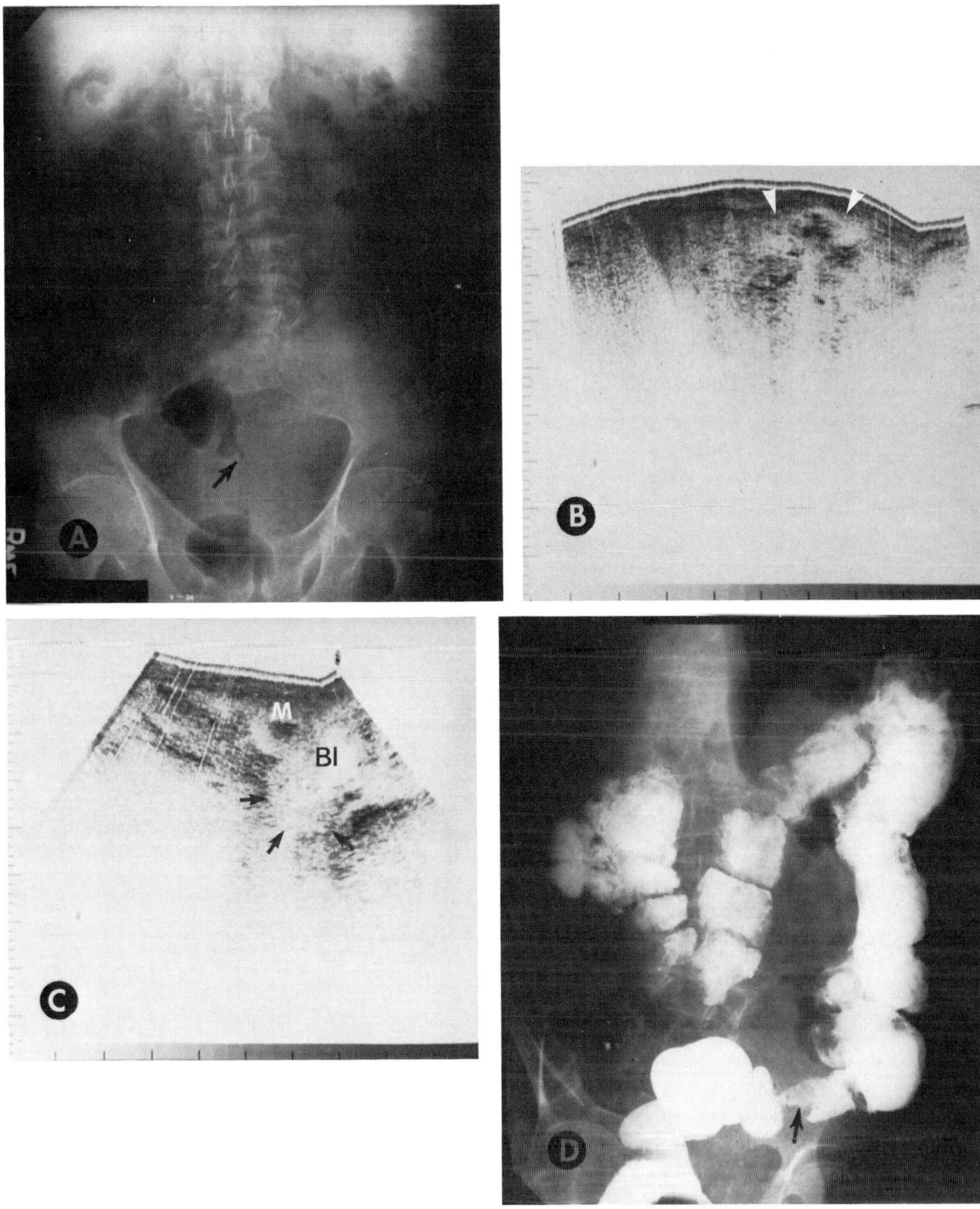

Fig 46–12.—Sigmoid colon carcinoma. Man, age 82, with 40- to 50-lb weight loss over 3 months. **A,** plain film of abdomen. Tapered column of intracolonic air *(arrow)* suggestive of malignancy. **B,** transverse ultrasound scan of lower pelvis. Persistent 6×3 cm mass *(arrowheads)* with thick sonolucent mantle, central strong echoes and acoustic shadowing. **C,** longitudinal scan 1 cm to left of midline. Mass *(M)* seen, ill-defined posterior extension *(arrows)*. *Bl* = partially filled bladder. **D,** barium enema: Annular constricting lesion of transverse sigmoid colon *(arrow)*. Surgery revealed adenocarcinoma of sigmoid colon with posterior and lateral extracolonic extension.

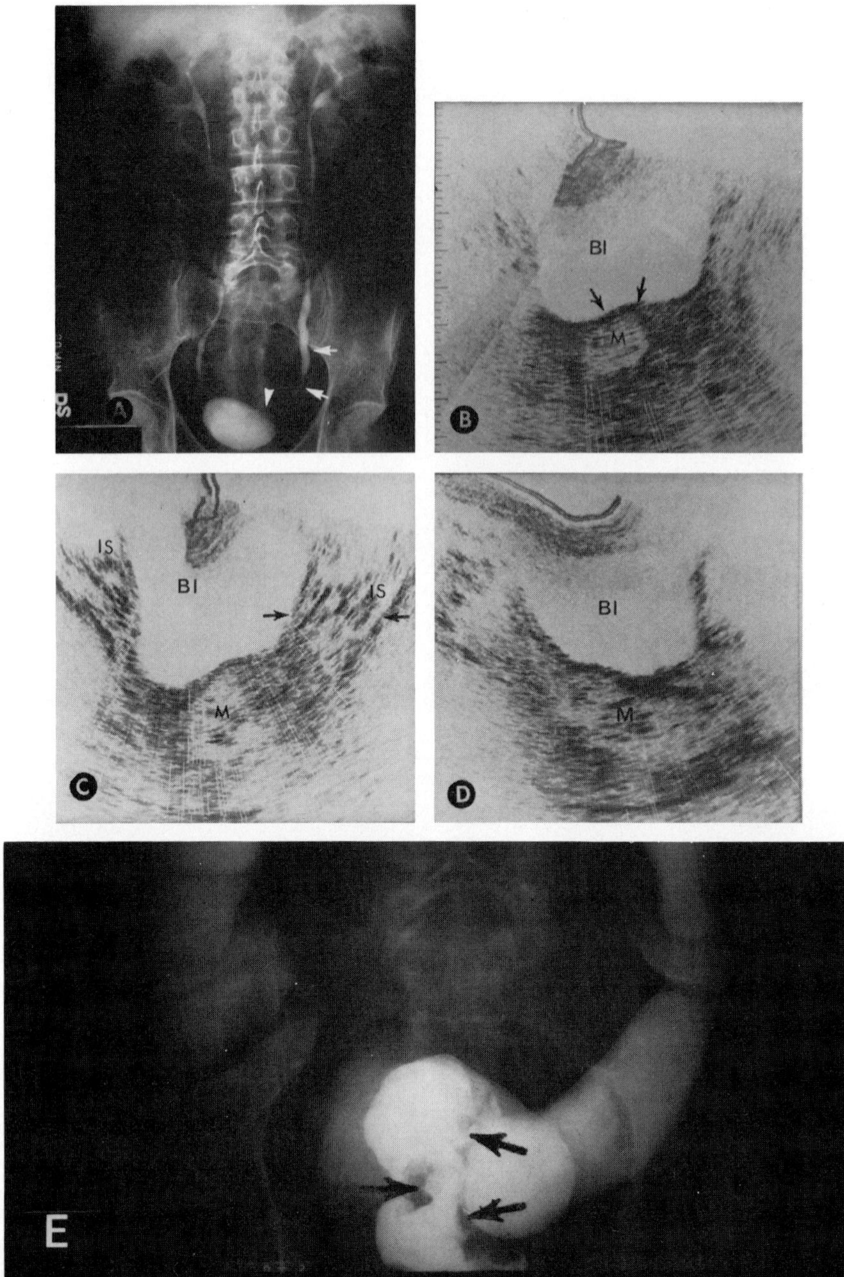

Fig 46–13. – Rectal carcinoma. Man, age 55, with 4-month history of 20-lb weight loss, bleeding, tenesmus. Rectal mass on physical examination. **A,** 20-minute intravenous urogram. Distal one third of ureter shows proximal dilatation with abrupt distal narrowing *(arrows).* Note extrinsic deformity of left superolateral portion of bladder *(arrowhead).* **B,** transverse scan just superior to prostate. Note well-defined 3-cm complex mass *(M)* posterior to bladder *(Bl)* and extrinsically impressing bladder floor *(arrows).* (Bladder impression abnormal in this case but can also be due to feces-filled bowel. **C,** transverse scan 4 cm superior to **B.** Rectal mass *(M)* with central sonodense echoes with sonolucent mantle. Region of left iliopsoas muscle markedly widened *(arrows),* compared to right side (also slightly widened). Highly suggestive of tumor extension. *IS* = iliopsoas muscle; *Bl* = bladder. **D,** longitudinal scan 1 cm left of midline. Large fusiform rectal mass (6×3×4). *Bl* = bladder; *M* = mass. **E,** barium enema. Annular carcinoma of rectum *(single arrow)* with extensive involvement of left lateral wall *(arrows).* At surgery, adenocarcinoma of rectum with bilateral extension to iliac nodes, metastasis to liver.

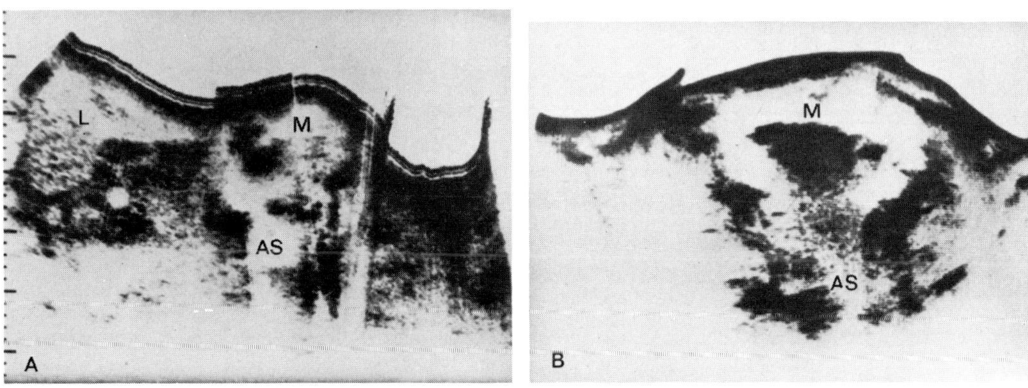

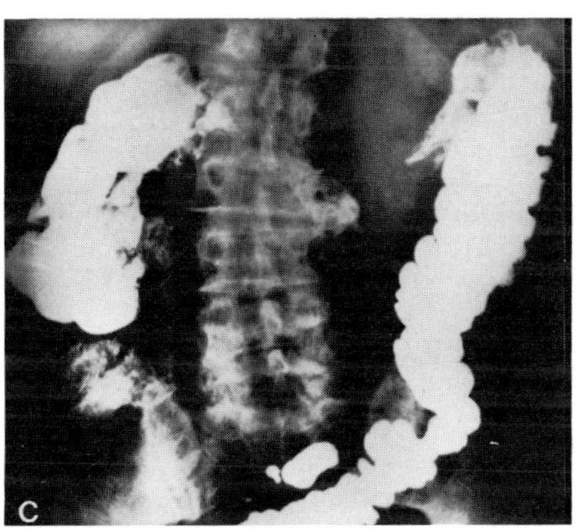

Fig 46–14.—Adenocarcinoma of transverse colon. **A,** longitudinal, and **B** transverse sonograms showing mass *(M)* 6×7×8 cm with dark echogenic area centrally. L = liver, AS = acoustic shadowing. **C,** delayed film following barium meal showing long constricting lesion with soft tissue mass in transverse colon. (From Peterson and Cooperberg, Gastrointest. Radiol. 3:303, 1978, with permission.)

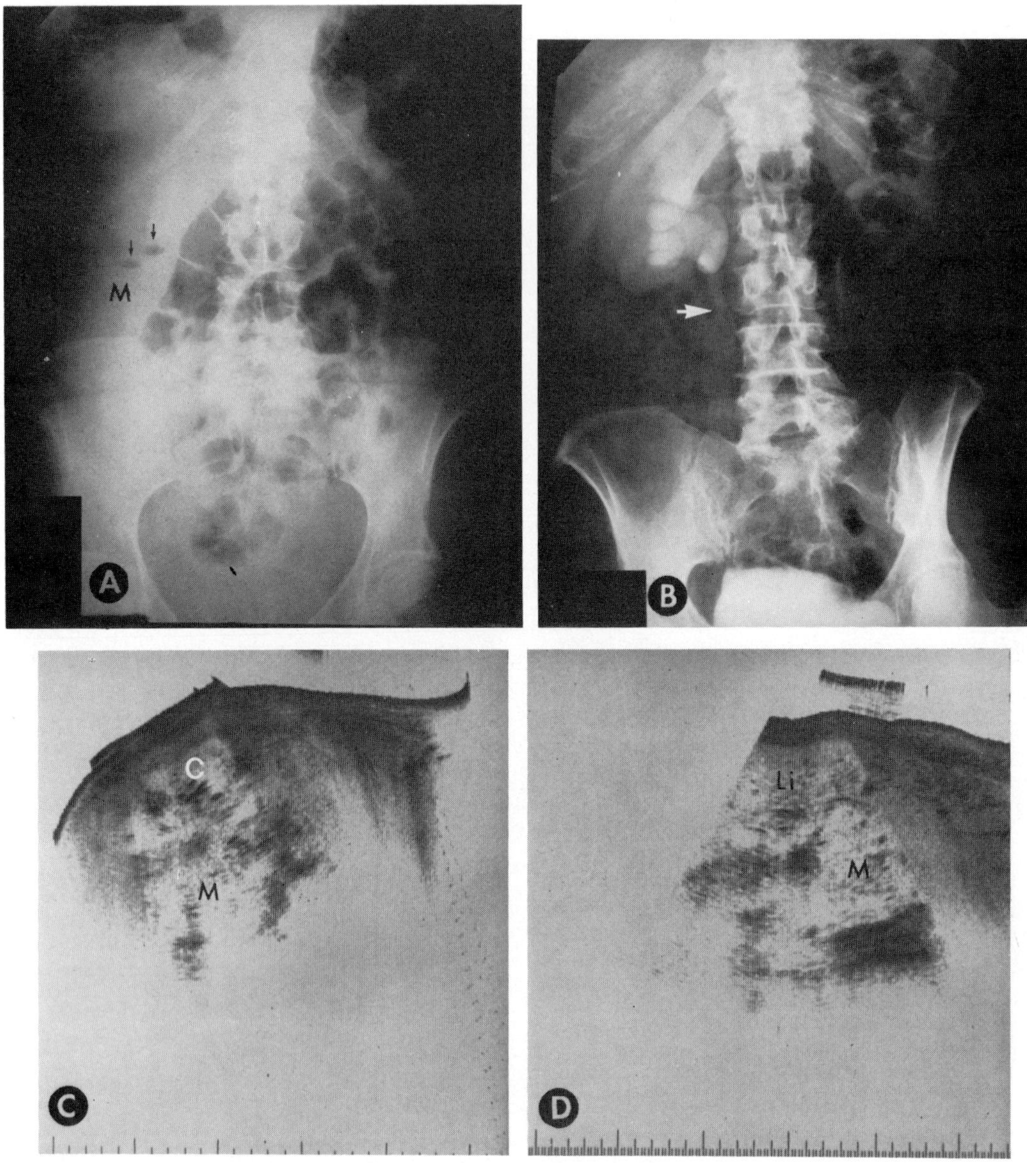

Fig 46–15. – Perforated cecal carcinoma. Woman, age 71, presenting with acute right lower quadrant pain. **A,** plain film of abdomen. Soft tissue mass *(M)* with air-fluid levels *(arrows)* in right midabdomen. Ascending colon displaced medially. **B,** intravenous urogram. Right pyelocaliectasis and hydroureter with obstruction at level of proximal ureter *(arrow).* **C,** transverse ultrasound scan of right midabdomen, inferior to right kidney. Complex (predominantly solid) mass *(C)* with dark central echoes representing cecum. Possible second mass *(M)* posterior to *C.* **D,** longitudinal scan lateral to right kidney. Complex mass *(M)* with good through-transmission: same mass *(M)* seen in **C,** consistent with an abscess. *Li* = liver.

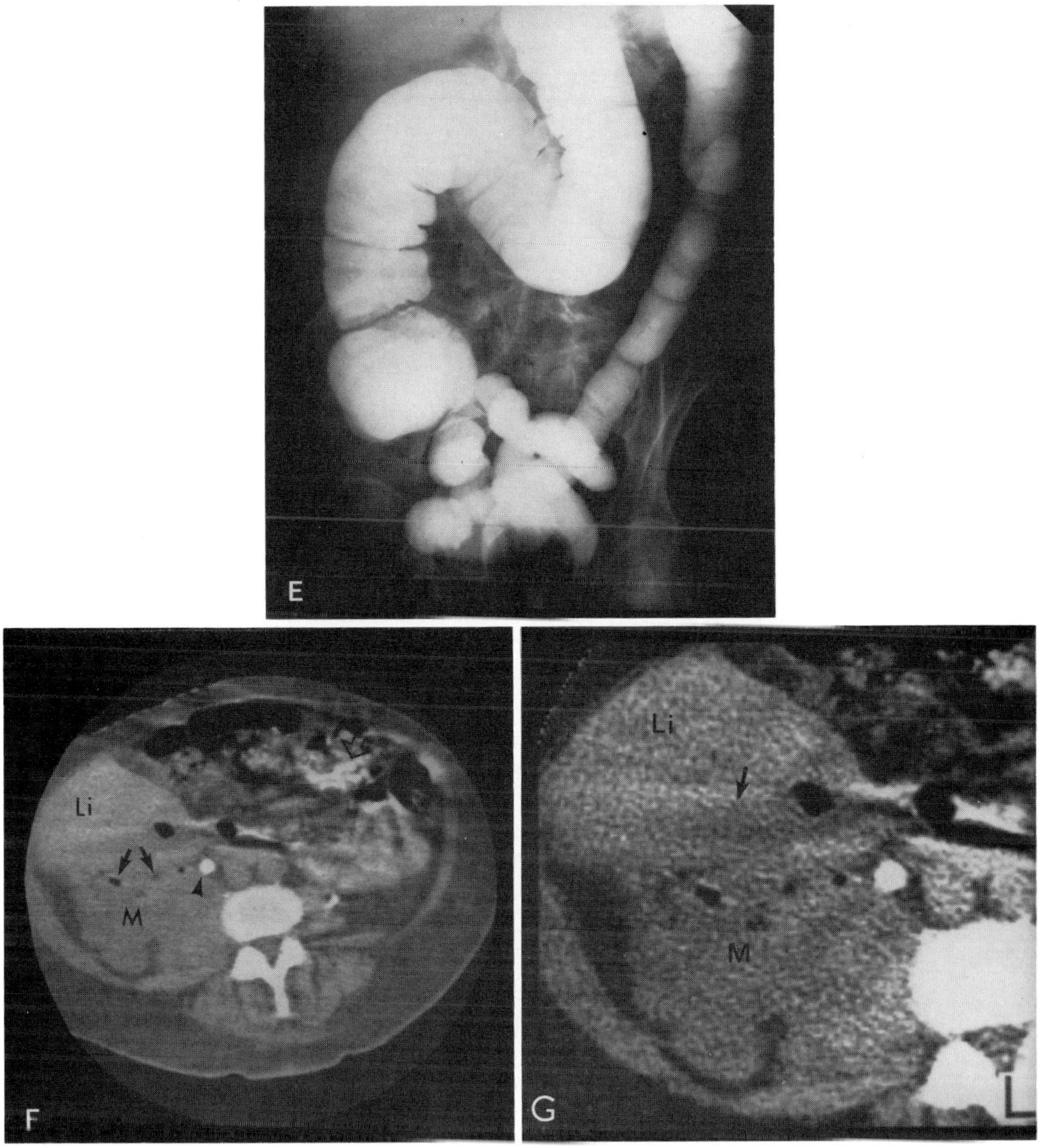

Fig 46–15 (continued).—**E,** barium enema. Cecum and ascending colon displaced medially; otherwise normal. **F,** CT below level of kidneys (intravenous and oral contrast used). Large retroperitoneal low-density mass with air-fluid levels. *M* = abscess; *arrows* = air-fluid levels; *arrowhead* = right hydroureter; *Li* = liver; *open arrow* = contrast in bowel. **G,** magnified view of abscess in **F,** window width and level adjusted for increased contrast. Better edge effect separates liver *(Li)* from abscess *(M)*. *Arrow* = demarcation of liver from abscess. (Courtesy of Drs. Lee Secrist and Kenneth Brown, Torrance, Calif.)

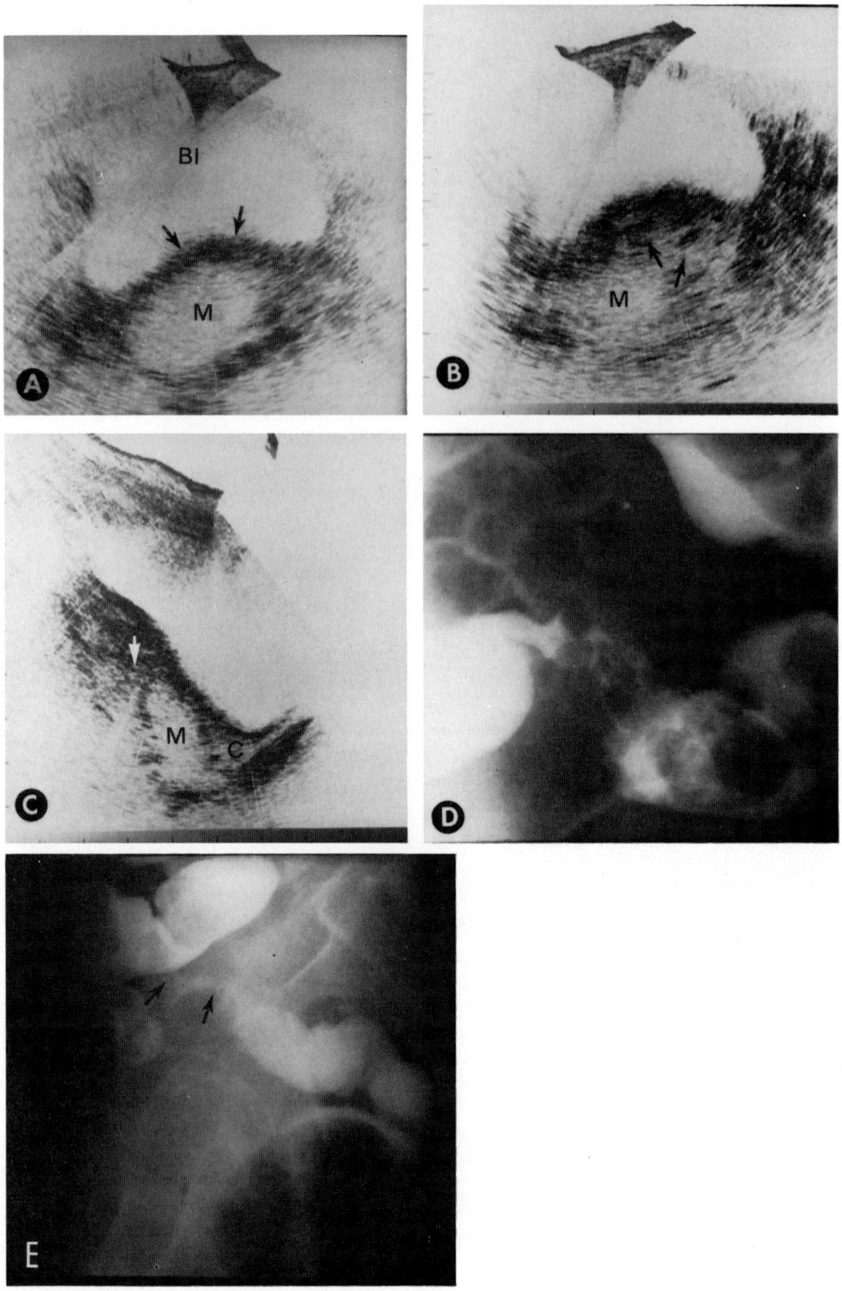

Fig 46–16.—Perforated sigmoid carcinoma. Woman, age 52, presenting with fever, left lower quadrant pain, and left adnexal mass. **A,** transverse scan of midpelvis. A 5×6 cm sonolucent mass *(M)* with good through-transmission thought to represent large abscess. Note bladder *(Bl)* floor impression by mass and thickened posterior bladder wall *(arrows),* indicating infiltration. **B,** transverse scan of upper pelvis. Mass *(M)* still present. Two loops of bowel *(arrows)* situated between mass and posterior wall of bladder. **C,** longitudinal scan 1 cm left of midline. Mass *(M)* in cul-de-sac, extending superiorly *(arrow).* Atrophic uterus separate from mass (seen in other scans). *C* = cervix. **D,** spot film barium enema. Long segment of sigmoid colon with infiltrated-appearing mucosa. **E,** lateral film barium enema. Lobulated intramural mass affecting sigmoid colon *(arrows)* and widening of presacral space. At surgery, perforated sigmoid adenocarcinoma with abscess collection surrounding and involving bladder and uterus. Loops of small bowel and colon adherent to bladder.

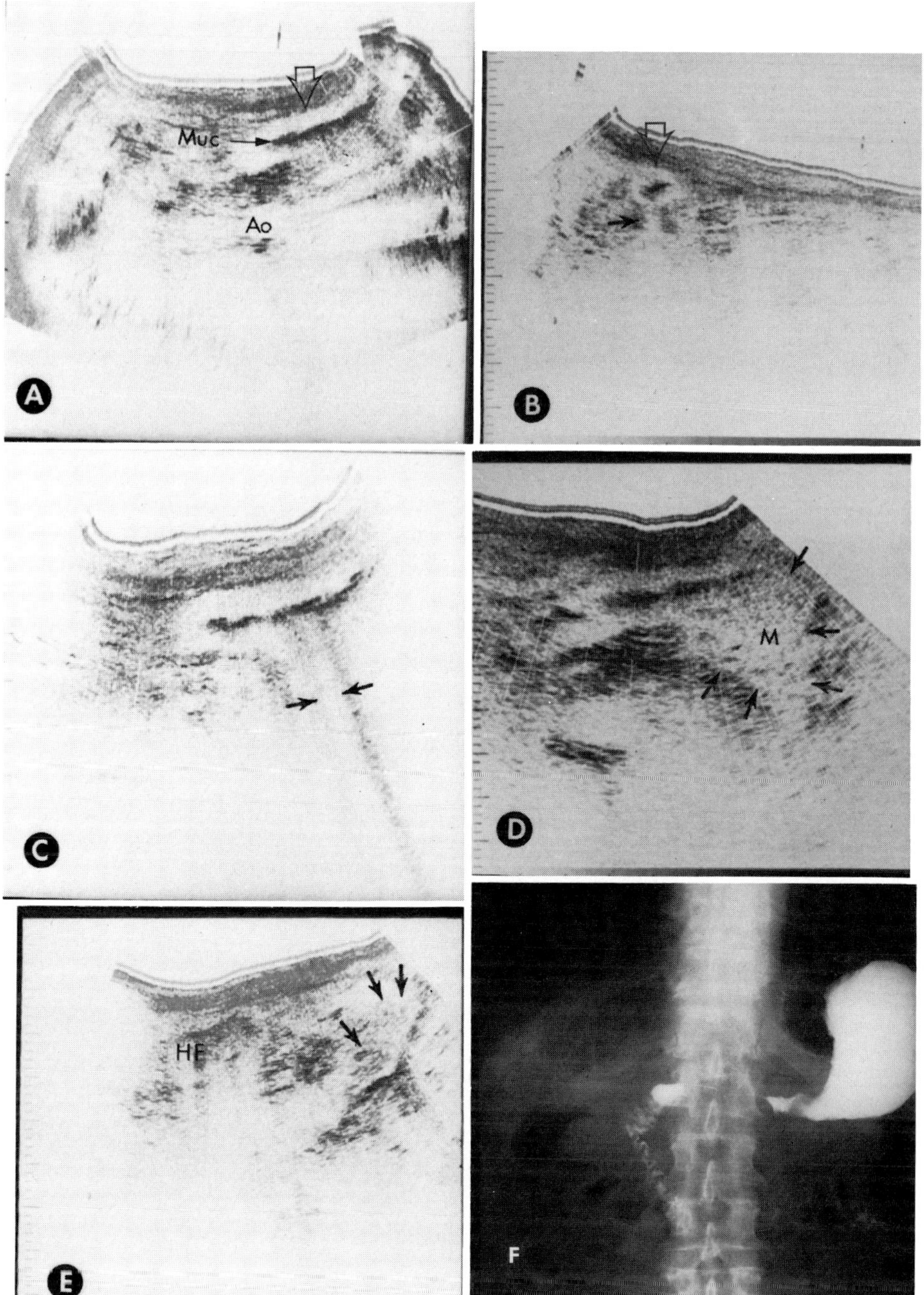

Fig 46–17.—Gastric carcinoma with exophytic extension. White male, age 72, with crampy epigastric pain and 30-lb weight loss. Ultrasound was first diagnostic examination. **A,** transverse scan just inferior to the xiphoid demonstrates left upper quadrant mass, with thickened sonolucent walls and intraluminal air and mucus *(Muc)*. *Open arrow* = abnormal stomach; *Ao* = aorta. **B,** longitudinal scan 3 cm to left of midline. Persistent unchanging and thickened loop of bowel *(closed arrow)*. *Open arrow* = stomach. **C,** magnified view of **A.** Note thickened walls and shadowing from microbubble effect[22] of gastric contents. *Arrows* = acoustic shadowing. **D,** transverse scan just inferior to **C** shows exophytic component extending into lesser sac and transverse mesocolon. *M* = mass; *arrows* = exophytic extension. **E,** oblique scan of left lobe of liver. Three metastatic or bull's-eye lesions seen. *Arrows* = metastases; *HF* = hepatic flexure. **F,** upper gastrointestinal series. Elongated segment of gastric antral carcinoma. Surgery confirmed adenocarcinoma of stomach with extension into transverse mesocolon. Following total gastrectomy and transverse colostomy, patient had ultrasound examination because of fever of undetermined origin.

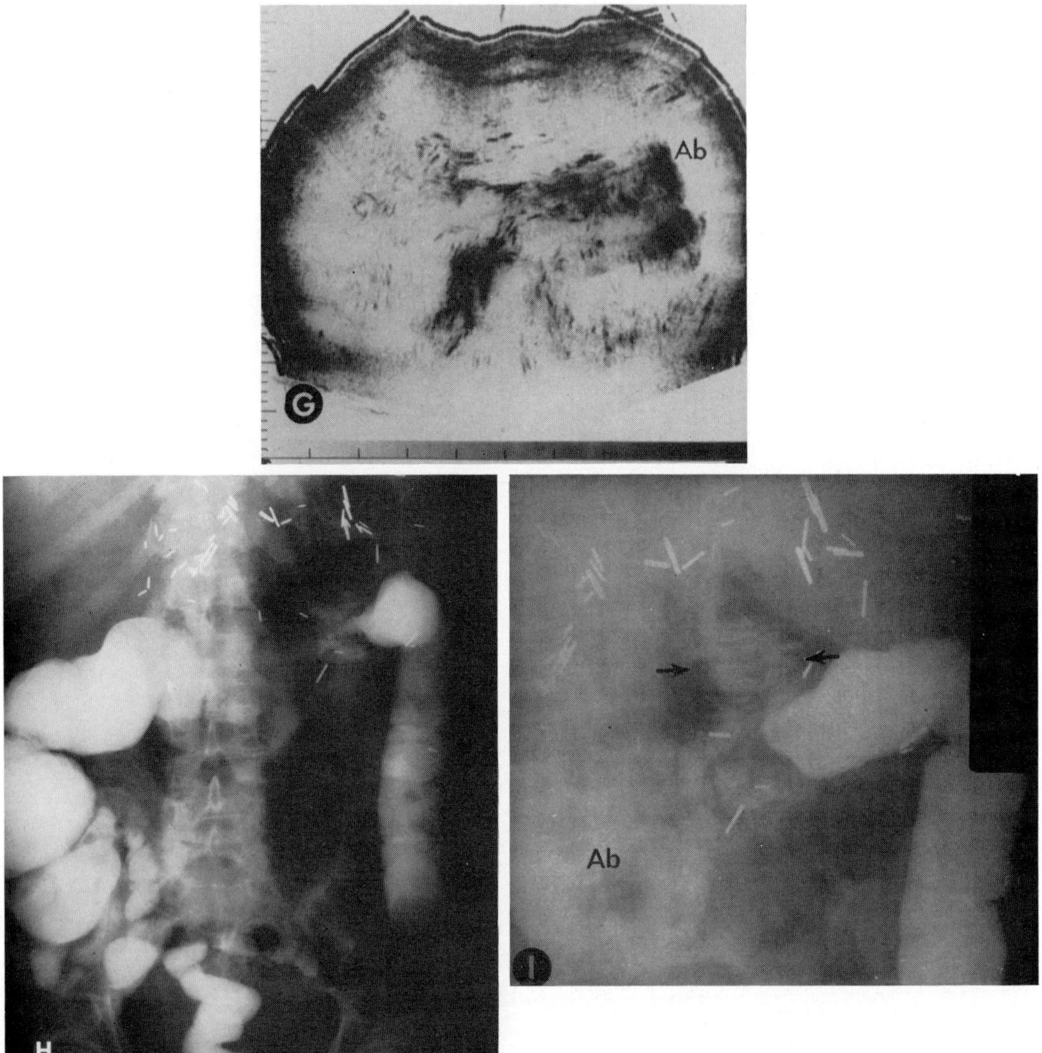

Fig 47–17 (continued). – **G,** transverse ultrasound scan 2 cm below xiphoid process. Left upper quadrant sonolucent cavity with occasional internal echoes. *Ab* = abscess cavity, extending into left subphrenic region. **H,** water-soluble contrast enema showing abnormal segment of transverse colon at anastomotic site. **I,** cone-down spot film from water-soluble contrast enema. Extravasation and contrast pooling. *Arrows* = coloenteric fistula; *Ab* = abscess cavity.

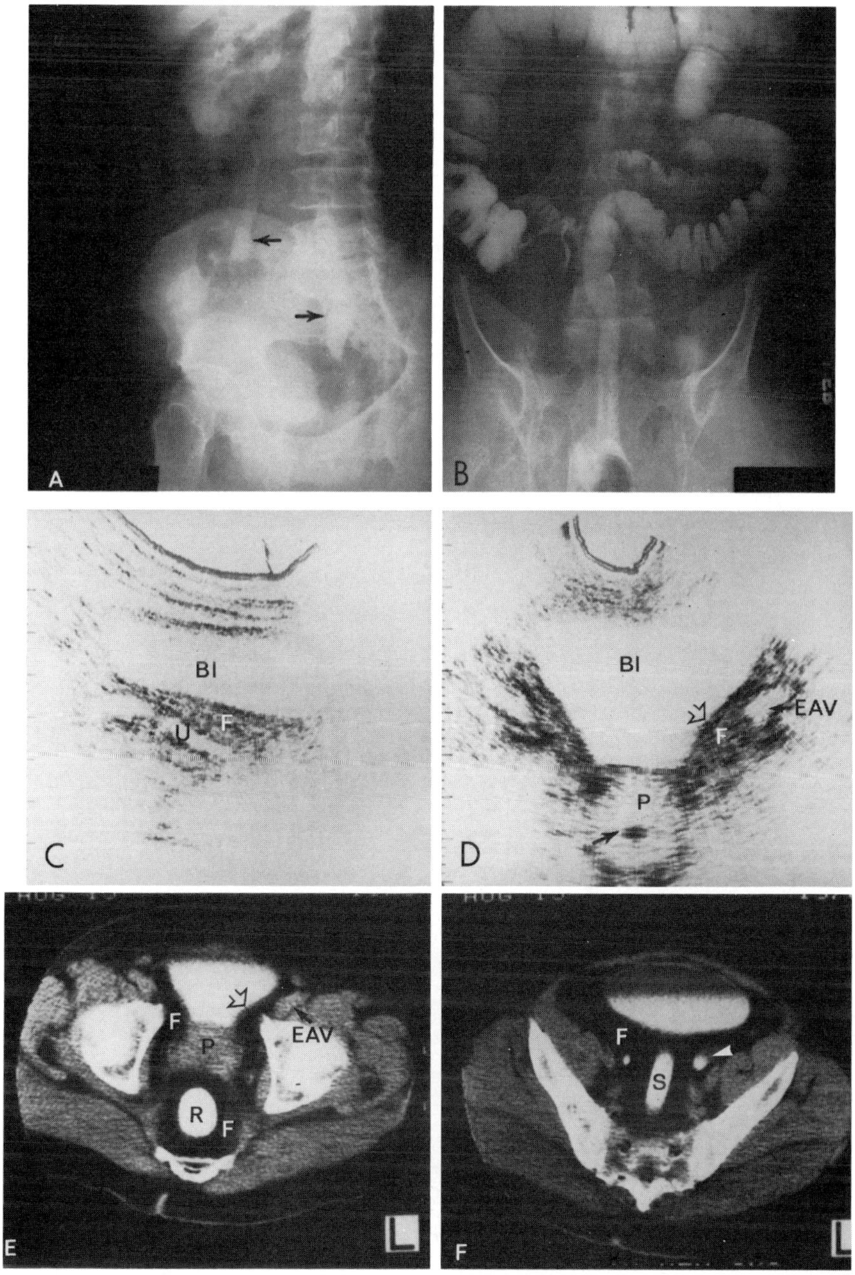

Fig 46–18.—Pelvic lipomatosis. Black man, age 57, presenting with hypertension; prostate was more superiorly located than usual on physical examination. **A,** intravenous urogram, RPO. Bilateral hydroureter *(arrows),* with bladder displaced superiorly and anteriorly out of pelvis. Tumor could not be ruled out. **B,** barium enema. Elevated, narrowed straightened sigmoid colon. **C,** longitudinal view, angled slightly to patient's left. Note sonolucent tubular structure coursing within echogenic material, presenting left ureter *(U).* Left ureter could be followed into bladder *(Bl). F* = pelvic fat. **D,** transverse ultrasound scan at level of prostate. Note asymmetrically deformed bladder wall on left, caused by very echogenic material *(F). F* = pelvic fat; *P* = prostate (enlarged); *closed arrow* = prostatic urethra; *EAV* = external iliac artery and vein; *open arrow* = bladder deformity; *Bl* = bladder. **E,** CT scan, same level as in **B.** Note similarity and plethora of low density material *(F)* surrounding contrast-filled bladder and rectum. *F* = pelvic fat; *open arrow* = bladder deformity; *P* = enlarged prostate; *EAV* = external iliac artery and vein, *R* = rectum. **F,** CT scan, midsacrum. Bladder totally surrounded by fat *(F)* and elevated out of pelvis. Sigmoid colon *(S)* is compressed. *Arrowhead* = left hydroureter.

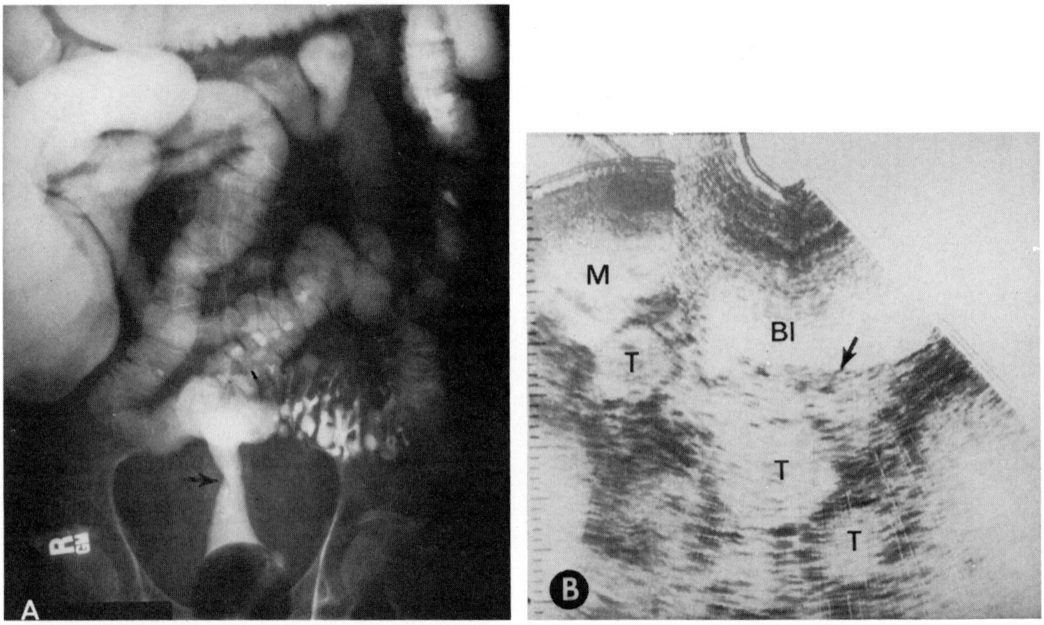

Fig 46–19.—Prostatic carcinoma with extrinsic compression of rectum. **A,** barium enema. Narrowing of rectum *(arrow);* diverticulosis of sigmoid colon. **B,** transverse ultrasound scan of pelvis. Extensive tumor spread *(T)* throughout pelvis. Palpable anterior abdominal mass *(M)* on right. *Bl* = bladder; *arrow* = bladder extension. Biopsy confirmed adenocarcinoma of prostate with widespread pelvic extension.

Fig 46–20.—Recurrent leiomyosarcoma of small bowel. **A,** barium enema. Annular constricting lesion *(arrow)* of rectosigmoid colon. **B,** transverse ultrasound scan of lower pelvis. Large mass *(M)* with sonolucent necrotic center compressing bladder *(arrowheads).* At surgery, recurrent leiomyosarcoma constricting rectosigmoid colon found.

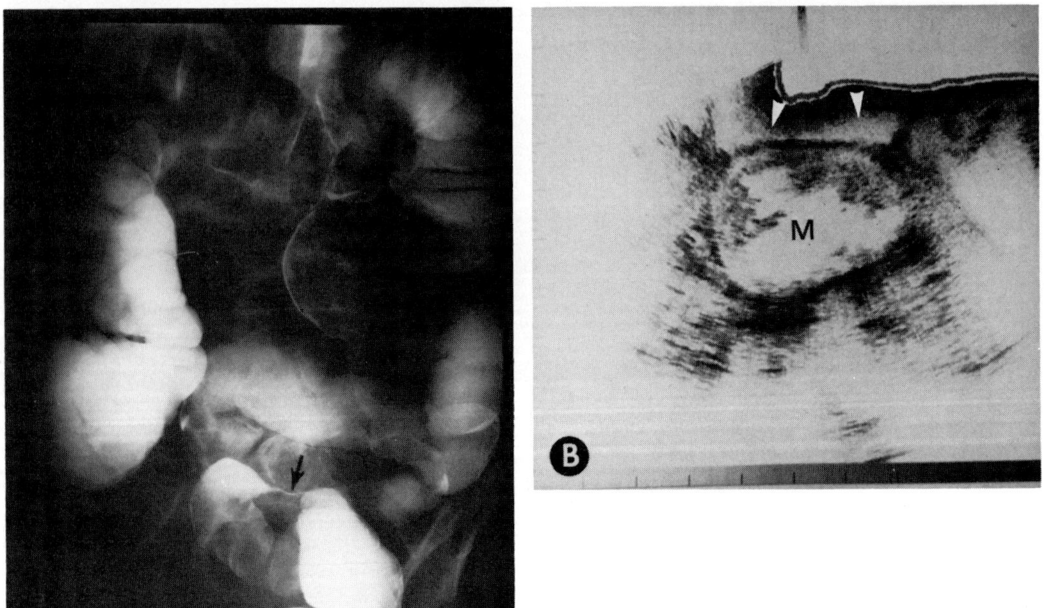

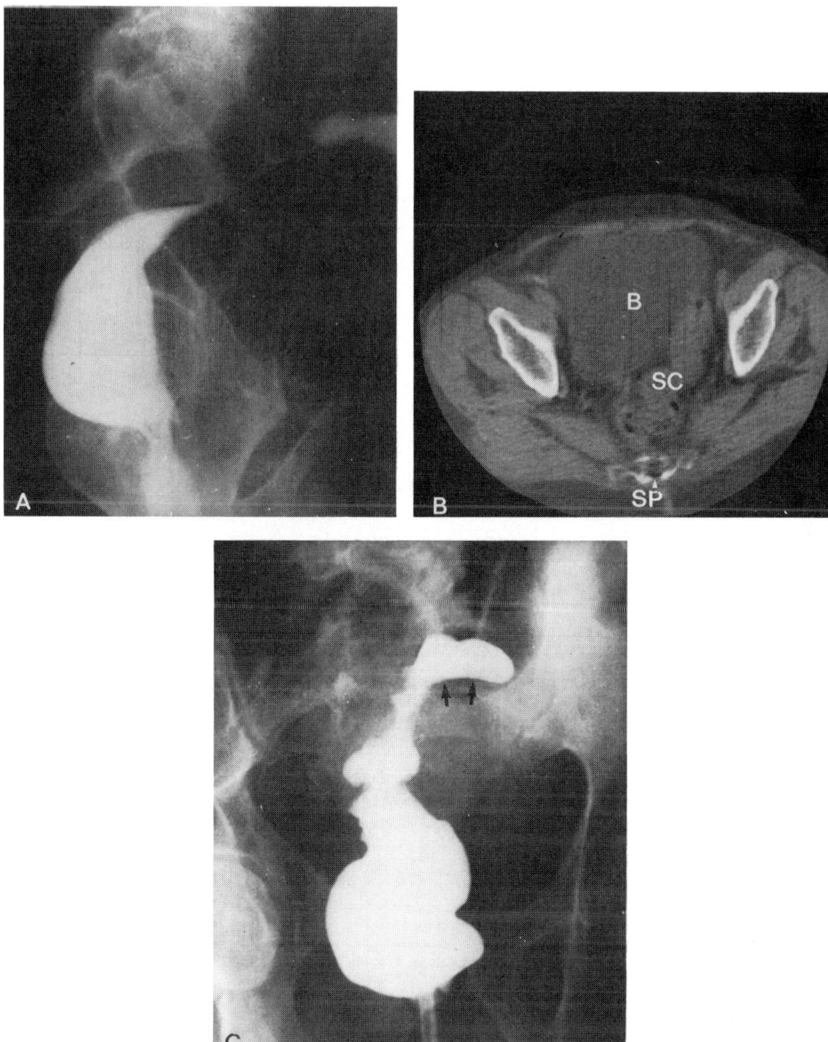

Fig 46–21.—Rectosigmoid pseudostenosis due to urinary retention. **A,** lateral projection on barium enema shows long, tapering, smooth-margined, narrow segment of rectosigmoid with maximal narrowing at sacral promontory, caused by distended bladder. **B,** CT of pelvis demonstrates anatomical relationship between distended urine-filled bladder *(B)* and sigmoid colon *(SC)*. Note region of sacral promontory *(SP)*. (Courtesy of Dr. Robert T. Reinke, Long Beach, Calif.) **C,** frontal projection shows ragged lateral margins of narrow segment due to incomplete filling. Note also characteristic smooth concave lower margin of sigmoid proximal to narrowing *(arrows)*. After drainage of bladder, colon returned to normal. (From Kleinhaus and Kaftori, Radiology 127:645, 1978, with permission.)

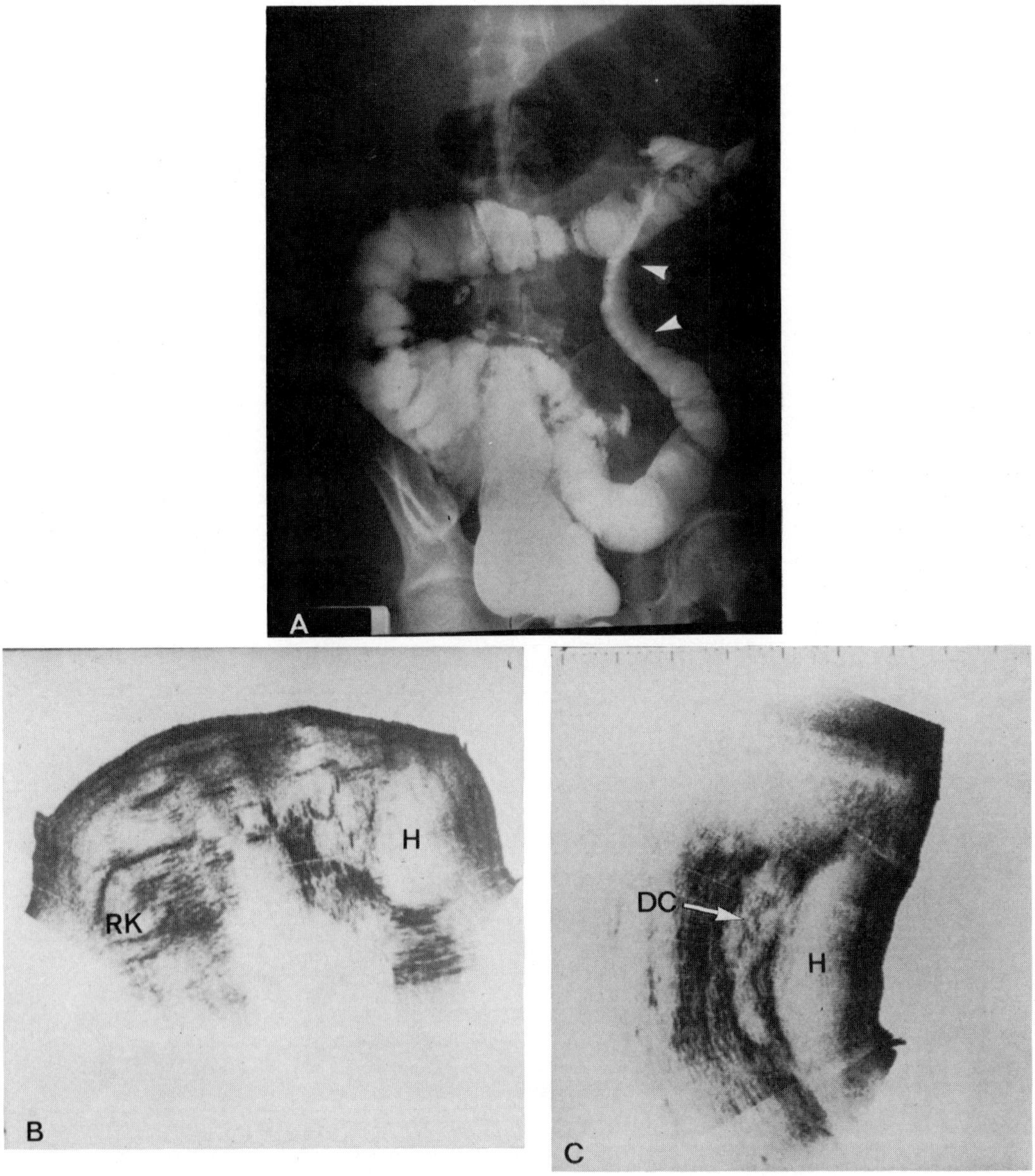

Fig 46–22.—Left upper quadrant hematoma. Young black male, 3 days post operation, with left upper quadrant pain and mass. **A,** barium enema. Smooth extrinsic mass *(arrowheads)* displacing descending colon. **B,** transverse ultrasound scan in upper abdomen. Left upper quadrant sonolucent mass with good through-transmission. *H* = hematoma; *RK* = right kidney. **C,** coronal scan, left upper quadrant. Normal descending colon *(DC)* is displaced by lateral hematoma *(H).* Corresponds to barium enema in **A.** Aspiration performed under ultrasound guidance yielded 300 cc of hemorrhagic fluid.

Chapter 47

Vascular Ectasias

JEANNE W. BAER, M.D.

THE DEVELOPMENT of selective visceral angiography by Margulis in 1960 made possible the identification of vascular ectasias of the cecum as an important source of lower gastrointestinal bleeding.[1] Since this date multiple reports have alerted the clinician to the high incidence of these ectasias. Since the causal factors are unknown, the lesion has been given various descriptive names: angiodysplasia, vascular dysplasia, angioma, vascular malformation and arteriovenous malformation.[2-7] It seems most appropriate to use the name "vascular ectasia," since there is evidence to support an acquired rather than a congenital cause, as suggested by the other terms. Moore and coworkers[5] have reclassified the various types of arteriovenous malformations in such a way that vascular ectasia of the cecum constitutes an entity unto itself, unrelated to (1) large congenital vascular malformations of the small bowel or (2) angiomas seen in hereditary hemorrhagic telangiectasia.

Incidence

Vascular ectasias of the cecum and ascending colon are the second most common cause of lower intestinal bleeding in the older population.[7,8] They occur predominantly on the antimesenteric border of the cecum or ascending colon.[3] In an angiographic evaluation of 88 patients with chronic intestinal blood loss, 25% of patients had vascular malformations. One half of these malformations were located in the cecum or ascending colon.[6] In another study, seven of 17 patients with arteriovenous malformations had ectasias of the cecum or ascending colon.[5] Ectasias may be single or multiple.[9] The highest number of ectasias per specimen (25) has been seen in patients over age 80, supporting the hypothesis that ectasias represent a degenerative process.[9] In addition, there is a high frequency of these lesions in the older population.[3,9] Angiographic examinations of 15 right colon specimens, removed for lesions other than vascular ectasias in a series of patients over age 60 without a history of bleeding, disclosed submucosal ectasias in 53%. One half of these also had mucosal capillary engorgement.[9] In seven of 24 patients operated on for vascular ectasia of the cecum, other lesions were responsible for the bleeding.[4] This should caution the clinician to exclude other sources of bleeding before removing the cecum and ascending colon.[4,6]

Clinical Presentation

Patients present between the 5th and 9th decades with anemia, and episodes of painless melena or maroon-colored stools initially, which may not require blood transfusions. However, with time, these episodes become more frequent and more impressive, requiring an increasing number of transfusions for stabilization. Analysis of the patients bleeding from vascular ectasias has disclosed a disproportionally high number with aortic stenosis, 20–25%; however, a causal relationship has not been shown.[4, 9, 10] The medical records are replete with recurrent admissions for bleeding in which the diagnosis is not made in spite of repeated barium examinations and even exploratory laparotomy. This is easily explained by the pathologic appearance (Figs 47–4 and 47–6).

Pathophysiology

The normal anatomy of the cecum is illustrated in Figure 47–1. There are three current hypotheses concerning the pathophysiology of vascular ectasias.

1. Baum et al.[4] postulate that a focal ectasia results from mucosal ischemia secondary to increased intraluminal pressure or poor perfusion pressure, which leads to submucosal shunting of blood from artery to vein. However, even though there is mucosal atrophy owing to encroachment by enlarged submucosal veins, there also are dilated mucosal capillaries adjacent to the mucosal ulcers without evidence of inflammation (see Fig 47–4).

2. Localized increased blood flow, with breakdown of the precapillary sphincters, may occur adjacent to ischemic areas in patients with occlusion of submucosal arteries, often by cholesterol emboli. This represents shunting away from the ischemic area to the adjacent mucosal segment. The incidence of cholesterol emboli has ranged from 18% to 25%[2, 3, 9] (see Fig 47–6, B).

3. The most plausible hypothesis has been proposed by Boley and co-workers,[11] who have carefully analyzed serial angiograms performed in 25 patients with surgically proved vascular ectasias. The earliest angiographic sign is a late-draining ileocecal vein, seen in 92% of cases. This is a result of chronic intermittent obstruction of the submucosal vein by muscular contraction as this vein obliquely passes between the circular muscles of the bowel wall to emerge on the serosa along the juxtamesenteric borders of the colon. The submucosal vein, being a low-pressure system, dilates and becomes tortuous. Eventually the venous engorgement is transmitted to the mucosal capillary rings, which also dilate. When the precapillary sphincter becomes incompetent, shunting of blood occurs among submucosal artery, mucosal capillaries and submucosal vein. This latter phenomenon is documented angiographically 50% of the time as an early-draining vein. The dilated tortuous submucosal veins form the identifiable vascular tuft, seen in 70–75% of angiograms[8, 11] (Figs 47–2, 47–5 to 47–7). Mucosal capillary ectasias measure less than 0.5 cm in more than 90% of cases.[3]

Baer and Ryan[3] were impressed by the similarity of the localized changes in vascular ectasias and the more generalized vascular engorgement seen in all layers of the bowel in congestive failure and portal hypertension. Is it possible for increased central venous pressure to cause localized vascular lesions, as seen in Figure 47–8?

REFERENCES

1. Margulis, A. R., Heinbecker, P., and Bernard, H. R.: Operative mesenteric arteriography in the search for the site of bleeding in unexplained gastrointestinal hemorrhage, Surgery 48:534, 1960.
2. Klein, H. J., Alfidi, R. J., Meany, T. F., and Poirer, V. C.: Angiography in the diagnosis of chronic gastrointestinal bleeding, Radiology 98:83, 1971.
3. Baer, J. W., and Ryan, S.: Analysis of cecal vasculature in the search for vascular malformations, Am J. Roentgenol. 126:394, 1976.
4. Baum, S., Athanasoulis, C. A., Waltman, A. C., Galdabini, J., Schapiro, R. H., Warshaw, A. L., and Ottinger, L. W.: Angiodysplasia of the right colon: A cause of gastro-intestinal bleeding, Am. J. Roentgenol. 129:789, 1977.
5. Moore, J. D., Thompson, N. W., Appelman, H. D., and Foley, D.: Arteriovenous malformations of the gastrointestinal tract, Arch. Surg. 111:381, 1976.

6. Sheedy, P. F. II, Fulton, R. E., and Atwell, D. T.: Angiographic evaluation of patients with chronic gastrointestinal bleeding, Am. J. Roentgenol. 123: 338, 1975.
7. Casarella, W. J., Galloway, S. J., Taxin, R. N., Follet, D. A., Pollock, E. J., and Seaman, W. B.: "Lower" gastrointestinal tract hemorrhage: New concepts based on arteriography, Am. J. Roentgenol. 121:357, 1974.
8. Sprayregen, S., and Boley, S. J.: Vascular ectasias of the right colon, J.A.M.A. 239:962, 1978.
9. Boley, S. J., Sammartano, R., Adams, A., DiBiase, A., Kleinhaus, S., and Sprayregen, S.: On the nature and etiology of vascular ectasias of the colon degenerative lesions of aging, Gastroenterology 72: 650, 1977.
10. Galloway, S. J., Cassarella, W. J., and Shimkin, P. M.: Vascular malformations of the right colon as a cause of bleeding in patients with aortic stenosis, Radiology 113:11, 1974.
11. Boley, S. J., Sprayregen, S., Sammartano, R. J., Adams, A., and Kleinhaus, S. K.: The pathophysiologic basis for the angiographic signs of vascular ectasias of the colon, Radiology 125:615, 1977.
12. Case records of Massachusetts General Hospital (Case 36-1974), N. Engl. J. Med. 291:569, 1974.
13. Boor, S. L., Parker, H. W., Ganesphappa, K. P., Komaki, S., and Dodds, W. J.: Vascular dysplasia of the right colon—An important cause of unexplained gastrointestinal bleeding, Dig. Dis. 23:89, 1978.
14. Rogers, B. H. G., and Adler, F.: Hemangiomas of the cecum: colonoscopic diagnosis and therapy, Gastroenterology 71:1079, 1976.

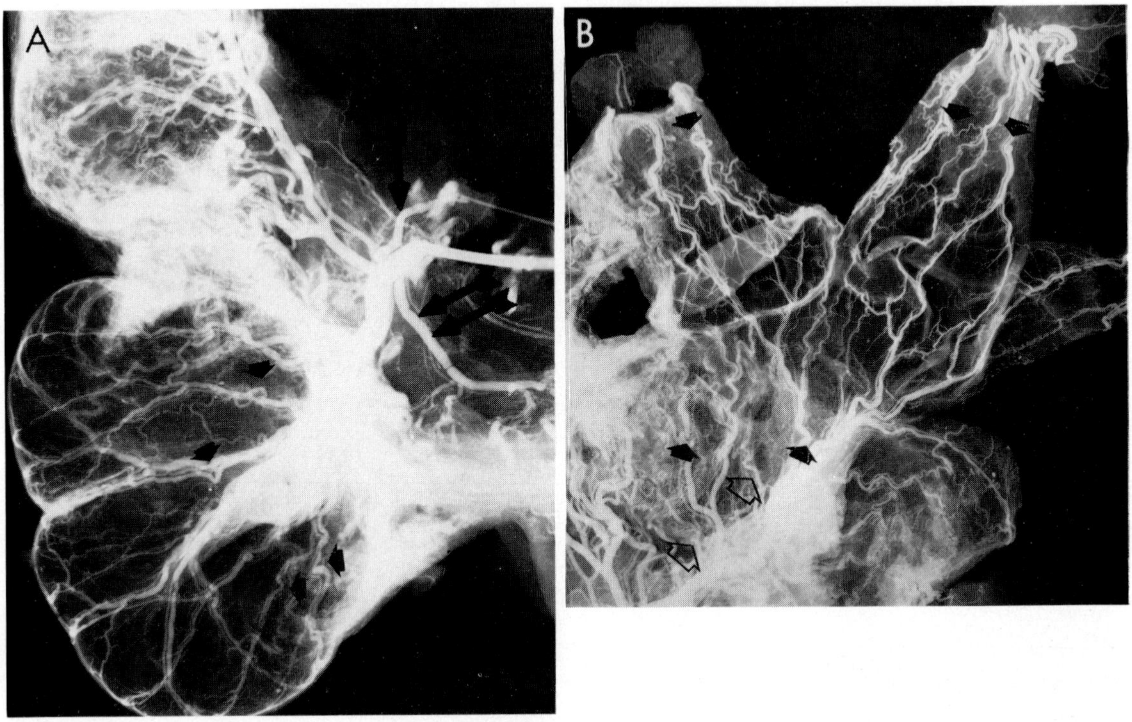

Fig 47–1. – **A,** normal anatomy. Specimen of right colon and cecum has been inflated with air, and vessels injected with barium gelatin mixture, in order to better demonstrate vascular anatomy. Vasa recta originate in pairs at mesenteric border from arcades of ileocolic artery or its ascending branch. Anterior and posterior vasa recta course subserosally for variable distances until proximal to antimesenteric teniae. Here the artery *(single long arrow)* and its companion vein *(double arrows),* about twice the caliber of the artery, penetrate bowel wall obliquely between bundles of circular muscle to reach submucosa *(short black arrows).* Vasa recta, which taper toward antimesenteric border, arborize and anastomose with similar branches from opposite wall and with branches of adjacent vasa recta. **B,** cecum has been opened along mesenteric border to better demonstrate arborization and anastomosis in **A.** *Open arrows* indicate vasa brevia, which arise from vascular arcades in mesentery to supply muscularis and mucosa of juxtamesenteric bowel. (From Baer and Ryan, Am. J. Roentgenol. 126:394, 1976, with permission.)

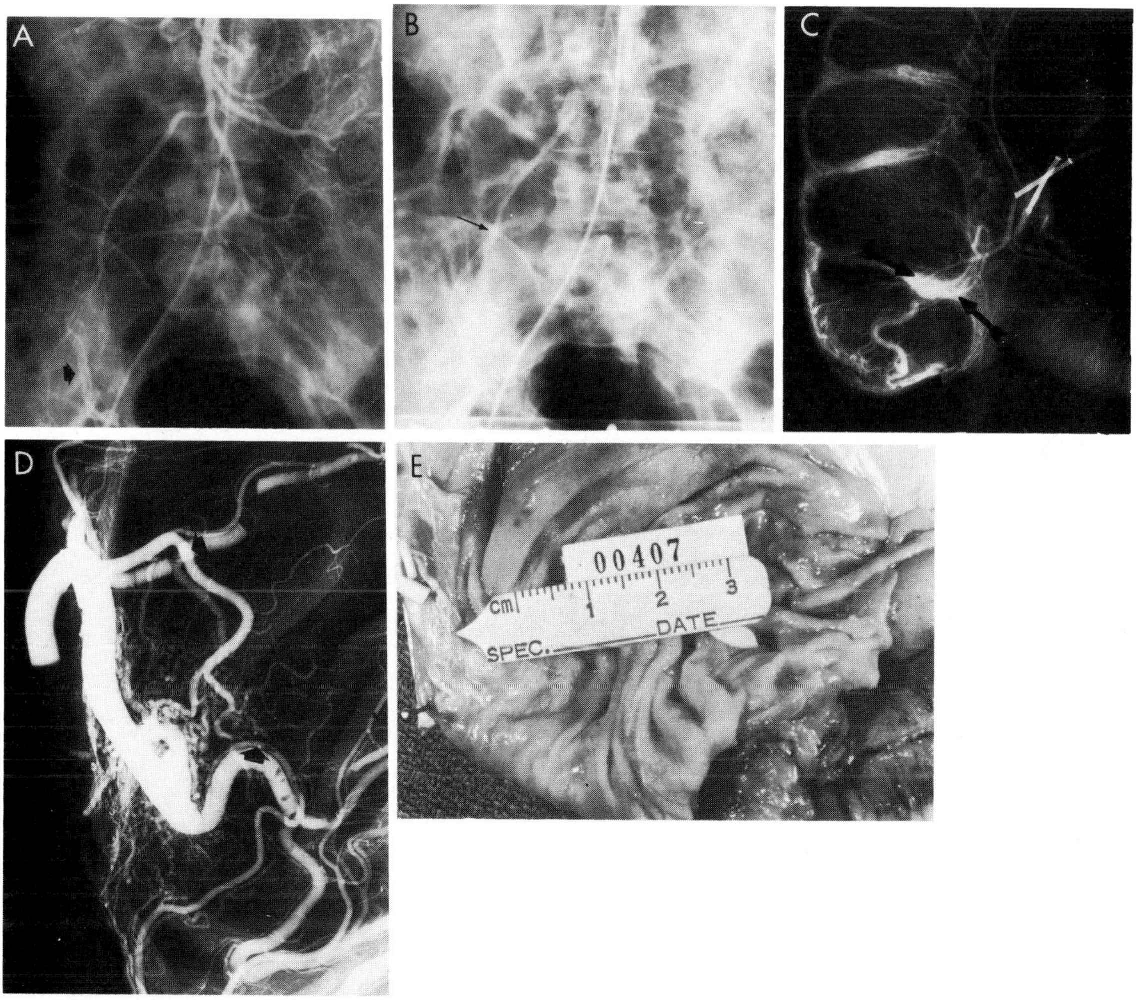

Fig 47–2.—Woman, age 48, with typical angiographic findings of vascular ectasia of cecum (biopsy proved cirrhosis without portal hypertension). She had been admitted 10 times for moderately severe hematochezia. Conventional radiographic examinations of gastrointestinal tract, upper endoscopy and exploratory laparotomy were normal. **A,** superior mesenteric arteriogram after air insufflation of colon demonstrates conglomeration of vessels overlying arterial catheter, which represents submucosal venous plexus or tuft. During early arterial phase (up to 6 seconds, depending on rate of injection of contrast material), there is simultaneous filling of draining ileocolic vein *(arrow)*. **B,** note prolonged intense opacification of ileocolic vein *(arrow)* after all other mesenteric veins have cleared. **C,** angioarchitecture of surgical specimen demonstrates slight enlargement of feeding vasa recta *(arrows)* from both juxtamesenteric borders with marked enlargement of draining vein. **D,** magnification (×3.6) shows extent of dilated tortuous veins, which arborize like a medusa's head around large draining vein. Accompanying vasa recta *(arrows)* supply vascular ectasia. **E,** vascular ectasias are not visible from serosal surface and only rarely seen at endoscopy on mucosal surface,[13, 14] because extensive venous plexus is submucosal (see Fig 47–4). In this case ectasia can be seen through mucosa, which has become very attenuated in 2.5-cm lesional area. Note normal velvety mucosa beneath pointer. (From Baer and Ryan, Am. J. Roentgenol. 126:394, 1976, with permission.)

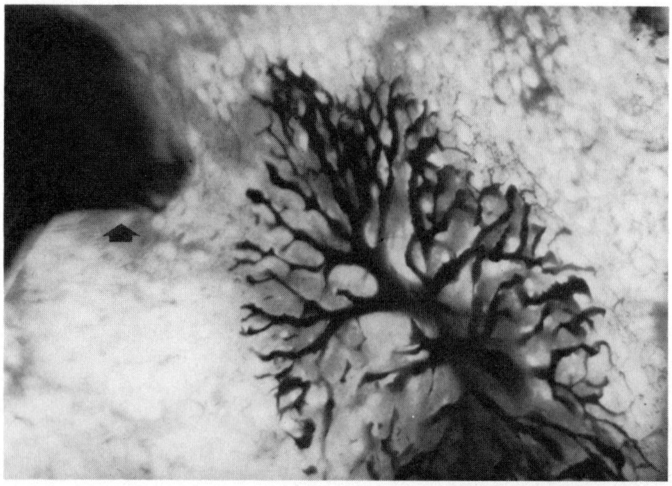

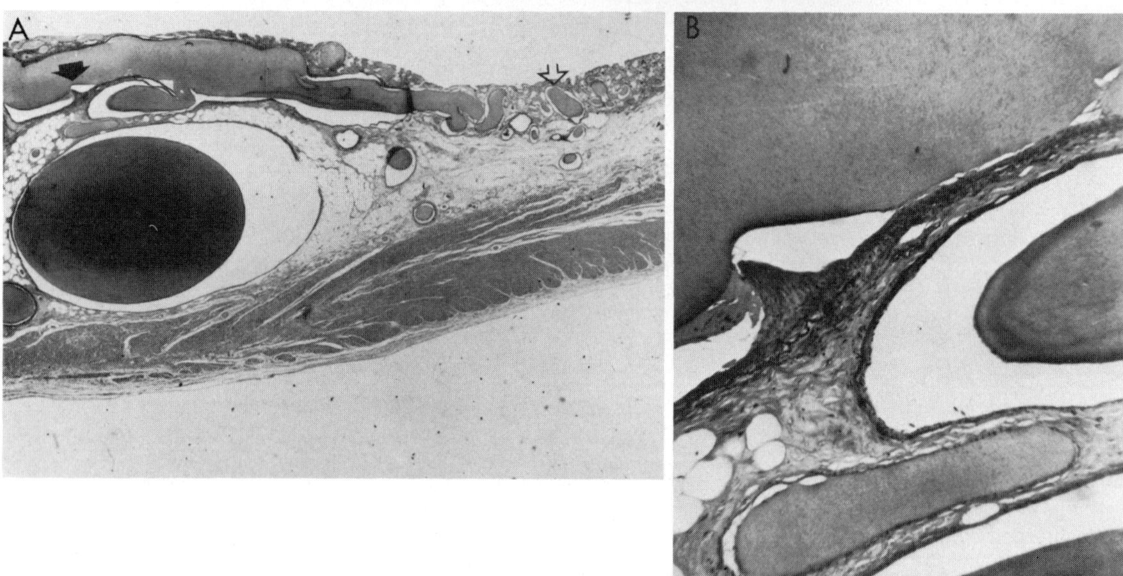

Fig 47–3 (top).—Another more sensitive method of identifying these lesions is to inject blood vessels with silicone rubber compound. Specimen is then dehydrated with increasing concentrations of ethyl alcohol and cleared with methyl salicylate.[4] Examination of this transparent specimen with dissecting microscope visualizes only opaque blood vessels. Honeycombed capillary network of mucosa is seen as background to darker medulla of ectatic capillaries. Size is compared to head of a pin *(arrow)*. (Mucosal capillary ectasias measure less than 0.5 cm in more than 90% of cases.[3]) (From Sprayregen and Boley, J.A.M.A. 239:962, 1978, with permission. Copyright 1978, American Medical Association.)

Fig 47–4 (bottom).—Microscopic (×10) examination demonstrates dilated mucosal capillaries *(open arrow)*. Mucosa is encroached on by thin-walled ectatic veins *(closed arrow)*, which in **B** show fragmentation of elastic lamina and occasional patches of normal smooth muscle (×50). (From Baer and Ryan, Am. J. Roentgenol. 126:394, 1976, with permission.)

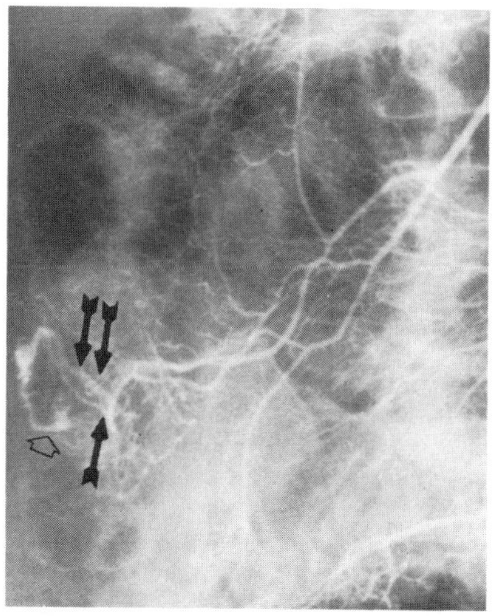

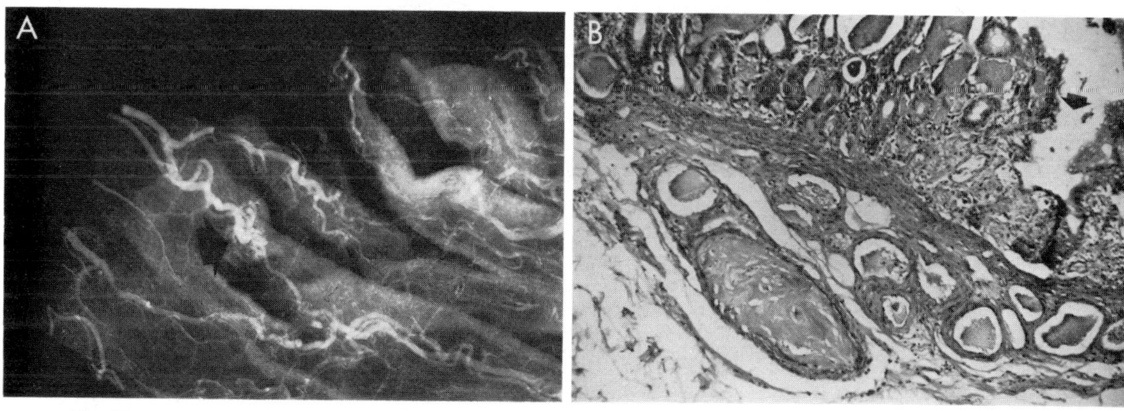

Fig 47–5 (top).—Woman, age 48, had two episodes of hematochezia in 10 years until 6 weeks prior to angiogram, when episodes became quite frequent, requiring two transfusions to maintain Hb of 10 gm%. Patient was unable to hold air enema. Nevertheless, lesion as well as extravasation *(open arrow)* into lumen, is well seen. Feeding artery *(arrow)* is enlarged due to increased flow. Early draining vein *(double arrows)*, which falls to taper along antimesenteric border, is identified. (From Baer and Ryan, Am. J. Roentgenol. 126:394, 1976, with permission.)

Fig 47–6 (bottom).—**A,** vascular ectasia in man, age 86, with murmur of aortic stenosis was identified only on superior mesenteric arteriogram during bleeding episode. Persistent stain along lateral wall of cecum in association with prolonged visualization of ileocolic vein. Angiogram of opened specimen demonstrates 4 mm ectasia *(arrow)* (×5). **B,** microscopic (×100) examination discloses thrombosed artery in muscularis mucosa beneath 4×0.5-mm ulceration of mucosa *(arrow)*. Markedly ectatic mucosal capillaries filled with contrast material seen around ulcer. (From Baer and Ryan, Am. J. Roentgenol. 126:394, 1976, with permission.)

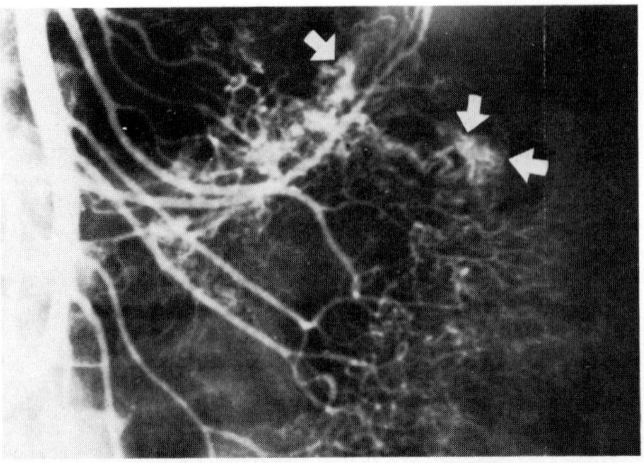

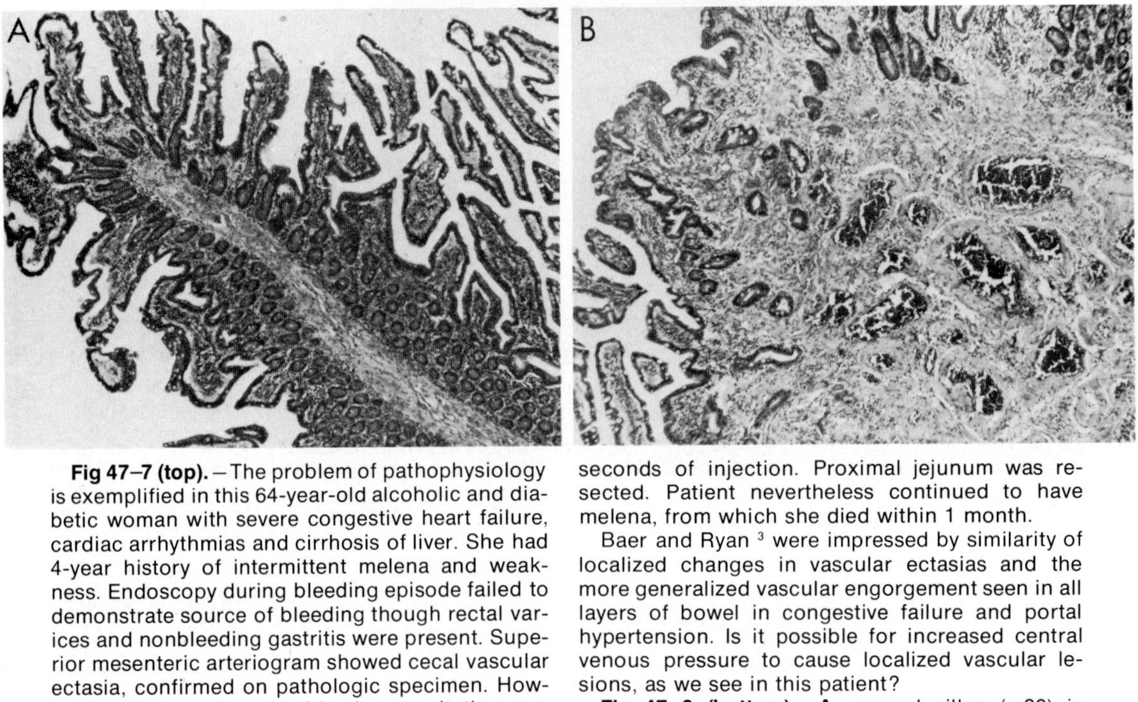

Fig 47–7 (top). – The problem of pathophysiology is exemplified in this 64-year-old alcoholic and diabetic woman with severe congestive heart failure, cardiac arrhythmias and cirrhosis of liver. She had 4-year history of intermittent melena and weakness. Endoscopy during bleeding episode failed to demonstrate source of bleeding though rectal varices and nonbleeding gastritis were present. Superior mesenteric arteriogram showed cecal vascular ectasia, confirmed on pathologic specimen. However, patient continued to bleed, necessitating second angiogram within 2 weeks of surgery. Case demonstrates vascular ectasia in proximal jejunum. Conglomerate of small arterioles *(arrows)* present in association with early draining vein within 2.5 seconds of injection. Proximal jejunum was resected. Patient nevertheless continued to have melena, from which she died within 1 month.

Baer and Ryan [3] were impressed by similarity of localized changes in vascular ectasias and the more generalized vascular engorgement seen in all layers of bowel in congestive failure and portal hypertension. Is it possible for increased central venous pressure to cause localized vascular lesions, as we see in this patient?

Fig 47–8 (bottom). – **A,** normal villus (×80) is compared to one involved with vascular ectasia **(B).** Note thickening of stalk by numerous ectatic veins, which lie beneath muscularis mucosa.

Chapter 48

Villous Adenoma of the Colon

DAVID G. BRAGG, M.D.
P. RUBEN KOEHLER, M.D.

COLONIC VILLOUS ADENOMAS provide the radiologist with an opportunity to specifically recognize a histologic entity on radiographic examination. Villous adenomas, which are uncommon, most frequently occur in the colon and have characteristics important both in specific recognition and in subsequent evaluation of the patient. Villous adenomas represent about 1.5–2.5% of all colonic neoplasms.[7]

Several important points need emphasis. (1) As will be demonstrated, most colonic villous tumors are found in the left colon. Rarely will they be recognized specifically on barium enema examination when they occur in the right colon. (2) Size is an important feature in estimating the probability that these tumors will contain invasive carcinomas. (3) Villous adenomas frequently occur in association with other malignant tumors of the gastrointestinal tract.[1, 12]

Distribution

Villous adenomas are rarely reported in the right colon. They are said to occur proximal to the peritoneal reflection in 78–98% of cases.[1, 9, 10]

A review of 70 cases of villous adenomas of the colon showed that 71.3% occurred in the sigmoid colon or proximally[8] (Fig 48–1). Figure 48–2 emphasizes the frequency with which the radiologist should expect to find the classic appearance of a villous adenoma in the right colon. Only three examples with recognizable patterns were encountered proximal to the splenic flexure, most being concentrated in the left colon. More often the right colon villous tumors presented as smoothly marginated or lobular polypoid filling defects.[8]

Clinical Features

Bright red rectal bleeding is the most common presenting feature. The percentage approached 50% in one series.[8] In another series, however, no specific clinical or laboratory findings reliably indicated the presence of a villous adenoma.[10]

Bright red rectal bleeding, of course, was more commonly noted in patients with left than right colon villous tumors. Right-sided lesions more often were associated with melena.

Diarrhea was more often found in patients with left-sided tumors and in those with malignant tumors.[8] Similarly, larger tumors were more often associated with diarrhea than were smaller ones. Finally, in the series of 70 patients, there was no instance in which the acute fluid and electrolyte depletion syndrome, often associated with villous adenomas, was observed.[8] This interesting clinical problem has received more attention than its frequency would warrant. One would expect that the electrolyte depletion syndrome would occur more frequently with large tumors of the left colon than with smaller ones of the right colon.[2]

Pathologic Features

Diagnosis of villous adenomas is based pathologically on their gross features.[5, 11] On gross examination these tumors usually are sessile and soft, with easily observed papillary and frondlike projections, imparting a very delicate gross appearance.

Size appears to have a prognostic influence on the likelihood of a villous tumor containing a focus of invasive carcinoma or being a frank cancer. In the reported series of 70 patients, 91% of all villous tumors less than 5 cm in diameter were found to be benign; 66% of tumors 8 cm or more, on the other hand, showed invasive carcinoma, and all tumors 9 cm or larger contained sites of cancer.[8] However, small lesions cannot reliably be assumed to be benign. Invasive tumors were noted in lesions as small as 2 cm in diameter[8] but rarely in those under 2 cm[8] (Fig 48–3).

The incidence of invasive carcinoma varies between 8% and 16%, according to reported previous series.[3, 4, 6, 7] In the series of 70 cases, the incidence of invasive carcinoma in villous adenomas was 24.2%.[8] In spite of the different radiographic appearances between right- and left-sided villous tumors, no significant difference was found pathologically in their gross appearance.

Villous tumors are commonly associated with additional benign or malignant gastrointestinal neoplasms.[4] Additional tumors of the colon were found in 34.3% of the 70 patients previously mentioned.[8] At least one additional malignant lesion was found in the gastrointestinal tract in 22.9%, and 8.6% had multiple villous adenomas of the colon.[8]

Radiographic Features

Emphasis in the radiographic literature has been on the classic appearance of villous adenomas since the original description by Wolf[13] in 1958. This classic appearance is dramatically demonstrated in Figures 48–4 and 48–5.

Double contrast examinations enhance the radiologist's ability to specifically recognize these tumors.

Even an annular pattern, consistent with an invasive, annular carcinoma of the colon, may on occasion prove to be a benign villous tumor of the colon. One such example was observed in the series of 70 cases.[8]

Kaye and Bragg[8] believed that the diagnosis of villous adenoma was justified retrospectively in 35.3% of 70 patients. In another 45.1%, the lesions could be recognized but did not suggest their true pathologic nature; and in almost 20%, the tumor found at surgery could not be detected on review of the barium enema examination, even with knowledge of its location. Size appeared to be the most critical determinant in predictability of the true nature of these lesions, as well as in correlation of those noted subsequently to contain sites of invasive tumor. Unusual examples of villous tumors, even large ones, are illustrated in Figures 48–6 and 48–7.

Examples of villous tumors of the proximal colon may vary in their radiographic appearance. As stated earlier, they can be recognized only infrequently as of villous origin. An exception to this is shown in Figure 48–8.

Figure 48–9 is a more typical example of the nonspecific appearance of villous adenomas of the right colon. This lesion presented as a polypoid filling defect, nonspecific in radiographic features, but was found histologically to be a villous tumor of the colon.

An example of multiplicity of tumors of villous origin is shown in Figure 48–10.

Three tumors, two of which are large, are located in the right colon. The more distal one is suggestive of its villous origin; the others appeared to be polypoid lesions.

Summary

Villous tumors of the colon usually can be recognized radiographically when they appear in the left colon. The radiologist's ability to recognize this lesion probably is based on size, the larger lesions more frequently revealing their villous origins. In addition, size appears to have a significant predictive value in judging which tumors will contain invasive carcinoma. Double contrast techniques should improve the diagnostic accuracy. Special attention should be paid to any margin of the colon with frondlike irregularities, which occasionally mimic inflammatory bowel disease. The radiologist should not only be alert to the tendency of villous tumors to be multiple, but should screen the gastrointestinal tract for additional benign and malignant gastrointestinal lesions when a villous adenoma is found.

Editor's Note.—Morson* studied 2,506 adenomatous polyps, villous adenomas and tumors of intermediate type (papillary, villoglandular or tubulovillous adenomas—all terms are synonomous). The frequency of villous adenomas was 9.7%. In 243 villous adenomas studied, there was a malignancy rate of 41%. Morson further states that even small villous adenomas (1–2 cm) have a malignancy rate of 9.5%, and cancer is found in 46% of those over 2 cm in diameter. Villous adenomas have a considerably greater malignant potential than adenomatous polyps. Apart from the important issue of size, it has been shown that the cancer rate increases with the degree of epithelial dysplasia, and severe dysplasia is more common in villous adenomas than in adenomatous polyps.—E. G.

*Morson, B.: The polyp-cancer sequence in the large bowel, Proc. R. Soc. Med. 67:451, 1974.

REFERENCES

1. Bacon, H. E., Lowell, E. J., Jr., and Trimpi, H. D.: Villous papillomas of the colon and rectum: Study of 28 cases with end results of treatment over five year period, Surgery 35:77, 1954.
2. Barbior, B. M.: Villous adenoma of the colon. Study of the patient with severe fluid and electrolyte disturbances, Am. J. Med. 41:615, 1966.
3. Dreese, W. C., et al.: Villous tumors of the rectum and sigmoid, Surg. Gynecol. Obstet. 115:182, 1962.
4. Enterline, H. T., et al.: Malignant potential of adenomas of the colon and rectum, J.A.M.A. 179:322, 1962.
5. Fisher, E. R., and Castro, A. F.: Diffuse papillomatous polyps (villous tumors) of the colon and rectum: Pathologic and clinical observations, Am. J. Surg. 85:146, 1953.
6. Hanley, P. H., et al.: Villous tumors: Experience with 163 patients, South. Med. J. 65:233, 1962.
7. Hines, M. O., et al.: Villous tumors of the colon and rectum, Dis. Colon Rectum 1:128, 1958.
8. Kaye, J., and Bragg, D. G.: Unusual roentgenologic and clinicopathologic features of villous adenomas of the colon, Radiology 91:799, 1968.
9. Liechty, R. D., and Raterman, L.: Villous adenoma, a surgical dilemma, Arch. Surg. 87:107, 1963.
10. Sunderland, D. A., and Binkley, G. E.: Papillary adenomas of the large intestine: Clinical and morphologic study of 48 cases, Cancer 1:184, 1948.
11. Swinton, N. W., Meissner, W. A., and Soland, W. A., Jr.: Papillary adenomas of the colon and rectum: Clinical and pathologic study, Arch. Intern. Med. 96:544, 1955.
12. Turek, R. E., Davis, W. C., Wilson, W. J., Olson, R. O., Jr.: The roentgenographic diagnosis of villous tumors of the colon, Am. J. Roentgenol. 113:349, 1971.
13. Wolf, B. S.: Roentgen diagnosis of villous adenoma of the colon, Mt. Sinai J. Med. NY 25:604, 1958.

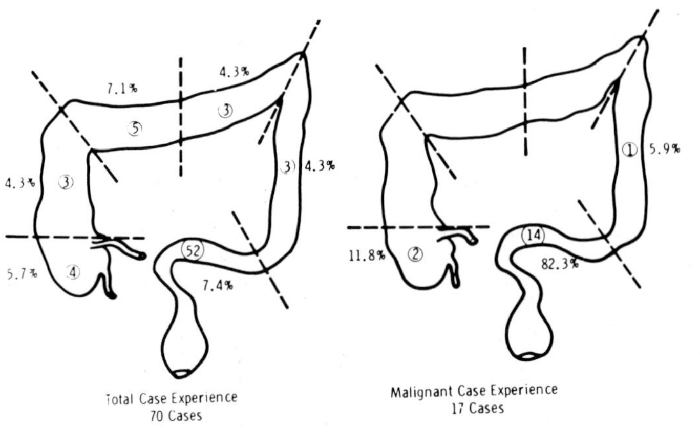

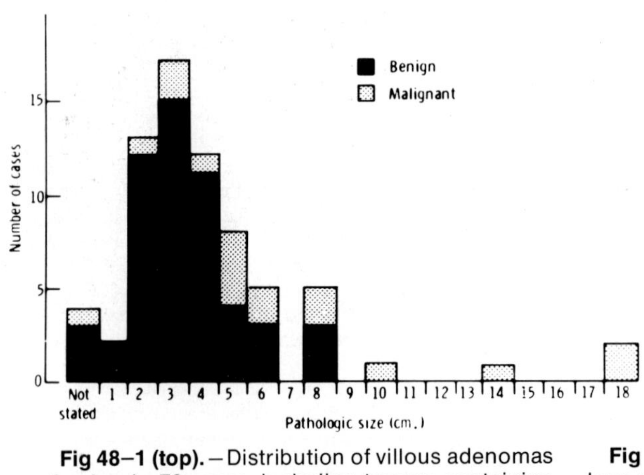

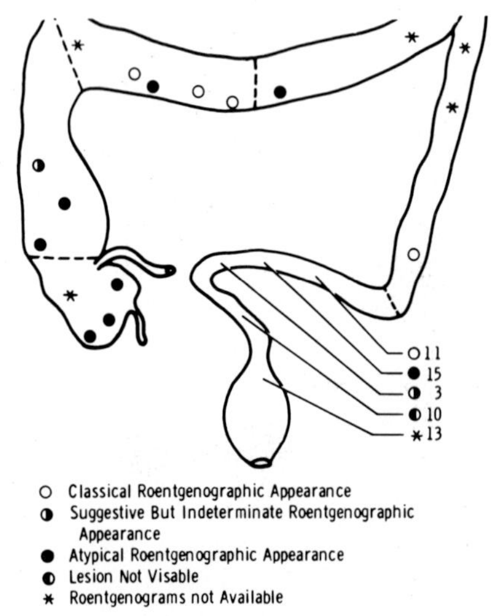

Fig 48–1 (top).—Distribution of villous adenomas of colon in 70 cases, including tumors containing invasive carcinoma (17 cases). (From Kaye and Bragg, Radiology 91:799, 1968, with permission.)

Fig 48–2 (right).—Appearance of villous adenomas of colon related to site. (From Kaye and Bragg, Radiology 91:799, 1968, with permission.)

Fig 48–3 (bottom).—Relationship of size of villous adenoma to malignant potential. (From Kaye and Bragg, Radiology 91:799, 1968, with permission.)

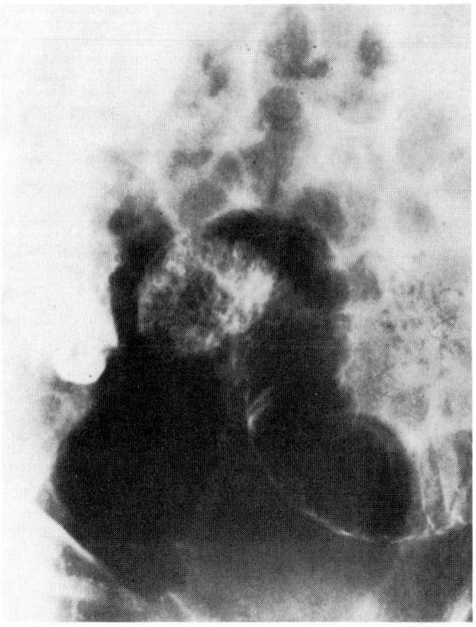

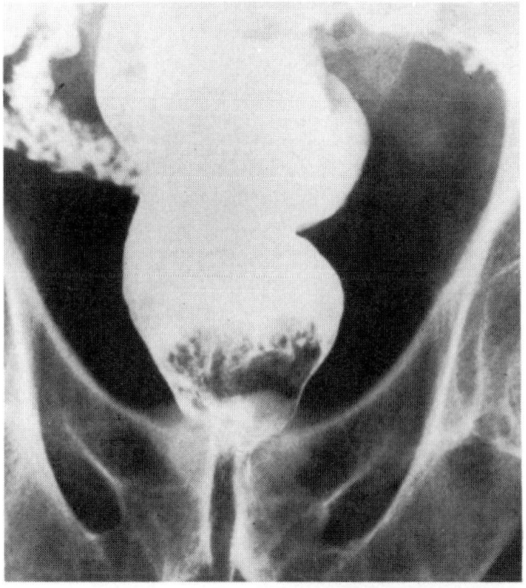

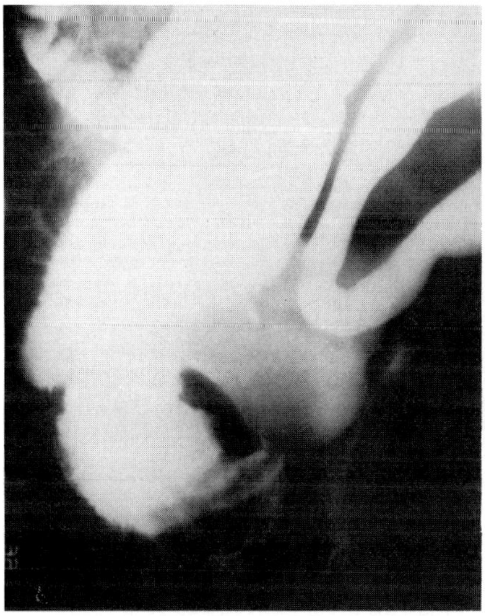

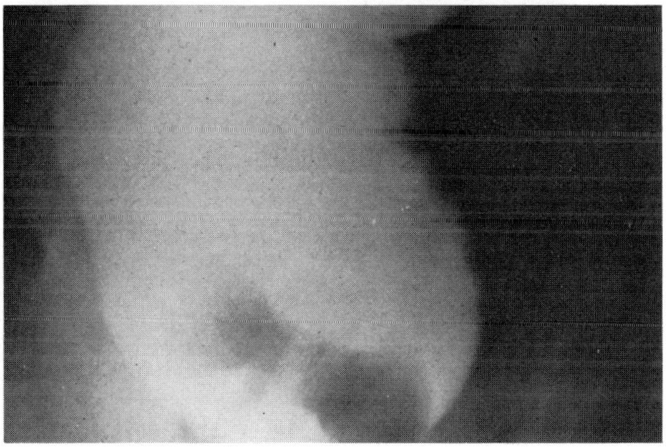

Fig 48–4 (top left). – Villous adenoma. Note classic appearance with barium within interstices of frondlike projections of villous mass. Air contrast examination shows typical frondlike appearance of villous tumor on double contrast examination of sigmoid colon.

Fig 48–5 (top right). – Typical appearance of rectal villous adenoma. AP view of distal rectum. (From Kaye and Bragg, Radiology 91:799, 1968, with permission.)

Fig 48–6 (bottom left). – Oblique view of barium enema, single contrast technique, in which spiculated margins of colon can be seen throughout rectum and extending into distal sigmoid. Very large villous adenoma found endoscopically and subsequently surgically, with sites of frank invasive carcinoma.

Fig 48–7 (bottom right). – Oblique view of barium enema, single contrast technique, shows on left anterior wall of rectum irregular contours of flat, long segment type of villous tumor. Radiographically this is typical of invasive carcinoma but at surgery was found to represent villous adenoma of colon. (Courtesy of Dr. James A. Nelson, Salt Lake City, Utah.)

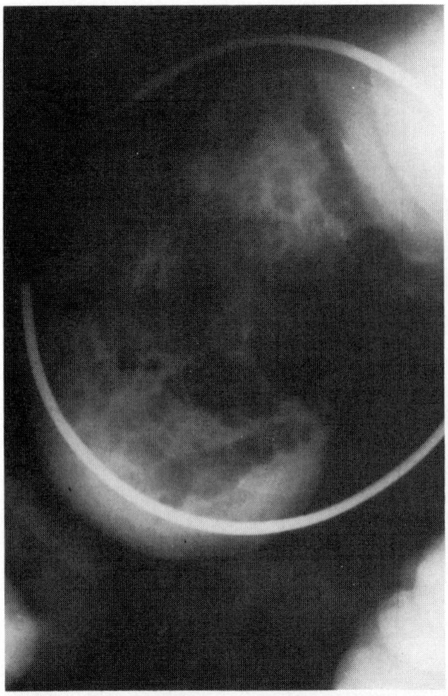

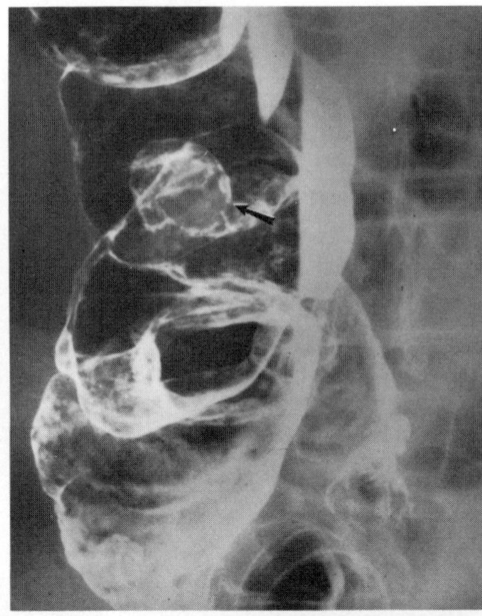

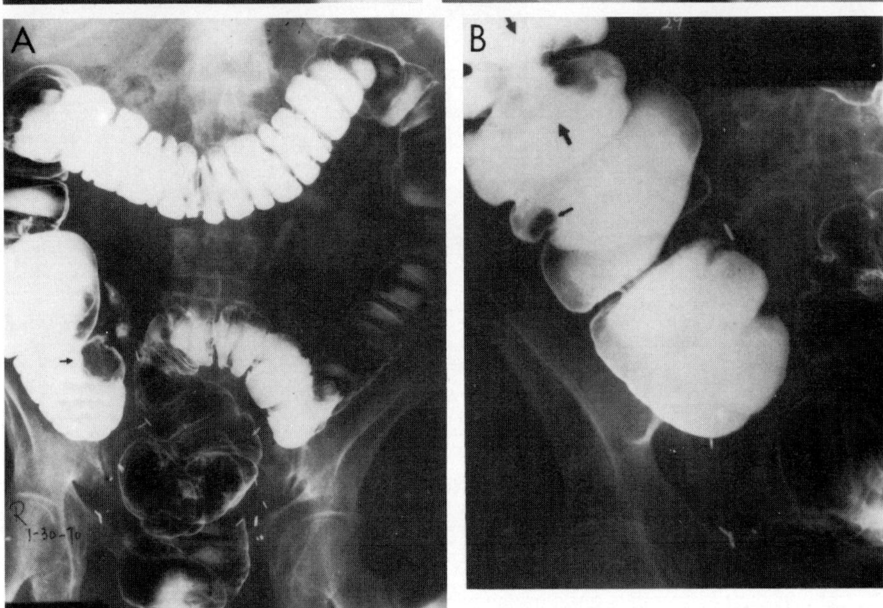

Fig 48–8 (top left).—Villous adenoma, proximal transverse colon. Spot film shows large multilobulated tumor of right colon, a classic villous adenoma by gross inspection. Tumor contained invasive cancer.

Fig 48–9 (top right).—Polypoid villous adenoma, right colon. This small polypoid filling defect *(arrow)* was found to be benign histologically. (From Kaye and Bragg, Radiology 91:799, 1968, with permission.)

Fig 48–10 (bottom).—Three villous tumors in one patient. **A,** large villous adenoma *(single arrow)* in region of ileocecal valve. This latter seen only on prone (PA) view. **B,** small lateral ascending colon lesion *(small arrow).* Bulky, lobular distal ascending colon lesion *(large opposed arrows).* (Courtesy of Dr. Edward I. Greenbaum, Los Angeles, Calif.)

Chapter 49

Volvulus

VOLVULUS OF THE CECUM AND RIGHT COLON

LEO S. FIGIEL, M.D., F.A.C.R.
STEVEN J. FIGIEL, M.D., F.A.C.R.

ALTHOUGH VOLVULUS of the right colon is a thoroughly documented roentgenologic entity, with highly specific findings on scout studies of the abdomen, rarely will a practicing radiologist have had the personal experience necessary to appreciate the variability in the obstructive patterns possible in this condition. If there is, in addition, a lack of familiarity with the older literature, it is possible that the radiologist will fail to diagnose this important mechanical form of obstruction, which is estimated to account for about 1% of acute obstructions of the colon.

Most of the important roentgenologic literature on this subject was published in the 1940s and 1950s. Even a cursory review of the articles by Courty,[3] Frimann–Dahl,[8] Ritvo et al.,[10] the authors[5-7] and others will provide a roentgenologic foundation for the understanding of this important form of obstruction. Excellent bibliographies are contained in the above references.

During the past 20 to 25 years, sporadic reports have been published, mostly in the surgical literature. These usually were concerned with the clinical and surgical aspects of this entity. Emphasis was properly made in these articles on the high mortality and morbidity associated with this form of obstruction when diagnosis and treatment were delayed for any reason.

Some of the developments since our studies in 1953–1954 have focused attention on the possibility of volvulus of the right colon, occurring in association with an obstructive lesion elsewhere in the colon, usually the left colon.[10] We have chosen to label this combination of events "double obstructions of the colon."[7] The "cecal bascule" form of volvulus also has been emphasized in the surgical and radiologic literature.[1, 2] Both situations will be covered later in this section.

Anatomical Considerations

To understand possible mechanisms of volvulus of the right colon, one should be familiar with the original work by Dott,[4] "Anomalies of Intestinal Rotation," and with autopsy studies by Wolfer, Beaton and Anson,[11] which analyze the peritoneal attachments and degree of fixation of the right colon and their relationship to volvulus. Recent studies by Balthazar[1] stress roentgenologic aspects of defective or abnormal fixation of the right colon and implications of these.

Summarized briefly, defective peritoneal fixation of the cecum and ascending colon is normally present in approximately 10% of all people.[11] The presence of defective fixation permits abnormal mobility. With the potential for abnormal mobility, displacement of the cecum and ascending colon into any portion of the abdominal cavity is possible. Depending on the length of the right colon, which is mobile, a great variety of obstructive patterns will be encountered.

In addition, most authors mention the association of bands, membranes or adhesions, which provide a fulcrum on which the mobile right colon can twist. Although these are frequently present, they are not a necessary prerequisite for volvulus of the right colon.

Precipitating Causes

Precipitating causes of volvulus of the right colon described in the literature are varied. Among those indicated are excess roughage in the diet, excessive gas in the cecum and ascending colon, traction due to disease of the appendix, meteorism occurring in unpressurized air flight, abdominal masses and others. For the greater part, these so-called exciting causes are not well understood and are probably not specific.

Importantly, one can make a case for the association of volvulus of the right colon and pregnancy, including the postpartum abdomen; volvulus occurring secondary to obstructing lesions in the left colon; volvulus of the postoperative abdomen; and volvulus occurring as a complication of colonic ileus. The association of volvulus of the right colon in this type of case occurs with sufficient frequency that special consideration must be given to it.

In pregnancy one can anticipate the possibility of cecal displacement by an enlarging, gravid uterus. Displacement may, in the presence of progressive distention, result in an acute torsion accident. By the same token, volvulus of the right colon occurring in the postpartum patient can be explained by a similar mechanism. Following delivery, a displaced, ectopically located right colon may distend with gas and be trapped between the anterior and posterior abdominal walls. When symptoms become manifest clinically, a state of acute volvulus may be said to exist. In both pregnancy and the postpartum state, movements of the patient from side to side, especially when she is recumbent, may be a factor in displacement of the cecum and ascending colon to abnormal positions.

Ritvo et al.[10] were the first to associate volvulus of the right colon with obstructive lesions elsewhere in the colon, usually the left colon. Carcinoma and diverticulitis were implicated. We have, in addition, found the postoperative abdomen—especially following closed, segmental resections of the left colon, presumably with stenosis—to be a precipitating cause of volvulus of the right colon when it is mobile. In these cases of double obstructions of the colon, a diagnosis of volvulus may have to be made on the basis of cecal displacement, since the barium enema study may demonstrate a complete or high-grade obstruction of the left colon. Complete evaluation of the colon during barium enema examination may be impossible. Furthermore, in instances of postoperative colon following resection and anastomosis, it may be undesirable to attempt evaluation of the colon by enema examination, no matter how carefully this is done. In most cases radiologic features will be characteristic of volvulus of the right colon, particularly when the cecum and ascending colon are ectopic. An interesting observation in four such cases reported by Figiel and Figiel was the actual demonstration of changes in position of the cecum and ascending colon as earlier scout and barium enema studies were reviewed.

We have also noted the occurrence of volvulus of the right colon as a complication of paralytic ileus with severe distention of the colon in which, owing to defective fixation, changes in cecal position took place. Such obstructions often are of the cecal bascule type;[1,2] however, a true volvulus is possible. The same mechanism also may apply in the postoperative abdomen.

We are inclined to believe that most cases of volvulus of the right colon occur when a patient with a mobile, defectively fixed right colon is asleep. Normal restless movements of the patient from side to side during sleep may result in displacement of the right colon to an ectopic or abnormal location. When meteorism occurs, trapping of the displaced right colon is possible, and symptomatic acute volvulus may be said to exist. It has been shown that in most instances the mobile right colon in instances of volvulus is found in the mid- or left upper abdomen. Almost uniformly this displacement is associated with a simple 180-degree twist, which occurs at the site of torsion. This is a type of displacement that could result simply from changes in position of the patient when recumbent and could hardly occur when the patient is in the upright position.

Roentgenographic Findings

From the roentgenographic standpoint, very little new information has been added since the 1950s.[3,5,7,10,11] The thrust of this section will be directed toward clarification of the mechanism of volvulus as it relates to the length of the right colon that is defective in its peritoneal attachment and to the various displacements that may occur. Considerations will be given to the various patterns possible when the cecum and ascending colon are normally located but freely mobile and to displacement patterns possible when abnormal mobility occurs in nonrotation or a hyperdescended cecum. We have indicated that the obstructed cecum and ascending colon may be encountered in any quadrant or portion of the abdominal cavity. This can be readily verified by study of case material presented in earlier publications.[3,5-7,10] We shall diagrammatically illustrate variations in fixation, length and mobility of the right colon, with displacement patterns seen under given conditions. The mechanism of displacement and torsion is based on correlations with 45 cases encountered in about 30 years of practice in radiology.

Fortunately in volvulus of the right colon, the roentgenographic findings usually are characteristic. Although the cecum and ascending colon may be found in any portion of the abdominal cavity, the most common displacement is into the epigastrium and left upper quadrant (Figs 49–5 to 49–8). An obliquely oriented cecum and ascending colon will be identified extending across the abdominal cavity, with the caput cecum located in the left upper or midabdomen. Colonic haustral pattern is maintained, and the anatomical characteristics of the cecum and ascending colon are readily identifiable. Variations in colonic diameter, from the ascending colon into the cecum, are readily appreciated. Rarely a dilated, displaced cecum and ascending colon located in the left upper quadrant may be confused with a normal or abnormally dilated stomach.

When shorter segments of the cecum and ascending colon are involved secondary to volvulus, the obstructed cecum and ascending colon generally will be found near the normal location, i.e., in the right half of the abdomen (Fig 49–9). Sometimes the cecum will be located in the right upper quadrant. We have noted a greater tendency toward obliteration of the haustral pattern in such displacements. This is probably due to the shorter length of colon involved and probably has a direct relationship to increased intraluminal gaseous pressure. Competency of the ileocecal valve may also be a factor.

When longer, more redundant portions of the right colon are implicated in volvulus, the displaced cecum and ascending colon may be found in any portion of the abdominal cavity. In some instances of malrotation, a vertically oriented, massively distended cecum and ascending colon occupy almost the entire vertical dimension of the abdominal cavity (Fig 49–8). The cecum may then be found in the upper abdomen or, in some instances, in the pelvic cavity. In some cases redundant, looplike presentations of the obstructed cecum and ascending colon may be present (Figs 49–9 to 49–11). These presentations may occur throughout the abdominal cavity, the cecal location being variable. Confusion of looplike right colon volvulus with sigmoid volvulus may be settled by barium enema when plain films are not diagnostic.

In almost all instances of cecal displacement associated with twisting, the obstruction is generally complete or of such magnitude that practically no gas or fecal matter is seen in the colon distal to the obstruction. Obviously, in cecal displacement the cecum and ascending colon will not be visualized in normal position, once again providing a clue to diagnosis of torsion-displacement or volvulus.

Upright or decubitus films usually demonstrate one large fluid level in the cecum and ascending colon. However two air fluid levels may be seen with marked redundancy of the involved right colon or when the point of volvulus is more distally placed, as in the hepatic flexure or transverse colon.

The combination of findings on AP and upright or decubitus studies is generally so characteristic that, in our opinion, the diagnosis of volvulus of the cecum and ascending colon usually is pathognomonic.

Occasionally small bowel loops may be identified to the right of the rotated and displaced cecum and ascending colon; ileocecal valve insertion often may be recognizable. At times, the point of torsion in the colon may be outlined by gas, visualized as an area of narrowing or conization.

Of considerable interest is the demonstration of changes in position of the cecum while the patient is under observation. Review of earlier scout studies or barium enema studies may show changes in position of the right colon. Change in position is indicative of abnormal mobility; abnormal mobility associated with abnormal distention is indicative of volvulus. For these reasons we often refer to volvulus of the right colon as a torsion-displacement accident.

In a previous publication we[5] indicated that sometimes torsion in the long axis of the colon may be associated with signs of incomplete obstruction. We noted several times that barium enema studies showed a rounded point of termination in the ascending colon and proximity to a dilated cecum. We indicated that this diagnosis was extremely difficult and probably could not be made without recourse to barium enema study.

Presently this form of obstruction is being referred to as a cecal bascule form of volvulus. It is thought that anterior folding of a movable cecum and ascending colon results in formation of a flap-valve obstruction at the folded point on the ascending colon. It is stressed that frequently in such instances adhesions are present and are a factor in the obstructive process. It is recommended that barium enema study be undertaken for diagnosis of problem cases of this type. Colonoscopy for purposes of decompression also should be considered.

Barium enema studies are always indicated when volvulus is suspected. A classic beaklike appearance is usually encountered (see Fig 49–5, B). There may be crossing or twisting of mucosal folds. In cecal bascule volvulus, a rounded termination of the barium column may be present. A rounded termination may also be seen elsewhere in volvulus. Such a rounded termination in the right lower quadrant, especially when a large gas-distended viscus is present in its proximity, should alert the radiologist to the diagnosis of volvulus.

We[6] have previously reported volvulus of the right colon being spontaneously reducible during the expulsion phase of the barium enema study. Obstructive symptoms were present and barium enema was undertaken for diagnostic purposes. Initial studies demonstrated abnormal orientation of a gas-distended cecum and ascending colon in the right flank or right upper quadrant, with complete obstruction demonstrated during the filling phase of the barium enema. During expulsion of the enema, the cecum and ascending colon returned to normal position in the right lower quadrant and the previously noted gas-filled viscus disappeared. This is an important observation, and the sequence of events is characteristic of spontaneous detorsion during the expulsion phase of the enema.

Special mention should be made of volvulus occurring in the postpartum patient. We[6] were successful in reducing a volvulus of the cecum and ascending colon with proved obstruction in the ascending colon on barium enema study. The cecum and ascending colon were located ectopically in the umbilical portion of the abdomen. The patient was placed in the knee-chest position with supports beneath chest and thighs. The relaxed musculature of the abdominal wall permitted changes in position of the cecum and ascending colon, with resultant decompression of the gas-distended viscus. Subsequently we demonstrated complete detorsion, with cure of the patient.

Once again we must emphasize that in double obstructions of the colon, it may be impossible to evaluate the right colon by barium enema study and the diagnosis of volvulus may have to be made on the basis of roentgenographic findings on scout studies.

Summary

Roentgenologic features of volvulus of the right colon are discussed. The mechanism of volvulus is correlated with anatomical variations in length and mobility of the right colon. Defective fixation of the right colon is correlated with various displacement patterns that can occur under given conditions. These are illustrated diagrammatically and are based on a review of roentgenographic surgical material in 45 cases encountered during a 30-year practice in radiology.

REFERENCES

1. Balthazar, E. J.: Congenital positional anomalies of the colon, radiographic diagnosis and clinical implications, I and II, Gastrointest. Radiol. 2:41, 1977.
2. Bobroff, L. M., Messinger, N. H., Subbarao, K., and Beneventano, T. C.: The cecal bascule, Am. J. Roentgenol. 115:249, 1972.
3. Courty, A.: *Les Volvulus Aigus du Colon Droit,* (Paris: Masson and Cie, 1950).
4. Dott, N. M.: Anomalies of intestinal rotation: Their embryological and surgical aspects, with report of five cases, Br. J. Surg. 11:251, 1923.
5. Figiel, L. S., and Figiel, S. J.: Volvulus of the cecum and ascending colon, Radiology 61:496, 1953.
6. Figiel, L. S., and Figiel, S. J.: Detorsion of volvulus of the right colon, roentgenographic considerations, Am. J. Roentgenol. 72:192, 1954.
7. Figiel, L. S., and Figiel, S. J.: Double obstructions of the colon, J. Abd. Surg. 13:244, 1971.
8. Frimann-Dahl, J.: *Roentgen Examinations in Acute Abdominal Diseases* (Springfield, Ill.: Charles C Thomas, 1974).
9. Füth, H., and Obladen: Weiterer Beitrag zur Frage der Verlagerung des Zökums in der Schwangerschaft, Dtsch. Med. Wochenschr. 54:819, 1928.
10. Ritvo, M., Farrell, G. E., and Schauffer, I. A.: The association of volvulus of the cecum and ascending colon with other obstructive colonic lesions, Am. J. Roentgenol. 78:587, 1957.
11. Wolfer, J. A., Beaton, L. E., and Anson, B. J.: Volvulus of the cecum: Anatomical factors in its etiology, Surg Gynecol. Obstet. 74:882, 1942.

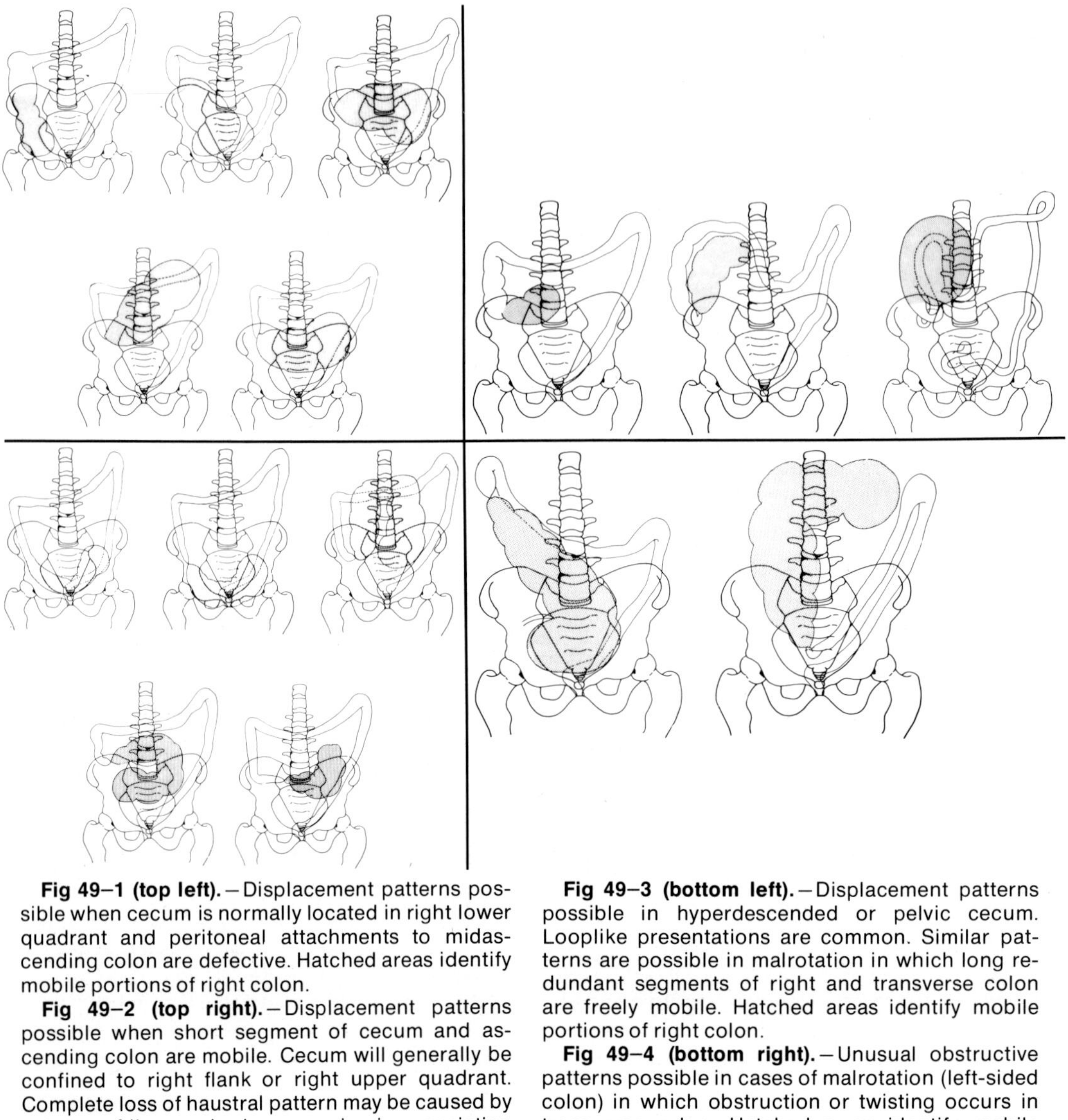

Fig 49–1 (top left).—Displacement patterns possible when cecum is normally located in right lower quadrant and peritoneal attachments to midascending colon are defective. Hatched areas identify mobile portions of right colon.

Fig 49–2 (top right).—Displacement patterns possible when short segment of cecum and ascending colon are mobile. Cecum will generally be confined to right flank or right upper quadrant. Complete loss of haustral pattern may be caused by patency of ileocecal valve occurring in association with short segment involved in volvulus. Hatched areas identify mobile portions of right colon.

Fig 49–3 (bottom left).—Displacement patterns possible in hyperdescended or pelvic cecum. Looplike presentations are common. Similar patterns are possible in malrotation in which long redundant segments of right and transverse colon are freely mobile. Hatched areas identify mobile portions of right colon.

Fig 49–4 (bottom right).—Unusual obstructive patterns possible in cases of malrotation (left-sided colon) in which obstruction or twisting occurs in transverse colon. Hatched areas identify mobile portions of right colon.

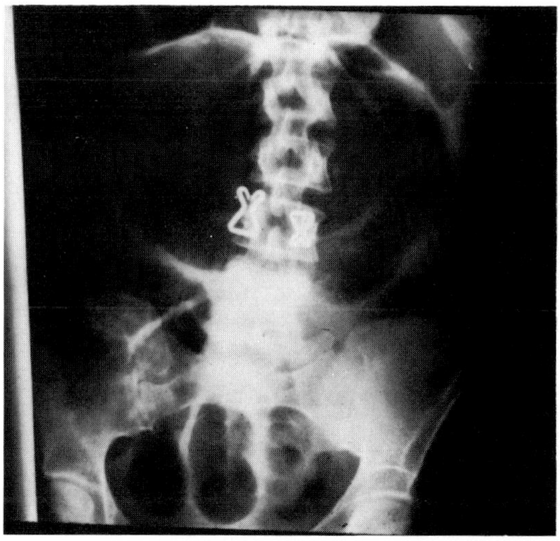

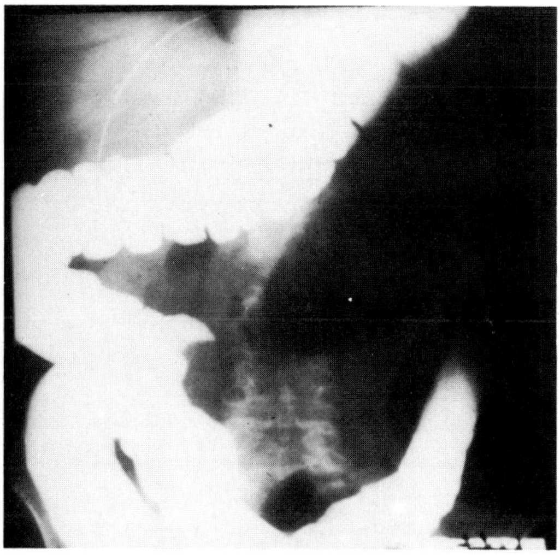

Fig 49–5 (top left). – Volvulus of cecum. Cecum is grossly distended and has rotated 180 degrees to lie within epigastrium. (Courtesy of Dr. Edward I Greenbaum, Los Angeles, Calif.)

Fig 49–6 (top right). – Cecal volvulus presenting in left upper quadrant. Barium enema shows complete obstruction with typical bird-of-prey appearance at point of obstruction. (Courtesy of Dr. Edward I. Greenbaum, Los Angeles, Calif.)

Fig 49–7 (bottom). – **A,** volvulus of cecum. Cecum is rotated 180 degrees and occupies epigastrium and left upper quadrant. Tip of cecum is noted to lie slightly above left iliac crest *(arrow).* **B,** upright view reveals long single air-fluid level in distended cecum. (Courtesy of Dr. Edward I. Greenbaum, Los Angeles, Calif.)

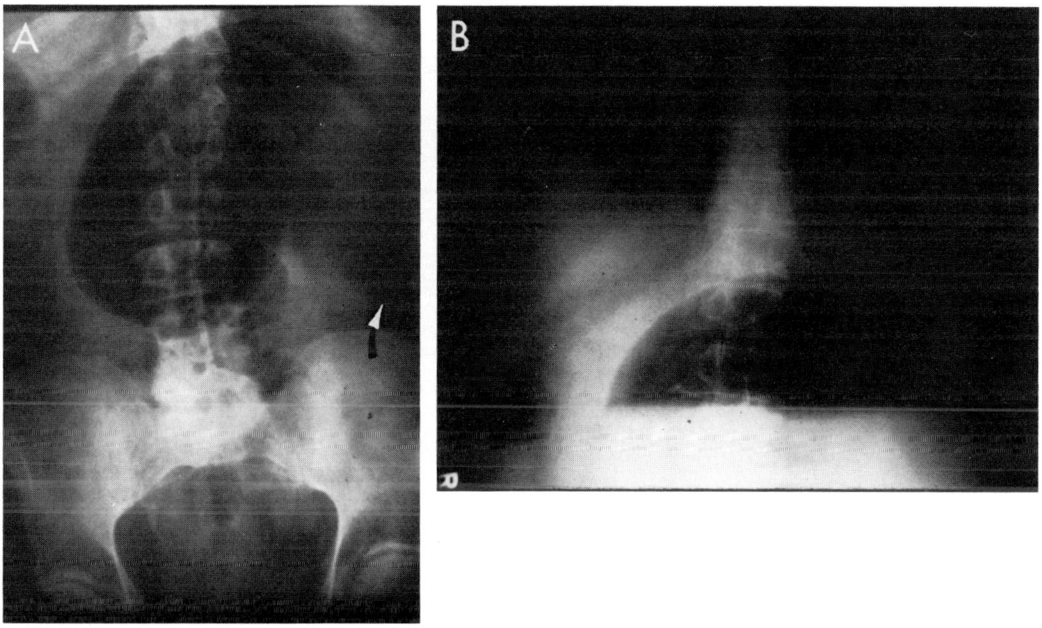

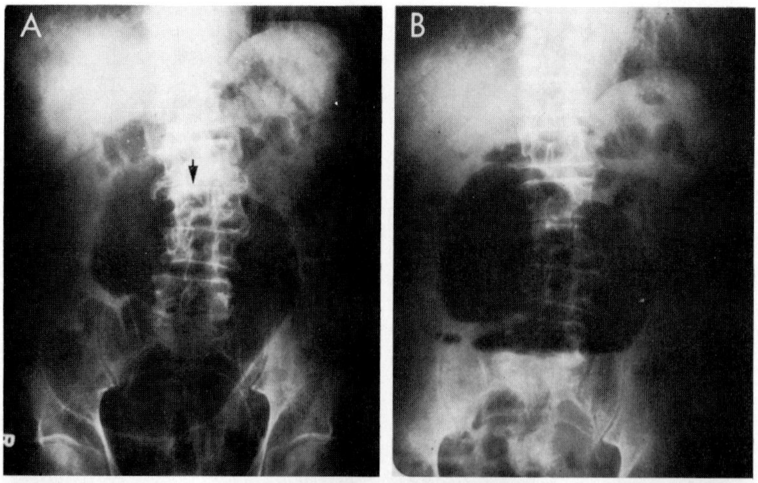

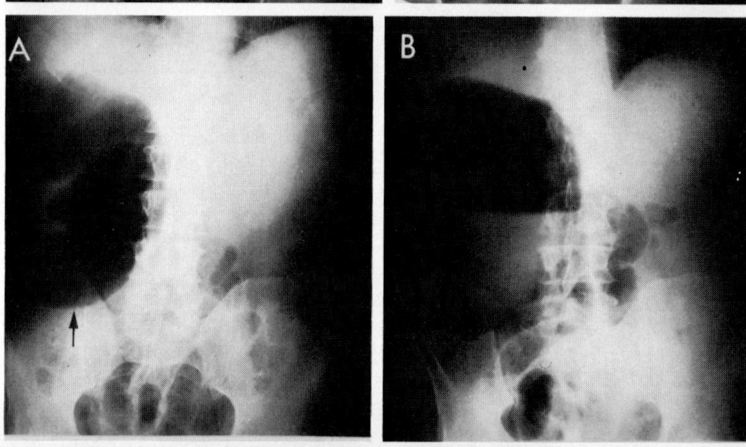

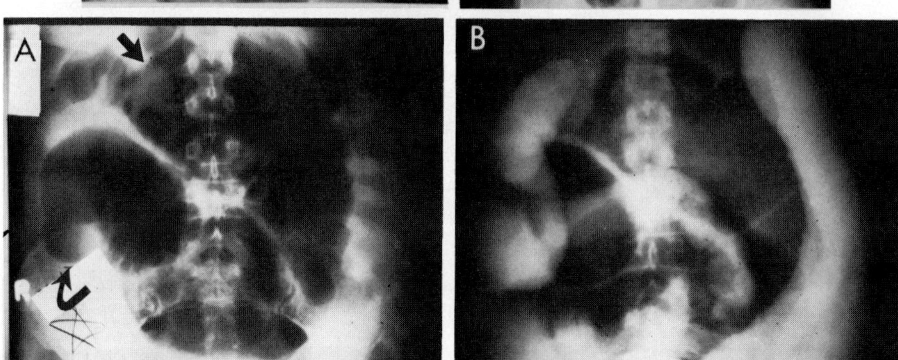

Fig 49–8 (top). – **A,** volvulus of ascending colon. There is a 180 degree twist in region of ascending colon with tip of cecum pointing toward epigastrium *(arrow)*. **B,** upright view shows single air-fluid level. (Courtesy of Dr. Edward I. Greenbaum, Los Angeles, Calif.)

Fig 49–9 (middle). – **A,** volvulus of ascending colon in right abdomen. Cecum *(arrow)* is situated in right lower quadrant, although it is turned 180 degrees from normal position, with ileocecal valve and medial wall of cecum now lying on right. **B,** upright views reveal two air-fluid levels in cecum and ascending colon. (Courtesy of Dr. Edward I. Greenbaum, Los Angeles, Calif.)

Fig 49–10 (bottom). – **A,** volvulus of right colon. Grossly distended cecum *(straight arrow)* and ascending colon seen in midabdomen. Point of obstruction *(curved arrow)* seen high in ascending colon. **B,** Gastrografin enema shows redundant sigmoid, which projects to right. Transverse colon overlaps sigmoid. On subsequent views, hepatic flexure could be seen, and point of obstruction corresponded to area noted above. (Courtesy of Dr. Edward I. Greenbaum, Los Angeles, Calif.)

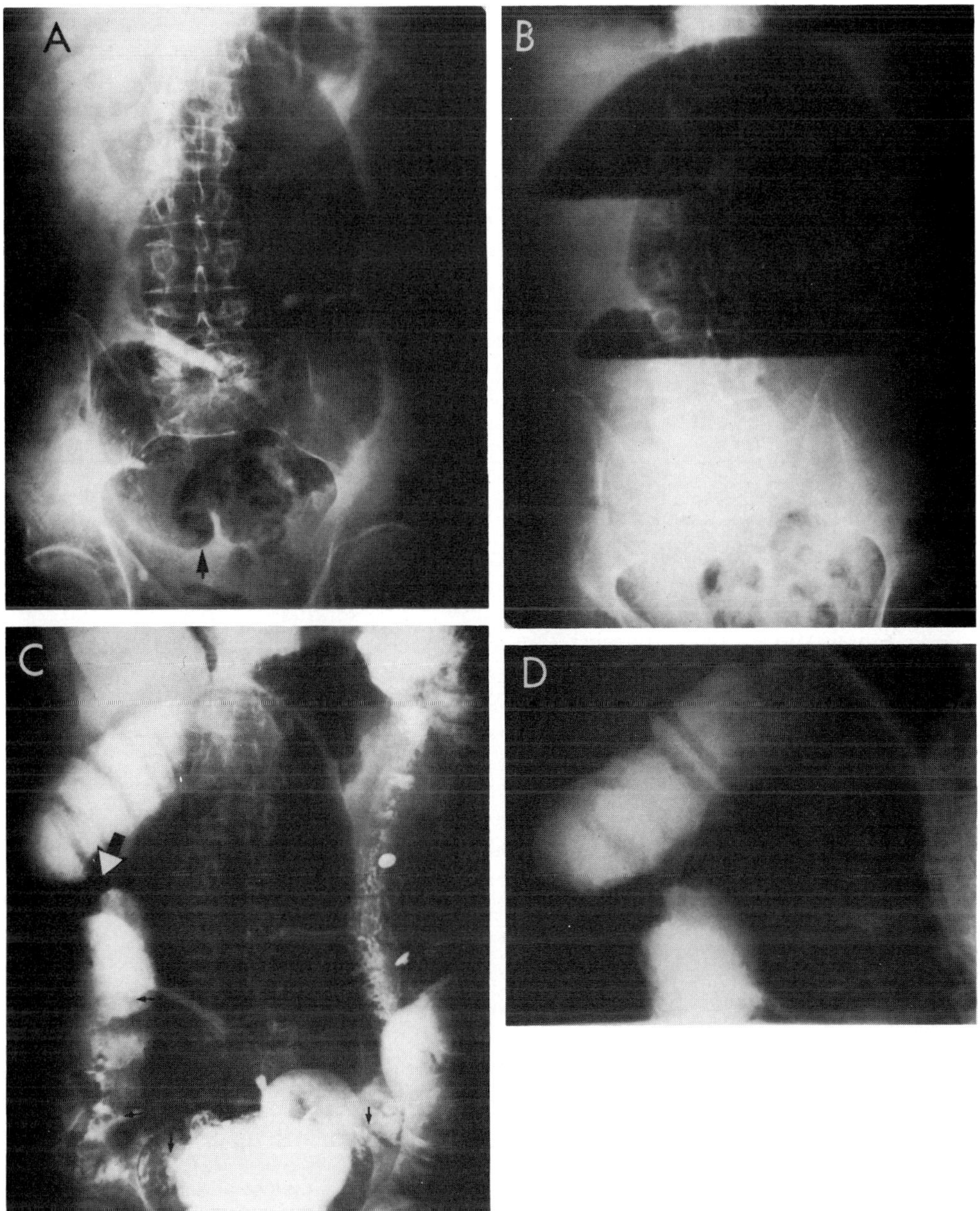

Fig 49–11.—A, volvulus of transverse colon. A 180-degree twist in transverse colon, with hepatic flexure flip-flopped so that it is now directed to left. Ascending colon and cecum *(arrow)* are left of midline. **B,** upright view of abdomen shows two air-fluid levels. Uppermost and shorter of air-fluid levels is in transverse colon; long air-fluid level is in midabdomen and is seen within cecum. **C,** barium enema shows filling of colon to point of obstruction *(large arrow)*. There is a bird of prey appearance at obstructed point, with barium entering dilated transverse colon, which is part of right-sided volvulus. *Small arrows* mark course of redundant transverse colon in pelvis where it overlaps sigmoid. **D,** spot film shows twisted mucosa and tapered margin of barium column, forming bird of prey appearance. Barium, also seen entering obstructed loop, fills dilated transverse colon in region of hepatic flexure. (Courtesy of Dr. Edward I. Greenbaum, Los Angeles, Calif.)

VOLVULUS OF THE SIGMOID COLON

EDWARD I. GREENBAUM, M.D.

VOLVULUS OF THE SIGMOID occurs with about the same frequency as volvulus of the cecum; together they represent about 18% of all colon obstructions.[1] Although this disease is seen mostly in the over 50 age group, cases in the pediatric age group have also been reported.[2] Mentally defective patients have a higher incidence, with constipation seemingly the link between this and the geriatric group. There is also a geographic distribution that relates to high cereal intake.[3] Predisposing causes include a redundant, mobile sigmoid that is increased in length, the so-called megasigmoid. Although most patients present with lower abdominal pain, about 16% of patients with volvulus of the sigmoid may have "chronic volvulus" without pain, and these patients present with distention, constipation and vomiting.[4] On physical examination the abdomen is tympanitic, and a palpable mass may be present. Shock and temperature elevation may be concomitant findings.

Plain films show a grossly distended sigmoid colon, which assumes a "bent inner tube" or inverted U appearance, the limbs of the sigmoid directed toward the pelvis (Figs 49–12 to 49–14). The sigmoid loop walls are usually ahaustral, and the medial walls are approximated to form a thick white line. Less frequently the medial walls overlap to show a central black band. The apex of the sigmoid loop usually lies to the left of midline. If the degree of proximal colon dilatation is marked, there is often difficulty in identifying the sigmoid loop, impeding reaching a diagnosis. This same difficulty may be encountered when there is an unusual amount of fluid and diminished amounts of air in the sigmoid. This causes a poorly defined image on the supine film, and the high position of air-fluid levels may be inadequate to define the sigmoid loop.[3]

Barium enema demonstrates the point of twist, and one sees tapering of the barium column, causing the bird-beak or bird-of-prey appearance. When barium traverses the point of obstruction, spiraling of the mucosal folds may be seen (see Fig 49–14). Barium enema should not be done in patients suspected of having gangrenous bowel or when pneumoperitoneum is noted.

Conservative treatment by proctosigmoidoscopy and placement of a rectal tube is controversial because of an associated high incidence of recurrence and mortality. If, however, this "conservative program" is utilized, the patient should be observed for persistence of abdominal pain and blood-stained stools. These clinical findings strongly suggest the possibility of superimposed ischemic colitis (Fig 49–15 to 49–18), and a barium enema may then show the telltale signs of ischemia, with thumbprinting, transverse ridging and mucosal ulcerations. Thickening and rigidity of the colon may be a result of intramural hemorrhage.[5] The extent of ischemic changes in the sigmoid colon should be determined prior to resection to prevent anastomosis of the ischemic colon and subsequent stenosis.

REFERENCES

1. Kerry, R. L., Lee, F., and Ransom, H. K.: Roentgenologic examination in the diagnosis and treatment of colon volvulus, Am. J. Roentgenol. 113:343, 1971.
2. Campbell, J. R., and Blank, E.: Sigmoid volvulus in children, Pediatrics 53:702, 1974.
3. Young, W. S., Engelbrecht, and Stoker, A.: Plain film analysis in sigmoid volvulus, Clin. Radiol. 29:553, 1978.
4. Kerry, R. L., and Ransom, H. K.: Volvulus of the colon, etiology, diagnosis and treatment, Arch. Surg. 99:215, 1969.
5. Meyers, M. A., Ghahremani, G. G., and Govoni, A. F.: Ischemic colitis associated with sigmoid volvulus: New observations, Am. J. Roentgenol. 128:591, 1977.

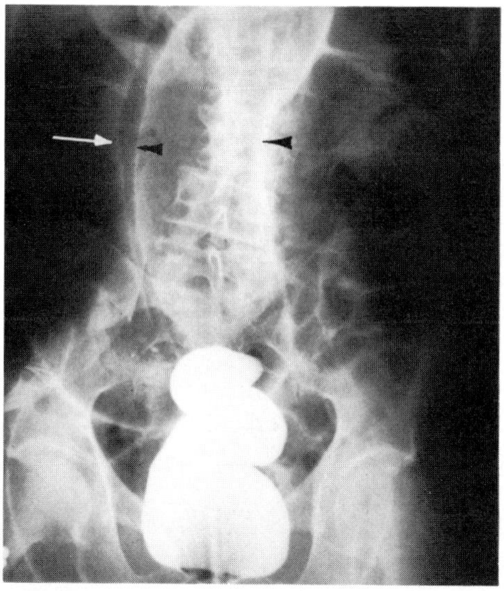

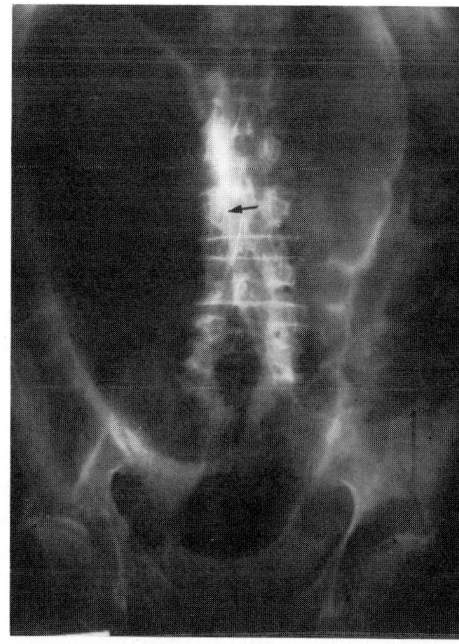

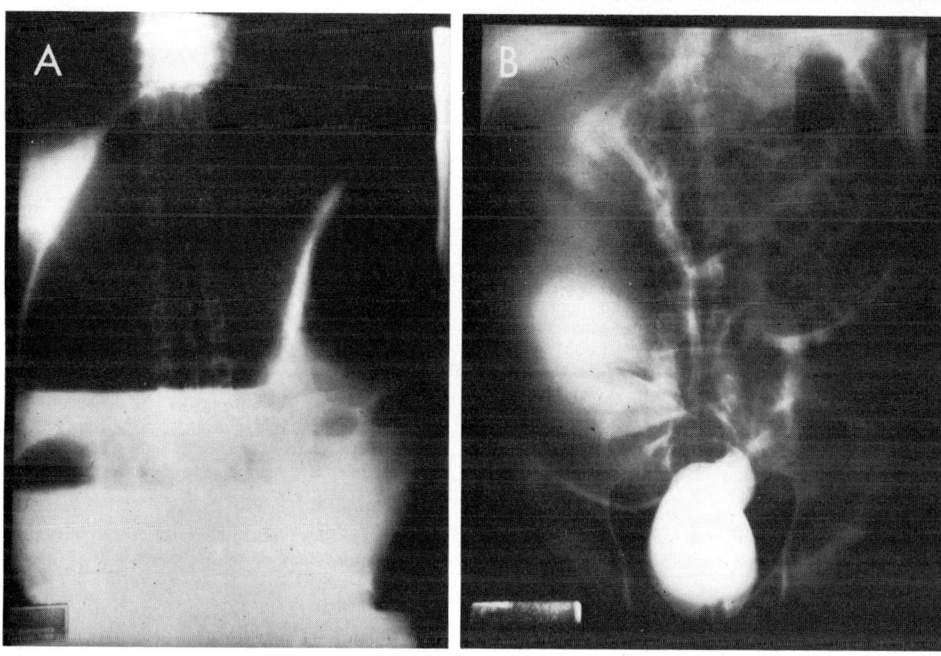

Fig 49–12 (top left). —Sigmoid volvulus. Grossly distended sigmoid colon has bent inner tube appearance. Medial walls overlap to show central black band *(opposing arrows)*. Left lateral wall of distended sigmoid marked by *single arrowhead*. Barium enema revealed obstruction to retrograde flow, with abrupt termination to barium column in region of sigmoid.

Fig 49–13 (top right). Volvulus of sigmoid. Sigmoid shows marked gaseous distention and assumes an inverted U, limbs pointing to pelvis. Margins are smooth except for short segment of limb on left where haustral markings persist. Medial walls are approximated to form thick white line *(arrow)*.

Fig 49–14 (bottom).—A, marked volvulus sigmoid presenting with bent inner-tube appearance. Both limbs point to pelvis. Apex is seen projecting to left of midline. **B,** barium enema shows partial obstruction at rectosigmoid, with small amount of barium entering grossly distended sigmoid loop. Barium outlines twisted mucosal folds, which have spiraled appearance.

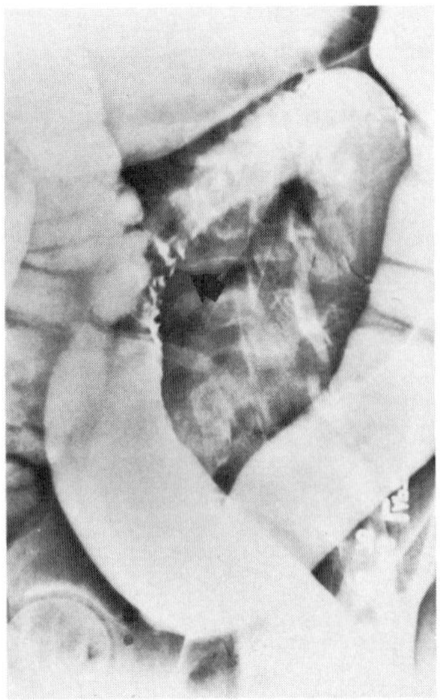

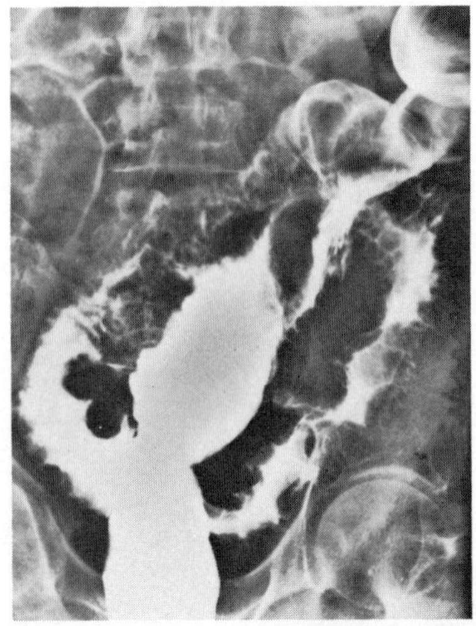

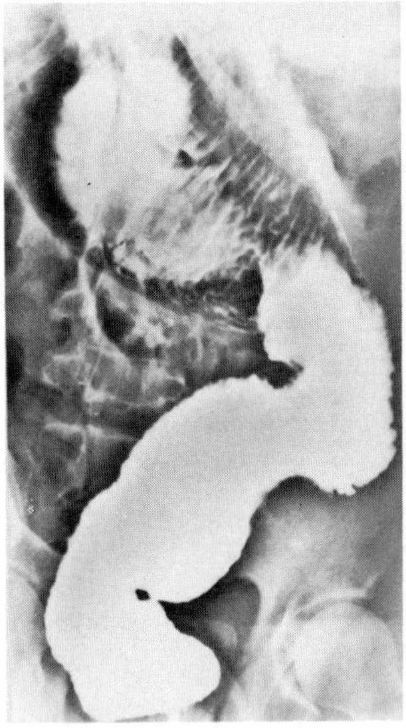

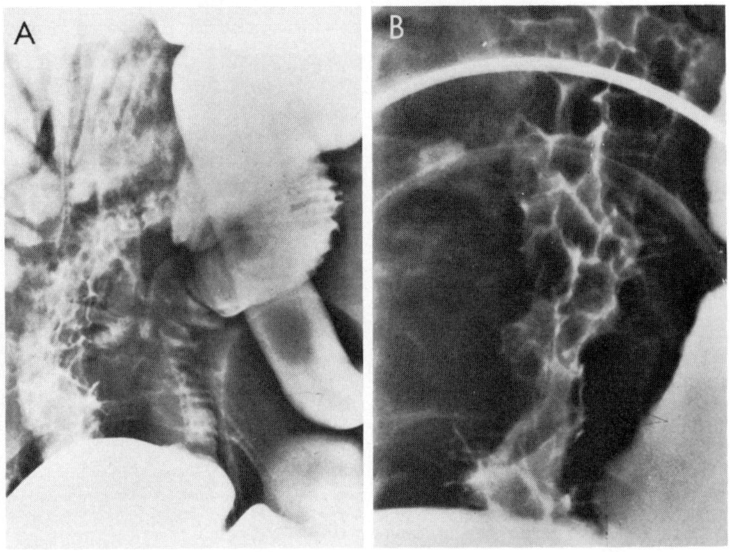

Fig 49–15 (top left).—Barium enema study showing ischemic colitis localized to 10-cm segment *(arrow)* at rectosigmoid junction, corresponding to distal point of fixation and torsion in sigmoid volvulus. (From Meyers and Ghahremani, Am. J. Roentgenol. 128:591, 1977, with permission.)

Fig 49–16 (top right).—Barium enema study 2 days after detorsion of sigmoid volvulus showing diffuse mucosal ulceration and submucosal hemorrhage manifested as thumbprints in redundant sigmoid colon. Note marked thickening and rigidity of colon due to intramural hemorrhage. Ischemic changes also involve adjacent segments of descending colon and rectum. (From Meyers and Ghahremani, Am. J. Roentgenol. 128:591, 1977, with permission.)

Fig 49–17 (bottom left).—Barium enema study 7 days after detorsion of volvulus showing marked transverse ridging secondary to intramural hemorrhage, due to ischemic change in rectum and sigmoid colon. (From Meyers and Ghahremani, Am. J. Roentgenol. 128:591, 1977, with permission.)

Fig 49–18 (bottom middle and right).—**A,** barium enema examination showing mucosal ulceration and edema involving distal limb of sigmoid colon. **B,** close-up of rectosigmoid junction showing abnormal mucosal pattern associated with extensive intramural hemorrhage. (From Meyers and Ghahremani, Am. J. Roentgenol. 128:591, 1977, with permission.)

VOLVULUS OF THE SPLENIC FLEXURE

EDWARD I. GREENBAUM, M.D.

VOLVULUS of the splenic flexure is rare, only 16 cases reported to date. Predisposing causes include absence of the phrenicolic, splenocolic and gastrocolic ligaments. In other instances there is a long mesenteric attachment with a redundant splenic flexure. Symptoms include cramping abdominal pain, distention, constipation and vomiting. On plain films there frequently is evidence of a large bowel obstruction with the point of obstruction in the region of the splenic flexure. An inordinately distended loop of splenic flexure will also be seen. Barium enema shows obstruction to retrograde flow (Fig 49–19), with a blunted or bird beak appearance at the point of obstruction. Barium enema may cause partial detorsion, and in this instance spiraling mucosal folds may be seen. Complete detorsion may follow passage of a long rectal tube or may occur spontaneously. To prevent recurrence, a primary resection with end-to-end anastomosis is the treatment of choice.[1, 2]

REFERENCES

1. Ghahremani, G. G., and Bowie, J. D.: Volvulus of the splenic flexure, Dis. Colon Rectum 17:100, 1974.
2. Lantieri, R., Teplick, S. K., and Labell, M. J.: Splenic flexure volvulus, Am. J. Roentgenol. 132:463, 1979.

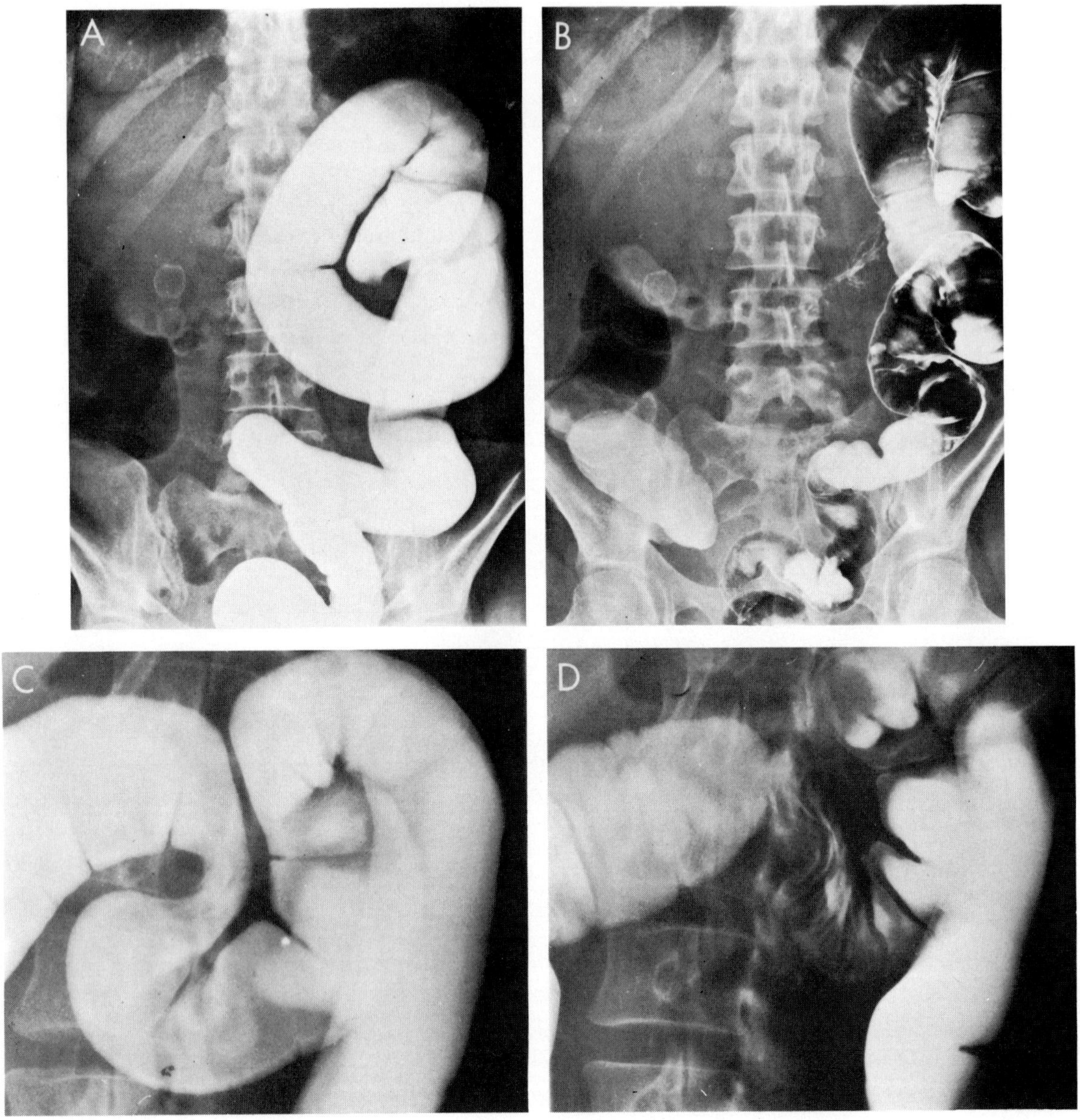

Fig 49–19. – Volvulus of splenic flexure. **A,** initial barium enema examination reveals complete obstruction to retrograde flow of barium in region of splenic flexure. Absence of distention of bowel proximal to obstruction indicated an acute or intermittant process. **B,** complete examination 2 hours later shows partial reduction of volvulus and spiraling mucosal folds in distal transverse colon. **C** and **D,** spot films obtained during study 6 days later illustrate extreme mobility of splenic flexure, with no further evidence of volvulus. (From Ghahremani and Bowie, Dis. Colon Rectum 17:100, 1974, with permission.)

Index

Numbers in *italics* are page references to illustrations.

R